Principles and Practice
of Nurse Anesthesia

Principles and Practice
of Nurse Anesthesia

Edited by

Wynne R. Waugaman, CRNA, Ph.D.
Assistant Professor and Director, Nurse Anesthesia Division, College of Medicine, The Ohio State University, Columbus, Ohio

Benjamin M. Rigor, M.D.
Professor and Chairman, Department of Anesthesiology, School of Medicine, University of Louisville, Louisville, Kentucky

Leah E. Katz, CRNA, Ed.D., J.D.
Adjunct Associate Professor, Department of Anesthesiology, School of Medicine, University of California, Los Angeles, Los Angeles, California

John F. Garde, CRNA, M.S.
Executive Director, American Association of Nurse Anesthetists, Park Ridge, Illinois

Hershal W. Bradshaw, CRNA, M.Ed.
Founder and Program Director for Nurse Anesthesia Education, University of Texas, Health Science Center at Houston, Houston, Texas

Endorsed by the Board of Directors of the American Association of Nurse Anesthetists 1987

APPLETON & LANGE
Norwalk, Connecticut/San Mateo, California

0-8385-7940-X

Copyright © 1988 by Appleton & Lange
A Publishing Division of Prentice Hall

88 89 90 91 92 / 10 9 8 7 6 5 4 3 2 1

Prentice-Hall of Australia, Pty. Ltd., Sydney
Prentice-Hall Canada, Inc.
Prentice-Hall Hispanoamericana, S.A., Mexico
Prentice-Hall of India Private Limited, New Delhi
Prentice-Hall International (UK) Limited, London
Prentice-Hall of Japan, Inc., Tokyo
Prentice-Hall of Southeast Asia (Pte.) Ltd., Singapore
Whitehall Books Ltd., Wellington, New Zealand
Editora Prentice-Hall do Brasil Ltda., Rio de Janeiro

Library of Congress Cataloging-in-Publication Data

Principles and practice of nurse anesthesia.

Includes index.
1. Anesthesiology. 2. Nurse anesthetists.
I. Waugaman, Wynne R. [DNLM: 1. Nurse Anesthetists.
WY 151 P957]
RD82.P755 1987   617'.96   87–17552
ISBN 0–8385–7940–X

Production Editors: Robin Millay, Karen Davis
Designer: M. Chandler Martylewski

PRINTED IN THE UNITED STATES OF AMERICA

**This Book Is Dedicated to Our Friend, Mentor,
and Colleague**

Hershal W. Bradshaw, CRNA, M.Ed.

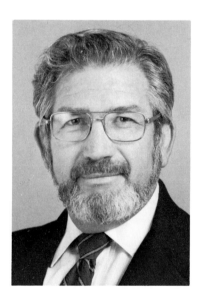

His motivation, love of life and profession,
and his unforgettable sense of humor live on with us

Contents

Contributors

Gerald D. Allen, M.D.
Professor, Department of Anesthesiology
School of Medicine
University of California, Los Angeles
Los Angeles, California

Roy Aston, Ph.D.
Professor, Department of Physiology and
   Pharmacology
School of Dentistry
University of Detroit
Detroit, Michigan

Sidney L. Barlow, CRNA, M.A.
Bar Medical Products
Louisville, Kentucky

Colleen Lynch Beesinger, CRNA
Anesthesiology Associates
Bryan, Texas

David E. Beesinger, M.D., F.A.C.S.
Former Director, Hermann Hospital for Thermal
   Injuries
Houston, Texas
Preceptor, General Surgery
School of Medicine
Texas A & M University
College Station, Texas

Jeffery M. Beutler, CRNA, M.S.
Director, Anesthesia and Surgical Services
Rose Medical Center
Denver, Colorado

Hollis E. Bivens, M.D.
Professor and Chairman, Department of
   Anesthesiology
The University of Texas System Cancer Center
M. D. Anderson Hospital and Tumor Institute
Houston, Texas

Norman H. Blass, M.D.
Professor of Anesthesia, Obstetrics and Gynecology
Medical College of Virginia
Richmond, Virginia

Lawrence L. Ciccarelli, M.D.
Instructor
Department of Anesthesiology
University of Louisville School of Medicine
Louisville, Kentucky

Lewis A. Coveler, M.D.
Associate Professor of Anesthesiology
Baylor College of Medicine
Houston, Texas

Lida S. Dahm, M.D.
Clinical Assistant Professor, Departments of
   Anesthesiology and Pediatrics
Baylor College of Medicine
Texas Medical Center
Houston, Texas

Cecil B. Drain, CRNA, Ph.D.
Lieutenant Colonel, U.S. Army Nurse Corps
Brooke Army Medical Center
San Antonio, Texas

Francis R. Gerbasi, CRNA, Ph.D.
Faculty, Wayne State University College of
   Pharmacy and Allied Health
Coordinator, Anesthesia Services, Hutzel Hospital,
   Detroit Medical Center
Detroit, Michigan

Stephen Hays, CRNA
Anesthesiology Associates
Bryan, Texas

Everard R. Hicks, M.Ed., CRNA
Professor Emeritus, Anesthesia for Nurses
   Educational Department
College of Health Related Professions
Medical University of South Carolina
Charleston, South Carolina

Philip B. Hollander, Ph.D.
Professor, Department of Pharmacology
College of Medicine
Professor, Divisions of Biomedical Engineering,
   Biophysics
Colleges of Engineering, Biological Sciences
The Ohio State University
Columbus, Ohio

James M. Hunn, CRNA, M.S.
Colonel, U.S. Army Nurse Corps (Ret.)
Formerly Anesthesia Nursing Consultant to the
   Surgeon General of the Army
Paragould, AR

Lorraine M. Jordan, CRNA, M.S.
Instructor, Nurse Anesthesia Division
College of Medicine
The Ohio State University
Columbus, Ohio

Joseph T. Kanusky, CRNA, M.S.
Lieutenant Colonel, U.S. Army Nurse Corps
Consultant to the Commanding General, 7th
   Medical Command, for Anesthesiology Nursing
Chief Anesthesia Nursing Section
97th General Hospital
New York, New York

Leah E. Katz, CRNA, Ed.D., J.D.
Adjunct Associate Professor, Department of
   Anesthesiology
School of Medicine
University of California, Los Angeles
Los Angeles, California

Ronald L. Katz, M.D.
Professor and Chairman, Department of
   Anesthesiology
School of Medicine
University of California, Los Angeles
Los Angeles, California

Kathleen C. Koerbacher, M.A., CRNA
Clinical Associate Professor, Anesthesia for Nurses
   Educational Department
College of Health Related Professions
Medical University of South Carolina
Charleston, South Carolina

Leo A. Le Bel, CRNA, M.S.N., J.D.
Lieutenant Colonel, U.S. Army Nurse Corps (Ret.)
Former Director, U.S. Army Anesthesiology Course
   for Army Nurse Corps Officers
Madigan Army Medical Center
Tacoma, Washington

Jerrold H. Levy, M.D.
Assistant Professor, Department of Anesthesiology
Emory University School of Medicine
Atlanta, Georgia

Stanley L. Loftness, M.D., F.A.A.P.
Associate Director, PICU
The Children's Hospital
Denver, Colorado

Mary Jeanette Mannino, CRNA, J.D.
Medical Resources Consulting Service
Irvine, California
Anesthesia Associates of Orange County
Tustin, California

Cathy A. Mastropietro, CRNA, M.Ed.
Director, School for Nurse Anesthetists
St. Elizabeth Hospital Medical Center
Youngstown, Ohio

Dean H. Morrow, M.D.
Professor and Chairman, Department of
   Anesthesiology
Baylor College of Medicine
Houston, Texas

Paul B. Oppenheimer, M.D.
Clinical Assistant Professor, Nurse Anesthesia
   Division
College of Medicine
The Ohio State University
Columbus, Ohio

Jeanette F. Peter, CRNA, M.A.Ed.
Adjunct Assistant Professor, Department of
   Anesthesiology
School of Medicine
University of California, Los Angeles
Los Angeles, California

Joseph T. Rando, CRNA, M.N.
Nurse Anesthetist Supervisor, Department of
   Anesthesiology
The University of Texas System Cancer Center
   M. D. Anderson Hospital & Tumor Institute
Clinical Assistant Professor Nurse Anesthesia
Education School of Nursing
University of Texas
Houston, Texas

Leslie Rendell-Baker, M.D.
Professor of Anesthesiology
School of Medicine
Loma Linda University
Loma Linda, California

Robert C. Reynolds, M.D., Ph.D.
Associate Professor, Department of Anesthesiology
School of Medicine
University of California, Los Angeles
Los Angeles, California

Benjamin M. Rigor, M.D.
Professor and Chairman, Department of
   Anesthesiology
School of Medicine
University of Louisville
Louisville, Kentucky

John J. Savarese, M.D.
Associate Professor, Department of Anaesthesia
Harvard Medical School
Boston, Massachusetts

Sister Mary Arthur Schramm, CRNA, Ph.D.
Professor, Nurse Anesthesia Program
Mount Marty College
Yankton, South Dakota

Barbara Shwiry, CRNA, B.S.
Staff Nurse Anesthetist
Beekman Hospital, New York Infirmary
New York, New York

Jonathan H. Skerman, B.D. Sc, M.SCD, D.S.C.
Associate Professor Anesthesia Obstetrics,
   Gynecology
Louisiana State University at Shreveport
Shreveport, Louisiana

Bruce Skolnick, Ph.D.
Adjunct Assistant Professor, Department of
   Anesthesiology
School of Medicine
University of California, Los Angeles
Los Angeles, California

Michael d'A. Stanton-Hicks, M.D.
Professor of Anesthesiology
Institut fur Anasthesiologie
Johannes Gutenberg Universitat
Mainz
West Germany

Doris J. Tanaka, CRNA, M.S.
Assistant Professor, Program in Nurse Anesthesia
School of Nursing
University of Texas, Health Science Center at
   Houston
Houston, Texas

Anastasios N. Triantafillou, M.D.
Instructor, Department of Anesthesiology
School of Medicine
University of Louisville
Louisville, Kentucky

Susan A. Ward, D.Phil.
Associate Professor, Departments of Anesthesiology
   and Physiology
School of Medicine
University of California, Los Angeles
Los Angeles, California

Marian Waterhouse, CRNA, M.Ed.
Colonel, U.S. Army Nurse Corps (Ret.)
Former Director, U.S. Army Anesthesiology
Program of Instruction for Army Nurse Corps
   Officers
San Antonia, Texas

Wynne R. Waugaman, CRNA, Ph.D.
Assistant Professor and Director, Nurse Anesthesia
   Division
College of Medicine
The Ohio State University
Columbus, Ohio

Joel M. Weaver, D.D.S., Ph.D.
Associate Professor, Section of Oral and
   Maxillofacial Surgery
College of Dentistry
Associate Professor, Department of Anesthesiology
College of Medicine
The Ohio State University
Columbus, Ohio

Rebecca S. Williams, CRNA
Associate Professor, Program in Nurse Anesthesia
   Education (Emeritus)
The University of Texas System Cancer Center
M.D. Anderson Hospital and Tumor Institute
Houston, Texas

Karen L. Zaglaniczny, CRNA, M.S.
Instructor, Wayne State University
Coordinator Anesthesia Services
Detroit Receiving Hospital—University Health
   Clinic
Detroit, Michigan

Christine S. Zambricki, CRNA, M.S.
Administrative Director of Nurse Anesthesiology
Mount Carmel Mercy Hospital
Program Director, Graduate Program of Nurse
   Anesthesiology
Mercy College of Detroit
Detroit, Michigan

Preface

While there is evidence that nurses were involved in administering anesthesia dating back to the American Civil War and the Franco-Prussian War in Europe, this clinical nursing specialty became formalized during the first two decades of the twentieth century. The history of this specialty demonstrates the dedication of nurse anesthetists to the advancement of the art and science of anesthesia through their involvement in pioneering new anesthetic techniques and working with physicians and engineers to develop new and better equipment. One of the major purposes for these nursing pioneers to come together and found the American Association of Nurse Anesthetists in 1931 was to share their knowledge and develop standards for high quality education for nurses entering this specialty. Their commitment and dedication to this purpose has served as an inspiration throughout the years to succeeding generations of nurse anesthetists.

This book represents no less of a milestone in the history of nurse anesthesia, than did many of the individual accomplishments of persons such as Alice McGaw, Agatha Hodgins, Helen Lamb, Hilda Soloman, Olive Berger, and others too numerous to mention. It is the first, multi-authored, comprehensive anesthesia textbook written principally by CRNAs for nurse anesthesia students and their CRNA colleagues. These CRNA authors have been joined by some basic scientists and physicians who have been directly involved in nurse anesthesia education and/or their practice. The contributors to this book have distilled the essence of the basic sciences and meshed them with concepts from the clinical and behavioral sciences in a manner which allows the learner to unify diverse knowledge components into a specific anesthesia care plan to meet the needs of an individual patient. As such, this book primarily deals with anesthesia practice, its concepts and its reality. In addition, the book addresses the environment within which anesthesia is practiced and the necessary management styles, programs, and resources to assess and assure the quality of anesthesia services.

While anesthesia practice is a dynamic, constantly changing field, this textbook provides those basic fundamentals that serve as a sound foundation for future growth and development in this field. It also may serve as a reference book for nurses in other specialties who care for the anesthetized patient. And finally, it will also be of interest to those nurses who have yet to decide upon a nursing specialty, allowing them to become more knowledgeable about this field, its educational requirements, and the clinical demands placed upon CRNAs.

The authors have kept faith with nurse anesthetist pioneers in accepting responsibility for putting something back into the specialty, rather than merely taking from those who were our predecessors. This book should serve as an incentive for other CRNA authors to undertake the writing of other needed texts or reference books from which we all can benefit.

John F. Garde, CRNA, M.S.

Acknowledgments

The identification of subject experts by the editors and the expertise and dedication of these contributors have been the heart of this project. Without the continued interest, support, and participation of these individuals in this project, this book never could have been completed. My deepest appreciation and admiration are extended to my fellow contributors and editors.

I would like to give special thanks to Dr. Ben Rigor who first sparked our interest and enthusiasm in this venture. It is he who identified the editors and first arranged for us to get together so many years ago. I would like to thank my other editors, Leah Katz, John Garde, and the late Hershal Bradshaw who helped to see this project through. I appreciate the help and guidance provided by the staff of Appleton and Lange especially Marion Kalstein Welch who continually encouraged me with this book. Lastly, I wish to express my deepest love and gratitude to my husband, Dr. Philip Hollander, and our daughters, Rachel, and Sara, for their unending patience and understanding during the preparation of *Principles and Practice of Nurse Anesthesia*.

Wynne R. Waugaman, CRNA, Ph.D.

Part I

FOUNDATIONS

1

From Nurse to Nurse Anesthetist

Wynne R. Waugaman

The circumstances under which a person enters a profession are highly predictive of the way that person will view the profession for the rest of his or her life. Most people enter preparation for their chosen careers only vaguely understanding the implications for change in behavior associated with their educational endeavors. The professional educational programs that people select greatly influence the type and quality of their career commitment.

Students entering nurse anesthesia programs, degree or certificate, have a more profound awareness of their chosen careers than do most students entering other professions. Student nurse anesthetists have been preparing for this career often for several years before actual enrollment through employment experience in critical care nursing, through additional coursework beyond the nursing credential, and by observing nurse anesthetist and physician anesthetist role models. Thus, the decision to enter the field of nurse anesthesia has not been a snap decision but rather one that has been thought out thoroughly.

Nurses seek a career in nurse anesthesia for many reasons. Some identify a need for increased autonomy as their impetus; others seek more challenges in their work setting and view nurse anesthesia as a means of enhancing their knowledge base in nursing.

PROFESSIONAL SOCIALIZATION

Sociologically, the development of a profession involves more than developing a distinct body of knowledge. It involves the realization that professionals are part of an ethical and moral community. They have social links not only to their patients and colleagues in the profession but also to all groups with whose activities their skills must interface. The legitimacy of their professional contribution must be acknowledged inclusively by all groups with whom they work as well as other professions.

What happens during the nurse anesthesia program to transform a nurse into a nurse anesthetist? The transformation process that occurs is professional socialization. Professional socialization, that process of developing skills, knowledge, professional behavior, and career commitment, occurs concurrently with the educational process, i.e., the clinical and didactic educational program. It is reported that not only does the socialization process adjust students to their educational roles but also, unlike adjustments to specific situations, it persists across status transitions and situational changes.

Socialization is time and space multidimensional. It encompasses occupational knowledge and skills in addition to occupational orientations such as collegialism, working within the hospital organizational structure, and views concerning leadership and authority. Socialization also enables the student nurse anesthetist to form personal relatedness to the field through developing career commitment and self-identification as a nurse anesthetist.

This socialization process is dynamic. A person's view of the work role may shift to fit the circumstances and demands of a work situation without any effect on job commitment. On the other hand, with changing family situations, social roles, and social orientations, commitment to the job itself may decline while views of the work role and the occupation of nurse anesthesia remain stable. This is the ever-changing face of professional socialization. Professional roles adapt to meet the necessary situation.

Early exposure to clinical practicum and learning the work of the profession facilitates all aspects of professional socialization in nurse anesthesia. Role modeling by nurse and physician anesthetists throughout the educational program is a valuable tool of professional socialization. The emphasis in nurse anesthesia education on practical experience during the curriculum enables students to visualize their professional roles with a high degree of realism from early in the program.

Educational program content, design, and faculty and practitioner role models all play a vital role in the professional socialization of nurse anesthetists. All of these factors influence the degree to which students are socialized into the profession, and the continuation of the socialization process influences the degree of professional career commitment as people mature from nurses to nurse anesthetists. The process of professional socialization is enhanced through the succeeding chapters of this book by the imparting of the occupational knowledge necessary to acquire the skills to practice the art and science of nurse anesthesia.

BIBLIOGRAPHY

Becker H, Hughes E, et al: Boys in White. Chicago, University of Chicago Press, 1961.

Christman L: Educational standards versus professional performance. Nurs Dig 6:27–44, 1978.

Cohen H: Authoritarianism and dependency: Problems in nursing socialization. In Flynn B, Miller M (eds): Current Perspectives in Nursing: Social Issues and Trends. St. Louis, Mosby, 1980, Vol. 2, pp. 160–167.

Corwin R: The professional employee, a study of conflicting nursing. Am J Sociol 66:604–615, 1961.

Corwin R, Traves M, Haas J: Professional disillusionment. Nurs Res 10:141–144, 1961.

Eli I, Shuval J: Professional socialization in dentistry. Soc Sci Med 16:951–955, 1982.

Keen MF, Dear MR: Mastery of role transition: Clinical teaching strategies. J Nurs Ed 22:183–186, 1983.

Merton R, Reader G, Kendall P: The Student-Physician. Cambridge, MA, Harvard University Press, 1957.

Pelligrino ED: What is a profession? J Allied Health 12:168–177, 1983.

Simpson I: From Student to Nurse. New York, Cambridge University Press, 1979.

Waugaman W: From Nurse to Nurse Anesthetist: Effects of Professional Socialization on Career Commitment, unpublished doctoral dissertation. University of Pittsburgh, PA, 1981.

2

History of Anesthesia

Sidney L. Barlow

Anesthesia is one of the most rapidly advancing fields of medicine. The degree of its development can be used as one index of social progress throughout history.

The value of anesthesia goes beyond the relief of pain as an end in itself. It has made possible the development of the modern science and art of surgery and has saved and is saving millions of lives. Because we live in a scientific age, further advances will continue to develop as anesthesia experts discover new applications and equipment in this and other branches of science. As our knowledge of anesthesia becomes more exact, the science itself will save more lives and alleviate suffering; but no matter how exact the science becomes, it will always reflect the words of S. Wier Mitchell in "The Birth and Death of Pain" when he wrote:

> . . . The Birth of Pain! Let centuries roll
> away; Come back with me to nature's primal day.
> What mighty forces pledged the dust of life!
> What awful will decreed its silent strife!
> When writhes the child beneath the surgeon's hand,
> What soul shall hope that pain to understand?
> Lo! Science falters o'er the hopeless task,
> And Love and Faith in vain an answer ask,
> When thrilling nerves demand what good is wrought
> Where torture clogs the very source of thought. . . .
> Recall this memory. Let the curtain fall,
> For gladder days shall know this storied hall! . . .
> Then radiant morning broke, and ampler hope
> To Art and Science gave illuminated scope.
> What angel bore the Christ-like gift inspired! . . .
> Made pain a dream, and suffering gently dumb!
> This heaven-sent answer to the cry of prayer
> This priceless gift which all mankind may share. . . .
> God's highest mercy brought by man to man.

The shortage of anesthetists may well have started the day after Dr. Crawford Long anesthetized James Venable on March 31, 1842. In the early days, the administration of anesthesia was haphazard. In most hospitals the interns were the anesthetists, a role for which they were given no training in medical school. Physicians were not interested in learning the newly developed art. The work of the anesthetist was considered subservient to that of the surgeon, and the pay was very low.

Surgeons started looking for more competent people to administer anesthesia. In America the trend was established early for the administration of anesthesia by persons who were not physicians, thus leading to the development of the nurse as anesthetist.

In 1877, Sister Mary Bernard entered St. Vincent's Hospital in Erie, Pennsylvania, to train as a nurse. She assumed the responsibilities of an anesthetist and did not complete her training as a nurse. In 1880 the administration of ether and chloroform was taught to Sister Aldoza Eltrich at St. John's Hospital in Springfield, Illinois. By 1889, nine more sisters of the Third Order of the Hospital Sisters of St. Francis had become anesthetists.

In 1889, St. Mary's, a small hospital with thirteen patients, three surgeons—the Mayos—and five sisters, was opened by the Sisters of St. Francis in Rochester, Minnesota. The anesthesia was administered by Edith and Dinah Graham, two sisters who graduated from nurses' training in Chicago, Illinois. They were succeeded by Alice McGaw in 1893. Miss McGaw brought fame to the nurse anesthetists and St. Mary's Hospital by being the first nurse anesthetist to publish articles on anesthesia. Her first paper, "Observations on 1092 Cases of Anesthesia from January 1, 1899, to January 1, 1900," was published in the *St. Paul Medical Journal*. She gained national fame when, in December 1906, she published "A Review of Over 14,000 Surgical Anesthetics" in *Surgery, Gynecology, and Obstetrics*. In the article she reported on the use of the open drop method of administering ether without a death being attributed to anesthesia.

The Mayo surgeons performed with outstanding skill, and soon the Mayo Clinic became a place for surgeons to come and observe the three in action. While observing the impressive surgical work, something else caught their eye—the anesthesia being administered by Miss Alice McGaw. The technique of using open drop chloroform and ether satisfied the surgeons and provided comfort and safety for the patients.

Miss Florence Henderson gained experience in the administration of anesthesia while working as superintendent of nurses at St Mary's Hospital from 1900 to 1903. In 1903 she became Dr. Charles H. Mayo's anesthetist. Miss Henderson published an article in the *American Journal of Nursing* in September 1909. In her article, which was read before the 12th annual convention of the American Nursing Association, Miss Henderson discussed the drawbacks of administration of anesthetic by interns, the reasons surgeons were turning to nurse anesthetists, and some factors the nurse anesthetist must bear in mind while administering anesthesia. She observed that the nurse's lack of self-confidence is one of her chief recommendations because it keeps her alert to the patient's condition at all times. She also stated that if the patient is watched carefully, the jaw properly handled, and plenty of air given, it is surprising how seldom trouble will be encountered. Miss Henderson felt the nurse was better able to establish rapport with the patient than the doctor because nurses are free of the aura of mystery that still clings to the surgeon, and so patients are apt to yield themselves much more readily to their suggestive influence. To establish a good anesthesia plan and maximum comfort for the patient, the nurse anesthetist must win the patient's confidence.

Ethel Baxter was one of the first nurse anesthetists in the South. After graduation from nursing school in 1899 she traveled with Dr. Eugene Johnson who was performing surgery throughout rural Mississippi. They traveled by any conveyance, even oxcart, sterilizing instruments in the oven, scrubbing floors, dousing the furniture with antiseptic solution, and on one occasion constructing an operating table from two planks pulled off a barn and laid across two casks, the operation being performed on the porch rather than in the house because the flies swarmed less viciously there.

In 1908, Dr. George Crile of Cleveland selected Miss Agatha Hodgins as his anesthetist. She was from Toronto, Canada, and a graduate of the Boston Hospital Training School for Nurses. Dr. Crile and Miss Hodgins had their own experimental school in which Miss Hodgins, under the supervision of Dr. Crile, anesthetized dogs and rabbits to familiarize her with the symptoms of death. According to Dr. Crile, Miss Hodgins had a special way of anesthetizing babies. With extraordinary skill she would amuse a child with toys or the doctor's watch while she allowed the gas to play gently over the child's face until the sandman closed his eyes and he slipped back on the pillow.

Miss Hodgins believed that the nurse anesthetist should administer other agents besides ether. She used nitrous oxide and oxygen. They were considered harder to administer because they require a special mechanical apparatus, and the proper mixture of nitrous oxide and oxygen must be adjusted to meet the needs of the individual patient.

Miss Hodgins deplored overconfidence but she stated that a nurse anesthetist should have a certain amount of confidence to ensure a calmness of conduct. She also felt that a nurse must never encroach on a doctor's province in regard to prescribing and ordering drugs.

The early training of nurse anesthetists varied from program to program. In 1909, the nurses in the Massachusetts General Hospital anesthesia training program received some didactic instruction along with practical instruction. A lecture was given on the fundamental principles of surgical anesthesia and the methods of its production. At least twice during her training each nurse received individual instruction in the actual administration of ether for surgical procedures.

In 1909, Agnes McGee organized the anesthesia course at St. Vincent's Hospital in Portland, Oregon. This course, which included instruction in anatomy and physiology of the respiratory system, pharmacology of anesthetic drugs, and the administration of the commonly used anesthetic drugs, lasted six months.

Ida Cain, writing in 1912, stated "The matter of proper instruction has not been settled. There is no place where a nurse may take an authorized course, though a few hospitals are teaching anesthesia as postgraduate courses to their own nurses. This may be very satisfactory in some cases but may be subject to abuse should certain unqualified individuals or hospitals take it up for financial profit, without regard to thorough instruction." The national nursing organization refused to become involved because the issue was one of controversy within the medical societies.

In 1913, the students at the New York Post Graduate Hospital attended heart clinics and lectures by physicians. Experimental work, such as the passing of laryngeal tubes, was practiced on cadavers. Two textbooks were used: *Anesthetics and Their Administration,* by Fredrick W. Hewett, and *Anesthetics: Their Uses and Administration,* by Dudley W. Buxton. By graduation, each student had administered ether anesthesia 400 times.

When the United States entered World War I, the nurse anesthetist became an important part of the personnel of the base hospital unit. The Army and Navy trained nurse anesthetists. The Army was able to have some of their nurses train at the Mayo Clinic for six weeks. The nurse anesthetist contributed to the improvement of anesthesia abroad, not only by administering the anesthesia, but also by teaching the techniques, especially the administration of nitrous oxide. Because of the ability displayed by nurse anesthetists during World War I, the demand for nurse anesthetists increased rapidly after the war.

Between 1914 and 1922, programs were organized in quite a few hospitals. Lakeside General Hospital School of Anesthesia, in Cleveland, Ohio, was established in 1915, when Agatha Hodgins returned from France. The course was open to graduate nurses who had passed their state boards and to qualified physicians and dentists. The duration of the courses was six months. The students had to pay their own living expenses and a tuition of $50. The same fee but a shorter course was required of physicians and dentists. In 1917, a controversy with the Ohio State Board of Medical Examiners closed the school. The program was reopened in 1918. In 1919, didactic instruction was incorporated into the program, with Miss Hodgins delivering the lectures.

The school of anesthesia at Charity Hospital in New Orleans, Louisiana, was established in 1917. The fee for the course was $100.

Another program was opened in 1917 at Johns Hopkins Hospital in Baltimore. This course lasted six months and was under the direction of Margaret Boise. The nurses received a certificate at the completion of the program.

Grady Memorial Hospital, in Atlanta, organized the first school for nurse anesthetists in the southeastern United States. The students were taught how to administer chloroform, ether, nitrous oxide, and oxygen anesthesia. Theoretic instruction consisted of about ten hours of lectures, mostly on pharmacology.

The need for continuous study and improvement in

technique was first emphasized by Julia Strebs, in 1920, who urged that the nurse anesthetist study and keep on studying and aim to give each anesthetic better than the previous one. Agatha Hodgins, in an article in 1930, wrote "A technical training may do very well for the handling of problems involving inanimate objects, but never for work involving human life; education, more of it and better in quality, is what we desire for the nurse anesthetist." The need continues for better education and improved methods of imparting knowledge so that, by generating enthusiasm for the subject, we encourage the student to become if not a scholar, at least a seeker after truth. Educational requirements for this work should be defined and standardized by those most concerned—surgeons, hospitals, and educators of nurse anesthetists, who show by their attitude the desire to create not a class of minimally instructed mechanical helpers but a group of educated, dedicated practitioners who will enhance and protect this vital and humanitarian work by their efforts.

ANESTHESIA IN ANTIQUITY

Nature has given us pain for protection. It is the instinctive cry of the body at the onset of injury and disease. The word "pain" comes from the Latin word *poena*, which means punishment or penalty.

It has been claimed that the deep sleep that the Creator caused to fall upon Adam is the germ of the idea of anesthesia. Primitive peoples, in an effort to eradicate pain, treated it as a demon and tried to frighten the demon away from their bodies. They often tattooed their skins to keep the demons outside the body. They wore rings in the ears and nose, as well as various ornaments on their person, such as talismans, amulets, tiger claws, and charms to ward off evil spirits. Primitive people also probably employed digital compression of the carotid arteries to produce a form of anesthesia. Indeed, the Greek and Roman words for the carotid artery mean "the artery of sleep."

Although the Egyptians had a well-developed legal code and considerable understanding of medicine, little evidence exists to show that they developed any real proficiency in the science of anesthesia, although scattered references came down through the writings of the Greeks. About 2000 B.C., the Babylonians had a well-developed legal code, the so-called Hamurabi Code. Admixed with rules governing daily life of the people and punishments for crimes were rules and regulations relating to the practice of medicine. It provided for severe penalties to be inflicted upon individuals who committed quackery and malpractice. These early cultures had little regard for the relief of pain and suffering, although there can be seen a gradual development of science and general medicine.

The Egyptians of the New Kingdom used Indian hemp and the juice of the poppy to cause a patient to become drowsy before surgical procedures. And the "sorrow-easing drug" that Ulysses' comrades gave him may have consisted of a similar substance. The ancient Egyptians also wrote of a species of rock brought from Memphis, which they used, powdered and moistened with sour wine, to apply to painful wounds. This was the first known record of the use of carbonic acid as a local anesthetic.

Early Hindus inhaled the fumes of burning Indian hemp to produce a stupor. In that condition, they used it as a mind relaxant to endure pain. Cannabis is the botanical term for hemp. According to H. R. Raper, the mental effect of cannabis is that ". . . the mind is immediately filled by a delicious succession of pleasant ideas." Cannabis is better known to modern Americans as marijuana.

The Greeks worshiped Hypnos, the god of sleep, the fatherless child of night and the twin brother of death. Hypnos was the father of Morpheus, the god of dreams. Therefore, Hypnos came to be the most longed-for of the Greek gods during times of sorrow, sickness, and especially during the pain of surgery. During these times, Hypnos was said to sleep and not hear the prayers of the suffering patient.

The Greeks first used the term *anesthesia*, a term derived from two Greek words meaning the absence of feeling. Plato used the word in his writings. Unfortunately, Greek poets and dramatists made more use of the term in the literary works than the medical men made use of pain-killing procedures in their practices. Not a single example of the use of anesthesia during an operation survived in known Greek medical writings, although Theocritus alluded to Lucina, the goddess of the obstetric art, as "pouring on insensibility to the throes of labor." From the Greek word *narkē*, meaning "stupor," stemmed our word "narcotic."

But the Greeks were not the only ones to make literary references to anesthesia. The Talmud contains several passages that mention that the practice of easing pain of torture and death by stupefying the sufferer was quite ancient. In China, a physician named Hau T'o, who lived about A.D. 230, came to hold a unique position in Chinese annals; he introduced surgery to that nation.

Until Hau T'o began his work, Confucian doctrine prevented the development of surgery in China because the priests considered the human body too sacred to be mutilated. However, Hau T'o developed into a surgeon so skillful that the Chinese people erected temples to him and he came to be worshiped as the god of surgery. Further, he discovered an effervescent powder called *ma-yo*, which when dissolved in wine produced complete insensibility, thus enabling him to operate on any portion of the body without the patient's knowledge. Unfortunately, he did not leave the formula for his soporific powder to posterity.

Ibn Sina, known to the western world as Avicenna, was a dominant figure among the Arabian practitioners of medicine. His canon of medicine, after being translated into Latin, became the medical authority in Europe for six centuries. He listed the types of anesthetic agents to alleviate pain as follows:

1. Those contrary to the cause of pain, which remove the pain; examples: fennel, linseed made into a poultice.
2. Those counteracting the acrimony of the humors, soothing, inducing sleep, or dulling the sensitive faculties and lessening their activity; examples: inebriants, milk, oil, sweet water.
3. Narcotics and somniferous drugs; the first of these is the most certain.

With the birth of Christianity came the concept of the relief of pain based upon divine healing through touch and prayer. Some theologians believed mandragora to be the *myrrh* which, according to Mark, the Romans offered with wine to Christ before they nailed him to the cross. Indeed, narcotic draughts were sometimes given to persons about to be crucified to lessen their sensibility to the agony.

The Greeks believed an evil spirit dwelt in the plant mandragora; Theophrastus, in his early writings on botany, alluded to its virtues when he wrote:

> Of all the roots nourished at the breast of Mother Earth, none was so mysterious as the mandragora (mandrake). The man-like form of the outspread, two legged root was awe-inspiring. It grew beneath the gallows, feeding on the flesh of felons; its pain-easing, sensation-destroying death wine (wine of the condemned) was given on a sponge to those about to be tortured and hanged.

Dioscorides, in about A.D. 100, first mentioned mandragora as an anesthetic. He recognized the difference between the hypnotic and anesthetic effects of the drug.

During the centuries that followed the fall of the Roman Empire, little progress was made in the sciences or humanities. With civilization and culture at a low ebb, anesthesia as a science also remained immature. The Renaissance, although a period of an awakening of science and the arts, contributed little to humanity's search for an effective anesthesia. St. Hilary, in the fourth century, distinguished between anesthesia caused by disease and anesthesia resulting from drugs. Otherwise, there emerged no significant writings on the subject.

In 1490, Theodoric of Lucca mentioned a preparation that he called *aleum de lateribus*. He described it as "most caustic, and a soporific which, by means of smelling alone, could put patients to sleep on occasion of painful operations which they were to suffer."

The mixture was placed on a sponge in hot water and then applied to the nostrils of the patient. He called it the *spongia somnifera* and described his recipe for it:

> Take of opium, or the juice of unripe mulberry, of hyoscyamus, of the juice of hemlock, of the juice of the leaf of mandragora, of the juice of the woody wig, of the juice of the forest mulberry, of the seed of lettuce, of the seeds of dock, which has round apples, and of the water-hemlock, each an ounce; mix all these in a brazen vessel, and then place in it a new sponge, let the whole boil as long as the sun lasts on the dog-days, until the sponge consumes it all, and has boiled away in it. . . . As oft as there shall be need of it, place this sponge in hot water for an hour, and let it be applied to the nostrils to him who is to be operated on until he has fallen asleep and so let the surgery be performed.

When later tested by modern scientists, it was found the result would not "even make a guinea pig nod."

In Brooke's *Tragical History of Romelus and Julietta*, printed in 1562, which has been suggested to be Shakespeare's source for *Romeo and Juliet*, the character Friar Laurence spoke to Julietta: "I have learned and proved of long time the composition of a certain paste which I make of divers somferous samples, which beated afterward to powdere and dronke with a quantitie of water, within a quarter of an houre after, bringeth the receiver into such a sleep, and burieth so deeply the senses and other spirits of life that the cunningest phistian will judge the party died." And the character continued, "And, besides that, it hath a more marvellous effect, for the person which useth the same feeleth no kind of grief and, according to the quantitie of draught, the patient remaineth in a sweet sleepe; but when the operation is perfect and done, he returneth unto his first estate." In Shakespeare's *Romeo and Juliet*, the lovely Juliet took a mysterious unnamed drug that produced such a profound sleep and such a perfect simulation of death that she was put into her tomb.

Thus, over the years, anesthetic agents have played a part in literature, but very little influence was derived from the actual practice of inducing sleep in the operating room. The Egyptians and Greeks placed a practical value on pain-killing drugs. One method of pain relief for surgery was strangulation, used first by the Assyrians for the circumcision of their children. Anesthesia by strangulation to the point of unconsciousness was practiced until the seventeenth century. Another method was cerebral concussion, achieved by placing a wooden bowl over the patient's head and striking it until the patient became unconscious. The directions were simple. The surgeon merely had to strike the bowl with sufficient strength to crack an almond, but lightly enough to leave the skull intact. Other medical doctors diminished pain by the application of intense cold or by the compression of nerve roots. These were all primitive and less-than-effective methods of rendering the victim unconscious of pain. Anesthesia progressed over the years at about the same rate as surgery—slowly. It was not until modern times that rapid development was accomplished in both fields.

Yet modern anesthetic agents and operating-room instruments may be considered by future generations to be primeval as the use of hemp appears to our modern medical personnel. The scientific use of anesthesia is still evolving. To better understand the current and future developments, we must consider that period of time during which there was a distinct change from ancient medicine to current scientific approaches to anesthesia.

INHALATION AGENTS

Present-day choices of agents mirror the progress of the evolution of anesthesia. Ether, an early agent, continued to be used until the 1960s. Nitrous oxide, another early agent, is currently one of the most frequently used agents. The popularity of chloroform and ethyl chloride was short-lived. The twentieth century brought us divinyl ether (Vinethene), ethylene, trichloroethylene (Trimar), fluroxene (Fluoromar), and cyclopropane. None of these agents are used today because they are either toxic or explosive. In the 1930s work began on the halogenated hydrocarbons. The first one released for clinical use was halothane, in the late 1950s. It was followed a year later by methoxyflurane (Penthrane), and in 1972 enflurane (Ethrane) was released for general use. The most recent inhalation agent released for use is isoflurane (Forane). Much research led to the development of these agents and to those not yet released.

Nitrous Oxide

Although many people worked toward the development of modern anesthesia, the early scientific investigations were performed by individuals in Great Britain. Joseph Priestly was a nonconformist minister who amused himself by experimenting with "fixed air" in a brewery next to his home in Leeds. There he isolated and described nine different gases. In 1772 he obtained nitrous oxide from metals heated with nitric acid. Nitrous oxide is also called protoxide of nitrogen, nitrogen monoxide, or "laughing gas." It is one of several oxides of nitrogen but the only one that exhibits anesthetic properties.

It was not until 1799 that Sir Humphrey Davy, at the age of 17, experimented with nitrous oxide and discovered that it had the ability to mask pain and suggested that it be used as an anesthetic agent. Also in 1799, James Wyatt designed a nitrous oxide container to assist in Davy's research. Davy was the first to refer to nitrous oxide as "laughing gas." He published a book on its effects entitled *Research, Chemical and Philosophic—Chiefly Concerning Nitrous Oxide and Respiration*. In it are described methods for obtaining the gas and its effects on human beings.

But Davy's suggestions lay unheeded for 45 years. Then on December 10, 1844, a traveling chemist-lecturer, Gardner Q. Colton, visited Hartford, Connecticut, and gave a public demonstration of nitrous oxide. During the course of the demonstration a man named Cooley, who had just inhaled the nitrous oxide, fell over a bench. When he came to his senses, he noted his leg was lacerated and bleeding but stated he felt no pain. Horace Wells, a dentist who was attending the lecture, asked Colton to administer him some nitrous oxide the next day for a dental extraction. Colton did so and, following this successful experiment, Wells had Colton teach him the method for producing nitrous oxide and used it in his dental practice for work on fifteen patients. In January 1845, Wells attempted to introduce nitrous oxide as an anesthetic by giving a demonstration at the Massachusetts General Hospital. Unfortunately, the patient cried out and his colleagues ridiculed the experiment, thereby causing nitrous oxide to fall into disrepute. Wells eventually became deranged and an ether addict. He later committed suicide in a New York City prison by cutting his cubital vein. Ironically, he inhaled ether while he did it, perhaps to relieve the pain of the incision.

In 1863, Colton revived the use of nitrous oxide when J. H. Smith, a dentist, heard his lecture and used the gas in his practice. Nitrous oxide was finally accepted, became widely used, and continues to be the most widely used inhalation agent in anesthesia practice today.

Edmund Andrews introduced the use of oxygen and nitrous oxide in 1868. He published *The Oxygen Mixture: A New Anesthetic Combination*, in which he described the efficacy of adding 20 percent of oxygen to nitrous oxide. He concluded the mixture was safer and more pleasant. The techniques of administration were worked out by him and by Paul Bert in 1879. Bert used positive-pressure administration. As a result of Bert's investigation, the first accurate knowledge of the action of nitrous oxide became available.

The Johnstone Brothers, a medical supply business, began in 1872 to supply liquid nitrous oxide in metal cylinders. At a pressure of 30 atmospheres the gas condenses into a liquid, thus requiring the measurement of pressure and flow rate of gases. An eventual result was the development of the anesthesia machine.

Diethyl Ether

The accidental mixing of two known substances gave the world ether. Its use and value was not fully realized for 600 years. In the 13th century, Raymundus Lillius, a Spanish chemist, mixed sulfuric acid and ethyl alcohol. The result, when heated, produced a product with a pleasant odor and was, therefore, called "sweet vitriol."

In 1540, Valerius Cordus of Germany described the synthesis and properties of ether. Among its uses he included treatment of upset stomach, phlegm, dysentery, colic, flatulence, hiccups, and whooping cough. In the same century, Paracelsus also experimented with ether by combining ethyl alcohol and sulfuric acid. He described the synthesized substance as a sweet sulfur compound. He told of how his chickens consumed the compound, fell asleep, and later awakened without any apparent ill effects. This inspired Paracelsus to hypothesize that this substance "quiets all suffering without any harm, relieves all pain, quenches all fevers, and prevents complications in any illness."

The name ether is attributed to a German scientist, Frobenius, who carried on experiments in 1730. The value of ether as an anesthetic was not appreciated until 1818, when Michael Faraday called attention to the profound lethargic state that resulted from the imprudent inhalation of ether. By 1824, a surgeon, Henry Hill Hickman, had advanced the idea of using the gas to produce insensibility during operations.

Crawford Long first witnessed the effects of ether at an "ether frolic" in Philadelphia. This seems to have been an accepted pastime of well-to-do of the day. In January 1842, Long first used ether clinically. He gave a patient named James Venable ether before removing a tumor from his neck. Long continued using ether for minor surgery but not without causing a stir in his community. The townspeople of Jefferson, Georgia, were so excited and afraid of the gas that there were threats to lynch him. Faced with this opposition, he ceased performing operations under ether and later moved his office to Athens, Georgia. His work there received little recognition until publicized by Marion Sims.

Another pioneer of ether, William Morton, unable to afford medical school, had become a successful dentist. But disturbed by the suffering of patients undergoing dental operations, he was driven to seek a means to alleviate the pain. Given a degree of financial security by his dental practice, he decided to attend medical school at Harvard University.

While at that august school, Morton consulted with Professor Charles J. Jackson and learned that sulfuric ether had some effect in producing unconsciousness. Morton experimented on his dog, his fish, himself, and his friends. He finally convinced a friend to permit him to extract a tooth painlessly under ether.

As a second-year medical student, he obtained permission from John Collins Warren, professor of surgery at Harvard, to make a public trial of ether on October 16, 1846. This was a turning point in the history of anesthesia. The event was brief, but dramatic and world-shaking.

Morton arrived late because he was working until the last minute to develop a suitable inhaler. He arrived at the amphitheater of the Massachusetts General Hospital, now named the Ether Dome in honor of the event, and proceeded to anesthetize Gilbert Abbott. When the patient was unconscious, Morton said "Sir, your patient is ready."

The procedure progressed quietly, without any struggling or screaming. At the conclusion of the procedure, Dr. Warren turned to the observers and said, "Gentlemen, this is no humbug." Dr. Henry J. Bigelow, an eminent surgeon of the day, declared "I have seen something today which will go around the world."

After Morton's demonstration of the effectiveness of ether anesthesia, the practice was generally accepted. Despite his experiments, Morton never received full recognition for the development of ether anesthesia during his lifetime. But the inscription on his tombstone reads:

Inventor and Revealor of Inhalation Anesthesia: Before Whom in All Time, Surgery was Agony: By Whom, Science had Control of Pain

Ether continued to be widely used until the early 1960s.

Chloroform

Chloroform was prepared in 1831 by Justus von Lerby in Germany, by Samuel Guthrie in the United States, and by Soubeiran in France. Jean-Baptiste Dumas described its physical and chemical properties in 1835 and gave it the name chloroform because of its relationship to chlorine and formic acid. Flourens discovered its anesthetic properties in 1847.

James Simpson and his associates introduced chloroform to clinical practice in Great Britain in November 1847. Simpson's use of chloroform to relieve the pain of childbirth came under attack because it was felt by the Calvinist clergy that he acted in defiance of divine will. However, the opposition received a serious blow when John Snow administered chloroform to Queen Victoria for the birth of her eighth child, Prince Leopold. A wag of the day suggested an obstetrician's coat of arms, which consisted of a newborn baby with the legend underneath, "Does your mother know you're out?"

Many deaths occurred with the use of chloroform, apparently because of improper administration based upon misconceptions and incomplete knowledge of the drug's direct effect on the heart and circulation. The incidence of death with chloroform came to be at least twice that of ether; yet its extreme potency, which made it lethal in unskilled hands, was the reason for chloroform's potential superiority as an anesthetic agent. Most of the black marks against it were the result of maladministration and lack of supportive therapy rather than of any inherent property of the drug itself. Until 1890, the deaths were considered consequences of overdosage. After 1890, the incidence of deaths in the postoperative period increased sharply. Liver damage or delayed chloroform poisoning were thought to be the reason. But several other factors were operating concurrently and may have influenced these results. These were

1. Introduction of opiates as premedication.
2. Increasing length of surgical procedures.
3. Change in usage, according to surgical demand, from borderline analgesia to surgical anesthesia.

That the number of deaths was not larger can be attributed to the skills and acute observations of these early physicians. It is remarkable that they were able to apply chloroform even as successfully as they did. Chloroform, with the exception of halothane, relaxes a laboring uterus better than any other known drug. It is the possibility of sudden inhalation of a strong concentration that makes chloroform extremely dangerous and a cause of cardiac depression.

Ethyl Chloride

Ethyl chloride was the last general anesthetic adopted in the nineteenth century. It was first prepared by Valentine in the seventeenth century and later by Flourens, who described its anesthetic properties in February 1847. Heyfelder first used it clinically in 1848; he found its action to be similar to ether and concluded that its extreme volatility, the difficulty of obtaining the pure compound, and the high price would preclude its frequent use.

The "Glasgow Committee" of the British Medical Association examined its action upon lower animals and in their report published in 1880 concluded that it was unsuitable for human beings because it produced convulsions and respiratory failure. The disrepute into which ethyl chloride fell was largely due to impurities in the samples examined. As a local anesthetic, the drug leaves much to be desired. It has limited use today in dental practice.

Ethylene

The anesthetic properties of ethylene were first noted by Hermann in 1864. It was not used clinically until 1923 when administered by Luckhardt, Carter, and Brown. Isabella Herb carried out the first clinical study in 1924. Even after that date, few hospitals used it because of its high combustibility. Its explosive nature offset its slight advantage over nitrous oxide.

Divinyl Ether

In 1897, Semmler prepared the first divinyl ether (Vinethene). In an attempt to make a hybrid molecule that would have the characteristics of parent agents ethyl ether and ethylene, Leake and Chen discovered its anesthetic properties in 1930. Ruigh and Major first successfully synthesized it in 1931 and Gelfen and Bell used it clinically at the University of Alberta in 1932. Many objections to this agent were associated with its breakdown products rather than with the original molecule.

Trichlorethylene

Fisher first described trichlorethylene (Trimar) in 1864. Originally the drug was used in medicine to control the pain of tic douloureux; researchers found in 1935 that its analgesic effect was general and not specific on the trigeminal nerve. Jackson described its anesthetic properties after experiments with dogs. Striker used it to anesthetize 300 patients in 1935. After an unenthusiastic report by the American Medical Association in 1936, its popularity as an inhaled agent waned.

Fluroxene

Fluroxene (Fluoromar) came to be the first inhalation agent to emerge from the group of fluorine-containing hydrocarbons and ethers that Krantz developed and evaluated extensively. He first described it after initial investigation in 1953. The drug was introduced for clinical trial in 1954. This drug is no longer used. It had no apparent advantages over other agents that were available.

Cyclopropane

August von Freund first produced cyclopropane in 1882. Its anesthetic properties were not discovered for 50 years and then quite by accident. Professor V. E. Henderson and his staff in Toronto, Canada, were working with propylene in an attempt to find an anesthetic agent that would be potent and less toxic than ether. They stored the propylene in metal alloy tanks, which consistently produced impurities. They believed these pollutions caused the myocardial depression and nausea associated with the use of the gas in general anesthesia. In 1927, a new member of Professor Henderson's staff, Dr. G. H. Lucas, was assigned to determine the toxic substances in the propylene storage tanks. He found mostly hexenes but also an isomer of propylene, formed during the preparation of propylene. He discovered cyclopropane and its anesthetic properties during tests for the contamination of propylene. He expected it to have toxic effects, but when it was tested on kittens, they went nicely to sleep and recovered rapidly without any significant problems. he concluded these tests during November 1928. Subsequently, Professor Henderson volunteered to be anesthetized with cyclopropane, first administered by a Dr. Brown. In spite of excellent results, their first attempts to introduce the drug clinically failed.

Later, Dr. Ralph Waters attended a meeting where an unknown physician suggested the use of cyclopropane as a general anesthetic. After some correspondence, Dr. Waters became convinced of its effectiveness and started clinical studies at the University of Wisconsin, where cyclopropane proved to have great promise. Waters and Rovenetine anesthetized the first three patients in August 1930. The studies continued for three years, with Waters and Schmidt publishing the first clinical report in 1934. Cyclopropane came to be used clinically until the advent of the nonexplosive agents.

The Search for an Ideal Agent

The initial work in the development of halothane began in the late 1920s. Scientists were looking for an "ideal agent" that would be nonexplosive, nonflammable, safe, potent, economical, compatible with other compounds, and have no deleterious effect on equipment. They felt it should provide a rapid pleasant induction, have little or no depressant effect on vital organs, and be easily and rapidly eliminated unchanged from the body with no side effects. Their agent was well termed "ideal."

Initial studies began with halogenated hydrocarbons. In 1929, Frederick Swatz discovered that fluorination added stability to the aliphatic hydrocarbons. He placed one fluo-

rine atom on a carbon molecule. In 1932, Booth, Bixby, Gnong, and Birchfield showed that by increasing the temperature and pressure they could put three fluorine atoms on a carbon molecule. But from 1932 to 1946, fluorocarbons came to be used primarily with vehicular gases for aerosols and refrigerants. Progress in developing anesthetic uses remained slow because of the difficulty of producing pure gases. Impurities were often present and caused more problems than the gas itself. The development of the gas spectrograph in the early 1940s proved to be a great asset for the development of pure gases. During this period most anesthesia research was concerned with the treatment of trauma caused by World War II.

In 1937, Henne developed a method for combining fluorinated hydrocarbons with other aliphatic chains, thus increasing the number of possible compounds that could be formed. Subsequently Brue began to add other halogenated chains and discovered some important relationships between fluorine, bromine, and chlorine. He found that increased fluorination produced agents with decreased boiling points and that decreasing the boiling point of an agent caused a greater incidence of convulsions in animal studies. The addition of chlorine or bromine increased the boiling point and decreased the seizure activity. He also found the bromination caused a greater increase in potency than did chlorination.

During the middle 1940s Benjamin Robbins published a report on results of two years of testing of 46 fluorinated compounds for their anesthesia activity. Of these he felt only four warranted further investigation. He reported four important discoveries:

1. There was increased potency with increased boiling point.
2. The introduction of a second halogen atom (chlorine, bromine, or iodine) to a fluorocarbon greatly increased the potency.
3. Most of the agents did not support the blood pressure in dogs.
4. Abnormalities in cardiac rhythm were frequently produced.

One of the agents that Robbins felt warranted further investigation was trifluorobromethane. It had good anesthesia properties and resembled the compound that was to become halothane ten years later.

Halothane

Suckling, a researcher working for Imperial Chemical Industries Laboratory, synthesized a series of compounds in 1951; bromochlorotrifluorethane was one of these. It was introduced as an anesthetic under the aegis of the Committee on Non-Explosive Anesthetics, formed by the British Medical Research Council. In 1956, Raventous investigated the pharmacologic use of the gas and its actions on animals.

The Imperial Chemical Industries Laboratory did not release halothane but hired the highly qualified anesthesiologists Johnstone, Bryce, Smith, and O'Bryan to test it and establish guidelines for its use. Johnstone and his associates published the findings of their research in October 1956. They listed the advantages and disadvantages of halothane. These studies led to the development of the Fluotec and other out-of-circuit vaporizers because they found halothane too potent to be used in the conventional in-circuit vaporizers. They also determined that the various side effects could be decreased if lower concentrations were used. Halothane was released in Great Britain in 1957 and in the United States and Canada in late 1958.

Between 1960 and 1962 a number of case studies reported halothane as the suspected cause of severe hepatic necrosis and postoperative hepatitis. This circumstance created a great deal of concern and led to the largest research project ever undertaken to investigate an anesthetic agent.

In 1961, the Committee on Anesthesia of the National Academy of Sciences National Research Council designated a study group to report periodically on all clinical aspects of halothane anesthesia and to give special attention to any evidence of association with fatal postoperative hepatic necrosis. The primary objectives were (1) to compare halothane with other general anesthetics regarding the incidence of fatal massive hepatic necrosis within six weeks of an anesthetic and (2) to compare total hospital mortality within six weeks of anesthesia.

The National Halothane Study produced facts and figures on over 800,000 anesthetic administrations. The conclusions indicated halothane to be safe or safer than other commonly used anesthetics. The effects of halothane on the liver, if any, are clinically negligible. It has become the most widely used, potent inhalation agent we identify with the 1960s and is still an extremely popular agent today.

Methoxyflurane

Methoxyflurane (Penthrane) a relatively modern anesthetic agent, is a halogen-substituted methyl ethyl ether. It is the first unsymmetrical methyl ether used in clinical anesthesia.

Larsen first synthesized it in 1958, and Artusia used it clinically as early as 1959. He and his associates published the first pharmacologic and clinical results in 1960. They found methoxyflurane (Penthrane) to be more susceptible to biogradation than halothane and to produce renal and hepatic injury. Also, its high blood and tissue solubility rendered it less flexible and more likely to be toxic. This agent is rarely used today.

For some time the success of halothane discouraged the search for new and better anesthetics. With time, scientists found that halothane, too, had its limitations. It caused respiratory depression, sensitized the myocardium to arrhythmias induced by epinephrine and isoproterenol, and caused uterine relaxation, which led to increased bleeding during delivery.

The primary criteria researchers sought in a new agent were nonflammability and chemical stability. Many researchers believed that stable chemicals would not be metabolized; therefore, possible toxic effects attributed to their metabolites would be eliminated. Other desirable criteria were minimal respiratory and cardiovascular depression, rapid and pleasant induction and recovery, good muscle relation, no sensitization of the myocardium to catecholamines, no cellular toxicity, and economy of production. Both enflurane—compound 347—and its isomer isoflurane—compound 469—satisfied most of these criteria.

Enflurane

Enflurane (Ethrane) was synthesized by Terrell in 1963. It was the second methyl ethyl ether made available to the anesthesia community.

Enflurane differed from halothane and methoxyflurane in its resistance to biogradation; as a consequence, organ injury is minimal. Rapid changes in alveolar concentrations are possible because of its low blood solubility. It provides heart rhythm stability and excellent muscle relaxation.

Isoflurane

Terrell synthesized isoflurane (Forane) in 1965. Because of the difficulty of synthesizing and purifying isoflurane, he developed it after the isomer enflurane. The problem of purifying isoflurane was so great that the compound was almost abandoned. Spears first accomplished a separation of isoflurane from the contaminants introduced during manufacturing; this permitted biologic testing. Initial testing in mice showed promise. Further studies by Rudo in 1967, by Dobkin and Byles in 1975, and by Stevens and Eger in 1975 were positive in outcome and suggested that no significant injury to the liver or kidneys would follow its use. Other studies of toxicity were negative. These findings led to trials in volunteers and the use of isoflurane with patients.

Isoflurane was scheduled for introduction in 1975. However, a study by Corbett using mice suggested that isoflurane might be a hepatocarcinogen. A larger study with better controls failed to confirm Corbett's findings, and the FDA released it for clinical use in 1980. Isoflurane (Forane) may constitute a major advance in the search for an "ideal" anesthetic.

ADJUNCTS TO ANESTHESIA

Over the years, various drugs have been used in conjunction with the inhalation agents. The barbiturates are still used today, with thiopental sodium (Pentothal) being the primary drug. The other group of drugs that are of significance are the neuromuscular blockers. They play a very important role in the practice of anesthesia.

Thiopental Sodium

In 1903, a German chemist, Emil Fisher, discovered barbiturates. The barbiturate first synthesized was barbital. At the beginning of the intravenous barbiturate era, several long-acting drugs were investigated for clinical use. Zerfes and Lundy investigated amobarbital in 1929, and Lundy experimented with pentobarbital in 1930. None of these drugs proved clinically satisfactory. Knopp and Taubb discovered the first ultra-short-acting barbiturate, hexobarbital. Weese and Scharpff tested it clinically in 1932, and Lundy tested it clinically at the Mayo Clinic in 1934.

Researchers also maintained an early desire to develop a drug that would produce profound hypnosis, but from which emergence would be prompt. As early as 1908, scientists detected that substituting sulfur for an oxygen atom on the carbon in the barbituric acid molecule produced less stable and shorter-acting drugs called thiobarbiturates. Thiopental came to be the sulfur analog of sodium pentobarbital. It was first prepared in the laboratory in 1929. Clinical trials with thiopental were begun in 1934, and it was first marketed in the United States in 1936.

A study covering the period 1934 through 1955 revealed that one-third of all surgical cases received thiopental (Pentothal). In 1950, an estimated 70 percent of all patients receiving general anesthesia were induced with thiopental. Thiopental suffered only one major decline in popularity. This occurred in 1941, in the early months of World War II. The problem was caused primarily by administration of the drug by untrained personnel. Thiopental is still used today as the main induction agent for general anesthesia. It can be found in all modern hospital operating rooms.

D-Tubocurarine

Indians along the Amazon and Orinoco Rivers in South America used blowpipes to shoot darts with tips that were covered with curare, which they used for killing wild animals and in warfare. Curare can be derived from about 30 species of plants that are found throughout northern and western South America. The Indians obtained the poison by soaking the roots and stalks in cold water, dissolving out the contents, and heating the mixture until it concentrated into a black paste.

In 1811, Sir Benjamin Brodie, an English scientist, while doing experiments on different modes of death from vegetable poisons, found that curare altered respirations and that the heart continued to beat for some time after respirations ceased. Artificial respiration by means of a bellows revived some of the experimental animals. Brodie and Watterton, in 1815, found that asphyxia was the cause of death in curare poisoning.

In 1856, Claude Bernard demonstrated that curare exerted its paralyzing action by blocking the nerve impulses at the neuromuscular junction. Bernard showed that curare did not act on central or peripheral nerves but on skeletal muscles. Dr. Carlos Chagus, of the University of Brazil, used electric eels, which have large neuronal endings, and radioactive carbon 14 to establish that curare attaches to a transmitter substance in the end plate, making this substance insensitive to the actions of acetylcholine.

Initial clinical use of curare was in the fields of psychiatry and neurology. Fiercelin and Benedict, French physicians, used curare in 1866 to prevent epileptic seizures in human beings. They had to discontinue their project because of a shortage of curare. Tubocurarine chloride (Intocostrin), the stable preparation of curare, was manufactured by Sembil Laboratories in 1939. Richard Gill, with the help of a Dr. McIntyre, developed a dependable curare product. Curare evolved into an extremely useful drug in the practice of modern anesthesia following its introduction into clinical anesthesia in 1942 by Griffiths and Johnson.

Succinylcholine

In 1906, Reid, Hunt, and Traveau first described the pharmacologic action of succinylcholine. Though they studied its effect on blood pressure, they failed to observe that it caused neuromuscular block because they were using a previously curarized animal. Gluk established in 1941 that the hydrolysis rate for succinylcholine was high and that it was broken down by cholinesterase in horse serum. Bovet and his colleagues in Italy and Phillips in the United States independently described the neuromuscular blocking properties of succinylcholine in 1949. The drug was first used on humans as a neuromuscular blocking agent by Thesleff at the Karolinska Institute in Stockholm in 1951. Foldes and his associates introduced it to the United States in 1952. Succinylcholine chloride is a very important adjunct to anesthesia today. It is widely used in most hospitals.

Gallamine Triethiodide

After the introduction of curare into clinical anesthesia, pharmacologists throughout the world sought to develop a synthetic drug with a similar action. In 1947, Bovet and his coworkers described the muscle relaxant properties of a synthetic product—gallamine triethiodide (Flaxedil). This drug is rarely used today. It has no advantages over other muscle relaxants that are available.

Pancuronium Bromide

While investigating a series of aminosteroids, Hervitt and Savage observed in 1964 that when they added an acetylcholine-like group to these biologically active compounds, Pancuronium bromide (Pavulon) appeared to be a very effective neuromuscular blocking agent. The pharmacology was studied extensively in animals by Bucket and Bonita in 1966. Boud and Reid introduced it into clinical practice in 1967. As a new muscle relaxant available to the anesthetist, this drug has developed great popularity in recent years.

Recently some intermediate-acting muscle relaxants have been introduced into clinical practice. These drugs, atracurium and vecuronium, will be discussed in Chapter 17.

BIBLIOGRAPHY

Abbott Laboratories: A Professional Guide to the Use of Pentothal. North Chicago, Ill., 1971.

Adriani J: The Chemistry and Physics of Anesthesia, 2nd ed. Springfield, Ill. Chas. C Thomas, 1962.

Ayerst Pharmaceutical Research Laboratories: Anesthesia. Montreal, 1962.

Artusio F Jr: Clinical Anesthesia Series, Halogenated Anesthetics. Philadelphia, Davis, 1963.

Bakutes AR: History of Anesthesia and the Role of the Nurse Specialist. Unpublished manuscript, 1971.

Bauer LH (ed): 75 Years of Medical Progress 1875–1953. Philadelphia, Lea & Febiger, 1954.

Buxton W: Anesthesia: Their Uses and Administration. Philadelphia, P. Blankinston's Son, 1907.

Cole F: Milestones in Anesthesia. Lincoln, Neb., University of Nebraska Press, 1965.

Collins VJ: Principles of Anesthesiology, 2nd ed. Philadelphia, Lea & Febiger, 1976.

Cullen SC: Curare: Its past and present. Anesthesiology 8:479–488, 1947.

Curtis RH: Triumph Over Pain. New York, McKay, 1972.

Dripps RD, Eckenhoff JE, Vandam LD: Introduction to Anesthesia, 6th ed. Philadelphia, Saunders, 1967.

Eger EI: Isoflurane (Forane). Madison, Wis., Airco, 1981.

Gill RC: Curare: Misconceptions regarding the discovery and development of present form of the drug. Anesthesiology 7:14–23, 1946.

Goodman LS, Gilman A: The Pharmacologic Basis of Therapeutics. New York, Macmillan, 1975.

Green NM: Clinical Anesthesia Series, Halothane. Philadelphia, Davis, 1968.

Keys TE: The History of Surgical Anesthesia. New York, Schuman, 1945.

Lee AJ: A Synopsis of Anesthesia, 7th ed. Baltimore, Williams & Wilkins, 1973.

Robinson V: Victory Over Pain. New York, McKay, 1942.

Raper HR: Man Against Pain. Englewood Cliffs, N.J., Prentice-Hall, 1945.

Salove MS, Wallace VE: Halothane. Philadelphia, Davis, 1962.

Thatcher VS: History of Anesthesia. Philadelphia, Lippincott, 1953.

U.S. Department of Health, Education, and Welfare, The Public Health Service: The National Halothane Study. Bethesda, Md., National Institutes of Health, National Institute of General Medical Sciences, 1969.

Vitcha JF: A history of Forane. Anesthesiology 35:4–7, 1971.

Wellcome HS: Anesthetics Ancient and Modern. New York, Burroughs Wellcome, 1907.

Wylie WD, Churchill-Davidson HC: A Practice of Anesthesia, 5th ed. Chicago, Year Book Med, Pub, 1984.

3

Legal Aspects of Nurse Anesthesia Practice

Mary Jeanette Mannino

"Ignorance of the law is no excuse" is an old adage that still holds true today. It applies equally in all areas: drivers are required to know traffic laws, and professionals are expected to know the laws that govern their practice. The nurse anesthetist faces a constant challenge to be aware of legal changes and advances in anesthesia and medicine in general. Although the legal process appears to move at a slower pace than medicine, the true professional must keep abreast of the emerging legal climate that reflects the trends and advances in society. Of immediate concern to health care professionals are the great number of malpractice suits and the extremely high damage awards in evidence today. It is incumbent on those in the medical field, including nurse anesthetists, to be knowledgeable about the law as it relates to their individual practices.

Nurse anesthetists should know that the practice of anesthesia has a firm basis in law. The legal basis of nurse anesthesia practice is derived from nurse practice acts, health and safety codes, judicial opinions, and a tradition of over 50 years of anesthesia service. Judicial opinions that authenticate the legality of nurse anesthesia practice were handed down in two landmark California cases. In Chalmers Francis vs Nelson (6 Cal 2d 402, 1936), nurse anesthesia practice was verified from a common-law perspective. In Magit vs Board of Medical Examiners (57 C 2d 17 Cal App 488, 1956), the court held that anesthesia is a medically delegated act: "It is generally recognized that the functions of nurses and physicians overlap to some extent, and a licensed nurse, when acting under some direction and supervision of a licensed physician, is permitted to perform certain tasks which without such direction and supervision would constitute the illegal practice of medicine or surgery."

Nurse anesthetists practice under the sphere of the Nurse Practice Act and the rules and regulations established by the nursing boards of individual states. In recent years, nursing laws have recognized the expanded role of nursing, particularly in such special functions as nurse anesthetists, nurse midwives, and nurse practitioners. The amount of recognition of these specialty groups varies from state to state. As the groups are recognized, educational and certification requirements are formulated, standards of practice are set, and the scope of practice is defined.

At one time it was assumed that the surgeon was responsible for the acts of the other health care professionals in the operating room. The myth that the surgeon is captain of the ship, and therefore responsible for the actions of nurses, is not supported by modern law. On the contrary, legal opinions and judicial decisions specifically support the nonliability of physicians for the negligent acts of others. In a leading case in New Jersey, the court held that the nurse anesthetist did not become the servant or agent of the obstetrician merely because she received instructions from him as to the work to be performed during the patient's childbirth (Susselman vs Muhlenberg Hospital, 1973).

Some courts have imposed vicarious liability on surgeons using nurse anesthetists based upon the degree of supervision or control the surgeon exerts. In general, it seems that the courts take a "common sense" approach to the issue by finding liability where the surgeon caused or could have prevented the damage to the patient either because of exerting control or because of failing to take remedial measures (Blumenreich and Benkov, 1984).

The liability of a hospital or clinic for an anesthesia injury is usually based on the doctrine of respondeat superior, in which the hospital, as an employer, must assume responsibility for its employees. In recent legal decisions, hospital liability has been expanded to include the acts of independent contractors and others who use the hospital facilities. The liability of the hospital does not relieve the nurse anesthetist of responsibility for negligent actions. It merely enlarges the scope of a lawsuit to allow the plaintiff to name both the hospital and the anesthetist in an action for negligence.

MALPRACTICE

The term *malpractice* has been used to encompass all liability-producing conduct by professionals. *Professional negligence* is the term most often used in current legal actions. If a patient suffers harm from the professional actions of a nurse anesthetist, the legal theory that would most likely apply

15

is the tort concept of negligence. Tort law recognizes the responsibility of a person to act as "an ordinary, prudent person" would under similar circumstances. A deviation from or breach of this reasonable-person standard is considered actionable under the legal rules of evidence. In an action for negligence the following components must be established by the plaintiff: duty, standard of care, causation, and damages.

Duty

To be held for professional negligence, it must be established that the anesthetist owed a duty to the injured party. A professional duty may be established under either the contract theory or a traditional professional relationship. When an anesthetist assumes the anesthesia management of a patient, a contract is in effect; that is, the anesthetist contracts to care for the patient through the entire anesthesia process, and the patient contracts to pay for this service. At the same time, a professional relationship is established. A professional relationship implies trust, in which a layperson, who does not have the expertise of the professional, relies on the professional for services to be performed at the highest level of that professional's knowledge and experience.

If this professional relationship is prematurely terminated, the professional may be liable for abandonment. In a judicial opinion based on facts in a Washington, D.C., case, the court ruled that once a professional relationship between a patient and a health care professional has been established, it cannot be terminated at will. The court stated: The relationship will continue until it is ended in one of the following circumstances: (1) the patient's lack of need for further care and (2) withdrawal of the physician upon being replaced by an equally qualified physician. Withdrawal from the case under any other circumstances constitutes a wrongful abandonment of the patient (*Ascher vs Gutierrez*, 1976).

Standard of Care

Negligence law presupposes uniform standards of behavior against which a defendant's conduct can be measured. The courts recognize that a health care professional has education and training above that of a layperson and is expected to act in a manner consistent with that knowledge and training. The standard of care by which a nurse anesthetist is evaluated is complex. The American Association of Nurse Anesthetists (AANA), exercising its inherent right to direct and control the activities of its membership, has established and published standards of practice for nurse anesthetists. In a lawsuit, these standards may be used to establish current standards of nurse anesthesia practice.

Another method of establishing the standard of care is through expert witnesses. The judicial system recognizes that the medical knowledge of lay jurors is limited, and therefore expert witnesses, who are members of the same profession, are asked to testify about the standard of care. The plaintiff and the defendant may both call expert witnesses to testify. To be an expert witness, a person must possess qualifications and knowledge in the area in question. The *Federal Rules of Evidence* state that an expert witness must be qualified by "knowledge, skill, experience, training, and education."

Historically, the defined standards of care for the medical profession were limited to a geographic area. This narrow ruling indicated that professionals had to practice only in a manner that was acceptable in their own community. This strict locality rule proved to be impractical and limited the pool of expert witnesses. Modern communications have expanded access to knowledge, and the courts have reasoned that with this expanded access to knowledge, all health care professionals should be able to keep up with medical advances, and they have modified the rule to include a national standard.

Package inserts on drugs and manufacturers' instructions regarding the manner in which drugs are to be administered or equipment used may also be admissible as evidence of the standard of care. Most courts, however, require that the information in these inserts and instructions be validated or refuted by expert witnesses. A Louisiana case illustrates how one court viewed the use of package inserts as evidence of the standard of care in a lawsuit involving a nurse anesthetist:

> A nurse anesthetist was sued by a patient for physical complications including phlebitis and thrombosis of the arm, alleging the injury was the result of improper administration of diazepam (Valium). At the trial, the manufacturer's recommendations for the administration of the drug were admitted into evidence.
>
> Expert testimony verified that the drug had been administered according to the standard of practice, rather than the manufacturer's directions. The court ruled that even if the anesthetist did not administer the diazepam in the precise way directed in the manufacturer's insert, her degree of precision and care did not vary from that adhered to in her specialty (*Mohr vs Jenkins*, 1980).

Causation

In a malpractice action the plaintiff must establish that the injury was caused by the alleged negligent acts of the defendant. This element of negligence, causation, is an important factor in a malpractice case and must be proved either by direct or expert testimony. The standard most commonly used to establish causation is whether or not the patient's injury is "more likely than not" the result of the defendant's conduct.

Multiple causation is often seen in malpractice cases, where frequently it cannot be determined that the injury was caused by one single factor or one person's acts. The plaintiff will name as defendants all those who were involved in any phase of the incident that could have caused injury. The following case illustrates causation in an anesthesia lawsuit:

> In June 1975, the patient underwent surgery to excise lymph nodes in his right groin and right armpit. As a result of the surgery, he alleged that he suffered damages to the median ulnar nerves caused by the surgeon's negligence. He also named the anesthetist, recovery room nurse, and the hospital in the suit, alleging that his left eye had been injured when

a foreign substance was dropped into it by the anesthetist before or during surgery.

The court trial resulted in a divided verdict in favor of all the defendants and the case was dismissed. The appellate court upheld the defense verdict and said that ". . . plaintiff produced no proof of any causal connection between his alleged eye injury and [the defendant's actions. . . . We] conclude that the evidence offered was woefully insufficient to connect the patient's eye injury to the defendants" (*Regas vs Argonaut Southern Insurance Co et al,* 1980).

Damages

The final element necessary for actionable negligence is damages, which refers to the amount of money or other compensation the plaintiff may receive for the loss or injury suffered. Categories of damages are nominal, compensatory, and punitive.

Nominal damages are usually awarded when the injury or loss is small or the question of liability is debatable. The award of nominal damages states, in essence, that the plaintiff's suit is justified, but the right recovery is minimal because of the nature of the injury or failure to prove gross loss or injury, the culpability of the defendants, or both. An example of nominal damages would be an award of only court costs or partial medical expenses.

Compensatory damages are awarded in an attempt to make appropriate and counterbalancing payment to the plaintiff for a loss or injury sustained through the acts or default of the defendant, with the desire to, insofar as possible, "make the plaintiff whole." Compensatory damages could include a judgment based on the plaintiff's loss of income, need for continuing medical care or rehabilitation, or loss of ability to enjoy life in the same manner as before the incident. These damages are usually large and can include payments to the defendant for the rest of his or her life.

Punitive damages are awarded as punishment to the defendant when it has been decided that his or her negligence was willful, aggravated, or wanton. Punitive damages, in a sense, carry the admonition to the defendant to "cease and desist" from such negligent behavior.

If a patient dies as the result of the negligent acts of a defendant, the survivors may collect for wrongful death. Damages can be based on the estimated time the deceased would have lived and the amount of money he or she could have earned in that length of time. These damages could include a lump sum payment to the surviving spouse and children and support for their lifetime. The surviving spouse could also be awarded damages for "loss of marital companionship." These damages are usually very large, although some states have statutes that establish the basis of recovery in a wrongful death suit and the maximum amount of damages that may be awarded.

INFORMED CONSENT

A common practice in malpractice lawsuits is to claim lack of informed consent. Plaintiffs allege that they were not informed of the anesthetic regimen planned or of any risks involved and that the consent obtained from them is therefore invalid. Consent for anesthesia and surgery is a defense

for the intentional tort of assault and battery. Express consent is consent given in writing by the patient or a person legally authorized to sign. Written consent is generally required when the proposed procedure carries some risk to the patient or when the patient's body is to be invaded. Express written consent should be as specific as possible.

Each state has enacted laws concerning consent. Competent adults can give their own consent. For this purpose, competency is defined as the ability to understand the nature and consequences of the action to which one is asked to consent. Justice Cardozo wrote in 1914, "Every human being of adult years and sound mind has a right to determine what shall be done with his body, and a surgeon who performs an operation without his patient's consent commits a battery for which he is liable in damages" (*Schoendorf vs Society of New York Hospital,* 1914).

The doctrine of informed consent dictates that the patient must receive sufficient information about the contemplated medical procedure so that any decision will be made with knowledge of the risks, complications, and alternatives. Recent cases in which lack of informed consent was a cause of action have been decided under negligence rather than battery. Medical and legal experts recommend that there be detailed documentation on the patient's permanent record that all aspects of the informed consent (nature of the treatment, risks, complications and expected benefits, and alternative forms of treatment) have been discussed with the patient and the patient has agreed to them.

Consent can be implied when a patient's actions indicate consent or when an emergency exists. Such emergencies, however, must endanger the life or health of the patient and require immediate emergency medical intervention. The following case illustrates judicial interpretation of the need for proper consent:

> A patient was admitted to the hospital for observation because of abdominal pain. An exploratory operation was agreed upon. The surgeon obtained written consent from the patient's husband for both the operation and the administration of anesthesia. After the operation, the patient allegedly suffered from phlebitis, bladder trouble, and partial paralysis.
>
> The patient alleged that she had never been advised that surgery was necessary and the use of an anesthetic had not been discussed with her. She said that she had had two previous spinal anesthetics and for that reason would not have agreed to the administration of a spinal anesthetic. Both the surgeon and the anesthesiologist claimed they had talked to her at least 2 hours before the surgery at a time when she was in full possession of her mental faculties and capable of giving consent.
>
> The court ruled that since no emergency existed, the patient's consent should have been obtained. The record failed to establish circumstances that would have justified an operation without the patient's consent for herself. The husband–wife relationship does not in itself make one the agent of the other (*Gravis vs Physicians and Surgeons Hospital of Alice,* 1967).

OBSTETRICS AND LAWSUITS

There are numerous lawsuits in the area of obstetrics and obstetric anesthesia. Bad results in an obstetric case usually involve both the mother and the baby, with resultant emotional impact. Nurse anesthetists administering obstetric anesthesia have a special need to maintain state-of-the-art skills, including maternal and fetal monitoring and endotracheal intubation for all parturients receiving general anesthesia and to be knowledgeable about advances in continuous epidural anesthesia.

REGIONAL VERSUS GENERAL ANESTHESIA

There is currently no evidence that there are more lawsuits after complications from regional anesthesia than from general anesthesia. The available statistics indicate, however, that there appear to be more serious side effects from general anesthesia than from regional anesthesia. A Department of Health, Education, and Welfare insurance survey recommended, because of the very large malpractice awards that have been given for brain damage resulting from general anesthesia accidents, that hospitals should support the use of local or spinal anesthetics wherever possible. Lawsuits arising from administration of regional anesthesia usually relate to complications from these blocks. However, these complications and side effects, while unfortunate, are not necessarily indicative of negligence.

There is currently some controversy about the legality of nurse anesthetists administering regional anesthesia. Although there is no state in the nation where it is illegal for nurse anesthetists to administer regional anesthesia, it is highly recommended that nurse anesthetists have clinical privileges approved by the appropriate committee of the medical staff. These privileges should delineate the scope of practice and should specifically mention regional anesthesia techniques if they are part of the CRNA service.

OVERVIEW OF THE U.S. LEGAL SYSTEM

Modern law is derived from four basic sources: statutes, regulations of government agencies, court decisions, and attorney general opinions. The basis of our legal system is common law, which is a system of jurisprudence inherited from the British. It is a system of judge-made laws that applies the principle of precedent rather than legislative enactment. The concept of precedent uses the rules and principles applied to a previous case to decide a current case. A court may recognize distinctions between the precedent and the current case or may conclude that a particular common-law rule is no longer in accord with the needs of society, thus departing from precedent.

The U.S. court system is divided into two divisions, federal and state, and each division hears cases that fall within its specific jurisdiction. On the state level, trial courts are courts of record and decisions from these lower courts may be appealed to the higher courts of the state. The decisions of the appellate courts are regarded as precedent-setting and are recorded in the books of law.

U.S. courts operate on the adversary system, which provides that both sides of a controversy will be represented by legal counsel and will have the right to present their case in the most forceful and favorable manner possible. The essence of the adversary system is that each side will have its day in court and it is hoped truth will be defined and justice realized.

The ultimate function of the legal system in a civil suit is to resolve disputes between the parties in a manner consistent with the law and to do so within a time frame that will make any relief granted meaningful. A typical negligence civil suit can be divided into three parts: preliminary (discovery), trial, and appeal.

In the discovery phase, legal papers are served, and both sides investigate the pertinent facts. Medical record reviews, interrogations, depositions, and use of experts are part of this phase of the legal action. Depositions from prospective witnesses may be taken by both sides of the controversy. Depositions are taken to acquaint legal counsel with the facts the witness is prepared to testify to, which enable counsel to prepare a knowledgeable suit or defense. Witnesses need to exercise great care in their statements and answers to questions when giving a deposition, and they must be aware that they will be held to these statements and answers at the time of trial. It is helpful at this time to refer to the patient's chart, or to any notes taken at the time of the incident, to assist in recall of the facts as they occurred. Witnesses are given a copy of their deposition and allowed to make changes and corrections before signing it.

When a case goes to trial, rules of civil procedure and evidence guide the proceedings. After hearing the evidence, testimony, and arguments, a verdict will be rendered by either the judge or a jury, and damages, if any, will be awarded. Either side of the controversy may appeal the verdict to one of the higher courts. Most malpractice cases that result in a high monetary award are appealed.

There are times when the dispute may be settled out of court. Settlements are determined on the basis of medical legal analysis of the facts, the severity of the injury, and the experience and judgment of the attorneys. A settlement is not to be considered an admission of guilt but simply as the best and most economical way of resolving the dispute.

PREVENTION AND DEFENSE OF LAWSUITS

Prevention of lawsuits and the defense of lawsuits are areas in which the nurse anesthetist should be knowledgeable. Although modern technology has been instrumental in streamlining the administration of anesthesia, there are risks in depending solely on mechanical devices. The nurse anesthetist must be well trained in the use of these devices, must know what each machine can and cannot do, and must be aware of malfunction possibilities. Keeping alive the human element by maintaining contact with the patient and monitoring the patient under anesthesia will help to keep the anesthetist alert to potential mishaps.

Accurate, timely, and legible reporting of events occurring during anesthesia is essential to the defense of a lawsuit. From a legal standpoint, documentation should be legible and accurate. Entries should be made as concurrently with the patient's care as possible. Erasures and white-outs should never be made on these records, nor should records be modified, be added to, or sustain deletions after the patient's discharge. Defense attorneys who specialize in malpractice cases often comment on the difficulty of defending a case because of the poor documentation on the patient's chart. The information on the anesthesia record must be consistent with other notations on the patient's chart. For example, if the recovery room nurse charts that the patient was unreactive on arrival in the recovery room and the anesthesia record shows that the patient was awake, this inconsistency would be difficult to defend in a lawsuit. Many juries place a greater weight on the documentation than on witnesses' recall, because of the time lapse of from 3 to 5 years from incident to trial. The importance of proper charting, therefore, cannot be overemphasized.

PREANESTHESIA EVALUATION

One of the most important acts an anesthetist can perform in the prevention of lawsuits is the preanesthesia evaluation. The anesthetist should explain to the patient the anesthesia program planned and give the reasons why that particular program is best suited to the patient's needs and the medical procedure to be performed. It is the anesthetist's responsibility to inform the patient of any risks involved and possible alternatives. A patient with whom the anesthetist has established rapport is less likely to initiate a lawsuit in the event of a mishap. At the time of the preanesthesia visit, it is the anesthetist's duty to ensure that all laboratory results and diagnostic information are recorded on the patient's chart. Communication among the anesthetist, the surgeon, and other members of the surgical team about the planned procedure and anesthesia regimen will also help to avoid incidents that could lead to a lawsuit.

PROFESSIONALISM

The nurse anesthetist who displays a high degree of professionalism will have an advantage in a legal action. Membership and participation in professional activities and evidence of maintaining the state of the art by continuing education activities are important factors in supporting the professional competence and credibility of the nurse anesthetist.

All certified registered nurse anesthetists should assess their employment status in regard to malpractice insurance coverage. Anesthetists employed by a hospital, clinic, or professional corporation should ascertain that insurance coverage is in existence and should be aware of the limits and terms of the liability coverage.

Independently practicing anesthetists are wise to carry their own professional liability insurance. It is foolhardy for any anesthetist to practice without insurance or without clarification, preferably in writing, of the terms and coverage of the insurance policy.

When an incident or unexpected problem develops with a patient, an incident report should be completed. This will serve to put the hospital administration and malpractice insurance company on notice of a potential legal action. An incident report is simply a statement of what happened and is not an admission of negligence or responsibility. In most jurisdictions these reports may not be subpoenaed and are protected from discovery in malpractice cases.

It is no longer sufficient for a nurse anesthetist to know only the scientific principles of the profession and to be skilled in the administration of anesthetics. Nurse anesthetists who are aware of the legal aspects of anesthesia practice, because they delineate both rights and responsibilities, and conduct their professional lives accordingly will reflect a high professionalism that will be recognized by coworkers in the health care field and by the general public.

REFERENCES

Ascher vs Gutierrez (U.S. Court of Appeals 175 U.S. App DC 100 F 2a 1235, 1976).

Blumenreich G, Benkov D: Liability of a surgeon when working with a nurse anesthetist. AANAJ 52:355–356, 1984.

Gravis vs Physicians and Surgeons Hospital of Alice (415 SW 2d 647 Tex, 1967).

Mohr vs Jenkins (393 So 2d 245 La, 1980).

Regas vs Argonaut Southern Insurance Co. et al (Cal App 379 So 2d 822, 1980).

Schoendorf vs Society of New York Hospital (211 NY 125 NE 92, 1914).

Susselman vs Muhlenberg Hospital (124 NJ Super. 1973).

4

Metric Medical Mathematics

Marian Waterhouse

RELATIONSHIPS OF MATHEMATICAL EQUIVALENTS

There are four common ways to express mathematical equivalents: fractions, ratios, decimals, and percent.

Changing Fractions to Ratios

A ratio is a fraction. The fraction ½ may be expressed as the ratio 1:2. A ratio of 1:2, or the fraction ½, means one of two equal parts, or 1 ÷ 2.

Changing Fractions or Ratios to Decimals

A decimal is a fraction whose denominator is 10, or any power of 10, i.e., 100, 1000, 10,000, etc. The denominator of a decimal is signified by the placement of the number to the right of a decimal point. A fraction is changed to a decimal by dividing the numerator by the denominator.

$$1:2 = \frac{1}{2} = \frac{5}{10} = 5 \div 10 = 0.5$$
$$1:4 = \frac{1}{4} = \frac{25}{100} = 25 \div 100 = 0.25$$
$$1:8 = \frac{1}{8} = 1 \div 8 = 0.125$$

Changing Decimals to Percent

Percent means "per hundred," or "divided by 100."

$$1:2 = \frac{1}{2} = \frac{50}{100} = 50\%$$
$$1:4 = \frac{1}{4} = \frac{25}{100} = 25\%$$
$$1:100 = \frac{1}{100} = 1\%$$

APPLICATION OF METRIC EQUIVALENTS TO DRUGS AND SOLUTIONS

Metric Units of Weight and Volume

Many mathematical errors made in calculating measurements of drugs and solutions occur because people do not remember that *milli-* means "thousandths" (not hundredths). To avoid such errors, it is imperative to remember the following relationships:

1 gram (g)	= 1000 milligrams (mg)
1 kilogram (kg)	= 1000 grams (g)
1 liter (L)	= 1000 milliliters (ml)
	= 1000 cubic centimeters (cc)
1 mg	= 0.001 g
1 ml or 1 cc	= 0.001 L

For the purpose of this text, 1 gram of drug dissolved in 1 milliliter of liquid solvent is a 100 percent solution. Therefore: 1 g = 1 ml, or 1 cc. All mathematics problems involving drugs and solutions can be quickly calculated if the number of milligrams per milliliter desired after dilution (or the percentage of the solution) and the total dosage (or total volume) of solution required are known.

Example. Make 20 milliliters of a 2 percent solution from a pure (100 percent) liquid drug.

> *Step 1:* Make a table of the mathematical equivalents for 2 percent and 100 percent, as illustrated in Table 4–1. Any one of the columns in Table 4–1 can be used to figure the grams per milliliter of a solution. For a 2 percent solution:
>
> a. Percent means grams per 100 milliliters. Therefore, a 2 percent solution has 2 g/100 ml of solution.
> b. The decimal means grams per milliliter. If there are 2 g/100 ml, there are 0.02 g/ml of solution.
> c. The fraction and the ratio also mean grams per milliliter. A 2 percent solution has 2 g/100 ml, or 1 g/50 ml. A 1:50, or 1/50th solution contains 1 gram of drug in 50 milliliters of solution, or 0.02 g/ml.
> d. The milligram per milliliter column means the number of milligrams dissolved per milliliter of solution. To change grams to milligrams, multiply the decimal by 1000.
>
> $$0.02 \text{ g/ml} \times 1000 \text{ mg/g} = 20 \text{ mg/ml}$$
> of solution

TABLE 4–1. MATHEMATICAL EQUIVALENTS FOR 2% AND 100% SOLUTIONS

Ratio (g/ml)	Fraction (g/ml)	Decimal (g/ml)	Percent (g/100 ml)	mg/ml	g/L
1:50	1/50, or 2/100	0.02	2	20	20
1:1	1/1, or 100/100	1.00	100	1000	1000

Step 2: The problem calls for 20 milliliters of a 2 percent solution. It is shown in the table that a 2 percent solution contains 20 mg/ml.

$$20 \text{ mg/ml} \times 20 \text{ ml} = 400 \text{ mg},$$
total amount drug needed

Step 3: The table shows that a pure (100 percent) drug contains 1 g/ml of solution, or 1000 mg/ml. A total of 400 milligrams of drug is needed.

$$400 \text{ mg} \div 1000 \text{ mg/ml} = 400 \text{ mg} \times \frac{\text{ml}}{1000 \text{ mg}}$$
$$= \tfrac{4}{10} \text{ ml, or } 0.4 \text{ ml}$$

The amount of 100 percent drug needed is 0.4 ml.

Answer: Take 0.4 milliliters of stock 100 percent drug and add 19.6 milliliters of solvent; 20 milliliters of a 2 percent solution, containing 20 mg/ml, will have been made.

Multiplication and Division of Grams, Milligrams, Liters, and Milliliters

The multiplication and division of the units are used extensively when figuring drug problems. They are fractions and therefore must be treated as such. Cancellation is usually possible, as illustrated here.

$$500 \text{ mg} \div 100 \text{ mg/ml} = 500 \text{ mg} \div \frac{100 \text{ mg}}{\text{ml}}$$
$$= 500 \text{ mg} \times \frac{\text{ml}}{100 \text{ mg}} = 5 \text{ ml}$$

(See Example 1.) Labeling all parts of the equations is very important so that the meaning will be clear. In any one equation, figures must all be in the same unit or measure, i.e.:

- If grams are used, all weight terms must be in grams.
- If milligrams are used, all weight terms must be in milligrams.
- If milliliters are used, all volume terms must be in milliliters.
- If liters are used, all volume terms must be in liters.

Only when one unit can be cancelled out while converting from one unit to another may both units appear in the same problem:

$$\frac{1 \text{ g}}{5 \text{ ml}} \times \frac{1000 \text{ mg}}{\text{g}} = \frac{1000 \text{ mg}}{5 \text{ ml}} = 200 \text{ mg/ml}$$

Example 1. Make 50 milliliters of a 1 percent solution from a 10 percent solution.

Step 1: Use the applicable parts of Table 4–1.

$$1\% = 1 \text{ g/100 ml} = 1000 \text{ mg/100 ml} = 10 \text{ mg/ml}$$
$$10 \text{ mg/ml} \times 50 \text{ ml} = 500 \text{ mg},$$
total amount drug needed

Step 2:

$$10\% = 10 \text{ g/100 ml} = 10,000 \text{ mg/100 ml}$$
$$= 100 \text{ mg/ml}$$

Step 3:

$$500 \text{ mg} \div 100 \text{ mg/ml} = 500 \text{ mg} \times \text{ml/100 mg}$$
$$= 5 \text{ ml}$$

Answer: Take 5 milliliters of a 10 percent solution and add solvent to 50 milliliters; 50 ml of a 1 percent solution, containing 10 mg/ml, will have been made.

Example 2. Make 20 milliliters of epinephrine 1:200,000. Available are 1-milliliter ampules of 1:1000 epinephrine and 50-milliliter vials of saline.

Step 1:

$$1:200,000 = 1 \text{ g/200,000 ml}$$
$$= 1000 \text{ mg/200,000 ml}$$
$$= 1 \text{ mg/200 ml}$$
$$= 0.005 \text{ mg/ml}$$
$$0.005 \text{ mg/ml} \times 20 \text{ ml} = 0.1 \text{ mg, total amount of}$$
epinephrine needed

Step 2:
Stock epinephrine 1:1000
$$= 1 \text{ g/1000 ml} = 1000 \text{ mg/1000 ml}$$
$$= 1 \text{ mg/ml} = 0.1 \text{ mg/0.1 ml}$$

Answer: Add 0.1 milliliter of epinephrine 1:1000 to 19.9 milliliters of saline; 20 milliliters of a 1:200,000 solution of epinephrine, containing 0.005 mg/ml, will have been made.

Example 3. What percentage is a 1:100,000 solution? Percent means g/100 ml.

$$1:100,000 = 1 \text{ g/100,000 ml} = 0.001 \text{ g/100 ml} = 0.001\%$$

Example 4. The label on the ampule reads "0.25 g pentobarbital, 5-ml ampule." The desired dosage is 25 milligrams of pentobarbital to be given intravenously. How much of this ampule should be given to the patient?

$$0.25 \text{ g} = 250 \text{ mg}$$

The ampule contains 250 mg/5 ml, or 50 mg/ml.

$$25 \text{ mg} \div \frac{50 \text{ mg}}{\text{ml}} = 25 \text{ mg} \times \frac{\text{ml}}{50 \text{ mg}} = \frac{1}{2} \text{ ml}$$

Answer: Give 0.5 milliliters of the drug. Because there are 50 mg/ml, there are 25 mg/0.5 ml.

Example 5. Make a 2.5 percent thiopental sodium (Pentothal) solution. Available are 5-gram powdered ampules of Pentothal, and 1000-milliliter bottles of solvent.

$$2.5\% = 2.5 \text{ g}/100 \text{ ml} = 25 \text{ g}/1000 \text{ ml}$$

Answer: Add 5 ampules of thiopental sodium (Pentothal), powdered 5-gram ampules, to 1000 milliliters of solvent.

Example 6. The patient's blood pressure is falling rapidly. An intravenous infusion of phenylephrine (Neo-Synephrine), 0.002 percent, is indicated. The drug will be added to the remaining 250 milliliters of an infusion already running. The phenylephrine ampule is a 1 percent solution. How much of the drug should be added to the bottle?

Step 1:

$$0.002\% = 0.002 \text{ g}/100 \text{ ml} = 2 \text{ mg}/100 \text{ ml}$$
$$= 0.02 \text{ mg}/\text{ml}$$

$$0.02 \text{ mg}/\text{ml} \times 250 \text{ ml} = 5 \text{ mg phenylephrine required}$$

Step 2:

$$1\% = 1 \text{ g}/100 \text{ ml} = 1000 \text{ mg}/100 \text{ ml}$$
$$= 10 \text{ mg}/\text{ml}$$

$$5 \text{ mg} \div 10 \text{ mg}/\text{ml} = 0.5 \text{ ml}$$

Answer: Add 0.5 milliliters of 1 percent phenylephrine to the 250 milliliter infusion; a 0.002-percent solution of phenylephrine (Neo-Synephrine) containing 0.02 mg/ml will have been made.

Example 7. Give neostigmine (Prostigmin), 1 milligram. Neostigmine, 1:4000, 2-milliliter ampules are available.

$$1:4000 = 1 \text{ g}/4000 \text{ ml} = 1000 \text{ mg}/4000 \text{ ml} = 1 \text{ mg}/4 \text{ ml}$$
$$= 0.5 \text{ mg}/2 \text{ ml}$$

Answer: A neostigmine, 1:4000, 2-milliliter ampule contains 0.5 mg of drug. To give 1 milligram of neostigmine, two 2-milliliter ampules of 1:4000 neostigmine (Prostigmin) should be administered.

Example 8. If 1 milliliter of 1 percent tetracaine hydrochloride (Pontocaine) is added to 1 milliliter of 10 percent dextrose in preparation for a spinal anesthetic, what percentage and how many milligrams per milliliter will result for each drug?

Step 1: The tetracaine hydrochloride problem:

$$1\% = 1 \text{ g}/100 \text{ ml} = 1000 \text{ mg}/100 \text{ ml}$$
$$= 10 \text{ mg}/\text{ml}$$

Answer: After adding 1 milliliter of 1 percent tetracaine hydrochloride to 1 milliliter of another solution, there will be 10 mg tetracaine hydrochloride/2 ml, or 5 mg/ml.

$$5 \text{ mg}/\text{ml} = 500 \text{ mg}/100 \text{ ml}$$
$$= 0.5 \text{ g}/100 \text{ ml}$$
$$= 0.5\% \text{ tetracaine hydrochloride}$$
$$\text{(Pontocaine) solution}$$

Step 2: The dextrose problem:

$$10\% = 10 \text{ g}/100 \text{ ml} = 10,000 \text{ mg}/100 \text{ ml}$$
$$= 100 \text{ mg}/\text{ml}$$

Answer: After adding 1 milliliter of 10 percent dextrose to 1 milliliter of another solution, there will be 100 mg dextrose/2 ml, or 50 mg/ml.

$$50 \text{ mg}/\text{ml} = 5000 \text{ mg}/100 \text{ ml} = 5 \text{ g}/100 \text{ ml}$$
$$= 5\% \text{ dextrose}$$
$$\text{solution}$$

Example 9. Pentobarbital, 10 milligrams, is to be given to a child. Available is pentobarbital 0.25 g/5-ml ampule. How should this medication be given?

$$0.25 \text{ g}/5 \text{ ml} = 250 \text{ mg}/5 \text{ ml} = 50 \text{ mg}/\text{ml}$$

Dilute the drug so that it is easy to give 10 milligrams. A satisfactory way to do this would be to add to 1 milliliter (50 milligrams) of the pentobarbital ampule enough saline to make 10 milliliters. Then there would be 50 mg/10 ml, or 5 mg/ml.

Answer: To receive 10 milligrams of pentobarbital, the child should be given 2 milliliters of the pentobarbital solution that has been diluted to 5 mg/ml.

MATHEMATICS OF BIOCHEMISTRY

A study of the nature of electrolytes is fundamental to understanding the biochemistry of the living body. There are two ways molecules behave in solutions:

1. The molecules may split or dissociate to form ions. This process is known as ionization, and chemical compounds that behave in this way are known as electrolytes. Sodium chloride is an example of an electrolyte in body water. In solution, each molecule ionizes into one positive sodium ion and one negative chloride ion.

$$NaCl \longrightarrow Na^+ + Cl^-$$

2. If molecules in solution do not ionize, they are known as nonelectrolytes. Dextrose and urea are examples of nonelectrolytes in body water.

Gram Atomic Weights

Definition. The atomic weight of an element, expressed in grams, is called the gram atomic weight (GAW) of that element. Hydrogen is used as a standard because it has a GAW of 1 gram. Note in Table 4–2 that

- 1 GAW of hydrogen weighs 1 gram.
- 1 GAW of sodium weighs 23 grams.
- 1 GAW of potassium weighs 39 grams.

The combining ability of 1 GAW of sodium or potassium is identical to that of 1 GAW of hydrogen, although 1 GAW of potassium weighs 39 times as much as does 1 GAW of hydrogen, and 1 GAW of sodium weighs 23 times as much as 1 GAW of hydrogen.

Gram Molecular Weights

Definition. The molecular weight of a compound, expressed in grams, is called the gram molecular weight (GMW) of that compound. 1 GMW is commonly known as 1 mole, or 1 mol.

Gram Equivalent Weights

The number of milligrams per milliliter of an electrolyte solution yields no information regarding its potential for maintaining electrical neutrality within the body. The *number* of ions or molecules in a solution must be counted. An equivalent weight counts the number of ions, i.e., the number of positive and negative charges possessed by an element or radical. Note in the table of GAWs that 1 GAW of hydrogen weighs 1 gram, the least of all the elements, and hydrogen ionizes to H^+ (it has only one positive charge).

TABLE 4–2. COMMON GRAM ATOMIC WEIGHTS AND VALENCES

Elements	Symbol	Gram Atomic Weight	Valence
Bromine	Br	80	−1, −3, −5, −7
Calcium	Ca	40	+2
Carbon	C	12	+4, −4
Chlorine	Cl	35	−1
Hydrogen	H	1	+1
Iron	Fe	56	+2, +3
Magnesium	Mg	24	+2
Nitrogen	N	14	+3, +5
Oxygen	O	16	−2
Potassium	K	39	+1
Phosphorus	P	31	+3, +5
Sodium	Na	23	+1
Sulfur	S	32	−2, +4, +6
Radicals			
Ammonium	NH_4		+1
Bicarbonate	HCO_3		−1
Carbonate	CO_3		−2
Chlorate	ClO_3		−1
Hydroxyl	OH		−1
Nitrate	NO_3		−1
Phosphate	PO_4		−3
Sulfate	SO_4		−2

For these two reasons, hydrogen is used as the element with which all other elements are compared.

One ion of each of the other elements weighs more than does one ion of hydrogen; however, the relative weight of each ion is *not* a factor involved in the *combining* ability of each ion. It is the *number of charges*, positive or negative, possessed by the individual ion (or radical) that is counted when comparing its combining ability with that of one ion of hydrogen.

Definition. An equivalent weight of an element is its weight in grams that is equivalent to, or equal in combining weight to, that of 1 gram of hydrogen. The gram equivalent weight (GEW) of an element (or radical) is the number of GAWs, or the *fraction* of 1 GAW of that element that exactly combines with, or replaces 1 GAW of hydrogen.

One ion of hydrogen has the same combining ability as one ion of sodium or potassium.

$$H^+ + Cl^- \rightarrow HCl$$
$$Na^+ + Cl^- \rightarrow NaCl$$
$$K^+ + Cl^- \rightarrow KCl$$

In each of these equations, one ion of H^+, one ion of Na^+, or one ion of K^+ combines exactly with one ion of Cl^-.

$$1 \text{ GAW (or 1 g) } H^+ + 1 \text{ GAW (or 35 g) } Cl^-$$
$$\rightarrow 1 \text{ GMW (or 36 g) HCl}$$

$$1 \text{ GAW (or 23 g) } Na^+ + 1 \text{ GAW (or 35 g) } Cl^-$$
$$\rightarrow 1 \text{ GMW (or 58 g) NaCl}$$

$$1 \text{ GAW (or 39 g) } K^+ + 1 \text{ GAW (or 35 g) } Cl^-$$
$$\rightarrow 1 \text{ GMW (or 74 g) KCl}$$

These equations illustrate the meaning not only of GAW and GMW, but also of GEW. It can be seen that 1 GAW of sodium, weighing 23 grams, can exactly replace 1 GAW of hydrogen, weighing 1 gram. Also, 1 GAW of potassium, weighing 39 grams, can exactly replace 1 GAW of hydrogen, or 1 GAW of sodium. 1 GAW of H^+ or Na^+ or K^+ can exactly combine with 1 GAW of Cl^-. Also demonstrated is the fact that, because 1 GAW of Na^+ or 1 GAW of K^+ exactly replaces 1 GAW of H^+, the GEW of Na^+, or K^+ is the same as its respective GAW.

Elements with a Valence of Two. An element with a valence of two, or more, presents a different situation. Table 4–2 indicates that sulfur has a valence of −2. This means that one ion of sulfur can combine with 2 ions of H^+. Therefore, one ion of H^+ combines exactly with one half an ion of S^{2-}.

$$1 \text{ GAW (or 32 g) } S^{2-} + 2 \text{ GAW (or 2 g) } H^+$$
$$\rightarrow 1 \text{ GMW (or 34 g) } H_2S$$

The GEW of S^{2-} (or the amount of sulfur that combines with 1 GAW or 1 gram of hydrogen) is equal to half its GAW. Thus

$$GEW\ S^{2-} = \frac{1 \text{ GAW (or 32 g) } S^{2-}}{2} = 16 \text{ g}$$

Referring to the definition of GEW, it is evident that the GEW of sulfur is the *fraction* of its GAW that combines exactly with 1 GAW (or 1 gram) of H^+.

1 GEW (or 16 g) S^{2-} + 1 GEW (or 1 g) H^+
$\rightarrow$ 1 GEW (or 17 g) H_2S

N.B.   1 GEW S^{2-} + GEW H^+ $\rightarrow$ 1 GEW H_2S

Avogadro's Law and Number

Avogadro's Law. Avogadro's law states that 1 GMW of any compound contains the same number of molecules as 1 GMW of any other compound. Similarly 1 GAW of any element contains the same number of atoms as 1 GAW of any other element.

Avogadro's Number. Avogadro's number describes 1 GMW of any substance as containing

6.02×10^{23} (or 602,000,000,000,000,000,000,000) molecules

Similarly, there are 6.02×10^{23} atoms in 1 GAW of any element. In 1 GAW or 1 GEW of hydrogen, there are 6.02×10^{23} ions. In 1 GAW or 1 GEW of chloride, there are 6.02×10^{23} ions. Therefore

6.02×10^{23} ions of H^+ + 6.02×10^{23} ions of Cl^-
$\rightarrow 6.02 \times 10^{23}$ molecules of HCl

In 1 GAW of sulfur there are 6.02×10^{23} ions. In 1 GEW of S^{2-} there are 3.01×10^{23} ions.

1 GEW (or 6.02×10^{23} ions) H^+
+ 1 GEW (or 3.01×10^{23} ions) S^{2-}
$\rightarrow$ 1 GEW (or 3.01×10^{23}) molecules H_2S

Figure 4–1 shows that only 0.5 GAW of S^{2-} is needed to neutralize 1 GAW of H^+.

Milliequivalent Weights

Definition. A milliequivalent weight of an element is its weight in milligrams that is equivalent to or equal in combining weight to that of 1 milligram of hydrogen.

As explained earlier, "milli" means "thousandths."

1000.0 milligrams (mg) = 1.0 grams (g)
1.0 mg = 0.001 g
1000.0 milliequivalent weights (mEq)
= 1.0 equivalent weight (GEW)
1.0 mEq = 0.001 GEW

Example. For NaCl

1.0 GEW weighs 58 grams
0.001 GEW weighs 0.058 grams
1.0 mEq (weight) weighs 0.058 grams
1.0 mEq weighs 58.0 mg

For H_2S

1.0 GEW weighs 16 grams
0.001 GEW weighs 0.016 grams
1.0 mEq (weight) weighs 0.016 grams
1.0 mEq weighs 16.0 mg

Milliequivalents measure body concentrations of specific ions known as electrolytes. There is an optimum concentra-

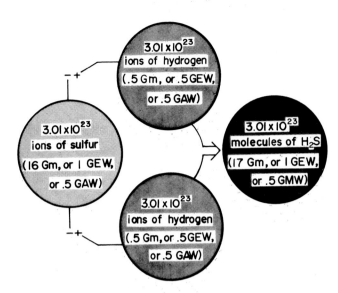

Figure 4–1. Diagram showing how 3.01×10^{23} ions of sulfur combine with 6.02×10^{23} ions of hydrogen to make 3.01×10^{23} molecules of H_2S. (*From Waterhouse, M. Practical Mathematics in Allied Health, 1979. Courtesy of Urban & Schwarzenberg.*)

tion of each electrolyte in each tissue or fluid compartment. Various laboratory tests of electrolytes are reported in milliequivalents because this is the only method by which specific laboratory results can be compared meaningfully to normal body electrolyte concentrations. In addition, electrolyte replacement therapy with drugs or by intravenous fluids can be accurately determined by assessing the milliequivalent concentration of the various body fluids.

Osmotic Pressure of Solutions

Figure 4–2 illustrates osmotic pressure, which can be defined as the pressure developed when two solutions of different concentrations of the same solute are separated by a membrane permeable to the solvent only. For example, Figure 4–2 shows that a 5-percent dextrose in water (D_5W) solution requires a certain amount of mechanical or hydrostatic pressure (illustrated by the plunger) to prevent osmosis of water from compartment B into compartment A. If there were only a 1-percent solution in the A side, just one-fifth as much pressure by the plunger would be required to prevent osmosis of water from compartment B into compartment A. Conversely, if $D_{10}W$ were in compartment A, twice as much pressure by the plunger would be required to prevent osmosis of water from compartment B into compartment A.

If compartment B were a 1-percent solution, and compartment A were a 5-percent solution, and there were no plunger, water would diffuse by osmosis from compartment B into compartment A until an equilibrium was reached and the solutes on both sides of the membrane were of equal concentration.

Individual molecules and individual ions that are too large to go through a semipermeable membrane exert osmotic pressure. The amount of osmotic pressure that one molecule of a nonionizing, nondiffusible substance exerts

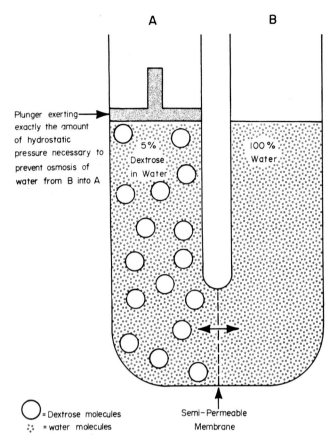

A   B

Plunger exerting
exactly the amount
of hydrostatic
pressure necessary to
prevent osmosis of
water from B into A

5%
Dextrose
in Water

100%
Water

○ = Dextrose molecules
∴ = water molecules

Semi-Permeable
Membrane

Figure 4–2. Osmotic pressure. The exact amount of mechanical or hydrostatic pressure required by the plunger to stop the water from flowing from compartment B into compartment A through a membrane that is impermeable to dextrose molecules is known as the osmotic pressure of that solution. (*From Waterhouse, M. Practical Mathematics in Allied Health, 1979. Courtesy of Urban & Schwarzenberg.*)

is the same amount of osmotic pressure as that of one molecule of any other nonionizing, nondiffusible substance.

Example 1. One nonionizing protein molecule with a GMW of 70,000 grams has the same osmotic effect as one molecule of dextrose with a GMW of 180 grams. Each molecule of dextrose plugs a pore in the semipermeable membrane as effectively as does one molecule of protein. (Compare the weights of a golf ball and a Ping-Pong ball. If they are the same size, each one can effectively plug the same hole.)

Example 2. One ion of a nondiffusible electrolyte has the same osmotic effect as one molecule of any nonionizing, nondiffusible substance, or the same as that of one ion of any other ionizing, nondiffusible substance. One molecule of a nondiffusible, nonionizing substance or one ion of a nondiffusible electrolyte is known as one solute particle that exerts osmotic pressure.

Osmoles and Osmolality

Osmoles. The *number* of ions or molecules in a solution must be counted if osmotic pressure is to be measured because it is the *number* of particles of solute that creates

the osmotic pressure of a solution. The unit of measure for osmotic activity is the osmole (osm). An osmole equals 6.02×10^{23} particles of dissolved solute that cannot diffuse through a semipermeable membrane. These particles of solute may be a combination of several different kinds of nondiffusible ions and molecules in a given solution.

One GMW of a dissolved, nonionizing, nondiffusible solute equals 1 osmole. One GMW of such a solute contains 6.02×10^{23} molecules (Avogadro's number). One GAW of an electrolyte that ionizes in solution equals 1 osmole. One GAW of such a solute contains 6.02×10^{23} ions.

Osmotic pressure is calculated by adding all the nondiffusible molecules and ions in a solution. For example, one Na^+ ion, or one Ca^{2+} ion, or one dextrose molecule exerts one particle of osmotic pressure. The concentration of all the added particles of osmotic pressure in a solution is generally given in osmoles per liter (osm/L) of solution.

Osmolality

- Osmotic pressure of 1 GAW Na^+/L = 1 osm/L.
- Osmotic pressure of 1 GAW Cl^-/L = 1 osm/L.
- Osmotic pressure of 1 GMW NaCl/L = 2 osm/L.
- Osmotic pressure of 1 GMW dextrose/L = 1 osm/L.

The osmolality of a solution is the number of osmoles or the fraction of one osmole that is dissolved in a given unit of solvent; osmolality is generally expressed as osmoles per liter of solvent. (It is the multiple of 6.02×10^{23} particles or the fraction of 6.02×10^{23} particles that exists in one liter of solvent.)

Relationship of Osmolality to Osmotic Pressure

Definition of Osmotic Pressure. The osmotic pressure of a solution is that pressure in millimeters of mercury (mm Hg) that when applied to a solution will just prevent osmosis of solvent into it through a semipermeable membrane (like the plunger in Figure 4–2).

Nonionizing Solutions. One GMW of any nonionizing, nondiffusible solute dissolved in 22.4 liters of water at 0C has an osmotic pressure of 760 mm Hg and contains 6.02×10^{23} particles. The osmolality of this solution is 1 GMW/22.4 L, or 1 osm/22.4 L of solvent.

The osmotic pressure of 1 osm/22.4 L is 760 mm Hg; 760 mm Hg pressure equals one atmosphere (atm). Therefore, the osmotic pressure of 1 osm/22.4 L of solvent = 1 atmosphere, or 760 mm Hg. If 1 osmole of any solute is dissolved in one liter of solvent, the osmotic pressure equals 22.4×760 mm Hg, which equals 17,024 mm Hg or 22.4 atmospheres (Fig. 4–3). The solute has been concentrated 22.4 times.

Ionizing Solutions. One GMW of an ionizing, nondiffusible solute, such as NaCl, dissolved in 22.4 liters of water at 0C has an osmotic pressure of 760 mm Hg × 2, which equals 1520 mm Hg, or 2 atmospheres.

One GMW of NaCl contains 6.02×10^{23} molecules. Each molecule ionizes into two ions. The number of particles has doubled. Therefore 1 GMW NaCl = 2 osm, or 12.04×10^{23} particles, each of which exerts osmotic pressure.

2 osm dissolved in 1 L H$_2$O = 2 × 760 mm Hg × 22.4
= 34,048 mm Hg or 44.8 atm

To summarize:

- 1 osm = 1 GMW nonionizing substance.
- 1 osm = 0.5 GMW ionizing monovalent substance.
- 1 osm = 0.33 GMW ionizing bivalent substance.

Osmolality of Body Fluids at Body Temperature

The osmotic pressure of 1 GMW/22.4 L at 0C is 760 mm Hg. Absolute zero is −273C. Zero degrees centigrade is 273 degrees warmer than absolute zero. Human beings have a normal body temperature of +37C. Gay-Lussac's law states that, if the volume of a gas remains constant, the pressure varies directly with the absolute temperature 1/273 for each degree centigrade. Solutes in solution abide by this law. At 0C, the osmotic pressure exerted by 1 osm of solute per liter of water is

273/273 × 760 mm Hg × 22.4 L = 17,024 mm Hg

(see Fig. 4–3).

At 37C, the osmotic pressure exerted by 1 osm solute/ L of water is

$$\frac{273 + 37}{273} \times 760 \text{ mm Hg} \times 22.4 \text{ L} = 19{,}331 \text{ mm Hg}$$

To reduce these figures to a useful size, milliosmoles (mosm) are used. Just as 1000 milligrams = 1 gram and 1 milli-

gram = 0.001 gram, so 1000 milliosmoles = 1 osmole and 1 milliosmole = 0.001 osmole.

At 37C the osmotic pressure of

- 1 osm of solute/L = 19,331 mm Hg.
- 1000 mosm of solute/L = 19,331 mm Hg.
- 1 mosm of solute/L = 19.3 mm Hg.

Osmotic Pressure of Body Fluids

The round figure 300 mosm/L (or 0.3 osm/L) osmotic concentration is used for convenience when discussing the osmotic pressure of body fluids. Since 1 mosm/L of water creates an osmotic pressure of 19.3 mm Hg at 37C, the osmotic pressure of

300 mosm/L = 19.3 mm Hg × 300 = 5790 mm Hg

Summary

- 1 GMW (or 1 GEW) glucose (180 g) = 1 osm (does not ionize).
- 1 GMW (or 1 GEW) NaCl (58 g) = 2 osm (ionizes into two particles).
- 1 mEq Na$^+$ (23 mg) = 1 mosm.
- 1 mEq Cl$^-$ (35 mg) = 1 mosm.
- 1 mEq NaCl (58 mg) = 2 mosm.
- 0.5 mEq Na$^+$ (11.5 mg) = 0.5 mosm.
- 0.5 mEq Cl$^-$ (17.5 mg) = 0.5 mosm.
- 0.5 mEq NaCl (29 mg) = 1 mosm.

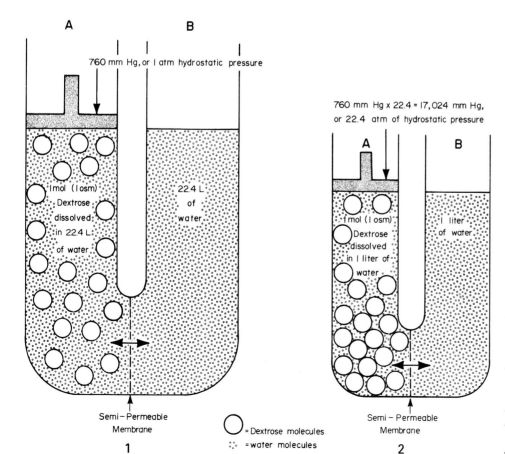

Figure 4–3. Osmotic pressure exerted by 1 GMW of dextrose dissolved in 22.4 L of water **(diagram 1)**, and by 1 GMW of dextrose dissolved in 1 L of water **(diagram 2)** when compartments A and B are separated by a membrane that is impermeable to dextrose molecules. (*From Waterhouse, M. Practical Mathematics in Allied Health, 1979. Courtesy of Urban & Schwarzenberg.*)

Therefore

> 1 mEq (or 1 mosm, or 23 mg) Na^+
> + 1 mEq (or 1 mosm, or 35 mg) Cl^-
> → 1 mEq (or 2 mosm, or 58 mg) NaCl

- 1 GMW $CaCl_2$ (110 g) = 3 osm (ionizes into three particles).
- 1 GEW $CaCl_2$ (55 g) = 1.5 osm.
- 1 mEq $CaCl_2$ (55 mg) = 1.5 mosm.
- 1 GAW Ca^{2+} (40 g) = 1 osm.
- 1 GEW Ca^{2+} (20 g) = 0.5 osm.
- 1 mEq Ca^{2+} (20 mg) = 0.5 mosm.
- 1 mEq Cl^- (35 mg) = 1 mosm.

Therefore

> 1 mEq (or 0.5 mosm, or 20 mg) Ca^{2+}
> + 1 mEq (or 1 mosm, or 35 mg) Cl^-
> → 1 mEq (or 1.5 mosm, or 55 mg) $CaCl_2$

N.B.

> 1 mEq Ca^{2+} + 1 mEq Cl^- → 1 mEq $CaCl_2$
>
> 0.5 mosm Ca^{2+} + 1 mosm Cl^- → 1.5 mosm $CaCl_2$

Solutions

Molar Solutions. A one-molar solution of any solute contains 1 GMW, or 1 mole/L of solution. The molar concentration of a solution is the number of moles (mol) or the *fraction* of 1 mole of solute present in 1 liter of solution.

One GMW of dextrose ($C_6H_{12}O_6$) weighs 180 grams; 180 g/L is an 18-percent solution. (See the discussion of drugs and solutions and Table 4–1.) An 18-percent solution of dextrose in water ($D_{18}W$) is a 1-molar dextrose solution. Therefore

> 0.3-molar dextrose solution = 0.3(180 g)/L
> = 54 g/L = 5.4% DW

One GMW NaCl weighs 58 grams; a one-molar NaCl solution = 58 g/L = 5.8 percent NaCl. Therefore

> 0.3-molar NaCl solution = 0.3(58 g/L) = 17.4 g/L
> = 1.74% NaCl

or

> 0.15-molar NaCl solution = 0.15(58 g/L) = 8.7 g/L
> = 0.87% NaCl

Normal Solutions. A 1-normal solution of any solute contains 1 GEW/L of solution; a 0.5 normal solution contains 0.5 GEW/L, or 0.5 mEq/ml of solution.

One GEW NaCl weighs 58 g; 58 g NaCl/L = 5.8 percent NaCl. One molar solution of NaCl equals one normal solution of NaCl.

One GEW $CaCl_2$ weighs 55 grams because it is a bivalent electrolyte. Therefore, a one-normal solution of $CaCl_2$ contains 55 g/L, or 5.5 percent $CaCl_2$.

The concentration of a one-normal solution of $CaCl_2$ is only half that of a one-molar $CaCl_2$ solution, which weighs 110 grams. Therefore, 0.5 molar $CaCl_2$ equals one normal $CaCl_2$.

Tonicity of Solutions. Tonicity refers to the osmotic pressure of a solution relative to that of body fluids. Isotonic, isoosmotic, or physiologic, solutions have an osmotic pressure similar to that of body fluids, or about 300 mosm/L. Hypertonic solutions, or hyperosmotic solutions, have an osmotic pressure greater than 300 mosm/L. Hypotonic, or hypoosmotic, solutions have an osmotic pressure less than 300 mosm/L.

Osmolality of Solutions. To calculate the osmolality of a solution, all the solute particles in a given volume of that solution must be counted.

Example 1. What is the osmolality of 5.4 percent DW?

> 5.4% DW = 54 g of dextrose/liter of solution
>
> 1 molar DW = 180 g/L

Therefore, the molarity of

$$5.4\% \text{ DW} = \frac{54\text{ g}}{L} \div \frac{180\text{ g}}{mol} = \frac{54\text{ g}}{L} \times \frac{mol}{180\text{ g}} = \frac{0.3\text{ mol}}{L}$$

As shown above, one molar dextrose = one osmolar dextrose; 0.3 molar dextrose = 0.3 osmolar dextrose, or 300 mosm/L, an isotonic solution.

Example 2. What is the osmolality of 5.4 percent dextrose in 0.87 percent NaCl? As shown in Example 1, the osmotic pressure of 5.4 percent DW is 300 mosm/L.

> 0.87% NaCl = 8.7 g NaCl/L
>
> 1 molar NaCl = 58 g/L

The molarity of

$$0.87\% \text{ NaCl} = \frac{8.7\text{ g}}{L} \div \frac{58\text{ g}}{mol} = \frac{8.7\text{ g}}{L} \times \frac{mol}{58\text{ g}} = \frac{0.15\text{ mol}}{L}$$

One molar NaCl equals two osmolar NaCl. Each molecule ionizes into two ions. Therefore, 0.15 molar NaCl = 0.3 osmolar NaCl, or 300 mosm/L. The osmotic pressure of 5.4 percent dextrose in 0.87 percent NaCl is

```
  300   mosm of dextrose/liter
+ 300   mosm of NaCl/liter
  600   mosm/L, a hypertonic solution.
```

Avogadro's Law and Solutions. Avogadro's law states that equal volumes of solutions of equal molarity contain the same number of moles and equal numbers of molecules. Avogadro's law is illustrated in Table 4–3. The table shows that ionizing solutions such as NaCl and $CaCl_2$ contain many more particles that exert osmotic pressure than do nonionizing solutions such as glucose.

The pH Concept

The number of hydrogen ions in one liter of a solution is called the hydrogen ion concentration per liter, commonly abbreviated $[H^+]$. The pH scale is used to simplify the expression of astronomical numbers of hydrogen ions. Hydrogen ions must be counted because it is the *number* of free H^+ in a solution that determines its acidity: the more H^+

TABLE 4–3. AVOGADRO'S LAW AND SOLUTIONS[a]

		1 molar solutions			
NaCl					**Glucose**
1 L H_2O 1 GMW 1 mol NaCl	Volume (1 L) 1 GMW (1 mol) 58 g/L 5.8% (5.8 g/100 ml) 6.02×10^{23} molecules 12.04×10^{23} ions or particles	$=$ $=$ $\neq$ $\neq$ $=$ $\neq$	Volume (1 L) 1 GMW (1 mol) 180 g/L 18% (18 g/100 ml) 6.02×10^{23} molecules Does not ionize		1 L H_2O 1 GMW 1 mol glucose
		0.5 molar solutions			
$CaCl_2$					**Glucose**
1 L H_2O 0.5 GMW 0.5 mol $CaCl_2$	Volume (1 L) 0.5 GMW (0.5 mol) 55 g/L 5.5% 3.01×10^{23} molecules 9.03×10^{23} ions or particles	$=$ $=$ $\neq$ $\neq$ $=$ $\neq$	Volume (1 L) 0.5 GMW (0.5 mol) 90 g/L 9.0% 3.01×10^{23} molecules Does not ionize		1 L H_2O 0.5 GMW 0.5 mol glucose

[a] Equal volumes of solutions of equal molarity contain the same number of moles (GMW), and equal number of molecules (Avogadro's law).
(*From Waterhouse, M: Practical Mathematics in Allied Health, 1979. Courtesy of Urban & Schwarzenberg.*)

in a solution, the more acid it is. There are 6.02×10^{23} atoms in 1 GAW (or 1 GEW) of hydrogen. The abbreviation pH means power of the hydrogen ion concentration. The pH is the power to which the number 10 must be raised to find the exact number of hydrogen ions that exist in a liter of a given solution. The pH of a solution is, therefore, an exponent of the number 10. The pH is also a logarithm because logarithms express powers of 10. (A log is the power to which the fixed number, 10, must be raised to produce a given number.) The pH of a solution is derived by converting the value of the $[H^+]$ to a single exponent of 10 by calculating its logarithm. The logarithm, or exponent of 10, of the $[H^+]$ will always be negative because the number of hydrogen ions being counted is a fraction of 1 GEW of hydrogen, i.e., a fraction of 6.02×10^{23} hydrogen ions. (The log of a fraction is always negative.) To avoid the constant use of a negative number, the sign of the negative exponent is arbitrarily changed to positive and called pH.

Any one of the following equations can be used to find the pH of a solution:

$$\text{pH} = -\log \text{ of the } [H^+] \quad (1)$$

$$\text{pH} = \log 1/[H^+] \quad (2)$$

$$\text{pH} = \log \text{ of the } [H^+] \text{ expressed as positive number} \quad (3)$$

To find the $[H^+]$ of a solution when the pH is known:

$$[H^+] = 1 \times 10^{-\text{pH}} \text{ equivalents (Eq) of hydrogen/L} \quad (4)$$

$$[H^+] = 1/10^{\text{pH}} \text{ Eq of hydrogen/L} \quad (5)$$

Examples. pH of pure water

$$[H^+] \text{ of pure water} = 1 \times 10^{-7} \text{ Eq/L}$$
$$= 0.000,000,1 \text{ Eq/L}$$

Using equation 1:

$$\log (0.000,000,1) = -7$$
$$\text{pH} = -(-7)$$
$$\text{pH of water} = +7$$

Using equation 2:

$$\text{pH} = \log 1/0.000,000,1$$
$$\text{pH} = \log 10,000,000 = 7$$

Using equation 3:

$$\log (0.000,000,1) = -7$$
$$\text{pH of water} = +7$$

Using equation 4:

$$[H^+] \text{ of water} = 1 \times 10^{-7} \text{ Eq of hydrogen/L}$$
$$[H^+] \text{ of water} = 0.000,000,1 \text{ Eq/L}$$

Using equation 5:

$$[H^+] \text{ of water} = 1/10,000,000 \text{ Eq/L} = 0.000,000,1 \text{ Eq/L}$$

Pure water is neutral. This means that it is neither acidic nor basic. There are identical numbers of H^+ and hydroxyl ions, $(OH)^-$, in pure water (Table 4–4).

$$0.000,000, 1 \text{ Eq } H^+ + 0.000,000,1 \text{ Eq } (OH)^-$$
$$\rightarrow 0.000,000,1 \text{ Eq H(OH)}$$

The pH of Acids and Bases. The hydrogen ion concentration of an acid is greater than 0.000,000,1 Eq/L. Because pH is, in reality, a negative number, the pH of acids is always less than 7. If a solution has more free hydrogen ions than pure water, it is acidic. If it has an $[H^+]$ of 8.7×10^{-6} (or 0.000,008,7) Eq/L, it has a higher $[H^+]$ than pure water. Therefore it is an acidic solution. Its pH is 5.06, a value less than 7, signifying an acid solution. Because the $[H^+]$ of a base is less than 0.000,000,1 Eq/L, the pH of a base is always more than 7. If a solution has an $[H^+]$ of 6.7×10^{-9} (or 0.000,000,006,7) Eq/L, it has a lower $[H^+]$ than pure water. It is an alkaline solution with a pH of 8.17, a value more than 7.

Blood pH. The normal $[H^+]$ of human blood is 0.000,000,040 Eq/L, or 40 nanoequivalents (nEq)/L, or 4×10^{-8} Eq/L. To express the pH of blood, any one of the above equations may be used.

TABLE 4–4. pH SCALE ILLUSTRATING THE RELATIONSHIP BETWEEN THE [H⁺], pH, AND THE [(OH)⁻]

When: [H⁺] =	pH =	[(OH)⁻] =
1.0 GEW/L of free H⁺	0	.000,000,000,000,01 Eq/L
.1	1	.000,000,000,000,1
.01	2	.000,000,000,001
.001	3	.000,000,000,01
.000,1	4	.000,000,000,1
.000,01	5	.000,000,001
.000,001	6	.000,000,01
.000,000,1	7	.000,000,1
.000,000,04	7.4	.000,000,25
.000,000,01	8	.000,001
.000,000,001	9	.000,01
.000,000,000,1	10	.000,1
.000,000,000,01	11	.001
.000,000,000,001	12	.01
.000,000,000,000,1	13	.1
.000,000,000,000,01 Eq/L	14	1.0 GEW/L of free (OH)⁻

Using equation 1:

$$pH \text{ of blood} = -(\log 0.000,000,04)$$
$$= \log 0.000,000,04 = -7.4$$
$$pH \text{ of blood} = -(-7.4)$$
$$= +7.4$$

Using equation 2:

$$pH \text{ of blood} = \log 1/0.000,000,04$$
$$= \log 25,000,000$$
$$pH \text{ of blood} = 7.4$$

Using equation 3:

$$pH \text{ of blood} = \log 0.000,000,04 \text{ expressed as}$$
$$\text{positive number}$$
$$= \log 0.000,000,04 = -7.4$$
$$pH \text{ of blood} = +7.4$$

Equations 4 and 5 *prove* that the pH of blood is 7.4.

Using equation 4:

$$[H⁺] \text{ of blood} = 1 \times 10^{-7.4} \text{ Eq/L} = 0.000,000,04 \text{ Eq/L}$$

Using equation 5:

$$[H⁺] \text{ of blood} = 1/10^{7.4} \text{ Eq/L} = 1/25,118,864 \text{ Eq/L}$$
$$[H⁺] \text{ of blood} = 0.000,000,04 \text{ Eq/L}$$

Because the pH of blood is more than 7, the [H⁺] of blood is less than that of water, so blood is slightly alkaline.

The pH of Normal Solutions of HCl. The [H⁺] of 1.0 normal solution of HCl is 1 Eq/L.

$$pH \text{ of 1.0 normal HCl} = \log 1/1.0 = \log 1 = 0$$

$$[H⁺] \text{ of 0.1 normal HCl} = 0.1 \text{ Eq/L}$$

$$pH \text{ of 0.1 normal HCl} = \log 1/0.1 = \log 10 = 1$$

$$[H⁺] \text{ of 0.01 normal HCl} = 0.01 \text{ Eq/L}$$

$$pH \text{ of 0.01 normal HCl} = \log 1/0.01 = \log 100 = 2$$

$$[H⁺] \text{ of 0.000,000,1 normal HCl} = 0.000,000,1 \text{ Eq/L}$$

$$pH \text{ of 0.000,000,1 Eq/L HCl} = \log 1/0.000,000,1$$
$$= \log 10,000,000 = 7$$

Summary of pH Concept. The relationships between [H⁺], pH, and [(OH)⁻] are illustrated in Table 4–4.

1. pH is an exponent of 10 used to express the [H⁺]. It is the log of the [H⁺] expressed as a positive number.
2. Table 4–4 shows that, at a pH of 7, both the [H⁺] and the [(OH)⁻] have the same value. The solution is neither acidic nor basic. It is a neutral solution.
3. A *decrease* of 1.0 on the pH scale means that the [H⁺] has been multiplied by 10. Example: If the pH of a solution is 4, the [H⁺] is 10 times greater than that of a solution with a pH of 5. If the pH of a solution is 9, the [H⁺] is 100 times less than that of a solution with a pH of 7.
4. The [H⁺] multiplied by the [(OH)⁻] always has 14 decimal places.

$$[H⁺] \times [(OH)⁻] = 1 \times 10^{-14} = 0.000,000,000,000,01$$

Application of pH to Human Life. The range of [H⁺] compatible with human life is extremely narrow. Table 4–5

TABLE 4–5. pH SCALE AND HUMAN LIFE

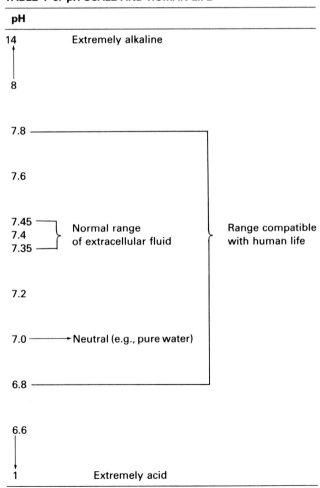

(Waterhouse, M. *Practical Mathematics in Allied Health*, 1979. Courtesy of Urban & Schwarzenberg.)

shows that the pH range compatible with human life lies between 6.8 and 7.8, with a *normal* range of 7.35 to 7.45. Note that a solution with a pH of 6.8 contains ten times as many hydrogen ions as does a solution with a pH of 7.8.

The pH concept is widely used in science and medicine today. If the mathematics behind its use is understood, it can be very useful as a tool for interpreting blood gases, pulmonary function studies, respiratory care, and some laboratory or diagnostic studies. The pH must also be considered in the manufacture of drugs and of the solutions used in all fields of medicine and biologic science.

ANESTHETIC VAPORIZER CALCULATIONS

A thorough mastery of the physics of gases and vapors is essential before the mathematics behind anesthetic vaporizer calculations can be understood (see Chapter 5).

Vaporizer flowmeters are designed specifically to direct oxygen through volatile anesthetic agent vaporizers. These vaporizer flowmeters may indicate either the milliliters per minute, expressed as cubic centimeters per minute, of saturated anesthetic *vapor* that emerge *from* the vaporizer, or they may indicate the amount of *oxygen* flow (cc/min) *into* the vaporizer. It is imperative that the anesthetist fully understand the calculations involved for each type of flowmeter because the results are very different. The accompanying vapor pressure-temperature graph (Fig. 4–4) illustrates the varying vapor pressure-temperature curves for enflurane,

halothane, and isoflurane. This discussion will include examples for calculating various concentrations of these three agents when using each type of vaporizer.

Direct-Metering Vaporization (Ohio Heidbrink DM 5000 Anesthesia Machines)

Direct-metering vaporizer flowmeters are calibrated to indicate, in cubic centimeters per minute, the amount of anesthetic *vapor* that is being introduced into the patient's circuit. Part or all of the life-sustaining (diluent) oxygen is diverted into the vaporizer, picks up the vapor, and conducts it to join the total mixture of anesthetic gases. The oxygen that is diverted into the vaporizer comes out 100 percent saturated with the agent at 23 to 24C. The vaporizer is heated to ensure a stable temperature.

The total output of the DM 5000 Ohio vaporizer is the sum of the flowmeter readings. The agent concentration is the direct ratio of the vaporized agent flow rate to the total flow rate of agent, oxygen, and other diluent gases. (See the manufacturer's literature for a discussion of computing agent concentrations at ambient temperature extremes or change in altitude.) Anesthetic vaporizer percentages and flow rates can be calculated just as easily as the drugs and solutions discussed in the first section of this chapter. Use a table, such as Table 4–1, substituting a column for

$$\frac{\text{cc/min vapor flow rate}}{\text{cc/min total flow rate}}$$

in place of mg/ml.

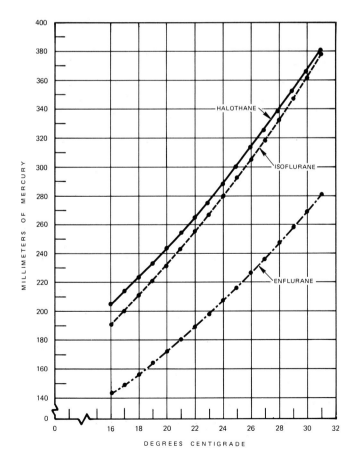

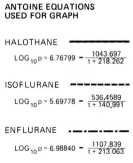

ANTOINE EQUATIONS
USED FOR GRAPH

HALOTHANE ———————

$$\text{LOG}_{10} p = 6.76799 - \frac{1043.697}{t + 218.262}$$

ISOFLURANE – – – – – – –

$$\text{LOG}_{10} p = 5.69778 - \frac{536.4589}{t + 140.991}$$

ENFLURANE –·–·–·–·–

$$\text{LOG}_{10} p = 6.98840 - \frac{1107.839}{t + 213.063}$$

Figure 4–4. Vapor pressure-temperature graph for enflurane, halothane, and isoflurane.

Calculating Percentages Using a Direct-Metering Machine at 24C

Example 1. What percentage halothane (or any volatile agent such as enflurane, isoflurane, methoxyflurane) is being conducted to the patient when the vaporizer flow rate is 100 cc/min halothane vapor, and the diluent gas flow rates are 2500 cc/min nitrous oxide and 2500 cc/min oxygen?

Step 1: Make a table such as Table 4–1.

$$\frac{100 \text{ cc/min halothane vapor}}{5000 \text{ cc/min} + 100 \text{ cc/min, total flow}}$$

$$= \frac{1}{51} \text{ (the fraction) or } 1:51 \text{ (the ratio)}$$

(For practical purposes, round figures are used. This machine setting would be a 1:50 concentration. Only when very high flow rates are required would the additional gas add significantly to the total flow rate, and it should then be included in the calculations. See Example 11.)

Step 2:

$$\frac{1}{50} = 0.02, \text{ the decimal}$$

Step 3: Percent means per hundred. Thus:

$$0.02 \times 100 = 2\%$$

Answer: Two percent halothane is being conducted to the patient.

Example 2. What percent halothane (or any volatile agent, such as enflurane or isoflurane) is being conducted to the patient when the vaporizer flow rate is 100 cc/min halothane vapor, and the diluent gas flow rates total 6 L/min?

Step 1: Determine the ratio or fraction. It is

$$\frac{100 \text{ cc/min vapor}}{6000 \text{ cc/min} + 100 \text{ cc/min vapor}}$$

Step 2: Reduced, the fraction is $\frac{1}{60}$ or 0.016, the decimal.
Step 3: The percent is 0.016 × 100, or 1.6%.
Answer: Percent halothane = 1.6.

Example 3. What percent halothane is being conducted to the patient when the vaporizer flow rate is 40 cc/min and the diluent gas flow rates total 4 L/min?

Step 1: The ratio or fraction is

$$\frac{40 \text{ cc/min vapor}}{4000 \text{ cc/min} + 40 \text{ cc/min vapor}} = 1/100$$

Step 2: The decimal is 0.01.
Step 3: The percent is 0.01 × 100 or 1%.
Answer: Percent halothane is 1.

Calculating Vaporizer Flow Rates Using a Direct-Metering Machine at 24C. It is often necessary to calculate the agent flow rate for a desired concentration and diluent flow rate.

Step 1: Convert the percentage to a decimal, as in Table 4–1.
Step 2: Multiply the decimal by the total flow rate.

Example 4. What should the cubic centimeter-per-minute agent flow rate be when a 2 percent enflurane concentration is desired with a 5 L/min diluent flow rate?

Step 1:

$$2\% = 0.02, \text{ the decimal}$$

$$(2\% \text{ means } 2/100 = 2 \div 100 = 0.02)$$

Step 2:

$$\text{Enflurane flow rate} = 0.02 \times 5000 \text{ cc/min}$$
$$= 100 \text{ cc/min}$$

Answer: The flow rate should be 100 cc/min.

Example 5. What should the vaporizer flow rate be when a 1.5 percent enflurane concentration is desired with a 6 L/min diluent flow rate?

Step 1:

$$1.5\% = 0.015$$

Step 2:

$$\text{Enflurane flow rate} = 0.015 \times 6000 \text{ cc/min}$$
$$= 90 \text{ cc/min}$$

Answer: The vaporizer flow rate should be 90 cc/min.

Example 6. What should the vaporizer flow rate be when 1 percent isoflurane concentration is desired with 4 L/min diluent gas flow rate?

Step 1:

$$1\% = 0.01$$

Step 2:

$$\text{Isoflurane flow rate} = 0.01 \times 4000 \text{ cc/min}$$
$$= 40 \text{ cc/min}$$

Answer: The vaporizer flow rate should be 40 cc/min.

Carrier Oxygen Vaporizer Flowmeters (Classic Verni-Trol and Side-Arm Vaporizers)

There are several differences between the direct-metering vaporizer just discussed and vaporizers such as the Ohio 2000 machine and Side-Arm Verni-Trol anesthetic vaporizer (Fig. 4–5).

1. Some vaporizers are heated to maintain a 23 to 25C temperature; some are not heated.
2. The vaporizer flowmeters have a separate oxygen source; they do not utilize part of the diluent oxygen.

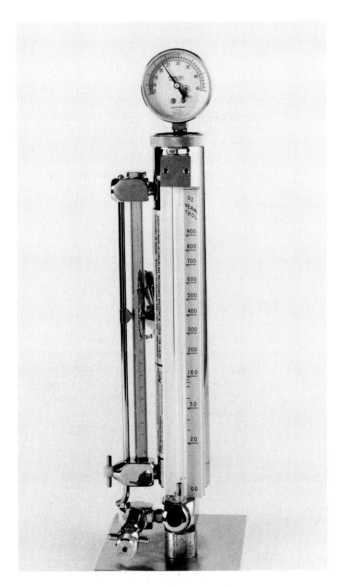

Figure 4–5. Ohio Side-Arm Verni-Trol Anesthetic Vaporizer. (*Courtesy of Anaquest, BOC, Madison, Wisconsin.*)

3. The vaporizer flowmeters indicate the amount of oxygen flowing into the vaporizer, and *not* the amount of anesthetic vapor coming out of it.
4. The anesthetist must calculate the cubic centimeters per minute of actual vapor coming out of the vaporizer into the patient's circuit.

Calculating Percentages Using the Side-Arm or Classic Verni-Trol Machine at 24C. Refer to a vapor pressure-temperature graph for the agent in use. Assume, in the following examples, that the vaporizer temperature is about 24C. Read the vapor pressure of the agent for that temperature. This vapor pressure (VP), divided by the ambient pressure (AP) (which is 760 mm Hg at sea level) minus the vapor pressure, equals the fraction of the carrier oxygen flow rate that is pure vapor being carried into the patient's circuit. This relationship expressed as equation is

$$\frac{VP}{AP - VP} = \text{fraction of carrier oxygen flow rate that is pure vapor carried}$$

Halothane

The vapor pressure of halothane at 24C is 288 mm Hg (see Fig. 4–4). Thus:

$$\frac{288 \text{ mm Hg}}{760 \text{ mm Hg} - 288 \text{ mm Hg}} = \frac{288 \text{ mm Hg}}{472 \text{ mm Hg}} = 0.6$$

This equation shows that every cubic centimeter of oxygen flowing into the halothane vaporizer carries 0.6 cc of pure halothane vapor out of the vaporizer with it.

Example 7. What percentage of halothane is being conducted to the patient when the carrier oxygen flow rate through the vaporizer is 100 cc/min, and the diluent gas flow rates total 5 L/min?

Step 1: 0.6×100 cc/min = 60 cc/min of halothane vapor being carried by the 100 cc of oxygen. The total amount of gas emerging from the vaporizer is 100 cc of oxygen plus 60 cc of halothane vapor, or 160 cc/min.

Step 2: Once the amount of actual vapor has been established, the rest of the calculations are identical to those discussed earlier for the direct-metering vaporizers, i.e., the agent concentration is the direct ratio of the agent flow rate, just calculated, to the total flow rate. Make a table to determine the fraction or ratio.

$$\frac{60 \text{ cc/min halothane vapor}}{5000 \text{ cc/min} + 100 \text{ cc/min oxygen} + 60 \text{ cc/min vapor}}$$

$$= \frac{60 \text{ cc/min}}{5160 \text{ cc/min}} = 0.0116$$

Step 3: Percent = $0.0116 \times 100 = 1.16\%$, or about 1.2%.

Answer: The percentage of halothane being conducted to the patient is about 1.2. (The same answer will be obtained if round figures are used:

$$\frac{60 \text{ cc/min}}{5000 \text{ cc/min}} = 0.012; \quad 0.012 \times 100 = 1.2\%.)$$

Compare this answer with that of Example 1.

Example 8. What percentage of halothane is being conducted to the patient when the carrier oxygen flow rate through the vaporizer is 80 cc/min, and the diluent gas flow rates total 6 L/min?

Step 1: Calculate the amount of halothane vapor 80 cc of oxygen will carry at 24C.

$$0.6 \times 80 \text{ cc} = 48 \text{ cc halothane vapor carried by 80 cc of oxygen}$$

Step 2:

$$\frac{48 \text{ cc/min}}{6000 \text{ cc/min} + 80 \text{ cc/min} + 48 \text{ cc/min}}$$

$$= \frac{48}{6128} = 0.0078$$

Step 3: Percent = 0.0078 × 100 = 0.78%, or about 0.8%

Answer: The percentage of halothane being conducted to the patient is about 0.8. (The same answer will be obtained if round figures are used: 48 cc/min ÷ 6000 cc/min = 0.008; 0.008 × 100 = 0.8%.)

Example 9. What percentage of halothane is being conducted to the patient when the carrier oxygen flow rate through the vaporizer is 40 cc/min, and the diluent gas flow rates total 4 L/min?

Step 1: 0.6 × 40 cc = 24 cc halothane vapor carried by 40 cc of oxygen at 24C.

Step 2:

$$\frac{24 \text{ cc/min}}{4000 \text{ cc/min} + 40 \text{ cc/min} + 24 \text{ cc/min}}$$

$$= \frac{24}{4064} = 0.0059$$

Step 3: Percent = 0.0059 × 100 = 0.59%, or about 0.6%

Compare this answer with that of Example 3.

Enflurane

The vapor pressure of enflurane at 24C is 207 mm Hg (see Fig. 4–4).

$$\frac{VP}{AP - VP} = \frac{\text{fraction of carrier oxygen flow rate}}{\text{that is pure vapor carried}}$$

$$\frac{207 \text{ mm Hg}}{760 \text{ mm Hg} - 207 \text{ mm Hg}} = \frac{207}{553} = 0.37$$

Thus, every cubic centimeter of oxygen flowing into the enflurane vaporizer carries 0.37 cc of pure enflurane vapor out of the vaporizer with it.

Example 10. What percentage of enflurane is being conducted to the patient when the carrier oxygen flow rate through the vaporizer is 250 cc/min, and the diluent flow rates total 5000 cc/min?

Step 1: 0.37 × 250 cc/min = 93 cc/min enflurane vapor carried by the 250 cc of carrier oxygen. The total amount of gas emerging from the vaporizer is 250 cc/min carrier oxygen plus 93 cc/min enflurane vapor, or 343 cc/min.

Step 2: The enflurane concentration is the direct ratio of the agent flow rate to the total flow rate. The percentage of enflurane equals this direct ratio times 100.

% Enflurane

$$= \frac{93 \text{ cc/min} \times 100}{5000 \text{ cc/min} + 250 \text{ cc/min} + 93 \text{ cc/min}}$$

$$= \frac{9300 \text{ cc/min}}{5343 \text{ cc/min}}$$

$$= 1.74\%$$

Answer: The percentage of enflurane being conducted to the patient is 1.74. (If round figures had been used, 9300/5000 = 1.9%.)

Example 11. What percentage of enflurane is being conducted to the patient when the carrier oxygen flow rate is 700 cc/min, and the diluent flow rate totals 6000 cc/min?

Step 1: 0.37 × 700 cc/min = 259 cc/min enflurane vapor carried by the 700 cc of carrier oxygen. The total amount of gas emerging from the vaporizer is 700 cc/min carrier oxygen plus 259 cc/min enflurane vapor, or 959 cc/min.

Step 2:

% Enflurane

$$= \frac{259 \text{ cc/min} \times 100}{6000 \text{ cc/min} + 700 \text{ cc/min} + 259 \text{ cc/min}}$$

$$= \frac{25,900 \text{ cc/min}}{6,959 \text{ cc/min}}$$

$$= 3.7\%$$

Answer: The percentage of enflurane being conducted to the patient is 3.7. (If round figures had been used, 25,900/6000 = 4.3%. This equation illustrates a situation where accurate calculations should be made. The difference between accurate calculations and round figures is too great to be ignored.)

Calculating Vaporizer Flow Rates for Desired Percentages, Using the Side-Arm, or Classic Verni-Trol Machine at 24C

Halothane

Since, at 24C, each cubic centimeter of carrier oxygen from the Side-Arm vaporizer picks up 6/10 cc of halothane vapor, the carrier oxygen flow rate must be 10/6 times that of the vapor actually carried.

Example 12. What should the carrier oxygen flow rate be when a 1 percent halothane concentration and a 4 L/min diluent gas flow rate is desired?

Step 1:

1% = 0.01 cc/min halothane vapor
= 0.01 × 4000 cc/min
= 40 cc/min

Step 2:

Carrier oxygen flow rate
= 10/6 × 40 cc/min halothane vapor
$$= \frac{400 \text{ cc/min}}{6} = 66 \text{ cc/min}$$

Answer: The carrier oxygen flow rate should be 66 cc/min.

Proof: Since each cubic centimeter of oxygen carries 0.6 cc of halothane vapor,

66 cc oxygen × 0.6 = 40 cc/min halothane vapor

$$\% = \frac{40 \text{ cc halothane vapor/min} \times 100}{\dfrac{4000 \text{ cc}}{\text{min}} + \dfrac{66 \text{ cc}}{\text{min oxygen}} + \dfrac{40 \text{ cc}}{\text{min vapor}}}$$

$$= \frac{4000 \text{ cc/min}}{4106 \text{ cc/min}} = 0.97\%, \text{ or about } 1\%$$

Example 13. What should the carrier oxygen flow rate be when a 1.5 percent halothane concentration and a 6 L/min diluent gas flow rate are desired?

Step 1:

$$1.5\% = 0.015 \text{ cc/min halothane vapor}$$
$$= 6000 \text{ cc/min} \times 0.015 = 90 \text{ cc/min}$$

Step 2:

$$\text{Carrier oxygen flow rate} = 10/6 \times 90 \text{ cc/min}$$
$$\tfrac{1}{6}(900) \text{ cc/min} = 150 \text{ cc/min}$$

Answer: The carrier oxygen flow rate should be 150 cc/min.

Proof: Since each cubic centimeter of oxygen carries 0.6 cc of halothane vapor,

$$150 \text{ cc oxygen} \times 0.6 = 90 \text{ cc halothane vapor}$$

$$\% = \frac{90 \text{ cc halothane vapor/min} \times 100}{6000 \text{ cc/min} + 150 \text{ cc/min} + 90 \text{ cc/min}}$$
$$= \frac{9000 \text{ cc/min}}{6240 \text{ cc/min}} = 1.44\%$$

(If round figures had been used:

$$\% = \frac{9000 \text{ cc/min}}{6000 \text{ cc/min}} = 1.5\%.)$$

Enflurane

Since, at 24C, each cubic centimeter of carrier oxygen from the Side-Arm vaporizer picks up 37/100 cc of enflurane vapor, carrier oxygen flow rate must be 100/37 times that of the vapor actually carried.

Example 14. What should the carrier oxygen flow rate be when a 1.5 percent enflurane concentration is desired with a 6 L/min diluent flow rate?

Step 1:

$$1.5\% = 0.015 \text{ cc/min enflurane vapor}$$
$$= 0.015 \times 6000 \text{ cc/min} = 90 \text{ cc/min}$$

Step 2:

$$\text{Carrier oxygen flow rate}$$
$$= 100/37 \times 90 \text{ cc/min enflurane vapor}$$
$$= (9000 \text{ cc/min})/37 = 243 \text{ cc/min}$$

Answer: The carrier oxygen flow rate should be 243 cc/min.

Compare this answer with that of Example 5.

Proof: Since each cubic centimeter of oxygen carries 0.37 cc of enflurane vapor,

$$243 \text{ cc of oxygen} \times 0.37$$
$$= 90 \text{ cc of enflurane vapor}$$

$$\% = \frac{90 \text{ cc/min enflurane vapor} \times 100}{6000 \text{ cc/min} + 243 \text{ cc/min} + 90 \text{ cc/min}}$$
$$= \frac{9000 \text{ cc/min}}{6333 \text{ cc/min}} = 1.42\%, \text{ accurate answer}$$

(If round figures had been used:

$$\% = \frac{90 \text{ cc/min enflurane vapor} \times 100}{6000 \text{ cc/min}} = 1.5\%.)$$

Example 15. What should the carrier oxygen flow rate be when a 3.5 percent enflurane concentration is desired with a 5 L/min diluent flow rate?

Step 1:

$$3.5\% = 0.035 \text{ cc/min enflurane vapor}$$
$$= 0.035 \times 5000 \text{ cc/min} = 175 \text{ cc/min}$$

Step 2:

$$\text{Carrier oxygen flow rate} = \frac{100}{37} \times 175 \text{ cc/min}$$
$$= \frac{17,500 \text{ cc/min}}{37}$$
$$= 473 \text{ cc/min}$$

Answer: The carrier oxygen flow rate should be 473 cc/min.

Proof: Since each cubic centimeter of oxygen carries 0.37 cc of enflurane vapor,

$$473 \text{ cc of oxygen} \times 0.37$$
$$= 175 \text{ cc enflurane vapor}$$

$$\% \text{ Enflurane}$$
$$= \frac{175 \text{ cc/min enflurane vapor} \times 100}{5000 \text{ cc/min} + 473 \text{ cc/min} + 175 \text{ cc/min}}$$
$$= \frac{17,500 \text{ cc/min}}{5,648 \text{ cc/min}} = 3.1\%, \text{ accurate answer}$$

(If round figures had been used:

$$\% = \frac{175 \text{ cc/min enflurane vapor} \times 100}{5000 \text{ cc/min}} = 3.5\%.)$$

Isoflurane

The vapor pressure of isoflurane at 24C is 280 mm Hg (see Fig. 4–4).

$$\frac{280 \text{ mm Hg}}{760 \text{ mm Hg} - 280 \text{ mm Hg}} = \frac{280 \text{ mm Hg}}{480 \text{ mm Hg}} = 0.583, \text{ or } 0.6$$

This equation shows that every cubic centimeter of oxygen flowing into the isoflurane vaporizer carries about 0.6 cc of pure isoflurane vapor out of the vaporizer with it. The vapor pressure curve of isoflurane is so close to that of halothane that, for practical purposes, isoflurane calculations for the Side-Arm or classic Verni-Trol vaporizers are the same as those for halothane. Anesthetists who use other well-known agents should be able to calculate percentages and agent flow rates through various vaporizers by referring to appropriate vapor pressure-temperature graphs.

BIBLIOGRAPHY

Guyton AC: Textbook of Medical Physiology, 6th ed. Philadelphia, Saunders, 1981.

Hill DW: Physics Applied to Anaesthesia. London, Butterworth, 1980.

Operation and maintenance manuals, Heidbrink series 2000 and series DM 5000. Ohio Medical Products, PO Box 7550, 3030 Airco Drive, Madison, Wisconsin 53707, 1978.

Rogers RC, Hill GE: Equations for vapour-pressure versus tempera- ture derivation and uses of the Antoine equation on a hand-held programmable calculator. Br J Anaesth 50:415–430, 1978.

Shapiro BA: Clinical Applications of Blood Gases, 2nd ed. Chicago, Year Book Med Pub, 1977.

Waterhouse M: Practical Mathematics in Allied Health. Baltimore, Urban & Schwarzenberg, 1979.

Wilson CO: Textbook of Organic, Medicinal, and Pharmaceutical Chemistry, 6th ed. Philadelphia, Lippincott, 1971.

Wylie WD, Churchill-Davidson HC: A Practice of Anaesthesia. 4th ed. Philadelphia, Saunders, 1978.

5

Principles of Chemistry and Physics in Anesthesia

Leo A. Le Bel

Anesthesia practice represents a superb example of the pragmatic application of science for the betterment of humanity. The "hard" sciences of physics and chemistry are joined with the "soft" sciences of psychology and sociology. The former provide an understanding of the fundamental processes by which nature operates; the latter provide the basis for the "art" of the specialty. This chapter addresses those "hard" science concepts and principles that impact on daily practice; a sound understanding of them is required of all nurse anesthetists.

Historically, the various scientific disciplines arose and developed independently. Only recently have we begun to appreciate that many natural processes are common to both chemistry and physics. The distinction between the two has become blurred, and this makes it more difficult to organize concepts systematically. A strong effort has been made to keep the presentation logically organized. Similar or related concepts are kept together; at the same time an attempt has been made to preserve a traditional approach by separating concepts on the basis of their primary association with either physics or chemistry. The important point to remember is that many of the concepts are valid for both sciences.

GENERAL CONCEPTS

Every material item possessing mass and occupying space represents a form of *matter*. Matter exists in three states: gases, liquids, and solids. All matter is composed of one or more basic parts referred to as *elements* (Table 5–1). Eighty-eight of these occur naturally. Some, most radioactive substances for instance, occur only under specific conditions. Of the naturally occurring elements, most are solids, eleven are gases, and two are liquids. Twenty elements are com- monly abundant and fifteen occur in the body. Elements cannot normally be further decomposed. When two or more elements are chemically combined, the substance is referred to as a *compound*.

Mass designates the quantity of matter and is generally characterized in terms of weight units (e.g., ounces, pounds, grams). However, *weight* is a measure of the forces of attraction between two bodies (e.g., you and the earth or you and the moon), expressed in terms of a scale. Therefore, in terms of a given scale—i.e., pounds—you will have a different weight depending upon whether you are stand- ing on earth or on the moon. This is because the frame of reference between the two objects is different. Because the mass of the earth and moon are different, your weight (mass) compared to each of them will vary.

This force of attraction between two bodies is called *gravity*. It varies inversely with the square of the distance between the two objects. Gravity is a basic force in nature. Other forces we commonly observe include mechanical, electrical, and chemical. Force is merely one way of talking about energy.

Energy is defined as the ability to do work, or to produce a change in matter. *Work* is performed when a force is exerted over a distance, such as moving a weight of 1 g a distance of 1 cm. Converting water to steam, a change in matter, also requires energy. Energy is thought of in two forms: *kinetic energy*, which is energy in motion, and *latent energy*, which is stored for later use.

Applying some form of energy to matter can result in either physical or chemical change. An example from anesthesia practice is the vaporization of a liquid to a gas by the application of heat. This represents a *physical change*. The state, but not the composition, of the substance is changed. In a *chemical change* a new substance is formed.

What force does depends on the form of the force (heat, gravity, etc.) and the manner in which it is applied to matter. For example, force may displace a stable object, accelerate a moving object, or change the direction (vector) of a moving object. The basic units of measurement for

TABLE 5-1. TABLE OF ELEMENTS: INTERNATIONAL ATOMIC WEIGHTS BASED ON CARBON-12 ISOTOPE[a]

Name	Symbol	Atomic Number	Atomic Weight	Name	Symbol	Atomic Number	Atomic Weight
Actinium	Ac	89	(227)	Mendelevium	Md	101	(256)
Aluminum	Al	13	26.98154	Mercury	Hg	80	200.59
Americum	Am	95	(243)	Molybdenum	Mo	42	95.94
Antimony	Sb	51	121.75	Neodymium	Nd	60	144.24
Argon	Ar	18	39.948	Neon	Ne	10	20.179
Arsenic	As	33	74.9216	Neptunium	Np	93	237.0482
Astatine	At	85	(210)	Nickel	Ni	28	58.71
Barium	Ba	56	137.34	Niobium	Nb	41	92.9064
Berkelium	Bk	97	(247)	Nitrogen	N	7	14.0067
Beryllium	Be	4	9.0118	Nobelium	No	102	(254)
Bismuth	Bi	83	208.9804	Osmium	Os	76	190.2
Boron	B	5	10.81	Oxygen	O	8	15.9994
Bromine	Br	35	79.904	Palladium	Pd	46	106.4
Cadmium	Cd	48	112.40	Phosphorus	P	15	30.97376
Calcium	Ca	20	40.08	Platinum	Pt	78	195.09
Californium	Cf	98	(251)	Plutonium	Pu	94	(242)
Carbon	C	6	12.011	Polonium	Po	84	(210)
Cerium	Ce	58	140.12	Potassium	K	19	39.098
Cesium	Cs	55	132.9054	Praseodymium	Pr	59	140.9077
Chlorine	Cl	17	35.453	Promethium	Pm	61	(145)
Chromium	Cr	24	51.996	Protactinum	Pa	91	231.0359
Cobalt	Co	27	58.9332	Radium	Ra	88	226.0254
Copper	Cu	29	63.546	Radon	Rn	86	(222)
Curium	Cm	96	(247)	Rhenium	Re	75	186.2
Dysprosium	Dy	66	162.50	Rhodium	Rh	45	102.9055
Einsteinium	Es	99	(254)	Rubidium	Rb	37	85.4678
Erbium	Er	68	167.26	Ruthenium	Ru	44	101.07
Europium	Eu	63	151.96	Samarium	Sm	62	150.4
Fermium	Fm	100	(253)	Scandium	Sc	21	44.9559
Fluorine	F	9	18.99840	Selenium	Se	34	78.96
Francium	Fr	87	(223)	Silicon	Si	14	28.086
Gadolinium	Gd	64	157.25	Silver	Ag	47	107.868
Gallium	Ga	31	69.72	Sodium	Na	11	22.98977
Germanium	Ge	32	72.59	Strontium	Sr	38	87.62
Gold	Au	79	196.9665	Sulfur	S	16	32.06
Hafnium	Hf	72	178.49	Tantalum	Ta	73	180.9479
Hahnium	Ha	105	(260)	Technetium	Tc	43	98.9062
Helium	He	2	4.00260	Tellurium	Te	52	127.60
Holmium	Ho	67	164.9304	Terbium	Tb	65	158.9254
Hydrogen	H	1	1.0079	Thallium	Tl	81	204.37
Indium	In	49	114.82	Thorium	Th	90	232.0381
Iodine	I	53	126.9045	Thulium	Tm	69	168.9342
Iridium	Ir	77	192.22	Tin	Sn	50	118.69
Iron	Fe	26	55.847	Titanium	Ti	22	47.90
Krypton	Kr	36	83.80	Tungsten	W	74	183.85
Lanthanum	La	57	138.9055	Uranium	U	92	238.029
Lawrencium	Lr	103	(257)	Vanadium	V	23	50.9414
Lead	Pb	82	207.2	Xenon	Xe	54	131.30
Lithium	Li	3	6.941	Ytterbium	Yb	70	173.04
Lutetium	Lu	71	174.97	Yttrium	Y	39	88.9059
Magnesium	Mg	12	24.305	Zinc	Zn	30	65.38
Manganese	Mn	25	54.9380	Zirconium	Zr	40	91.22

[a] Numbers in parentheses are mass numbers of most stable isotope of that element.

From King GB, Caldwell WE, et al: College Chemistry, 7th ed. Belmont, CA, Litton Educational Pub., 1977. Reprinted with permission of Wadsworth Publishing.

force are the dyne and the newton; they are defined as follows:

Dyne (dyn): Force required to move a 1-g mass 1 cm/sec

Newton (N): Force required to move a 1-kg mass 1 m/sec

Notice that each is defined in terms of moving a mass of given weight, a given distance, in a specified unit of time. Movement over a given distance in a specified time is called *acceleration*. Thus, the general formula for force can be expressed as

Force (f) = mass (m) × acceleration (a)

The force required to expand the lungs of an anesthetized patient can be expressed in terms of dynes, although it is more common to express it as centimeters of water pressure:

1 cm H_2O = (approx.) 980.7 dynes
20 cm H_2O = 19,614 dynes

the approximate amount of force normally required to inflate adult lungs.

The concepts of mass and energy are basic to an understanding of chemistry and physics. Energy acts upon mass (matter), and a change in mass involves the addition or release of energy. Indeed, mass and energy are interchangeable concepts, a truth recognized first by Albert Einstein in his formulation of the equation

$E = mc^2$

in which c^2 equals the speed of light—the acceleration point at which mass becomes nonexistent, and all is pure energy.

The universe contains a finite amount of matter, and therefore the amount of energy present in the universe is also finite. Matter and energy can neither be created nor destroyed. These two concepts are referred to as the *law of conservation of mass* and the *law of conservation of energy*.

TABLE 5–2. BASIC SI UNITS

Physical Quantity	Name	Symbol
Length	Meter	m
Mass	Kilogram	kg
Time	Second[a]	s
Electric current	Ampere	A
Thermodynamic temperature	Kelvin	K
Luminous intensity	Candela	cd
Amount of substance	Mole	mol

[a] Minute (min), hour (h), and day (d) will remain in use although they are not official SI units.
From Can Anaesth Soc J 29(6):652–654, 1982.

Measurement

The aforementioned dyne and newton are examples of how natural phenomena can be defined and measured. A common method for making those measurements facilitates communication between scientists and ensures that observations are made in a standardized and reproducible fashion. In 1960, the international scientific community adopted a new system for measuring physical and chemical events. It is known as the international system, or *SI system*. The SI system replaces the older and less precise English and metric systems, although some of their components have been retained. Conversion to the new system is not yet complete, but in the near future all scientific measurements, including those related to medicine, will be expressed in terms of SI units. SI units are of two types: basic units and derived units. (See Tables 5–2 and 5–3.) In addition, prefixes derived from the metric system are used to denote fractions or multiples of base units. For example, the basic unit of length, the meter, can, by use of the prefixes, be expressed in either fractions or multiples:

1 kilometer = 1000 meters
1 millimeter = 1/1000 meter

The commonly used prefixes are listed in Table 5–4.

TABLE 5–3. DERIVED SI UNITS

Quantity	SI unit	Symbol	Expression in Terms of SI Base Units or Derived Units
Frequency	Hertz	Hz	1 Hz = 1 cycle /s (1 cs^{-1})
Force	Newton	N	1 N = 1 kg × m/s^2 (1 kg × ms^{-2})
Work, energy, quantity of heat	Joule	J	1 J = 1 N × m
Power	Watt	W	1 W = 1 J/s (1 J × s^{-1})
Quantity of electricity	Coulomb	C	1 C = 1 A × s
Electric potential, potential difference, tension, electromotive force	Volt	V	1 V = 1 W/A (1 W × A^{-1})
Electric capacitance	Farad	F	1 F = 1 A × s/V (1 A × s × V^{-1})
Electric resistance	Ohm	Ω	1 Ω = 1 V/A (V × A^{-1})
Flux of magnetic induction, magnetic flux	Weber	Wb	1 Wb = 1 V × s
Magnetic flux density, magnetic induction	Tesla	T	1 T = Wb/m^2 (1 Wb × m^{-2})
Inductance	Henry	H	1 H = 1 V × s/A (1 V × s × A^{-1})
Pressure	Pascal	Pa	1 Pa = 1 N/m^2 (1 N × m^{-2}) = 1 kg/m × s^2 (1 kg × m^{-1} × s^{-2})

The liter (10^{-3}m^3 = dm^3), though not official, will remain in use as a unit of volume as also will the dyne (dyn) as a unit of force (1 dyn = 10—5N).
From Can Anaesth Soc J 29(6):652–654, 1982.

TABLE 5–4. PREFIXES FOR SI UNITS

Factor	Name	Symbol	Factor	Name	Symbol
10^{18}	Exa-	E	10^{-18}	Atto-	a
10^{15}	Peta-	P	10^{-15}	Femto-	f
10^{12}	Tera-	T	10^{-12}	Pico-	p
10^{9}	Giga-	G	10^{-9}	Nano-	n
10^{6}	Mega-	M	10^{-6}	Micro-	μ
10^{3}	Kilo-	k	10^{-3}	Milli-	m
10^{2}	Hecto-	h	10^{-2}	Centi-	c
10^{1}	Deca-	da	10^{-1}	Deci-	d

From Can Anaesth Soc J 29(6):652–654, 1982.

For the present, the use of several measurement systems generates confusion. For example, blood pressures are still reported as 120/80 millimeters of mercury (1 mm Hg = 1 torr). Under the SI system this would be expressed as 16/11 kPa (kPa = kilopascal, the basic unit for measuring pressure).

It is important to select the prefix appropriate to the idea to be conveyed. Using millimeters when one really wishes to express kilometers results in a millionfold error. Such errors are certainly intolerable in both science and medicine. The same caution applies to the expression of numbers where the misplacement of the decimal point by one number results in a tenfold difference. Administering 0.1 mg of a potent drug is not the same as administering 0.01 mg.

Many of the measurement units of the SI system are applicable in medicine as is demonstrated in Tables 5–5 through 5–9. Conversion factors are included to facilitate the interpretation of data expressed by the older measurement systems.

States of Matter

Much of what has been discussed regarding general concepts also applies on the atomic, subatomic, and molecular level as well as on the large scale of everyday existence. The three states of matter (gases, liquids, and solids) are distinguished by specific characteristics: Solids have volume and shape and cannot be compressed, e.g., a cube of ice. Liquids have volume but no specific shape; rather, they assume the shape of their container, e.g., water. Gases have neither shape nor volume; they expand indefinitely, e.g., steam.

Notice that in our example we do not have three different substances ice, water, and steam, but three different physical states of the same substance. The difference between states is related to the activity of the molecules that make up the substance and the forces that act upon it. For example, removing heat (energy) by cooling causes water molecules to draw closer together, because of gravitational and other forces, and to become solidified. If additional energy is added to water—say, by the application of heat—the additional energy accelerates molecular activity and makes it easier for the molecules to overcome the forces that draw them together. As the forces are overcome, the molecules are dispersed and the water becomes steam.

This same principle also applies to liquid anesthetics, which, through the addition of heat energy, are vaporized to gases that can be administered to patients. Before taking a closer look at how atoms, subatomic particles, and molecules interact, there are two additional concepts that require discussion because they have applications to anesthesia practice.

Density shows the relationship between the weight and volume of a substance. The formula for density is

$$\text{Density} = \frac{\text{Weight}}{\text{Volume}}$$

In most cases density is expressed in grams per cubic centimeter, but for gases it is expressed as grams per liter.

The density of air is 1.3 g/L. Hydrogen has a density of 0.09 g/L; therefore hydrogen rises in air. Similarly, the

TABLE 5–5. SI CONVERSION FACTORS

SI Unit	Old Unit	Conversion Factors	
		Old to SI (Exact)	SI to Old (Approximate)
kPa	mm Hg[a]	0.133	7.5
kPa	1 standard atmosphere[b] (approx. 1 bar)	101.3	0.01
kPa	cm H_2O	0.0981	10.0
kPa	lb/sq in	6.89	0.145

[a] E.g., systolic blood pressure of 120 mm Hg = 16 kPa and diastolic blood pressure of 80 mm Hg = 11 kPa.
[b] 760 mm Hg.
From Can Anaesth Soc J 29(6):652–654, 1982.

TABLE 5–6. BLOOD CHEMISTRY: UNITS AND CONVERSION FACTORS

Measurement	SI Unit	Old Unit	Conversion Factors Old to SI (Exact)	SI to Old (Approximate)
Blood				
Acid-base				
P_{CO_2}	kPa	mm Hg	0.133	7.5
P_{O_2}	kPa	mm Hg	0.133	7.5
Standard bicarbonate	mmol/L	mEq/L	Numerically equivalent	
Base excess	mmol/L	mEq/L	Numerically equivalent	
Glucose	mmol/L	mg/100 ml	0.0555	18.0
Plasma				
Sodium	mmol/L	mEq/L	Numerically equivalent	
Potassium	mmol/L	mEq/L	Numerically equivalent	
Magnesium	mmol/L	mEq/L	0.5	2.0
Chloride	mmol/L	mEq/L	Numerically equivalent	
Phosphate (inorganic)	mmol/L	mEq/L	0.323	3.0
Creatinine	μmol/L	mg/100 ml	88.4	0.01
Urea	mmol/L	mg/100 ml	0.166	6.0
Serum				
Calcium	mmol/L	mg/100 ml	0.25	4.0
Iron	μmol/L	μg/100 mol	0.179	5.6
Bilirubin	μmol/L	mg/100 ml	17.1	0.06
Cholesterol	mmol/L	mg/100 ml	0.1259	39.0
Total proteins	g/L	g/100 ml	10.0	0.1
Albumin	g/L	g/100 ml	10.0	0.1
Globulin	g/L	g/100 ml	10.0	0.1

From Can Anaesth Soc J 29(6):652–654, 1982.

TABLE 5–7. BIOCHEMICAL CONTENT OF OTHER BODY FLUIDS

Measurement	SI Unit	Old Unit	Conversion Factors Old to SI (Exact)	SI to Old (Approximate)
Urine	mmol/24 h	mg/24 h	0.025	40.0
Creatinine	mmol/24 h	mg/24 h	0.00884	113.0
Potassium	mmol/L	mEq/L	Numerically equivalent	
Sodium	mmol/L	mEq/L	Numerically equivalent	
Cerebrospinal fluid				
Protein	g/L	mg/100 ml	0.01	100.0
Glucose	mmol/L	mg/100 ml	0.0555	18.0

From Can Anaesth Soc J 29(6):652–654, 1982.

TABLE 5–8. HEMATOLOGY

Measurement	SI Units	Old Unit	Conversion Factors Old to SI	SI to Old
Hemoglobin (Hb)	g/dl	g/100	Numerically equivalent	
Packed cell volume	No unit[a]	Percent	0.01	100
Mean cell Hb concentration	g/dl	Percent	Numerically equivalent	
Mean cell Hb	pg	μμg	Numerically equivalent	
Red cell count	Cells/L	Cells/mm^3	10^6	10^{-6}
White cell count	Cells/L	Cells/mm^3	10^6	10^{-6}
Reticulocytes	Percent	Percent	Numerically equivalent	
Platelets	Cells/L	Cells/mm^3	10^6	10^{-6}

[a] Expressed as decimal fraction, e.g., normal adult-male value 0.40 to 0.54.
From Can Anaesth Soc 29(6):652–654, 1982.

TABLE 5–9. pH AND nmol/liter OF H⁺ ACTIVITY

pH	nmol/L
6.80	158
6.90	126
7.00	100
7.10	79
7.20	63
7.25	56
7.30	50
7.35	45
7.40	40
7.45	36
7.50	32
7.55	28
7.60	25
7.70	20

From Can Anaesth Soc J 29(6):652–654, 1982.

density of water is 1.0 g/cc, and that of ice 0.92 g/cc. Therefore ice floats in water.

Specific gravity (sp gr) expresses the ratio between two densities. It does not have measuring units of its own, but is merely used to make comparisons. For example:

$$\text{Specific gravity} = \frac{\text{Density of substance } X}{\text{Density of water (or air)}}.$$

The standard of comparison normally used is the density of water. For gases air is the comparison standard. Specific gravity tells us how much lighter or heavier a substance is than the standard to which it is compared. Both substances must be compared under similar conditions of temperature and pressure. The concept of specific gravity is important to anesthesia because it tells us which gases will be heavier than room air. Nitrogen, helium, and water vapor are all lighter than air, whereas carbon dioxide and nitrous oxide are about 1.5 times heavier. Oxygen is only slightly heavier than air (sp gr = 1.1).

ATOMIC STRUCTURE OF MATTER

Elements exist as discrete atoms of specific configuration. Combining two or more atoms of the same element or two or more atoms of different elements produces a molecule. Many millions of molecules are required to provide enough volume for a substance to be visible because of the infinitesimal size of atoms.

A single atom of an element retains all of the properties of the element; and all atoms of the same element are identically configured. Atoms of different elements differ not only in their configuration, but also in size, weight, and chemical properties.

We now know atoms are themselves made up of smaller parts. The nucleus, or central core, of the atom is made up of protons and neutrons. Circling in orbits around the nucleus are the electrons. Additional subatomic particles have been identified (e.g., positron, muon, neutrino, and pion—each with its corresponding antiparticle) but their importance lies in the field of high-energy physics, and they are not essential to understanding atomic structure

as it relates to anesthesia practice. Therefore, the following discussion will be limited to the proton, neutron, and electron. The three differ from each other in two respects: mass and electric charge. Hydrogen, the simplest, lightest, and most abundant element in the universe can illustrate the basic configuration of atoms. The hydrogen ion has one proton of positive charge and a neutron with no charge that make up its nucleus. The mass of both proton and neutron are the same. The electron that orbits the nucleus has a negative charge equal to the charge of the proton, but with a mass only 1/1800 that of the nucleus.

The *atomic weight* of an atom is determined by the masses of the protons and neutrons contained in its nucleus. Because protons and neutrons are equal in mass, they are each said to represent one *atomic mass unit* (amu). The electrical charge of the nucleus is determined by the number of protons. This is called the *atomic number*. As the number of protons in the nucleus is increased by one, the next heavier element is obtained. For example, hydrogen has one proton, helium has two protons, lithium has three protons, etc.

As protons are increased in number, the number of positive charges goes up correspondingly. To maintain electrical balance, the number of electrons must go up by the same number. In this way the atom remains electrically neutral because all positive charges are balanced by an equal number of negative charges.

As electrons travel about the nucleus, they do not all travel the same path; rather, they travel different paths (directions) in orbits of varying distance from the nucleus. In helium, for instance, the two electrons travel different paths in the same orbit (that is, at essentially the same distance from the nucleus). For other atoms with more electrons, the electrons of the same orbital distance from the nucleus travel at different angles (paths) from each other; and electrons at other orbital distances do the same.

Each succeeding electron orbit is not only farther in distance from the nucleus, but each orbit can contain only a specific number of electrons. Each succeeding orbit is filled, in turn, from the next innermost orbit. These orbits are also referred to as *energy levels*, since each orbit varies in the energy its electrons possess relative to electrons in the other orbits. (There are actually some variations within orbits, referred to as suborbits, but for our purposes, these can be ignored.) The first energy level contains a maximum of two electrons, the second can have eight, as can the third. Up to element number 20 (calcium), the two-eight-eight configuration is retained. After that, electrons move randomly between energy levels—that is they can skip from orbit to orbit. The outermost level can contain any number of electrons up to eight but may have any number between one and eight. To understand the operations of atoms, it is important to recognize that: (1) the outermost energy level of an atom is most important because it is the number of electrons in this orbit that determines the chemical activity of the atom; (2) each atom desires stability to achieve a configuration of a complete (eight-electron) outer orbit—the basis for chemical reactions between elements.

The number of protons and neutrons in an atom is not always equal. When the number of neutrons in the nucleus is less or greater than the number of protons, the weight of the nucleus will be different. The element retains its chemical properties because the number of protons and electrons determines these; but, because of the change in weight caused by the loss or gain of neutrons, the element will have different physical properties. Such elements are called *isotopes*. Many of the radioactive isotopes are useful diagnostic tools in medicine.

It is because an element can exist as different isotopes that atomic weights cannot be given as whole numbers. Instead, the weight of an element given in a periodic table represents the balance of weights in a mixture of that element's basic and isotope atoms.

As mentioned previously, combining two or more atoms of the same or different elements produces a molecule. When atoms of different elements are combined we call the molecular substance a *compound*. Because we deal mostly with compounds rather than lone elements in anesthesia, it is often more practical to discuss molecules than atoms.

Generally, a molecule of a compound is made up of atoms of several elements. By adding the atomic weights of all elements in a moelcule, we obtain the compound's *molecular weight*. Sodium (Na) has an atomic weight of 22.989, and chlorine (Cl), 35.453. Since an atom of each, chemically combined, produces a molecule of sodium chloride (NaCl) the molecular weight of sodium chloride is 58.442. (In reality, sodium chloride, common table salt, exists in crystal form, where each chloride ion is surrounded by six sodium ions, and vice versa. These concepts are dealt with later, but the example of adding atomic weights to obtain molecular weight remains valid.)

A molecule of a substance is always made up of the same number of the same atoms, in the same configuration. This is known as the *law of definite composition*. For this reason, the molecular weight of a given compound always remains the same. Because a single molecule is so small and lightweight, it is preferable to speak of a large number of them together—1 gram's worth. This is known as the *gram molecular weight* (GMW). It is also called 1 mole. One mole is equal to the total of the atomic weights of each and every atom in the compound and is expressed in grams.

When speaking of atomic or molecular weights, we are really comparing the mass of one atom or molecule to that of an equal unit of carbon (C-12). Carbon-12 serves as the standard against which other elements are compared. It would take 6.02×10^{23} carbon-12 atoms to add up to 12 grams of carbon. The number of atoms required to provide the gram molecular weight of any element is always 6.02×10^{23}. This is known as *Avogadro's number*. It is the basis for expression of the mole. Atomic weights of different elements must always contain the same number of atoms. Therefore, the mole is Avogadro's number of formula units of a substance. Avogadro's number applies to molecular weights as well as atomic weights. Hence, 1 GMW of a compound always contains 6.02×10^{23} molecules.

VOLUME, PRESSURE, AND FORCES

Volume is the expanse of space occupied by a given number of atoms or molecules. One atom or molecule occupies little space, but a large collection of them can occupy enough space to enable measurement. For solids, the basic units of measurement are the cubic meter and the cubic centimeter (cm^3 or cc). For liquids and gases, volumes are measured in liters (L) and milliliters (ml).

Any aggregate collection (volume) of atoms or molecules also exerts pressure. *Pressure* arises from two primary sources: from the gravitational pull on the atoms or molecules and from the energy forces that operate within the atoms themselves.

Sea-level atmospheric pressure results from the earth's gravitational pull on the atoms and molecules that make up the surrounding air. Similarly, hydrostatic pressure at ocean depths results from gravitational influences upon the molecules of water. Density also plays a role in determining pressure. A column of mercury will exert more pressure than an equal column of water because mercury is denser. This fact makes measuring blood pressure with a mercury manometer more practical than using a water manometer. By the contraction or expansion of a given volume of molecules, the density of those molecules is changed and more or less pressure will be exerted. This will be discussed in the section on gas laws.

The other primary factor by which atoms or molecules are able to exert pressure relates to the *kinetic theory of matter*, which states that *all matter consists of atoms or molecules in constant motion*. Therefore, pressure is also generated by the force of atoms or molecules striking a surface as they move about. An example is the pressure exerted against the walls of a cylinder containing anesthetic gases. An appreciation for the importance of the kinetic theory of matter is essential to a proper understanding of other concepts such as vaporization, temperature, and the behavior of gases. An additional concept related to the kinetic theory of matter is that of *momentum*. If two atoms of given mass travel at a certain rate, they are said to have momentum. Their masses and velocities represent a sum of energy. If they collided, and were perfectly "elastic," they would each leave the collision with the same mass and velocities or energy as they had before the collision. In reality, perfect elasticity does not exist, so atomic or molecular collisions result in a loss of momentum. The concomitant release (loss) of energy produces heat.

In the SI system, pressure is measured in pascals (Pa) and perhaps someday all pressure measurements will be expressed in this fashion. For the present, pressure is measured in a number of ways. This stems from both historical and practical considerations. In anesthesia practice measurements include millimeters of mercury (also known as torr pressure), centimeters of water, pounds per square inch, and others.

Molecules have an inherent capacity to interact with each other. There are four principal forces of interaction important enough to deserve mention: adhesion, cohesion, surface tension, and van der Waals forces.

Adhesion is the force of attraction between unlike molecules. In a liquid flowing through a glass tube, adhesive forces slow the passage of liquid molecules traveling next to the glass walls, whereas liquid molecules in the center of the fluid column travel at a faster rate. This is because of the attraction between the dissimilar molecules of the liquid and the glass. The concept of adhesive force is utilized in anesthesia draw-over vaporizers in which liquid anesthetic is drawn onto a cloth wick by adhesion. This is called *capillary action*. Gas flowing over and through the wick causes vaporization of the liquid and allows the anesthetic to be delivered as a gas.

Cohesion, on the other hand, is the force of attraction between like molecules. The outward bulge of water in a container filled to the brim is called a meniscus. This bulge is due to the cohesive forces of the water molecules. They gather together above the container rim where adhesive forces are working. If the water level is below the vessel rim, the meniscus is inverted, since adhesive forces are still operating and are stronger than the water's cohesive forces.

In addition to being affected by adhesion and cohesion, molecules at the surface of a liquid, the liquid-gas interface, are subject to unequal stresses. This difference in molecular forces between the air and water creates a high-force level, called *surface tension*, at the very top layer of liquid molecules. Cleaning agents, such as soaps, alter surface tension. This concept is used to improve cleaning of anesthesia equipment. Cohesive forces influence vapor pressure, boiling point, heat of vaporization, and viscosity as well as surface tension.

Both adhesion and cohesion result from the electrical properties of molecules, which in turn stem from the atomic configuration of the elements that make up the molecule. This will be discussed in more detail later.

The fourth type of intermolecular force has extensive and important implications for anesthesia practice. When molecules, because of their shape and the pattern of their electrical charges (caused by electron travel around the nuclei), are aligned in such a way that the molecule has a relatively positive end and a relatively negative end, they are said to be in a "dipole" configuration. The molecule is electrically polarized.

This situation sets up the molecule to interact electrically with surrounding molecules. Though such forces operate only over a short distance, they are relatively strong, and they increase with the size of the molecule. They affect the boiling point, surface tension, and viscosity of the substance. They also affect the amount of energy (heat) required to vaporize that substance. All of these are concepts important to anesthesia practice.

Polar molecules have a higher intermolecular force than nonpolar ones. But even nonpolar molecules, if by chance properly ordered, assume a brief polar configuration. This "induced" dipole configuration causes the surrounding molecules also to assume a dipole configuration. Adjacent atoms then begin to act synchronously rather than independently. These induced dipole configurations are termed London dispersion forces—after the German who first theorized them. They are also termed *van der Waals forces*—although this latter term is more often used to denote all types of intermolecular forces. All intermolecular forces, especially dispersion forces, greatly influence the behavior of a substance.

HEAT AND TEMPERATURE

Heat is a form of energy. The intensity of heat is indicated by temperature. As mentioned previously, physical changes in a substance are often induced by reductions or additions of heat, and temperature has important implications for the action of solids, liquids, and gases.

Temperature Scales

Scientifically, temperature is measured on the Kelvin (K) or absolute (A) temperature scale. More common to everyday life and anesthesia practice are the Fahrenheit (F) and Celsius or centigrade (C) scales. Converting from one scale to the other is relatively easy.

$$F = (C \times 1.8) + 32$$
$$F = ([K - 273] \times 1.8) + 32$$
$$C = (F - 32) \div 1.8$$
$$C = K - 273$$
$$K = C + 273$$
$$K = ([F - 32] \div 1.8) + 273$$

Note that conversions between Fahrenheit and Kelvin scales first required conversion to the centigrade scale. The 1.8 conversion factor results from the fact that both Fahrenheit and centigrade scales are based on the freezing point and boiling point of water. The temperature variation between these two points is divided into 100 degrees on the centigrade scale and 180 degrees on the Fahrenheit scale, or a ratio of 1.8 to 1. Since the freezing point "baseline" differs by 32 degrees, this conversion factor is required to achieve comparable numerical equivalency between the two scales. The 273 conversion factor represents the difference between the 0C freezing point of water and the equivalent point on the Kelvin scale. The Kelvin scale begins at "absolute zero" (approximately −273C), that point at which, at least theoretically, all molecular motion stops.

Measurement of Heat Capacity

Although temperature scales are useful indices of the changes wrought by heat, they do not measure the amount (capacity) of heat expended in working that change. For measuring the amount of work performed by heat, other work units are used. The amount of heat required to raise the temperature of 1 gram of water 1 degree centigrade is called the *calorie* (also known as the gram calorie or small calorie).

To raise the temperature of the same 1 g of water to 5C would require 5 times as much heat; to raise it to 100C would require 100 times as much heat. One thousand small calories equals 1 kilocalorie. The small calorie is abbreviated c; the large, or kilocalorie, is abbreviated with a large C. This large caloric measurement is the one used by nutritionists when referring to the amount of calories contained in food or expended by exercise. The *British thermal unit*, or *BTU*, is the amount of heat required to raise the temperature of 1 pound of water 1 degree Fahrenheit. It is equivalent to 252 small calories.

It is also useful to be able to equate work performed by other means, such as mechanical, to work performed by heat. The joule is used to make such comparisons. A gram calorie is approximately equal to 4.185 joules. Other measures of work, such as the foot-pound, can be converted to joules also (1 joule = 1.355 foot-pounds of work). This makes it possible to compare work performed by various means. The amount of heat that raises the temperature of a given mass of substance (at atmospheric pressure) by 1 degree unit is called the *thermal heat capacity* of the substance. In most cases, this is expressed as calories per gram per degree centigrade.

A term often confused with thermal capacity is that of specific heat. The *specific heat* of a substance is the ratio of the amount of heat needed to raise the temperature of one unit mass by 1 degree centigrade compared with the quantity of heat needed to raise the temperature of an equivalent mass of water by 1 degree centigrade. To obtain the amount of energy required to change x grams of a substance y degrees of temperature, multiply the total weight in grams by the number of degrees of temperature change desired and multiply again by its specific heat.

Of interest to anesthetists is the fact that gases have two specific heats: one at which the gas maintains the same volume, and one at which the gas maintains the same pressure. (As will be seen later, one cannot change the volume of a gas without affecting the pressure it exerts or change the pressure without changing the gas's volume.) In general, gases have low specific heats, whereas solids and liquids have high specific heats. Inhaled cold gases must therefore depend on external sources of heat if they are to be warmed to body temperature. Also, vaporization quickly ceases as a spontaneous process in bubble vaporizers unless external heat is applied. This is because gases possess low specific heats. Water has a very high specific heat compared to most substances.

The rapidity of heat exchange between molecules varies with each substance. Substances whose molecules exchange heat readily are said to be thermally conductive. This *conduction* is one of three means by which heat may be transferred from one place to another. The other ways by which heat may be transferred are convection and radiation. *Convection* is the transfer of heat by means of air currents. The surrounding air transports and dissipates the heat absorbed from a substance to other areas. *Radiant heat* is the transfer of heat energy in the form of waves, usually by electromagnetic means. Microwave ovens are an example of radiant heat.

Gases composed of single atoms are free to travel in three paths: (1) back and forth, (2) vertically, and (3) sideways. Polyatomic gases have a greater degree of freedom, that is, the various atoms may be traveling in several directions at once. The more directions in which a given gas can travel, the more the heat that will be required to raise the temperature of that gas. The heat required to raise the temperature of 1 mole of a gas 1 degree centigrade is called the *molal heat capacity*, and it increases as the number and weight of atoms in the gas molecule increase. This makes the gas less susceptible to combustion. If inert gases, especially those with high thermal capacities, are mixed with combustible gases, the mixture is less likely to become ignited. The high thermal capacity inert gases absorb ignition heat and therefore "cool" the mixture so that it doesn't readily ignite. They are therefore called "quenching agents" and are discussed in the section on combustion.

Converting a substance from the solid to liquid state or liquid to gas state (or vice versa) requires a gain or loss of additional heat (energy). These are referred to as *latent heats of vaporization, condensation, crystallization*, and *melting*. To convert 1 g of boiling water at 100C requires almost

540 additional calories to break the molecular forces and allow the liquid to become a gas (heat of vaporization). When cooling steam, an additional 540 calories of heat energy must be lost to allow the molecules to come close enough for the intermolecular forces to take over and change the gas to a liquid (heat of condensation). Similarly, extra energy (heat) must be extracted for a gram of water at zero degrees centigrade to be converted to ice (heat of crystallization), since removal of the heat allows greater action by the intermolecular forces that draw the molecules into a solid. Melting ice to water (heat of melting) requires that a similar amount of energy be added.

Contraction or expansion of molecules that accompanies a change in the state of matter is dependent on two factors: temperature and pressure. For gases with very high molecular velocities, the change to the liquid state cannot be accomplished without first cooling the gas substantially. After cooling, pressurizing the gas will force it into the liquid state. For all gases, a temperature exists above which liquefaction is impossible regardless of the amount of pressure applied. This is known as the *critical temperature*. The pressure required to cause liquefaction at the critical temperature is known as the *critical pressure*. At the critical temperature and pressure, one gram molecular weight of the gas will occupy a specific volume termed the *critical volume* and have a density that is termed the *critical density*. By the proper application of temperature and pressure it is possible to store large amounts of gas as very much smaller amounts of liquid. These principles are utilized in the storage of bulk volumes of oxygen for hospital use.

THE PERIODIC TABLE

All chemical elements can be grouped on the basis of their similarities in properties (Table 5–10). This was first recognized by the Russian chemist Mendeleyev. He arranged the then-known elements in a chart in order of their increasing atomic weights. He noted that elements with similar properties recurred at regular intervals or "periods," and he placed these in vertical groupings. Some inconsistencies were noted and later resolved by reordering the tables on the basis of increasing atomic numbers. Gaps in the original chart led Mendeleev to predict, rightly, that vacant spaces represented as yet undiscovered elements—elements whose properties he could predict on the basis of the grouping to which they belonged. Periodic tables provide the chemical symbols commonly used for each element. For each element, two numbers are given: a whole number representing the atomic number of the element (number of nuclear protons), and a decimal number that gives the element's atomic weight. Some tables also provide the arrangement of electrons according to their energy level, e.g., two-eight-eight-two.

Group numbers are provided at the very top of the chart. They indicate the number of electrons in the outer shell. Knowing this, one can predict the chemical behavior of the element. For example, elements in group I have one electron in the outermost shell, those in group VII have seven, and so forth.

Most charts have the metals listed on the left, nonmetals on the right, and the transition elements that can act as either metals or nonmetals in the middle. Therefore, as

TABLE 5–10. PERIODIC TABLE

PERIODIC TABLE OF THE ELEMENTS [a]

KEY TO CHART

Atomic Number → 50 +2 ← Oxidation States
Symbol → Sn +4
1983 Atomic Weight → 118.71
18 18 4 ← Electron Configuration

[a] Numbers in parentheses are mass numbers of most stable isotope of that element.
Reprinted with permission from Weast, RC (ed): CRC Handbook of Chemistry and Physics, 65th ed. Boca Raton, CRC Press, 1984–1985.

one scans the table from left to right, the elements have decreasingly fewer metallic properties and increasingly more nonmetallic properties.

The families of elements, those that behave similarly both chemically and physically, are given in vertical columns. Knowing the properties of one element in the family tells you the properties of the other elements in that family, properties that depend upon the number of electrons in the outer shell. Within each family, there will be variations in activity level. In general, elements on the left-hand side increase in activity as one reads down the table. For nonmetals, activity generally increases as one reads up the table. The transition elements vary in activity depending upon circumstances. Group VIII elements are nonreactive with the other elements.

The horizontal rows of elements are termed periods because each element in the row differs in chemical properties.

All of the elements can be categorized in one of four main classes: metals, nonmetals, transition elements, or inert gases. Metals tend to have a shiny appearance, be soft, have low melting points, and be good conductors of heat and electricity. The metals in group I A are called the alkali metal group, those in group II A are called the alkaline earth metal group.

Nonmetals vary greatly in properties; most are gases, some are solids, and one is a liquid. Except for carbon,

they conduct heat and electricity poorly. They tend toward dullness. Group VII A, which contains chlorine, fluorine, bromine, iodine, and astatine, is called the *halogen*, or salt-former group, because they are found in many salt compounds.

Transition elements are able to act as either metals or nonmetals (or as acids or bases as will be discussed later). They are also termed *amphoteric* elements. Carbon is the premier example of this group. The fact that it contains four electrons in its outer orbit means that it readily loses or gains electrons in trying to achieve stability. It is for this reason that carbon is so valuable to organic chemistry.

Inert gases are also known as the "rare" or "noble" gases. They are chemically inert, not reacting with any of the other elements. Except for helium, which has two electrons in its outer shell, all of the elements in this category have eight electrons in their outer shell. They are therefore stable because their outer shell is completely filled.

Of all the elements known today, only about a dozen have special importance to the human body and anesthesia practice. They include oxygen, carbon, hydrogen, sodium, potassium, calcium, iron, phosphorus, chlorine, sulfur, and less important, the trace elements, such as iodine and cobalt. Knowing the information provided in a periodic table enables one to understand more easily and group like elements on the basis of their properties and to gain a better understanding of how chemical reactions take place.

CHEMICAL BONDING

Compounds are formed by combining and recombining the various elements, excluding those of the inert group. The joining together of elements into molecules and compounds is termed *chemical bonding*. Bonding is primarily dependent upon the configuration of atoms of each involved element, especially the distribution of electrons in the outer shell. Only elements with eight electrons in their outer shells are stable (helium excepted—being stable with two electrons). Elements with one to seven electrons in their outer shells will react, almost always in a way that helps them become more stable—that is, by trying to achieve an eight-electron-outer-shell configuration. Achieving stability requires one of two things to occur: either outer-shell electrons are lost, enabling the element to achieve eight-electron stability in the next innermost shell; or enough electrons are gained from another element to obtain the required eight-electron configuration. Therefore, elements normally having one, two, or three electrons in their outer shells tend to lose them readily, whereas elements having five, six, or seven electrons tend to take on additional electrons to achieve stability. Each of these patterns is energy efficient; that is, less energy is required to remove two electrons from an element's outer shell than would be required to add the necessary six needed for stability. Conversely, less energy is required to gain one electron for an element having seven electrons in its outer shell than would be required to lose the seven electrons.

Remember, each atom by itself is electrically neutral, proton charges balancing electron charges. In bonding chemically with other elements this electrical neutrality is lost, and the resulting particles are called *ions*. Where electrons are lost, the particle will have a positive charge because more protons than electrons are present—and these are called *cations*. Conversely, if electrons are gained, the particle will have more negative charge. These particles are called *anions*. In all chemical reactions, it is always electrons, never protons, that are lost or gained. In becoming ions, atoms lose their original physical and chemical properties and develop new ones. For example, the poisonous gas chlorine reacts with sodium to become common table salt, sodium chloride, a solid with entirely different physical and chemical properties.

From the preceding discussion on the periodic table, it can be seen that metals, to the left of the table and having one to three electrons in their outer shells, tend to lose electrons—becoming cations in the process. The nonmetals, to the right of the chart and configured with five, six, or seven electrons in their outer shells, tend to gain electrons and become anions. Metals and nonmetals react well together, one losing, the other gaining electrons. The transfer of electrons between the two results in what is termed an *electrovalent* compound. The process is also termed *ionic bonding* because each atom has, in effect, become an ion. In each case of ionic bonding, the number of electrons lost by one element is always equal to the number gained by the other element. Electrovalence means simply that a given number of electrons have been transferred to form the new compound and that the two ions thus created have opposite, and therefore mutually attracted, electrical

charges (anion/cation) that enable the new compound to maintain stability.

As mentioned previously, elements with four electrons in their outer shell tend to share electrons with other elements but may lose or gain them to achieve stability.

In naming ionically bonded compounds, the name of the metal is used first, followed by the name of the nonmetal modified to *-ide* to indicate that it is part of a compound. For example, combining sodium and chlorine produces sodium chlor*ide*. Most diatomic (two-atom) compounds are named in this fashion. (The naming of more complex compounds is covered later.) In some cases, one of the ions cannot yield or gain the same number of electrons as the element with which it is reacted. In these cases, two or more atoms of one element may combine with one atom of the other element. In this way, electrical balance is achieved. If instead of reacting chlorine with sodium, we react it with calcium, we get calcium chloride, but the chemical formula ($CaCl_2$) indicates that two chlorine atoms have been combined with one atom of calcium to achieve the necessary electrical balance. Polyatomic compounds must always be electrically balanced.

In a discussion of chemical reactions, several terms are frequently encountered: oxidation number or state, radical, valence, and covalence. The *oxidation number* denotes the electrical state of the atom: positive, negative, or neutral. A positive state exists when electrons have been given up; a negative state when electrons have been accepted. Plus or minus signs denote the state, the number denotes the number of electrons shifted. Oxidation numbers refer only to one atom of the element in the compound. Elemental atoms, being electrically balanced and neutral, have a zero oxidation number. The algebraic sum of any compound must always equal zero. Some elements can exist in any of several states. That is why the exact number and state must be specified. Iron, for example, can exist in either a two plus or a three plus state. To correctly name the compound in written or spoken form, the metal of the compound is given the ending *-ous* for lower states and *-ic* for higher states. Therefore, Fe^{+2} is a ferr*ous* compound, whereas Fe^{+3} is a ferr*ic* compound. For elements having more than two possible oxidative states (e.g., tin [Sn]), the correct state is described by Roman numerals: tin (IV) chloride.

The term *radical* describes a group of atoms that have bonded together but act as an individual atom in chemical reactions. Radicals exhibit specific behaviors not characteristic of the atoms that constitute them. Many radicals are involved in bodily reactions and are thus important in anesthesia. These include the hydroxyl (OH), bicarbonate (HCO_3), phosphate (PO_4), ammonium (NH_4), carbonate (CO_3), sulfate (SO_4), and nitrate (NO_3) radicals. The *-ate* ending indicates a radical of higher oxidative states. An *-ite* ending is used for lower-state radicals: e.g., nitrites and sulfites (NO_2 and SO_3). So radicals, too, can have different oxidative states. Radicals are often written within parentheses, a subscript indicating the number of radicals in the compound, e.g., $Ca(OH)_2$. The term *valence* was originally used to denote the number of electrons in an atom's outer shell that could be shifted in chemical reactions. The term has largely been replaced by the more correct *oxidation* *number.* Covalence is a term that denotes the number of electron *pairs* that are shared by atoms in a compound. In covalent compounds, electrons are fully shared between the atoms; in electrovalent compounds, electrons are shared only in that one element loses electrons and the other gains them, more an exchange than a sharing. Rules for determining oxidation numbers of compounds may be found in standard chemistry texts.

WRITING CHEMICAL FORMULAS

Chemical formulas are a shorthand method of expressing the changes taking place in chemical reactions. Using symbols for each element (found in periodic tables) and taking into account radicals, oxidation states, and electrical balance, complex reactions can be written in a manner that will precisely explain what has occurred in the reaction. It will also be expressed in a way that can be universally understood. Care must be taken to write equations correctly, using proper symbols. Sodium chloride and sodium chlorate are not the same compound. *Empirical formulas* indicate the ratio of each type of atom in a compound, but they do not indicate the specific number of atoms in it. Their usefulness is limited. *Chemical equations* (formulas) are more practical. When properly written, they indicate the proper amounts and electrical balance of reactants and their end products. In writing equations, reactants are written to the left, products to the right, the direction of reaction being indicated by an arrow. Where reactions proceed in both directions, double arrows are used, each in the opposite direction, the length of each arrow indicating the relative degree to which the reaction proceeds in that direction. Virtually all chemical reactions, including those that occur within the body, involve one or more of the following: emission or absorption of heat, emission of an odor, formation of a gas or precipitate, a change in color, fluorescence, or luminescence. These are sometimes indicated in a chemical formula by symbols that help clarify what can be expected from the reaction. In all cases, either the reactants or the product will be known.

Writing the equation begins by setting down each of the component elements. The next step is to write each molecule's oxidation number as a superscript and to check to be sure that their algebraic sum equals zero.

Reactants: Sodium (Na) and sulfate (SO_4)

Step 1. $Na \ + SO_4 \longrightarrow ?$

Step 2. $Na^{1+} + SO_4^{2-} \longrightarrow$? Algebraic sum is not equal to zero $(1+) + (2-)$

Checking the equation, we find an imbalance in the oxidative states. To rectify this, a procedure analogous to obtaining an arithmetic lowest common denominator is used. It simply involves crisscrossing the oxidation numbers. Superscripts may then be erased.

Step 3. $Na^{1+} \diagdown\!\!\!\diagup SO_4^{2-} \longrightarrow Na_2(SO_4)$

The final step is to balance the complete equation to ensure that an equal quantity of each element is shown on both sides of the equation. This may involve trial and error to determine the proper coefficient(s) needed to balance the equation. A coefficient is the number placed in front of the chemical symbol to denote the number of molecules undergoing reaction. In this example the coefficient 2 must be placed in front of the Na to balance the equation.

Step 4. $2Na + SO_4 \longrightarrow Na_2(SO_4)$ sodium sulfate

In this final equation, we express the idea that two atoms of sodium combined with one radical of sulfate produces one molecule of sodium sulfate. This is but one type of chemical reaction, but the same general principles are used in writing equations for other reactions.

There are four basic types of chemical reactions: *synthesis, decomposition, single displacement,* and *double displacement.* The previous example typifies a synthesis reaction wherein simple elements are combined into a more complex compound. In a decomposition reaction, a complex substance is broken down into less complex ones. In a single displacement reaction, one element replaces another in a compound. Reacting zinc with hydrochloric acid produces zinc chloride and the release of hydrogen. The hydrogen atom in the hydrochloric acid molecule is replaced by a zinc atom. This type of reaction is also known as a substitution or replacement reaction. In a double displacement reaction, parts of two compounds are exchanged for one another. Reacting silver nitrate and sodium chloride yields silver chloride and sodium nitrate, sodium and silver having both been exchanged.

Another type of chemical reaction is one termed *oxidation-reduction.* Atoms losing electrons are said to be oxidized; atoms gaining electrons are said to be reduced. Such processes are essential to the chemistry of living tissues. Body energy is gained by oxidation of carbohydrates, fats, and proteins, each oxidation reaction being balanced by an equal number of reduction reactions. Chemical compounds, such as Dakin's solution and hydrogen peroxide, have antiseptic and cleaning uses because of their strong oxidizing properties.

PROPERTIES OF SOLUTIONS

Water

Water is called a universal solvent because so many substances may be dissolved in or combined with it. A large proportion of the human body is made up of water and virtually all bodily chemical reactions depend on its presence. A gain or loss of body water characterizes many disease states. Even healthy adults fasting for 24 hours may lose 5 percent of their body water. Infants and children can lose twice that amount in the same period, enough water loss to produce neurologic and other symptoms. For these reasons, understanding the properties of water is important to anesthesia practice.

The density of water is considered to be 1 g/ml, and this concept will suffice for most practical applications, although it is important to realize that the density of water is dependent upon temperature (and, under some circumstances, pressure). As water is warmed, its volume increases and its density decreases. This is in keeping with what has previously been discussed regarding the effect of temperature on molecular action. At atmospheric pressure, cooling water contracts its volume and increases its density. But as the temperature reaches 4C, additional cooling results in volume expansion, about a 10 percent increase by the time the freezing point of 0C is reached. In winter, exposed water pipes rupture because of this volume expansion. In the same way, water-laden body cells exposed to extreme cold expand and rupture causing the tissue damage associated with frostbite.

Water, like all liquids, is subject to certain forces and exhibits certain properties. These include *cohesion, adhesion,* and *capillary action,* all of which have been previously discussed. When water is placed in a glass capillary tube, the central portion of the water level will be drawn downward. The smaller the tube bore, the more noticeable the central downward depression. For this reason, calibrated tubes (manometers) containing aqueous solutions should be read at the bottom of the liquid depression. Along the edges of the tube, the water can be seen to rise noticeably because of adhesive forces. Adhesive forces help account for the "wetting" properties of water and other liquids. They also account for the creeping of a liquid up the sides of a tube, as when blood is drawn with a capillary tube.

With aqueous solutions, cohesive forces are usually overcome by adhesive forces. However, certain liquids have cohesive forces so strong that adhesive forces become negligible. Mercury is such a liquid. Placing mercury in a glass blood-pressure manometer results in a meniscus (liquid level) that is raised in the center. Such manometers should be read at the liquid's highest point.

Water can exert a vapor pressure. As with all liquids, its molecules are constantly in motion, the extent of motion being dependent on the energy they possess and whether additional energy in the form of heat is absorbed from the surrounding atmosphere. In their random motion, some molecules gather enough energy to break free from the liquid and enter the atmosphere as a vapor. The more heat applied, the greater the number of molecules released. When the molecules escape, they exert a vapor pressure. That pressure also rises with increasing temperature. When the vapor pressure of escaping molecules is high enough to displace the air above it, the water boils. At sea level atmospheric pressure (760 torr), water boils at 100C. Below sea level, where atmospheric pressure is higher, water boils at a higher temperature. More escaping molecules are required to reach a specific vapor pressure. At high altitudes, the converse is true because atmospheric pressure is lessened. The boiling point of water is therefore dependent upon the pressure exerted by the surrounding atmosphere, and vapor pressure always equals atmospheric pressure at the boiling point. As more external heat is applied to the water, the liquid's temperature remains stable. The extra energy just allows more of the molecules to escape, thereby increasing the speed of the evaporation process. Steam sterilizers, by increasing their internal atmospheric pressure, allow water temperature to exceed 100C and thus kill bacteria that might otherwise survive that temperature.

Vaporization continually occurs at any liquid-air interface, although not rapidly. A pan of water left open to the atmosphere will eventually be fully evaporated. In anesthesia vaporizers, liquid anesthetic is continually vaporized within the chamber. But since the chamber is a closed one, the enclosed atmosphere becomes fully saturated, a state of equilibrium is achieved, and vaporization slows. Opening the circuit allows vapor to escape into the anesthetic delivery system and vaporization again becomes a continuous process. The process is driven by heat absorbed from the room atmosphere and conducted through the metal framework of the machine to the vaporizer. High ambient temperatures allow vaporization to proceed at a faster rate. If room temperature drops, less energy (heat) is conducted to the vaporizer and the process slows. For this reason thermometers that read vaporizer temperature are included on most new anesthesia machines. They allow the anesthetist to be cognizant of temperature changes that affect the concentration of the agent being administered. Some vaporizers, by virtue of their internal design, allow the same concentration of agent to be delivered despite temperature fluctuation of several degrees. These are known as temperature-compensated vaporizers. Another evaporation process of concern in anesthesia practice is the continuous evaporation of body water from skin surfaces and exposed abdominal and thoracic organs. Because they are barely noticeable, they are termed insensible losses. The volume of fluid a patient may lose in this manner can be substantial and must be accounted for by the anesthetist in calculating fluid replacement. Fever substantially increases the amount of insensible fluid lost. Of less frequent concern, yet another evaporative process seen in anesthesia practice relates to those substances that have low boiling points and thus evaporate readily when applied to the skin. Ethyl chloride, a topical anesthetic, typifies such substances.

One especially important property of water relates to its molecular structure and is termed *hydrogen bonding.* Water is composed of one oxygen and two hydrogen atoms. Although a molecule of water is electrically neutral, its structure is such that the molecule assumes an asymmetrical distribution. Rather than the hydrogen atoms being located to either side of the oxygen atom, they both align to one side of the oxygen, being separated by an angle of approximately 104 degrees. This configuration is assumed because it allows the hydrogens and oxygen to combine with the least expenditure of energy. It also makes one side of the molecule relatively positive, the other side relatively negative. In other words, the molecule assumes a dipolar configuration. This facilitates development of attractive forces *between* water molecules, and the hydrogen atoms of one water molecule become oriented toward the oxygen atom of another water molecule. This occurs with all the molecules so that a latticework arrangement develops. These hydrogen bonds, though weak when compared to covalent bonds, are biologically important. They account for the relative instability of complex proteins and help maintain amino acid peptide integrity for synthesis of new proteins. Because water has polarity, it is an excellent solvent for other polar molecules, such as alcohols, but not for nonpolar substances, such as oils. Hydrogen bonding helps account for many properties of water, such as its high boiling point and surface tension. Dissolving solutes in water not only produces anions, cations, undissociated molecules, or radicals, but it also changes what are termed the colligative properties of water. Colligative changes are alterations in physical properties wrought by disruption of water's normal structure. This results in elevation of the boiling point, depression of the freezing point, lowering of the vapor pressure, and a change in osmotic pressure.

A final property of water important to anesthesia practice is its ability to combine with other elements directly to form crystalline structures known as *hydrates*. Baralyme, a mixture of barium and calcium hydroxide used in anesthesia circuits to absorb exhaled carbon dioxide, contains water as a hydrate. Hydrates always contain water in a definite proportion, the water of crystallization. Barium hydroxide is an octahydrate, containing eight water molecules in its structure. When hydrates are exposed to excessive heat, the water portion is evaporated and the remaining substance is referred to as an *anhydrate*. Hydrates that spontaneously lose their water content on exposure to air are called *efflorescent compounds*. *Hygroscopic compounds* are those that absorb water from the surrounding air. If they actually become dissolved in the absorbed water they are termed *deliquescent*. Surgical casts made from plaster of Paris (calcium sulfate) are efflorescent hydrates. When the water evaporates, the remaining anhydrate, gypsum, expands and hardens into whatever shape has been formed.

Natural water contains many impurities. If large amounts of calcium and magnesium bicarbonate are present it is referred to as "hard" water. Water that contains primarily sodium ions is termed "soft" water. Natural water is not pure enough for medicinal use, which requires ion-free water. Purifying water requires demineralization and distillation. Distillation involves boiling, followed by cooling and condensation of the steam. Dissolved gases are evaporated off and particulate matter is left as residue. Distilled water for injection normally undergoes triple distillation to assure purity.

Solutions

A *solution* may be defined as a uniformly distributed, homogeneous mixture of two or more substances, which can vary in proportion. Dissolving instant coffee crystals in a cup of hot water results in a solution, and solutions are one of the main ways by which the body absorbs nutrients it needs for sustenance. Under some conditions, chemical reactions proceed more quickly in a solution. Substances dissolved in a solution are termed *solutes*; the dissolving medium is termed the *solvent*. For a given temperature, only a limited amount of solute can be dissolved per volume of solvent. This limit is termed its *solubility*. Dissolving solids in liquids forms one type of solution. Other combinations are also possible: gases may be dissolved in gases or liquids in other liquids. This latter type of solution is the one most often encountered and one in which the distinctions between solute and solvent become blurred. Solvents may be classed as either polar or nonpolar based on their molecular structure. Polar solvents, like water, are excellent for dissolving ionic compounds. Nonpolar solvents are better for dissolving covalent and nonpolar compounds. Solutes placed in dissolving media become uniformly distributed. At first, the solution is *unsaturated*; that is, more solute can be dissolved without precipitating. At the point at which

addition of more solute results in precipitation, the mixture is said to be *saturated*. Saturation occurs because the equilibrium point between particles going into solution and those being forced out of solution has been reached. Heating the mixture allows for more solute to be added, whereas cooling it increases precipitation. However, under some conditions, it is possible to cool a mixture without creating precipitation. The mixture is then said to be *supersaturated*; such solutions are very unstable.

Gases in Solution

Solubility varies with the solute, nature of the solvent, and temperature. Solubility of gases in liquids, e.g., in blood, is similar to that of solids dissolved in liquids, except that the amount (weight) of gas dissolved per volume of blood (at constant temperature) is directly proportional to the pressure of the gas over the liquid (Henry's law). The pressure (tension) of gas in solution is always equal to that of the gas above the air-liquid interface. If a mixture of gases is dissolved, each gas comes to its own equilibrium. (It is assumed that gases will not combine with the blood or solvent.)

Because the number of gas molecules in solution varies directly with pressure, the *volume* of dissolved gas is independent of pressure (if temperature is constant). This is in keeping with Boyle's law, covered in more detail later. Hence, dissolved gas "bubbles" expand or contract as necessary to maintain equilibrium pressure with undissolved gas.

What about the situation where temperature is changed? Increasing heat, as occurs with a rise in body temperature, displaces gases from solution. Cooling allows more gas to go into solution. So, in terms of gas solubilities in the body, solubility varies inversely with temperature. Therefore, a patient who is allowed to become hypothermic during anesthesia develops a higher relative blood concentration. The same is not true for solids dissolved in liquids, where addition of heat allows an increased amount of solute to be dissolved.

Henry's law has daily application in anesthesia practice because it accounts for gas tensions that develop between alveoli and blood and between blood and other body tissues. The potentially hazardous implication of this principle is seen with caisson disease (decompression sickness) where a sudden decrease in "atmospheric" pressure causes rapid expansion of dissolved gases that then occlude small blood vessels.

Solubility Coefficients

The volume of gas dissolved (absorbed) in a given volume of liquid can be measured by a variety of means. One method, in which measurements are reported under conditions of standard temperature and pressure (STP), is the Bunsen absorption coefficient. Another, the Ostwald solubility coefficient, is usually reported at the temperature and pressure of the experiment, frequently at body temperature. Other methods are also available.

Because solubility of a gas varies with the tissues in which it is dissolved, it has become common practice to speak of the relative ratios of dissolved gas between body compartments. These are termed *distribution* or *partition coefficients*. They are useful tools for comparing anesthetic agent distribution between body tissues and for predicting the clinical effects of those agents.

Although anesthetists are often concerned with solubility of gases in blood and other body tissues, there are times when they may be more concerned with the solubility of nonvolatile solutes. It then becomes important to know that addition of solute to a liquid (like our coffee crystals placed in a cup of hot water) lowers the liquid's vapor pressure. This is because the solute lowers the fraction of solvent present. The decrease in vapor pressure is proportional to the concentration of solute in solution (Raoult's law).

ACIDS, BASES, AND SALTS

Earlier, in the discussion pertaining to organization of the periodic table, metals, nonmetals, and transition elements were discussed. A related and important topic is that of acid-base balance. The entire body chemistry is aimed at maintaining homeostasis by balancing acids against bases, a process termed *neutralization*. An *acid* can be any substance that separates into ions, at least one of which must be hydrogen. The other ions can be nonmetals or radicals. Hydrogen ions are really protons, the atom having given up its electron. It therefore has a positive charge. This is why acids are said to be proton donors. In solution, they tend to attach themselves to water molecules as hydronium ions by a bond that is easily broken, releasing the hydrogen for other chemical reactions.

Acids ionize in water to form an electrolyte solution capable of conducting electricity, a property of acids. Other properties include a sour, tart taste; corrosiveness; an ability to change the colors of dyes; and an ability to react with some (but not all) metals. Acids react with metallic oxides to form a salt and water, and with carbonates and bicarbonates to produce carbonic acid. Carbonic acid, in turn, can be decomposed to carbon dioxide and water. A common reaction for acids is neutralization of bases. This, too, forms a salt plus water. Acids are classed as either strong or weak depending upon the extent of ionization. Some are relatively stable, while others, such as carbonic acid, decompose readily. Concentrated acids are more corrosive than dilute ones. Important acids to body chemistry are the amino acids used for building proteins and lactic acid produced by metabolism within muscles. Acids are also important pharmacologically. Salicylic acid, the essential ingredient in aspirin, is a good example.

A *base* is any substance that can neutralize an acid and, in water, ionize to produce hydroxyl ions $(OH)^-$. Though not producing hydroxyl ions on dissociation, carbonates and bicarbonates are also considered bases because they effectively neutralize acids. In contradistinction to acids, bases are proton acceptors. They often have greasy consistencies in solution and possess metallic, bitter tastes. Like acids, bases can be corrosive and change the color of dyes. They react with soluble salts to form an insoluble hydroxide, which precipitates. Bases can react with some metals to release hydrogen just as acids can. Two bases important to anesthesia practice are sodium bicarbonate,

used to treat acute metabolic acidosis, and calcium hydroxide, important for chemical absorption of carbon dioxide from breathing circuits. Strong and weak bases are also distinguished by the extent to which they ionize in solution.

Salts are formed by neutralization reactions between acids and bases. Through such reactions, body cations and anions are kept in a narrow range of ever-changing concentrations. Salts are of three types: *normal salts*, which have no replaceable hydrogen or hydroxyl groups; *acidic salts*, which contain partly neutralized hydrogen; and *basic salts*, in which only part of the hydroxyl group has been replaced. This last group maintains the properties of both a salt and a base. Salts have physiologic importance: maintaining osmotic pressure, body-tissue building, nerve and muscle functioning, and maintenance of body fluid pH.

The term *pH* indicates the concentration of hydrogen ion in the body (relative acidity or alkalinity). It is expressed as a whole number plus a decimal fraction (e.g., pH 7.45) representing the reciprocal logarithm (negative logarithm) of the hydrogen ion concentration in moles per liter. A pH of 7.00 indicates neutrality, acids and bases being in balance. Readings from 7 to 14 indicate increasing alkalinity. Readings from 7 downward indicate increasing acidity. Because the numbers indicate a logarithmic change (based on powers of 10) a pH change from 6.00 to 5.00 is really a tenfold increase in the number of circulating hydrogen ions. Certain body fluids may normally be either acidic or basic (e.g., urine and gastric juice are typically quite acidic) but it is blood pH with which anesthetists are most often concerned. Blood pH is normally 7.40. A drop to 7.20 is considered severely acidotic, and below 7.00 is immediately life-threatening without treatment. When pH rises to 8.00 or higher, a similar situation ensues. Indeed, treating acute acidotic states by excessive administration of intravenous sodium bicarbonate can result in death from acute alkalosis.

If a 7.00 pH is considered neutral, why is normal blood pH 7.40? Neutrality (pH 7.00) is most ideally required at the cellular level, where all metabolic activity occurs. Blood, like urine and gastric juice, has a somewhat different normal pH. However, blood quickly reflects changes occurring at cellular level, so pH analysis and blood gas measurements remain the best current indicators of cellular metabolic states. In an attempt to measure cellular pH changes directly, increasing use has been made of transcutaneous analyzers. Research substantiates that this technique may be more useful for early detection of tissue acidosis or alkalosis. Cost and technical factors have limited routine employment of such devices, but as these problems are solved, transcutaneous electrode monitoring is likely to become an important aspect of anesthesia management.

A concept allied to pH, and one important to pharmacologic aspects of anesthesia practice, is that of the drug dissociation constant, pKa. This constant expresses the pH at which a drug is dissociated so that bound and unbound ions are chemically balanced. Changes in pH increase or decrease the amount of drug available to perform a specific action. More detailed information on this concept can be found in pharmacology texts.

A last topic important to any discussion of acids and bases is that of buffers. Buffer systems are important in helping maintain normal pH, and they can neutralize either acids or bases. Most often, buffers are composed of a weak acid and the sodium or potassium salt of that acid, called the conjugate base. If a strong acid is added to any buffer pair, a weak acid and a neutral salt is produced. Buffer pairs reacting with strong alkalis form a weak alkaline salt and water.

The carbonate-bicarbonate buffer system illustrates how buffers act. Carbon dioxide produced by cellular metabolism combines with water in the blood to form carbonic acid. Being weak, carbonic acid dissociates only slightly so that few hydrogen ions are released. Those that are released leave behind a bicarbonate radical, so that both carbonic acid and bicarbonate are present in solution. As additional hydrogen is added (increasing acidosis), it combines with the bicarbonate to form additional carbonic acid. The bicarbonate has, in effect, tied up the excess hydrogen and thus reduced acidity.

If extra base had been added instead of hydrogen, it would be neutralized by the carbonic acid that is present. This removes (buffers) excess hydroxyl ions so that pH is again restored. The body maintains a bicarbonate-ion-to-carbonic-acid ratio of 20:1. This is in keeping with the Henderson-Hasselbalch equation:

$$pH = pKa + \log \frac{(HCO_3^-)}{(H_2CO_3)}$$

The pKa of carbonic acid (H_2CO_3) at body temperature is 6.10, and the normal concentrations of bicarbonate and carbonic acid are 24.0 and 1.2 mM or a ratio of 20:1. Therefore,

$$pH = 6.10 + \log 20$$
$$pH = 6.10 + 1.30$$
$$pH = 7.40$$

The body's other buffers operate in a similar fashion; they include the phosphate, protein, and hemoglobin buffer systems. Regulation of acid-base status is a function of both respiratory and renal systems. Disruptions of regulation produce either acidosis or alkalosis, whose components may be respiratory, metabolic, or mixed. Although regulation of acid-base status constitutes an important aspect of anesthesia practice, the complexity of these disorders places the topic beyond the scope of the present discussion. For additional information, the reader is referred to special texts dealing exclusively with acid-base disorders.

OSMOSIS

For a gas to reach blood from the surrounding atmosphere, it has to pass through the lung's alveolar-capillary membrane. Diffusion of a dissolved substance through a semipermeable membrane is termed osmosis. An example occurs at the cellular level, where gases and other substances pass into and out of the cell, whose wall is, in effect, semipermeable membrane. This diffusion (passage of substances from one side of the membrane to the other) depends upon the selectivity of the membrane and relative concentrations of substance on either side. Osmosis is an important body process, being necessary for urine formation, distribution of water to various body compartments, and maintenance of blood volume.

Membrane *permeability* refers to the ease or difficulty with which substances may pass through it. In the body, membranes usually separate two aqueous compartments having different concentrations of ions and molecules. The membrane selectively allows passage of water but not of solutes. The direction of water flow is from the area of low solute concentration to the area of high concentration. The force that moves the water is *osmotic pressure*. Water movement will continue until concentrations on both sides of the membrane equilibrate. Osmosis then stops. Further loss or addition of solute will restart the osmotic process. Osmosis allows for fluid shifts between intracellular and extracellular fluid compartments. Alterations in the fluids' ionic content occur as the individual takes in more salt by ingestion or as water losses occur through urine formation. There is, therefore, a constant flux in water level and ion concentration between each compartment.

Two solutions exerting the same osmotic pressure are isotonic to each other; that is, pressure is being exerted in equal but opposing directions. Physiologic intravenous solution of 0.9 percent sodium chloride in sterile water is isotonic compared with blood. Solutions containing smaller concentrations of solutes are termed *hypotonic*. Their administration causes additional water to flow into red cells (the area of higher solute concentration), causing them to swell and rupture (hemolyze). Intravenous solutions containing more solutes (salts) than blood cause red cells to lose water. This red-cell shrinking is called crenation or plasmolysis, and fluids that cause it are said to be *hypertonic*. Any two fluids separated by a semipermeable membrane can be iso-, hypo-, or hypertonic relative to one another.

Suspensions and Colloids

Dissolved salts in water represent a true solution, but some substances cannot dissolve in a solvent. Rather, they remain intact as fine particles. When placed in water, they give it a milky appearance. Particles are merely suspended in the solvent and such mixtures are termed *suspensions*. Between suspensions and true solutions, we have *colloids* or colloidal solutions. Colloidal solutions occur when solutes are too small to be suspended but too large to form a true solution. Colloids disrupt and disperse light (the *Tyndall effect*). Particles in such a solution move about in random fashion as if colliding with invisible molecules of solvent. This zigzag motion of colloidal particles describes *Brownian movement*.

Concentrations of Solutions

The ratio of dissolved solute to volume of solvent determines solution concentration. Most often, this information is presented in terms of how many grams of solute are dissolved per 100 ml of solvent (percent solutions). A 0.9 percent physiologic saline solution contains 0.9 g of salt in each 100 ml. As mentioned earlier, the molecular weight of a compound is termed a mole (mol). One mole of a compound dissolved in 1 liter of solution results in a one-molar solution, abbreviated 1M. Doubling or tripling the amount of dissolved substance in the same volume makes it a two-molar (2M) or three-molar (3M) solution. The same holds true for fractions of a mole, e.g., 0.3M. A *molal* solution is identical to a molar solution except that the temperature of the solution is at 4C, at which 1 liter of water equals 1000 g. At other temperatures the weight of water varies slightly from the 1000 g. Molal solutions are based on the amount of solute per 1000 g.

The number of particles in a solution, not their size or weight, determines the amount of osmotic pressure generated. An ionized substance exerts more pressure than a nonionized one. This is because, in ionizing, a greater number of discrete particles is formed. Osmotic activity of a given molar solution is expressed in *osmoles*. One dissolved GMW of a substance per liter is equal to 1 osmole. If the substance does not ionize, molarity and osmolarity are equal. But if the substance ionizes, osmolarity equals the solution molarity multiplied by the number of ionized particles. A 1M solution of substance that ionizes into two particles exerts 2 osmoles of pressure. If the substance ionizes into three particles, as does calcium chloride, a 1M solution will exert 3 osmoles of pressure.

According to Avogadro's law, 1 GMW of a substance contains 6.02×10^{23} molecules. If vaporized, that substance would occupy, at STP, a volume of 22.4 liters, the *gram molecular volume*. If 1 GMW of nonionizing substance is placed in a volume of 22.4 liters of solution on one side of a semipermeable membrane, it would take a force of 1 atmosphere to prevent water migration across the membrane. With a substance ionized into two particles, osmolarity would be doubled, and two atmospheres of pressure would be required to prevent transmigration of water. It is thus possible to visualize how much pressure osmolarity actually involves. However, osmoles are too large a unit for discussion of the osmotic activities in human biology, so osmolarity of body fluids is expressed in terms of milliosmoles (mOsm) per liter. A milliosmole exerts a pressure equal to 1/1000 of an osmole. Average osmolarity of body fluids is approximately 300 mOsm. Milliosmoles should not be confused with a millimole, which is 1/1000 of a mole. Sodium, potassium, and chloride contribute the most to osmolarity of body fluids.

Normality

In discussing the concepts of molarity and osmolarity, emphasis was on GMW and number of particles formed in dissociation. GMW per liter determined molar concentration, whereas the number of particles determined osmolarity (osmotic force). Neither of these concepts addresses the chemical activity (reactivity) of the dissolved substance. The *equivalent* expresses the ability of a substance to react or combine chemically with other substances. *Equivalent weight* of a substance is the weight in grams (*gram equivalent weight* or *GEW*) that will react with 1 g of hydrogen (or 8 g of oxygen). GEW is calculated by dividing GMW by the positive oxidation number of the substance. Placing a GEW of a substance in 1 liter of solution creates a one *normal* (N) *solution*. Doubling that amount of substance in 1 liter produces a twice normal solution, while halving the amount produces a half normal solution. (*Caution:* the terms "normality" and "normal solution" as discussed here refer to definitions of chemical concepts. They should not be confused with medical use of the term normal, e.g., normal

saline solution, which implies that a solution is physiologically compatible with body fluids. So-called "normal" saline is not a one normal solution.) In terms of chemical reactivity, one GEW of any one substance is equal (in combining power) to one GEW of any other substance, even though their GMWs might vary substantially. *Normality* expresses the concentration of a solution in terms of chemical reactivity.

Equivalent weights are too large to express concentrations found in body tissues, so a more useful term is used—the *milliequivalent*. One milliequivalent (mEq) is 1/1000 of an equivalent weight. It is a more useful term for expressing concentration of body ions than milligrams per volume of fluid, which provides no useful information about electrical balance. When necessary, milligram percent may be converted to milliequivalents by using the formula:

$$\frac{mg \% \times 10}{\text{Atomic weight}} \times \text{Valence}$$

It also is occasionally necessary to convert molarity to normality. This is accomplished by multiplying molarity by valence, since with normality we are considering the influence of positive valences. Reversing the procedure enables us to change normality to molarity: normality divided by valence equals molarity. The relationship of milliequivalents and milliosmoles can be summarized as follows:

1. For univalent cations (e.g., sodium or potassium)

    1 mEq of cation = 1 mOsm

2. For nonionizing substances (e.g., sugars)

    1 mEq = 1 mOsm

3. For bivalent cations (e.g., calcium)

    (mEq ÷ valence)—therefore 1 mEq of cation = 0.5 mOsm

    2 mEq of cation = 1 mOsm

4. For trivalent cations

    1 mEq = 0.33 mOsm

    3 mEq = 1 mOsm

GASES

As discussed earlier, gases are notable in that their molecules are widely dispersed. Intermolecular forces are slight compared with liquids and solids. Therefore, gases may easily be compressed. Lacking strong intermolecular attraction and possessing high velocities, gases tend to expand indefinitely. These two characteristics, compressibility and expandability, distinguish gases from liquids and solids. Gases also have a high degree of freedom (random motion), enabling them to travel large distances quickly. This accounts for our ability to detect odors at a distance. Random movement of gas molecules resembles that of Brownian movement in colloidal solutions. (Watch dust particles in a beam of sunlight move in random directions.) Because of random motion and high velocity, gases in a container collide with the walls of that container, exerting a pressure against it. The smaller the container is made (compression), the more often molecules collide. This exerts an increasing amount of pressure against container walls. Heating the container accelerates molecular motion (according to the kinetic theory of matter discussed earlier) and this, too, serves to increase the pressure exerted by the gas. The ability of gases to vary in pressure or volume as the container is changed is an important concept for understanding the gas laws that are discussed later.

Weight of a volume of gas can be expressed in several ways. It may be expressed as density: molecular weight (at STP) divided by gram molecular volume (22.4 liters). But more often, we are interested in its specific gravity; that is, how much lighter or heavier it is than another gas. By convention, this is calculated by comparing the weight of a volume of the gas to the weight of an equal volume of dry air (taken to be a weight of one). Gases with a specific gravity less than one will rise in room air, while those with a specific gravity greater than one will flow toward the floor. This fact is used clinically in doing gas inductions, especially for children. Using gases heavier than the atmosphere, the anesthetist can hold the mask above a child's face, yet gases will still flow down over his nose and mouth, where he breathes them in.

Diffusion

Diffusion is the process whereby gases move from an area of high concentration to one of low concentration. Movement of oxygen from the alveoli to blood and of carbon dioxide from blood to alveoli is, in part, the result of diffusion processes. By diffusion, a volume of gas will uniformly distribute throughout a container. If two or more gases are mixed, they each will mix and distribute uniformly. How quickly the process comes to equilibration depends on the molecular weight of the gas and its temperature, diffusion occurring more rapidly with increasing temperatures. Lighter gases diffuse more rapidly than heavy ones. This principle underlies *Graham's law*, which states that the rate of gas diffusion varies inversely with the square root of its molecular weight. Therefore, in a mixture of gases A and B, where B has a molecular weight four times greater than A, A will diffuse twice as rapidly as B. Conversely, gas B will take twice as long to diffuse as will gas A. ($A = \sqrt{1} = 1$; $B = \sqrt{4} = 2$.)

As gas moves from an area of high concentration to an area of lesser concentration, a difference develops in the pressure (pressure gradient) exerted by the gas at those two sites (concentrations). At first, when the pressure gradient is large, diffusion proceeds rapidly. As concentrations and pressures become equalized, the rate of diffusion slows. This is known as *Fick's law*: diffusion rate is proportional to the difference in partial pressures. At the start of a general anesthetic, the anesthetist uses high delivered gas concentrations and high pressures (generated by compression of the breathing bag). This accelerates the diffusion process and contributes to the patient becoming anesthetized more quickly.

The atmosphere we breathe is a mixture of gases (oxygen, nitrogen, and smaller amounts of carbon dioxide, inert gases, and water vapor). At sea level, this mixture exerts a pressure equal to 760 mm Hg (torr) or 1 atmospheric pressure (atm). Each gas contributes a portion of this total pressure, the *partial pressure*. If our atmosphere consisted of equal amounts of four gases, each would contribute 25 percent of the total pressure, or 190 torr. So the total pressure exerted by any mixture of gases is equal to the sum of all the partial pressures (*Dalton's law*). Any volatile liquid anesthetic converted into a vapor acts as a constituent gas of the mixture and adheres to the principle expressed by Dalton's law. Diffusion becomes a clinically important phenomenon when hyperbaric pressures are used. By using higher than atmospheric pressures, more oxygen can be delivered into a patient's blood.

The Gas Laws

An *ideal* gas would be one existing in a very rarified environment where no intermolecular forces are exerted. *Boyle's law* (formulated on the basis of an ideal gas) expresses the compressibility of such gases. It states that at constant temperature, the volume of a gas varies inversely with its pressure. Therefore, multiplying the gas volume by its pressure would (for a fixed weight of gas) always equal a constant. But with *real* gases, especially when at low temperatures and subjected to high pressures, there are intermolecular forces that must be taken into account. This is why Van der Waals' modification of Boyle's law has greater applicability in explaining the behavior of real gases because it takes into account forces of cohesion and the volume occupied by gas molecules. In this formulation, the reduction in pressure caused by cohesive forces is added to the molecular motion pressure. This is then multiplied by the total volume occupied by the gas less the maximum compressible volume occupied by the molecules. In this way, the pressure-volume constant more clearly expresses the behavior of real gases. However, at low pressures and high temperatures, real gases behave more like ideal gases.

Heating a gas expands it. If pressure is held constant, the amount (volume) of expansion is proportional to the increase in absolute temperature. This is *Charles' law*. Cooling the gas makes the converse true also. For every degree centigrade decrease in temperature, gas volume will change by 1/273 so that at absolute zero temperature ($-273C$, $0K$), the gas would theoretically have no pressure or volume. The volume change expressed in Charles' law is based on changes in absolute (Kelvin scale) temperature. That same scale is important to the formulation of *Gay-Lussac's law*, which states that when volume is kept constant, gas pressure varies directly with absolute temperature. Charles' law and Gay-Lussac's law are similar in that they both serve to explain the effect of (absolute) temperature changes on volume and pressure of a gas.

The foregoing gas laws have been formulated into a *general gas law*: $PV = nRT$, where pressure multiplied by volume is equal to the number of molecules times a constant (R), which is the same for all ideal gases, times absolute temperature. This general gas law is useful for explaining the behavior of ideal gases. A modified version is more relevant to clinical practice when one wants to determine the effects of changes in volume, temperature, or pressure. The modified formula is

$$P_1V_1A_2 = P_2V_2A_1$$

where P_1 = initial pressure, V_1 = initial volume, A_1 = initial temperature (Kelvin), P_2 = new pressure, V_2 = new volume, and A_2 = new temperature (Kelvin). For example, if one starts with a 100-liter volume of gas at 273K (0C), which exerts a pressure of 1000 pounds per square inch (psi), and doubling the temperature ($273 \times 2 = 546$) causes a fourfold increase in pressure, what will be the new volume of gas?

$$100 \times 1000 \times 546 = x \times 4000 \times 273$$
$$54,600,000 = x \times 1,092,000$$

$$x = \frac{54,600,000}{1,092,000}$$
$$x = 50 \text{ liters}$$

According to Charles' law, doubling the temperature could be expected to double the volume, making it 200 liters. But, by Boyle's law, a quadrupling of pressure would decrease volume to one-quarter. The net change in volume then must be ¼ of 200 or 50 liters. This simple example serves to exemplify how the formula can be used to solve practical problems in the clinical setting, e.g., calculating the volume of gas in a cylinder transported from a cold outdoor environment to a warm indoor one. It must be remembered, however, that (1) temperatures must be converted to the Kelvin scale and (2) all volumes and (3) all pressures must be in the same measurement units.

Vapor Pressures and Vaporization

Vaporization is the conversion of a volatile liquid to a gas or vapor. Within anesthesia vaporizers, the end atmospheric pressure is typically composed of carrier gas (usually oxygen) and the vaporized anesthetic. If 50 ml of vapor is produced for each 100-ml flow of oxygen into the vaporizer, then the final atmosphere consists of 150 ml exerting a total of 760 torr pressure. The partial pressure of the anesthetic is one third (50/150) of 760 torr, or 253.33 torr (the vapor pressure). This example is very close to the 243 torr vapor pressure exerted by the anesthetic halothane (at 20C). When the combination of anesthetic vapor and carrier gas is added to the nitrous oxide and additional oxygen of the diluent flows, the partial pressure of the anesthetic vapor (at point of delivery to the patient) will be less than it exerted coming out of the vaporizer. Assuming 50 percent concentrations of nitrous oxide and oxygen at a total diluent flow of 5 liters, the final delivered atmosphere will consist of: 2500 ml oxygen (diluent) + 2500 ml nitrous oxide (diluent) + 100 ml (carrier gas) + 50 ml of anesthetic vapor—a total of 5150 ml. Since the anesthetic vapor is only 50 ml of this total or 0.97 percent ($5150:100\% :: 50/x$), the final delivered anesthetic concentration will be 0.97 percent. It will also exert that portion of the total pressure, or $0.0097 \times 760 = 7.3$ torr. So partial pressure gradients apply to both gases and vapors. Knowing this makes rapid calculation of the amount of vapor produced, required carrier gas flow, required diluent flow, or delivered concentration very easy. They may be calculated as follows:

1. Calculation of amount of vapor being produced (knowing the vapor pressure of the agent at the temperature at which vaporization is occurring)
   a. Agent vapor pressure:total pressure (760 torr)* $:: x:100\%$
   b. $100\% - x\% = \%$ exerted by carrier gas ($y\%$)
   c. Carrier gas milliliter (known):$x\%$ (from step a)::vapor milliliter:$y\%$ (from step b) (Calculate for the vapor milliliter produced)
2. Knowing the vapor pressure of the agent at use temperature, calculate the amount of carrier gas required to produce a specific amount of vapor. Use the same calculations as in (1) above, making the assumption that 100 ml of carrier gas is to be used. Then, knowing the amount of vapor being produced for each 100 ml of carrier gas, the amount of carrier gas required to produce other vapor pressures can be calculated by

$$\frac{100 \text{ ml carrier gas}}{\text{Amount of vapor produced}} :: \frac{x \text{ (amount of carrier gas required)}}{\text{Vapor amount desired}}$$

3. Calculate the diluent flow required to achieve a desired concentration, knowing the amount of anesthetic vapor being produced (i.e., knowing the information from (1) and (2), which are calculated only from the known vapor pressure of the agent). Multiply the amount of vapor being produced by 100. This will tell you the amount of diluent flow required to achieve a 1 percent concentration. Halving the diluent flow doubles the concentration. Doubling the diluent flow halves the concentration. Knowing how much diluent flow is required to produce a 1 percent concentration, one can calculate the desired concentration diluent flow as

$$\frac{1\%}{\text{Required diluent flow } (1\% \times 100)} :: \frac{\text{Desired concentration}}{(x) \text{ required diluent flow}}$$

4. Delivered concentration of agent can be calculated by the formula:

$$\frac{[\text{Vapor pressure of agent/(atmospheric pressure} - \text{vapor pressure of agent)}] \times \text{flow of carrier gas} \times 100\dagger}{\text{Total flow}}$$

Clinically, total flow is often taken to be only the diluent flow because this makes mental calculation simpler and errs on the safe side; that is, actual delivered concentration will be slightly less than the calculated delivered concentration. To be more correct, total flow should include diluent flow amount, carrier gas amount, and amount of vapor

---

* *Note: At other than sea level, total pressure (atmospheric pressure) will be other than 760 torr. Pressure decreases with altitude.*
† *100 = percent conversion to move decimal point.*

produced. It must be remembered that these calculations are based on knowing the vapor pressure of the agent at the temperature at which it is being used. Changes in ambient temperature, either up or down, will vary the vapor pressure. Fortunately, the change in vapor pressure over the range of clinically used temperatures (20 to 25C) is minimal in terms of the effects on the final concentration delivered to the patient. Wide variations in temperature must, however, be accounted for.

Unless additional heat is provided, vaporization has a cooling effect, so that over time, less concentration is delivered. If additional heat is provided, vapor pressure of the agent is increased, producing a greater delivered concentration. Traditionally, anesthesia machines have been manufactured from highly conductive metals that allow heat from the ambient atmosphere to be continually drawn to the vaporizer, thus providing continued energy for vaporization. Today, most machines use temperature-compensated draw-over vaporizers to minimize the impact of temperature variations.

Depending on the vaporizer used, several other factors play a role in vaporization efficiency. The amount of contact carrier gas has with liquid anesthetic is one. Failure to keep a vaporizer adequately filled results in low delivered concentrations and the patient awakens, despite the fact that carrier gas flow is adequate. Rapid gas flow through a vaporizer may outpace the vaporization process and also result in low delivered concentrations, because carrier gas-liquid contact is brief. Contamination of wicks by moisture prevents mixing of volatile agents and carrier gas so no anesthetic vapor is produced. In certain equipment designs, pressure on the breathing bag creates negative pressures within the vaporizer that vacuums liquid anesthetic into the delivery circuit, a potentially hazardous occurrence. Adding baffles that prevent liquid from entering the breathing circuit is helpful in minimizing this problem. These problems point out the fact that anesthetists must be thoroughly familiar with the design and operation of vaporizers and circuits they use. Sudden malfunctions are cause for removing equipment from service until the cause is identified and remedied.

Principles engendered by the gas laws, laws of diffusion, and vaporization process have wide application in clinical settings because they help explain how gases behave. They help explain ventilation, internal and external respiration, the behavior of gases in closed body cavities, and the usefulness of therapeutic gases.

The Therapeutic Gases

Therapeutic gases find their principal medical applications in anesthesia and respiratory therapy. Some, nitrous oxide and oxygen for instance, are widely used each day. Others have more limited uses. The following discussion reviews basic properties of the more useful gaseous agents.

Oxygen. Oxygen is by far the most widely used medical gas. This colorless, tasteless, odorless gas constitutes one-fifth of our atmosphere and is an essential requirement for survival because it is the primary element used by the body as an oxidant for metabolic reactions. It is transported in the body combined with hemoglobin and, to a lesser extent, in simple solution within blood. (The amount in solution can be increased by hyperbaric administration.) Disease states that interfere with delivery or utilization of oxygen require treatment by administration of increased oxygen levels up to 100 percent by mask, nasal catheter, or endotracheal tube. Some substances, e.g., cyanide and carbon monoxide, interfere with oxygen-hemoglobin binding. Sodium nitroprusside, a hypotension-producing drug used in anesthesia, can produce such a block because it contains significant amounts of cyanide.

Oxygen occurs naturally in three isotopic forms, the most common being O-16. Here, one atom combines readily with another atom to form molecular oxygen (O_2). It can also combine to O_3, ozone, a constituent of the upper atmosphere that helps protect the earth from the sun's radiations. Molecular oxygen used for medicinal purposes is 98 to 99 percent pure. When cooled below its boiling point (−183C), it becomes a light-blue liquid. Further cooling to −217C solidifies the liquid. Oxygen is a paramagnetic substance and is drawn to magnetic fields. Under proper conditions, it may form free radicals (superoxide anions) thought to be implicated in oxygen toxicity. Oxygen is highly reactive, combining with a wide range of substances. It spontaneously reacts to discolor (oxidize) many metals, makes fats or oils rancid, and supports combustion of flammable substances. It also forms peroxides (H_2O_2).

Molecular oxygen has a weight of 32, a density just over 1.4 at STP, and a specific gravity of 1.105 compared to air. Its critical temperature is −118.4C. Oxygen has a low specific heat and is readily soluble in water (about 5 ml per every 100 ml at 0C). Under normal conditions, approximately 0.3 ml of oxygen is in simple solution in each 100 ml of blood. Each gram of hemoglobin chemically combines with 1.34 ml of oxygen. The gas is commercially prepared by fractional distillation of liquified air. Its concentration in a mixture of gases, as from anesthesia machines, can be measured by oxygen analyzers, of which there are several types. Oxygen saturation of hemoglobin can be detected by oximeters. The gas is most commonly stored as a compressed gas in green or green-and-white cylinders of various sizes at pressures around 2000 psi. For large-use facilities, such as hospitals, bulk liquid storage is used. As the liquid is warmed and decompressed, it converts to the gaseous form. Prolonged administration of high oxygen concentrations can produce changes in lung tissue, producing symptoms of oxygen toxicity. The exact cause is not yet known. Several mechanisms may be involved.

Nitrogen. Nitrogen, as an inert element, does not readily combine with other substances. It, too, is prepared by fractional distillation of liquid air and is odorless, colorless, and tasteless. Atomic weight is 14, but like oxygen, nitrogen exists primarily as a diatomic structure (N_2) with a molecular weight of 28, the two atoms held together by a triple bond. Nitrogen has a density of 1.205 at STP and is lighter than air, having a specific gravity of 0.967. Under appropriate conditions it can combine with hydrogen, or with oxygen, with which five oxide combinations are possible. One is nitric oxide (NO), a possible impurity of nitrous oxide gas that is used to formulate nitric acid. Nitrous oxide, another oxide, is widely used as an anesthetic. It is the only nontoxic oxide of nitrogen. Large amounts of nitrogen are in simple solution in blood and other body fluids. Introduction of anesthetic agents into the body requires displacement of nitrogen, a process termed *denitrogenation.* Under conditions of sudden atmospheric decompression, expansion of nitrogen bubbles within the body gives rise to gaseous emboli that occlude blood vessels and disrupt circulation ("bends" or caisson disease). Treatment is by rapid recompression followed by slow decompression. Untreated, patients will develop symptoms of narcotization. Severe symptoms can produce death. Detection of nitrogen in a gas mixture is accomplished by gas chromatography or mass spectography.

Nitrogen can also be liquified (boiling point, −196C) and used as a cooling agent, as for cryosurgery. (Caution should be exercised because contact with liquid nitrogen can produce "cold burns.") Freezing tissue samples for microscopic analysis is sometimes accomplished with this agent. It is also used as a compressed gas for powering various tools used in surgery. Combined with oxygen, it serves as a breathing mixture for deep-sea diving and flying, and for medicinal uses where administration of pure oxygen is contraindicated. Its low reactivity makes it useful for adjusting atmospheres where combustible materials are kept or where the chance for fires is great. It is noncombustible and is stored in either liquid form or as a compressed gas in black cylinders at a pressure of approximately 2000 psi. (Compressed air, the mixture of nitrogen and oxygen used medically, is stored in yellow containers. Oxygen-nitrogen mixtures for nonmedicinal purposes are stored in black-and-green cylinders.)

Nitrous Oxide. Nitrous oxide is the most important inorganic gas used in clinical anesthesia practice. It has a molecular weight of 44.02 and is roughly 1.5 times as heavy as air (sp gr = 1.527). Nitrous oxide is colorless but possesses a slight taste and odor. It is not considered irritating when inhaled. Its boiling point is −89C (the critical temperature). Manufacture is by decomposition of ammonium nitrate. Nitrous oxide is stored as a liquid in blue cylinders. Cylinder pressure varies with room temperature but averages 750 to 800 psi. If moisture is present around the cylinder outlet, condensation and freezing can occur. This is no longer a common problem with modern preparation of the gas. To prevent contamination of cylinders by higher oxides of nitrogen that can cause epithelial damage to lungs, commercial production is carried out in multiple stages, which ensures purity. Nitrous oxide is relatively insoluble (blood solubility is 0.47), so that it enters and exits the body quickly and relatively unchanged. It does, however, rapidly diffuse into endotracheal tube cuffs and closed body compartments. This can be a problem during certain types of pneumoencephalograms or when patients have a bowel obstruction. Expansion of the gas generates detrimental increases in pressures. Providing analgesia requires relatively high concentrations (50 to 70 percent), and the minimum alveolar concentration (MAC) required to provide complete anesthesia would exceed 100 percent, so nitrous oxide is regarded as an incomplete anesthetic. (The concept of MAC and its

importance to anesthesia practice is discussed elsewhere in this text.)

Nitrous oxide is nonflammable; but, containing oxygen, it supports combustion. Under most conditions, however, the gas is stable, neither decomposing nor polymerizing. It maintains its stability even when passed through carbon dioxide absorption canisters.

Carbon Dioxide. Carbon dioxide is an organic compound. Its main importance lies in the fact that it is the end product of the body's biochemical respiration. It also has some limited use as a respiratory stimulant.

Carbon may combine with oxygen to form either carbon monoxide or carbon dioxide. The former is lethal when inhaled because it prevents oxygen from combining with hemoglobin. Carbon dioxide (CO_2) also forms a small part of our atmosphere (0.03 percent). It combines readily with water to form carbonic acid, important in acid-base regulation. But in general, it is a stable chemical. Similar to nitrous oxide in molecular weight (44) and specific gravity (1.54), it too is easily compressed to a colorless liquid and is stored as such in gray cylinders. Carbon dioxide is absorbed and neutralized by alkalis to form carbonates or, if large amounts of CO_2 are present, bicarbonates. Having a very high molal heat capacity, carbon dioxide is an excellent quenching agent for reducing flammability of combustible mixtures or for extinguishing fires. Absorption techniques are used to detect its presence in a mixture of gases because it absorbs infrared waves. Measurement of end-expired carbon dioxide has become a more widely used clinical tool in the past few years. Carbon dioxide is also used for calibrating blood gas analysis machines. A 5 percent carbon dioxide and oxygen mixture has been used as a respiratory stimulant in the past, especially for postoperative patients. The technique has largely fallen out of use because disadvantages often outweigh possible benefits, but it may have limited application. Exhaled carbon dioxide collecting in anesthesia breathing circuits, especially circle systems, must be disposed of physically or chemically to prevent rebreathing of CO_2 and development of hypercarbia. This topic is discussed separately later.

Helium. As one of the "rare" gases, helium is an inert, stable gas. Its principle anesthesia use has been as a diluent for other gas mixtures. The second lightest known element, helium exists as a single atom (atomic number 2, molecular weight 4) and diffuses readily, almost three times faster than oxygen. It is this property that makes helium useful for patients with severe respiratory obstruction, because less respiratory effort is required to breathe a helium-oxygen mixture than a pure oxygen atmosphere. An additional advantage is that helium is only slowly absorbed from occluded alveoli, minimizing development of atelectasis. Both properties facilitate oxygen delivery to patients with respiratory obstruction from airway narrowing.

Helium is also tasteless, odorless, and colorless. It liquifies only at extremely cold temperatures, below −269C, which is almost to the absolute zero point. It is quite insoluble, about 0.87 ml/100 ml at body temperature, so that it is readily eliminated from the body when administration is discontinued. Possessing a high degree of heat conductivity, helium used to be used as a quenching agent to reduce flammability of explosive or flammable anesthetic mixtures. Elimination of flammable agents from anesthesia practice has eliminated the need for quenching agents, but helium used as a carrier gas for delivery of oxygen in cases of respiratory obstruction still finds limited application.

HUMIDITY

The gases just described are dry, having no moisture content of their own. When administered to patients, they exert a drying effect that may damage tissues of the respiratory system. To overcome this problem, gases may be humidified. Adding water to dry gases (humidification) is a technique often employed during long surgical cases, not only to prevent respiratory system damage, but also to reduce loss of body heat and moisture. Having a GMW of 18 g, water added to an atmosphere of dry gas lightens the atmosphere because it replaces diatomic molecules, e.g., oxygen and nitrogen, which are considerably heavier. The effect is to reduce barometric (atmospheric) pressure. How well saturated with moisture dry gases become depends on the temperature of the environment and the amount of water present.

Dry air entering the lungs must be humidified by the respiratory passages. At normal body temperature, this creates a stable *water vapor tension (partial pressure)* of about 47 torr. Even when the atmosphere is highly saturated with water, it is cooler and less saturated than alveoli air. So body heat and water are lost in heating even this air. When patients breathe gases within a closed system where carbon dioxide is absorbed chemically (to be discussed later), the relative humidity approaches 100 percent. The patient's exhaled air, coupled with water liberated by the chemical reactions of carbon dioxide absorption, provides the moisture-building mechanism. But even then, the water gradient is from the lungs to the atmosphere, because of the temperature difference. If water particles are large enough, they are seen as a mist or fog. Clinically, humidification is provided by bubble-through vaporizers or by nebulization. Some anesthesia humidifiers electrically warm and humidify the air passing through in an attempt to minimize body water loss. Temperature monitors should then be used in the delivery circuit to prevent delivered gas temperatures from exceeding that of body temperature. If delivered anesthetic gases are not humidified, large amounts of body water are lost as lungs work to moisten the incoming air by evaporation of their cellular water. Humidity may be classed as either *absolute* (the maximum saturation of a given volume of air in grams per liter possible at a given temperature) or *relative* (the saturation actually present compared to the maximum possible saturation). Relative humidity is expressed as a percent of the possible total. Dew point is the temperature at which, if a volume of air is cooled, excess moisture precipitates out. Measurement of humidity is termed *hygrometry*. One method uses a combination of two thermometers, one attached to a capillary-action wick soaked in water—which, in a dry atmosphere, evaporates quickly to cause a marked fall in temperature—and one exposed to room air. The temperature difference between the two thermometers will be small if humidity is high. A

greater difference occurs when humidity is low. Other methods, including electrically operated devices, are available for measuring humidity.

Barometers are used for recording atmospheric pressures. Several types are used. One is a closed *liquid-type* manometer consisting of a long, calibrated tube placed in a pool of mercury open to atmospheric pressure. Changes in pressure are transmitted against the mercury, which rises or falls in the tube. Variations of this type include both open and closed U-tube devices. *Aneroid* types (e.g., Bourdon gauges) transmit changes in pressure exerted against a diaphragm, through levers and gears, to a needle, which registers on a calibrated scale. Similar manometers are used in a variety of anesthesia settings for measuring tank pressures, blood pressures, etc.

FLOW OF FLUIDS

Both gases and liquids may be thought of as fluid in that both are capable of flow through tubes or orifices. A *tube* is defined as a pathway whose length is greater than its diameter. An *orifice* is considered to have diameter but no length (or negligible length). Flow through tubes or orifices occurs when a pressure differential develops on either side of the pathway, the direction of flow being from high to low pressure. *Steady flow* occurs when all molecules of fluid pass through the pathway in the same direction and at the same velocity. Flow may be one of two types: *laminar flow*, where all molecules travel a parallel path within the tube, or *turbulent flow*, where some molecules take on a nonparallel path with respect to the other molecules (eddy currents). This concept is important to anesthesia practice because more energy is required to pass fluid through a tube in which flow is turbulent. An excellent example is the turbulence created in breathing circuits by kinking tubes or use of right-angle connectors. These reduce the efficiency of gas delivery. High flows increase the velocity of the molecules and thus create turbulence. This occurs when critical flow rates are exceeded. Laminar flows are typically associated with low velocities. Velocity will vary with the cross-sectional area of the tube pathway. The volume of flow per unit of time is a function of the cross-sectional area times velocity. Volume passed by a tube (per unit of time) is not only dependent upon cross-sectional area, but also tube length, pressure differential, and viscosity of the fluid. These relationships are summarized by *Poiseuille's law*, which states that (for laminar flow in a cylindrical tube) volume of discharge is directly proportional to pressure gradient, inversely proportional with viscosity, inversely proportional to tube length, and directly proportional to the fourth power of the radius. This means that doubling the length halves the output, requiring an increase to twice the driving pressure to maintain the same output. Halving the length doubles output, so half the driving pressure is required to maintain output per unit of time. Of greater importance in most applications is the fourth power of the radius. Doubling or halving radius size results in sixteenfold change in flow. This is because a number of changes occur including a redirection of molecular velocities. Poiseuille's law finds numerous applications in anesthesia: in breathing circuits, use of intravenous tubing, changes in airway size, blood flow through constricted vessels, etc.

For liquids in a confined pathway, *Pascal's law* applies. It states that, for confined liquids, any applied pressure is transmitted undiminished to all parts of the liquid. This accounts for the fact that a driving pressure may be developed in a closed system (e.g., water pipes), such that when the system is opened, flow begins immediately.

Fluid flows encounter resistance because traveling molecules create friction along pathway walls. Some of the driving pressure is directed toward overcoming forces of friction. It is friction that accounts for a drop in pressure as tube length is increased, usually as the square of the rate of flow. Friction is always higher with turbulent flows. For any given liquid, at any given temperature, a point exists, known as the *critical flow rate*, beyond which flow cannot be laminar because frictional forces limit laminar flow and create turbulence. This situation is analogous to the concept of electrical resistance found in Ohm's law.

Friction arises from two sources. One was described before where molecules of the flowing fluid are impeded by contact with molecules of the container walls. The other arises as internal friction within the flowing fluid caused by molecules passing alongside other molecules. This internal friction is termed *viscosity*. Molecules flow fastest in the center of the fluid, slowest at the edges nearest the container walls. Viscosity is dependent upon the nature of the substance and its temperature. Liquids generally become less viscous as temperature increases, whereas gases usually increase in viscosity. Viscosity is not related to the density of the substance. Carbon dioxide, which is heavier and denser than oxygen, nonetheless flows faster through a tube of the same size. This is because its coefficient of viscosity is less. Mixing of gases or liquids alters viscosity. The ratio of viscosity to density (of a gas) does influence critical flow rate. This ratio is termed the *Reynold's number*.

When liquids flow through a tube, a side pressure is exerted against the wall of the tube. The faster the flow through the tube, the less side pressure generated against the walls. This is known as *Bernoulli's law*. If the pathway varies in cross-sectional diameter, then at the point of greatest constriction, speed of flow will be greatest, and side pressure least. Conversely, at the widest point, side pressure is greatest and speed of flow the slowest.

It is Bernoulli's theory that underlies the operation of a Venturi tube. The tube consists of a constricted path along which calibrated manometers are placed, proximal, at, and distal to the constriction. The tube is used to measure volumes and flow rates of passing fluids. Venturi found that

if the tube constriction gradually widened out in cone fashion at an angle less than 15 degrees, distal pressures and flow rates reverted to what they were proximally. For constrictions that abruptly returned to the size and shape of the proximal tubing, pressures stayed below what they were proximally. By constructing a tube with a cone-shaped constriction and placing a right-angle port at the point of greatest constriction (where pressure is least, possibly even subatmospheric), it becomes possible to draw a fluid, either gas or liquid, into the main tube. There it mixes with the primary fluid for delivery to the distal opening. This device is called an injector (Fig. 5–1). The principle is used in atomizers and nebulizers for delivering drugs and aerosols or for humidifying anesthetic gases. With injectors, the ratio of aspirated fluid remains constant despite changes in primary fluid flow (the Venturi effect).

To summarize what has thus far been presented regarding fluid flow through tubes and orifices:

- Flow through tubes is primarily dependent upon viscosity and hardly affected by density.
- Flow through orifices is primarily dependent upon density, viscosity playing a minor role.

However, the picture is somewhat more complex in that orifices may be of two types: *fixed* and *variable*. In the former, the size of the opening remains fixed, so that as more gas arrives from the source, pressure builds on the proximal side. Flow rate for any gas of given density will be dependent upon, and proportional to, the square root of the proximal/distal pressure differential.

Initially, both pressures will be equal, and flow rate will equal one unit of the appropriate measurement, e.g., L/min, ml/min. As proximal pressure is increased fourfold, flow rate doubles. Quadrupling proximal pressure again results in a fourfold flow rate increase from the initial flow rate. These changes are summarized as follows:

Proximal Pressure	Flow Rate	Distal Pressure	Pressure Difference
1	1	1	1:1
4	$\sqrt{4} = 2$	1	4:1
16	$\sqrt{16} = 4$	1	16:1

But what happens when two different gases having dissimilar densities flow through the same fixed orifice? They will develop different pressure gradients, less pressure being generated by the less dense (lighter) gas. The pressure differential of two gases compared in this fashion will vary inversely with the square root of their densities. For exam-

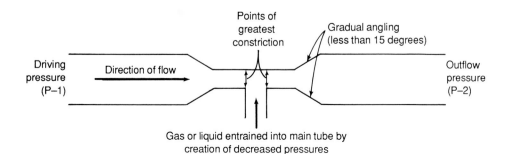

Figure 5–1. Venturi tube injector.

ple: hydrogen is $\frac{1}{16}$ as dense as oxygen ($H_2 = \sqrt{MW}$ 2; $O_2 = \sqrt{MW}$ 32; or a ratio of 1:16). Taking the square root of this density difference ($\sqrt{16} = 4$) tells us that oxygen, the heavier gas, will create a fourfold pressure difference compared to hydrogen. Therefore, proximal and distal pressures for hydrogen and oxygen are always in a ratio of 1:4; flow rate (column 2) doubles with each fourfold increase in pressure differential; but actual flow rate for oxygen will be double that of hydrogen (column 4) because the net proximal-distal pressure differences for oxygen are always greater because of the density difference between the two gases.

	Proximal Pressure	Flow Rate*	Distal Pressure	Actual Flow Rate†
H_2	1	1	1	1
O_2	4	1	4	2
H_2	4	2	1	2
O_2	16	2	4	4
H_2	16	4	1	4
O_2	64	4	4	8

* Discounts density, flow rate is equal to the square root of pressure differential only.
† Actual flow rate considering pressure differential and gas densities.

From the foregoing table:

	Proximal Pressure	Distal Pressure	Net Difference	Actual Flow Rate
H_2	4	1	3	2
O_2	16	4	12	4

If oxygen could be reduced to the same net difference as hydrogen, oxygen's actual flow rate would be $\frac{3}{12}$ of 4. Then, oxygen would flow only $\frac{1}{4}$ as fast: 1 L/min against hydrogen's 2 L/min.

	Proximal Pressure	Distal Pressure	Net Difference	Actual Flow Rate
H_2	4	1	3	2
O_2	4	1	3	1 ($\frac{3}{12}$ of 4)

This demonstrates the next point about flow through fixed orifices: the flow rate per unit of time of a light (less dense) gas can be accomplished through a smaller orifice than can the same flow rate for a heavy gas. Lastly, if the proximal-distal pressure difference is kept constant, flow rate will be directly related to the orifice diameter squared, a concept underlying the operation of anesthesia machine variable-orifice flowmeters. In reality, the flowmeter is internally tapered so that when placed vertically, the tapered end is at the bottom. Within the tube, a floating bobbin (rotameter or float) moves up and down against a calibrated scale to indicate flow rate. A brief glance at the calibration scale will indicate that flow rates are not uniformly linear as one moves up or down the scale. A further comparison of flowmeters for the same gas from several machines will also reveal slight differences between supposedly similar flowmeters. This is because flowmeters must be individually calibrated against a standard, and the scale for each tube must take into account slight variations that have occurred in the manufacturing process. For this reason, broken

flowmeters should have both the tube and corresponding scale replaced by another matched set. There are also wide variations, not always easily noticeable to the naked eye, between flow tubes for different gases. Each tube must take into account the density and viscosity of the gas for which it was designed. It also makes interchanging flow tubes between agents extremely hazardous because readings will no longer be accurate. Catastrophes have occurred in the past because of failure to appreciate these differences. Tapered tube/rotameter devices are known as Thorpe tubes.

Within a Thorpe tube, gas flows up from the source, around the bobbin, to the mixing manifold. The ring (annular) area around the bobbin increases as it moves up the tube because the cross-sectional area is greater (less tube tapering). The increase in annular opening is such that, relative to the length of the bobbin, more of an orifice is created. At low flows near the bottom of the tube, the ratio of bobbin length to annular opening more approaches the configuration of a tube. Therefore, low gas flow is a function of viscosity, in line with Poiseuille's law. At high flows, where the opening is more of an orifice, flow rate depends on gas density. This is in keeping with Graham's law. Some flowmeters utilize a double taper within the tube to improve their accuracy at low flows.

With variable-orifice flowmeters, gas flow pushes the bobbin upward and gravity pulls it down. These flowmeters have an advantage over fixed-orifice meters in that the pressure difference across the orifice remains constant, and flow rate is measured against changes in the effective diameter of the orifice. This allows for all flowmeter tubes to be of approximately the same size, a mechanical advantage in machine design. Other types of flowmeters have been and are being used, but variable-orifice flowmeters are by far the most widely used. These principles have application to other types of flowmeters also.

CARBON DIOXIDE ABSORPTION

Hypercarbia (excess blood levels of carbon dioxide) and respiratory acidosis develop whenever the body is unable to rid itself of end products of metabolism, or whenever a patient is allowed to breathe from an atmosphere high in CO_2 content. The latter situation can develop whenever a person rebreathes from an anesthesia circuit unless means are taken either to disperse exhaled CO_2 or to remove it by chemical means. In nonrebreathing anesthesia circuits, exhaled carbon dioxide is eliminated by diverting it to room atmosphere or into a scavenging device that removes it from the operating room environment. High fresh gas flows, in effect, blow the carbon dioxide out of the system.

With circuits that allow rebreathing of exhaled gases, such as a circle system, chemical removal provides a means of eliminating excess carbon dioxide. The amount chemically removed will depend on whether the circuit is fully closed, allowing rebreathing of all exhaled gases, or partially closed, when only a fraction of exhaled gases are rebreathed (semiclosed system). The rate of fresh gas inflow relative to production of exhaled CO_2 will also be a factor.

Chemical absorption depends on the fact that carbon dioxide is a gaseous, nonmetal oxide, forming carbonic acid when in contact with water, and is capable of reacting with metal oxides. Metal oxides in contact with water form hydroxides (bases), which can neutralize acids. How effective a metal oxide will be in neutralizing acids depends upon the metal's reactivity (position on the periodic table). Alkali metals are the most active. Of this group, potassium and sodium hydroxides are most commonly used. Alkaline earth metals are less reactive than the alkali metals but may also be used. Of this group, barium and calcium hydroxides are used most often. As neutralization occurs, the reaction produces water and the carbonate of the metal hydroxide involved, e.g., calcium hydroxide becomes calcium carbonate. Additional exposure of the carbonate to the acid produces a bicarbonate. Sodium, potassium, calcium, and barium hydroxides can all eventually be converted to bicarbonates. Although some bicarbonate may form in CO_2 absorption canisters, complete conversion is usually not seen because canister efficiency is depleted before the conversion is complete. The canister must then be changed to maintain efficient CO_2 absorption. The carbonates formed are quite stable, decomposition occurring only under unusual conditions. As neutralization proceeds, the canister heats because of exothermic reactions produced by the hydroxides dissolving in water (heat of solution). Hydroxides have such affinity for water that they are termed hygroscopic; that is, they are substances that absorb, even become dissolved in, water from the surrounding environment. Yet a small amount of water is added as a film to soda lime granules to allow for ionization. The amount of water has to be controlled because too much reduces absorption efficiency.

Size, shape, and consistency of absorbent granules is important in maximizing efficiency. Granules are of a size termed 4–8 mesh because they must pass through a mesh screening having four to eight openings per inch. Because hydroxides are normally soft and easily pulverized, a small amount of silica is added to increase hardness. Granules should have a hardness number greater than 75, a number determined by agitating the granules with steel ball bearings prior to passing them through the sizing mesh. The shape of each granule, which looks like a small piece of lava rock with many indentations, maximizes the surface area available for chemical reactions.

Soda lime is composed of 4 percent sodium hydroxide, 1 percent potassium hydroxide, and 14 to 19 percent water, the balance being calcium hydroxide. This is known as the "wet" variety and is the most commonly used absorbent today. Silica may be added in small amounts to increase hardness. The amount of sodium hydroxide is limited, to prevent caking caused by hygroscopic absorption of water. Caking reduces absorption efficiency and increases resistance to gas flow within the circuit. With older forms of soda lime, a phenomenon known as "peaking" or "regeneration" occurred. After prolonged use, soda lime efficiency would fall. Removing the canister from use allowed for some carbonate to be reconverted to soda lime. The canister could again be reused with high efficiency but only for short periods of time. With modern canisters, peaking is of little clinical importance.

Because soda lime is used in the presence of dry gases, one might think that absorption efficiency is reduced. This is not the case, provided the moisture content of granules is high (above 14 percent). Besides water adhered to gran-

ules, additional water for chemical reactions is provided by exhaled moisture (minimal) and by chemical release of hydrogen and hydroxyl ions, which combine to form water (see the subsequent numbered chemical reactions). Production of water by chemical reactions liberates heat (13,700 calories per mole of carbon dioxide absorbed), which warms gases within the absorber. If excessive heat develops, the canister may feel warm to the touch. Excessive temperatures may have an adverse impact upon patients by preventing dissipation of body heat.

Barium hydroxide granules are not as widely used. These granules differ in some respects from those of soda lime. Because barium hydroxide is an octahydrate $(Ba(OH)_2 \cdot 8\,H_2O)$, additional water is not required. The barium hydroxide type of absorbent also contains calcium (about 80 percent) and potassium hydroxide (1 percent). It too is 4–8 mesh in size, but no hardening material is added. The water of crystallization keeps dust formation to a minimum. Heat production and additional water formation are essentially the same as with soda lime. As with soda lime, a color indicator is used to indicate expenditure of the granules. However, barium hydroxide does not regenerate to any appreciable extent.

Color indicators (dyes) are added to both soda lime and barium hydroxide to indicate the extent to which absorbent has been exhausted. Those indicators are themselves either acids or bases that react to hydrogen ion concentration with a color change. With regeneration, dye color disappears. But any change in absorbent coloration indicates reduced efficiency with further use and one should consider changing the canister element. A number of indicator dyes are used including ethyl violet, Clayton yellow, ethyl orange, mimosa Z, and phenolphthalein. Package inserts generally describe the color change to be expected from a particular brand of absorbent. Indicators are not absolutely reflective of the extent to which absorbent has been used because a number of factors may impact on dye color changes.

Absorbers used today utilize a dual-canister configuration. Fresh canisters come packaged in airtight containers to prevent moisture contamination prior to use. Each has a baffle at the top and bottom, which some manufacturers seal with an adhesive label. Failure to remove the label will obstruct gas flow within the absorber. Typically, modern absorbers are designed to allow a flow of gases exceeding expected tidal volumes breathed by patients. They also minimize mechanical resistance to breathing. A number of factors influence the efficiency of absorbers including the rate and pattern of ventilation, amount of carbon dioxide produced by the patient, rate of fresh gas flows used, and the pattern of gas flow through the absorber. This last factor results in what is termed channeling. As gases pass through the canister, they take the path of least resistance. This is usually along the sides of the canister where granules are less tightly packed. The effect is to funnel flows over the same areas of absorbent. Because of channeling, absorbent around the walls of the container is used up first, one factor responsible for rapid indicator dye changes along easily visible canister outer walls.

The chemical steps involved in carbon dioxide absorption may be summarized as follows:

1. Exhaled carbon dioxide combines with available water to form carbonic acid:

$$CO_2 + H_2O \longrightarrow H_2CO_3$$

2. Carbonic acid dissociates into hydrogen and bicarbonate ions:

$$H_2CO_3 \longrightarrow H^+ + HCO_3^-$$

3. The metal oxides dissociate to their respective ions. Soda lime absorbent includes sodium, calcium, and potassium hydroxides. Barium hydroxide lime includes calcium, potassium, and barium hydroxides.

Sodium: $\quad NaOH \longrightarrow Na^+ + OH^-$

Calcium: $\quad Ca(OH)_2 \longrightarrow Ca^{++} + 2\,OH^-$

Potassium: $\quad KOH \longrightarrow K^+ + OH^-$

Barium:

$$Ba(OH)_2 \cdot 8\,H_2O \longrightarrow Ba^{++} + 2\,OH^- + 8\,H_2O$$

4. Hydroxides react with carbonic acid to produce carbonates:
Sodium:

$$2\,NaOH + H_2CO_3 \longrightarrow Na_2CO_3 + 2\,H_2O + heat$$

Calcium:

$$Ca(OH)_2 + H_2CO_3 \longrightarrow CaCO_3 + 2\,H_2O + heat$$

Potassium:

$$2\,KOH + H_2CO_3 \longrightarrow K_2CO_3 + 2\,H_2O + heat$$

Barium: Here four reactions are involved.
  a. Barium hydroxide directly reacts with carbon dioxide:

$$Ba(OH)_2 \cdot 8\,H_2O + CO_2 \longrightarrow BaCO_3 + 9\,H_2O + heat$$

  b. Water from (a) combines with carbon dioxide to form carbonic acid.

$$9\,H_2O + 9\,CO_2 \longrightarrow 9\,H_2CO_3 + heat$$

  c. and d. The carbonic acid reacts with the available calcium and potassium hydroxides.

$$9\,H_2CO_3 + 9\,Ca(OH)_2 \longrightarrow 9\,CaCO_3 + 18\,H_2O + heat$$

$$2\,KOH + H_2CO_3 \longrightarrow K_2CO_3 + 2\,H_2O + heat$$

When regeneration reactions are allowed to occur, only sodium and potassium carbonates are reconverted to their respective hydroxides by reacting with unused calcium hydroxide. This is because both carbonates are soluble. Barium carbonate and calcium carbonate, being insoluble, cannot be reconverted to hydroxides. The two regenerative reactions thus possible are

$$K_2CO_3 + Ca(OH)_2 \longrightarrow CaCO_3 + 2\,KOH$$

$$Na_2CO_3 + Ca(OH)_2 \longrightarrow CaCO_3 + 2\,NaOH$$

Regenerative reactions further deplete available calcium hydroxide and contribute to additional formation of calcium carbonate.

SOUND, OPTICS, AND NUCLEAR FORCES

Sound

These three topics are grouped together for two reasons. First, all of them relate more to physics than to chemistry. Second, they each have only an indirect or peripheral relationship to anesthesia practice.

Sound waves are longitudinal waves created by molecular displacement within the conducting medium. They can travel through solids, liquids, or gases, the rate of conduction being fastest in solids and least in gas mediums. As the waves make contact with the tympanic membrane, secondary oscillations are developed that, through the auditory mechanism, are perceived as sound.

As with any wave phenomena, the waves occur with varying frequency per unit of time. Wave frequency determines the perceived tone so that changes in frequency are detected as changes in pitch. However, pitch and frequency are not truly synonymous because pitch is a subjective interpretation. Frequency can also be expressed and measured as the number of cycles (waves) per second. The older measurement term cycles per second (cps) has been replaced by the *hertz* (1 hertz [Hz] equals 1 cps). Doubling a given base frequency produces a *harmonic* of that frequency. Tuning forks used for testing auditory acuity are set to vibrate as harmonics of a two-cycles-per-second base, so that a fork vibrating at 512 Hz represents an eighth harmonic. Sound-wave velocity in air is 1089 ft/sec, (331 m/sec), accounting for sound's rapid dispersion. Stethoscopes used for listening to heart tones help diminish the otherwise rapid loss of those sounds. Loudness, or sound intensity, depends upon the level of energy expended in generating the sound. A yell generates more loudness than a whisper of similar frequency because energy expenditure is greater. Sound intensity is measured in decibels (db). Quiet breathing produces a sound level of about 10 db, the lower threshold for audible sound. Normal conversation tone generates about 60 db, and loud noises such as clatter caused by a metal operating room tray being dropped can exceed 100 db. Levels above 120 db may cause pain. The Occupations, Safety, and Health Act sets a maximum average exposure level of 90 db. Continuous exposure to higher levels can result in hearing impairment. In addition, a number of physiologic responses to noise are known to occur. These include sleep alterations, depressed mental functioning, changes in endocrine function including glucocorticoid and catecholamine release, and cardiovascular vasoconstriction. Chronic exposure to high levels of background noise is now considered a form of nonspecific stress. Since most operating rooms have highly sound-reflective walls, floors, and ceilings, anesthetists and other operating room personnel risk chronic exposure to high noise "pollution." Use of soundproofing materials within operating rooms is limited by the need for facilities that can be made bacteriostatic.

As a noise source moves toward a listener, the sound's frequency appears to change, even though the sound is being generated at a constant frequency. This difference between perceived and actual sound frequencies is known as the Doppler effect and is due to the fact that the number of sound wave fronts converging upon the listener (per unit of time) increases as the noise source moves toward him or her. The Doppler principle is used in anesthesia monitoring devices able to emit sound and also receive the reflected waves. Such devices are used for blood pressure monitoring and detecting blood flow changes through the heart. Pulsations cause heart or blood vessel position to change with respect to the sensing device. The reflected sound waves change correspondingly, and this frequency change is detected by the sensor, which emits the altered tones from a built-in speaker. Such Doppler devices allow more accurate blood pressure readings and detection of heart sound changes caused by air emboli. As little as 0.5 ml of air passing through the heart can be detected in this way.

Sound waves are often thought of in terms of the frequency range perceptible to human ears, but they exist above and below that range as well. Those under normal range (below 20 Hz) are referred to as subsonic. Those above the range of normal hearing (about 20,000 Hz) are termed ultrasonic. The ultrasound range has several useful applications in medicine. Newly developed ultrasonic detectors are important as diagnostic tools. Their growing popularity stems from the fact that they can be used noninvasively. Ultrasonic waves are also used for cleaning. Often found in operating rooms, ultrasonic cleaners are highly efficient in removing tenacious debris from difficult-to-clean areas, such as removing mucous from inside a bronchoscope. They operate on the basis of a cavitation process. As sound waves are transmitted through the cleaning medium (water), pressure changes create numerous small bubbles. Rupture of the bubbles creates negative pressure, which acts as a vacuum to break up and disperse dirt or colloidal proteinaceous material.

Optics

The term optics refers to the science concerned with study of light. Visible light forms but a small portion of a continuum of radiant energies known as the electromagnetic spectrum. At the low end of the spectrum are electrical waves of long wavelength. Above this range we have, in order of decreasing wavelength: long and short radio waves, infrared light waves, visible light, the ultraviolet light range, x-rays, gamma rays, and cosmic rays. The nature of these radiations is controversial. Early light theories postulated a continuous wave form. Later, light was thought a particle, and later yet, a form of electromagnetic wave. The wave-particle controversy continued for decades, with adherents and scientific "proof" abundant on both sides. The controversy stemmed from the fact that wave theories are generally correct for explaining the behavior of light but cannot explain all its properties. For example, the photoelectric effect (electron emission from substances exposed to light) was first described by Hertz. But it was Einstein who later explained the phenomena on the basis of light being a particle. Einstein also first postulated that light is quantified into small bundles called photons, each possessing an energy

proportional to its wave frequency. Today it is generally accepted that light has a dual nature and that other electromagnetic radiations also represent *quanta* of energy. This quantum of light energy, the photon, is now assumed to be a massless particle capable of carrying energy and momentum from place to place. Light is subject to gravitational bending, but being massless, it can never itself come to rest. That is, it can never be stopped, so that it becomes impossible to ever capture (detect) a photon.

Light travels at a phenomenal speed: 2.98×10^8 km/sec (about 186,000 miles per second); yet it can easily be refracted (bent) as it moves from one medium to another, as from air to water. Prism laryngoscopes use this principle. Light travels in two planes, horizontal and vertical, so it is said to be polarized, and one or the other plane may be blocked by polarized filters. If light is directed upon a reflective surface at an angle, it is reflected from that surface at an equal angle. It is thus possible to concentrate light where it is needed. Fiberoptic laryngoscopes and microscopes use this principle. Shining white light through a prism separates it into individual colors (frequencies) by dispersion, a property underlying the operating of spectroscopes. The candela (cd) is the SI unit of measurement for light intensity.

Lasers are a form of light energy increasingly utilized as a surgical tool. Atoms exposed to an energy source have their electrons forced into a higher energy state, a process called excitation. As the electron returns to its normal energy state, a photon is released. That photon may then collide with other "excited" atoms, causing release of another photon of the same frequency. This process repeats and is termed stimulated emission. The photons multiply as a chain reaction. If the reaction takes place inside a substance with a crystalline configuration, such as a ruby crystal, a large number of photons pass down the crystal's axis. Mirrors are used to deflect additional photons into traveling the same axis, so that as more and more photons are released, all are of the same frequency (wavelength) and travel in the same direction. A partially transparent mirror allows the laser light to be emitted. As it leaves, beam intensity can be controlled and focused to allow its use as a surgical tool.

The term "laser" itself describes the process: *L*ight *A*mplification by *S*timulated *E*mission of *R*adiation. Laser light differs from other forms of light not only in the manner by which it is produced, but also in its nature. It is monochromatic (all of one color), coherent (all photons in phase), and parallel (all photons traveling in the same direction). Because each photon represents a packet of energy, concentrating the sum energies of all the photons makes lasers extremely powerful.

Besides solid lasers, such as those employing a ruby, there are also gas lasers. These have more surgical applications. Generally they use carbon dioxide, argon, or helium-neon. Carbon dioxide lasers, in particular, find wide application. They deliver a beam in the infrared range (10.6 microns), which destroys tissue and coagulates blood by a thermal effect. The amount of tissue destroyed depends on its moisture content and the amount of laser energy used. Lasers have some important implications for anesthesia. The light may be reflected, so all personnel must use eyewear to protect delicate eye tissue from beam contact. Endotracheal tubes or other equipment may be damaged by the high energies of a misdirected laser beam. When used in the presence of high delivered oxygen concentrations, flash fires can occur as endotracheal tubes or other items are heated to the combustion point and fueled by the oxygen.

Nuclear Forces

Nuclear forces are those energies associated with substances whose atomic nuclei spontaneously decompose (radioactivity) to transmute the substance into another element. This spontaneous degeneration releases three forms of energy particles: alpha, beta, and gamma. An alpha particle is essentially the nucleus of the helium atom stripped of its electrons, leaving it with two positive charges and an atomic mass unit of 4. Beta particles are massless electrons possessing a negative charge. Gamma radiation is a nonparticle electromagnetic radiation of shorter wavelength (higher frequency) than x-rays. Radioactive elements are typically unstable isotopes (substances with altered atomic masses because of a change in neutron number within the nucleus). Cobalt-60, sodium-24, phosphorus-32, iodine-131, and radioactive iron and gold are all isotopes with useful diagnostic and therapeutic applications in medicine.

The rate at which a radioactive substance decomposes is its *half-life*, the length of time required for a given mass to be reduced by half. Half-life can vary in time from minutes to thousands of years, depending upon which substance is involved. A similar term, *biologic half-life* refers to the time required for half a given dose of radioactive isotope to be eliminated from the body.

Alpha, beta, and gamma radiations vary in both the speed at which they travel and in the amount of ionizing potential they possess. Ionization occurs as the particles interact with either the orbital electrons or nuclei of other atoms, including those in body tissues. Alpha particles are highly ionizing but travel slowly and can be stopped by skin so that their biologic importance is limited. Beta particles have higher velocities and are more penetrating but have a lower ionizing potential. Gamma radiations travel at the speed of light and are extremely penetrating, but they have the least energy. However, all are capable of causing ionization, thereby converting other substances into ions or radicals. Proteins become altered, and genes may be changed so that cellular growth becomes abnormal. These changes produce radiation sickness, the symptoms of which vary with the dose of radiation received.

Radiation is measured in several forms. The curie (Ci) is a measure of the activity of radioactive substances. The roentgen measures exposure to x-rays or gamma radiation. But it is the rad (radiation absorbed dose) that has great biologic importance because it measures the dose absorbed by body tissues. The rem (roentgen-equivalent-man) is the amount of any absorbed radiation equivalent to one roentgen. The RBE (relative biological effectiveness) is used to compare an absorbed dose of radiation to that of cobalt-60. It is primarily used in radiation therapy to measure tissue effects of a given radiation dose.

Radiation can be detected in a variety of ways including radiation badges, dosimeters, and radiation counter devices. The maximum permissible dose (MPD) is a calculated value indicating how much radiation may be absorbed before exerting detrimental effects on important body organs (genitals, heart, blood-forming organs, etc.). How much radiation a person receives depends upon a number of factors including type of radiation, length of exposure, distance from the source, previous level of exposure, and the amount of shielding.

In terms of a single exposure, total absorbed dose determines the extent and severity of radiation illness produced. Less than 100 rad produces minimal biologic injury. Above that level, three recognized syndromes may occur. At up to 600 rad, patients develop a hematopoietic syndrome characterized by anemia and hemorrhage caused by suppression of blood-forming organs. With 600 to 1000 rad, a gastrointestinal syndrome occurs with accompanying symptoms of nausea, vomiting, diarrhea, fever, abdominal pain, and loss of hair. At doses exceeding 1000 rad, patients develop a central nervous system syndrome, which is inevitably fatal. Symptoms include lethargy, ataxia, and convulsions. Doses of 3000 rad or greater are usually fatal within a few hours to days.

BIBLIOGRAPHY

Adriani JA: The Chemistry and Physics of Anesthesia. Springfield, IL, Chas. C Thomas, 1962.

Alberty RA: Physical Chemistry, 6h ed. New York, Wiley, 1983.

Beiser A, Cummings B: Physics 4th ed. Menlo Park, CA, Bubco, 1986.

Blatt FJ: Principles of Physics, 2nd ed. Boston, Allyn and Bacon, 1986.

Brown TL, Lemay HE: Chemistry: The Central Science. Englewood Cliffs, NJ Prentice-Hall, 1977.

Dorsch JA, Dorsch SE: Understanding Anesthesia Equipment. Baltimore, Williams & Wilkins, 1975.

Dorsch JA, Dorsch SE: Understanding Anesthesia Equipment, 2nd ed. Baltimore, Williams & Wilkins, 1984.

Huheey JE: Inorganic Chemistry: Principles of Structure and Reactivity, 3rd ed. New York, Harper & Row, 1986.

King GB, Caldwell WE, et al: College Chemistry. New York, Van Nostrand, 1977.

Oxtoby DW, Nachtrieb NH: Principles of Modern Chemistry. New York, CBS, 1986.

Shugar G, Shugar R, et al: Health Sciences Chemistry. Philadelphia, Davis, 1978.

Tipler PA: Physics. New York, Worth Publishers, 1976.

6

Principles of Organic Chemistry and Biochemistry in Anesthesia

Leo A. Le Bel

Until 1828, scientists thought the chemistry of living organisms distinct from that of inorganic substances. In that year, a German chemist named Wohler prepared urea, a supposed organic substance, from ammonium cyanate. By demonstrating that organic compounds were not dependent upon bodily chemistry for their production, Wohler opened up a whole new branch of chemistry. Organic chemistry is devoted to the study of compounds formulated from a base of carbon atoms. The diversity of organic compounds is almost beyond belief. Drugs, petroleum products, plastics, and numerous other substances we encounter daily in every sphere of life depend on the versatile atomic structure of the carbon atom.

The Carbon Atoms and the Alkanes

Carbon has six protons and six electrons in its atomic structure. The electrons are distributed according to the theory of octet: two in the first orbit and the remaining four in the outer orbit. It is carbon's four outer electrons that give it is unique properties. Carbon shares its outer electrons with other atoms, in pairs, forming a *covalent bond*. In covalent bonding, sharing of electrons benefits each basic atom. Carbon forms such bonds with many elements, including other carbon atoms. In particular, it readily combines with hydrogen atoms having one outer orbit electron. This provides needed stability for both atoms. By sharing carbon's electrons, hydrogen assumes the stable configuration of a helium atom. Carbon and hydrogen so readily come together that they form a whole group of distinct compounds—the hydrocarbons.

Simplest of the hydrocarbon structures is one carbon atom surrounded by four of hydrogen, the gas methane (CH_4).

The next most complex hydrocarbon structure is called ethane. It contains two carbon atoms that each share one electron; the remaining carbon electrons pair with hydrogen electrons (CH_3—CH_3).

After ethane comes propane. Propane has three carbon atoms linked together, hydrogen filling the remaining binding sites. In order of increasing complexity, propane is followed by:

Hydrocarbon Structure	No. of Carbon Atoms
Butane	4
Pentane	5
Hexane	6
Heptane	7
Octane	8
Nonane	9
Decane	10

The list continues, but these are the more commonly encountered compounds. Note that in each case the next higher compound in the series differs from the preceding one by C—H_2. This means the number of hydrogens is always twice the number of carbon atoms plus two ($2n + 2$). For example, decane with 10 carbons contains 22 hydrogens ($2 \times 10 + 2 = 22$). In this series of straight-chain hydrocarbons, known as the alkane series, each bond is accounted for by an individual atom. The hydrocarbons of this group are therefore said to be saturated. Removing a hydrogen results in the substance becoming a radical. For example, removing a hydrogen from methane (CH_4) leaves the methyl radical (CH_3). The methyl group is often encountered in organic chemistry and biochemistry. Radicals are named by converting the *-ane* ending of the parent compound to a *-yl* ending: methane becomes methyl, propane becomes propyl, etc. Most saturated hydrocarbons are formed from fractional distillation of petroleum products. Compounds having fewer than 5 carbon atoms are gases, those having 5 to 16 are liquids, and those containing more than 16 carbons are solids. Alkanes are not extremely active chemically, although they burn readily and react with the halogens, especially chlorine and bromine, a fact important to the development of halogenated anesthetics. When burned, straight-chain hydrocarbons form water and carbon dioxide. Because of its limited chemical reactivity, the alkane series was formerly known as the paraffin group, paraffin meaning "little activity." They tend to be insoluble in water, though they are soluble in weakly polar solvents, such as the ethers. Isomers may be formed from many, but not all, alkanes having three carbon atoms or more. Isomers are discussed later.

The IUPAC (Geneva) System. Organic compounds can become exceedingly complex in structure. To simplify the naming of substances, the International Union of Pure and Applied Chemistry (IUPAC) developed a system for naming organic compounds known as the Geneva system. The more common or important rules are summarized here:

1. For branched-chain alkanes, the name is based on the longest continuous (i.e., unbranched) chain of carbons in the compound. For example:

$$CH_3-CH-CH_2-CH_2-CH_2 \atop CH_3 \quad CH_3 \quad CH_3$$

when straightened becomes:

$$CH_3-CH_2-\underset{CH_3}{CH}CH_2-CH_2-CH_2-CH_3$$
$$1 \quad 2 \quad 3 \ 4 \quad 5 \quad 6 \quad 7$$

The longest continuous chain totals seven carbons. The compound will therefore be a heptane.

2. When naming positions of chains (e.g., methyl group in the example), beginning at either end of the longest continuous chain, assign a number to each long-chain carbon so that the first branching occurs at the carbon with the lowest number. In the example, numbering from the right would put the methyl group at carbon 5. Numbering from the left puts it at carbon 3. Branching is named from the lowest numbered carbon atom at which branching occurs (3-methylheptane). If another methyl group occurred at carbon 4, the compound would be 3,4-methylheptane.

3. The terms primary, secondary, and tertiary are used to differentiate different forms of the same compound. It can also designate the number of direct bonds to other carbon atoms. For example, a tertiary butyl would have one carbon attached directly to three carbons of the group:

$$CH_3-\overset{CH_3}{\underset{CH_3}{\overset{|}{C}}}-$$

4. Substituents (atoms of groups) may be indicated by a prefix and a number showing their position relative to the long chain. For example: 1,3,7-dimethyl nonane indicates that two methyl groups are located on each carbon at positions 1, 3, and 7 of the longest chain.

5. When identical groups are located on the same carbon of the main chain, numbers are supplied for each group. For example: 2,2-dimethylhexane says that two methyl groups are attached to the same carbon atom. Hyphens and commas are used to organize the parts of the name of the substance. Hyphens always separate numbers from word parts, and commas separate numbers from numbers. The intent is to make the final name one word.

6. Whenever two or more different groups are attached to the chain, several ways are acceptable for organizing the name of the compound. The last portion of the compound name will be the main-chain alkane. Other parts can be ordered in terms of their increasing complexity, e.g., methyl, ethyl, propyl, or they can be listed in alphabetical order.

The Geneva system has other rules, but these basics should suffice for most compounds the anesthetist is apt to encounter. Radicals formed from alkane structures are sometimes termed alkyls. Beside the methyl radical, other common radicals are ethyl (C_2H_5) and propyl (C_3H_7).

In addition to straight-chain alkanes, there are also ring-structured saturated hydrocarbons. The one of most interest to anesthetists is cyclopropane (C_3H_6). These ring structures are called *cycloalkanes.*

$$\begin{array}{c} H \quad H \\ \diagdown \diagup \\ H \diagdown \overset{C}{\diagup} \diagdown H \\ H \diagdown \overset{\diagup}{C}-\overset{\diagdown}{C} \diagup H \\ \diagup \qquad \diagdown \\ H \qquad\quad H \end{array}$$

Ring structures require additional energy to maintain their configurations, and this explains their instability. Cyclopropane is explosive for this reason.

New compounds can be obtained by substituting other atoms for hydrogen in straight-chain alkanes. Substituting chlorine for a hydrogen in methane produces methyl chloride. Such substitution compounds are termed derivatives. Other important nonalkyl substitutes include fluorine, chlorine, bromine, iodine, and the nitro (NO_2) and amino (NH_2) groups. It is also possible to combine several organic substances into new complex molecules with new properties. The process is known as polymerization and the new substance as a polymer.

Alkenes and Alkynes. Chemically treating saturated hydrocarbons to remove hydrogen atoms produces unsaturated hydrocarbons that contain either two or three bonds between carbons. Those containing two bonds are called alkenes, those with three bonds alkynes. Because of their unsaturated double or triple bonding, these substances tend to be chemically reactive.

Alkenes have the general formula C_nH_{2n}. The ring structures previously described known as cycloalkanes also have the general formula C_nH_{2n}. Alkenes and cycloalkanes have two hydrogen atoms less than alkanes. The first member of the alkene group is ethylene, and the series is sometimes called the ethylene series. Older terminology referred to them as the olefin series. The gas ethylene has been used in anesthesia, but it was never extremely popular. It does form the basis for the production of many compounds including polyethylene, from which certain types of surgical suture are made.

Alkynes have the general formula C_nH_{2n-2}. They contain one triple bond. Just as alkene compounds end their names in *-ene*, alkynes have names ending in *-yne*. The first of the series is ethyne, more commonly known as acetylene.

Dienes and *trienes* are organic compounds that contain two or three double bonds within their structure. They are not members of the alkene series, which contains only one double bond.

Isomers. Compounds having the same molecular formula but different structures are termed *isomers*. Carbon compounds facilitate isomeric structures because the carbon atom possesses the characteristic of being able to rotate its bonds about its central axis. Isomers are of two main types: structural and stereoisomers. The latter is further divided into two types: optical isomers and geometric isomers. *Structural isomers* usually differ in both physical and chemical properties from one another. The straight-chain form is known as the *normal isomer*. When one methyl group is branched off the major chain, the compound is called an *isoisomer*.

Normal   Isoisomer

Stereoisomers have identical structural formulas but differ in their spatial arrangement. *Optical isomers* occur when the groups attached to the carbon atom differ from one another. This causes a bending (rotation) of light passing through the substance's vertical axis. Light polarized to the right produces a *dextro isomer*. When the light is polarized to the left, the *levo* (or sinister) *isomer* is formed. The two forms are mirror images of one another. Dextro and levo isomers are also known as enantiomorphs. Where a mixture of both forms is such that no polarization of light occurs, the mixture is termed *racemic*.

Geometric isomers are formed from compounds containing two carbon atoms joined by a double bond. The double bond locks the carbons so that no axial rotation can occur. Two forms are possible: *cis* isomers and *trans* isomers. In the *cis isomer* form, groupings are arranged on the same side of the double bond. With *trans isomers* they are located on opposite sides of the bond. Their spatial configuration is therefore different.

Cis isomer   Trans isomer

A variation of structural isomerism occurs when, in certain compounds, atoms are able to shift from one position to another. This ability is known as *tautomerism*. Such shifts are often found in barbiturate drug structures. Isomers thus formed are known as *tautomers*, also called *ketoenol isomers*, because one group of compounds, ketones, are often able to shift a hydrogen bond from the attached carbon (the keto form) to the carbonyl portion of the structure (the enol form). In the following example, R represents any given radical.

Keto form   Enol form

Some compounds, notably proteins, are capable of temporarily reorganizing their shapes so that the spatial orientation of any part of the structure changes in relation to its other parts. These so called *conformational changes* are often induced by other physical or chemical factors. Removing the causative factor allows the compound to revert to its original shape.

Class Divisions of Organic Compounds. Organic compounds are normally divided into specific classes on the basis of identifiable structural groupings. The general formula for each group provides the common configuration for the class. R is used to represent any base group or radical.

Halogen Compounds. Halogen compounds have the general formula R—X, in which X can be any halogen atom, i.e., chlorine, bromine, etc. Alkyl halogen compounds (alkyl halides) are formed by replacing one or more hydrogen atoms of an aliphatic (straight-chain) compound with a halogen. Chloroform ($CHCl_3$), though no longer used as an anesthetic, is an example. It was prepared by chlorination of methane, three hydrogen atoms being replaced by chlorine.

Also used as an organic solvent, chloroform easily decomposes in the presence of light and air to phosgene, a poisonous gas. Ethyl chloride (C_2H_5Cl), a topically applied skin anesthetic, is another halide. Yet another halogenated compound used in anesthesia was trichlorethylene. Being double bonded (unsaturated), trichlorethylene was very unstable, especially in the presence of soda lime, where it decomposed to toxic by-products (dichloracetylene, phosgene, and carbon monoxide) to produce neuritis of cranial nerves and other problems. Despite such previous difficulties, most modern inhalation anesthetics have resulted from halide conversion of aliphatic or ether compounds.

Alcohols. Alcohols are derived from hydrocarbons in which a hydrogen is replaced by an OH group (general formula: R—OH). Thus, replacing hydrogen in methane produces methyl alcohol. Similarly, ethyl alcohol is derived from ethane, propyl alcohol from propane, etc. Alcohols have a distinctive taste, burn readily, and enter into many chemical reactions. The simpler alcohols are readily soluble in water. Alcohols are classed as *primary, secondary,* or *tertiary* depending upon the position of the radical(s). With a primary alcohol, the OH group is attached to the carbon atom at the end of a straight chain. In secondary alcohols, two radicals are joined to the carbon atom holding the OH group. Similarly, a tertiary alcohol has three organic radicals attached to the carbon having the OH group. The following illustrates the differences:

Propyl alcohol (primary)   Isopropyl (secondary)   Tert-butyl alcohol (tertiary)

Although often neutral in chemical reactions, alcohols may behave as weak acids under appropriate conditions, and all are readily oxidized. When a primary alcohol is oxidized, an aldehyde is formed:

Methyl alcohol + oxygen ⟶ formaldehyde.

Oxidizing a secondary alcohol produces a ketone:

Isopropyl alcohol + oxygen ⟶ acetone + water.

Both aldehydes and ketones are discussed later. Oxidation of tertiary alcohols can produce a variety of compounds. Complex alcohols form the basis for such substances as glycol (ethylene glycol), commonly used as antifreeze and poisonous if taken internally. Most alcohols contain some water, but an anhydrous form is sometimes used to perform a permanent neurolytic block in the treatment of intractable pain.

Aldehydes. Aldehydes have the functional group

which gives the group its characteristic properties. As previously mentioned, aldehydes are formed from oxidation of primary alcohols. This process involves removal of two hydrogen atoms from the hydrocarbon. The molecular oxygen that oxidizes the hydrocarbon splits, one atom of oxygen joining the two hydrogens to form water. The remaining oxygen becomes double-bonded to the carbon atom. Oxidation of hydrocarbons normally produces a new compound (in this case, aldehyde) and water. Two important aldehydes encountered in medicine are formaldehyde and acetaldehyde. Both are gases at room temperature, have suffocating odors, and are strong reducing agents. Formaldehyde is used as a tissue preservative. Acetaldehyde is a breakdown product of ethyl alcohol, which forms the basis of commercial liquors. Aldehydes have a marked tendency to combine with themselves (polymerization). Acetaldehyde polymerizes to the hypnotic drug paraldehyde.

Ketones. Ketones are formed by oxidation of secondary alcohols. They have the general configuration

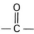

known as the carbonyl group. The best example is acetone. It is derived from isopropyl alcohol in the same manner as aldehydes, discussed in the preceding section. Acetone is a colorless liquid with a pleasant odor. An excellent solvent, acetone is particularly useful for removing residual adhesive tape from patients' skin. Diabetic ketoacidosis is a condition in which the body produces excessive amounts of ketones.

Organic acids. Organic acids are hydrocarbons in which one or more hydrogen has been replaced by a COOH group (carboxyl group). The carboxyl grouping is really a combination of the carbonyl and hydroxyl groups already discussed and is characteristic of all organic acids. The hydrogen atom of the group ionizes in solution to give the compound acidic properties. Organic acids may be formed in one of two ways. They may be produced by oxidation of a primary alcohol to an aldehyde, which is further oxidized to the acid; or they may be produced by treating an organic acid salt with a strong mineral acid (e.g., sodium acetate when reacted with sulfuric acid yields acetic acid and sodium hydrosulfate). Because the hydrogen of the functional group is ionizable, it is replaceable by all metals above it in the electromotive series. As with other acids, the organic acids react with bases to form salts and water. One important organic acid is acetic acid (also known as ethanoic acid because it is derived from ethane), formed in the body by further oxidation of acetaldehyde. Organic acids are also important to the formation of body fats.

Esters. Esters are produced by the interaction of an alcohol with an acid. They are very volatile and have pleasant odors. Esters have the general formula R—COO—R. Isoamyl nitrite, used in a breakable ampule to treat angina pectoris by relaxing smooth muscles of the cardiovascular system, is an example. The drug is inhaled and enters the bloodstream where it dilates vessels and lowers blood pressure. A whole series of local anesthetic compounds are classed as esters. Most are esters of *para*-aminobenzoic acid. Tetracaine, used for subarachnoid block anesthesia, is an example of this group. Cocaine, a benzoic acid ester, is another local anesthetic. Primarily used for topical anesthesia of mucous membranes, it is also associated with a high incidence of illegal abuse. Benzoates and *para*-aminobenzoic acid are discussed later.

Ethers. Ethers are organic oxides having the general formula R—O—R. They consist of two hydrocarbon radicals joined by an atom of oxygen, which is the functional group. Although diethyl and divinyl (C_2H_5—O—C_2H_5 and C_2H_3—O—C_2H_3 respectively) ethers have largely been removed from anesthesia practice because of their volatility and explosiveness, they were anesthetic mainstays for decades. Even today, the public associates the practice of anesthesia with administration of ether. However, the explosive ethers have been replaced by halogenated, nonexplosive ones.

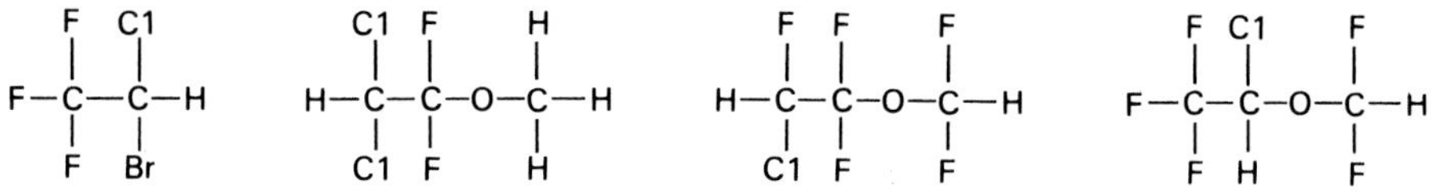

```
    F  Cl              Cl  F   H            F   F   F            F  Cl   F
    |   |               |   |   |            |   |   |            |   |   |
  F-C - C - H       H - C - C - O - C - H  H-C - C - O - C - H  F-C - C - O - C - H
    |   |               |   |   |            |   |   |            |   |   |
    F  Br              Cl   F   H           Cl   F   F            F   H   F
   Halothane         Methoxyflurane          Enflurane             Isoflurane
```

Figure 6–1. Structural formulas for commonly used anesthetic agents.

Methoxyflurane (2,2-dichloro-1,1-difluoroethyl methyl ether) is a pungent, sweet-smelling, potent anesthetic. Its use has diminished since discovery of the fact that fluoride ions released during breakdown can contribute to high output renal failure. Accumulation of the ions is both time- and dose-related.

Enflurane (2-chloro-1,1,2-trifluoroethyl difluoromethyl ether) is another sweet-smelling, nonflammable ether anesthetic. Still widely used, it is chemically very stable and does not require a preservative. While it, too, may produce some renal dysfunction by ion accumulation during metabolism, the incidence is significantly less than with methoxyflurane.

Isoflurane (1-chloro-2,2,2-trifluoroethyl difluoromethyl ether) is the newest halogenated ether to be introduced into practice. Its properties are similar to that of enflurane, but induction and recovery periods are slightly shorter.

Halothane. Halothane (2-bromo-2-chloro-1,1,1-trifluoroethane) is another halogenated anesthetic compound, but it is *not* a halogenated ether. Halothane rightfully belongs in the class of halogenated hydrocarbons. It is a saturated compound with a pleasant odor and is still widely used despite its rare implication as a possible cause of hepatic damage. The structural formulas for the commonly used anesthetic agents are grouped together in Figure 6–1. Characteristics of the agents are listed in Table 6–1.

Amines. Amines have the general formula $R-NH_2$ and may be regarded as derivatives of ammonia (NH_3). The functional group is the nitrogen atom. Like alcohols, amines are also divided into primary, secondary, and tertiary forms. A primary amine has one hydrogen of ammonia replaced by an organic radical such as a methyl or ethyl grouping.

In secondary amines, two hydrogens are replaced by organic radicals, while tertiary amines have all hydrogens replaced by a radical. Amines confer hydrophilic properties to a molecule, making it more water soluble. They react chemically with water to form a base and with acids to form ammonium (NH_4) salts. Combined with a benzene ring structure, they become aromatic amines. Many vasopressor drugs used in anesthesia, including phenylephrine, epinephrine, and norepinephrine, have such a structure.

Quaternary Bases. Quaternary bases are formed from ammonium hydroxide (NH_4OH), the hydrogen atoms around the nitrogen being replaced by alkyl radicals. They have bacteriostatic and germicidal properties. More important to anesthesia, they form an essential part of the structure of muscle relaxants, ganglionic blocking agents, and cholinergic compounds. An example is succinylcholine:

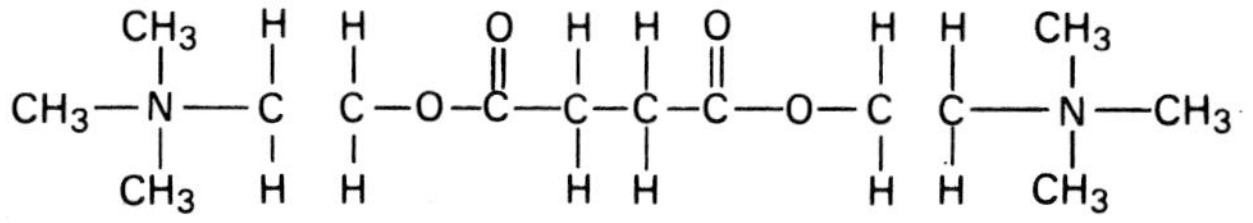

```
    CH3   H  H        O  H  H  O        H  H   CH3
     |    |  |         ||  |  |  ||      |  |    |
CH3-N --- C  C-O-C-C-C-C-O-C  C --- N-CH3
     |    |  |             |  |      |  |    |
    CH3   H  H            H  H      H  H   CH3
```

Amides. Amides are characterized by the functional group

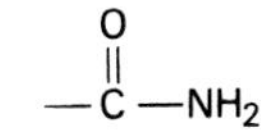

$$\overset{O}{\overset{\|}{-C}}-NH_2$$

sometimes written as $-CONH_2$. They are related to carboxylic acid. Urea, the body's end product of protein metabolism, is the best example. Amides constitute the second main group of local anesthetic compounds. Lidocaine is the most prominent example. Amines and amides are frequently confused. They may be distinguished by remembering that amines retain their hydrogen atoms intact, whereas

TABLE 6–1. CHEMICAL CHARACTERISTICS OF COMMONLY USED ANESTHETIC AGENTS

Characteristic	Halothane	Methoxyflurane	Enflurane	Isoflurane
Molecular weight	197.39	164.97	184.50	184.50
Boiling point (degrees C)	50.30	104.60	56.50	48.50
Specific gravity of liquid	1.86	1.40	1.51	1.50
Specific gravity of vapor	8.86	6.13	6.40	—
Vapor pressure at 20C	243.00	23.00	174.50	238.00
MAC (minimum alveolar concentration)	0.74	0.16	1.68	1.15
Solubility coefficients				
Blood/gas	2.30	13.00	1.91	1.40
Brain/blood	2.60	1.70	1.40	2.60
Muscle/blood	3.50	1.30	1.70	4.00
Fat/blood	60.00	49.00	36.00	45.00
Oil/gas	224.00	890.00	98.50	99.00
Rubber/gas	120.00	630.00	74.00	62.00
Induction concentrations	2.0–3.0%	1.0–1.5%	3.4–4.5%	1.5–3.0%
Maintenance concentrations	0.4–1.5%	0.2–0.5%	1.5–3.0%	1.0–2.5%

amides have the hydrogens surrounding the nitrogen atom replaced by radicals.

Amino Acids. Amino acids contain both an amino group ($-NH_2$) and an acid group ($-COOH$). Proteins are built by combining amino acids; and conversely, hydrolysis splits a protein into its constituent amino acids. The amino group can react with carboxyl groups to form acid amides. This reaction results in the liberation of water and formation of *peptides.* Polypeptides are long chains of cojoined peptides. By these processes, amino acids can be combined and recombined into thousands of protein combinations, each differing in chemical properties. Of the approximately 20 known fundamental amino acids, 10 are essential to life. One of these, alanine, typifies the basic structure of amino acids:

$$CH_3-CH-COOH$$
$$|$$
$$NH_2$$

Because amino acids possess both an acidic and basic group, they act as either. This accounts for their amphoteric nature and allows them to become self-neutralized. When this occurs, a dipolar ion is formed called a zwitterion. Self-neutralization also means that amino acid molecules are themselves electrically neutral. This facilitates their combination with other acids or bases, a trait that allows them to function as a body buffer system.

Besides amines, amides, and amino acids, other nitrogen-containing compounds are possible. Reacting alcohols with *nitrous* acid forms nitroso groups ($-NO_2$). Substituting *nitric* acid results in formation of nitro groups ($-NO_3$). Nitroso compounds are referred to as nitrites, whereas nitro compounds form nitrates. Amyl nitrite exemplifies the former, and glycerol trinitrate (nitroglycerin) typifies the latter. Both have useful medicinal properties as coronary vasodilators.

Nitrogen-containing heterocyclic ring structures form the basis for pyrroles, pyridines, and purines. Pyrroles are one component of hemoglobin, pyridines form part of nicotinic acid and vitamin B, and purines form part of the genetically important RNA and DNA molecules. Other heterocyclic nitrogen-containing compounds are important for formulation of a number of alkaloids encountered in anesthesia practice, including morphine, codeine, cocaine, atropine, quinine, reserpine, and LSD (lysergic acid).

Thio Compounds. Thio compounds occur when oxygen-containing organic molecules have their oxygen replaced by an atom of sulfur—the functional group. This exchange occurs readily because both oxygen and sulfur are within the same periodic table. Sulfur-containing substances are distinguished by a number of terms: thio-, sulfhydryl-, mercapto-, and sulfides. Alcohols, ethers, acids, or amides may all contain sulfur. Thiourea, condensed with malonic acid, helps form the thiobarbiturates. Widely used as anesthesia induction agents, thiobarbiturates are bitter-tasting yellow powders, whose sodium salts are highly alkaline (pH 9 to 11) and soluble in water. A number of these ultra-short-acting barbiturates are used clinically, all derived from the basic barbiturate acid (keto) structure:

Keto form   Enol form

Note: Position numbers of the ring are in parentheses.

1. Hydrogens at (1) and (3) are referred to as imide hydrogens. They confer acidity on the compound. When one or the other or both imide hydrogens are replaced by a methyl or ethyl group, a nitrogen-substituted barbiturate is formed. Such drugs excite the central nervous system.
2. An oxygen at position (2) characterizes oxybarbiturates. Substitution of this oxygen with sulfur forms thiobarbiturates.
3. R_1 and R_2 are aliphatic compounds (one long and one short chain), which confer hypnotic potency to the compound.
4. The migrated hydrogen (*) may be substituted with an alkaline metal (e.g., sodium) to form a salt, making the drug more water-soluble.

The ultra-short-acting thiobarbiturate sodium thiopental (sodium 5-ethyl-5-(1-methylbutyl)-2-thiobarbiturate) best exemplifies the structure of these compounds:

Sodium thiopental

Like other thiobarbiturates, this drug is stable in dry form but subject to decomposition when in solution. Concurrent administration with an acidic drug may cause precipitation. Thiopental is normally used in a 2.5 percent concentration prepared by adding 5 g of powder to 200 ml of diluent. The diluent may be sterile water, sodium chloride, or dextrose solution. Thiopental is the thio analogue of another useful drug, pentobarbital, one of the oxybarbiturates. Although several groups of barbiturates exist, most clinically useful ones are either oxy- or thiobarbiturates.

Two other sulfur-containing groups are medicinally useful: *sulfonamides* and *sulfones.* The former are derived from sulfonic acid (SO_2OH). An acid amide member of this group, sulfanilamide ($-SO_2 NH_2$), was the first systemic antimicrobial drug to gain wide use. Sulfones have the identifying group

Phenolsulfonphthalein dye is a member of this group. It is used to measure the excretory ability of the renal system.

Aromatic   Compounds. Aromatic   hydrocarbons   are formed when six carbon atoms are placed in a ring configuration containing three double bonds attached to alternate carbon atoms. Such double bonds are not the same as those in alkene structures. Rather, they represent oscillating electrons that are dispersed over the entire ring structure. This is often indicated by drawing the structure as a hexagon with an enclosed circle. Benzene (C_6H_6) is the simplest and most characteristic compound of the aromatic hydrocarbons. Its structure is:

often drawn simply as:

In these compounds only one hydrogen is attached to each carbon atom. New compounds are formed by replacing one or more hydrogens with radicals. If only one substitution is made, the position of the radical need not be stated. However, if two or more substitutions are made, some means of distinguishing their locations is necessary. This is done using the terms *ortho, meta,* or *para* isomers. In an *ortho* isomer, the two radicals are attached to adjacent carbon atoms. With a *meta* isomer, the radicals containing carbon atoms are separated by an intervening carbon atom; with *para* isomers there are two intervening carbon atoms. Generally, aromatic compounds are poorly reactive but highly flammable and volatile, their fumes often being toxic. They are also insoluble in water.

Multiple benzene rings can be joined to form *polynuclear aromatic compounds.* Two rings form naphthalene, three rings, anthracene. Another tribenzene ring, in which the third ring is moved out of the horizontal arrangement to an angled position, is called phenanthrene. It forms the basic structure for vitamin D, cholesterol, and sex hormones. Polynuclear aromatic structures are important to the formation of numerous pharmacologic preparations used in medicine. Producing these drugs usually involves converting single or polynuclear aromatic compounds to aromatic radicals. Virtually all the same radicals are possible with aromatic compounds as were possible with straight-chain hydrocarbons. Removing a hydrogen from benzene forms the phenyl radical. Radicals exist only in combination with other radicals or functional groups, never alone. A few of the more pertinent aromatic radicals are reviewed next.

Halogen aromatics are formed by substituting a halogen for a benzene hydrogen. Chlorobenzene is formed by substituting a chloride atom for one of benzene's hydrogens. A more complex structure, hexachlorophene, used as a surgical preparing solution, contains two halogenated benzene rings joined by a methylene group. Both rings also contain an —OH group, which makes them a hydroxy aromatic structure as well.

Hydroxy aromatic compounds are called *phenols,* from the combination of *phenyl* and the *ol* ending of alcohol. As the name implies, they contain both a phenyl and hydroxyl group. Phenol, known also as hydroxybenzene or carbolic acid, was the first widely used antiseptic solution. Though no longer used, it remains the germicide against which all others are compared.

Carboxylic acid derivatives are formed when a benzene hydrogen is replaced by a —COOH grouping. Simplest of these structures is benzoic acid. The aromatic esters are produced in the same manner as other esters, and a number of salicylate compounds are formed from them. The structures for hydroxy and carboxylic acid molecules can be diagrammed as

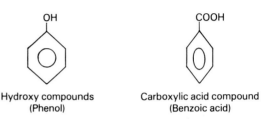

Hydroxy compounds   Carboxylic acid compound
(Phenol)   (Benzoic acid)

As previously mentioned, aromatic nitro compounds, aldehydes, ketones, amines, and amides are also possible. A number of more complex medicinal compounds (e.g., phenacetin) are drawn from these variations, and each group is formed in the same manner as already described for their nonaromatic counterparts.

Two other ring structure types are important in organic chemistry. The first is the heterocyclic compounds, such as the thiobarbiturates, which contain elements other than carbon in the main structure. The second group is the cycloalkanes, ring structures in which each carbon has two hydrogen atoms or radicals attached to each carbon. These differ from benzene in which each ring carbon has only one hydrogen attached and the entire structure shares oscillating electrons. Cyclopropane, the highly unstable and explosive anesthetic agent widely used in past years, typifies the cycloalkanes. (The terms alicyclic compound, cyclic hydrocarbon, and carbocyclic are used interchangeably with cycloalkane.)

There are certain generalizations that can be made regarding the relationship of hydrocarbon structures to their chemical and pharmacologic activity.

1. Volatility, flammability, and water solubility decrease as molecular weight increases. However, the higher the molecular weight, the more likely the substance will split into smaller, lighter compounds.
2. As carbon atoms are added to a saturated hydrocarbon series, pharmacologic potency usually increases and the margin of safety decreases.
3. As molecular weight increases, so too does lipid solubility and the magnitude of the oil/water distribution coefficient.
4. Potency also increases with the degree of unsaturation. Substances containing double or triple bonds are more unstable and therefore more willing to react. The more easily they react, the more potent they are likely to be.
5. Replacing hydrogen atoms with an —OH (hydroxyl) group usually decreases potency.

Most pharmacologic agents have extremely complex structures encompassing multiples of the components discussed in this section. Detailed structures of specific drugs can be obtained from pharmacology texts, but primary groupings presented here should allow identification of a drug's class and major molecular components. Understanding these enables the anesthetist to better judge the clinical effects of drugs and agents.

BIOCHEMISTRY

Introduction. Biochemistry is the branch of science concerned with chemical reactions and substrates necessary to the life of biologic organisms. Biologic substrates can be loosely classed as water, carbohydrates, lipids, proteins and nucleic acids, enzymes, vitamins, and hormones. These help build cell structures for organs and systems. In turn, structure will determine function, enabling muscles to contract, nerves to conduct impulses, etc. In addition, substrates are involved in chemical reactions that provide the organism with energy. Bioenergetic processes allow the body systems to perform work and maintain a homeostatic environment.

The Substrates

Water. Water is the most abundant material constituting living organisms, accounting for 60 percent of total weight in human adults, 80 percent in infants. It serves as a solvent, lubricant, chemical reactant, and coolant for the body. The major portion of body water is chemically bound to cell constituents, but a smaller portion exists as "free" water, mostly in the blood and urine. The chemical properties of water make it the ideal physiologic solvent. It has a high dielectric constant (D = 80.4), which allows it to carry other substances as ions without allowing the substances to combine. Since most nutrients and wastes which enter and leave the body do so as molecules in ionic form, water serves as a transport system. Water's high heat of vaporization (540 cal/g) and high heat capacity allow the body to dissipate or absorb large amounts of heat readily, thus maintaining body temperature within a narrow range. As a conductor of electricity, water facilitates nerve impulse transmission. Its dipolar configuration (see previous material on the chemical properties of water) gives water the capacity for hydrogen bonding. This property is physiologically important because it gives appreciable structure to water and other substances such as proteins. Water is necessary for hydrolysis reactions (reaction of a salt ion with water to form an acid plus a base). This, along with its limited ability to dissociate to H^+ and OH^- ions, allows it to play a role in acid-base balance.

Carbohydrates. Carbohydrates are another substrate. They are produced in plants by the interaction of photosynthesis and light on carbon dioxide and water. The term implies that carbon is attached to water in hydrate form. In reality, the carbon is attached to a number of separate hydrogen and hydroxyl groups. Moreover, an aldehyde or ketone group is often present because sugars are derived from polyhydric alcohols, those containing multiple OH^- groups. All have the general formula CHO, and four classes of sugars exist: mono-, di-, oligo-, and polysaccharides. *Monosaccharides*, the simplest sugars, cannot be further hydrolyzed. They have the formula $C_nH_{2n}O_n$. Simple sugars are further classed as *trioses*, *tetroses*, *pentoses*, or *hexoses* based upon the number of carbon atoms present. Each may also be an aldose or ketose depending upon which functional group it contains. For example, glucose is an *aldose* whereas fructose is a *ketose*. Carbohydrate chemical structures are often drawn in straight-chain form, but such a form cannot account for all of their chemical properties. A cyclic hemiacetyl structure suffices to explain their chemical properties, but diffraction studies using x-ray analysis show them to have a bent-ring configuration resembling a chair. For most discussion purposes, the straight-chain formulation is adequate.

$$
\begin{array}{cc}
\underset{\text{D-glucose}}{
\begin{array}{c}
\text{O} \\
\parallel \\
\text{C}-\text{H} \\
| \\
\text{H}-\text{C}-\text{OH} \\
| \\
\text{OH}-\text{C}-\text{H} \\
| \\
\text{H}-\text{C}-\text{OH} \\
| \\
\text{H}-\text{C}-\text{OH} \\
| \\
\text{CH}_2\text{OH}
\end{array}}
&
\underset{\text{D-fructose}}{
\begin{array}{c}
\text{CH}_2\text{OH} \\
| \\
\text{CO} \\
| \\
\text{HO}-\text{C}-\text{H} \\
| \\
\text{H}-\text{C}-\text{OH} \\
| \\
\text{H}-\text{C}-\text{OH} \\
| \\
\text{CH}_2\text{OH}
\end{array}}
\end{array}
$$

Disaccharides are those sugars that, when hydrolyzed, yield two monosaccharides of either identical or dissimilar configuration. Sometimes included with the *oligosaccharides*, this class includes maltose and sucrose. Oligo-sugars yield two to six simple sugars when hydrolyzed, whereas *polysaccharides* yield more than six. Starches and dextrins are polysaccharides. Along with glycogen, they represent carbohydrates that are normally stored by the body for later use, whereas simple sugars are readily available for energy processes. Oxidation of carbohydrates produces carbon dioxide, water, and energy. The process is discussed later. As may be discernable from the two structures diagrammed earlier, carbohydrates are capable of forming isomers. (See the discussion of isomers in the section on carbon compounds.) Most, but not all, biologically important sugars are dextro isomers. In addition, alpha and beta *anomers* occur when groups attached to the first carbon become rotated in position. Alterations in the positions of hydrogen and hydroxyl groups on carbon atoms 2, 3, or 4 results in *epimers*. Galactose, for example, is an epimer of glucose, the change occurring on the fourth carbon atom.

Of the monosaccharide subclasses, several are biologically important. D-Glyceraldehyde is a triose sugar that results from oxidation of glucose. Ribose and deoxyribose, both pentoses, are important to the structure of RNA and DNA. Hexoses are the physiologically most important simple sugars. This group includes glucose, galactose, and fructose.

Glucose, always present in human blood, is the principle carbohydrate to pass into cells. Once there, it is readily oxidized for energy. Galactose, a glucose isomer, is produced from hydrolysis of milk sugar (lactose). Fructose, obtained from the same foodstuffs as glucose, is often chemically interchangeable with it.

Sucrose, lactose, and maltose are classed as disaccharides. They are isomers of one another. The first, sucrose, is table sugar. When hydrolyzed by the body enzyme sucrase, it breaks down to invert sugar—a mixture of glucose and fructose. Lactose, principle ingredient of breast milk, hydrolyzes to glucose and galactose under the influence of the enzyme lactase. Malt sugar, or maltose, is broken down by maltase to two molecules of glucose.

When a number of monosaccharides are joined together (polymerized), a polysaccharide is formed. Important members of this group are cellulose, starch, and dextrins. Cellulose constitutes the fiber portion of many foods providing the diet with bulk necessary for stimulating intestinal peristalsis. It passes through the body essentially unchanged because it cannot be hydrolyzed by body enzymes. Starch, on the other hand, can be hydrolyzed, first to dextrin, then maltose, and finally glucose. Dextrin is formed by partial hydrolysis of starch. Adhesive tape adheres to the skin because of its dextrin base. Spilling an iodine-based reagent such as povidone-iodine on the tape causes it to turn a blue-black color. The reaction indicates the presence of hydrolyzed starch. Starch is actually a composition of straight and branched structures (amylose and amylopectin). Glycogen resembles amylopectin but is more branched. It is produced in the liver and stored both there and in muscle. As blood glucose level is depleted by exercise, the glucose is replenished by hydrolysis of glycogen. This process helps the body maintain a constant blood sugar level of narrow range.

Polysaccharides contribute to tissue structure. The *mucopolysaccharides* or glucosaminoglycans are an example. They consist of amino sugars and uronic acids and help build skin, bones, and other tissues. One mucopolysaccharide of particular importance to anesthetists during surgery is the anticoagulant heparin. Heparin is composed of two compounds derived from glucose—glucuronic acid and glucosamine. Dextran, a plasma substitute sometimes used to treat severe hypovolemic shock, is a high-molecular-weight polysaccharide compound. *Glycoproteins* (mucoproteins) combine protein and polysaccharide structures. They contribute to the composition of mucous secretions and plasma alpha-globulins. The substances (isoagglutinogens) of red blood cells responsible for determining blood type and pituitary hormones (like luteinizing hormone and human chorionic gonadotropin) also have glycoproteins in their composition. Glycoproteins, along with glycolipids, contribute to the structure of cell membranes.

Sugars that can be easily oxidized by Benedict's or Fehling's solutions or Tollen's reagent are known as reducing sugars. All mono and disaccharide sugars except sucrose have this property because they contain an easily oxidized aldehyde group. The CH_2OH group in sugars can also be oxidized, either alone or with the aldehyde group. The latter produces a carboxyl group. It is also possible for the hydroxyl group to react with acids to produce esters. This occurs with phosphoric acid, the esters of which, when hydrolyzed, produce high-energy bonds for bioenergetics. Oxidation facilitates conversion of chemical energy within

sugars to other forms more easily stored or utilized by cells to perform work.

Lipids. *Lipids* are related to fatty acids and have two distinguishing properties; they are (1) relatively insoluble in water and (2) easily soluble in nonpolar solvents. All are greasy to the touch and have a glistening appearance. Fats, oils, and waxes are included in the class. Having a specific gravity less than one, they float on water. Dissolving lipids in water forms an emulsion, which separates into layers on standing. Like carbohydrates, they are composed of carbon, oxygen, and hydrogen but may also contain nitrogen and phosphorus. Lipids are the major constituent of adipose tissue. Colorless, odorless, and tasteless, lipids perform a multiplicity of functions for the body, acting as sources of energy and as insulation and protection for organs and the body as a whole. Ingested lipids are emulsified by bile in the intestines and carried in that form to body cells.

Hydrolysis of fats produces fatty acids normally containing an even number of carbon atoms and having a straight-chain configuration. *Saturated fats* contain no double bonds whereas *unsaturated fats* contain one or more such bonds. Under the Geneva system, fatty acids are named by substituting *-oic* for the final *e* in the name of the hydrocarbon containing the same number of carbon atoms. Saturated acids thus end in *anoic* while unsaturated ones end in *enoic*. An eight-carbon fatty acid would be named octanoic—derived from octane. Carbon atoms are numbered from the carbon that helps form the carboxyl group. Superscripts are used with unsaturated lipids to indicate the number of carbons, number of double bonds, and their position, e.g. $C^{20:1;10}$.

Lipids are classed on the basis of their solubility and their hydrolysis products. *Simple lipids* are esters formed by reacting fatty acids with alcohols. Those that contain another group in addition to the ester are termed *compound lipids*. Two specialized groups in this class are the *phospholipids*—containing a fatty acid, alcohol, and phosphoric acid residue—and *cerebrosides*, which contain fatty acids, carbohydrates, and nitrogen, but no phosphoric acid. Lipoproteins are also a compound lipid. Derived lipids or fatty acids are formed by hydrolyzing the other groups. Glycerols, sterols, aldehydes, and ketone bodies are included in this category.

Acetic acid (vinegar, CH_3COOH) is the fatty acid forming the basis for the *saturated series* of lipids. They have the general formula $C_nH_{2n+1}COOH$. Acetic acid's structure is

$$\begin{array}{c} O \\ \| \\ C-OH \\ | \\ H-C-H \\ | \\ H \end{array}$$

Propionic, butyric, and caproic acids are also important saturated fatty acids. Respectively, their formulas are C_2H_5COOH, C_3H_7COOH, and $C_5H_{11}COOH$. Palmitic, stearic, and arachidic fatty acids have dietary importance, and lignoceric acid is important to the structure of brain and nervous tissues.

In addition *unsaturated* fatty acids are classed on the

basis of their degree of unsaturation. *Monounsaturated* acids have the general formula: $C_nH_{2n-3}COOH$. Oleic acid is an example of this group. It is found in nearly all fats. *Polyunsaturates* can have two or more double bonds. Linoleic, linolenic, and arachidonic acids have, respectively, two, three, and four double bonds. Prostaglandins, compounds that exert a number of physiologic effects on blood vessels, muscles, and other tissues, are derived from arachidonic acid. Unsaturated fatty acids may have a number of geometric isomers.

The alcohols in more complex lipid structures include glycerol and cholesterol. Triacylglycerols, more commonly known as *triglycerides* or neutral fats, are esters formed from glycerol and fatty acids. Hydrolysis splits the triglycerides to the alcohol and fatty acid that formed them. Neutral fats can be oxidized for energy, and most body cells except the brain can use broken-down triglycerides interchangeably with glucose for energy. Breakdown of fatty acids occurs in cell mitochondria by a process termed *beta oxidation*. The acid is first combined with coenzyme A (CoA) (discussed in the section on enzymes) to form a molecule known as fatty acyl-CoA. This process is energized by the degradation of adenosine triphosphate (ATP) to adenosine monophosphate (AMP) with concurrent loss of two high-energy phosphate bonds. The second step of the process involves removal of two hydrogen atoms from carbons of the fatty acyl-CoA, leaving a residual double bond. The hydrogens are joined to FAD (flavin adenine dinucleotide) and are later oxidized. The remaining double bond joins with water so that one hydrogen attaches to one carbon and a hydroxyl radical attaches to the other carbon. Next, two more hydrogen atoms are removed by NAD (nicotinamide adenine dinucleotide), which combines with one hydrogen and the hydrogen from the hydroxyl group. The two removed hydrogens are later oxidized. The process breaks the alpha and beta carbons of the compound to form a long and short chain. The long chain combines with new CoA and the process is repeated from step two onward. The short chain is really acetyl-CoA since it remains bound to the original coenzyme A that started the process. The entire process is repeated over and over again until the entire fatty acid has been converted to acetyl-CoA.

In turn, some acetyl-CoA combines with oxaloacetic acid and joins in the citric acid cycle, a process discussed later. Those molecules that do not, pair and condense to form molecules of acetoacetic acid. This acid is then converted to beta-hydroxybutyric acid and lesser amounts of acetone. Small amounts of hydroxybutyric acid and acetone are always present in the blood, but their accumulation can cause a condition known as *ketosis*. Acetoacetic acid is a keto acid; it and beta-hydroxybutyric acid and acetone are known as ketone bodies. Ketosis occurs with starvation and certain diseases that derange metabolism (e.g., diabetes mellitus). Carbohydrates and proteins can also be converted to acetyl-CoA and in turn be built into triglycerides, thus adding to stored body fats.

Along with hydrolysis (reacting lipids in the presence of catalytic enzymes to produce glycerol and fatty acids) lipids may be split by *saponification*—a process that involves splitting a glyceride with a base, such as sodium hydroxide, to produce glycerol and the salt of a fatty acid. This process

is not important physiologically but is used in making soaps. Volatile fatty acids often turn rancid and develop a foul odor. The process is like the one that converts lipids to body energy, that is, hydrolysis of the ester followed by oxidation to aldehydes and ketones, which are then acted upon by bacteria to produce butyric acid.

The *iodine number* of a lipid substance indicates the degree of unsaturation. A high number indicates a high degree of unsaturation and vice versa. Hydrogenation is the process of adding hydrogen atoms to unsaturated lipids to produce saturated compounds.

Phospholipids include phosphatidic acid, phosphatidylglycerols, phosphatidylcholine, phosphatidylethanolamine, phosphatidylinositol, phosphatidylserine, lysophospholipids, plasmalogens, and sphingomyelins. The first is an important intermediate in triglyceride production. The second helps form cardiolipin, a phospholipid found in mitochondria. The third, phosphatidylcholine, also known as lecithin, is widely dispersed throughout the body and has both metabolic and structural functions; e.g., dipalmityl lecithin is a surface-active agent responsible for alveolar surface tension; its destruction results in respiratory disease. Cephalins, formed from ethanolamine phospholipids, are similar to the lecithins. Plasmalogens also resemble lecithins and cephalins. They constitute as much as a tenth of the phospholipids found in brain and muscle. Sphingomyelins are also found in large quantities in the brain and other parts of the nervous system.

Cerebrosides, or glycolipids, contain a combination of galactose and sphingosine (derived from the amino acid serine). They are therefore often grouped with sphingomyelins as sphingolipids. Found in large quantities in the brain and nervous system, especially in medullated nerve fibers, they are also present in the spleen and other reticuloendothelial tissues. Upon hydrolysis, many phospholipids produce phosphoric acid and a nitrogen-containing compound.

Steroids are often found in association with fats. All are formed from a cyclic nucleus similar to that of phenanthrene. (See the section on organic chemistry.) Like other compounds previously mentioned, they, too, are capable of forming a number of isomers. Steroids that contain at least one hydroxyl group and no carbonyl or carboxyl groups are called sterols. One, cholesterol, has been implicated in cardiovascular disease and the development of gallstones. Steroids help form a number of biologically important substances including sex hormones, vitamin D, adrenocortical hormones, and the bile acids (cholic acid). In addition, cardiac glycosides and some alkaloid drugs may also contain steroidal structures.

Lipids are insoluble in water because they contain a large number of nonpolar hydrocarbon groups. Those lipids that do contain some polar groups (e.g., sphingolipids, phospholipids, and fatty acids) may be partly soluble. At oil-water interfaces these molecules will become oriented in a particular direction. Polar groups will orient to the water, nonpolar to the lipid. Cell membranes are considered to consist of a bilayer of such polar lipids. Aggregation of these polar groups containing lipids in a highly aqueous medium causes formation of micelles—groups of molecules that orient their polar sides to the water, thus forming a ball-like arrangement. The nonpolar portion of the molecules become pointed in toward the center of the ball. Larger micelles arrange themselves in the same manner but are usually stabilized by emulsifying agents, which help form a surface layer that separates the aqueous phase from the nonpolar ends of the molecules. Danielli and Davson (1935) proposed that cell membranes were composed of lipid bilayers sandwiched between proteins. Later, this description was modified to include protein "pores" embedded in the bilayer. Singer and Nicolson (1972) proposed that the entire structure constituted a fluid mosaic capable of temporary restructuring to allow for entry of drugs and other substances. This fit in well with the earlier observation of Overton (circa 1900) that many compounds penetrated cells on the basis of their lipid solubility rather than molecular size. Current thinking postulates that anesthetics may work by temporarily, and reversibly, disrupting bimolecular lipoprotein cell membranes. Several recent experiments support this view, but it remains unclear whether anesthesia is produced by membrane disruption only, or as a result of yet undiscovered intracellular processes, or by a combination of mechanisms. Other theories of narcosis have been advanced, but the one described appears the best model, based on current evidence.

Proteins and Nucleic Acids. Proteins and nucleic acids are the next important groups of substrates. Both are important for forming protoplasm, building new body tissues, and repairing damaged tissues. Protein buffer systems act to maintain normal pH in cells, body fluids, and lymph. They also help maintain water balance between those tissues. Proteins provide amino acids for synthesis of new nitrogen-containing compounds and can furnish energy stores when both carbohydrate and lipid mechanisms are depleted or fail to function. They also supply ingredients for building enzymes, hormones, and oxygen-carrying hemoglobin.

Proteins are large molecules built by polymerization of various combinations of the 21 known amino acids. Generally, they contain carbon, hydrogen, oxygen, nitrogen, and sulfur. In amino acids, the amino group (NH_2) is attached to the carbon atom of the first CH_2 group that in turn is attached to the —COOH group. Those amino acids the body can synthesize only to a slight extent or not at all are referred to as essential amino acids. The remainder are termed nonessential. The simplest amino acid is glycine. Its structure is

$$H-\underset{\underset{NH_2}{|}}{\overset{\overset{H}{|}}{C}}-COOH$$

Nonessential amino acids include alanine, aspargine, aspartic acid, cysteine, cystine, glutamic acid, glutamine, glycine, proline, serine, and tyrosine. The essential group includes arginine, histidine, isoleucine, leucine, lysine, methionine, phenylalanine, threonine, tryptophan, and valine. Like the simplest sugars, all amino acids except glycine contain an asymmetric carbon and thus polarize light so that isomers could exist. However, all naturally occurring ones have the same L- configuration, comparable with D-glyceralde-

hyde. Serine has been shown to be convertible to L-glyceraldehyde; therefore, other amino acids are referenced to serine, e.g., L_s−leucine. A plus or minus sign is used to indicate the plane in which the light is polarized.

Conjugated proteins consist of both protein and nonprotein substructures. The latter are termed *nucleic acids*. Nucleic acids are polymers of *nucleotides*, low-molecular-weight molecules that participate in a number of biochemical reactions. Nucleotides are composed of a nucleoside and phosphate (H_3PO_4). *Nucleosides* are made up of a pentose sugar (either ribose or deoxyribose) and a purine or pyrimidine ring. Cytosine, uracil, and thymine are the main pyrimidine rings used, while adenine and guanine are the usually encountered purine rings. Nucleotides serve as precursors for ribonucleic acid (RNA) and deoxyribonucleic acid (DNA). In addition, purine ribonucleotides participate in high-energy and messenger mechanisms in the body. ATP is an example of the former, whereas AMP exemplifies the latter. They are also components of some coenzymes. The pyrimidine nucleotides play a role as high-energy intermediates in carbohydrate metabolism.

Proteins may be classed as simple and conjugated. *Simple proteins* produce only alpha-amino acids when hydrolyzed. They include albumins, globulins, globins, and albuminoids (scleroproteins). *Conjugated proteins* hydrolyze to other amino acid types and include phosphoproteins, glycoproteins, chromoproteins, and nucleoproteins. Proteins may also be classed according to structure (see the next paragraph) or functionally as structural proteins, enzymes, hormones, antibodies, blood proteins, or contractile proteins. This latter group includes actin and myosin, which allow muscles to contract. Since proteins are composed of amino acids, it is not surprising that their chemistry is essentially that of amino acids. As pointed out earlier, amino acids contain both an amino group, which is basic, and an acid carboxyl group. They can therefore act as either acids or bases and for this reason are said to have an amphoteric nature. Building of proteins from amino acids involves combining the amino group of one molecule with the carboxyl group of another. When two amino acids are combined in this way, a molecule of water is lost, and the two amino acids become a dipeptide. As additional molecules are added, the structure becomes a tripeptide or polypeptide. The *peptide linkage* (—CO—NH—) is also known as the amide grouping. As each amino acid is added, another peptide bond is formed. If the amino acid contains sulfur, as does cysteine, there may be an oxidation reaction between two cysteine residues, which produces a cystine residue and water. This is known as a *disulfide bond*. Another bond found in amino acid structures is known as a *salt bridge*. This type occurs when the ionic bond between an acid group and a base, or amino, group forms a salt. *Hydrogen bonds* may form between hydrogen and either carbonyl oxygen or nitrogen atoms within a protein structure. These may occur within the main chain as well as in side chains. Electrostatic bonds are those that form between salt bonds of opposite electrical charges. Of the various types of bonds that may occur, peptide bonds are the strongest.

From a biochemical viewpoint, proteins may have four structures, referred to as primary, secondary, tertiary, and quaternary. Primary structures show the amino-acid/peptide-bond chain in ordered sequence with radical groups running to the sides of the chain. Secondary types depend on hydrogen bonding within the molecule and may take one of two forms: a coil-shaped helical arrangement or a pleated sheet in which hydrogen bonds exist between chains. Tertiary structures occur when the protein molecule is folded on itself and held together by various types of bonds. Fibrous collagen tissue is an example. Quaternary structures are formed by bringing the protein's chains together. In hemoglobin, four chains are held together by various bonds giving the molecule an overall convoluted appearance.

Hemoglobin has two pairs of chains, alpha and beta. The first pair has 141 amino acids per chain, the second pair 146 each. Each chain also contains a heme group. Sequence of the amino acids on each chain is genetically determined. Hemoglobin's function is to transport oxygen necessary for respiration. This is accomplished by hemoglobin altering its structure in such a manner as to envelop the oxygen. When the oxygen is released to the tissues, the hemoglobin returns to its original form. Such conformational alterations of structure are characteristic of proteins.

Proteins are high-molecular-weight compounds, sometimes exceeding a molecular weight of 1,000,000. Most are water-soluble, though they tend to form colloidal solutions rather than a true solution. Their size and number enable them to exert considerable osmotic effect. However, they do not traverse membranes well, which accounts for the fact that proteins are not normally recoverable in urine.

Because they can carry electrical charges, proteins readily interact with other charged substances. Although peptide chains bind up the greater portion of amino and carboxyl groups, the presence of these groups on side chains means that they will ionize in solution and carry a net charge, which varies with the pH of the solution. At one specific pH point, the *isoelectric point*, all charges are balanced. The protein will not travel to either the cathode or the anode because its electric charge is equal to zero. (See Chapter 7.) To either side of the isoelectric point, the protein will migrate to one or the other pole depending upon its electrical charge. This property is useful for separating proteins from one another by electrophoresis, as in the diagnosis of sickle cell disease, where any abnormal hemoglobin will have a different isoelectric point from normal hemoglobin.

Proteins may be broken down or destroyed by a number of processes. Within the body, chemical hydrolysis is facilitated by the presence of enzymes called proteases. The resulting amino acids can be recombined into new proteins. Proteins may also be destroyed by heat and other sterilizing processes. This principle is used in destroying bacteria protein to kill microorganisms and to render items sterile for surgical use. The process is called *denaturation* and consists of physical disruption of the protein's helical structure by disruption of the weak bonds linking various protein chain sections together. This disruption causes the protein to coagulate. Only the weak bonds, not the peptide ones, are broken. Nonetheless, the protein is effectively destroyed. Certain chemicals may also denature proteins. Examples include an alkaloid, tannic acid, which has been used to cauterize bleeding tissues. Other examples are alcohols—

used as disinfectants—and heavy metals, which cause poisoning by destroying tissue proteins. Strong acids and bases also denature proteins.

The body is incapable of storing proteins and has only a limited capability for building them. Essential amino acids cannot be provided by the body itself and must be provided exogenously by dietary intake. Postsurgery, protein supplements may be useful in hastening tissue healing and recovery. When patients must remain fasting for prolonged periods of time, supplemental proteins may be given parenterally in solutions that contain amino acids, trace minerals, and other supplements.

Protein metabolism results in salvage of any purine-based structures, which can then be used for rebuilding, but pyrimidine-based structures are degraded to urea and ammonia. Diseases that upset protein metabolism can result in elevated blood urea levels, tissue wasting, and other detrimental changes.

Other Substrates: Enzymes, Vitamins, and Hormones.
Enzymes, vitamins, and hormones are three additional substrates necessary for biochemical reactions.

Enzymes. Enzymes function as catalysts for a variety of chemical activities. As catalysts, they reduce the amount of energy required to initiate or sustain a reaction but are themselves not part of it. Enzyme facilitation of reactions is very specific. Proteases act only on proteins, not on carbohydrates or lipids. Each enzyme has two constituents: a protein portion called the *apoenzyme* and a nonprotein portion termed the *coenzyme*. Enzymes fall into six categories. Those that facilitate oxidation-reduction reactions are called oxidoreductases. Transferases move chemical groups between molecules. Hydrolases catalyze reactions between substrates and water. Lysases help form double bonds, and isomerases facilitate production of isomers. Ligases break molecular couplings.

The important coenzymes include adenosine mono-, di-, and triphosphate (AMP, ADP, and ATP), cyclic adenosine monophosphate (3', 5'-cyclic AMP, often abbreviated cAMP), nicotinamide adenine dinucleotide with and without phosphate (NAD^+ and $NADP^+$), flavin adenine dinucleotide (FAD), and coenzyme A (CoA). Coenzymes are all involved in transfer reactions and may be functionally classed into those that transfer hydrogen (NAD^+ and $NADP^+$) and those that transfer other groups (ATP and associated compounds). Most contain an adenine ring coupled to a ribose sugar and phosphate. This gives them a strong resemblence to AMP. They differ only in the attached radical group.

Enzymes are important in electron transport and phosphate bond energy mechanisms. They are named by using the substrate name followed by the type of reaction catalyzed, e.g., cytochrome c: O_2 oxido-reductase (cytochrome c oxidase). The suffix -ase identifies enzymes. Interestingly, enzyme activity is temperature-dependent, optimum temperature being that found at cellular level. Enzyme action may also be altered by changes in pH. Enzyme activity can be diminished or blocked altogether by inhibitors, of which there are two types: competitive and noncompetitive. Competitive inhibitors are so named because they compete with substrates. Generally, they have a similar chemical configuration. Noncompetitive inhibitors disable the enzyme by reacting with one or more of its functional groups. For example, cyanide binds iron to render cytochrome c oxidase ineffective. Some enzymes, such as serum glutamic-pyruvic transaminase (SGPT) and serum glutamic-oxalo-acetic transaminase (SGOT), can be diagnostic for disease states, often indicating liver or heart muscle damage. A few diseases, phenylketonuria (PKU) for instance, are caused by hereditary enzyme disorders.

Vitamins. Vitamins are important in regulating a number of biochemical reactions. They also serve as essential components of many, though not all, coenzymes. All are classed as either water- or fat-soluble. Fat-soluble vitamins are associated with lipids found in natural foods and include vitamins A, D, E, and K. Vitamin C and all B-complex members constitute the water-soluble group.

Recognition that particular foods possessed essential nutrients necessary for disease prevention came well before chemical identification of vitamin compounds. For this reason, vitamins have common names based on the alphabet—vitamins A, B, C, D, etc. Each differs substantially in chemical structure, but all play a role in normal growth and health. Vitamins can be prepared in pure form by pharmaceutical companies, but an average balanced diet generally supplies all recommended daily allowances. Some vitamins have species-specific effects; and lack of even minute amounts of a particular vitamin can sometimes make a life-or-death difference to the organism. Fortunately, severe deficiencies in humans are rare and often easily correctable. When they do occur, they produce symptoms deleterious to optimum health. For example, lack of vitamin C alters formation of collagen-based connective tissues. This results in bleeding gums, loss of teeth, and other pathologic changes. Like essential amino acids, vitamins cannot be synthesized by the body. They must therefore be provided in the diet. Even today, many of their exact functions are not entirely clear. The following briefly summarizes the important points to be noted about each vitamin.

Vitamin A (retinal) is derived from beta-carotene, a plant pigment, which serves as a provitamin. The vitamin plays a role in maintaining epithelial tissue. Ocular tissues are especially susceptible to damage if the vitamin is lacking from the diet. This is because light striking the eye causes a splitting of the eye pigment rhodopsin (visual purple) to a protein portion called opsin and the nonprotein retinal. Retinal is also called vitamin A_1 aldehyde or retinene. The light further decomposes the aldehyde to an alcohol, retinol. Then the enzyme, retinene reductase, with NAD acting as coenzyme, causes regeneration of retinal from retinol and, under conditions of darkness, new rhodopsin is formed. Lack of vitamin A retards this regeneration and a prolonged deficiency can result in night blindness or keratinization of the ocular tissues. Keratinization can, over time, result in permanent blindness. Lack of vitamin A also causes a number of other toxic effects, including decreased skeletal and soft-tissue growth, damage to the brain and spinal cord, altered collagen formation, decreased mucopolysaccharide production, changes in cell membrane stability, and disturbances of liver cell mitochondria. Excess

vitamin A intake can present problems as well. These include periosteal thickening of long bones, loss of hair, and painful joints. Zinc may play a role in maintaining plasma levels of the vitamin. Intestinal diseases such as sprue and dysentary decrease the amount of vitamin A absorbed by the body.

Vitamin D is, in reality, a group of sterol compounds. Some are provitamins. Under the influence of ultraviolet light, they undergo changes that help prevent rickets, a disease characterized by skeletal malformations and decreased bone calcification. The two most important members of the vitamin D group are ergocalciferol (D_2) and activated 7-dehydrocholesterol, also known as cholecalciferol or vitamin D_3. The latter can be synthesized and activated in humans through the action of sunlight. The reaction takes place in the skin. The main functions of vitamin D are to increase absorption of calcium and phosphorus by the intestines and to maintain phosphate regulation in the kidney. Cholecalciferol must first be converted to 1,25-dihydroxycholecalciferol to be metabolically active. This compound enables vitamin D to exert a major impact on calcium mobilization from storage sites in bone. Conversion takes place because of a number of chemical reactions in both the liver and kidneys. Apart from its effects on bone development and calcium absorption and mobilization, vitamin D plays a role in formation of messenger-RNA and protein biosynthesis. Excess intake produces hypercalcemia and nephrocalcinosis (renal stone formation).

Vitamin E is derived from tocopherols and tocotrienols in plant oils. The principle ingredient, alpha-tocopherol, is present in many foods, but its absorption from the intestines is decreased in malabsorption syndromes, especially those involving lipids. Premature infants are susceptible to increased hemolysis, preventable by vitamin E administration. In adults, deficiency often occurs with a concurrent decrease in polyunsaturated fatty acid intake. Macrocytic anemia and decreased survival time of erythrocytes results. Low-birth-weight infants fed vitamin-E-deficient formulas develop a syndrome characterized by anemia, thrombosis, edema, and reticulocytosis. Exogenous vitamin E therapy prevents the syndrome. The most important chemical role for vitamin E in the body is as an antioxidant. Since polyunsaturated fatty acids easily react with molecular oxygen to form peroxides, it is beneficial that the vitamin prevents their toxic accumulation in tissues. By the same mechanism, it may also prevent lung damage associated with oxidant-containing atmospheres, such as smog. Other antioxidant biologic properties of the vitamin are being discovered. Vitamin E's properties possibly depend upon the presence of selenium. Selenium is an essential component of the enzyme glutathione peroxidase, which scavenges hydroperoxides and converts them to primary and secondary alcohols. The vitamin exhibits notable species specificity. Tocopherol deficiency produces infertility in rats, muscular dystrophy in guinea pigs, and vascular degeneration in chickens. No comparable changes have been proven to occur in humans.

Vitamin K's primary physiologic function is to catalyze synthesis of prothrombin by the liver. Its absence causes development of hypoprothrombinemia and prolonged blood-clotting times. For vitamin K to be effective, it is necessary that liver parenchymal tissues be intact and functioning. No effect occurs when the liver has been damaged by cirrhosis or tumor. Its action is also blocked by agents such as dicumarol. (Conversely, bleeding caused by overtreatment with the anticoagulant dicumarol can be treated with vitamin K.) Prothrombin formation and clotting factors VII, IX, and X are all, to some extent, controlled by the presence of the vitamin. One of its two variations, K_1, may play a role in oxidative phosphorylation within mitochondria of tissue cells, though this has not been conclusively proven. Coenzyme Q, important in electron transport and oxidative phosphorylation, is similar in chemical structure to vitamin K and has been observed to exert many of the same effects.

Vitamin K deficiency is very unlikely, given its wide distribution in food and the fact that intestinal microorganisms are capable of producing it. In theory, prolonged fasting combined with administration of agents that destroy intestinal flora could produce a deficiency state. A somewhat analogous situation occurs in newborns where the sterility of the intestines predisposes to hypoprothrombinemia for several days until bacterial flora start producing the vitamin. For this reason, vitamin K may be administered prophylactically at the time of birth to prevent development of hypoprothrombinemia-induced hemorrhage within vital organs. Anesthetists should be aware of this and other aspects of vitamin K therapy. One such aspect is that, like dicumarol, salicylates antagonize the vitamin's effects. Another is that the vitamin is sometimes used in treatment of uncontrolled bleeding at surgery. This may be especially true for surgery of the biliary tract because normal absorption of the vitamin is dependent upon bile, and resection of the intestine may alter its bacterial production, even into the postoperative period. In such situations, treatment with water-soluble preparations of the vitamin may be preferred.

Vitamin C, first of the water-soluble vitamins to be discussed, is called ascorbic acid. Its biochemical function is not yet entirely clear. It is known to play a role in maintaining teeth, cartilage, bone, and collagen synthesis. In addition, there are postulated nonspecific roles in oxidation-reduction systems and in metabolism of tyrosine, drugs, and adrenal steroids. It is found in large amounts in the adrenal cortex, where levels are quickly depleted by adrenocorticotropic hormone (ACTH) stimulation. Infectious processes increase the rapidity with which the vitamin is lost. On this basis, it has been suggested that vitamin C may have a role in stress reactions. Ascorbic acid is available in a number of foods, notably citrus fruits, but it is easily destroyed by cooking or oxidation. It is stored throughout the body in amounts corresponding to the metabolic activity of the tissues.

The *B vitamins* include thiamine (B_1), riboflavin (B_2), niacin, pyridoxine (B_6), pantothenic acid, lipoic acid, biotin (also known as vitamin H), inositol, *para*-aminobenzoic acid, cyanocobalamin (B_{12}), and the folic acid group.

Thiamine acts as coenzyme in a number of systems including the oxidative pathway for glucose. Lack of this vitamin impacts on cardiovascular, gastrointestinal, and peripheral nervous systems. Though it is readily absorbed by the body, it cannot be stored to any appreciable extent. The amount available to the body depends on overall dietary intake of fats, carbohydrates, and proteins. It has been used to treat various neuritic conditions.

Riboflavin occurs naturally as a coenzyme with two flavoproteins: flavin mononucleotide (FMN) and flavin adenine dinucleotide (FAD). Both are involved in hydrogen transport. Riboflavin is combined with phosphate prior to its absorption. This occurs in intestinal mucosa. Phosphate activates the compound to enable it to participate in oxidation-reduction reactions. Deficiencies in humans are rare, and symptoms are similar to those of niacin deficiency.

Niacin helps form nicotinamide nucleotide coenzymes such as NAD^+ or the phosphate form $NADP^+$. Deficiency causes pellagra, whose symptoms include dermatitis, cheilosis (fissuring of the lips), and a dark-red tongue. Niacin compounds serve as coenzymes for dehydrogenases and are involved in oxidation-reduction reactions. However, these reactions are not decreased when the vitamin is lacking. Niacin, or nicotinic acid, can be synthesized in small quantities from the amino acid tryptophan.

Pyridoxine is not, of itself, an extremely potent vitamin, but it can be readily converted to two other more active forms: pyridoxal phosphate and pyridoxamine phosphate. All three are generally present in any natural food containing vitamin B_6. Pyridoxal phosphate is involved with enzymes that decarboxylate or dehydrate amino acids and those involved in transamination. It is also involved in some transulfuration reactions. Vitamin B_6 is required for growth and maturation. Deficiency produces a hypochromic, microcytic anemia, which can be reversed with treatment. Infants and pregnant women are most prone to severe deficiency, which may produce a convulsive disorder. This fact, along with other recent evidence, points to a role for pyridoxine in maintaining the integrity of the central nervous system. Demyelination and axonal degeneration of nerves has been demonstrated in animals. Other evidence points to a possible influence on gamma-aminobutyric acid (GABA). This substance, found in brain gray matter, seems to exert some control over both central and peripheral neuronal activity.

Pantothenic acid is a constituent of CoA. The A, which stands for acetyl, indicates that the coenzyme is involved in acetylation reactions by contributing the acyl group. These reactions normally involve fatty acid oxidation or synthesis. Deficiency in humans has not been demonstrated, but in animals it produces a number of symptoms including alopecia, gastritis, and skin conditions. Acetyl-coA is formed from oxidation of pyruvate or fatty acids. A major function of acetyl-CoA is to join with oxaloacetic acid to form citric acid, which initiates the citric acid cycle. Another reaction important to anesthetists is the enzymatic reaction with compounds that are acyl-group receptors, such as choline. The two join to form acetylcholine. This reaction also forms CoA-SH, a thio compound capable of providing high-energy bonds much like high-energy phosphate bonds.

Lipoic acid is involved in a number of oxidative decarboxylation reactions, such as for pyruvic acid. In general it functions much like other vitamins involved in the same reactions (e.g., thiamine, riboflavin, etc.). Deficiency is unknown and the vitamin plays no outstanding biochemical role.

Biotin functions in carboxylation reactions, attaching and translocating carbon dioxide. It possibly plays a role in purine synthesis and may influence other enzymes, especially deaminases.

Folic acid is composed of three parts: glutamic acid, *para*-aminobenzoic acid, and a pteridine nucleus. Variations in the number of glutamic acid structures produces three chemically related substances. All are termed pteroyl glutamates. These coenzymes are primarily involved in reactions requiring transfer or utilization of single-carbon groups. Indirectly, they influence synthesis of purines and other compounds and may play a role in cell development. Folic acid deficiency is rare. It seems to induce changes in red cell production and anemia, but these changes are more likely due to concomitant deficiencies of other vitamins. Folic acid can be antagonized by some substances, notably antimetabolites like methotrexate.

Inositol has nine isomers, but only one exerts biologic activity and its importance has not been established.

Para-aminobenzoic acid's prime role is as a member of the folic acid molecule, which has already been discussed.

Vitamin B$_{12}$ has a unique chemical configuration. Consisting of four reduced and substituted pyrrole rings surrounding a cobalt atom, it somewhat resembles the porphyrins. Attached to the cobalt atom is a cyanide group. For this reason, vitamin B$_{12}$ is also known as cyanocobalamin. The cyano- portion may be removed or substituted to form other compounds. Absorption of B$_{12}$ occurs in the ileum, a process that depends on the presence of hydrochloric acid and a substance called intrinsic factor (IF). Prevention of pernicious anemia is dependent upon the presence of both IF and B$_{12}$. The vitamin is sometimes called extrinsic factor. Pernicious anemia is characterized by a macrocytic anemia and neurologic symptoms. Though important for nucleic acid formation, the vitamin's major impact is on the hematopoietic system.

Hormones. Hormones act as chemical messengers for the body and thus augment neuronal pathways in providing integration of bodily functions. They may be produced by either exocrine glands, which secrete into ducts, or by endocrine organs, which secrete the hormone directly into the blood, which then transports it to the target organ. In some respects, hormones resemble both enzymes and vitamins. Like enzymes, they catalyze chemical reactions without participating in them. They are like vitamins in that minute amounts can exert profound effects on the growth, development, and survival of the organism.

Chemically hormones may be proteins, polypeptides, amino acids, or steroids. Protein hormones are associated with the pituitary and parathyroid glands, and with the pancreas, whereas thyroid and adrenal gland medullary hormones are mainly amino acids. Hormones associated with the ovaries, testes, and adrenal cortex are steroidal in nature. Hormone secretion is often an autoregulated process involving feedback mechanisms. Some hormones also require conversion to more active forms to exert their effects. The liver and kidneys are the most common sites of degradation. Hormones can change the synthesis rate of enzymes and proteins, alter the catalytic rates of enzymes, and render cell membranes more permeable. They thus influence cellular membrane transport, protein synthesis, and enzyme and coenzyme activity.

Cyclic adenosine 3',5'-monophosphate (cAMP) is an important mediator of hormonal action. It is sometimes called the second messenger for this reason. cAMP is synthesized from ATP by the action of adenyl cyclase, and it is destroyed by hydrolysis to AMP. The hydrolysis reaction is caused by the action of phosphodiesterase.

Target organs of nonsteroidal hormones usually have receptors on the plasma membrane of their cells. The hormone, also called the first messenger, never enters the cell. Instead, it binds with the receptor to stimulate adenyl cyclase, which is also present in the membrane. The adenyl cyclase activity increases the amount of cAMP within the cell, enabling it to change the rate of one or more reactions within the cell, thus providing the terminal effect of the originally secreted hormone.

Receptor sites are quite specific so that only one hormone is capable of initiating a particular second messenger effect. Receptors of different target organs can be triggered by the same hormone. However, each organ will respond differently because internal second messenger effects will vary with the target organ. Phosphodiesterase inhibitors such as caffeine and theophylline can, at least theoretically, act synergistically with those hormones dependent upon a second messenger effect. These include epinephrine, norepinephrine, glucagon, vasopressin, thyroxine, parathyroid hormone, luteinizing hormone, and thyroid- and melanocyte-stimulating hormones. In turn, second messenger effects produced by cAMP include ketogenesis, gluconeogenesis, glycolysis, lipolysis, insulin release, and renin and gastric hydrochloric acid production. To produce these effects, cAMP must activate protein kinases, which consist of two subunits. One binds with the cAMP, leaving the other free to catalyze reactions within the cell. Prostaglandins may also modulate the effects of hormones, but except for a few instances, their roles have not been clearly defined. Secretion of a number of hormones is dependent upon the presence of releasing or inhibiting factors at the secreting gland. Most are associated with the hypothalamus.

Steroidal hormones, such as cortisone, must enter target cells to exert their effect, which tends to be one of gene expression rather than enzymatic alteration. These hormones act at the cell nucleus rather than at its membrane. Steroidal hormones generally take hours to produce their effects, compared with the few minutes required for second messenger mechanisms. This is because their actions depend upon formation of new proteins. As the hormone enters the cell, it binds to a receptor in the cellular cytoplasm. The conjoined hormone and receptor travel to the nucleus to interact with DNA. Messenger RNA may play a role in this interaction, which ends with formation of new proteins. The new protein is, in effect, an induced enzyme. The induced enzyme contributes the terminal action of the hormone. Additional information on hormones is provided elsewhere in this text.

Bioenergetics

The study of energy changes resulting from chemical reactions within living organisms is called bioenergetics. Foods provide basic nutrient substrates for energy. Their assimilation occurs in the alimentary tract, where complex foods are reduced by digestive enzymes, hydrochloric acid, and bile to amino acids, fatty acids, and simple sugars. These are next converted to acetyl groups, phosphoric acid, and other essential compounds necessary for cellular metabolism. Several metabolic pathways use these essential compounds to produce energy. The two main pathways are oxidative phosphorylation and the citric acid cycle. Though proteins and fats can be used for energy, glucose is the foremost energy substrate. (Fructose and galactose are essentially converted to glucose early after ingestion.) The glucose is oxidized to carbon dioxide and water. Metabolic processes concomitantly build ATP, the chemical fuel allowing the body to perform work. Contraction of muscles, nerve conduction, active transport of chemicals, and synthesis of new molecular compounds would not be possible without a continued supply of ATP. Enzymes control the rate of metabolic reactions, but how much energy is produced depends on the amount of available substrate, the amount of free energy involved in each chemical reaction, and a process called electron transport. These last two concepts are discussed next.

The Concept of Free Energy. Reactions that convert high-binding-energy compounds to ones of a lower energy state must, of necessity, yield up their excess energy. This excess is beyond that required to drive the reaction. It may be lost as body heat or coupled to oxidative reactions for transfer and use elsewhere in the body. Because it is freely available to do work elsewhere, it is also called "free" energy. Reactions that generate free energy are called *exergonic,* whereas those that require it for fuel are termed *endergonic.* Excess free heat energy used to be measured in calories or kilocalories. The newer scientific designations are joules and kilojoules per mole.

Exergonic and endergonic reactions can be coupled by various methods. The transfer can be effected by use of a common intermediate capable of interacting in both reactions. This is not a common process in the body, because the intermediate would have to be specific for both reactions. A more efficient method is to synthesize a high-energy compound from the exergonic reaction that can then participate in the endergonic reaction. Given this mechanism, it is possible for the synthesized compound to participate in a number of endergonic reactions. ATP serves as the major, though not exclusive, transfer substance in most biochemical reactions.

The amount of energy freed by a chemical reaction is determined by the laws of thermodynamics. Essentially, the first law is that of conservation of energy. It states that the total energy of a chemical system remains unchanged, energy being neither lost nor gained. The second law states that the extent of molecular disorder or randomness (entropy) in a chemical system must increase if a spontaneous reaction is to occur. This randomness reaches a maximum as the equilibrium point of the reaction is reached. For a reaction occurring under conditions of constant temperature and pressure, the relationship of the change in free energy and the change in randomness is given by the Gibbs equation, which combines both thermodynamic principles. According to the Gibbs equation:

$$\Delta G = \Delta H - T\Delta S$$

in which G = the free energy change, H = the thermodynamic potential at constant pressure, and S = the change in randomness. If the change in G is equal to zero, the reaction is at equilibrium. When the change in G is negative, a spontaneous reaction can occur and free energy will be available. The reaction will be exergonic. A positive change in G means that additional input of energy will be required as fuel and that the reaction is therefore endergonic.

For laboratory reactions, free energy is standardized at absolute temperature using 1.0 M concentrations of each reactant. This type of free energy is expressed with the designation: G^o. Because biochemical reactions occur under conditions found within the body, the standard state of biochemical reactions has been defined by convention to be based on a pH of 7, with a value of 1 being assigned to both the free energy of water and the activity of hydrogen ions. This is called the free energy change at pH 7 and is abbreviated $G^{o'}$. The total free energy available through a series of reactions is equivalent to the algebraic sum of the free energy changes provided by individual steps in the series.

Organophosphate compounds are especially suited for energy transfer. The body possesses two groups of these compounds: a high-energy group and a low-energy one. ATP has a standard free energy at pH 7 ($\Delta G^{o'}$) midway between the groups. The high-energy group includes (in decreasing order of standard free energy): phosphoenolpyruvate, carbonyl phosphate, 1,3-biphosphoglycerate, creatine phosphate, acetyl phosphate, and arginine phosphate. After ATP, the list continues (low-energy group): glucose-1-phosphate, fructose-6-phosphate, glucose-6-phosphate, and glycerol-3-phosphate. By virtue of its position, ATP is able to donate a high-energy phosphate bond to compounds lower on the list. Since ATP breaks down to ADP and a phosphate bond, the ADP can receive a high-energy phosphate bond from compounds in the first part of the list (providing that appropriate enzymes are available to catalyze the process). ATP and ADP can therefore join processes that generate high energy with those requiring energy input.

As was previously discussed, ATP is a nucleotide composed of adenine, a ribose sugar, and three phosphate units. In its active form ATP is part of a complex with magnesium. For energy purposes, the important parts of the molecule are the two phosphoanhydride bonds that make up the last part of the molecule. Hydrolysis releases a large amount of energy as the end bond is split to produce ADP and orthophosphate (P_i). A similar energy release occurs when ADP has its terminal bond split to produce AMP and pyrophosphate (PP_i). Simplified structural formulas for ATP, ADP, and AMP are

High-energy phosphate bonds are sometimes also drawn as: (P)~(P). The amount of energy liberated by these hydrolysis reactions depends to some extent on the concentration of magnesium and the ionic strength of the medium. Other biochemical reactions rely on compounds analogous to ATP. These include guanosine triphosphate (GTP), uridine triphosphate (UTP), and cytidine triphosphate (CTP). Each, in turn, is degraded to a diphosphate—GDP, UDP, and CDP. Enzymes can transfer the phosphoryl group from one nucleotide to another.

Four processes contribute high-energy phosphate bonds to the ATP/ADP cycle. Most come from intracellular mitochondrial reactions involving ATP synthetase known as oxidative phosphorylation. This process acts to capture energy. Another mechanism involves breakdown of glucose to lactic acid via a glycolytic action known as the Embden-Meyerhof pathway. This pathway is capable of forming a net gain of two high-energy phosphate groups per mole of glucose catabolized. A third mechanism is the citric acid cycle, and the last occurs in muscle. It involves both creatine and arginine phosphate.

Electron Transfer and Oxidative Phosphorylation. Oxidation involves loss of electrons whereas reduction involves electron gain. Activation of one reaction is always matched by an opposing reaction. Hence, the terms oxidation-reduction and redox are used to describe them. For redox reactions, the amount of free energy available is proportional to the ability of reactants to accept or donate electrons, termed their redox potential. Biologically, oxygen is the prime electron acceptor, but the process is not a direct one. Instead, electrons are carried (transferred) by pyridine nucleotides or flavins. The reduced forms of these carriers transfer electrons to oxygen by way of an electron transport chain within the inner membrane of mitochondria. It is the flow of electrons down the chain that helps combine ADP and P_i into ATP. This process, known as oxidative phosphorylation, is the major source of ATP for aerobic organisms. The major electron carriers are NADH, NADPH, and $FADH_2$. These were discussed earlier in the sections on enzymes and vitamins where it was pointed out that the dinucleotide is a carrier of hydrogen ($FADH_2$ carries two). NAD^+ can carry a hydrogen ion and two electrons. This is equivalent to a hydride ion. NADH is the reduced form. NADPH's role is in ATP production. Enzymes control the rate at which ATP-producing reactions occur. Without these catalysts, such reactions would proceed slowly, if at all. Whereas ATP functions as the prime carrier of phosphoryl groups, coenzyme A functions as the main carrier of acyl groups. The acetyl-CoA thus formed is, like ATP, a major essential ingredient in metabolic processes.

Metabolic Pathways of Glucose. Human bodies use three main glycolytic mechanisms. These are the Embden-Meyerhof pathway, the hexose-monophosphate shunt, and the Krebs cycle.

The Embden-Meyerhof pathway (E-M pathway) consists of a series of non-oxygen-dependent reactions. As an anaerobic process, it can provide energy to meet emergency situations where oxygen might be lacking. But under normal conditions, it feeds into the aerobic Krebs cycle that serves as the final common path for oxidation of ingested nutrients. The E-M pathway is also known as the lactic acid cycle, anaerobic glycolysis, or the Cori cycle. It is but one intermediate path in the metabolism of carbohydrates. Two other intermediate processes, glycogenesis and glycogenolysis, relate to storage of glucose as glycogen and are discussed later. The function of the E-M pathway is to convert glucose to pyruvate or, in the absence of oxygen, to lactic acid. A buildup of lactic acid occurs during periods of strenuous exercise when metabolic processes outstrip available oxygen, causing muscles to become fatigued.

Intermediate substances in the E-M pathway have either three or six carbons, the latter being derived from glucose and fructose whereas those with three carbons derive from glyceraldehyde, glycerate, pyruvate, or dihydroxyacetone. As the process converts glucose to pyruvate, a repeated number of phosphorylation reactions occur, which result in phosphoryl groups that have ester or anhydride linkages. Five types of reactions occur:

1. Transfer of phosphoryl groups from ATP.
2. Shifting of phosphoryl groups from one oxygen molecule to another.
3. Interconversion (isomerization) of ketoses and aldoses.
4. Dehydration and removal of a molecule of water.
5. Splitting of aldol linkages.

There are ten steps in the glycolytic pathway. All occur in cell cytosol. The process both consumes and produces energy. Two ATP molecules are lost, one in the conversion of glucose to glucose-6-phosphate (G-6-P) and one in the conversion of fructose-6-phosphate to fructose-1,6-diphosphate. However, four ATP molecules are produced by the pathway so that there is a net gain of two ATP molecules for the entire process. This gain occurs by conversion of two molecules of 1,3-diphosphoglycerate to two of 3-phosphoglycerate, and by that of two molecules of phosphoenolpyruvate to two of pyruvate. Each pathway step involves an enzyme, but the enzyme phosphofructokinase is the major determinant of the rate of glycolysis. Steps in the E-M pathway are given in Table 6–2.

Pyruvate formed by the E-M process can be converted to either lactate or acetyl-CoA. When oxygen is limited, pyruvate is reduced by NADH to form lactate, a process catalyzed by lactate dehydrogenase. The reduction reaction causes regeneration of NAD^+ needed to allow the E-M pathway to function past the point at which glyceraldehyde-3-phosphate is formed. Where this not possible, no ATP would be produced. Pyruvate reduction thereby provides energy for a limited period of time until oxygen becomes available. Obviously, there is a limit to how long the body can function under anaerobic conditions alone, but the process does provide a safeguard for survival. Once oxygen becomes available, the lactate is reconverted to pyruvate and the acidosis quickly dissipates. Formation of acetyl-CoA occurs when pyruvate combines with NAD^+ and CoA to produce carbon dioxide, NADH, H^+, and acetyl-CoA. The acetyl-CoA then enters the citric acid cycle.

One offshoot of the glycolytic pathway carries additional importance for anesthesia practice. A mutase may convert 1,3-diphosphoglycerate (1,3-DPG) to 2,3-diphos-

TABLE 6-2. THE EMBDEN-MEYERHOF PATHWAY

Substrate	Enzyme	Product
*Glucose + ATP	Hexokinase	Glucose-6-phosphate + ADP + H^+
Glucose-6-phosphate	Phosphoglucose isomerase	Fructose-6-phosphate
*Fructose-6-phosphate + ATP	Phosphofructokinase	Fructose-1,6-diphosphate + ADP + H^+
Fructose-1,6-diphosphate	Aldolase	Dihydroxyacetone phosphate + glyceraldehyde 3-phosphate
Dihydroxyacetone phosphate	Triose phosphate isomerase	Glyceraldehyde 3-phosphate
Glyceraldehyde-3-phosphate + P_i + NAD^+	Glyceraldehyde 3-phosphate dehydrogenase	1,3-Diphosphoglycerate + NADH + H^+
1,3-Diphosphoglycerate + ADP	Phosphoglycerate kinase	3-Phosphoglycerate + ATP
3-Phosphoglycerate	Phosphoglyceromutase	2-Phosphoglycerate
2-Phosphoglycerate	Enolase	Phosphoenolpyruvate + H_2O
Phosphoenolpyruvate + ADP + H^{+a}	Pyruvate kinase	Pyruvate + ATP

[a] Nonreversible reactions.
Adapted with permission from Stryer L: Biochemistry, 2nd ed. New York, Freeman, 1981.

phoglycerate (2,3-DPG). Large amounts of 2,3-DPG are found in hemoglobin of red cells, where it acts to control the transport of oxygen. Changes in hemoglobin oxygen-affinity caused by 2,3-DPG can hold important implications for patients.

The hexose-monophosphate shunt is an aerobic, enzyme-dependent series of reactions that generate ribose and NADPH. Ribose is used for synthesizing nucleic acids and NADPH is important to the formation of fatty acids. Basically, three molecules of glucose-6-phosphate are combined with six of NADP to form three molecules of carbon dioxide, two of fructose-6-phosphate, six molecules of NADPH, and one of glyceraldehyde-3-phosphate. Two compounds produced by the series, fructose-6-phosphate and glyceraldehyde 3-phosphate, may be shared with the Embden-Meyerhof pathway. The shunt pathway, sometimes called the direct oxidative pathway, functions mostly in the liver, adre-

nals, thyroid, erythrocytes, and adipose tissues. It operates only minimally in skeletal muscle. Shunt reactions begin with oxidation but eventually produce a number of sugars, which are enzymatically converted by nonoxidative means. Table 6-3 shows the steps of both groups of reactions. Sugars produced may contain four, five, or seven carbon atoms. Because two molecules of glyceraldehyde-3-phosphate can regenerate one molecule of glucose-6-phosphate, the shunt pathway can account for complete oxidation of glucose. The oxidative portion of the reactions relies on dehydrogenation, much like the E-M pathway; but NADP, rather than NAD, becomes the hydrogen carrier. Enzymes for shunt reactions are located in cell cytosol. The hexose-monophosphate shunt provides metabolic energy through its reducing powers. Unlike the E-M pathway or Krebs cycle, it is not concerned with ATP production.

The body's principle metabolic pathway is the *Krebs*

TABLE 6-3. THE HEXOSE-MONOPHOSPHATE SHUNT

Group I	Enzyme	Product
Glucose-6-phosphate + $NADP^+$	Glucose-6-phosphate dehydrogenase	6-Phosphogluconolactone + NADPH + H^+
6-Phosphogluconolactone + H_2O^a	Lactonase	6-Phosphogluconate + H^+
6-Phosphogluconate + $NADP^{+a}$	6-Phosphogluconate dehydrogenase	Ribulose-5-phosphate[c] + CO_2 + NADPH
Group II		
Ribulose-5-phosphate[c]	Phosphopentose isomerase	Ribose-5-phosphate[c]
Ribulose-5-phosphate[c]	Phosphopentose epimerase	Xylulose-5-phosphate[c]
Xylulose-5-phosphate[c] + ribose 5-phosphate[c]	Transketolase	Sedoheptulose-7-phosphate[d] + glyceraldehyde-3-phosphate
Sedoheptulose-7-phosphate[d] + glyceraldehyde-3-phosphate	Transaldolase	Fructose-6-phosphate + erythrose-4-phosphate[b]
Xylulose-5-phosphate[c] + erythrose-4-phosphate[b]	Transketolase	Fructose-6-phosphate + glyceraldehyde 3-phosphate

[a] Nonreversible reactions.
[b] Four-carbon sugar.
[c] Five-carbon sugar.
[d] Seven-carbon sugar.
Adapted with permission from Stryer L: Biochemistry, 2nd ed. New York, Freeman, 1981.

cycle, also called the citric acid or tricarboxylic cycle. When combined with Embden-Meyerhof reactions, the complete pathway is termed aerobic glycolysis. As with glycolytic and shunt pathways, each step is enzymatically controlled. Enzymes for the Krebs cycle are located within folded areas of mitochondria known as cristae. The cycle also serves to provide intermediate products for building other chemical components for the body (biosynthesis).

Acetyl-CoA formed from pyruvate during the last stages of glycolytic reactions feeds the cycle. The cycle starts with the combining of oxaloacetate, a four-carbon compound, to the two-carbon acetyl group of acetyl-CoA. The combined compound reacts with water to form CoA and citrate under the influence of citrate synthetase. The citrate is then isomerized to isocitrate through a dehydration-hydration reaction that allows for interchange of H^+ and OH^- groups. Isocitrate undergoes an oxidative-reduction reaction, which is facilitated by NAD^+ and the enzyme isocitrate dehydrogenase. This reaction produces an intermediate, oxalosuccinate. Loss of carbon dioxide from oxalosuccinate leads to formation of alpha-ketoglutarate. Formation of this compound determines the overall functioning of the cycle. A second oxidative reduction converts alpha-ketoglutarate to succinyl-CoA. This reaction, too, results in conversion of the NAD^+ to NADH and the release of CO_2, the reaction being much like the one that converted pyruvate to acetyl-CoA during glycolysis except that here a three-enzyme complex (alpha-ketoglutarate dehydrogenase complex) is required to achieve conversion. The succinyl-CoA contains an energy bond similar to ATP. In a dual reaction catalyzed by succinyl-CoA synthetase, the energy bond is released at the same time that GDP is phosphorylated. The reactions end with formation of GTP, succinate, and CoA, but the phosphoryl group of GTP can be transferred to ADP by nucleoside diphosphokinase to form ATP. Formation of the high-energy bond compares with oxidative phosphorylation discussed earlier. However, this energy-bond formation occurs only once in the tricarboxylic cycle. The last step in the cycle involves reforming oxaloacetate from succinate. Three substeps are required for this process, two of oxidation and one hydration reaction. When oxaloacetate has been reformed, the cycle may begin again. Steps in the Krebs cycle are outlined in Table 6–4.

In the Krebs cycle, hydrogen is lost through five reactions. The loss is mostly in the form of NADH, which then enters the electron transport chain. In the chain hydrogen is passed between compounds to facilitate oxidation-reduction reactions. A number of these reactions allow energy to be stored as ATP. Finally, the hydrogens combine with oxygen to form water. Three molecules of ATP are formed from each molecule of NADH, but the entire aerobic glycolysis process forms a net 38 molecules of ATP. This can be summarized as follows:

4	from E-M pathway
6	from two NADH released in E-M pathway
30*	from the two pyruvic acids in Krebs cycle
40	
− 2	used in E-M pathway
38	molecules of ATP total

Glycogen is a polymerized, storable form of glucose. Forming glycogen (*glycogenesis*) from excess glucose insures that the E-M, hexose-monophosphate, and Krebs pathways can continue to function during periods of decreased food intake. Glycogenesis occurs mainly in the liver, with some conversion occurring in muscle. Once stored, glycogen can later be split by hydrolysis to reform glucose, a process termed *glycogenolysis*.

Glycogenesis involves the following steps:

1. In the presence of magnesium and the enzyme glucokinase, glucose reacts with ATP. The latter is degraded to ADP and the glucose is converted to glucose-6-phosphate (G-6-P).
2. Phosphomutase converts G-6-P to glucose-1-phosphate (G-1-P).
3. The G-1-P reacts with the uracil-containing nucleotide, UTP, under the influence of the enzyme UDPG pyrophosphorylase. This forms UDP-glucose.

---

* Each glucose molecule yields two pyruvic acids in the E-M pathway, and each of these produces 5 NADH molecules, each capable of producing three molecules of ATP: $2 \times 5 \times 3 = 30$.

TABLE 6–4. THE KREBS CYCLE

	Enzyme[b]	
Acetyl-CoA + oxaloacetate + H_2O[a]	Citrate synthetase	Citrate + CoA + H^+
Citrate	Aconitase	*Cis*-aconitate + H_2O
Isocitrate + NAD^+	Isocitrate dehydrogenase	Alpha-ketoglutarate + CO_2 + NADH
Alpha-ketoglutarate + NAD^+ + CoA	Alpha-ketoglutarate dehydrogenase complex	Succinyl-CoA + CO_2 + NADH
Succinyl-CoA + P_i + GDP	Succinyl-CoA synthetase	Succinate + GTP + CoA
Succinate + FAD[c]	Succinate dehydrogenase	Fumarate + $FADH_2$
Fumarate + H_2O[c]	Fumarase	Maltate
Malate + NAD^+[c]	Malate dehydrogenase	Oxaloacetate + NADH + H^+

[a] Nonreversible reactions.
[b] Cofactors, as well as enzymes, are required for nearly all of the steps.
[c] The last three steps are aimed at reforming oxaloacetate from succinate.
Adapted with permission from Stryer L: Biochemistry, 2nd ed. New York, Freeman, 1981.

4. UDP-glucose is polymerized to glycogen under the influence of UDPG-glycogen-transglucolase. This reaction releases UDP.
5. UDP reacts with ATP to form ADP and allows regeneration of UTP. (Two molecules of ATP are required for every molecule of glucose stored.)

Glycogenolysis is not merely the reverse process of glycogenesis. It is a much more accelerated process. An (inactive) enzyme, phosphorylase (b), is changed to (active) phosphorylase (a) by a complex interaction termed the cascade reaction. Phosphorylase (a) is then able to split off a G-1-P from glycogen. The G-1-P is reconverted to G-6-P. Glucose-6-phosphatase then removes phosphate from G-6-P to form glucose. The cascade reaction is generated by a number of hormones including ACTH, glucagon, and epinephrine. Each step of the cascade accelerates the following step by as much as 100 times. Steps in the cascade are as follows:

1. The hormone (e.g., epinephrine) activates adenyl cyclase.
2. Adenyl cyclase converts AMP to cAMP.
3. cAMP activates protein kinase.
4. Protein kinase activates phosphorylase kinase.
5. Phosphorylase kinase converts phosphorylase (b) to phosphorylase (a).
6. Phosphorylase (a) acts on glycogen to split off G-1-P.
7. G-1-P is converted to G-6-P.
8. G-6-P is converted to glucose and enters the bloodstream or glycolytic pathways.

The above reaction occurs only in the liver, since muscles lack the enzyme necessary to convert G-6-P to glucose. The G-6-P of muscle must enter a glycolytic pathway.

The bioenergetic and other biochemical reactions discussed in this section impact, in one fashion or another, upon every patient who receives an anesthetic. An appreciation by the anesthetist of the often subtle yet complex biochemical balances required to maintain homeostasis contributes substantially to providing patients optimum safe care.

BIBLIOGRAPHY

Adriani JA: The Chemistry and Physics of Anesthesia. Springfield, IL, Chas C Thomas, 1962.

Baden JM, Rice SA: Metabolism and toxicity of inhaled anesthetics. In Miller RD (ed): Anesthesia. New York, Churchill-Livingstone, 1981.

Bohinski RC: Modern Concepts in Biochemistry. Boston, Allyn & Bacon, 1976.

Danielli JF, Davson H: A contribution to the theory of permeability of thin films. J Cell Comp Physiol 5: 495–508, 1935.

Harper HA, Rodwell VW, et al: Review of Physiologic Chemistry. Los Altos, CA, Lange, 1977.

Lehninger AL: Biochemistry, 2nd ed. New York, Worth Publishers, 1985.

Ruch T, Patton HD: Physiology and Biophysics, 20th ed. Philadelphia, Saunders, 1982.

Shugar G, Shugar R, et al: Health Sciences Chemistry. Philadelphia, Davis, 1978.

Singer SJ, Nicolson GL: The fluid mosaic model of the structure of cell membranes. Science 175: 720, 1972.

Solomons TW: Organic Chemistry, 3rd ed. New York, Wiley, 1984.

Zubay G: Biochemistry. Reading, MA, Addison-Wesley, 1983.

Stryer L: Biochemistry, 2nd ed. New York, Freeman, 1981.

7

Electronic and Other Principles Related to Anesthesia

Leo A. Le Bel

Growing use of sophisticated electronic devices in surgery and anesthesia practice makes a basic knowledge of electronic components and circuits virtually mandatory for today's practicing anesthetist. The purpose of the following section is to provide fundamental information about electrical laws and circuits and to show their relevance to anesthesia practice.

BASIC PRINCIPLES

Electricity is a phenomenon of nature that depends upon atomic structure and the difference in force between electrons and protons. Electrons have a negative charge, protons an equal but positive charge. The *charge* each possesses is a function of mass, and it is the gravitational force between their masses that keeps them bound in atomic configuration. Having opposite charges, electrons and protons are mutually attracted to one another. On the other hand, electrons repel other electrons and protons repel other protons. If one thinks of an aggregate of electrons or protons on the surface of two objects, it is easier to envision how electricity flows. If two objects of opposite charge are kept separate, they retain their relative charges. No electricity flows, and the charges are said to be *static*. As the objects are brought close to one another, forces of attraction build between the two into what is termed an *energy field*. At this point, the objects possess potential energy. But once the two are brought close together, the electricity becomes dynamic and electrons from the negatively charged object flow to the positively charged one. This is termed an *electric current*.

Quantity of charge is measured in *coulombs*. The rate at which the charge travels is measured as a function of time. A rate of one coulomb per second is called an *ampere*. While current flows, it also generates a kinetic energy force field, which is termed *magnetism*. The word electromagnetic reflects the close association between the two force fields. When electricity flows, the resulting energy can be used to perform work. In most cases, this involves converting the electrical energy to mechanical energy. Electric motors are one example by which the conversion is made.

In addition to *mass*, *force (charge)*, and *rate of flow*, a fourth factor, *distance*, will determine the sum effect of an electric current. All electrical quantities can be expressed as a function of one or more of these parameters.

When electricity flows, it is the electron that physically moves. Substances, such as metals, that have loosely attached and easily lost electrons in their atomic structure are called *conductors*. Those that have tightly bound electrons, such as glass and plastics, are called *nonconductors* or *insulators*. Positive charges may be thought of as holes in the atom(s) where electrons are missing and whose positions may be constantly changing, much like a ferris wheel with several of its gondolas missing. Substances whose electrical characteristics are determined by the motion of electrons and the position of holes are termed *semiconductors*. These include transistors and integrated circuits, so prevalent in modern solid-state electronic devices.

The *permittivity* of a substance is an indication of how well it conducts an electrical current compared with current flow in a vacuum. Permittivity is also termed the *dialectric constant* of a substance. It gives an indication of the velocity with which current will flow in that material. Dialectric constants are used for making comparisons between substances as to their current-carrying ability, e.g., copper versus silver.

As current flows, magnetic fields that can generate secondary current flows are developed. This process is termed *induction* and occurs when electricity flowing in one wire sets up a current in an adjoining wire. An electric *shield* is anything that prevents development of induced charges.

Devices that store a charge are termed *capacitors* or *condensers*. Devices that oppose current flow are called *resistors*. The term *electromotive force* (emf) describes any source of electrical energy. Electromotive force is measured in *volts*, 1 volt being equal to the potential required to flow a current of 1 ampere through a resistance of 1 *ohm* (the unit of resistance).

Charges that flow in an electric current have a force of given potential. When that potential is reduced to a zero point level, the charge is said to be *grounded*. Electrical grounds are used to reduce or eliminate unwanted electric charges. This concept has particular applicability to operating room floors, where grounding may be used to rapidly dispel excess charges before they build to levels high enough to cause "static shock." As electricity courses through an electronic circuit, its potential is progressively decreased. This is termed *voltage drop*.

Any combination of electrical source, resistors, capacitors, or other components is called an *electrical network* or *circuit*. All electronic equipment is made up of a number of such networks. A circuit may be designed to perform a unique function or to work in tandem with other circuits to effect multiple operations. Anesthesia monitors that simultaneously keep track of temperature, blood pressure, and other parameters require the integration of literally dozens of specific circuits made up of many discrete parts. Whether or not failure of a single component will result in failure of the entire unit depends on the manner in which the unit has been designed. Special diagrams, *schematics*, outline the entire circuitry of an electronic device by means of electronic symbols. A legend that identifies the symbols used is usually provided. By referring to the schematic diagram of an electronic device before using it, the anesthetist can gain some appreciation of how the unit functions. Many manufacturers also supply block diagrams, which provide information about how major circuits within the unit are functionally related.

Current can be described as one of two types: *alternating* (AC) or *direct* (DC). If one imagines looking at a single cross-sectional area of a conductor (wire) and seeing electrons flow first in one direction and then the other, the impression left by one back-and-forth movement would be that there was no net movement of electrons, merely one cycle of movement by the same electron. The observer would be left to conclude that there was no flow of electricity (net flow of charge). Yet, what has just been described is known commonly as AC. The answer to the illusion lies in the fact that different electrons were seen to be transversing the cross-sectional area. This is because the molecules of metal that make up the wire are constantly exchanging their loose electrons. With DC, movement of electrons would appear unidirectional. AC is more easily carried over large distances, but DC is generally more efficient and is therefore the primary form used in electronic circuits.

Changes that occur with alternating current can be visualized by use of a *sine wave*. With the conventional electricity we use (AC), the direction of travel of electrons is changed 120 times per second, or 60 back-and-forth cycles, hence the term 60-cycle electricity. Each cycle is identical, and a sine-wave pattern describes the algebraic sum of the movement of electrons through one cycle.

Alternating Current Sine Wave

Describing electricity as being 60 cycles/second (hertz) is to say something about its frequency. Certain electronic circuits operate at an optimum frequency, termed *resonance*, where forces that facilitate current flow through the circuit (*conductance*) are balanced by the forces that hamper current flow (*impedance*). Resonant circuits can be easily upset and flow through the circuit becomes asynchronous, but, if working properly, resonant circuits perform best at their designed frequency. With some circuits, it becomes possible to tune the resonant circuit over a range of frequencies. Radio receivers use this principle, as do certain medical devices, such as ultrasonic equipment and electrocardiographic telemetry units. Antennas also are a form of resonator; that is, the length or physical design of the antenna determines the best frequency range of operation.

Radiations that possess both electrical and magnetic properties are said to lie in the *electromagnetic spectrum*. These range from electrical waves that are very long in wavelength, relatively slow-moving, and relatively low-energy to very short, high-energy, rapidly moving cosmic rays. In between, the spectrum includes broadcast and short radio waves, very-high and ultra-high-frequency (VHF/UHF) radio waves, infrared, visible, and ultraviolet light spectrums, x-rays, and gamma radiation.

If current is flowing through a conductor (wire) and that conductor is formed into a coil, the electromagnetic field generated by each turn of the coil works in concert with those generated by all other turns. When an identical but nonconducting circuit is brought into close proximity, an induced current will begin to flow in the second circuit. This is the basis on which *transformers* work; that is, energy from one part of the circuit is transformed to energy within the second part of the circuit. Yet there is no direct linkage between the two. This transfer of energy represents work done by the electromotive source providing current to the first (primary) circuit. Energy lost by the first circuit can be measured as a voltage drop. Certain forces facilitate or inhibit the energy transfer. For example, placing an iron magnetic rod within the first coil makes it an electromagnet, making energy transfer easier. On the other hand, air between the turns of the first coil provides capacitance, thus restricting the energy transfer, air being a poor conductor of electricity. However, if the current generated through the coil creates enough charge, arcing (voltage breakdown) will occur between coil elements. The example just presented represents mutual inductance between circuits, but it is also possible for a single circuit to be self-inducting.

Electronic Circuits

Mechanical devices and electronic circuits are often conceptually similar. The former's efficiency is determined by the interaction of components that store energy, those that dissipate it (i.e., cause resistance), those capable of storing and using kinetic energy, and those that transform the system's energy in some way (e.g., gears). Electronic circuits have resistors that use up energy, capacitors that store it, inductors that can both store and use energy, and transformers that regulate voltage and current carried by the circuit.

The rate at which both systems perform work is termed *power*. In electrical terms, power is measured as *watts* and is equal to the electromotive force in volts multiplied by the current in amperes (P = EI). One watt is equal to 1 volt multiplied by 1 ampere. The same amount of power can therefore be obtained by using high voltage at low current or low voltage at high current. *Efficiency of an electronic circuit* can be measured by dividing its power output by its power input. A circuit that outputs 50 watts for every

100 watts input is operating at 50 percent efficiency. The rest of the power is dissipated in performing within the circuit or as heat loss.

Because any electronic circuit consists of imperfect components, there will always be some resistance to electrical flow. Indeed, just as pressure differences occur within anesthesia breathing circuits so, too, are there numerous factors within an electronic circuit that hamper electrical flow.

The simplest conceivable electric circuit would consist of a battery (electromotive force source) and a resistor in a closed circuit. (Placing a switch in the circuit breaks the current flow and the circuit is said to be open or broken.)

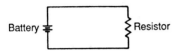

This simple circuit can illustrate basic interactions between voltage (E), current (I), and resistance (R). The relationships are expressed as *Ohm's law,* which states that current flowing in a circuit is directly proportional to applied electromotive force and inversely proportional to resistance; or,

$$I \text{ (amperes)} = \frac{E \text{ (volts)}}{R \text{ (ohms)}}$$

The formula can be transposed to solve for any needed value, given that two of the values are known. Therefore:

$$E = IR \quad \text{and} \quad R = \frac{E}{I}$$

Ohm's law applies to all parts of a circuit as well as to the circuit as a whole. If more than one resistance is present, total resistance will depend on whether the *resistances* are *in series* or *parallel*. For resistances in series, total resistance equals the sum of all resistors (R=R1+R2+R3 etc.). With serial resistances, current remains the same throughout the circuit. However, with parallel resistances the current becomes divided between the various parallel resistors. This causes total resistance for the circuit to be less than that of the lowest resistance value present. The formula for calculating parallel resistances is

$$R = \frac{1}{1/R1 + 1/R2 + 1/R3 + \cdots}$$

In calculating Ohm's law equations, it must be remembered to convert known figures to the measurements required by the law. For instance, milliamperes or millivolts must first be converted to their ampere or voltage equivalents by moving the decimal point appropriately. Obtaining values for voltage, current, and resistance normally involves direct measurement by means of voltmeters, ammeters, and ohmeters.

The importance of Ohm's law lies in the fact that it is equally applicable to other electronic components within the circuit. For example, capacitors in a circuit can be thought of as resistors and their effect on current and voltage can be calculated in the same manner. This also applies for series and parallel inductances.

Though electricity has been known since the dawn of humanity through the phenomenon of lightning, only in the past few hundred years have we come to understand its powers and how to control it. By 1900, electricity had some practical applications (e.g. telegraphy), but equipment had to be tied by direct connections. Even early radio frequency transmitters capable of sending signals over distances relied on broad emissions scattered over vast frequency ranges. They required high-energy inputs and were terribly inefficient.

The modern electrical era begin with invention of the *vacuum tube.* Vacuum tubes allowed the electricity flowing through a circuit to be carefully controlled and directed toward performing specific tasks. A tube contains active elements enclosed in a glass envelope from which air has been evacuated to provide an internal vacuum. Because electrons flow more freely in a vacuum, electrical flow is more efficient. The two primary active elements of a tube are a *cathode* (negative pole from which electrons flow) and an *anode* or plate (positive pole to which electrons flow). A wire filament provides a resistive pathway within the tube, which, by building up heat, enhances electron flow. Interspersed between cathode and anode may be one to several grids, which serve to control electron flux across the tube circuit. Tubes are named for the number of active elements present (excluding filament). A triode has a cathode, anode, and one grid, whereas a pentode has three grids. Connection of tube circuitry to the rest of the electronic circuit is by means of pins located in the base of the tube.

The advent of vacuum tubes meant that, for the first time, sophisticated circuits could be designed for controlling and using electricity. But a few short decades later, tubes gave way to *semiconductors,* electronic components that are part conductor and part insulator, hence their name. In this category are *diodes* and *transistors.* Diodes have only two active elements (cathode and anode) and are often named for the substance from which they are made (selenium, silicon, etc.). More sophisticated, transistor semiconductors contain multiple active elements. Basic elements of transistors are the emitter, base, and collector.

Semiconductors perform essentially the same functions as tubes, but their mode of operation is different. In vacuum tubes, electrons function as discrete charged solid particles. Semiconductors rely on the various energy states (levels) of the atoms that compose them. When orbital energy levels are such that energy flows, the device conducts. When energy levels prevent energy flow, the device acts as an insulator. The energy levels for both states are partly determined by the amount of electrical energy coming into the device. By the selection of appropriate construction materials and control of their physical assembly, semiconductors can be developed that have relatively positive or relatively negative "poles." These are not specific poles in the usual sense; rather they represent areas of preponderant negative or positive charges. These preponderant charges relate to the energy levels created within the various sections of the semiconductor, a factor of their design and construction materials. The "positive" charge carriers are the "holes" referred to earlier. The two sections of material within the semiconductor are called P type (for positive) and N type (for negative). When a P type is joined to an N-type material, a one-way current flow occurs. This PN junction is found in all semiconductor devices. A variation, the PNP (positive-negative-positive) transistor, uses a common emitter. Bipolar transistors combine two PN junctions and provide some power amplification for the circuit. A field effect transistor (FET) is another modification that can also amplify. In many respects, FETs resemble pentode vacuum tubes but require much less voltage. Because semiconductors are composed of solid materials, circuits in which they are used are called *solid-state circuits*. *Integrated circuits* (IC) are, as the name implies, devices that incorporate several interconnected components designed for a particular application. Through the process of microminiaturization it is possible to build complex ICs of very small size, much the way the size of photographs is reduced. Nearly invisible silicon chips now contain all the circuitry that formerly took multiple vacuum tubes, wiring, etc. to accomplish. By designing chips that function when electricity is "on" and don't function when electricity is "off," it is possible to develop what are termed *digital-logic ICs*. They are termed digital because they deal with discrete events, and logical because they operate in accordance with mathematical principles. Digital-logic ICs form the heart of the modern microcomputer.

With development of semiconductors and microcomputers we have entered the neomodern period of electronics. What are the advantages of solid-state devices besides size and production costs? Principle advantages lie in the fact that they use electricity much more efficiently. Substantially less voltage is required to perform work than was necessary with vacuum tubes. Less heat is generated, equipment operates efficiently for longer periods of time, repair costs are less, and work can be performed more rapidly. Virtually all electronic equipment used today in both surgery and anesthesia is of solid-state design.

A number of circuits are common to most electronic equipment and a brief description of these is presented next.

The *power supply circuit* receives electrical input from the available commercial power source. In most facilities, this is provided through standard two- or three-prong AC outlets that provide 117 volts at 60 hertz (range 110 to 125 volts). With three-prong outlets, one conductor serves as the neutral connection, one is grounded, and one provides the AC. Three-conductor power outlets are now fairly standard, but those used in operating rooms reserved for use of explosive anesthetic agents must have interlocking explosion-proof plugs. These are connected to the surgical suite's isolation transformer, a concept discussed later. As electricity enters the electronic device, a transformer is used to convert line voltage to a value suitable for the unit. A *rectifier circuit* then converts the AC to a pulsating DC. *Filtering circuits* may be used to decrease DC pulsations. This smoothes the voltage into a relatively constant current. Power supply filtering circuits serve to regulate voltage and eliminate unwanted (ripple) currents by grounding them through a *bleeder* circuit to ground. A bleeder circuit provides a safety measure for dissipating excess current when the device is turned off. The power supply of any unit normally contains a fuse at the site at which electricity enters the unit. This protects the unit from electrical overloading.

Frequency filtering circuits are used either to protect the unit from the effects of extraneous interference, or to keep the unit from generating a signal at a frequency that could cause interference to other nearby electronic equipment. Such filters are of four basic types: those that cut out all signals below a specified frequency; those that cut signals above a given frequency; those that pass certain frequency bands while filtering others; and those that inhibit passage of a block of frequencies while passing those above and below.

Oscillator circuits generate signals of either single or multiple frequencies. They are sometimes used to provide an internal standard for calibrating an electronic unit. *Multiplier circuits* multiply a given frequency, usually by two, three, or four times. *Divider circuits* break down a frequency into smaller units. *Mixer circuits* combine different frequencies.

Driver circuits generate signals that, in turn, feed into another stage of the circuit. *Amplifier circuits* enhance or increase signal strength. *Metering circuits* allow measurement of a specific function. For example, temperature-measuring devices used in the operating room read out on either a needle-and-scale device or on digital displays. Digital readout devices use light-emitting diodes (LEDs), which glow when activated by electrical energy within the circuit. Digital displays may use hundreds of transistors; the combination of energy flow through these determines what numbers appear on the display. Digital devices that read out both letters and numbers are termed alphanumeric. *Audio circuits* convert electrical signals into audible tones. Doppler and ultrasound devices often incorporate such circuits to allow the user to hear changes detected by the device. Another type of readout device is the oscilloscope on which electrical changes are seen as movement of a light beam across a television-like screen. For example, electrocardiographic (ECG) monitors used in surgery provide a readout of heart electrical impulses as they are transmitted across the body. The displayed pattern represents the algebraic sum of impulses traveling to and away from the monitoring electrodes. The pattern changes with the combination of electrodes used, that is, whatever ECG lead is being utilized. Two types of interference commonly may occur to disrupt the ECG pattern. The first is termed 60-cycle interference, which appears as a sine wave of even amplitude superimposed on the normally isoelectric (0 voltage) baseline of the ECG pattern. It occurs whenever line voltage AC enters the monitoring circuit, perhaps as the result of malfunctioning other electronic devices, improper grounding, or because of capacitive current flow. Complete disruption of the pattern with scattering of the oscilloscope electron beam occurs whenever the monitor is subjected to radio frequency interference (RFI). This is usually caused by electrocautery equipment that disperses energy throughout the operating room environment. This electrical energy enters the monitor to cause disruption of the normal circuitry, which in turn results in disruption of the oscilloscope pattern. Present-day monitoring devices contain circuits designed to dampen electrical interference. Still, high radiant energies may overload these to produce momentary disruptions. A normal pattern is quickly reestablished once the RFI source is eliminated.

Monitoring devices constitute the largest class of electronic devices used by anesthetists. Interestingly, a single circuit forms the basis for most monitors. Known as a *Wheat-*

stone bridge (Fig. 7–1), it operates by balancing voltages at two different points in such a fashion that a zero potential difference is established between them. Establishing this zero potential difference is termed balancing, zeroing, or nulling the circuit. Once calibrated in this way, any change in circuit balance can be read as a change in voltage. (This voltage change is typically read on a needle-and-scale, oscilloscope, or digital display in terms of the values being monitored, e.g., torr pressure, degrees of temperature, etc.) The circuit consists of four resistances, of which two are of a fixed, known value (R-1 and R-2 in Fig. 7–1). Once the resistance of standard (R-s) is zeroed, any change it experiences is reflective of the unknown resistance (R-x). To restate this in another fashion: if any three resistances are known, the fourth can be calculated, since:

$$R\text{-}x = R\text{-}s\,\frac{R\text{-}2}{R\text{-}1}.$$

It is important to note that resistance ratios, not actual resistor values, are the basis for the way a Wheatstone bridge functions.

Bridge circuits require a sensing device to provide input capable of changing the reference resistance. The sensing device may be a thermistor probe used for monitoring temperature. Change in heat is carried by cable to the monitor, where it elicits a change in R-s. Another sensing device is the pressure transducer. A transducer's pressure plate moves in response to mechanical alterations generated by a liquid column attached to an indwelling arterial line catheter. Such a device is often used for continuously measuring blood pressure. Fluctuations at the pressure-plate/liquid-dome assembly are carried by cable to the monitor to induce changes in R-s. When the monitor has previously been zeroed to air (no mechanical pressure) accurate blood pressure measurements can be made. The monitor may also provide a continuous oscilloscopic pressure wave tracing.

Movement of the transducer pressure plate causes nearly imperceptible alterations in cable wire length that act to change its resistance. This variation in electrical resistance is responsible for changing the value of R-s.

The foregoing examples are but two of the more common applications of a Wheatstone bridge circuit. Other circuits (e.g., electromagnetic induction circuits) are also employed in measurement and monitoring devices, but the Wheatstone bridge is the most widely used. Monitors may incorporate amplification and filtering circuits to enhance input to the bridge. They may also be coupled to recording devices to provide permanent recordings of measured changes.

Among the more recent significant advances in monitoring has been the integration of microcomputers, which can take raw measured data, analyze it, and predict trends. If it appears that the measured parameters (i.e., vital signs) are deteriorating, the monitor can trigger an alarm and thus warn the anesthetist to take corrective action. The more sophisticated computerized monitors identify likely problems (based on probability) and recommend corrective actions to be considered. This can be an invaluable aid clinically, especially if multiple parameters are simultaneously tracked. The fact that the monitor can produce a written record of all measurements will undoubtedly have a future impact upon the legal aspects of anesthesia practice.

ELECTRICAL HAZARDS IN THE OPERATING ROOM

Electrical energy, though a common and useful facet of daily life, is not an entirely benign force. In the high-technology environment of the modern operating room, failure to appreciate electricity's potential to maim and kill can lead to disaster for both patients and personnel. Indeed, carelessness has been found to be a major contributing factor to electrically related operating room mishaps.

To appreciate electricity's potential impact upon the human body, several concepts should be kept in mind. First, human bodies readily conduct electrical impulses. Second, bodies coming into contact with an electrical circuit become part of that circuit. Third, the extent of physical injury is dependent upon the type, amount, and path of electric current. Last, all electrical flow seeks the least resistive path to ground potential.

Major physiologic hazards of electricity include ventricular fibrillation, asphyxia, central nervous system disruption, and burns. Electric shock hazards are divided into two categories based on current density: macroshock and microshock. Current density refers to the cross-sectional distribution of the electric current. With *macroshock*, the current is typically distributed throughout the entire body, though not uniformly. Macroshock hazards are typically those to which we are exposed on a daily basis from faulty wiring or improper grounding of electric devices. The mass of the adult human body helps determine the body's resistance to electrical flow. Although various body tissues conduct electricity at different rates, the skin usually takes the brunt of the current, thus providing a protective measure for the body because dangerous currents are shifted away from the heart, the most susceptible organ. However, because currents travel in a conical fashion from the point

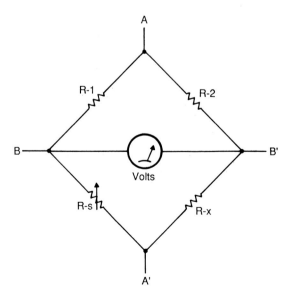

Figure 7–1. Wheatstone bridge circuit. R-1 = R-2; R-1, R-2, R-x = fixed resistances; R-2 = a variable resistance. A and A′ are connections to direct current power source; B and B′ are inputs from sensing device (transducer).

of entry, some macroshock current can almost always be expected to reach the heart. Happily, the current density or cross-sectional flow of current through the myocardium does not always entirely disrupt its normal electrical conducting system because flow per unit area has been diffused. It is for this reason that not every electric "shock" results in death and that relatively high current flows are required to produce cardiac arrest, compared with current flows associated with microshock. Still, in susceptible patients, currents of even a few hundred milliamperes can cause fibrillation of heart muscle.

Microshock injuries are most often produced by indwelling electrodes of conducting devices, such as cardiac pacemakers. Because the current is applied near or directly upon the heart, current densities are high. This means that very little current is required to produce ventricular fibrillation. Thus it is obvious that patients, not operating-room personnel, are at greatest risk from microshock. Even just a few dozen *micro*amperes have been known to produce death. Such injuries occur in part because the body's protective mechanisms are bypassed.

How much current flows through a body area determines the type and extent of physiologic injury. Several factors determine the current flow. It has already been mentioned that tissue conductivity plays a role. Dry skin, for example, is highly resistive. But, the presence of sweat can reduce skin resistance by nearly a hundredfold.

The type of current to which the body is exposed is also a determinant of the degree of injury. While the term *leakage current* is used to describe any unintended current flow, whether through a person or an electrical device, it can make a difference if the current is of the direct or alternating type; and, if the latter, what its frequency is. For example, while both high- and low-frequency ACs are capable of producing heat and burns, only low-frequency currents stimulate nerves and muscles. This can lead to asphyxia secondary to muscle paralysis caused by the electrical stimulus. This is why surgical electrocautery units use high-frequency AC. Almost any device that plugs into 60-hertz electrical outlets can be a source of low-frequency electric current. Unfortunately, 60-hertz current is nearly ideal for producing muscle paralysis.

Cautery units have frequently been implicated as sources of patient injury. The high current densities created by the surgeon's active electrode are supposed to be quickly dissipated through the unit's grounding pad. Safe use requires that the grounding pad be correctly placed, contain a liberal amount of conductive jelly, and be properly connected at all points. It should not be placed over bony prominences, scar areas, or near other electrical conducting points such as electrocardiographic electrodes. This is especially to be avoided if the electrodes are of the needle type with small surface areas. All wiring should be intact and connection plugs should be firmly placed in their receptacles. Cautery wiring should not cross or come into contact with wires from other electronic devices.

Electric shock requires two points of contact—the current source and a ground. Because many items within the operating room can serve as a ground, contact with only a current source can cause a person to experience shock. Surfaces wet with blood or irrigating solutions have a lower resistance and facilitate conduction of current, thus adding to the hazard. Virtually any electrical device emits some leakage current, typically below 1000 microamperes. This is below the threshold of perception, the current being quickly carried away by grounding connections. A current of 1 milliampere causes skin tingling. It is considered the lowest level of current that can be perceived. A 16-milliampere current normally causes an individual to let go of the source. However, this current causes paralysis of flexor muscles and a firm grasp of the source may prevent release. Currents of 50 milliamperes cause pain, loss of consciousness, and mechanical injury. A 0.1-ampere (100-milliampere) current is capable of inducing ventricular fibrillation. All of the foregoing (approximate) current values are associated with macroshock injuries from 60-hertz AC. Under microshock conditions, where current is delivered directly to the heart, 20 microamperes can induce ventricular fibrillation. To minimize the potential for electrical injury, all devices used within the operating room should be inspected and labeled by biomedical personnel prior to use. They should also be reexamined on a periodic basis. All items should be operated within the guidelines of manufacturer recommendations. *All suspect equipment should be removed from the operating room environment until repaired and reinspected by biomedical personnel.* Equipment should be inspected carefully before it is used, with particular attention to ensure that ground and other connections are made before the equipment is turned on.

Safety Regulations and Requirements

Although each government municipality is responsible for developing and enforcing its own construction and electrical codes, there exists a high degree of regulatory similarity across the United States. This is because most government agencies look to standards of the National Electrical Code (NEC) and the National Fire Protection Association (NFPA) for guidance in all aspects of electrical and other safety practices. NFPA standards address electrical safety and use of explosive and nonexplosive anesthetic and therapeutic gases and other hazardous substances capable of initiating a fire. Standards are developed by experts who periodically review, update, and publish them in pamphlet form. Though not enforceable as law except where they have been codified by legislative agencies, the standards are still highly regarded by accrediting bodies, which find them useful in making judgments about the quality of care rendered by a health-care facility. The governing board of each hospital is responsible for ensuring adherence to legal requirements and for developing internal safety policies and procedures. All anesthetists should be thoroughly familiar with those standards bearing on safe anesthesia practice.

Two primary areas encompassed by safety standards on electrical use by a health facility are testing and grounding. It will be remembered that electrical flow is dependent upon a charge difference between two objects. This occurs when a charge-producing substance is brought into contact with a nonconductor. Separation of the two leaves each with a charge of "static" electricity. Static electricity has often been implicated as an ignition source of operating room fires and explosions in the past, but the trend away from using explosive anesthetic agents has reduced the hazard. Nevertheless, the principles for dealing with static electricity remain valid for even the most modern of operating rooms because it, like electricity's other forms, can be a source of harm when circumstances allow. For example, a spark could ignite fumes from an open container of volatile cleaning fluid.

A considerable number of electrical items are used in operating rooms. On any given day, most of the following could be employed during just one case: electrocautery, monitors, x-ray equipment, electrical operating room table, microscopes, headlamps, endoscopic equipment, and fluid pumps. The growing use of lasers and other high-energy systems will add to the problem. Lasers have already been the source of several operating room fires. Outside the operating room items such as heating lamps and diathermy units can become dangerous sources of electricity. One cannot even consider psychiatric wards safe because electroconvulsive therapy performed in this area has been responsible for patient deaths (probably through cardiac arrhythmias accompanying central nervous system disruption and catecholamine release induced by the therapy). Indeed, no area of a health facility is totally free from the possibility of electrical injury to patients and personnel. For this reason, patient risks for electrical injury have now been classified. Surgical patients represent the highest risk group because they are exposed to both macro- and microshock hazards. All these considerations underscore the need for careful vigilance and attention to electrical safety requirements.

The most critical factor in operating room safety is electrical grounding. Proper grounding rapidly dissipates static charges and carries away dangerous currents that develop in equipment. As previously mentioned, a power source outlet in the United States consists of three conductors: one is a "live" wire that conducts current; one returns current from equipment back to the power source, at which point it is grounded to earth; and one is locally connected to an earth ground. Conducting wires are normally colored black, white, and green respectively. The redundant local ground is connected to the equipment chassis by way of the unit's three-conductor power cable. This third conductor serves to remove charges occurring as a result of component malfunction within the unit and as a backup ground should an electrical fault develop to prevent current from being returned via the normal pathway. Providing a redundant ground for equipment increases safety. Live current flowing through equipment as a result of malfunction presents a macroshock hazard, at least until fuse or circuit-breaker disruption interrupts power to the unit. With an intact redundant ground, current is dissipated quickly—before someone coming into contact with the unit is injured. Extension cords circumvent this safety precaution, and the use of such cords in the operating room is to be condemned.

Both NEC and NFPA standards require patient-care areas to use *equipotential grounding*. This type of grounding joins all equipment, conductive surfaces, and metal objects in the area in such a way that all are at the same voltage. The point at which these objects are electrically joined is called the *patient reference ground* because the patient is in contact with many of the conducting surfaces or items. The patient reference ground point is, in turn, connected

to the earth ground system of the electrical source. Equipotential environments provide a conductive path for any 60-hertz current accidentally entering a patient-connected system. Proper operation requires that all electrical and ground conductors be well insulated and correctly wired. There may also be specific ground points for special equipment and for a room's conductive metal framework. Potential differences between any two exposed conductive surfaces in an equipotential environment should not exceed 100 to 500 millivolts for frequencies below one kilohertz when measured across a 1000-ohm resistance. Specific requirements vary with the degree of patient risk.

Anesthetizing locations require a special type of high-resistance power-delivery circuit using what is called an isolation transformer. Isolated power circuits receive current from the normal electrical service lines by way of the transformer's primary winding. The operating room's electrical outlets are connected to the transformer's secondary winding. Therefore, no direct connection exists between the power source and outlets. Within the transformer, power is transferred from the primary to the secondary by means of magnetic inductance, a concept discussed earlier. Neither of the transformer's output connections is connected to ground. Because energy has been transferred magnetically and not carried as a pure current, the output wires are "isolated." No current will flow through a grounded person coming into contact with either of the wires; hence, the person is not "shocked." However, current can flow between the two isolated output conductors. Touching both outputs simultaneously will cause current flow through the individual's arms. Obviously, isolated power circuits increase safety by requiring the individual to make two contacts, rather than one, before receiving a shock. Although they increase safety, isolated power circuits are not perfect. Some capacitive coupling between transformer and person can occur and cause current to be perceived. An additional advantage of isolated power circuits is that a short circuit from either of the lines to a piece of grounded equipment does not disrupt power by activating circuit breakers or fuses. The equipment can be used until the short-circuit defect is repaired. Also, "free-floating" electricity from such a short circuit would not cause sparking that could serve as a fire ignition source.

Because it is possible for an isolated line to become directly shorted to ground and thus present the same hazard as a normal electrical outlet, line isolation monitoring devices are incorporated to warn of the defect. When the monitor detects current flowing to ground, it activates a visual and/or audible alarm. Line monitors are placed in each operating room served by an isolated power system, but they cannot identify a break in equipment grounding systems and should not be relied upon to ensure equipment safety.

Use of explosive agents in anesthesia practice has waned considerably, but some institutions still use them occasionally. For such facilities conductive floors are mandatory. The purpose for conductive materials, footwear, and flooring in operating rooms is the elimination of static electricity. In addition some protection is afforded against macroshock injury. Standards require conductive flooring to have a minimum resistance of 25,000 ohms. Maximum allowed resistance is 1,000,000 ohms. This range is best to allow dissipation of static charges, but it also creates enough resistance to reduce the likelihood of serious macroshock injury from currents typically encountered in the operating room environment. Resistance levels are measured with two electrodes placed three feet apart on the conductive floor. Testing should be performed at east monthly, and records kept to track any changes in resistance level. Other equipment is also checked for conductivity, including operating room tables and anesthesia machines. The presence of dirt, wax, plastics, and debris works to reduce conductivity and render conductive flooring ineffective. Table and equipment wheels should be made of conductive materials and periodically cleaned to insure firm contact with the floor. All rubber goods must be electrically conductive if explosive agents are administered.

Besides testing conductive flooring, biomedical personnel normally carry out inspection and testing of all operating room equipment; this includes checking wiring, plugs, electrical circuits, and other items. Any equipment needing repair is tagged and removed for servicing. Logs are kept of all test findings and repair work. New equipment should undergo a shakedown period before being placed in service within the operating room area.

Special Electrical Hazards

It is a common misconception that battery-operated devices present no hazard. Although battery operated equipment is typically at low voltage, malfunction under certain conditions can be dangerous. Endoscopic equipment has been responsible for detonating explosions within patient body cavities. Fuel for such explosions can be flammable anesthetics sequestered in the cavity or natural organic by-products. Arcing or heat caused by malfunction of an endoscope bulb can be enough to ignite volatile substances. Even laryngoscopes have caused anesthetic-agent explosions. Use of the electrocautery during laparoscopy is especially dangerous. Laparoscopy involves insufflating a gas into the abdominal cavity to distend it and allow passage of the laparoscope. Carbon dioxide can be the insufflating gas. More often, nitrous oxide is used because patients tolerate it better. Nitrous oxide supports combustion and readily diffuses into the gut to mix with highly explosive methane and hydrogen gas contained there. Heat generated by electrocautery forceps, if they are misapplied to the gut rather than the fallopian tubes, can ignite the gases to cause an explosion.

Another frequently overlooked hazard is that of burns caused by passage of an electric current through an area where electrolyte solution is present. If physiologic saline is pooled under an electrode or on a surface in contact with the patient's skin, passage of the current will ionize the solution to sodium hydroxide and chlorine gas. Contact of these substances with the skin for an extended period results in caustic burns. These are often deep and heal poorly. The anesthetist should always examine the patient's skin for evidence of such burns, particularly under electrode or grounding pads. Even without the presence of an electrolyte solution, leakage current applied to the skin for a long period of time will produce a thermal injury as current is carried through the patient's body to a grounding site.

Exposure to intense radio frequencies, even when no direct skin contact is made, also results in burns. Recently, questions about the long-term biologic effects of radio frequency exposure have been raised. Research in this area is underway, but no definite information is yet available. Given that nearly every person daily receives radio frequency radiation from the environment, the results of such research could hold important future implications.

In the event that one comes upon an electrocution victim, rapid intervention is necessary to prevent death. The following steps should be taken:

1. If possible, shut off the source of electricity.
2. If cutting off power is not possible, separate the victim from the electrical contact using a nonconducting lever (e.g., a piece of wood). *Do not touch the victim until this is accomplished.*
3. Summon aid.
4. Initiate cardiopulmonary resuscitation.
5. Transport the patient to a medical facility.

FIRE AND EXPLOSION HAZARDS

Operating room fires and explosions decreased substantially in the 1970s as anesthesia personnel abandoned the use of flammable anesthetics. Yet, a number of such incidents are still reported each year, and fire and explosion remain the most frightening and devastating events that can occur in an operating room.

Three factors are necessary for a fire to start: *fuel, oxygen, and an ignition source.* Any substance capable of chemically combining with oxygen can serve as fuel. This includes most organic compounds, which, because they contain carbon and hydrogen, will lend themselves to burning. A fuel's chemical nature determines the rapidity with which it burns (flammability). For this reason, volatile substances, whether gases, vapors, or liquids, usually burn more easily than solids. Burning involves an oxidative process, but not all oxidative reactions result in fire or explosion. Combustion is a term used to indicate those that do. Primary end products of combustion are carbon, carbon dioxide, and water. Oxygen for combustion reactions can be in either pure or combined form. For example, when nitrous oxide is dissociated to its components—nitrogen and oxygen—released oxygen becomes free to enter into oxidative reactions. Therefore, nitrous oxide can support combustion. In relative terms, fire is a slow oxidative process if contrasted with explosions which, upon detonation, occur instantly. Burning is an exothermic reaction; that is, heat is produced and liberated. As the reactants of a fire become sufficiently heated, they become luminescent. This glow is seen as the fire flame. Heat in any form can serve as a fire ignition source. This includes open flames, static sparks, electrical arcing, and chemical reactions. Under appropriate conditions, ignition sources need not be intense or applied for a long period.

The *oxidative process* involves transfer of electrons. As heat from the ignition source accelerates molecular motion within the fuel-oxygen mixture, molecular bonds are broken and electrons transfer from oxygen to the fuel substance. This results in a chemical reduction of the fuel. Heat released with the breaking of the first few bonds activates further molecular activity: more broken bonds bring about greater heat release, which accelerates electron transfer. Certain conditions that facilitate this process include: high ambient temperatures, compression of gases, availability of fuel and oxygen, and the extent to which fuel and oxygen are allowed to mix. Conditions that limit either the rate or extent of burning include: low fuel reactivity, a limited supply of either fuel or oxygen, effectiveness of heat dissipation, and the presence of quenching agents.

Combustible mixtures are of three types: *lean, rich,* and *stoichiometric.* With lean mixtures, oxygen is in greater abundance than fuel. For rich mixtures, the reverse is true—there being fuel still available after oxygen has been used up. Stoichiometric mixtures are those in which combustion is complete, there being neither fuel nor oxygen remaining. The proportions of fuel and oxygen in a mixture determine the flammability range for the mix. Outside the range, oxygen or fuel amounts are insufficient to allow significant combustion. Upper and lower limits of flammability have been determined for all explosive anesthetic agents in combination with oxygen, air, or nitrous oxide. Because of limited use of explosive agents today, flammability ranges are not covered here; they are available in standard texts for those desiring more information. Generally, flammable anesthetic concentrations of 1 to 80 percent are sufficiently volatile to cause explosions. With one exception, trichlorethylene, anesthetic concentrations of all explosive agents fall within this range. Mixtures in which oxygen is present at less than 10 percent by volume generally will not self-propagate if ignited. With metabolic oxygen requirements being more than double this amount, it is impossible to entirely eliminate the explosive hazard of flammable anesthetic mixtures.

The fire factor easiest to control is ignition source. A number of sources have already been identified in this chapter. Two ignition source terms that are sometimes confused are flashpoint and ignition temperature. *Flashpoint* is the temperature at which a mixture first burns. However, upon removing the ignition source, the flame goes out. At *ignition temperature,* the mixture continues to burn even after the ignition source has been removed. In most cases of fire and explosion, ignition temperatures are below 500C. Even heat from a small spark is enough to raise the temperature of a portion of flammable mixture above the ignition point. A mixture's *detonation point* is the temperature at which it explodes. Static electricity has been a major ignition source of operating room fires. The use of conductive flooring for removing static charges has been discussed. Another operating room factor serving the same purpose is environmental humidity. At a *relative humidity of 55 to 60 percent,* air moisture provides enough conductivity on open surfaces to carry away static charges to a ground point.

Halogenation of anesthetic compounds has been another approach to reducing operating room flammability hazards.

One ignition source peculiar to anesthesia and inhalation therapy practice is that of *adiabatic compression* or *expansion.* Under most conditions, compression increases and

expansion decreases the temperature of a gas. These temperature changes are transferred to the surrounding environment. However, when volume changes occur under conditions that do not allow gain or loss of heat from the environment, they are termed adiabatic. Because such volume changes occur very rapidly, high temperatures are generated instantaneously. This is the case within compressed gas cylinders when the tank valve is opened. Gas from the cylinder enters the valve where it is recompressed because of the valve's smaller volume. This creates extremely high temperatures capable of igniting particulate matter lodged in the valve outlet. A flash fire results. Oxygen from the surrounding air or within the gas mixture feeds the fire and adds to the hazard. It is for this reason that cylinder valves should always be kept capped until ready for use. In addition, no oil or other flammable substance should be used as a lubricant around the valve opening. Gas cylinders should be "cracked" (opened slowly to air) prior to attachment of regulating valves. This procedure is not recommended when attaching cylinders to the anesthesia machine. A strainer nipple is present in the machine to filter particulate matter. Adiabatic compression also presents a hazard when cylinders are being filled from bulk supplies. Manufacturers of compressed gas equipment must follow special safety precautions when transfilling cylinders, and anesthesia personnel should never attempt to transfill anesthetic gases themselves.

Another phenomenon seen when releasing gas from a compressed cylinder is the *Joule-Thomson effect.* As gas leaves the cylinder, its expansion cools the surrounding air, causing condensation of moisture on the tank. The Joule-Thomson effect per se does not represent a fire hazard. But hand contact with the cylinder as cooling takes place can result in a freeze burn to the skin.

The flammability range of explosive mixtures can be narrowed by addition of *quenching agents,* nonoxidizable inert gases, of which the three most prominent are carbon dioxide, helium, and nitrogen. Quenching agents reduce combustibility because they possess high molal heat capacities or high thermal conductivity. This means they either absorb large amounts of heat readily (thus increasing the amount of heat required for ignition) or they rapidly dispel heat, conducting it away before ignition can occur. These agents are often used in safety devices for hazardous locations. Carbon dioxide fire extinguishers are an example.

Using flammable anesthetics requires a number of special precautions. Electrical outlets are kept five feet above the floor to prevent contact with gases accumulating near the floor. All electrical connections have to be of the interlocking type. Explosion-proof switches are required. All precautions required when using explosive agents are explained in NFPA pamphlet 56-A, a current copy of which should be in every surgical suite.

Every operating room should have a fire emergency plan. Prior planning and training can save lives and prevent injury. The following outline reviews the major steps to be taken in the event of an operating room fire or explosion:

Phase I (Notification)

1. The senior operating room charge person initiates the plan at the first hint of a fire.

2. He or she sounds the fire alarm or calls the fire department. Many operating rooms are equipped with automatic alarms to notify firefighters of the emergency. It is possible for such systems to malfunction. A secondary notification system should also be used. Failure to summon help promptly can be catastrophic.
3. All traffic into the surgical suite is stopped and all personnel alerted to the emergency.
4. Fire doors are closed and emergency exits readied.
5. Personnel are assigned to operate fire-fighting equipment at all key locations.

Phase II (Preparation)
Within each operating room, personnel should take the following measures:

1. Unplug all unnecessary electrical equipment.
2. Remove all flammable agents (e.g., alcohols) to a nonpatient area such as a substerile room. Surgical procedures not yet begun should be aborted. Those underway require individual professional judgments as to whether or not to continue.
3. Disconnect piped-in anesthesia gases, turn on machine reserve cylinders, and lower delivered flows if feasible.
4. Disconnect all unnecessary equipment (e.g., blood warmers, humidifiers, etc.).
5. Gather essential drugs and equipment necessary for patient evacuation.
6. Plan for maintenance of the patient's vital functions during evacuation.

Phase III (Implementation)

1. Until an all-clear or evacuation signal is given, all personnel should remain at their assigned locations. When notified by the senior person to begin evacuation, proceed rapidly according to preplanned policies, using designated evacuation routes. How the patient is transported will vary with the circum-

stances; it may not be feasible to do more than carry the patient. All equipment may have to be abandoned. Patient vital functions may have to be maintained using cardiopulmonary resuscitation procedures. If abandoning the anesthesia machine, shut off all gas flows.
2. Disconnect main electrical and gas lines.

Every fire alarm should be treated with the utmost seriousness. Undoubtedly, many alarms will be either false or quickly handled. Callous disregard of an alarm can have dire consequences for both patients and operating room staffs.

CONCLUSION

The potential for electrical- and fire-related injuries found in the modern operating room is virtually unmatched by any other human work environment. Patients trust the nurse anesthetist to ensure their well-being while they are anesthetized. Meeting that responsibility requires an understanding and appreciation of the basic principles underlying operating room hazards. As in all other phases of anesthesia practice, safety resides in constant vigilance.

BIBLIOGRAPHY

Adriani JA: The Chemistry and Physics of Anesthesia. Springfield, IL, Chas. C. Thomas, 1962.

Beiser A, Cummings B: Physics, 4th ed. Menlo Park, CA, Bubco, 1986.

Blatt FJ: Principles of Physics, 2nd ed. Boston, Allyn & Bacon, 1986.

Collins VJ: Principles of Anesthesiology. Philadelphia, Lea & Febiger, 1976.

Neufeld GR: Fires and explosions. In Orkin FK, Cooperman LH (eds): Complications in Anesthesiology. Philadelphia, Lippincott, 1983.

Scurr C, Feldman S: Scientific Foundations of Anaesthesia, 3rd ed. Chicago, Year Book Med Pub, 1982.

8

The Care of Anesthesia Equipment

Leslie Rendell-Baker

The practice of anesthesia, once the simple dripping of ether on a mask while keeping a finger on the pulse, now depends on a wide range of mechanical, electronic, and plastic equipment. All of this is exposed daily to potential contamination with the patient's blood and secretions and with microorganisms carried on the users' hands.

Dr. Howard L. Zauder, in 1965 when he was Chairman of the American Society of Anesthesiologists' (ASA) Subcommittee on Sterilization, reported to the ASA Committee on Equipment and Standardization that "as part of a preventive routine, periodically cultures were taken from all equipment, anesthetic and other, used in the operating rooms" of his hospital. "The anesthesia machines—in spite of superficial cleaning—were not only contaminated, they were downright filthy!" (Fig. 8–1). After this report, all machines were washed daily by an aide, and Zauder commented that the machines were then cleaner, but the job was made difficult by the machines' design. "The multiple surfaces, the complex of semiexposed tubing, the knobs, yolks, wheels, and dials, while sound from an engineering viewpoint, were a housekeeping nightmare. The outside surfaces of gas cylinders are frequently quite dirty and should be cleaned before they are brought into the operating room." Zauder believed that the cylinders should be enclosed. "Manufacturers should be encouraged when present equipment is redesigned to eliminate all exposed dirt-collecting surfaces." This report was discussed in a 1965 symposium at Mt. Sinai Hospital (New York) in which manufacturers' engineers participated, and the Dupaco company later produced their Hygienic Model (Fig. 8–2), which eliminated many dirt traps and held the cylinders in a rear enclosure. Now that most machines operate from pipeline gas supplies and the cylinders are rarely changed, being kept solely as an emergency reserve, the argument for their enclosure on hygienic grounds should carry more weight. However, although the apparatus introduced since the publication in 1979 of the ANSI Z79.8* Standard on the safety and performance of anesthesia apparatus were much improved in safety, they were still as difficult to clean.

---

* The American National Standards Institute Committee Z79, which formerly worked on standards for anesthesia and ventilatory equipment has, since 1983, been replaced by the American Society for Testing and Materials Committee F29, which has the same functions.

STERILIZATION, DISINFECTION, AND ANTISEPSIS

The wide range of apparatus we use and their varying tolerance to cleaning and sterilizing procedures require that we have suitable alternatives available. Sterilization is any process that completely destroys all living organisms in or on an object. Disinfection is a process in which an agent is used to kill pathogenic microorganisms, usually on inanimate objects. Antisepsis is any process that prevents or combats infection by killing or inhibiting microorganisms usually on human tissue. Decontamination is the process that frees a person or object from soiling with an infectious material.

The type of sterilization or disinfection is selected contingent on the material of the item to be decontaminated, the microorganism to be destroyed, and the degree of decontamination to be attained. Items that penetrate the skin barrier or come in contact with mucous membranes must be sterilized, whereas equipment in a contaminated room can be properly decontaminated by washing with a germicidal detergent solution.

Cleaning is the first step in any decontamination method. Dirt, body secretions, or other extraneous material inhibits the action of the disinfectant by a mechanical blocking or neutralizing effect. The efficiency of any disinfectant is dependent on time and concentration and especially upon the acidity or alkalinity (pH) of the environment. Some disinfectants are more efficacious under neutral conditions. This is important to remember when using alkaline soaps and detergents for preliminary cleaning. If these alkaline solutions are not completely rinsed from the surface to be disinfected, they may neutralize or decrease the effectiveness of a disinfectant requiring an acid environment. Temperature is a determinant of the efficiency of disinfectants. As a general rule, the higher the temperature, the faster-acting will be the disinfectant.

Recommended Methods

    I. *Sterilization*
        A. Steam autoclaving
            1. Always the first choice
            2. Items must tolerate the heat and steam

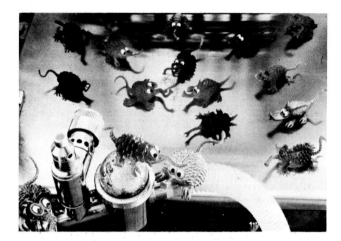

Figure 8–1. Bacterial contamination of the anesthesia apparatus. Unfortunately, microorganisms cannot be seen. If they were as visible as are these contaminants, we would be sure to clean our equipment properly. © *1987 L Rendell-Baker.*

B. Ethylene oxide gas autoclaving
  1. Large enough stock of items must be available to permit proper duration of aeration to eliminate residues of the gas
  2. Never gas autoclave any item that can be steam autoclaved

II. *Disinfection*
  A. Alkaline glutaraldehyde (e.g., Cidex)
    1. Mix solution as instructed
    2. Use solution no longer than 28 days
    3. Rinse disinfected items properly to remove residues
    4. Avoid contact with skin
    5. Use in well-ventilated area
    6. Flush splashes to eyes with water and report to employee health service for immediate care
  B. Phenolic solution (e.g., Wexcide)
    1. This solution is the hospital germicidal disinfectant of choice and should be supplied from the pharmacy diluted and ready for use
    2. Follow manufacturer's instructions when diluting concentrated product for use
    3. Avoid contact with skin by wearing gloves
    4. Solution is caustic; if splashed in eyes, flood with water and contact employee health service
  C. Sodium hypochlorite (chlorine bleach 1:5 to 1:10 dilution)
    1. First-choice disinfectant for destroying hepatitis virus
    2. Bleach solution will decolorize fabric

III. *Antisepsis*
  A. Iodophor (e.g., Betadine)
    1. The povidone-iodine surgical scrub, which incorporates liquid soap, is also recommended for hand washing
    2. The povidone-iodine solution is used in surgical preparation and wound cleaning

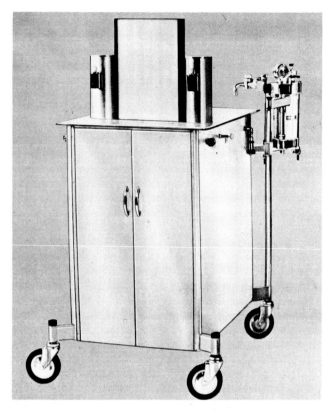

Figure 8–2. Dupaco Hygienic Machine. The cylinders were enclosed by doors, and many dirt traps were eliminated, greatly simplifying the task of cleaning. (*Illustration courtesy of the Dupaco Company.*)

  B. Chlorhexidine gluconate (e.g., Hibiclens)
    1. Recommended for hand washing
      a. Rinse thoroughly with water
  C. Hexachlorophene
    1. Recommended for hand washing for persons who are allergic to iodophor and chlorhexidine gluconate
  D. Alcohol, 70 percent
    1. Keep bottle tightly closed; alcohol is volatile
  E. Unsatisfactory agent: Benzalkonium chloride is not listed as a disinfectant or antiseptic because it is not effective against all gram-negative organisms, some of which can multiply in it. It may be used as a sanitizer only.

Infection Control Guidelines for Anesthesia Equipment

I. *Anesthesia machines and ventilators*
  A. Clean all surfaces, including flow control knobs, daily with a phenolic solution
  B. Cover machine counter with clean towel for each patient
  C. After use with an infectious patient, such as one with lung abcess or open pulmonary tuberculosis, clean all surfaces immediately with a phenolic solution

II. *Disposable equipment to be discarded after each use*
   A. Syringes and needles
   B. Breathing systems including breathing bags
   C. Tracheal tubes, polyvinyl chloride (PVC) plastic wire-reinforced tubes, plastic endobronchial tubes
   D. Esophageal stethoscopes[†]

III. *Equipment to be sterilized or pasteurized.* Whenever possible, use steam sterilization. It is simpler, safer, and quicker than ethylene oxide gas sterilization. Pasteurization can be used when clean rather than sterile equipment is acceptable.
   A. Rubber breathing systems[*†]
   B. Wire-reinforced latex tubes[*‡] Rubber endobronchial tubes[†]
   C. Face masks[*†]
   D. Oral airways[*]
   E. Temperature probes[*†]
   F. Laryngoscope blades[*§]
   G. Wash and gas sterilize ventilator bellows on a rotation basis and after use with a contaminated patient
   H. Autoclave the carbon dioxide absorber assembly whenever possible after anesthetizing patients with pulmonary tuberculosis and other pulmonary infections

Methods of Disinfection and Sterilization

Moist Heat. Moist heat is much more effective in causing coagulation of cellular proteins and death of organisms at lower temperatures than is dry heat, which is of little use for sterilization of anesthesia equipment.

Pasteurization. Louis Pasteur (1822–1895), the French chemist, discovered the bacteria that are responsible for fermentation and disease and developed the process of pasteurization to protect wine and milk against spoilage. Milk is heated to 62C and held there for 30 minutes, then rapidly cooled. Although pasteurization does not destroy spores, it kills *Mycobacterium tuberculosis*, salmonellae, brucellae, and streptococci, which were the cause of serious milk-borne diseases.

Pasteurization is now widely used to disinfect biologicals and plastic and rubber anesthesia equipment. It is most important that blood secretions and other soil be removed first by a thorough washing process. The equipment to be disinfected is then exposed to hot water at 170F (77C) for 30 minutes. This method does not produce sterility, since the outside of the equipment must be handled twice as it is transferred from the washer to the drier and again when it is removed from the drier to be packed into plastic bags. However, anesthesia breathing systems properly processed in this way are as clean as disposable breathing systems. Use of a mechanical rotary washer and pasteurizing equipment, such as the Olympic Pasteurmatic (Figs. 8–3A, B, 8–4) has proved to be an efficient and economical method of providing clean equipment in some busy anesthesia services. The Cidematic is a similar system that uses glutaraldehyde instead of heat to kill the bacteria. Glutaraldehyde is effective against *M. tuberculosis* and vegetative forms of bacteria even in the presence of blood and mucus. It is an irritant to the skin, so rubber gloves should be worn. The equipment must be rinsed thoroughly to remove the residues and odor. Glutaraldehyde solution has a limited stability and should be discarded after 2 weeks.

Boiling. Boiling was a widely used method of sterilization in earlier days. Boiling occurs at 100C at sea level (760 mm Hg) and at lower temperatures at higher altitudes, for example, at 94.4C in Denver, Colorado, at 5550 feet, and at 86.6C in LaPaz, Bolivia, at 13,600 feet. There is a drop of about 1C in the temperature at which water boils for each 1000 feet rise in altitude. Boiling at 100C for 30 minutes is lethal to all vegetative forms of bacteria, most spores, and most viruses. It is recommended that the boiling time be extended 5 minutes for each 1000 feet rise in altitude above sea level. These facts are of importance where high-pressure steam sterilization is not available.

Steam Autoclave. At sea level, water in a pan boils at 100C. However, if the water is heated in a pressure cooker, as the pressure rises so will the temperature at which the water boils. The change from liquid to vapor requires a considerable amount of heat (i.e., 580 calories for each milliliter of water). It is the availability of this latent heat in the steam that is given up when the steam condenses on the cool load in the sterilizer that so shortens the time required by steam to produce sterility, compared with hot air at the same temperature. The higher the pressure the higher will be the steam's temperature and with it the shorter the time required to heat everything within the sterilizer to the temperature required for sterility.

Before commencing the sterilizing cycle it is important to remove the air from the chamber by vacuum, for otherwise the air will reduce the amount of steam entering and, thus, the temperature achieved at any given pressure. Sterilization starts when steam flows into the chamber, penetrating the load and giving up its latent heat as it condenses on the cooler items. Once the desired temperature is achieved the required duration for sterilization is set. At the end of this period, to avoid residual condensation on the load when the cool air is admitted, the steam is exhausted from the chamber by vacuum.

Most modern autoclaves have automatic controls to ensure that the correct sequence is followed. Commonly used combinations are 15 minutes at 121C and 15 psi and 5 to 10 minutes at 132C and 30 psi.

Steam autoclaving is by far the quickest and most effective method of sterilization, provided the materials to be sterilized can tolerate steam and the temperature. Items that must be sterile for use should be packed in nylon bags or specially made packets that are easily permeable to steam.

---

[*] *May be pasteurized*
[†] *May be washed, packaged, and gas sterilized*
[‡] *May be autoclaved using liquid cycle only*
[§] *May be autoclaved*

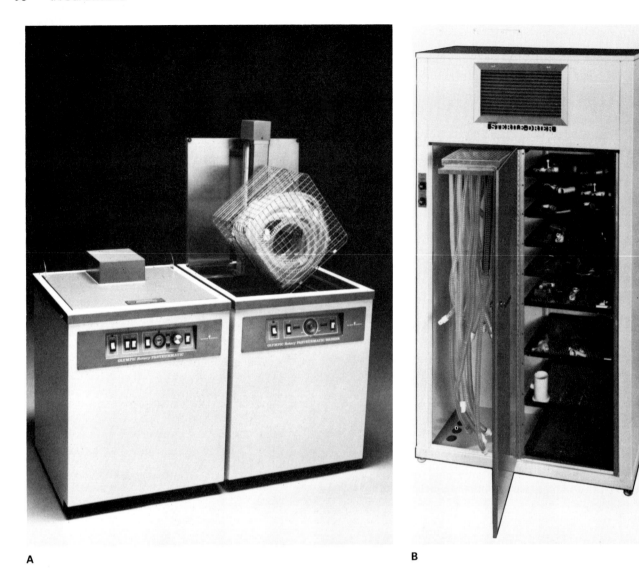

Figure 8–3. The Olympic Rotary Pasteurmatic system. **A.** Rotary washer (30-minute cycle) (*right*). Up to 20 anesthesia breathing system components are loaded into the stainless steel baskets, which are lowered into the washer. The baskets rotate as jets of hot water at 60C (140F) spray onto the contents. As the chamber fills, the equipment is repeatedly plunged into the hot detergent solution to dislodge the contaminating soil. At the end of the wash cycle the equipment is rinsed in hot water and allowed to drain. Rotary Pasteurmatic (30-minute cycle) (*left*). The same baskets are transferred to the pasteurizer, which contains hotter water (77C,170F), and are submerged for 30 minutes after a preliminary period of rotation to release trapped air. **B.** Drying Cabinet. Bacteria free HEPA-filtered air at 57C (135F) is blown over and through the equipment to speed up the drying process. On removal from the dryer, the equipment is sealed in plastic bags (Fig. 8–4) to prevent contamination before its next use.

Ethylene Oxide Gas Sterilization. Ethylene oxide was first used as a fumigant in 1928 and has been extensively used as a sterilizing agent since the technique for its use, introduced by Phillips and Kaye in 1949, was perfected by McDonald in 1962. It is particularly useful for sterilizing plastic and other equipment that would be damaged by the higher temperatures achieved in the steam autoclave. It was the availability of this convenient, low-temperature method of sterilization that made possible the provision of the sterile disposable equipment now so widely used in our hospitals.

The method was first used to sterilize anesthesia equipment by the anesthesia department of Buffalo General Hospital in 1960 and by Dr. John Snow of Boston in 1962. Very little information was available on the rate of elimination of the gas from sterilized plastic items, and no one knew how much ethylene oxide human tissues could tolerate. By 1968, reports of skin and tracheal burns and hemolysis of blood began to appear, which led the ANSI Z79 anesthesia standards committee to form a subcommittee to study this problem. This group has continued its work,

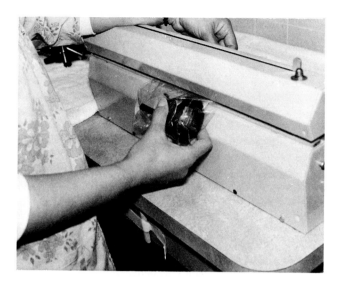

Figure 8–4. Anesthesia technician sealing clean equipment in plastic bag for storage. © *1987 L Rendell-Baker.*

now under the aegis of the Association for Advancement of Medical Instrumentation, from whom up-to-date advice on the safe use of ethylene oxide may be obtained (see Appendix at the end of this chapter).

It has become apparent that ethylene oxide, which would not be effective if it were not poisonous, is a much more serious danger to the operator's health than is nitrous oxide pollution in the operating room. As a result, the earlier maximum permitted level of 50 ppm (with a peak of 75 ppm), averaged over an 8-hour working day, has now been reduced by the Occupational Safety and Health Administration to a threshold limit value of 1 ppm over an 8-hour working day. The maximum permitted peak level has not yet been published. To maintain this low level and protect the employees' health, it is desirable that ethyl-

ene oxide sterilizers and aerators not be placed in work areas, but rather in a separate area. In any case they should be equipped with a dedicated air extraction system to remove the gas residues to the outside air.

Since ethylene oxide is highly explosive, the larger sterilizers use a mixture of 12 percent ethylene oxide and 88 percent Freon 12, a fluorocarbon gaseous quenching agent, or 10 percent ethylene oxide and 90 percent carbon dioxide, which has the same effect. Small sterilizers often use cartridges of 100 percent ethylene oxide.

Factors of importance in the use of ethylene oxide sterilization follow:

1. Unlike steam sterilization, the ethylene oxide process has two phases, one during which the gas is forced into the load, the other during which it slowly escapes from the load. Unfortunately, the second phase is much longer than the first. It may last from 8 hours to 7 days, depending upon the temperature and airflow. An aerator cabinet providing a flow of warm, bacterially filtered air at 140F produces satisfactory aeration in 8 hours. Contrast this with packets of polyvinyl chloride items left on a shelf at 70F, which will take 7 days to eliminate the large quantity of the gas absorbed by the plastic.
2. Before sterilization, clean and remove all gross water droplets; however, equipment must not be heat-dried, for ethylene oxide requires the presence of greater than 45 percent relative humidity for efficient penetration and sterilization of the load.
3. Pack the equipment in 3-mil-thick polyethylene bags or in specially designed gas sterilization packages. Nylon is impermeable to ethylene oxide and PVC retains the gas, hindering aeration, so neither material should be used with ethylene oxide sterilization. Place the items in the sterilizer and proceed (Fig. 8–5).

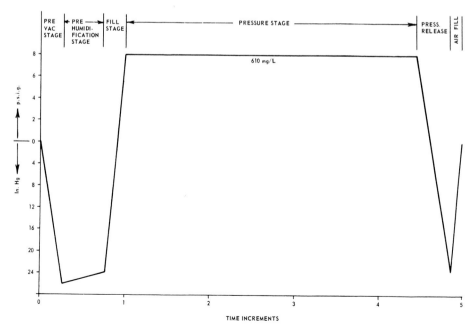

Figure 8–5. The McDonald ethylene oxide gaseous sterilization process. The graph shows the pressure changes during the sequential events of the cycle. Note the high degree of vacuum produced at the beginning and at the end of the sequence.

4. A vacuum of 29 inches Hg is required to remove the air from the chamber and the load.
5. Apply steam to humidify the load; this is necessary for the gas to penetrate and kill the bacteria.
6. An exposure to ethylene oxide for 4 to 5 hours at a pressure of 8 psi with Freon mixtures or 25 psig with carbon dioxide mixtures and a temperature of 130F is necessary. Freon 12 facilitates penetration of the gas through the packaging and into the depths of the plastic or rubber items being sterilized.
7. Even after exposure to a vacuum to remove the bulk of the gas from the sterilizer, a cloud of 2000 to 5000 ppm ethylene oxide is released when the sterilizer door is first opened. Therefore, open the sterilizer door and leave the room for 15 to 20 minutes until the gas has dissipated.
8. Transfer the load to an aerator through which a stream of bacterially filtered air at 120 to 140F is drawn. The standard aeration phase usually lasts 8 to 12 hours to remove the gas from such items as PVC plastic tubes, which retain the gas much longer than do any other materials.

An aeration time less than the 8 to 12 hours recommended by the manufacturer allows the risk of skin burns or mucosal irritation caused by retained residues of the gas in the equipment. Therefore, whenever equipment can withstand high temperatures, steam sterilization is preferred; it is quicker, simpler, and safer for both patient and technician.

Special Problems

Contamination of Apparatus with Mycobacteria. There have been no documented cases of transmission of tubercle bacilli via anesthesia equipment. However, of all bacteria, the acid-fast bacilli are the most adaptable and are particularly resistant to desiccation. duMoulin and colleagues report that in Massachusetts there has been a fivefold increase in the incidence of nontuberculous mycobacterial infections that are insidious and difficult to treat with antimycobacterial drugs (duMoulin and Stottmeier, 1986). Most lesions require surgical resection. Since 1972, there has been a fourfold increase in pulmonary infections in adults and lymphadenitis in children due to the *M. avium-intracellular* bacilli in Massachusetts (duMoulin and Hedley-Whyte, 1982). Transmission of these organisms is by environmental contact rather than person to person, with tap water implicated as the primary vehicle of transmission. These authors have documented infection of patients via the hospital water supply during the summer months, when the numbers of these chlorine-resistant organisms are high. Mycobacterium were isolated from a number of sites including heated nebulizers, ice machines, hot and cold faucets, bedside drinking water carafes, and water fountains in their hospital (duMoulin and Stottmeier, 1986). Unfortunately, hand washing can contaminate the anesthetist's hands with these organisms, which can thus be transferred to the patient. duMoulin and Hedley-Whyte advise a greater degree of vigilance by anesthesia staff when dealing with patients who have pulmonary disease than could be due to acid-fast organisms. This vigilance should include the following precautions:

1. Nondisposable equipment must be subjected to initial sterilization or disinfection with appropriate chemicals (e.g., glutaraldehyde) after use. Subsequently, equipment must be washed thoroughly. Keep in mind that washing with tap water will recontaminate the equipment with waterborne organisms that may include acid-fast bacilli. Finally, wrapping, labeling, and terminal sterilization (preferably with steam) should follow.
2. Use of a disposable circle system and absorber may be helpful.
3. All operating room staff should be aware that the patient is infectious.
4. Whenever possible, the patient should wear a mask.
5. All gowns, gloves, shoe covers, and masks should be discarded in the approved manner on leaving the operating theater.
6. Traffic and equipment within the operating room should be kept to a minimum.
7. The anesthesia staff should be gloved and should keep intraoral manipulations to a minimum.

Viral Infections and Contamination of Equipment

Hepatitis B. The practice of anesthesia requires that one have frequent contact with the patient's mucous membranes and saliva, and this poses the risk of transmission of hepatitis B, as does contact with the patient's blood when starting an infusion or drawing blood samples. It is important, therefore, to take precautions to guard one's health by wearing gloves and gown, in addition to a mask, when treating any of the following groups of patients who may be carriers: all patients with liver disease; patients on dialysis or with renal transplants; patients with leukemia, lymphoreticuloses, polyarteritis nodosa, or polymyositis; patients receiving radiotherapy or immunosuppressive drugs; immigrants or visitors or people who have recently returned from countries with high incidence of hepatitis B (tropical or subtropical areas, and Greenland); inmates of prisons or institutions for the mentally defective, drug addicts, prostitutes, homosexuals, and persons who have been tatooed (duMoulin and Hedley-Whyte, 1983). Surveys have shown that in an anesthesia staff tested for the presence of hepatitis B surface antibody and antigen, an indicator of prior exposure to the virus, 17 percent in the American Medical Association study and 31 percent in a German study tested positive. Fortunately, a hepatitis B vaccine is now available to provide protection. Immunization should be encouraged for all high-risk staff, such as surgical, anesthesia, laboratory, and hemodialysis personnel.

The hepatitis B surface antigen can survive for several days on stainless steel surfaces, needles, and gloves so that many of the items of equipment used in anesthesia are potential routes of transmission. The virus is resistant to phenol- and chlorine-containing disinfectants so that steam sterilization or disposable equipment should be used.

Acquired Immunodeficiency Syndrome. The precautions advised against hepatitis B will also be effective against infection with the aquired immunodeficiency syndrome (AIDS) virus, human immunodeficiency virus (HIV), and recently reported in the United States, the human T-cell leukemia virus-1 (HTLV-1) (Bishop, 1987). In spite of its greater prominence in the press, AIDS is at present a less prevalent hazard to anesthesia staff than hepatitis B. Also it is a less infectious virus and is not transmitted by casual contact with the patient's saliva or other secretion. The risk of nosocomial transmission of HIV is extremely low, provided adequate precautions are taken (Gerberding, 1986). The use of gloves, gown, and mask when in direct contact with the patient's blood or secretion, together with frequent hand washing and precautions against needle sticks and decontamination procedures used for hepatitis B are recommended (Scullon, 1986).

Other Viruses. As the techniques for the growth and isolation of viruses have improved, a new and unsuspected type of virus has been discovered by the laboratory that first described the AIDS virus in the United States (Salahuddin et al, 1986; Lancet, 1986; Barnes, 1986; Gallo, 1987; Josephs et al, 1986). This new human B-lymphotropic herpes virus (HBLV) is associated with malignant conditions of the lymphatic system and, unlike the AIDS virus, is fairly infectious by casual contact. HBLV resembles the Epstein-Barr virus associated with infectious mononucleosis and is being investigated as the possible cause of outbreaks of a "chronic mononucleosislike" disease reported from Lake Tahoe, Boston, New York, Houston, Fort Lauderdale, and Miami. Though not fatal, it is associated with disabling chronic fatigue, inability to concentrate, and memory impairment. As HBLV is more easily spread by casual contact with saliva or droplets from coughing and sneezing, it could pose a more serious problem to anesthesia staff in the future.

Wire-reinforced Latex Tracheal Tubes. Reinforced latex tracheal tubes, which can be recognized by their caramel color, are manufactured by sequentially dipping rods into liquid latex rubber and then allowing the latex to dry. Small bubbles of air may be trapped between the wire and the latex, and if the tubes are later sterilized in an ethylene oxide or steam sterilizer that uses vacuum to remove the air from the chamber, the bubbles may be greatly enlarged, separating the layers of latex. If the tubes are reused, nitrous oxide and volatile agents will diffuse into the air in the bubble, which may expand enough to obstruct the airway through the tube. Since the obstruction occurs gradually during anesthesia administration, its occurrence and its cause may be missed or incorrectly diagnosed until serious damage has been done.

For this reason, the manufacturer marks packets containing these tubes "Use once only (for North America only)." However, a review of the Willy Rusch Company's (Waiblingen, West Germany) original 1977 recommendations indicates that these tubes may be safely sterilized in a steam autoclave by using the liquid cycle at 121C (250F) *without the use of vacuum.* This recommendation was published in *Anesthesiology* in 1980 in response to additional reports of this problem (Rendell-Baker, 1980). Most ethylene

oxide sterilizers use one or two vacuum cycles and cannot, therefore, be used with safety to sterilize wire-reinforced tubes. If a clean rather than a sterile tube is acceptable, the Pasteurmatic system can be used.

Hand Washing. To an interested observer, the contrast between the careful hand scrubbing of surgeons and the often total absence of hand washing by the anesthesia personnel is marked. We expect dental surgeons to wash their hands before working in our mouths; should not our patients expect the same standard from us? Scrub sinks for anesthesia personnel should be provided in anesthesia induction areas.

Hepatitis B. Anesthetists should always protect themselves against infection from patients with a high risk of having infectious hepatitis B by wearing gloves throughout the administration. This applies to any patient when manipulation within the mouth is required, such as the passage of a nasogastric tube, or when extensive contact with the patient's blood may occur, such as the placement of a central venous pressure catheter. Careful attention to such precautions will reduce the risk of the anesthetist's contributing to the already high incidence of hepatitis B among anesthesia personnel.

USE OF DISPOSABLE EQUIPMENT

When the first disposable plastic blood and intravenous administration sets were introduced in 1947, they were such a major improvement over the reusable red rubber sets that they were rapidly accepted in the United States and, later, in other countries.

Modern hospitals at that time had a syringe service to clean and sterilize the syringes and needles used throughout the hospital. Needles were checked and sharpened each time before sterilization, although the standard of sharpness achieved would hardly be acceptable today. This service required considerable hand labor, so the introduction in 1957 of disposable plastic syringes and really sharp needles was generally welcomed. These were followed in 1959 by disposable trays for minor procedures, such as catheterization. Since then, the quality and variety of available disposable equipment have expanded so much that it is doubtful whether reusable products of the equivalent performance can be produced at a reasonable price, if at all.

Anesthesiology and respiratory therapy came to this field later, and it was not until 1969 that the first disposable breathing systems and humidifiers were introduced. R. Bryan Roberts, M.D., who played a leading role in their development, recounted that:

> their introduction is in great part, due to the foresight of a New Jersey businessman, Thomas J. Mahon, who in 1958, having just sold his pharmaceutical business, looked around for new medical problems to tackle. Concerned about the reported incidence of patients, both in hospital and at home, using ventilatory therapy equipment, who were crossinfecting each other and reinfecting themselves, he, with an engineering friend, Samuel Cherba, set about designing a low-cost disposable oxygen nebulizer and humidifier.

It soon became apparent that a length of disposable corrugated hose would be necessary to bridge the gap between nebulizer and patient. However, no company in the United States at that time had the technology to produce corrugated polyethylene hose of 22 mm standard diameter. Further search disclosed that a machine capable of this spiral blow-molding technique had been developed in West Germany, and one of these was imported into the United States. After considerable trial and error a hose of acceptable diameter, weight, flexibility, and distensibility was first made in 1967 (Roberts, 1972).

Bryan Roberts (Fig. 8–6A) told how he worked with Mahon to design a lightweight anesthesia breathing system with a plastic swivel mask and tube adapter, which was first shown at the ASA Convention in Washington, D.C., in October 1968 (Fig. 8–6B). Since that time, the use of such disposable breathing systems in anesthesia and respiratory care has expanded to a volume of $125 million per annum. In addition to the savings in labor costs, part of the attraction of disposable items for hospitals has been that they formed an easily identifiable cost item for reimbursement purposes, whereas the total cost of reusable items is more difficult to identify.

Problems with Disposable Breathing Systems

Standard 15 mm and 22 mm fittings were introduced by the American National Standards Institute's Z79 Anesthesia Standards Committee between 1960 and 1965. Standard "plug and ring" gauges were also designed to facilitate checking whether fittings were made to the correct dimensions. Before that time each manufacturer had its own size of fittings and the user had to buy the same size of bags, masks, and breathing tubes from the original manufacturer. Adoption of standard fittings by all manufacturers meant that the user had to stock only one supply of expendable rubber components that could be obtained from a number of suppliers.

Accidental Disconnection. Adoption of standard-sized fittings encouraged plastic molding firms to make tracheal tube connectors, Y-pieces, mask adaptors, and complete breathing systems from plastic. In metal the gradual 1-in-40 taper (1 unit increase in diameter for each 40 units of length) used for the conical fittings worked well, but for molded plastic fittings a much steeper taper of about 1 in 20 was better. It is much simpler to achieve the required accuracy in metal than in plastic, which tends to shrink after it leaves the mold. The characteristics of plastic also vary: Polycarbonate is rigid and can be given a highly polished surface that grips securely when the components are wrung together; at the other extreme is polyethylene, which is quite flexible and can have a slippery, waxy surface, which is the reason it is used in artificial hip joints. In addition, female fittings made from softer plastics tend to stretch, and the male fittings "creep" when wrung tightly

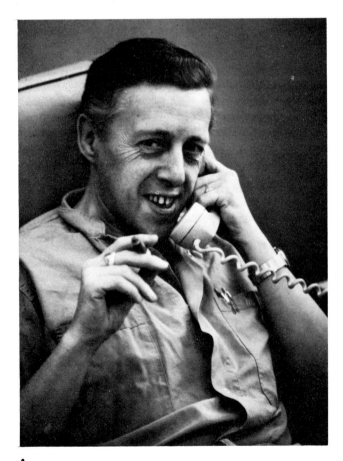

A

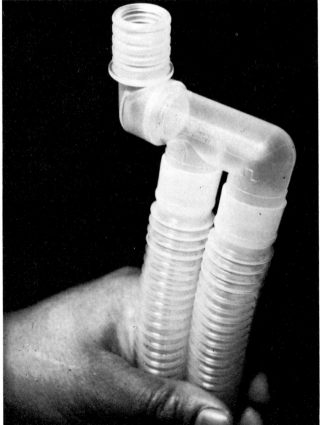

B

Figure 8–6. A. Robert Bryan Roberts, M.D., 1933–1983 (1974 photograph). **B.** U-Mid disposable anesthesia system and swivel Y designed by Bryan Roberts and Thomas J. Mahon in 1968. © *1987 L Rendell-Baker.*

together. Clearly, one's confidence in the ability of a breathing system to stay securely connected under the drapes will depend on the suitability of the plastic used and the accuracy achieved in the final product.

Unfortunately, manufacturers of plastic components were often unaware of the existence of standard dimensions and gauges to determine the accuracy of their fittings. As a result, they made their components to fit as many other makers' plastic items as possible, which were often incorrectly sized in the first place, so that the value of having all components of standard size and readily interchangeable was lost.

Accidental disconnection was the most frequent anesthesia problem reported to Cooper et al in their Boston "critical incident" surveys in 1978–1984 (Cooper et al, 1984; 1979; 1978). The poor retention of some plastic fittings received most of the blame. The problem of accidental disconnection became so widespread and troublesome that the Food and Drug Administration (FDA) funded a study to determine the cause and, if possible, a cure. The January 1986 final report found (1) that disconnection commonly occurred in anesthesia and critical care and resulted in preventable serious injuries and deaths; (2) that most disconnections occurred between the tracheal tube connector and the breathing system from several causes—the need of the user to make and undo the connection easily, which repeatedly inhibits the use of maximum force in making the engagement for fear of then being unable to disengage the components, and the fear that if the connection is made too securely, extubation might occur; (3) standards limited to dimensions are obsolete because of the variable properties of the materials; (4) a better connector design and a performance standard are required; and (5) users need to appreciate the importance of the rotatory movement while forcing the components together (FDA 86–4205).

New gauges specially designed to allow for the variable characteristics of plastics have now been adopted by the ASTM F29 Anesthesia Standards Committee (see Appendix II), so in the future plastic components should at least be correctly sized and, it is to be hoped, will provide more security from accidental disengagement—though a satisfactory test for the force necessary for disengagement has not yet been devised.

The security with which plastic components grip each other can be assessed by forcing them together while rotating them 45 degrees. Unsatisfactory components cannot be made to grip and will continue to rotate no matter how much force is applied. If the components make a cracking sound as they are wrung together and grip so firmly that they cannot be rotated further, it is unlikely they will come apart in use. In everyday use it is essential when attaching the plastic and metal components together to rotate them to obtain a secure fit.

Though the poor retention of some plastic fittings received most of the blame for the damage resulting from accidental disconnections, changes in anesthesia practice also played a part. When most patients breathed spontaneously or were hand ventilated, any accidental disconnection was quickly noted; but with the increasing use of volume ventilators with weighted *dependent* bellows, disconnection is less easily detected. The bellows of such ventilators will rise and fall in a normal manner whether attached to the patient or not. If the ventilator's bellows are designed to ascend only when filled with expired gas, the bellows will collapse and remain motionless if disconnection occurs, thus promptly alerting the anesthetist to the problem. For this reason, only ventilators designed with ascending bellows should be chosen for use in future.

Can We Reuse Disposable Equipment?

Much disposable equipment can be reused if it is carefully handled, cleaned, tested, repackaged, and resterilized, usually with ethylene oxide, and it is likely that most hospitals in the United States are reusing selected, disposable items, such as hemodialyzers, cardiovascular catheters, and respiratory therapy breathing circuits. If a hospital has the necessary staff and wants to reprocess disposables, it should follow the FDA guidelines and

> be able to demonstrate: (1) that the device can be adequately cleaned and sterilized; (2) that the physical characteristics or quality of the device will not be adversely affected; (3) that the device remains safe and effective for its intended use; and (4) they must accept full responsibility for the device's safety and effectiveness (FDA, 1981).

When a hospital reprocesses and reuses disposable equipment, the hospital, not the manufacturer, is responsible for its safety and effectiveness.

DISPOSABLES OR REUSABLES: WHICH TO USE?

The objective of either system is to provide each patient with:

1. A sterile tracheal tube
2. A clean breathing system—face mask, mask adapter, Y-piece, two breathing tubes, and breathing bag[*]
3. A clean oral airway[*]
4. A clean esophageal stethoscope[*]
5. A clean telethermometer probe[*]

Note: Hand washing of reusable equipment cannot satisfy these requirements.

Factors to Be Considered

1. Annual number of operations projected
2. Number of anesthetists
3. Number of anesthesia technicians
4. Space available in or near operating room suite

Resusables

In the past, reusable items were hand-washed, but technicians' hands cannot tolerate the high temperatures necessary, nor is the equipment exposed long enough to hot water at 170F, which is necessary to effect pasteurization. If reusable equipment is selected, a Pasteurmatic or similar system is required.

---

[*] *It may be desirable to provide these items in sterile packets for immunosuppressed patients.*

The Pasteurmatic system (see Figs. 8–3, 8–4) takes 20 anesthesia breathing systems per load, and a technician can process 5 loads in an 8-hour shift, that is, a total of 100 breathing systems per shift. This type of system produces a clean rather than a sterile final product. The process proceeds in four phases: washing, pasteurization, drying, and bagging. The most time-consuming part of the process is bagging the clean equipment. This system could handle the equipment for 20 to 25 operating rooms or more if an evening technician is employed.

Disposables

The small hospital with few operations per day and no anesthesia technicians to clean the equipment between patients can achieve the same hygienic standards by providing a clean, disposable system for each patient. Most hospitals now use disposable tracheal tubes, including disposable double-lumen endobronchial tubes.

Space in or near the operating room is essential for storing the bulky disposable breathing systems and other items. A local equipment dealer may agree to store major portions of a hospital's disposables if awarded the annual supply contract. The quantity required can be delivered once or twice a month to suit the hospital's storage capacity. However, remember that deliveries can be halted by strikes, bad weather, or other factors, and keep 2-week's supply in the hospital.

The features of the disposable items chosen should be at least as good as those of the reusable items. The plastic breathing systems are always lighter, and the clear ones permit easy monitoring of the amount of condensation in the system. A clear plastic system should always be chosen when a heated humidifier is to be used to help maintain the patient's body temperature.

If in doubt about whether to choose reusables or disposables, remember that the manufacturers of the Pasteurmatic and Cidematic equipment will produce a cost analysis comparing the cost to your hospital of using their equipment and reusable items to the cost of the use of disposable items.

CROSS-INFECTION FROM ANESTHESIA EQUIPMENT: IS IT A REAL PROBLEM?

Interest in possible cross-infection from anesthesia equipment was stimulated by a dramatic increase in nosocomial infections, particularly those caused by gram-negative bacilli. Studies clearly showed a link between the use of respiratory therapy equipment, particularly nebulizers, and the incidence of necrotizing pneumonia. Because of this correlation, the occurrence of postoperative chest infections was presumed by many clinicians to be due to the less-than-ideal standards of hygiene found in many anesthesia departments. However, although no good clinical studies demonstrated that anesthesia equipment was the cause of the infections, disposable breathing systems with bacterial filters were strongly advocated as the answer to the problem.

duMoulin and Saubermann showed that the anesthesia machine and breathing system are not likely to be sources of bacterial contamination, because the breathing system is an inhospitable environment for bacteria (duMoulin and Saubermann, 1977). They found that after 75 minutes of anesthesia administration to a patient colonized with *Pseudomonas aeruginosa*, although the expiratory tube nearest to the patient was contaminated, neither in this or any of their other patients was contamination of the expiratory valve on the carbon dioxide absorber observed. When the expiratory valve was deliberately inoculated with a bacterial culture and 3 L of nitrous oxide–oxygen flowed through the system for 3 hours, there was a progressive decrease in the bacteria present at the valve, and the organisms failed to propagate to other parts of the system. Feeley et al (1981) showed that the use of sterile breathing systems had no effect on the incidence of postoperative pulmonary infection, and Pace et al (1979) and Garibaldi et al (1981) reported that bacterial filters failed to reduce the incidence of pneumonia after inhalation anesthesia. Commenting on these studies, Mazze (1981) stated that bacterial filters in breathing systems probably add $20 to $30 million to the annual health care budget without any apparent influence on patients' outcome. He believes that we should stop using bacterial filters for breathing circuits until better-designed and executed experiments cause us to question the validity of the studies reviewed here.

The incidence of postoperative atelectasis and pneumonia is more directly influenced by the patient's preoperative pulmonary condition, the location and duration of surgery, the amount of postoperative pain and narcotics given, and the efficiency of the "stir up" regimen than by the presence of a small number of skin or surface contaminants in the breathing tubes.

Bacterial Filters

The work by duMoulin (1977), Feeley et al (1981), and Garibaldi et al (1981) convinced the Z79 standards committee that bacterial filters were not necessary in anesthesia breathing systems and should not be included in their standard on the safety and performance of these breathing systems. A concern about bacterial filters is that there is no single, universally accepted performance standard against which the efficiency of a filter can be measured. There is the dioctyl phthalate test, in which a fine dust of known particle size is blown through the filter to determine the proportion entrapped. Another test is the bacterial aerosol challenge test, in which a microbial aerosol is directed through the filter and bacteria in the effluent flow are collected on agar plates in an Anderson sampler. Although both tests appear efficient, they often give contradictory results, and filters that satisfy one test may not do well in the other. This situation hardly inspires confidence.

An additional problem with filters is that they add another source of leakage and increase the resistance to breathing. If a heated humidifier is used to help maintain the patient's body temperature during prolonged surgery, condensation within the filter may greatly increase its resistance. There is a tendency, because filters are expensive, to use them for more than one patient, thus increasing the chance that bacteria may accumulate in condensation within the filter. The filter, therefore, may become a bacterial accumulator rather than a bacterial eliminator.

DESIRABLE FEATURES OF ANESTHESIA APPARATUS

Anesthesia apparatus are potentially dangerous, and their internal mechanisms are becoming increasingly complicated. The quality of maintenance available locally should always be considered first in selecting anesthesia apparatus. Other features to be considered are as follows.

Hygiene

1. The apparatus should be easy to clean.
2. The absorber assembly and absorbent containers should be easily removable for cleaning and should be steam autoclavable (Fig. 8–7).
3. The ventilator's patient breathing system should be easily removable for cleaning and should withstand steam autoclaving or, if not that, ethylene oxide sterilization.
4. If disposable breathing systems are not to be used, the breathing system tubing, Y-piece, mask adapter, and mask should be able to withstand steam sterilization or pasteurization.
5. Because the cylinders are for emergency use only and are changed infrequently, they can be enclosed at the rear of the apparatus, as they were on the Dupaco Hygienic model (Fig. 8–2).

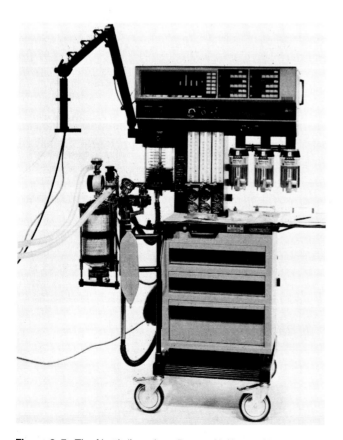

Figure 8–7. The North American Drager Narkomed 3 apparatus showing the autoclavable carbon dioxide absorber, the automatically switched-on oxygen analyzer and other monitors, and the integrated alarms system. © *1987 L Rendell-Baker.*

Gas Supply

1. Now that most apparatus are operated entirely from pipeline supplies of gases supplied through standard Diameter Index Safety System (DISS) (see Appendix III) pipeline inlet fittings on the machine, it is essential to have at least one, and preferably two, cylinder yokes for oxygen on the machine in case of interruption of pipeline supplies.
2. All apparatus have oxygen supply failure systems (so-called fail safe) that shut off the other gases if the oxygen pressure within the machine falls to less than 50 percent normal. (Note: this does not prevent the administration of a hypoxic mixture.) A further safety feature should be included in any apparatus chosen: automatic reduction of the flow of the other gases as the oxygen flow is reduced manually, to prevent the accidental administration of less than 30 percent oxygen.

Common Gas Outlet

1. The Z79.8 standard specified a 15-mm female/ 22-mm male coaxial fitting for the common gas outlet. There have been reports of the 15-mm male fitting accidentally becoming detached from the 15-mm female fitting within the common gas outlet, with resultant hypoxia. Some earlier 15-mm female common gas outlet fittings incorporated a rubber O ring that ensured secure retention of the male fitting. It is essential to see that a positive retention mechanism is fitted to prevent accidental disconnection at this position.

Flowmeters

1. The flow controls for oxygen and nitrous oxide should be linked mechanically, pneumatically, or electronically to prevent the accidental administration of a hypoxic mixture.
2. There should be only one flow control knob per gas to prevent the accidental use of milliliters of oxygen when liters were intended, as has happened in the past when two separate flowmeters with separate flow controls were fitted. If two flowmeters, one for milliliters and the other for liters, are desired, they can be placed in series and can be operated by a single control knob.
3. The flowmeter calibration should be etched onto the tube or the tube and its scale should be linked, to prevent accidental incorrect reassembly after cleaning.
4. A flowmeter for air should be provided for use:
   a. in anesthetizing neonates—to avoid too high an oxygen tension and with it the danger of retrolental fibroplasia;
   b. in surgery for bowel obstruction to avoid the diffusion of nitrous oxide into and consequent distension of the bowel;
   c. in laryngeal laser surgery to minimize the danger of fire—ever present when nitrous oxide-oxygen gas mixtures are used.

Vaporizers

1. Vaporizers should be permanently mounted between the flowmeters and the machine's fresh gas outlet. Mounting an extra vaporizer between the fresh gas outlet and the absorber or breathing system is a dangerous practice and should be avoided. Dangers include a wrong-way-around gas connection leading to a higher-than-intended vapor concentration (Marks and Bullard, 1976), tilting of a filled vaporizer, leading to excessive vapor delivery (Munson, 1965), disconnection of the gas flow to a vaporizer incorporating a check valve going undetected and resulting in hypoxia (Capan et al, 1980).

2. The vaporizers can be fitted with an agent-specific filling mechanism, to prevent errors in filling the vaporizer with the wrong agent and to reduce the chance of spillage.

3. Interlock or other mechanisms should be used to prevent gas passing through the vaporizing chamber of one vaporizer and then through that of another, thus contaminating the downstream vaporizer with the agent from the upstream one.

Ventilators

1. The ventilator controls can be conveniently built into the gas machine. The controls should be arranged so that they directly determine the parameters of importance in controlling the patient's respiration. Some ventilators require the user to adjust inspiratory flow rate, expiratory flow rate, expiratory pause, and tidal volume before counting the respiratory rate and measuring the minute volume to see if the result is satisfactory. The clinician needs to control (1) the minute volume ventilation, which controls carbon dioxide elimination, (2) the frequency of respiration, which with minute volume ventilation will determine a reasonable tidal volume, and (3) the inspiratory:expiratory time ratio to provide adequate expiratory time for the circulation to compensate for the abnormal rise in intrathoracic pressure during inspiration produced by the ventilator. On some simpler ventilators, this is fixed at 1:2, which is usually satisfactory.

2. The ventilator's patient breathing system should be easy to disassemble for cleaning and disinfection. For safety, the patient bellows should be designed to ascend as they fill with the patient's expired gas. These bellows will collapse should leakage or breathing-system disconnection occur.

Ventilator Alarm

1. The ventilator should have an alarm that sounds (1) if the normal pressure wave is not detected in the patient breathing system within a period of 12 seconds, or (2) if excessively high or sustained peak pressure is detected. It would be an advantage if the mechanism could also release the pressure in the breathing system promptly until the user can attend to the problem (Rendell-Baker and Meyer, 1983). The North American Drager MDM S monitor is an example of a device that satisfies all these requirements except for the pressure-release mechanism.

Scavenging System

The adjustable pressure-limiting valve (APL) or "pop-off" valve of the anesthesia breathing system and the ventilator gas overflow valve are designed to capture the surplus anesthetic gases and convey them to the scavenger interface system.

This interface system usually incorporates a reservoir bag to hold excess flows of gas, a needle valve to control the suction and with it the rate of gas outflow, together with two valves to limit the pressure within the system to a negative pressure of -0.5 cm H_2O) and a positive pressure of $+5$ cm H_2O). The interface is an essential safety feature, for it guards against either (1) excessive suction drawing all the gases from the breathing system or (2) a high degree of positive end-expiratory pressure (PEEP) if the scavenge system becomes blocked. The conical fittings in the scavenging system of 19-mm diameter are smaller than the breathing system's 22-mm diameter fittings. This is to limit the chance of wrong connection of the breathing tubing to the breathing-system scavenging valve.

It may be more convenient to dispose of the surplus anesthetic gases into the air-conditioning system, provided: (1) the operating rooms have efficient (20 air changes/hour) nonrecirculating air conditioning and (2) the air-conditioning exhaust grills are conveniently close to the anesthesia apparatus. In this case wide-bore tubing should be used between the interface and the air exhaust grill to reduce the resistance to gas flow.

No matter how good the scavenging system is, contamination of the operating room atmosphere will occur from time to time, e.g., during suction of the patient's airway or during inhalation inductions, so efficient air conditioning is essential to remove these gases.

Suction

An efficient suction system conveniently sited on the anesthesia apparatus is an essential safety feature. This should provide a reservoir container and an On/Off control that also permits the degree of suction to be adjusted.

Heated Humidifiers

1. The combination of high rates of laminar air flow of 20 to 25 changes per hour and prolonged surgery with wide exposure of abdominal viscera has made inadvertent hypothermia a serious problem in many modern operating rooms.

2. In addition to the use of a warming blanket under the patient, a heated humidifier in the patient's breathing system has proved invaluable. The humidifier should be controlled by a temperature sen-

sor placed close to the patient's airway with a servomechanism controlling the heater within the humidifier so that the patient receives gas 80 to 100 percent saturated with water vapor at body temperature. The problem of condensation caused by the temperature drop along the inspiratory tubing can be avoided if the servomechanism also controls a wire heating element within the inspiratory tubing to maintain the desired temperature of 37C within the tubing. The Fisher Paykel is an example of a servomechanism-controlled heated humidifier that has been found satisfactory. Maintaining the normal humidity within the bronchial tree helps maintain normal mucosiliary activity. The dry gases normally present in breathing systems, except during use of low-flow methods, have been shown to damage the cilia and superficial cells of the bronchial tree (Chalon et al, 1981). This impedes the clearance of secretions postoperatively and increases the incidence of atelectasis and pulmonary complications.

If the patient becomes hypothermic, a large-capacity warm-air blower (Fig. 8–8) has been found invaluable in rewarming such patients in the recovery room at Loma Linda University Medical Center (Loma Linda, Calif.).

CHECKING THE ANESTHESIA APPARATUS PRIOR TO USE

Before commencing each flight, the pilot of a commercial airplane goes through a series of checks to ensure that all systems are functioning correctly. The FDA published such a recommended checklist for anesthesia apparatus, which was subsequently endorsed by the American Association of Nurse Anesthetists (AANA J,1986), (Table 8–1). It is intended that each hospital's staff will evolve their own checklist tailored to the equipment they use in their practice.

STANDARDS FOR PATIENT MONITORING DURING ANESTHESIA

The Department of Anaesthesia of Harvard Medical School (Boston), as part of a patient safety risk management effort, devised detailed mandatory standards for minimal patient monitoring during anesthesia at its nine component teaching hospitals. (Eichorn et al, 1986) These standards were endorsed by the AANA in 1986 (AANA J, 1986), (Table 8–2). It should be noted that in addition to time-honored clinical monitoring, such as frequent checks of the blood pressure and continuous auscultation of the heart rate and breath sounds and observation of the electrocardiogram (ECG) and movement of the reservoir bag, the standard strongly recommends the following continuous monitoring:

- For ventilation, an end-tidal carbon dioxide monitor is strongly preferred;
- for circulation, pulse oximetry;
- for breathing system, oxygen analyzer with low-concentration alarm. A disconnection monitor is to be used when ventilation is controlled by a ventilator.

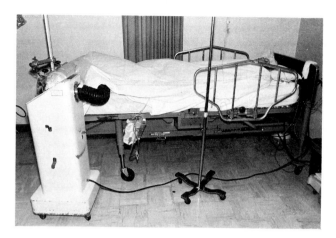

Figure 8–8. Large-capacity warm-air blower in use in recovery room, Loma Linda University Medical Center (Loma Linda, Calif.), to rewarm a patient who is hypothermic after surgery. © *1987 L Rendell-Baker.*

Monitors

Though emphasis in the past has been on monitoring of the circulation, i.e., blood pressure, pulse, and ECG, analysis of anesthetic accidents by Katz showed that most accidents stem from problems with the airway and unrecognized hypoxia (Katz, 1986). To minimize this risk the following monitors are of prime importance:

1. The oxygen analyzer is most important, as it is the only instrument that can give prompt indication that the gas supplied by the oxygen flowmeter is not oxygen. It will also give the earliest warning of any accidental reduction of oxygen percentage in the gas mixture. The oxygen analyzer should be so designed that it is switched on automatically as the machines gases are turned on. This is essential to avoid those hypoxic accidents that have occurred when the analyzer is switched on only when hypoxia is suspected.
2. The capnograph or mass spectrometer, by displaying the patient's end-tidal carbon dioxide, indicates the correct or incorrect placement of the tracheal tube and the adequacy of the minute ventilation.
3. The pulse oximeter indicates the adequacy of peripheral oxygen saturation and the circulation.
4. A disconnection monitor should be used whenever a ventilator is in use. This may detect either failure of the ventilator to achieve the preset minimum pressure or to achieve the minimum tidal exchange.

In addition there should be (1) an automatic blood pressure apparatus, which—if combined with an automatic chart recorder—will indicate what happened during induction and at other times when one is too busy to record these signs manually; (2) an ECG with numerical displays for pulse rate, temperature, and with channels for display of arterial and venous pressures; (3) a telethermometer if it is not included in the ECG; (4) a breathing spirometer and a pressure gauge, which are very useful as a cross-check on the influence of the breathing system's compliance on the minute volume delivered to the patient.

TABLE 8–1. ANESTHESIA APPARATUS CHECKOUT RECOMMENDATIONS

This checkout, or a reasonable equivalent, should be conducted before administering anesthesia. This is a guideline, which users are encouraged to modify to accommodate differences in equipment design and variations in local clinical practice. Such local modifications should have appropriate peer review. Users should refer to the operator's manual for special procedures or precautions.

*1. **Inspect anesthesia machine for:**
machine identification number;
valid inspection sticker;
undamaged flowmeters, vaporizers, gauges, supply hoses;
complete, undamaged breathing system with adequate carbon dioxide (CO_2) absorbent;
correct mounting of cylinders in yokes;
presence of cylinder wrench.

*2. **Inspect and turn on:**
electrical equipment requiring warm-up (ECG/pressure monitor, oxygen monitor, etc.).

*3. **Connect waste gas scavenging system:**
adjust vacuum as required.

*4. **Check that:**
flow-control valves are off;
vaporizers are off;
vaporizers are filled (not overfilled);
filler caps are sealed tightly;
CO_2 absorber bypass (if any) is off.

*5. **Check oxygen (O_2) cylinder supplies:**
  a. Disconnect pipeline supply (if connected) and return cylinder and pipeline pressure gauges to zero with O_2 flush valve.
  b. Open O_2 cylinder; check pressure; close cylinder and observe gauge for evidence of high-pressure leak.
  c. With the O_2 flush valve, flush to empty piping.
  d. Repeat as in b. and c. above for second O_2 cylinder, if present.
  e. Replace any cylinder less than about 600 psig. At least one should be nearly full.
  f. Open less full cylinder.

*6. **Turn on master switch (if present).**

*7. **Check nitrous oxide (N_2O) and other gas cylinder supplies:**
Use same procedure as described in 5a. and b. above, but open and *CLOSE* flow-control valve to empty piping.
Note: N_2O pressure below 745 psig indicates that the cylinder is less than ¼ full.

*8. **Test flowmeters:**
  a. Check that float is at bottom of tube with flow-control valves closed (or at min. O_2 flow if so equipped).
  b. Adjust flow of all gases through their full range and check for erratic movements of floats.

*9. **Test ratio protection/warning system (if present):**
Attempt to create hypoxic O_2/N_2O mixture, and verify correct change in gas flows and/or alarm.

*10. **Test O_2 pressure failure system:**
  a. Set O_2 and other gas flows to midrange.
  b. Close O_2 cylinder and flush to release O_2 pressure.
  c. Verify that all flows fall to zero. Open O_2 cylinder.
  d. Close all other cylinders and bleed piping pressures.
  e. Close O_2 cylinder and bleed piping pressure.
  f. CLOSE FLOW-CONTROL VALVES.

*11. **Test central pipeline gas supplies:**
  a. Inspect supply hoses (should not be cracked or worn).
  b. Connect supply hoses, verifying correct color coding.
  c. Adjust all flows to at least midrange.
  d. Verify that supply pressures hold (45–55 psig).
  e. Shut off flow-control valves.

*12. **Add any accessory equipment to the breathing system:**
Add PEEP valve, humidifier, etc., if they might be used (if necessary remove after step 18 until needed).

13. **Calibrate O_2 monitor:**
  *a. Calibrate O_2 monitor to read 21% in room air.
  *b. Test low alarm.
  c. Occlude breathing system at patient end; fill and empty system several times with 100% O_2.
  d. Check that monitor reading is nearly 100%.

14. **Sniff inspiratory gas:**
There should be no odor.

*15. **Check unidirectional valves:**
  a. Inhale and exhale through a surgical mask into the breathing system (each limb individually, if possible).
  b. Verify unidirectional flow in each limb.
  c. Reconnect tubing firmly.

†16. **Test for leaks in machine and breathing system:**
  a. Close APL (pop-off) valve and occlude system at patient end.
  b. Fill system via O_2 flush until bag just full, but negligible pressure in system. Set O_2 flow to 5 L/min.
  c. Slowly decrease O_2 flow until pressure *no longer rises* above about 20 cm H_2O. This approximates total leak rate, which should be no greater than a few hundred ml/min (less for closed-circuit techniques).
  CAUTION: Check valves in some machines make it imperative to measure flow in step c (above) when pressure *just stops rising*.
  d. Squeeze bag to pressure of about 50 cm H_2O and verify that system is tight.

17. **Exhaust valve and scavenger system:**
  a. Open APL valve and observe release of pressure.
  b. Occlude breathing system at patient end and verify that negligible positive or negative pressure appears with either zero or 5 L/min flow and exhaust relief valve (if present) opens with flush flow.

18. **Test ventilator:**
  a. If switching valve is present, test function in both bag and ventilator mode.
  b. Close APL valve if necessary and occlude system at patient end.
  c. Test for leaks and pressure relief by appropriate cycling (exact procedure will vary with type of ventilator).
  d. Attach reservoir bag at mask fitting, fill system and cycle ventilator. Assure filling/emptying of bag.

19. **Check for appropriate level of patient suction.**

20. **Check, connect, and calibrate other electronic monitors.**

21. **Check final position of all controls.**

22. **Turn on and set other appropriate alarms** for equipment to be used.
(Perform next two steps as soon as is practical.)

23. **Set O_2 monitor alarm limits.**

24. **Set airway pressure and/or volume monitor alarm limits** (if adjustable).

If an anesthetist uses the same machine in successive cases, the steps marked with an asterisk (*) need not be repeated or may be abbreviated after the initial checkout. †A vaporizer leak can only be detected if the vaporizer is turned on during this test. Even then, a relatively small but clinically significant leak may still be obscured. APL = adjustable pressure-limiting; ECG = electrocardiograph; PEEP = positive end-expiratory pressure.

TABLE 8–2. HARVARD MEDICAL SCHOOL STANDARDS FOR MINIMAL PATIENT MONITORING DURING ANESTHESIA

These standards apply for any administration of anesthesia involving department of anesthesia personnel and are specifically referable to preplanned anesthetics administered in designated anesthetizing locations (specific exclusion: administration of epidural analgesia for labor or pain management). In emergency circumstances in any location, immediate life support measures of whatever appropriate nature come first with attention turning to the measures described in these standards as soon as possible and practical. These are minimal standards that may be exceeded at any time based on the judgment of the involved anesthesia personnel. These standards encourage high-quality patient care, but observing them cannot guarantee any specific patient outcome. These standards are subject to revision from time to time, as warranted by the evolution of technology and practice.

Anesthesiologist's or Nurse Anesthetist's Presence in Operating Room
For all anesthetics initiated by or involving a member of the department of anaesthesia, an attending or resident anesthesiologist or nurse anesthetist shall be present in the room throughout the conduct of all general anesthetics, regional anesthetics, and monitored intravenous anesthetics. An exception is made when there is a direct known hazard, e.g., radiation, to the anesthesiologist or nurse anesthetist, in which case some provision for monitoring the patient must be made.

Blood Pressure and Heart Rate
Every patient receiving general anesthesia, regional anesthesia, or managed intravenous anesthesia shall have arterial blood pressure and heart rate measured at least every five minutes, where not clinically impractical.[a]

Electrocardiogram
Every patient shall have the electrocardiogram continuously displayed from the induction or institution of anesthesia until preparing to leave the anesthetizing location, where not clinically impractical.[a]

Continuous Monitoring
During every administration of general anesthesia, the anesthetist shall employ methods of continuously monitoring the patient's ventilation and circulation. The methods shall include, for ventilation and circulation each, at least one of the following or the equivalent.[b]

For Ventilation.—Palpation or observation of the reservoir breathing bag, auscultation of breath sounds, monitoring of respiratory gases such as end-tidal carbon dioxide, or monitoring of expiratory gas flow. Monitoring end-tidal carbon dioxide is an emerging standard and is strongly preferred.

For Circulation.—Palpation of a pulse, auscultation of heart sounds, monitoring of a tracing of intra-arterial pressure, pulse plethysmography/oximetry, or ultrasound peripheral pulse monitoring. It is recognized that brief interruptions of the continuous monitoring may be unavoidable.

Breathing System Disconnection Monitoring
When ventilation is controlled by an automatic mechanical ventilator, there shall be in continuous use a device that is capable of detecting disconnection of any component of the breathing system. The device must give an audible signal when its alarm threshold is exceeded. (It is recognized that there are certain rare or unusual circumstances in which such a device may fail to detect a disconnection.)

Oxygen Analyzer
During every administration of general anesthesia using an anesthesia machine, the concentration of oxygen in the patient breathing system will be measured by a functioning oxygen analyzer with a low-concentration-limit alarm in use. This device must conform to the American National Standards Institute Z79.10 standard.[a]

Ability to Measure Temperature
During every administration of general anesthesia, there shall be readily available a means to measure the patient's temperature.

Rationale.—A means of temperature measurement must be available as a potential aid in the diagnosis and treatment of suspected or actual intraoperative hypothermia and malignant hyperthermia. The measurement/monitoring of temperature during *every* general anesthetic is not specifically mandated because of the potential risks of such monitoring and because of the likelihood of other physical signs giving earlier indication of the development of malignant hyperthermia.

[a] Under extenuating circumstances, the attending anesthesiologist may waive this requirement after so stating (including the reasons) in a note in the patient's chart.
[b] Equivalence is to be defined by the chief of the individual hospital department after submission to and review by the department heads. Department of Anesthesia, Harvard Medical School, Boston.
From Eichhorn JH et al: Standards for patient monitoring during anesthesia at Harvard Medical School. JAMA 256:1019, 1986.

The ultimate monitor is the anesthetist, who stays in close contact with the patient via a precordial or esophageal stethoscope and whose trained ear will pick up instantly any significant change in heartbeat or respiration.

Monitor Confusion

As the design of anesthesia apparatus has progressed, especially during the last 10 years, more and more monitors have been added, each with its own audible and visual alarms (Fig. 8–9). There is a dangerous tendency to silence these alarms to avoid disturbing surgical composure. A better solution is for the manufacturer to combine all the alarms so that the tone of the single audible alarm indicates its urgency, and the visual display shows which function requires attention (Fig. 8–10).

VISIBILITY OF CONTROLS

The controls, gauges, and monitors on the apparatus should be arranged so that they can be seen with only a minumum movement of the head while looking at the patient. They

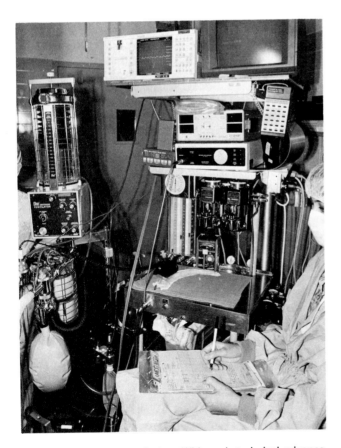

Figure 8–9. Monitor confusion. With each technical advance, more and more monitors have been added. The anesthetist closely monitoring the patient may easily miss changes on the mass spectrometer screen placed well above her line of sight. Good human engineering requires that all important items to be checked frequently occupy the space now taken by the anesthesia ventilator. © 1987 L Rendell-Baker.

should face the user (Fig. 8–11) as do the airplane pilot's instruments.

Though an apparatus built to achieve this objective was exhibited widely in the 1970s (Fig. 8–12), manufacturers have made little effort to incorporate good human engineering principles that would make their apparatus easier and safer to use. Maybe one reason for this is that they see users arrange their present apparatus so that the controls are least visible to them (Fig. 8–13).

Standardized Equipment and Layout

A policy to standardize widely used equipment in all hospital areas helps to eliminate mishaps, e.g., when, in an emergency, staff encounter equipment with which they are unfamiliar, or when intravenous sets or arterial line transducers are incompatible and have to be changed. I am familiar with one hospital where a patient may have an arterial line with its transducer set up in the coronary care unit and then, should the patient require cardiac surgery, the set and transducer are changed and the first ones are scrapped. After surgery, if the patient is sent to the surgical intensive care unit, another change is made, making a total of three transducers and arterial sets expended for one course of treatment. Clearly, adoption of one standard set of equipment would save time and money and would eliminate the inevitable hazards involved in these changes.

Similarly, if one manufacturer's intravenous cannulas are used, personnel will become familiar with that company's color code for the various sizes of cannula. There is, in fact, an International Standard Color Code ISO 6009 to distinguish needle and cannula sizes, which manufacturers in most countries other than the United States have adopted (Table 8–3). It is hoped that with sufficient user pressure, manufacturers in the United States, who supply needles and cannulas to the ISO standard to overseas customers, will be persuaded to adopt this standard in the United States also.

New ASTM standard approved emergency prefilled syringe labels will greatly simplify the identification of these syringes, which in the past were difficult to distinguish one from another because of their poor labels (Fig. 8–14).

SERVICING OF EQUIPMENT

The lives of our patients often depend on the correct functioning of our equipment, and to ensure this, gas machines, ventilators, and other devices should be serviced at regular intervals. In addition, it is essential for medicolegal reasons to be able to prove that such maintenance has been carried out. Most authorities advise that apparatus be serviced quarterly. The manufacturers of most equipment offer service contracts, and in addition there are biomedical servicing companies that service a wide range of hospital equipment. It may be advantageous to hire such a company, which can service most makes of equipment at a single visit, instead of the manufacturer's servicing agent, who handles only his make of equipment. Before signing a contract, seek bids from all companies offering this service in the

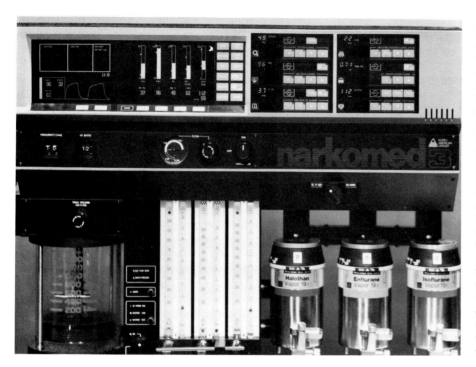

Figure 8–10. Centralized monitors and alarms on the NA Drager Narkomed 3 apparatus. Three levels of alert are displayed on the left-hand panel: Warning, requiring immediate action; Caution, requiring prompt action; and Advisory. The high-level warning always takes precedence over other competing alarms. Below this appear the pulse oximeter's pulse amplitude, oxygen saturation, and the pulse rate, together with the expired carbon dioxide value and wave forms and a digital clock. Bar graphs and figures in the center panel show the expired carbon dioxide, tissue oxygen saturation, inspired oxygen percentage in the gas mixture, pulse rate, and blood pressure. The information can be displayed in more detail numerically, in traces or trends. The right-hand panel contains the monitors and the controls for setting the alarm levels for breathing-system oxygen concentration, tissue oxygen saturation, expired carbon dioxide level, and breathing-system pressure together with the expired tidal volume. All monitors are activated automatically when the machine is turned on. © *1987 L Rendell-Baker.*

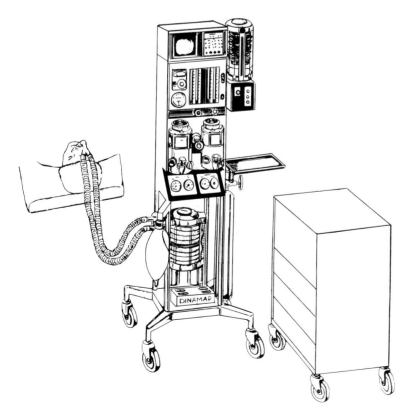

Figure 8–11. The gauges and controls should face the user. Ohio Modulus components are arranged as a compact apparatus that can be placed alongside the patient's head so that the anesthetist can see the controls at all times. © *1987 L Rendell-Baker.*

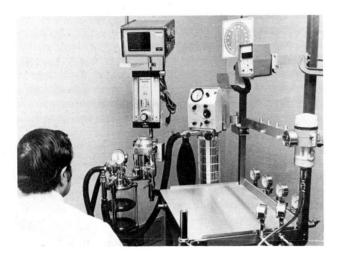

Figure 8–12. Harris-Lake "Line of Sight" anesthesia apparatus, designed by Chalmers Goodyear and Leslie Rendell-Baker, M.D., and built for the Department of Anesthesiology, Mt. Sinai Medical Center, New York. N.Y., in 1976. The engineer is seated to show how the machine's controls face the anesthetist seated at the head of the operating room table and looking at the patient. © *1987 L Rendell-Baker.*

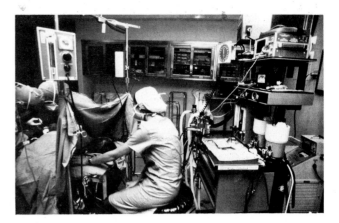

Figure 8–13. How not to arrange your apparatus for greatest safety. Would you fly with an airline who required the pilot to look over his shoulder to check his instruments while landing? Should not we also have our instruments in front of us like the pilot? © *1987 L Rendell-Baker.*

area and check with other hospitals to discuss their experience with the service provided.

Large medical centers with an efficient biomedical engineering department may wish to consider having the servicing of the equipment carried out by the center's own staff. In this way, the staff can become familiar with a wide range of equipment and can advise on the choice of apparatus and inspect it before purchase. Their opinion will be unbiased, unlike that of the local equipment supplier. A biomedical engineering department can help to unify the choice of equipment throughout the hospital, thus avoiding the purchase of incompatible pieces of equipment, all requiring their own specific attachments.

Final Preuse Check

Although some servicing companies check the apparatus after servicing and warrant it to be in good working order, some manufacturers give the user the responsibility for

the final check by attaching a prominent label to the apparatus warning that it should be checked before use.

ORGANIZATION OF DEPARTMENTAL ANCILLARY SERVICES

In a large hospital with many operating rooms, it can be difficult to know how the operations are progressing, where help may be needed, and which operating rooms are vacant. One method used successfully in a hospital with 22 operating rooms on three contiguous floors was to install a TV surveillance camera in each operating room. It was arranged so that the anesthetist and the anesthesia apparatus appeared on the screen in the foreground, and since the cameras had wide-angle lenses, the picture included the whole of the operating room. Small TV monitoring screens for each operating room were mounted at the operating room control desk, where they could be seen by the operating room and anesthesia supervisors (Fig. 8–15). A two-way speaker and microphone permitted instant communication with any operating room. The expense of this installation was modest, since the cameras and monitors were the type

TABLE 8–3. COLORS USED IN CATHETERS IN THE UNITED STATES AND THOSE USED IN OTHER COUNTRIES

	Present United States Catheter Colors				
	14 Gauge	*16 Gauge*	*18 Gauge*	*20 Gauge*	*22 Gauge*
Abbocath (Abbott)	Gold/tan	Gray	Green	Pink	Dark blue
Medicut (Argyle)	Orange/tan	Gray	Green	Dark pink	Blue
IV Cath (B-D)	Light gray	Lavender	Light pink	Light yellow	Dark gray
Longdwell (D-B)	Olive	Purple	Pink	Yellow	Black
Angiocath (Deseret)	Pink	Yellow	Tan	Light green	Light blue
Cathlon (Jelco)	Orange	Gray	Dark green	Pink	Dark blue
Quick Cath (Vicra)	Orange	Gray	Light green	Light pink	Light blue
	ISO 6009 International Standard Colors				
	2.0 mm	*1.6 mm*	*1.2 mm*	*0.9 mm*	*0.7 mm*
Equivalent ISO 6009 metric size	Light green/yellow	White	Pink	Yellow	Black

From Rendell-Baker L: Standard colors for intravenous catheters. Anesthesiology 58: 111, 1983.

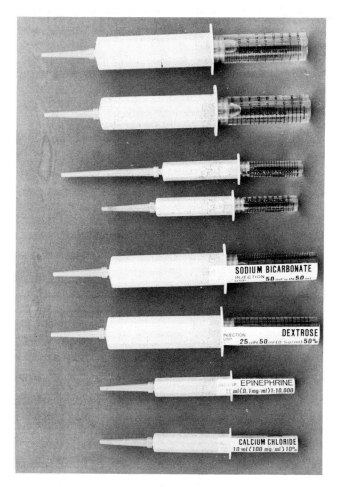

Figure 8–14. New, clearly legible labels for prefilled syringes are shown here on the lower four syringes. The ASTM standard (See Appendix II, A.3) requires that they be legible—through the barrel—at 5 feet, i.e., across the patient's bed or litter. They form a vivid contrast with the old, difficult-to-read labels seen on the four upper syringes. © *1987 L Rendell-Baker.*

used for security monitoring in shops and other commercial establishments. The ease of control provided was without price.

Operating Room Intercom System

Communication between the operating rooms and 30 locations, including the equipment rooms, blood banks, laboratories, and operating room supervisor's office, is greatly simplified by the use of a two-way speaker and microphone on the operating room wall behind the anesthetist (Fig. 8–16).

Anesthesia Technician Call System

A call button for the anesthesia technicians is placed beside the operating room door, where it can be activated as the anesthetist and surgeon move the patient from the operating room to the recovery room (Fig. 8–17). This button sounds a chime and illuminates a number on a call panel in the anesthesia equipment room (Fig. 8–18) to notify the technicians that the operating room is clear and ready for removal

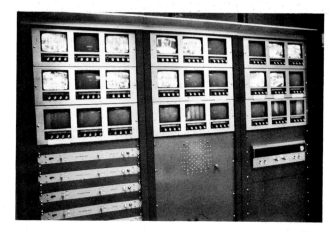

Figure 8–15. TV monitors provide at a glance the information needed from 22 operating rooms on three floors. © *1987 L Rendell-Baker.*

of used equipment and restocking of drugs and apparatus. This system reduces cleanup time between cases and makes the maximum use of the technician's time.

Organization of Anesthesia Supplies

The myriad of items we now need for our everyday practice of anesthesia no longer fits into the drawers in the anesthesia apparatus. A drug and equipment cart is essential (Fig. 8–19). Many anesthesia departments in the past used the tool cabinets sold by commercial firms. These cabinets, made from painted steel, are much less expensive. However, they are prone to rust if washed down with disinfectant solutions and are not easy to clean. The contrast between a large department without a well-organized disposal and cleaning system (Fig. 8–20) and one with an efficient system (Fig. 8–21) is immediately apparent. Providing one receptacle for contaminated equipment that is to be cleaned and another for trash greatly simplifies the work of the technicians, and the apparatus is quickly readied for the

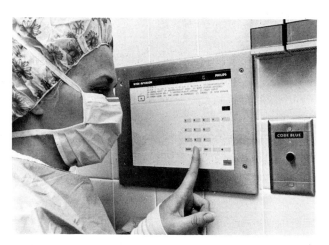

Figure 8–16. Anesthetist using two-way intercom in operating room. This provides direct contact with 30 locations, including the anesthesia equipment room, blood bank, blood gas laboratory, pathology frozen section laboratory, recovery room, and operating room switchboard. © *1987 L Rendell-Baker.*

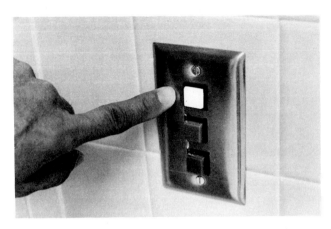

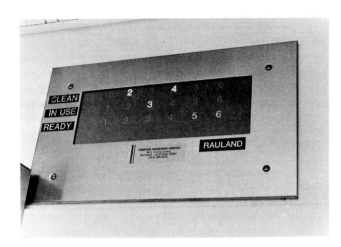

Figure 8–17. The operating room call system. By pressing the yellow top button the anesthetist tells the anesthesia technician and the operating room supervisor that the procedure is completed and that the operating room is ready to be cleaned. When the room is clean and ready to receive the next patient, the lowest green button is pressed. The center red button is pressed when the next patient enters the operating room. This tells the operating room supervisor and the anesthesia staff that the room is occupied. © *1987 L Rendell-Baker.*

Figure 8–18. Operating-room status monitor in anesthesia workroom and operating room supervisor's office. The yellow figures 2 and 4 in the top row indicate that those operating rooms are ready to be cleaned. The red figure 3 in the center row indicates that the room is in use, and the green figures 5 and 6 in the bottom row show that those operating rooms are ready for their next patients. © *1987 L Rendell-Baker.*

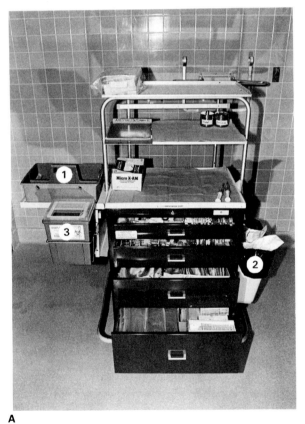

A

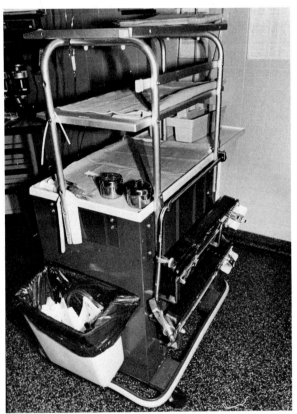

B

Figure 8–19. A. The anesthesia drug and equipment cart (Blue Bell Biomedical, Blue Bell, Pa. 19422) enables one to separate reusables (laryngoscopes, face masks, etc.), which are placed in the plastic basket (1) for cleaning, from the disposables, which are placed in the plastic trash bag in the basket (2). Syringes, needles, and ampules are placed in the plastic sharps collection system box (3) (Devon Industries Inc. 9530 DeSoto Avenue, Chatsworth Calif. 91311–5084). **B.** The back of the cart has hooks for patient screen and arm boards. © *1987 L Rendell-Baker.*

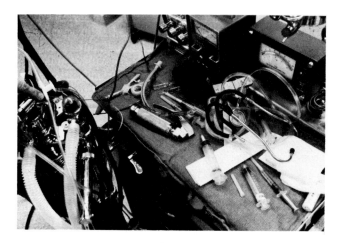

Figure 8–20. An anesthesia department with no cleanup system. This is the way many gas machines looked at the end of an operation before a proper system for the disposal of used equipment was introduced. Note the heavy contamination from used tracheal tube, suction catheter, and laryngoscope lying on the machine. © *1987 L Rendell-Baker.*

next operation (Fig. 8–22). There have become available modular plastic carts and cabinets (Fig. 8–23) that are more easily cleaned and do not rust or corrode. They can be assembled from interchangeable components to accommodate the specific equipment needed. However, one must check that their drawers slide easily.

Accidental Injection of the Wrong Drug

Because many drugs are drawn up into syringes before the commencement of anesthesia, it is important to ensure that they are clearly labeled. Unfortunately, confusion can easily arise when labels of similar colors are used for drugs as different as succinylcholine and fentanyl. The inadvertent injection of 5 ml of succinylcholine before thiopental when fentanyl was intended is an error that neither patient nor anesthetist is likely to forget. The label colors used in each hospital may vary, and anesthetists working in several hospitals can easily be misled. To bring order to this situation ASTM Standards Subcommittee DIO.34, comprising users, drug firms, and label manufacturers, has developed a range of standard colors, based upon a proposal from the South African Society of Anaesthetists Standards Committee (Fig. 8–24).

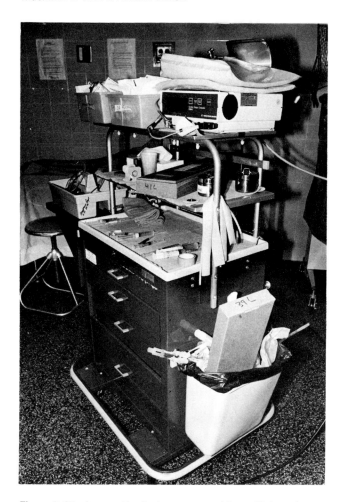

Figure 8–21. An anesthesia department with an efficient cleanup system. Anesthesia drug and equipment cart at the end of a thoracic operation. The reusable equipment to be cleaned has been placed in the plastic caddy on the far end of the cart, while the disposables and trash are overflowing the trash basket, indicating that a larger one is needed. © *1987 L Rendell-Baker.*

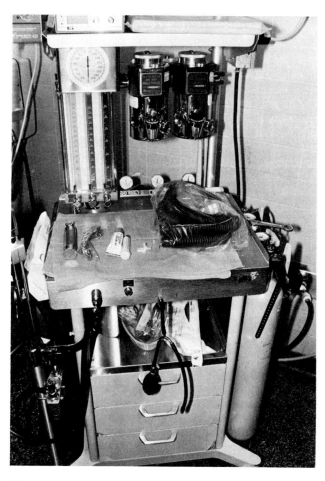

Figure 8–22. Anesthesia apparatus ready for use, with clean towel on table top, clean breathing system, and bag in plastic packet. A clean laryngoscope blade is in the plastic bag. © *1987 L Rendell-Baker.*

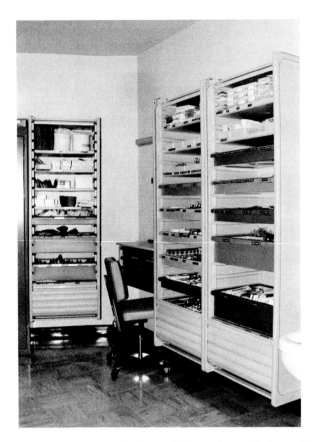

Figure 8–23. Modular plastic anesthesia equipment lockers with roll-up tambour doors are hung from the wall. The depth of the trays may be varied to suit the equipment. A charting desk with drawers forms part of the same equipment installation (Herman Miller Inc., Zeeland, Mich. 49464). © *1987 L Rendell-Baker.*

Dangerous Concentrated Solutions of Drugs

Drugs that must be diluted before use, such as potassium chloride 1 in 1000 epinephrine, dopamine, and 10 percent or 20 percent lidocaine are at present available in ampules, vials, and syringes. This makes a bolus overdose of the concentrated solution fatally easy to administer. Deaths from mistaken injection of potassium chloride when sodium chloride was intended would appear to occur with frightening regularity (as reported by Secretary, Medical Defense Union, London [U.K.] and personal reports in the United States) (Rendell-Baker, 1985). A recently adopted ASTM standard requires that such drugs be supplied as a powder or solution in a plastic container fitted with an injection spike (similar to the Anectine Flo-Pack) to facilitate their addition to a bag or bottle of diluent. However, it will doubtless be some time before these changes are reflected in the marketplace. In the meantime, as these solutions are rarely required at a moment's notice, this hazard can be greatly reduced if all containers of such concentrated solutions are kept in the pharmacy so that suitably diluted solutions can be dispensed upon request. In hospitals that do not provide 24-hour pharmacy service, these concentrated solutions should be kept under lock and key away from the rest of the drug supplies.

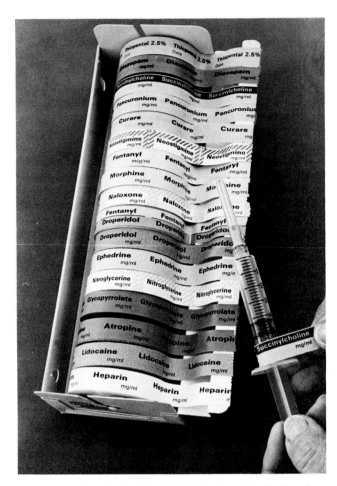

Figure 8–24. Standard syringe labels developed by the American Society for Testing and Materials Subcommittee D10.34 (see Appendix). Standard colors, defined by the Pantone Matching System for printers inks, are used to indicate the group to which a drug belongs. Examples are: induction agents, Pantone yellow; tranquilizers, PMS 151 orange; muscle relaxants, PMS 811 fluorescent red; narcotics, PMS 297 blue; vasopressors, PMS 256 violet; local anesthetics, PMS 401 gray; and anticholinergics, PMS 367 green. The antagonists are distinguished by diagonal stripes of the agonist color alternating with white stripes. © *1987 L Rendell-Baker.*

Anesthesia Equipment Room

Good storage facilities will greatly simplify the tasks of technicians and anesthetists. Small plastic bins of various sizes can be used for curved tracheal tube connectors and other small parts, and tracheal tubes can be stored in larger bins (Fig. 8–25). These bins hang on racks attached to the wall. Modular plastic lockers with roll-up doors that also hang from the wall (Fig. 8–23) provide excellent flexibility in arranging an equipment room. The depth of the shelves or drawers can be chosen to suit the size and type of equipment to be stored. When the requirements change, the lockers can be rearranged or relocated readily. The manufacturers of modular hospital furniture are always ready to help solve a storage problem or help plan a new facility.

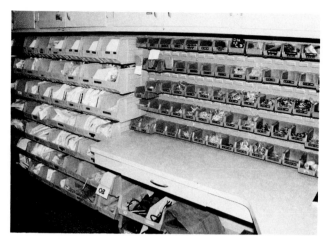

Figure 8–25. Plastic storage bins for tracheal tube connectors and tracheal tubes facilitate the orderly storage of these small parts in the anesthesia equipment room. © *1987 L Rendell-Baker.*

REFERENCES

American Association of Nurse Anesthetists: JAANA 54:494, 1986.

Barnes DM: Mystery disease at Lake Tahoe challenges virologists and clinicians. Science 234:541–542, 1986.

Bishop JE: Concerns grow that cancer virus is spreading in same way as AIDS. Wall Street Journal January 20:31, 1987.

Capal L, Ramanathan S, et al: A possible hazard with the use of the Ohio Ethrane vaporizer. Anesth Analg 59:65, 1980.

Chalon J, Mahgul A, et al: Humidification of Anesthetic Gases. Springfield, Ill.: Chas C Thomas, 1981.

Cooper JB, Newbower RS, et al: Preventable anesthesia mishaps: A study of human factors. Anesthesiology 49:399–406, 1978.

Cooper JB, Newbower RS, et al: An analysis of major errors and equipment failures in anesthesia; considerations for prevention and detection. Anesthesiology 60:34–42, 1984.

Cooper JB, Long CD, et al: Multi-hospital study of preventable anesthesia mishaps (abstract). Anesthesiology 51:S348, September, 1979.

duMoulin GC, Hedley-Whyte J: Bacterial interactions between anesthesiologists, their patients, and equipment. Anesthesiology 57:37–44, 1982.

duMoulin GC, Hedley-Whyte J: Hospital-associated viral infection and the anesthesiologist. Anesthesiology 59:51–65, 1983.

duMoulin GC, Saubermann AJ: The anesthesia machine and circle system are not likely to be sources of bacterial contamination. Anesthesiology 47:353–358, 1977.

duMoulin GC, Sherman IH, et al: Mycobacterium avium complex, an emerging pathenogen in Massachusetts. T Clin Microbiol 22:9–12, 1985.

duMoulin GC, Stottmeier KD: Waterborne mycobacteria: an increasing threat to health. ASM News 52:525–529, 1986.

Eichhorn JH, et al: Standards for patient monitoring during anesthesia at Harvard Medical School. JAMA 256:1017–1020, 1986.

FDA Compliance Policy Guide #7124–16. Reuse of medical devices. July 1, 1981.

Feeley WT, Hamilton WK, et al: Sterile anesthesia breathing circuits do not prevent postoperative pulmonary infections. Anesthesiology 54:369, 1981.

Gallo RC: The AIDS virus. Scientific American 256:47–56, 1987.

Garibaldi RA, Britt MR, et al: Failure of bacterial filters to reduce the incidence of pneumonia after inhalation anesthesia. Anesthesiology 54:364, 1981.

Gerberding JL: Recommended infection control policies for patients with human immunodeficiency virus infection. N Engl J Med 315:1562–1563, 1986.

HHS Publication FDA 86–4205: Accidental Breathing Systems Disconnections. NTSI Accession No PB86–185204/AS. National Technical Information Service, U.S. Dept. of Commerce, 5285 Port Royal Rd, Springfield, Va. 22161.

Josephs SF, et al: Genomic analysis of the human B-lymphotropic virus (HBLV). Science 234:601–603, 1986.

Katz R: Lessons learned from malpractice review. ASA Refresher Course Lecture 134A, 1986.

Marks WE, Bullard JR: Another hazard of free-standing vaporizers: Increased anesthetic concentration with reversed flow of vaporizing gas. Anesthesiology 45:445, 1976.

Mazze RI: Bacterial air filters (editorial). Anesthesiology 54:359, 1981.

Munson WM: Cardiac arrest: Hazard of tipping a vaporizer. Anesthesiology 26:235, 1965.

Pace NL, Webster C, et al: Failure of anesthetic circuit bacterial filters to reduce postoperative pulmonary infections. Anesthesiology 51(3):S362, 1979.

Rendell-Baker L: A hazard alert: Reinforced endotracheal tubes. Anesthesiology 53:268–269, 1980.

Rendell-Baker L: Paraplegia from accidental injection of potassium chloride. Anaesthesia 40:912–913, 1985.

Rendell-Baker L, Meyer JA: Accidental disconnection and pulmonary barotrauma. Anesthesiology 58:286, 1983.

Roberts RB: Infections and sterilization problems. Int Anesthesiol Clin 10:1–177, 1972.

Salahuddin SZ, et al: Isolation of a new virus, HBLV, in patients with lymphoproliferative disorders. Science 234:596–601, 1986.

Scullon DI: Anesthetic implications of the acquired immunodeficiency syndrome (AIDS). JAANA 54:400–410, 480–485, 1986.

An unexpected new human virus (editorial). Lancet ii:1430–1431, 1986.

BIBLIOGRAPHY

Dorsch JA, Dorsch SE: Understanding Anesthesia Equipment (2nd ed.). Baltimore, Williams & Wilkins, 1984.

Kaye S, Phillips CR: The sterilizing action of gaseous ethylene oxide: IV. The effects of moisture. Am J Hyg 50:296, 1949.

Lisbon A: Anesthetic considerations in setting up a new medical facility. Int Anesthesiol Clin 19, 1987.

Martin JT (ed). and Committee on Hospital Planning and Construction: Handbook of Hospital Facilities for the Anesthesiologist. Park Ridge, Ill., American Society of Anesthesiologists, 1974. (Available for reference in Wood Library–Museum.)

McDonald RL: Method of Sterilizing. U.S. Patent No. 3.068.064:1962.

Petty C: The Anesthesia Machine. New York, Churchill Livingstone, 1987.

Phillips CR: The sterilization action of gaseous ethylene oxide: II. Sterilization of contaminated objects and related compounds. Time, concentration and temperature relationships. Am J Hyg 50:280, 1949.

Rendell-Baker L: Problems with anesthetic and respiratory therapy equipment. Int Anesthesiol Clin 20:153–170, 1982.

Schreiber P: Safety Guidelines for Anesthesia Systems. North American Drager, 1985.

APPENDIX. INFORMATION RESOURCES FOR EQUIPMENT AND STANDARDS

I. The following documents on the performance of medical equipment and steam and ethylene oxide sterilization may be obtained from

> Elizabeth A. Bridgeman
> Manager for Technical Development
> Association for Advancement of Medical Instrumentation
> Suite 602, 1901 N. Fort Meyer Drive
> Arlington, Va. 22209
> (703) 525–4890

A. *Good Hospital Practices* on:
   1. Steam sterilization and sterility assurance
   2. Steam sterilization using the unwrapped method (flash sterilization)
   3. Ethylene oxide gas—ventilation recommendations and safe use
   4. Performance evaluation of ethylene oxide sterilizers

B. *Standards and Recommended Practices* on:
   1. Hospital steam sterilizers
   2. Automatic, general purpose ethylene oxide sterilizers and sterilant sources intended for use in health care facilities
   3. Determining residual ethylene oxide in medical devices
   4. Sphygmomanometers, electronic or automated
   5. Human engineering guidelines and preferred practice for design of medical devices

II. The following standards applicable to anesthesia practice may be obtained from

> American Society for Testing and Materials
> 1916 Race St.
> Philadelphia, Pa. 19103

A. Contact Brent Backus (216–299–5518) for these D10.34 documents:
   1. D4267–83 standard specifications for (the legibility of) labels for small-volume (less than 100 ml) parenteral drug containers
   2. Standard practice for user-applied drug labels in anesthesiology[a]
   3. Standard specifications for identification and configuration of prefilled syringes and delivery systems for drugs—excluding pharmacy bulk packages

B. Contact Raymond Sansone (215–299–5521) for these F29 documents:
   1. F920–85 Minimum performance and safety requirements for resuscitation intended for use with humans
   2. F927–86 Pediatric tracheostomy tubes
   3. F960–86 Medical and surgical suction and drainage systems
   4. F965–85 Rigid laryngoscopes for tracheal intubation—hook-on fittings for laryngoscope handles and blades with lamps
   5. F984–86 Cutaneous gas monitoring devices for oxygen and carbon dioxide
   6. Minimum performance and safety requirements for components and systems of continuous–flow anesthesia gas machines
   7. Minimum performance and safety requirements for anesthesia breathing systems
   8. Standard practice for conical fittings of 15-mm and 22-mm sizes
   9. Cuffed tracheostomy tubes
   10. Standard specification for breathing tubes/bags
   11. Standard specification for tracheal tube connectors
   12. Standard specification for ventilators intended for use in critical care
   13. Standard specification for ventilators intended for use during anesthesia
   14. Standard specification for blood gas analyzers
   15. Standard specification for humidifiers for medical use
   16. Standard specification for oxygen analyzers for monitoring patient breathing mixtures
   17. Standard specification for home-care ventilators
   18. Oxygen concentrators for medical use

III. The following pamphlet can be obtained from

> Don Slee
> Compressed Gas Association
> 1235 Jefferson Davis Hwy
> Arlington, Va. 22202

Pamphlet V5, Diameter
Index Safety System

---

[a] Syringe labels complying with this standard may be obtained from label manufacturers including the following:
- United Ad Label, Inc., P.O. Box 2165, 1035 S. Greenleaf Ave., Whittier, Calif. 90610
- Professional Tape Co., 144 Tower Drive, Hinsdale, Ill. 60521
- Shamrock Scientific Systems, Inc., 34 Davis Drive, Bellwood, Ill. 60104

Part II
PREOPERATIVE CONSIDERATIONS

9

Positioning for Anesthesia and Surgery

Everard R. Hicks and Kathleen C. Koerbacher

POSITIONING

Alterations in body physiology caused by positioning for surgical procedures are well documented but often ignored until a catastrophe occurs. Perhaps the earliest recorded death under anesthesia caused by posture change occurred on January 19, 1849. The patient was John Griffith, age 31, a seaman in the United States Navy. He received chloroform by open mask in the sitting position and as soon as he was anesthetized, he was placed in the lateral position for the removal of some hemorrhoids. History records that as soon as the posture change occurred, he ceased to breathe and was found to be pulseless. All efforts to restore the deceased failed (Little, 1960).

Obviously there is little comparison between anesthesia in the 1840s and anesthesia in the 1980s. Nevertheless, body physiology has changed little. Despite our advanced knowledge, profound changes in the circulatory and respiratory systems do occur as a result of posture changes. Nerve injuries associated with malpositioning of the patient on the operating table are not infrequent occurrences.

The purpose of this chapter is to present an overview of the alteration in the body physiology caused by posture changes, with special emphasis being placed on the circulatory and respiratory systems, and of common nerve injuries associated with the commonly used surgical positions.

Not only do we have a moral obligation to care properly for those we anesthetize, but we also have a legal one. The court has made a clear statement in this regard: "During general anesthesia, the patient is unconscious. The protective reflexes have now been attenuated and the patient is no longer able to protect himself against injury. The patient cannot cry out in pain. Responsibility for the patient then falls solely upon the anesthesia care provider." One is also reminded of the motto of the Canadian Anesthetists Society: "We watch closely those who sleep."

The type of surgery and the anatomic location of the surgery dictate the posture of the patient for that particular surgical intervention. Some of these positions do indeed "defy the muscular and skeletal mechanics possible to the human body" (Little, 1960).

It may be worthwhile for all anesthetists to be placed in each of the common postures to allow them to experience the discomfort associated with various surgical positions.

For example, in tests done on awake patients subjected to many of the modifications of the prone position, it was found that no subject could be made to feel comfortable, and these subjects complained of severe pain and numbness in various parts of their bodies within five to ten minutes (Smith, et al, 1961).

Because the role of anesthesia is to relieve the pain of surgery, the pain of positioning is also relieved. Often the patient has been heard to remark that he or she is not concerned with the surgical position because "I will be asleep and I will not feel any pain." These same patients in the conscious state, however, could not and would not tolerate this discomfort.

Circulation

The role of the pressoreceptors in the regulation of systemic blood pressure should be well known to all students of physiology.

These receptors—located in the carotid sinuses, the aortic arch, pulmonary arteries, and in other arteries—respond to pressure changes. An increase in blood pressure causes impulses to inhibit the medullary vasoconstrictor center and excite the vagus nerve. Once the vagus is stimulated, the heart rate slows, the peripheral vessels dilate, and the myocardial contractility is decreased, resulting in a compensatory fall in blood pressure.

A sudden fall in arterial blood pressure has somewhat the opposite effect. There is now a sympathetic effect that increases the heart rate, causes a constriction of peripheral vessels, and increases myocardial contraction.

The Bainbridge reflex, located in the right atrium, also responds to returning blood flow and pressure and adjusts the heart rate to allow for more effective filling.

All these compensatory reflexes attempt to regulate blood flow to the vital organs of the body, especially the brain, heart, and kidney, as well as other vessel-rich organs.

In the normal, healthy, awake person, these reflexes rapidly regulate blood pressure and tissue perfusion. The vigor of these protective mechanisms is impaired by disease, injury, and anesthesia. Postural changes that normally cause little or no change in blood pressure and tissue perfusion will cause a significant fall in both blood pressure and perfusion in the anesthetized patient.

Any drug producing a sympatholytic effect will seem to accentuate these changes to varying degrees. These depressant drugs usually can be considered dose related, so it becomes important to avoid deep or even moderate levels of anesthesia prior to position changes. Agents known for their circulation-depressing effects should be avoided until the posture change has been completed.

Most authorities agree that the safest anesthesia prior to position change would be a thiopental, nitrous oxide, oxygen, muscle relaxant technique. Use of the fluorinated agents prior to a posture change will almost always result in blood pressure drops caused by their sympatholytic action.

Caution should also be taken with postural changes at the termination of surgery. Blood pooling in body areas below heart level will reenter the general circulation; however, those areas above the heart level will rapidly receive a large volume of blood when lowered to heart level. Many times one will see a precipitous fall in blood pressure unless the rate of posture change is slow. Even rapid, rough movement from the operating room table to the stretcher can adversely influence circulatory homeostasis.

Alterations in positions from the horizontal to the upright or tilted to head down cause little or no alteration in blood pressure in the conscious person. The head-down tilt is extremely uncomfortable in conscious subjects because of increased pressure in the cranial veins, capillary distention with possible edema, and petechial hemorrhage.

In the 1950s, the importance of blood pressure and blood flow to the brain during anesthesia and surgery when the patient is tilted away from the horizontal position was noted. When blood pressure is taken in the arm, the blood pressure may stay the same after tilt, because the limb remains on the approximate level of the heart. If blood pressure were taken in both the elevated and lowered portion of the body, one would see a dramatic difference in pressure.

Wylie and Churchill-Davidson, in 1972, suggested that "As a general rule the difference in pressure in a particular area may be calculated on the basis of allowing plus or minus 2 mmHg for each one inch (2.5 cm) of tilt below or above the level of the heart."

Nerve Injuries Associated with Anesthesia

Stretching or direct compression of a nerve is the chief cause of nerve damage from positioning.

Either stretching or compression interferes with the blood supply to the nerve and can result in permanent damage and necrosis.

The blood supply to the peripheral nerves is via small arterioles that anastomose with each other at regular intervals. Because these vessels are so small, they are easily compressed, resulting in ischemia.

General anesthesia produces two conditions ideal for nerve damage: muscle tone is lost and perceptive power is no longer intact to warn the patient of impending danger.

Space limits a broad coverage here of each peripheral nerve subject to damage caused by improper posture. The reader is referred to Britt and Gordon's excellent article on this subject (1964).

Brachial Plexus. The brachial plexus is the group of nerves most vulnerable by far to damage from malpositioning.

Stretching is the chief cause of damage to the brachial plexus. This stretching can be produced by many factors, but one of the most common is abduction and dorsal extension of the arm on an arm board at an angle of more than 60 degrees to the operating table. With the arm extended to a maximum of 90 degrees and the hand forcibly pronated, the brachial plexus is stretched across the humeral-clavicular joint, leading to injury (Figs. 9–1 and 9–2).

Suspension of the arm from the ether screen in the lateral position, as well as any manner that causes the plexus to stretch, should be avoided (Fig. 9–3).

Ulnar Nerve. The ulnar nerve is especially vulnerable as it passes posteriorly under the medial epicondyle of the elbow. The ulnar nerve and the ulnar collateral artery pass through the cubital tunnel at the elbow as they course from the arm to the forearm. External compression on this cubital tunnel can produce the "cubital tunnel external compression syndrome" (Wadsworth, 1974). This syndrome can be the consequence of rest in an armchair, but more often it occurs because of external pressure during anesthesia and operation. Controversy exists as to whether the arm should be placed on the arm board with the hand in the pronated or supinated position (Britt & Gordon, 1964; Wadsworth,

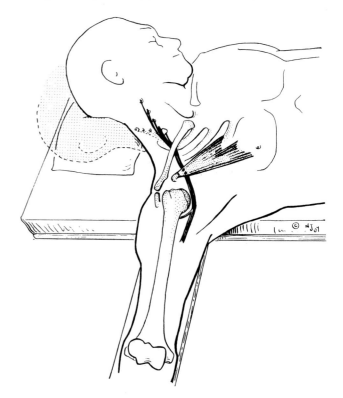

Figure 9–1. Nerve damage occurs when the brachial plexus is stretched when the arm is abducted, extended, and externally rotated, and the head is deviated to the opposite side. (*Department of Art as Applied to Medicine, Faculty of Medicine, University of Toronto.*)

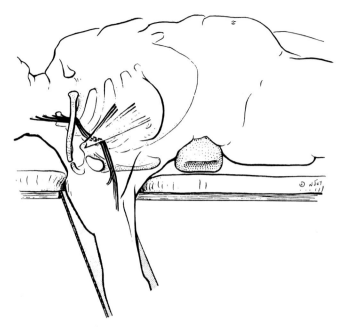

Figure 9–2. Damaging stretching of the brachial plexus around the tendon of pectoralis minor when the shoulder girdle falls back with the arm abducted, extended, and externally rotated. (*Department of Art as Applied to Medicine, Faculty of Medicine, University of Toronto.*)

1974). With the arm extended and supinated, the cubital tunnel is free from compression, but stretch is placed on the brachial plexus. If the hand is pronated, the cubital tunnel is exposed to compression. This tunnel must be protected with soft pads and judicious positioning to prevent pressure on the ulnar nerve.

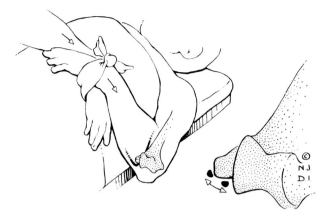

Figure 9–4. Ulnar nerve injury is caused by compression between the medial epicondyle of the humerus and the edge of the operating table. Inset: Anomalous position of ulnar nerve. (*Department of Art as Applied to Medicine, Faculty of Medicine, University of Toronto.*)

Compression of the ulnar nerve may also be caused by allowing the elbow to sag slightly over the side of the operating table or when the arms are folded across the abdomen or chest (Fig. 9–4).

A patient with damage to this nerve has clawing of the ring and little finger and sensory deficit in the ulnar nerve distribution.

Radial Nerve. When the arm is compressed between the body and ether screen there is danger of damage to the radial nerve if the nerve is pinched between the screen and spiral groove of the humerus (Fig. 9–5).

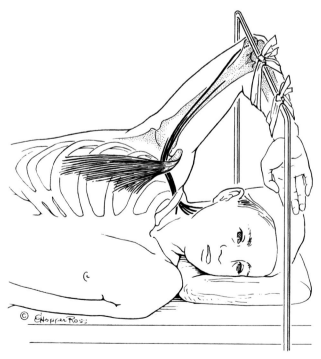

Figure 9–3. Stretching of the brachial plexus around the clavicle and tendon of pectoralis minor by fixation of the abducted arm to the frame of an ether screen is to be avoided.

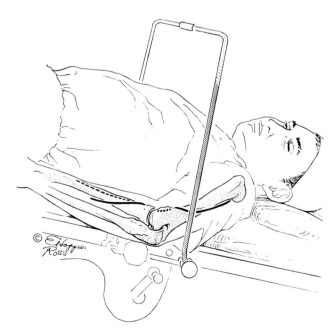

Figure 9–5. Damaging compression of the radial nerve between the humerus and an ether screen. (*Department of Art as Applied to Medicine, Faculty of Medicine, University of Toronto.*)

Clinically, with radial nerve injury there is wrist drop and inability to extend the metacarpophalangeal joints because of paralysis of the extensor muscles in the forearm.

Peroneal and Saphenous Nerves. The most frequently damaged nerves of the lower extremities are the common peroneal and the saphenous.

The common peroneal nerve is injured in the lithotomy position when the nerve is allowed to be compressed between the lithotomy stirrup and the neck of the fibula. This occurs when the legs are inside the stirrups in the lithotomy position. Soft padding should be used between the leg and the stirrup (Fig. 9–6).

The saphenous nerve is damaged in the lithotomy position when the legs are suspended lateral to the vertical braces or stirrups. This nerve can be compressed between the stirrup and tibia (Fig. 9–7). Soft padding between leg and stirrups can help prevent this nerve injury.

Malpositioning compression damage has also been reported on a host of other nerves, including the pudendal, femoral, and obturator. Others have been injured by injections and slippage of anesthesia airway equipment. These include the phrenic nerve, stellate ganglion, lumbar spinal, optic and supraorbital, facial, abducens, and trigeminal nerves (Britt & Gordon, 1964).

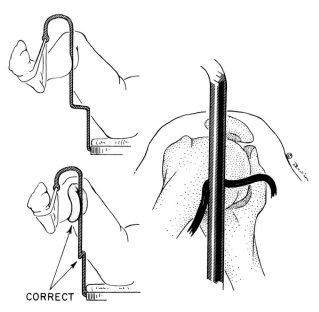

Figure 9–7. Saphenous nerve compressed between lithotomy stirrup and tibia. (*Department of Art as Applied to Medicine, Faculty of Medicine, University of Toronto.*)

Respiration

Mechanical interference with chest movement, which limits expansion of the lung, is perhaps the single most important effect of posture upon respiration.

In normal respiration the lung expands in an inferior-superior direction with movement of the diaphragm. The thorax expands in all directions, except posteriorly because it is prevented by the spine.

Because the diaphragm is responsible for movement of about 60 percent or more of intrathoracic volume, any limitation on this muscle's movement can become "the most significant postural influence on respiration [, one that] contributes most to the deleterious effects of posture" (Courington & Little 1968).

It is well documented that in the conscious subject any variation from the sitting position will produce decreases in vital capacity. These decreases are brought about by a variety of causes, but all surgical positions do mechanically restrict air flow into the lungs.

Little, in 1960, described these four effects of posture on respiration: (1) changes in pulmonary blood flow, (2) changes in lung compliance, (3) changes in intrapulmonary distribution of inspired air, and (4), most important, limitation of expansion of the lungs from simple mechanical interference with normal movements.

In his studies, Little compared the decrease in vital capacity from the sitting position to all of the common surgical positions. It is to be noted that all positions did restrict diaphragmatic movement and all positions, with the exception of supine and reverse Trendelenburg, restricted movements in the lateral as well as anterior-posterior expansion of the chest.

The following respiratory effects of surgical postures are all extracted from Little's chart. These figures show

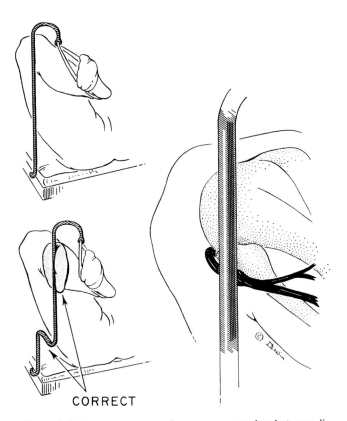

Figure 9–6. Common peroneal nerve compression between lithotomy stirrup and neck of fibula. This may be avoided by padding (see inset). (*Department of Art as Applied to Medicine, Faculty of Medicine, University of Toronto.*)

the decrease in vital capacity from the sitting position to common surgical positions in the normal, awake subject. These figures may be decreased further in the anesthetized patient.

Supine	9.5%
Reverse Trendelenburg	9.0%
Prone	10.0%
Lateral	10.0%
Jacknife	12.5%
Gall bladder	13.5%
Kidney	14.5%
Trendelenburg	14.5%
Lithotomy	18.0%

Because gravity influences the blood flow as well as the gas volume in the lungs, it is well to think of the lungs as two distinct areas functionally. There will always be a lower, or dependent, portion and an upper, or independent, portion.

In the lateral position, because of the weight of the viscera and increased hydrostatic pressure, the down or dependent side will afford the diaphragm on that side a markedly increased excursion. Radiologic evidence indicates that ventilation is always greater in the dependent portion of the lungs no matter what the surgical posture is (Jenkins, 1968).

With spontaneous breathing, both ventilation and perfusion are increased when the patient is in the lateral position. If the patient is paralyzed and artificially ventilated, the upper or independent lung now becomes preferentially ventilated; its compliance is greater because of less pressure from abdominal contents and partly because of less perfusion (Wylie & Churchill-Davidson, 1972). Anesthesia has a marked effect upon pulmonary compliance by decreasing it.

Men have a greater compliance than women in the awake state but also have a greater reduction in compliance in the anesthetized state. Men also have a greater incidence of postoperative pulmonary complications.

One should be constantly reminded that the most deadly and persistant enemy of the anesthetist is hypoxia. The clinical manifestations of hypoxia and hypercarbia are not always immediately recognized because of "masking" of signs and symptoms by the anesthetic drugs. Be assured that hypoventilation will eventually take its toll and will produce problems over a period of time. Any decrease in tidal volume should be avoided by assisted or controlled breathing.

Obesity

Obesity constitutes one of the gravest hazards in anesthesia today. Excess weight markedly restricts the diaphragm with a reduction of tidal exchange and functional residual capacity. "Extreme obesity, therefore, exaggerates all of the deleterious effects of surgical posture and accelerates the clinical manifestations of respiratory insufficiency" (Courington & Little 1968).

A study by Dr. Jenkins of one thousand obese surgical patients disclosed a precipitous drop in vital capacity, ex-

piratory reserve volume, and maximum inspiratory and expiratory reserves in the postoperative period. It took these obese patients five days to return even to sublevels of their preoperative values.

Judicious use of endotracheal tubes with assisted positive pressure is recommended for the postoperative period if obesity presents a ventilation problem. One patient in Dr. Jenkins' series was improved significantly by sitting up, which removed the weight that was restricting movement of the diaphragm.

Along with assisted or controlled respiration, it is recommended that arterial blood gases be monitored postoperatively as well as during surgery.

Intragastric Pressure

A potential complication associated with posture changes under anesthesia is the change in intragastric pressure.

If the patient is in a steep foot-down position during induction there is a lowering of intragastric pressure, helping to prevent regurgitation. If, however, gastric contents do get into the oropharynx, the chance of aspiration is enhanced. Use of a steep head-down position causes an increase in intragastric pressure, which encourages the flow of gastric contents into the oropharynx but makes aspiration into the trachea improbable. To some degree the supine horizontal position combines the disadvantages of the two positions described. The writer recommends a head-up position with cricoid pressure until the patient is intubated with a cuffed tube.

Muscular System

General anesthesia with the use of muscle relaxants produces complete muscle relaxation, as does spinal anesthesia. This profound muscle relaxation causes the legs to lie flat on the operating table and unduly stretches ligaments and muscles of the lower spine. This stretch is responsible for most cases of backache in the postoperative period. Soft padding should be placed under the legs and back to prevent this discomfort.

The use of the lithotomy position has been shown to cause backache in 37 percent of the patients whereas the lateral position caused backache in only 12 percent when compared to reported incidence of backache following surgery performed in the supine position.

The other important factor affecting the likelihood of backache was the duration of surgery. In cases lasting from 1 to 60 minutes, 18 percent of the patients developed postoperative backache whereas in those procedures lasting 181 to 240 minutes, 34 percent developed backache.

SUPINE

The supine is perhaps the position given least thought in anesthesia and surgery. Patients are moved onto the flat, minimally padded, cold operating table, adjusted so "you feel like you're in the middle of the table," and extensions placed to support heels and occiput as necessary. As he or she lies flat on the table, the patient's weight is distributed to occiput, shoulder, spine, hips, and heels, which are bone prominences. The skin on these areas receives minimal protection and maximum pressure, ideal conditions for rapid development of ischemia. In the harsh environment of the operating theater this ischemia can be more pronounced and occurs even more rapidly than otherwise.

Dr. James T. Martin advocates a "lawn chair" position that is more physiologic than the anatomic supine (Fig. 9–8). It incorporates hip and knee flexion, with slight head elevation on a small pillow. This position not only redistributes the weight, but it also brings the hips and knee joints into a more neutral position, thereby decreasing pull or tension on muscles and nerves. This position will alleviate some of the postoperative complaints of leg and back muscle pain often voiced by patients. If the procedure is long or drapes unduly heavy, the feet require support to prevent foot drop.

The leg strap should be applied across midthigh on top of a smooth sheet and around the table for maximum patient protection and safety. The arm, when positioned by the side, must fit on the mattress and not hang off. Touching the metal table causes pressure on the ulnar nerve at the elbow, and it is a possible site for unintentional cautery grounding. The arms, when positioned at the side, should not be tucked under the buttocks but should be placed under the lift sheet. This sheet should extend above the elbow to midupper arm for support and be tucked under the mattress. Anything placed beneath the patient should be smooth and wrinkle-free because wrinkles or any distortion will increase pressure areas (Fig. 9–9).

The arm when placed on an arm board must be in a neutral position to protect neural and vascular structures, as discussed earlier. During prolonged mask cases, damage can occur to the optic nerve from direct mask pressure or mask strap tension. The facial nerve as it passes around the mandibular rami is at risk from a tight mask strap or the hand supporting the upper airway and mask (Fig. 9–10).

PRONE

This position is most awkward for patients of all ages and sizes. Irrespective of size, the patient's abdominal wall must not touch or dig into the mattress. Support on two "shoulder rolls" that extend from the shoulder to the iliac crest not only frees the abdominal wall but the anterior thoracic wall as well. This markedly improves circulation and respiration. There are numerous variations of this position: Georgia

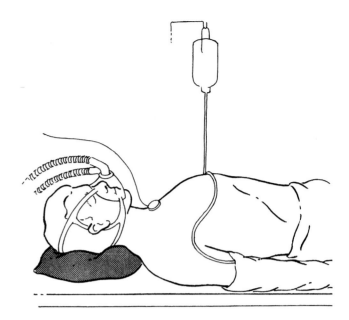

Figure 9–9. The supine position: head on small pillow, arm by side, well on mattress, with lift sheet extending above the elbow to provide support. (*Department of Art as Applied to Medicine, Faculty of Medicine, University of Toronto.*)

position, Smith's modification of the Georgia position, Overholt, and Sellor-Brown, to mention a few. In addition, there have been developed several tables that carry the inventor's name for the prone position. All these various modifications provide for free space between table and mattress and anterior abdominal wall to prevent resistance to respiration, compression of vena cava and lymphatic sys-

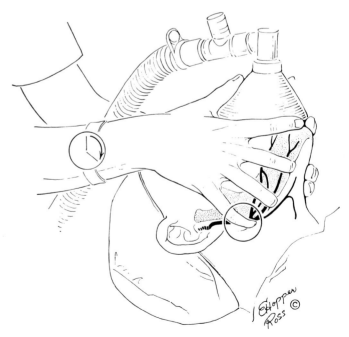

Figure 9–10. Motor root of facial nerve injured by traction on the angle of the mandible. (*From Martin J T: Positioning in Anesthesia and Surgery, 1978. Courtesy of Saunders.*)

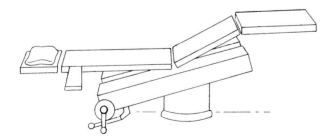

Figure 9–8. The supine position; "lawn chair" with hip and knee flexion and a pillow for the head. (*From Martin JT: Positioning in Anesthesia and Surgery, 1978. Courtesy of Saunders.*)

tem, and stability so that the patient does not give or slip during surgical procedures. The male genitalia must also be protected by ensuring that the patient is not lying on them, that they are not caught between patient and table, and that the electrosurgical ground pad is well away from the area. The female breasts can pose problems, especially the large pendulous ones and the high, firm breasts of the young. Large breasts, because of their elasticity, can be swept away from the midline so that the shoulder-to-hip roll can be placed between them. The arms of the patient must then be placed above her head. The arms must be rotated through the natural arch when positioning them overhead. The upper arm biceps-triceps area must be supported to the same elevation as the thorax to prevent pull and stretch on brachial plexus. If arms must be by the side, often the breasts are swept inward and the shoulder rolls placed distal to them. This way the arms can easily be accommodated at the side. The buxom nullipara often presents more of a challenge as these breasts are firm and immobile, offering little or no opportunity for movement. Though some of the mass may be shifted, it is often impossible to reduce the pressure on them significantly.

Obviously the dorsum of the foot is at grave risk and must be supported and protected by rolls or pillows or both. Injury to the eyes, ears, and nose can easily occur from protracted pressure from the weight of the head

against the table or mattress. The possibility of spinal cord and boney spine injury during the act of turning the patient exists because of the lack of muscular support. Consequently the head, neck, shoulders, hip, and thigh must be kept in alignment and the patient turned as a unit, logrolling. A minimum of three people is required to turn patients from the supine position: one to turn the head and neck, coordinate the team, and maintain the airway, one to turn shoulders and thorax, and one to turn the hips and legs (Fig. 9–11). There are many methods used to achieve the prone position; two are more desirable than the others. The first one is to anesthetize the patient on the stretcher and then logroll him or her onto the operating room table. The advantage is that shoulder rolls, head support, foot rolls, and arm board can be prepositioned, and the patient can be "rolled into the arms of the team," lifted and placed on the supports. Naturally some adjustments will be required. In those instances when the patient must be anesthetized on the operating room table, the second method is used. Again with the turning team of three, after the patient is anesthetized, he or she is turned to lateral and then to prone. Supports are placed one at a time—shoulder roll, head support, arm boards, foot rolls, etc. Final adjustments are made when all supports have been placed. This ensures that the extremities are in alignment and position of function, with no pressure areas,

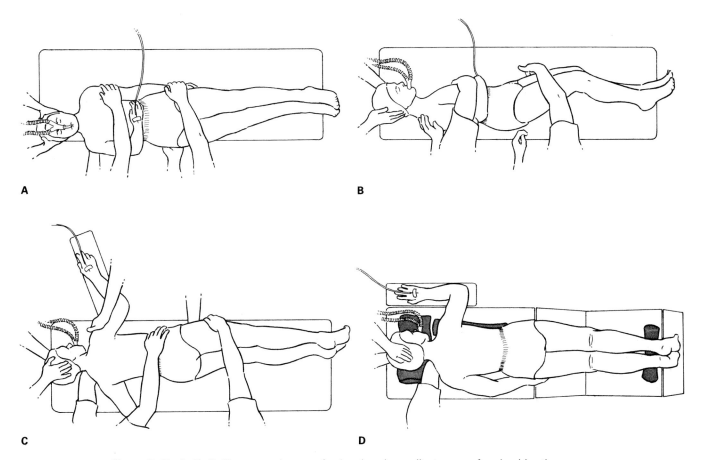

A

B

C

D

Figure 9–11. A, B, C. Three people—one for head and coordinator, one for shoulder thorax, and one for hips and legs—turn patient as a unit. **D.** Placement of supports. (*From Martin J T: Positioning in Anesthesia and Surgery, 1978. Courtesy of Saunders.*)

capillary refill is good, and distal pulse is present and easily palpable. A check is made to ensure that the eyes are closed, ears are flat, that anterior abdominal and thoracic walls are free, and that no instruments, tubes, or other objects are under the patient to cause pressure. The catheter drainage tubing, if a Foley is in place, can be run down between the legs and off the caudal end of the table or passed under the muscular anterior thigh and over the side of the table.

Because many anesthetic agents cause depression of the cardiovascular system, including diminished pressure response, the likelihood of acute protracted hypotension exists whenever an anesthetized patient's position is altered.

LITHOTOMY

Since ancient times the lithotomy position has been used by both obstetrician and urologist; it is only within the last century that this position has been used by gynecologists. To prevent injury it is imperative that the equipment fit the patient. Both legs must be flexed and extended simultaneously to prevent joint and spinal injury, including hip disarticulation. Whichever type of stirrups is chosen, the right and the left device must be a pair. The leg support with an adjustable foot plate is preferable because it evenly distributes the weight; however, it is time-consuming to adjust the angles of both the hip and knee joint and shorten or lengthen the foot plate. Consequently this stirrup is often abandoned in favor of the ankle strap or, more unfortunately, the leg support is misused. With the ankle strap, the upright rods are at right angles to the table and the leg is flexed inside the uprights. When more exposure is necessary the legs are placed outside the uprights which is one of the modified positions for radical peroneal surgery. When the ankle straps are used, the legs must not rest against the upright. The common peroneal nerve, running lateral and very superficial to the fibular head, is at risk from pressure of the upright support (Fig. 9–6). The superficial peroneal nerve, as the name implies, runs between the subcutaneous fat and muscles of the lateral calf. The surgical assistant will often push the calf against the rod to have a keener view of the surgical field, compressing the superficial peroneal nerve between the tibia and upright. With the legs on the outside of the upright, undue stretch is often placed upon the muscle, tendons, and joints by the surgical assistants who crowd in for a better view of the operative field. The saphenous nerve is at risk from assistants who stand outside and lean against the leg in an effort to obtain a better view of the surgical field from "above."

The obturator, saphenous, and femoral nerves are all at risk when the leg support stirrup is used because of the compression of the legs in the supports and accompanying straps. It goes without saying that venous pooling is a problem with this position, its severity depending upon patient condition, anesthetic management, position, and length of time requiring this surgical position. When the legs are returned to the supine position they should be lowered simultaneously and slowly in stages, to prevent hypotension secondary to filling the dilated peripheral vascular bed.

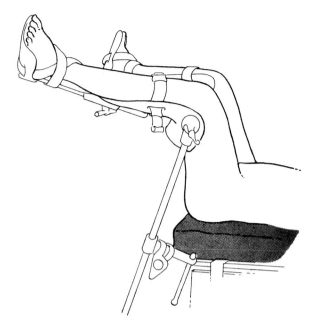

Figure 9–12. The lithotomy position. Note placement of legs into stirrups and buttocks on table. (*From Martin J T: Positioning in Anesthesia and Surgery, 1978. Courtesy of Saunders.*)

The arms may be positioned in several ways: both on arm boards, one on an arm board and one on the chest, or both on the chest; however, the precautions discussed regarding the supine position must be adhered to if either or both arms are extended on arm boards. When positioning the arm or arms on the chest, care must be taken that the elbow does not rest on the table. This causes pressure on the ulnar nerve and is an unintentional cautery ground site. The arm should not be acutely flexed across the chest. An angle of more than 100 degrees at the elbow can compromise the arterial supply to the lower arm and hand. The placement of the arm by the side is not recommended because the fingers can extend beyond the table break, becoming entrapped between the two table sections and, as the lower piece is raised after completion of the surgical procedure, resulting in damage to or even amputation of one or more fingers.

LATERAL

This position bears a number of labels, depending on the purpose for which it is used: thoracotomy, kidney, lateral, and decubitus. The position has been used by thoracic surgeons for a multitude of surgical procedures. The flexed lateral is used most frequently by urologists and nephrologists for access to the kidney via various types of incisions.

Essentially, the patient is turned 90 degrees to the horizontal surface of the table and stabilized. Flexion or extension of the extremities modifies this perpendicular position. Flexion of the lower leg causes the patient to roll backward to achieve a greater-than-90-degree angle, useful for the anterior thoracic incision. The upper arm then must be supported in an elevated position on an accessory or double-deck arm board, on a Mayo stand, or hung from the ether

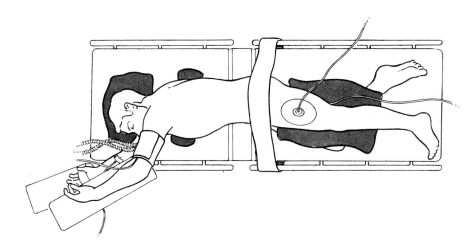

Figure 9–13. The lateral position. Note placement of support, flexion of lower leg, extension of upper leg, separation by pillow, placement of IV catheter, grounding pad, blood pressure cuff, and strap across iliac crest. (*From Martin J T: Positioning in Anesthesia and Surgery, 1978. Courtesy of Saunders.*)

screen (Fig. 9–13). The precautions that must be observed are the same as those previously discussed. The upper arm must be positioned to protect its arterial and nerve supply and must be in good body alignment; the nail beds should be checked for capillary refill; the radial pulse should be readily palpable before securing the patient. Care must be taken when using either an accessory arm board or Mayo stand that the edge does not press into the tissue causing pressure on the brachial artery or median or ulnar nerves. There must be a tunnel created for the lower arm to prevent compression of the dependent brachial artery and overstretching of the brachial plexus. A small rolled towel, a covered sandbag, or covered intravenous (IV) fluid bag placed under the upper chest, not in the axilla, all work nicely.

Flexion of the upper leg causes the patient to roll forward to achieve a less-than-90-degree angle. The upper arm can be supported on a small pillow in either an extended or flexed position. Again, the radial pulse should be checked along with capillary refill before securing the patient.

The flexed position used for approaches to the kidney is a modification of any of the three above-mentioned positions. The "kidney rest," or break in the table between upper and lower sections, must be at the level of the iliac crest (Fig. 9–14). The table sections are lower, causing the muscle to be stretched. The table can be placed in reverse Trendelenburg, making the operative sets parallel to the

floor. The lower leg is usually slightly flexed, the upper remaining extended. The legs must not overhang or touch the metal table and must be separated by a pillow. This removes the weight of the upper leg and promotes venous drainage. The upper arm is extended on a support (double arm board, Mayo, etc.). The head and neck are supported on folded sheets or pillows in line with the thoracic spine (Fig. 9–15).

Broad straps or strips of nonelastic adhesive tape, placed across the hips just below the iliac crest and across the shoulder, are secured to the undersides of the table to insure stability.

Again, as in prone positioning, the patient must be turned as a whole or unit ensuring that body alignment is maintained at all times. A minimum of three people is required, one a coordinator who also turns the head and maintains the airway, one to turn shoulders and thorax, and one to turn the hips and legs. It is highly desirable to have additional personnel to place the required folded sheets and pillows and support patients while straps are being secured.

OTHER POSITIONS

The sitting or "park-bench" position is used for posterior fossa craniotomies and some posterior cervical surgical procedures. The recent advent of the skeletal positioning device

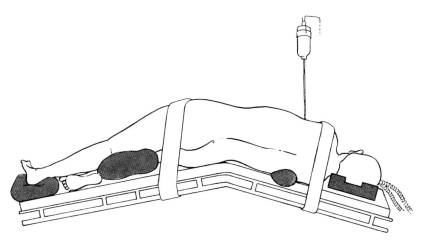

Figure 9–14. The kidney position. Note support of head, neck, and upper thorax, separation of legs by pillow and elevation of foot of upper leg, position of dependent flexed leg with foot on mattress, position of nonelastic adhesive tape across iliac crest and under table to provide stable positioning. (*From Martin J T: Positioning in Anesthesia and Surgery, 1978. Courtesy of Saunders.*)

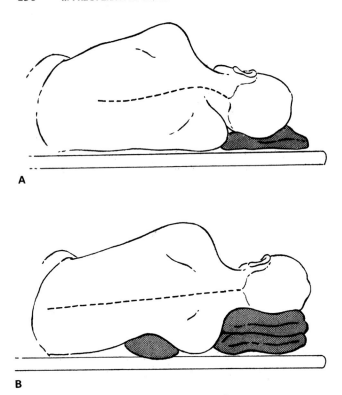

A

B

Figure 9–15. Spinal alignment in the lateral position. **A.** Note lack of support for head, upper thorax, and poor spinal alignment. **B.** Proper support of head and upper thorax.

has improved the stability and decreased complications of this position. The older horseshoe face masks and opposing pads offered little stability, and occular damage resulted from intraoperative movement. Skull-pin head holder assemblies are available from a number of surgical instrument

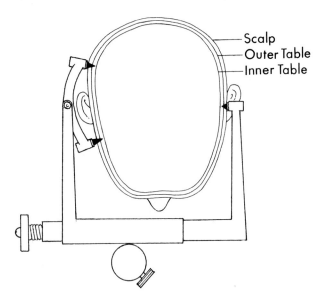

Scalp
Outer Table
Inner Table

Figure 9–16. Head holder. Typical of the variety commercially available. Note pin placement. Two pins equidistant from midpoint of opposing third pin also piercing the outer but not the inner table of skull. (*From Martin J T: Positioning in Anesthesia and Surgery, 1978. Courtesy of Saunders.*)

manufacturers (Fig. 9–16). All contain the same essentials including a bar or rod for table attachment, a connecting rod from the upright to the head-holding unit, the head-holding units, and three pins. The head-holding unit is a C-shaped clamp with two pins on one arm of the C and one pin on the opposite side. When placed, however, *no* two pins should be opposite each other; rather, the two closer pins should be equidistant from a point directly opposite the third pin in the same plane. These pins should pierce the outer table of the skull for maximum stability. Naturally for individuals with thin skulls, hydrocephalic infants, etc., the possibility of penetrating both tables of the skull contraindicates use of this device. It is also useful for positioning patients for surgical procedures requiring access to more than a single surgical plane, i.e., frontal and temporal, both temporal areas, etc., when prone position with marked neck flexion is necessary.

When the sitting position is used, the legs should be wrapped in woven elastic bandages or elastic stockings applied as far as the groin. Some institutions use "antigravity" units or "MAST" trousers to improve venous return. The legs are flexed at both hips and knees, with the lower legs and feet at the level of the heart (Fig. 9–17). The arms are crossed in the patient's lap. This provides access to peripheral lines, both arterial and venous. Care should be taken to see that the elbows are not touching the metal table. Access to the anterior thoracic wall is also provided, allowing access to the heart should percutaneous removal of air from the right ventricle become necessary. Because the head is securely supported by the skull pins and assembly, it can be flexed to accommodate surgical requirements.

The use of various "frames," "traction," or "fracture" tables to provide access to the operative sites pose potential problems and complications too numerous for the scope of this chapter. However, the basic principles of positioning apply, irrespective of the specific device required: stability; protection of boney prominences, superficial nerves, and extremities including ears and nose, as well as external male genitalia; and the maintenance of homeostasis.

SUMMARY

All surgical postures have been shown to be potentially harmful because they interfere with circulation, respiration, and the muscloskeletal system and may cause injury to peripheral nerves.

Postural interference with the circulatory system during anesthesia includes vasodilation, peripheral pooling of blood, obstruction to blood flow, and the obtundation of compensatory cardiovascular reflexes. These deleterious effects are increased by an increase in depth of anesthesia.

The effects of posture on respiration include changes in lung compliance, vital capacity, blood flow, and changes in distribution of inspired air, as well as mechanical interference with movements of the diaphragm. These changes will lead to respiratory fatigue, hypercapnea, and hypoxia secondary to hypoventilation.

The harmful effects of posture on the skeletal system, muscular system, and peripheral nerves are due to compression and stretch while the patient is relaxed and pain-free. All of these potentially harmful effects can be avoided or lessened by the judicious use of the following: (1) soft pads to prevent compression of peripheral nerves, (2) assisted or controlled breathing to ensure adequate ventilation, (3) the avoidance of deep anesthesia prior to postural changes to prevent cardiovascular collapse, and (4) modification of extreme positions whenever possible to prevent stretch of muscles, ligaments, and nerves.

BIBLIOGRAPHY

Britt BA, Gordon RA: Peripheral nerve injuries associated with anesthesia. Can Anaesth Soc J 11:514, 1964.

Castenacchi AJ, Anderson JD, Boersma D: Anesthetic hazards of obesity. JAMA 175:657, 1961.

Courington FW, Little DM Jr: The role of posture in anesthesia. Clin Anesth 3:24, 1968.

Ellis H, Feldman S, Anatomy for Anesthetists, 3rd ed. Oxford, Blackwell Scientific Publications, 1977.

Gray H, Goss CM: Anatomy of the Human Body, 25th ed. Philadelphia, Lea & Febiger, 1948.

Little DM: Posture and anesthesia. Can Anesth Soc J 7:2–15, 1960.

Martin JT: Positioning in Anesthesia and Surgery. Philadelphia, Saunders, 1978.

Millar RA: Neurosurgical anesthesia in the sitting position. Br J Anaesth 44:495, 1972.

Smith RH, Grambling ZW, et al: Problems related to the prone position for surgical operations. Anesthesiology 22:189, 1961.

Wadsworth TG: The cubital tunnel and the external compression syndrome. Anesth Analg 53:303, 1974.

Wylie WD, Churchill-Davidson HC: A Practice of Anesthesia, 3rd ed. Chicago, Year Book, Med Pub, 1972.

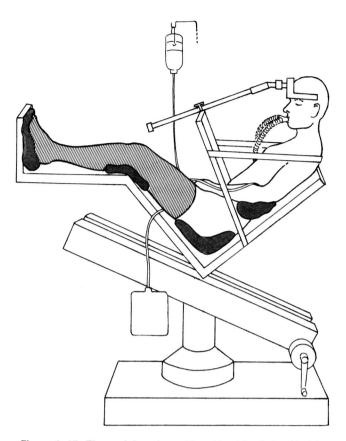

Figure 9-17. The park bench position. Head in skeletal holder, legs flexed and at heart level, with support hose to thigh level. Access to anterior thoracic wall.

10

Intraoperative Monitoring

Anastasios N. Triantafillou and Benjamin M. Rigor

The role of the physician or nurse anesthetist is to provide safe anesthesia. The definition of the term safe anesthesia includes the following:

   I. *Administration of the proper anesthetic, according to the patient's condition and the type of surgery.*
   II. *The ability, at any given moment, to be able to collect and put together the appropriate data and extrapolate meaningful information regarding the status and well-being of the vital organs. To be able to do this, the anesthetist should be*
      A. *Familiar with the various types of monitoring procedures and equipment, their functions, and their limitations.*
      B. *Able to apply them effectively.*
      C. *Able to obtain the appropriate information.*
      D. *Able to put together every piece of information and extrapolate the correct diagnosis.*
      E. *Able to apply the appropriate correcting measures.*

In the computerized days we live in, monitoring has become more and more sophisticated and complicated. Yesterday's luxury is a necessity tomorrow, and tomorrow is always closer than it seems to be.

In this chapter we deal with the various types of intraoperative monitoring applied today and emphasize some basic concepts.

PRECORDIAL/ESOPHAGEAL STETHOSCOPE

The precordial/esophageal stethoscope is a basic and inexpensive mode of monitoring and should be used with every patient. Changes in the sound of the airway or the heart sounds can be detected easily and early with this instrument. An esophageal or precordial stethoscope is particularly valuable in patients in whom the airway cannot be reached easily (e.g., head and neck surgery, prone position).

The precordial stethoscope should be bell shaped, with or without a diaphragm, and made of material of adequate weight to provide an airtight seal. The esophageal stetho-

scope should be a balloon-tipped tube used when endotracheal anesthesia is employed. Both devices can be reused after proper cleaning. Causes of failure of the device include improper placement, kinking or obstruction of the tubing, tubing that is too long, improper fitting of the earpiece, and, of course, hearing loss of the anesthetist.

ELECTROCARDIOGRAPHY

The electrocardiogram (ECG), a continuous recording of the heart's action currents, is another basic mode of intraoperative monitoring. With the ECG, the anesthetist can obtain valuable information about heart rate and rhythm and various electrocardiographic changes related to ischemia, electrolyte abnormalities, and impulse conduction.

In Figure 10–1, the classic Einthoven's triangle is shown. In most cases, lead II is monitored by the use of either a three-lead or a five-lead cable. Lead II is used to monitor heart rate, rhythm, P wave configuration, and ST segment morphology. Lead II can detect ischemia affecting the inferior wall of the heart. However, ischemia most often occurs in the lateral wall, which lead II is unable to see. Then it is obvious that a lead looking at the lateral wall must be used, such as precordial lead V_4 or V_5. If a five-lead cable is being used, it is easy to dial V_4 or V_5 and monitor this lateral wall lead. If a three-lead cable only is available, lead placement should be modified so one can obtain a precordial lead. For this, the placement of the three leads should be modified as follows:

   1. The left arm lead should be placed on the lateral chest wall.
   2. The right arm lead should remain on the right arm.
   3. The ground lead should be placed on the left shoulder.
   4. The monitor switch should be set for lead II (with a three-lead cable) or for lead II or aV_F (if there is such a capability).

Our recommendation is the use of leads II and V_5 simultaneously in patients with known preexisting coronary artery disease, because the ability of detecting ischemia in-

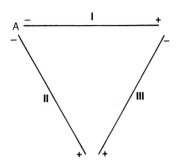

Figure 10–1. Einthoven's triangle.

creases significantly. If simultaneous monitoring of two electrocardiographic leads is not possible because appropriate equipment is not available, monitoring of the lead that shows the most significant changes on the reference baseline ECG is recommended.

ARTERIAL PRESSURE MONITORING

Blood pressure (BP) monitoring is mandatory in every instance of anesthesia. BP can be monitored either (1) noninvasively or (2) invasively.

Auscultatory Method

Noninvasive blood pressure measurement can be done using the auscultatory method of detection of the Korotkoff sounds using a standard BP cuff and a stethoscope. The cuff is applied on the upper arm and is inflated to a pressure greater than the patient's systolic BP, and the diaphragm of the stethoscope is placed distally over the brachial artery. The cuff is then slowly deflated, and the examiner detects the sounds of blood flowing through the brachial artery. As the cuff is deflated to a pressure just slightly less than the pressure necessary to impede blood flow, a small amount of blood passes through the obstruction and creates a turbulence that can be heard distally, indicating the systolic BP. As the cuff is further deflated, the sounds of turbulence progressively increase in intensity and the amount of blood allowed through increases, thus creating more arterial flutter. As the cuff pressure reaches diastolic pressure, the artery is no longer occluded, flow returns to laminar, and a change in the quality of the sounds occurs. This change (muffling) of the Korotkoff sounds indicates the diastolic BP.

Although the auscultatory method has been widely used over decades with good clinical results, it should be realized that several factors can influence the accuracy and reliability of the method. Its deficiency is the fact that the method measures pressure and flow, whereas the existence of pressure without flow is possible.

Generally, the clinical impression is that there is a pressure difference of about 20 mm Hg between a direct and indirect simultaneous BP measurement, although much wider variations can occasionally occur. Factors responsible for wide variations in pressure readings between direct and indirect measurements include (1) flow-related factors and (2) local or other factors.

Flow-related factors can occasionally be the cause of grossly false readings. In case of a low flow state due to hypovolemia and diminishing venous return or increased peripheral resistance, the auscultatory technique may be totally useless for determining systemic BP. In a high-output state (hyperdynamic circulation), the direct method usually gives a systolic arterial pressure that is much higher than that obtained by the auscultatory method. This is because of the abrupt hyperdynamic upstroke of the arterial waveform. Although it can be picked up by a transducer, it is associated with minimum or even no flow at all and therefore cannot be heard.

Local and other factors that can produce false readings by the auscultatory method include the following:

1. The size of the cuff. Cuff size is an important factor in accurate measurement. The American Heart Association recommends the following cuff sizes: adult arm, 12.5 × 23 cm; adult thigh, 18.0 × 35 cm; child arm, 9.4 × 21 cm; infant arm, 5.0 × 11.9 cm; and newborn arm, 2.5 × 5 cm.
2. The type of manometer used. Aneroid manometers, with time, tend to become inaccurate when compared with standard mercury column manometers.
3. Temperature. Temperature can in some instances influence accuracy. For example, if on the same arm there is a peripheral intravenous line administering fluids at room temperature or the arm is exposed and uncovered, blood vessels will constrict and the BP measurement will be inaccurate.
4. Acoustic acuity of the examiner. Loss of the ability to hear low-frequency sounds can affect the examiner's ability to detect the first or second squirt of blood during systole.
5. Speed of pressure release (deflation) of the BP cuff. The rate of cuff deflation has been standardized by the American Heart Association, which recommends 2 to 3 mm Hg of deflation per heart beat.

Electronic Detection of Korotkoff Sounds

Many devices have been designed for automatic electronic detection of BP (noninvasive BP monitors). The function of these devices is based on the Doppler effect. These devices can detect either (1) flow within a vessel or (2) motion of a vessel. All the devices are equipped with a pneumatic cuff and a Doppler sensor. Various units have been tested against a standard sphygmomanometer by different investigators. The results range from excellent to fair. We do not believe these units are more accurate than a standard mercury manometer, and they are much more expensive, although they can be of use in selected cases.

Direct Measurement

Direct measurement of arterial blood pressure, although it is an invasive procedure, affords many advantages to the anesthetist particularly in monitoring the hemodynamically unstable patient. Visual analysis of the arterial wave form and observed trends over a period of time yield valuable information beyond the traditional systolic/diastolic and/or mean readings. Invasive or direct blood pressure monitoring necessitates arterial cannulation and the use of a pressure measuring monitor.

Arterial cannulation not only permits direct measurement of arterial blood pressure and wave form analysis, but it facilitates the collection of arterial blood samples for gas, electrolyte, glucose, hematocrit, and other types of analyses. Arteries available for cannulation include the radial, ulner, brachial, axillary, dorsalis pedis, femoral, and superficial temporal. The radial artery is probably the most frequently used in anesthesia practice because of its ease of accessibility and the relatively low rate of complications. Cannulation of the dorsalis pedis artery is generally the second choice to the radial artery in adults for direct arterial measurement. Certain medical conditions such as Raynaud's disease or thromboembolitic disease in the limb may preclude arterial cannulation at one or more of the aforementioned sites.

Adequate collateral circulation should be assessed prior to arterial cannulation of the radial artery through use of the Allen's test. Occlusion of both the radial and ulnar arteries followed by release of the radial artery occlusion will provide an indication of the collateral blood flow available through the ulnar artery. If the radial arteries in both arms appear to be unsatisfactory after the Allen's test has been performed bilaterally, an alternative site should be considered.

Direct monitoring of arterial pressure can be accom-

plished with a pressure transducer which is attached to a signal processing monitor that displays the data. A less desirable system would be the use of an aneroid manometer that yields numerical data (mean arterial pressure) only. The arterial wave form displayed on the electronic monitor can provide information on myocardial contractility, systemic vascular resistance, stroke volume, circulating blood volume, and the hemodynamic significance of cardiac arrhythmias. See Figure 10–2.

THERMOMETRY

Thermometry is a basic mode of intraoperative monitoring that should be applied in every instance of anesthesia. It is absolutely essential in all pediatric cases. A number of commercially available units are designed for continuous temperature monitoring, and a number of different temperature probes are able to sense temperature from various sites. From the clinical point of view, the important factor is not which device is used, but which temperature is being monitored.

The use of air-conditioned operating rooms or hypothermic techniques, the massive administration of fluids and blood products, the lengthy major procedures, surgery for burns, or septic, febrile patients can be associated with wide temperature swings that we should be able to monitor reliably.

The sites most commonly used for temperature monitoring are the esophagus, rectum, skin, tympanic membrane, and muscle. The lower esophageal temperature, at the level of the left atrium, correlates closely with the core temperature, even when temperature changes rapidly. Thus esophageal temperature is useful to monitor core temperature. When a hypothermic technique is being used, however, esophageal temperature will not reflect the temperature of the muscle mass, which takes time to equilibrate. Rectal temperature has been found to correlate well with core temperature under steady-state conditions. If wide temperature swings occur, rectal sensors are significantly delayed in detecting the changes. Tympanic membrane temperature has also been found to correlate well with core temperature. Because it reflects temperature of the brain, it is useful during cardiopulmonary bypass. Skin and muscle temperatures do not accurately reflect core temperature changes. Muscle temperature can, however, be useful to determine if the core temperature recorded by one of the methods previously described has been equilibrated with the rest of the body.

VENOUS AND PULMONARY ARTERIAL PRESSURE MONITORING

Central venous catheterization and pressure monitoring have been widely used in the management of seriously ill patients. A central venous catheter facilitates central venous pressure (CVP) monitoring, blood sampling, and administration of various drugs.

Properly placed, a central venous catheter enables us to directly measure right atrial pressure, which, in the absence of tricuspid valve disease, will reflect right ventricular

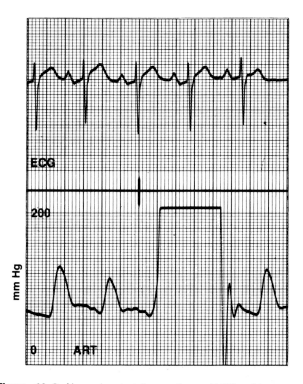

Figure 10–2. Normal arterial waveform (ART) with normal square wave response during rapid flushing with continuous flush system. (*From Kaye W: Invasive monitoring techniques. In McIntyre KM, Lewis AJ (eds): Textbook of Advanced Cardiac Life Support, American Heart Association, Dallas, Tx, 1981.*)

and diastolic pressures. It can thus furnish valuable information about volume status and right heart contractile state. In the absence of left ventricular disease, particularly in young patients, right atrial pressure correlates well with left atrial pressure, and thus a simple CVP line and pressure measurement can provide valuable information about the overall cardiac function.

All CVP lines can be placed percutaneously. The most commonly used sites of insertion are the antecubital fossae veins, neck veins (internal and external jugular), and subclavian veins. Each site of insertion is associated with particular advantages and disadvantages.

Antecubital Fossae Veins. These veins are very frequently used for central venous catheter insertion, because a CVP catheter through them causes minimum discomfort to the patient and introduction is relatively easy. Central venous catheters in antecubital veins are also very easy for nursing personnel to care for. The basilic (and midbasilic) vein is preferred over the cephalic vein, because when using the former, insertion is easier and the central position is easier to achieve, particularly if the right arm is used. The most significant disadvantages of the central venous catheterization of antecubital veins are a relatively high incidence of thrombophlebitis and failure to thread the catheter in a central position. If the CVP measurement is crucial and the antecubital approach has been chosen, x-ray verification of the position is recommended. After insertion and before the use of a central venous catheter (regardless of the site of insertion) free venous blood return should be assured.

Internal Jugular Vein. For internal jugular vein catheterization, Seldinger's technique should be applied with the use of a short catheter to initially cannulate the vein, a soft-tipped wire, and the appropriate size and length catheter. In the approach we use and recommend as the safest for insertion of a central venous catheter, the neck (or the antecubital fossae, or upper chest) should be prepared and draped in a sterile fashion. The use of cap, mask, gown, and gloves is also strongly recommended. Trendelenburg's position of the patient, if tolerated, could also facilitate the initial cannulation.

External Jugular Vein. Cannulation of the external jugular vein is probably easier than cannulation of the internal jugular vein. The final insertion of a long catheter to a central position is associated with a success rate of approximately 75 to 90 percent. The techniques of catheterization are similar, only a soft J-tipped wire should be used instead. Neck lines are easy to insert and to care for and are associated with a low complication rate, so their use should be considered safe.

Subclavian Vein. Catheterization of the subclavian is associated with a relatively high incidence of various complications but also with a high success rate. Subclavian vein catheterization is thought of as second choice. Subclavian central catheters are easy to care for.

Methods of Measuring Central Venous Pressure

CVP can be measured using a water column (in centimeters or millimeters of water) or using an electronic pressure device. A water column device (commercially provided or homemade) is easy to use and can be applied quickly in most places, but it has some serious disadvantages. First, it requires an extra set of stopcocks and pressure tubing and back-and-forth switching and thus compromises the sterility of a central line. Second and most important, it is associated with a high rate of false readings. Since the CVP tracing cannot be observed, if there is a malfunction of the line, the reading will be false. The best way to monitor CVP is by using a pressure transducer and an appropriate amplifier and screen monitor. With a well-calibrated transducer, the reading will be accurate and observation of the CVP tracing will give very valuable information on the functioning of the line. In addition, by observing the CVP waveform, one can obtain information on many aspects of the function of the cardiovascular system, from heart rhythm to function of the tricuspid valve. Whichever method is used, one should remember that right or left atrial pressure readings should always be made during end-expiration. It has long been recognized that if there is left ventricular dysfunction, left heart filling pressure does not correlate with CVP.

Flow-directed balloon-tipped pulmonary artery (PA) catheters were introduced into clinical practice in the early 1970s and have become very popular. From the anesthesiologist's point of view, history of preexisting heart disease, advanced age, and surgical procedures in which large volume shifts are anticipated are classic indications for PA catheter placement. The catheter can be placed through one of the commonly used sites for central line placement, described above. Neck veins and subclavian veins are the most convenient and popular sites. The placement of a PA catheter requires the use of the appropriate electronic devices for pressure monitoring. Obviously, a flow-directed catheter should not be placed if a screen monitor is not available. Complications associated with PA catheters include atrial or ventricular arrhythmias, right bundle branch block, thrombosis around the catheter, perforation of the pulmonary artery, balloon rupture, intracardiac knotting, and infection.

CARDIAC OUTPUT

Cardiac output is the amount of blood pumped out of the ventricle in a time unit. Under normal conditions, the output of the right ventricle equals that of the left. There are a number of methods to determine cardiac output. The most commonly used today are

    I. The Fick method
   II. The indicator dilution method
     A. Dye dilution
     B. Thermodilution
  III. The radioisotope method
  IV. The pulse contour method

It is to be noted that the two last methods are gaining greater popularity. Both the Fick and the dye dilution methods are rarely used at the bedside, whereas the thermodilution method is used widely at the bedside as well as in the operating room.

The invention and use of quadruple-lumen PA catheters has allowed fast and accurate determination of serial cardiac output. The principle of the method is based on the indicator dilution method, using a given volume of a known-temperature cold injectate as indicator. The indicator is injected into the right atrium, and the sampling is from the PA, from the thermistor attached to the PA catheter. The temperature gradient is fed into a computer that computes the cardiac output from the following formula:

$$V \cdot Di \cdot Si(Tb - Ti) = Q \cdot dT \cdot t \cdot Db \cdot Sb(1000/600)$$

where Q is cardiac output, Db and Di are the densities, Sb and Si are the specific heats, Tb and Ti are the temperatures, V is the volume of injectate, dT is the temperature differential, t is the duration of the change in temperature, and 1000/60 is a constant factor. Note that the most important variables are volume of injectate and temperature gradient.

The thermodilution method provides fast and accurate cardiac output determinations because of minimal recirculation of the indicator, and determination can be performed as frequently as every 1 minute. The injectate, theoretically, can be at any temperature lower than that of the blood, but since the temperature gradient is a major factor in the formula, the greater the temperature gradient, the more accurate will be the determination. Variance greater than ±20 percent between conservative measurements should raise the suspicion of mechanical or technical error.

MONITORING MUSCLE RELAXATION

The three classic components of anesthesia include hypnosis, amnesia, and muscle paralysis. Thus, provision of appropriate and adequate muscle relaxation is one of the many duties of an anesthesiologist, and the subsequent monitoring of this intervention is also essential. To monitor the effects of neuromuscular blocking agents, one can electrically stimulate a peripheral nerve (usually the ulnar nerve at the wrist) and visually observe or electronically record the adduction of the thumb. Use of a single twitch, which is an electrical stimulation at a rate of 1 Hz, or the train of four, which is supramaximal stimulation at a rate of 2 Hz, or a tetanic stimulus at 50 Hz for 5 seconds all are accepted ways of monitoring neuromuscular blockade. The two groups of muscle relaxants provoke different responses to both train of four and tetanic stimulation. In Figure 10–3, the effects of nondepolarizing and depolarizing muscle relaxants on the train of four and tetanic stimulation are shown. By monitoring the neuromuscular transmission, we are able not only to determine the depth of the neuromuscular blockade but to diagnose a phase 2 block and to judge the amount of reversal required.

The role of the anesthetist in the operating room is crucial and delicate. Physician and nurse anesthetists are probably the only healthcare givers who provide intensive

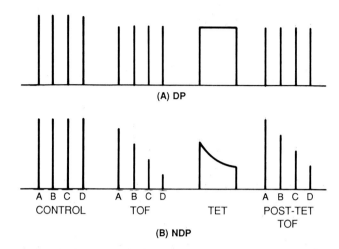

Figure 10–3. Train of four using (A) depolarizing muscle relaxants (DP) and (B) nondepolarizing muscle relaxants (NDP). Note the nonfade of train of four (TOF), the sustained tetanus, and the absence of post-tetanic facilitation when using depolarizing muscle relaxants as opposed to the use of nondepolarizing agents.

care to the patient on a minute-to-minute basis—obviously very responsible and complicated work. Our job is becoming even more complicated with the addition of numerous sophisticated electronic monitoring devices to our armamentarium. Common sense and in-depth knowledge of the patient are still essential to providing safe anesthesia.

BIBLIOGRAPHY

Ali HH, Savarese JJ: Monitoring of neuromuscular function. Anesthesiology 45:216–249, 1976.

Armstrong PW, Baigrie RS: Hemodynamic Monitoring in the Critically Ill. Philadelphia, Lippincott, 1986.

Cooper JB: Toward prevention of anesthetic mishaps. Int Anesthesiol Clin 22:167–183, 1984.

Daily BK, Schroeder JS: Technique in Bedside Hemodynamic Monitoring, 3rd ed. St. Louis, CV Mosby, 1985.

Grundy B: Intraoperative monitoring of sensory-evoked potentials. Anesthesiology 58:72–87, 1983.

Kaye W: Invasive monitoring techniques. In McIntyre KM, Lewis AJ (eds): Textbook of Advanced Cardiac Life Support. American Heart Association, Dallas, Tx, 1981.

McKenzie N, Forest AL: Patient monitoring in the operating theatre. A comparison of practice between 1976 and 1983. Anaesthesia 40:141–145, 1985.

Philip JH, Raemer DB: Selecting the optimal anesthesia monitoring array. Med Instrum 19:122–126, 1985.

Saidman L, Smith NT: Monitoring in Anesthesia, 2nd ed. London, Butterworth, 1984.

Silvay G (ed): Recent advances in monitoring during anesthesia. Mt Sinai J Med 51:559–599, 1984.

Watts RC, Mylrea KC: Monitoring the anesthetized patient in the operating room. Med Instrum 17:383–388, 1983.

Wynands JE: Hemodynamic monitoring: Cardiovascular system functions. Can Anaesth Soc J 32:288–293, 1985.

11

Preoperative Preparation and Evaluation

Christine S. Zambricki

The preanesthetic visit affords the anesthetist a unique opportunity to make a significant impact on patient response to surgery and anesthesia. Every patient should be seen by the anesthetist before arrival in the operating suite and the anesthetist's findings used to prepare the patient for surgery and to formulate the anesthetic care plan. The anesthetist needs to spend sufficient time with the patient to complete a thorough preoperative visit, and it should be done enough in advance that there is time for further diagnostic testing and preoperative preparation.

Within the holistic approach to patient care, preoperative assessment is as important to patient outcome as intraoperative or postanesthetic management. Although students in the field of anesthesiology acknowledge the value of the preanesthetic visit, in actual practice a surprising number of graduates secure positions in which they do not see their own patients preoperatively or do not see their patients until the day of surgery. It is expected that the reader will be convinced of the importance of a goal-directed preanesthetic assessment and insist on carrying out that responsibility with the same enthusiasm exhibited in other phases of anesthetic care.

Under certain circumstances the importance of the preanesthetic visit is magnified. Advances in surgery, coupled with the increasing life-span of our population, have accelerated the trend toward extensive surgical procedures for geriatric patients. Because of the high incidence of associated disease in the elderly, it is preferable to see these patients 48 hours before the scheduled date of surgery. Patients scheduled for major surgical procedures or those patients expected to have multiple medical problems should also be visited at least 48 hours preoperatively.

Some institutions use the team approach to anesthesia care. The team may consist of an anesthesiologist, certified registered nurse anesthetist, and a student or resident. If a team approach is used, every member of the team should become knowledgeable about the patient before surgery. One team member should be designated to do a thorough preanesthetic evaluation and complete a written summary, which is placed on the chart. All team members must be responsible for reviewing data preoperatively and for introducing themselves to the patient as part of the anesthetic care team. The patient can then recognize the anesthesia care providers in the operating room. In addition, the patient will not be surprised or frightened to find a "team" in attendance rather than one individual practitioner.

The anesthetist can most effectively direct the course of the preoperative visit by being cognizant of the goals to be achieved:

1. *Procurement of information*
2. *Reduction of patient anxiety: education of patient*
3. *Securing informed consent*
4. *Evaluation and documentation of anesthetic risk*
5. *Optimization of preoperative status: reduction of perioperative morbidity*
6. *Selection of premedication*
7. *Formulation of anesthetic care plan*

The text that follows discusses the goals of the preoperative visit and describes the format for a thorough preoperative assessment.

PROCUREMENT OF INFORMATION

The most obvious goal of the preoperative visit is the acquisition of factual information about the patient. This information can come from several sources including a chart review, careful health history, and a thorough physical and psychological assessment. Thus, a baseline of data is established for comparing intraoperative or postoperative abnormalities.

Chart Review

There are several reasons why the preanesthetic assessment begins with careful scrutiny of the patient's chart. The name and identification number found on the chart should be matched with information from the operating room schedule, and the anesthetist should note the surgeon's name and planned procedure to be sure that the visit is being made to the correct patient and to avoid having to obtain that information from the patient. Patients find it disquieting to be asked several times when and what type of surgery is to be performed. The release should be checked for completeness, and any question regarding the legality of the signatures should be checked at this time. The surgical procedure listed on the release should be compared with the operating schedule. Any questions in this regard should be clarified before the patient's arrival in the operating suite. Preliminary chart review provides the anesthetist with a basis for the patient interview and eliminates the need to return to question the patient again after stumbling on a contradiction or problem in the chart.

A preanesthetic assessment questionnaire may be part of the patient's chart. The questionnaire is given to the patient to complete as soon as surgery is scheduled so that it can be reviewed at an early date. Correctly completed, this document helps the anesthetist focus attention on the patient at risk and allows for efficient use of time available for the preoperative visit. The preanesthetic assessment questionnaire cannot, however, substitute for a careful health history and physical assessment of the patient. Drawbacks to the use of such a form include misinterpretation by the infirm or elderly patient resulting in omission or incorrect information and the operational difficulties of getting the form distributed, completed, and returned to the chart before the anesthetist's visit.

Valuable information about the course of the patient's illness can be obtained from the progress notes. The history and physical should be reviewed for any points that might indicate the need for special attention during patient assessment, e.g., thyroid disease is cause for detailed inquiry about endocrine disease and related sequelae during the preoperative interview. The progress notes describe the primary diagnosis as well as the patient's other coexisting disease states.

The nursing notes provide information related to a particular patient's disabilities that might affect the approach to the patient interview. Is the patient's hearing impaired? If so, a standard printed questionnaire can be supplemented with handwritten questions, and a translator for signing may be of help. If the patient can read lips, the anesthetist is careful to face the patient directly and speak slowly. Does the patient have sight in both eyes? If not, the anesthetist can help establish contact by taking the patient's hand during the introduction. The nursing portion of the patient record may include the date and reason for admission and descriptions of the patient's condition, progress, complaints, and ability to cope with the diagnosed condition. Nursing interventions using individually focused activities to promote support and their impact will be described. The graphic sheet is a source of information about daily temperature, weight, pulse, blood pressure, respiration, and possibly intake and output. This background data can be logged on the preanesthetic evaluation sheet before the patient is seen. The anesthetist is responsible for providing care consistent with the nursing care plan, within the limitations of the operating room environment.

The preoperative chart review includes attention to pharmacologic agents the patient currently receives or has taken in the past. These drugs should be considered in the development of the anesthetic care plan, because drug interactions with anesthetic agents are possible. Specifically, succinylcholine is potentiated by a wide range of drugs, including some antibiotics, lithium, quinidine, echothiophate iodide, cyclophosphamide, and other antineoplastic drugs. Augmentation of nondepolarizing neuromuscular

blockade has been reported in patients receiving local anesthetics, antibiotics, or antiarrhythmics, such as digitalis or quinidine, propranolol, and phenytoin. The drug history will help determine the focus of the interview. For example, the patient taking beta blockers will be questioned regarding the reason for the drug, relief of symptoms by the drug, and the person's cardiovascular history. A decision as to the continuance of drug therapy on the day of surgery must be made. Recent literature indicates that antihypertensives, antiseizure medication, and some cardiac drugs should be administered on the day of surgery. Attention to the patient's pharmacologic regimen may alert the anesthetist to request further diagnostic tests to complete the patient assessment, as is shown in Table 11–1.

Diagnostic Tests. The results of laboratory tests and diagnostic studies should be reviewed before seeing the patient. The selection of preoperative screening tests has been the subject of recent controversy in the field of anesthesiology. Health care providers have been scrutinized both by the federal government and by private insurers for cost efficiency, and as a result, the list of "routine" preoperative tests has dwindled. It has been estimated that approximately one-half of all surgical procedures performed in this country are performed on patients with no systematic disturbances—that is, no disease other than the surgical pathology. Unfortunately, there are few studies that evaluate the cost:benefit ratio of preoperative laboratory tests as a routine for healthy patients undergoing elective surgery.

Several criteria must be met if a preoperative study is to be considered routinely essential for the healthy patient. (1) The condition tested for must be asymptomatic and not apparent on the normal health history and physical assessment. (2) The condition must increase surgical morbidity or mortality or represent significant risk to those associated with the patient's care. (3) Preoperative diagnosis must be more beneficial in terms of patient outcome than a diagnosis established postoperatively, and (4) the abnormality should influence anesthetic approach. (5) The available tests must be specific and sensitive enough to allow for accurate detection of the condition, and (6) a test should not be used if there exists an alternative that compares in sensitivity at less cost.

Several tests are of value as routine indicators for apparently healthy people being considered for surgery. Both hematocrit and urinalysis are tests of low cost and moderate sensitivity. Abnormal results identify the need for further studies and possible preoperative intervention. A pregnancy test should be done if the female patient is susceptible

TABLE 11–1. A COMPARISON OF PHARMACOLOGIC AGENTS AND DIAGNOSTIC TESTS THAT MAY BE INDICATED

Drug	Test
Digitalis (Digoxin)	Digitalis level, electrolytes
Levothyroxine sodium (Synthroid)	Triiodothyronine, thyroxine
Antihypertensives/diuretics	Electrolytes
Phenytoin (Dilantin)	Dilatin level
Insulin	Fasting blood glucose

to pregnancy. Although the predictive value for hepatitis is low, the serum glutamic-oxaloactic transaminase (SGOT) has been recommended by some authors because of the serious risk of hepatitis to patients and staff. Tuberculosis screening is relatively inexpensive and should be used when a high-risk population may expose other patients and staff to the disease.

Many authors have questioned the value of routine preoperative chest x-ray and electrocardiogram (ECG). In one instance, 12,000 chest x-rays of pregnant women were examined, and there was no detection of clinical abnormalities that would not have been apparent from the physical examination and health history. Routine use of the preoperative chest x-ray is expensive and bears the risks of irradiation. In addition, interpretation of chest x-ray is often not available until after surgery, and the results may make no difference in anesthetic management in the asymptomatic patient. A chest x-ray is indicated after positive findings during the examination of the pulmonary patient.

Similarly, the ECG has not proven itself to be a cost-effective component of routine preanesthetic screening for the apparently healthy patient. Both the chest x-ray and ECG may, however, be indicated on the basis of findings during the preanesthetic visit.

The Health History

Talking with the patient and obtaining a health history are extremely important components of the preanesthetic process. The anesthetist is enabled to gather an organized, comprehensive set of data for the anesthetic care plan; moreover, this interview can establish trust and confidence. The anesthetist and patient can then proceed to define the therapeutic goals of the anesthetic plan of care.

The anesthetist sets the stage for a positive interaction by deliberate manipulation of the environment. The location of the interview should be quiet, private, and free from interruption. If the patient is eating or receiving therapy, a return visit should be made. Visitors can be asked to step out while the interview takes place unless a visitor functions as a history provider for pediatric or unreliable patients. Lighting should be adequate to provide for accurate visual inspection. Conducting the interview at eye level and several feet distant from the patient is recommended for patient comfort. The patient must be alert, without the influence of narcotics or tranquilizers. The clinician should avoid taking a position between the patient and a bright light, which would require the patient to talk to a silhouette.

Care taken with the initial approach can do much to create a good first impression. The anesthetist should appear tactful and unhurried, and clothing should be clean, neat, and professional. Under no circumstances should the preoperative visit be made in a bloodstained scrub suit or with a dirty tourniquet wrapped around the stethoscope. It has been demonstrated that the proper use of names is a critical determinant of the patient's attitude, and the patient who is treated with respect is more likely to be satisfied and comply with instructions. The patient should be greeted using proper names, i.e., Mrs. Katz, rather than impersonal nicknames such as "grannie" or "honey." Pediatric patients may be addressed by first name.

The anesthesia practitioner should always indicate what his or her title and role are in the anesthetic care of the patient. The patient has the right to know if the preoperative visitor is a student, certified registered nurse anesthetist, or anesthesiologist. Furthermore, the patient needs to know if there is a chance that the person making the preoperative assessment will not be the same person administering the anesthetic.

Because a significant amount of information is needed from the health history, it is useful to follow an organized interview schedule. Use of silence, posture, actions, and projection of an accepting attitude encourage the patient's response. Direct questions should proceed from the general to the specific. Leading questions should be avoided. A graded response is preferable to a yes or no answer, e.g., "how many pillows do you sleep with at night" rather than "do you sleep with your head up?" It is less confusing to the patient if one question is posed at a time, rather than a list of questions such as "have you ever had heart disease, lung disease, or liver disease?" Language must be clearly understood and appropriate to the patient. Current medical jargon can boggle the mind of even the brightest patient, but the anesthetist must also take pains to avoid any condescension.

The health history can be organized in many ways. Table 11–2 shows a suggested method of organizing the data. It should be kept in mind that the sequencing of information is not as important as thoroughness. The topics listed should be rephrased in layperson's terms.

The Physical Assessment

In practice, the physical assessment and health history can be obtained simultaneously; for the purposes of this discussion, however, the two areas are presented separately. Organization and thoroughness are the hallmarks of a good preanesthetic physical assessment.

A relaxed, unhurried, professional approach on the part of the anesthetist is imperative for the patient's comfort and confidence. The patient's privacy and freedom from interruption are of primary importance. Ideally the patient should sit on the edge of the bed for most of the examination, allowing examination of the front and back of the chest. As the physical assessment is carried out, the anesthetist explains the procedures to be done, gives appropriate instructions, and warns the patient of any maneuver that may produce discomfort.

The examination is conducted systematically, from head to foot. The following equipment may be used: flashlight, tongue depressor, stethoscope with diaphragm and bell, and a blood pressure cuff.

General Impression. The physical examination begins with an inspection of the patient's general appearance, including general observations such as the patient's age, race, development, skin color, overall state of health, weight, gait, and posture. Personality characteristics and emotional status can also be observed. Abnormalities in any of these areas deserve further exploration during the physical assessment.

TABLE 11–2. THE PREANESTHETIC HEALTH HISTORY

General Health History General state of health Activities of daily living/work Previous hospitalization/surgery/anesthesia Medications/dosage/efficiency Allergies Alcohol intake/drug use Nutrition **Personal or Family History of Surgical or Anesthetic Complications** Postoperative bleeding Perioperative cardiac arrest Cancellation of surgery Postoperative jaundice Prolonged apnea Malignant hyperthermia "Allergies" to anesthesia **Respiratory History** Dyspnea/orthopnea Exercise tolerance Asthma/bronchitis Tuberculosis Pneumothorax Smoking history Cough/wheezing Colds Epistaxis Hoarseness	**Cardiovascular History** Hypertension Myocardial infarction Heart failure Anemia Angina Exercise tolerance Paroxysmal nocturnal dyspnea Coagulopathy **Neuromuscular History** Headaches Seizures Transient ischemic attacks Paralysis/paresis Muscular disorders Back pain Syncope **Endocrine History** Diabetes Liver disease/jaundice Thyroid disease **Renal History** Kidney disease Genito-urinary disease **Gynecological History** Vaginal bleeding Pregnancy

Head and Neck. The head is inspected to evaluate size and shape, to note symmetry and normalcy of ears, and to identify the presence of maldistribution of hair. The eyes are examined for redness or drainage, and the pupils inspected with a flashlight for reaction to light and accommodation. Inspection of the nasal cavity through the anterior naris reveals the degree of nasal symmetry, septal position, patency of nares, and condition of the turbinates. This information is essential if nasoendotracheal intubation is planned. The patient is asked to breathe through each nostril independently to compare patency. Dark-red nasal mucosa indicates inflammation, rhinitis, or hemorrhage.

The mouth and pharynx are inspected, using a tongue depressor and flashlight. The tongue is evaluated for size, deviation, and the presence of lesions. The size of the tongue is an important consideration when use of a mask is planned. A large tongue is seen with conditions such as acromegaly, cretinism, and mongolism. Beyond the tongue and above it is an arch formed by the anterior and posterior pillars, soft palate, and uvula. A long, narrow oral cavity has minimal space within the dental arch, which makes intubation difficult because the laryngoscope blocks the anesthetist's view of the larynx. A narrow, V-shaped arch can compromise placement of the laryngoscope as well, because the blade catches on the maxillary teeth. The normal soft palate is pink, moist, and smooth without inflammation or masses. There are usually 32 teeth in the adult mouth. Dental abnormalities, such as missing, chipped, or diseased teeth, are identified. Incisors that are widely spread apart or protruding may present a problem with instrumentation,

and dental malocclusion can lead to difficulties with airway management.

The mouth is examined for the presence of loose teeth. Newly erupted deciduous teeth appear at approximately six months of age. At this time the roots are only partially formed. Permanent teeth begin to erupt at six years of age; therefore, we can expect loose deciduous teeth between the ages of six and twelve. The location of loose teeth is noted on the chart and the parents warned of possible damage. It is recommended that the patient or parent (in the case of minors) sign a sheet describing the condition of the teeth. Besides damage to the teeth, the possibility of a dislodged tooth migrating to the pharynx, larynx, or trachea is also a danger.

The existence and position of dental crowns and bridges are noted on the preoperative evaluation to minimize the possibility of damage. The patient is advised to remove any dentures preoperatively.

Some congenital anomalies result in unusual problems in airway management, which can be anticipated. Pierre Robin syndrome is characterized by a small mandible, micrognathia, and downward displacement or retraction of the tongue; Treacher Collins syndrome presents with a receding chin; and hemifacial microsomia is a deformity consisting of hypoplasia of the mandible and soft-tissue structures of the face and cranium.

Joint function is an additional anatomic factor that is important when considering airway management. Two distinct motions are involved in the joint function of the mouth. The hingelike action of the condyle allows the mouth to open partially whereas the wider opening of the mouth results from a motion of anterior displacement and forward gliding. Ankylosis of the temporomandibular joint or progressive arthritic changes may limit mandibular opening.

Mobility of the temporomandibular joint is assessed by asking the patient to open his or her mouth as wide as possible. The patient is then asked to touch chin to chest, to extend the head posteriorly as far as possible, and to turn the head to the right and to the left. Normally the chin can be touched to the chest and the head can be bent through at least 45 degrees and rotated 90 degrees to either side, parallel with the shoulder axis. The neck is examined for physical characteristics, keeping in mind that airway management is more difficult when the patient has a short, muscular neck. The neck is inspected for symmetry and abnormal swelling or masses and the trachea palpated. The presence of nodules or swelling of the thyroid gland is noted.

The mobility of the cervical vertebrae is dependent on 23 joints extending from the occiput to the thoracic vertebrae. The joint movement consists of sliding, rotation, flexion, and extension. The normal flexion and extension of the head varies from 165 to 190 degrees, with a 20 percent decrease in range of motion expected after the age of 75. Impaired cervical mobility may not be apparent upon casual observation, and the patient may be unaware of the disability because limited extension at the lower cervical vertebrae is possible.

The vasculature of the neck is inspected at this time. The jugular veins are the most visible veins proximal to the mediastinal and cardiac structures. The jugular veins are observed for venous congestion and for suitability for cannulation. The internal jugular veins and carotid artery cross superior to the neck just lateral to and slightly behind the trachea. Atherosclerosis frequently affects the carotid arteries, producing audible bruits that may be auscultated with a stethoscope. Carotid pulsations are palpated for quality and symmetry.

Lungs and Thorax. Examination of the lungs and thorax is accomplished by inspection, palpation, percussion, and auscultation. The posterior thorax is inspected while the patient is in the sitting position, with arms folded across the chest. Anterior thorax and lungs can be examined with the patient in Fowler's position.

The midsternal, midclavicular, and anterior axillary line provide imaginary vertical reference points for localization (Fig. 11–1). Ribs can be numbered by using the sternal angle to locate the adjacent second rib. The external measurement along the body surface from the upper border of the cricoid cartilage to the tip of the xiphoid process corresponds to the internal distance from the upper teeth to the carina. Knowing that the trachea bifurcates at the level of the second interspace is helpful when judging endotracheal tube length.

Assessment of the chest begins with observation of the rate, rhythm, and effort of respiration. The ratio of inspiration to expiration (normal approximately 1:2) is noted and the depth of respiration estimated. The slope of the ribs and shape of the chest are assessed. Abnormal retractions or a widened costal angle indicate the presence of obstructive disease.

Palpation is used to assess respiratory excursion and to evaluate tactile fremitus. The anesthetist places his or her hands parallel to the tenth rib posteriorly and the costal margin anteriorly (Fig. 11–2). The range and symmetry of respiratory movement are observed as the patient inhales deeply and exhales. The patient is then asked to repeat

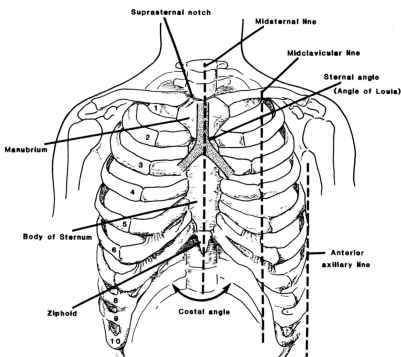

Figure 11–1. Anatomic relationships of surface and internal structures.

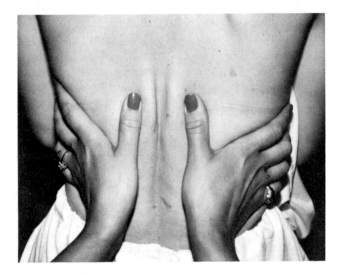

Figure 11–2. Palpation technique for respiratory excursion.

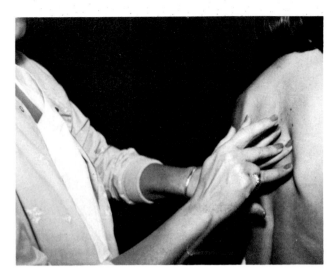

Figure 11–4. Indirect method of percussion.

the words "ninety-nine." Simultaneously the anesthetist uses the lateral aspect of his or her hand to palpate the vibration transmitted through the bronchopulmonary system to the chest wall (Fig. 11–3). Fremitus is decreased when a bronchus is obstructed or the pleural space is filled with fluid or air. Lung consolidation is manifested by increased fremitus.

Percussion causes vibration of the chest wall and underlying tissue, which produces audible sounds. Percussion can be done either directly or indirectly. Direct percussion is accomplished by striking the body surface with the tips of all four fingers held together; however, the indirect method is most commonly used (Fig. 11–4). The examiner hyperextends the middle finger of the left hand, firmly pressing the distal phalanx on the body surface to be percussed. This stationary finger is referred to as the pleximeter. The middle finger of the other hand (plexor) is used to strike the base of the distal phalanx of the left middle

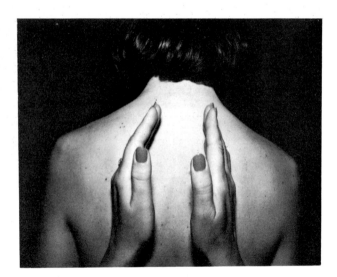

Figure 11–3. Palpation technique for transmission of bronchopulmonary vibrations.

finger. The sounds produced by percussion are described in Table 11–3.

Auscultation of the chest with the diaphragm of a stethoscope yields information about the quality of breath sounds and the presence of any abnormal sounds. The pitch, intensity, and duration of respirations are noted in all lung fields.

Adventitious sounds are superimposed on breath sounds and are not normally heard. Rales are discrete, crackling sounds heard most often on inspiration. They are caused by the bubbling of air through a fluid medium. Rales often disappear with deep breathing or coughing. Rhonchi and wheezes are more prominent during expiration and are caused by air passing through a partially obstructed airway. Pleural friction rubs are rough, multiphasic, rubbing sounds that are present when the pleura is inflamed. Adventitious sounds should be identified by type, where in the respiratory cycle they are heard, and where on the chest wall they are located.

There are several semiquantitative screening tests of pulmonary function that may be employed when bedside spirometry is not available. The anesthetist may accompany the patient walking down the hall or climbing one flight of stairs to quantify "breathlessness." A match test may be helpful for the patient with obstructive lung disease. In this test, the examiner lights a match and holds it approximately 6 inches from the patient's mouth. The patient is asked to blow out the match without pursing his or her lips. To blow out a match this way, the patient must exceed a maximum flow rate of 100 liters per minute (normal 300 liters per minute). If a person fails the match test, there is indication of obstructive pulmonary disease, requiring a more detailed assessment. The third semiquantitative test of pulmonary function is carried out with the anesthetist applying a stethoscope to the interscapular region and asking the patient to breathe in as much air as possible. The anesthetist times the expiratory effort until expirations are inaudible. A patient with obstructive lung disease will take considerable time to exhale, and expiratory sounds will be heard longer than 3 seconds. Vital capacity can be measured with a spirometer.

TABLE 11-3. QUALITIES OF PERCUSSION SOUNDS

Quality	Intensity	Pitch	Duration	Normal Location	Pathology
Resonant	Loud	Low	Long	Lung	
Hyperresonant	Very loud	Lower	Longer		Emphysema
Flat	Soft	High	Short	Thigh	Pleural effusion
Dull	Medium	Medium	Medium	Liver, diaphragm	Pneumonia, fluid in pleural space
Tympany	Loud	High	Long	Stomach, intestine	

A simple test to evaluate the presence of retained secretions is to ask the patient to take a deep breath and forcibly exhale a few times. In the patient with chronic bronchitis, this maneuver will usually produce an attack of paroxysmal coughing with rhonchi and wheezing.

Cardiovascular System. Physical examination of the heart requires that the patient be supine or with the upper body slightly elevated. The anterior chest is inspected for abnormal pulses, which can sometime be felt as "thrills." The point of maximum impulse is identified relative to superficial landmarks.

A stethoscope is used to auscultate the first and second heart sounds (S_1 and S_2). S_2 is normally louder than S_1 at the aortic (second right interspace close to sternum) and pulmonic (second left interspace close to sternum) areas. Extrasystolic or -diastolic sounds are identified and noted for location, timing, intensity, pitch, and effects of respirations on the sounds. The heart rate is counted for a minute and the heart rhythm evaluated.

The tricuspid (lower left sternal border) and mitral (fifth interspace medial to the midclavicular line) areas are auscultated for abnormal sounds. The patient is positioned with the left side down for accentuation of mitral murmurs and presence of S_3 or S_4. S_4 is common in the presence of coronary heart disease.

The clinical features of peripheral vascular disease of the lower extremities include diminution or absence of pulses, systolic bruits, ischemic skin changes, and muscle wasting. The anesthetist palpates peripheral pulses bilaterally and compares one side against the other. An Allen test is done if arterial catheterization is planned. The blood pressure is measured with a sphygmomanometer in both arms. Average mean arterial pressure is calculated based on readings for a 24-hour period.

Despite the number of systems to be reviewed, the preanesthetic physical assessment can be accomplished in fifteen minutes or less. Organization of the examination according to body systems will help to facilitate the development of thorough, efficient skills.

REDUCTION OF PATIENT ANXIETY: EDUCATION OF PATIENT

The short-term effects of psychological preparation and teaching before surgery are shown to reduce the need for pain medication in the postoperative period. This advantage could conceivably translate into a shorter hospital stay, mak-

ing the time spent in psychological preparation well worth it.

Despite the safeguards of modern medicine, many patients face thoughts of death when scheduled for surgery and are terrified or severely depressed. Because this anxiety continues through the operation and beyond it, there is an imperative need to decrease anxiety preoperatively. When properly done, the preoperative visit compares favorably with a purely pharmacologic approach. While demonstrating concern, the anesthetist can employ strategies aimed at reducing the patient's anxiety and educating the patient to strengthen his or her coping mechanisms.

The patient scheduled for surgery is likely to have many life changes and stresses. The patient is undergoing personal injury or illness and changing personal habits, however temporarily. Normal routines of sleeping, eating, recreation, and spiritual activities are disrupted. Socially the patient may undergo changes in marital relations or work setting, and his or her financial picture may be altered. The anesthetist must be sensitive to these possible stressors during the preanesthetic interview.

There is evidence that a striking relationship exists between preoperative fear and postoperative behavior. Three distinct coping patterns have been noted in patients facing surgery:

1. *High anticipatory fear.* Patients in this category manifest a heightened level of anxiety and fear of pain, multilation, and death. After surgery the patient continues to be extremely anxious.
2. *Moderate anticipatory fear.* Patients in this category worry occasionally and are anxious about specific details of the operation. After the operation they are cooperative and participate in their postoperative care.
3. *Low anticipatory fear.* Patients in this category exhibit an absence of anxiety coupled with an unrealistic, optimistic outlook. After surgery these patients are preoccupied and difficult, sometimes refusing postoperative treatments.

During the preoperative visit, the anesthetist looks at the anticipated effect of the surgery, as perceived by the patient, and the patient's attitude toward his or her illness. It may be helpful to elicit details of the surgical and anesthetic experiences of relatives and friends as perceived by the patient. Special attention is given to the patient's recall of previous surgical experiences and reaction to anesthesia.

The duration of the preoperative visit and characteristics of interview techniques have been compared as to their effectiveness in patients possessing difficult coping patterns. A cursory preoperative interview—one with minimal information and the absence of rapport—results in increased anxiety levels and increased thiopental sodium requirements in patients with low anticipatory fear. This same interview technique results in decreased anxiety and lower thiopental dosage in patients with high anticipatory fear. A supportive interview, of long duration and including the establishment of rapport and provision of information, has little effect on the patient with initial low anxiety levels. In the extremely anxious patient, this supportive interview also reduces the anxiety level. Clearly, the highly anxious patient needs a preoperative visit to reduce anxiety, regardless of the characteristics of that visit.

It appears that maximum benefit in the patient's psychological preparation will be derived if the anesthetist (1) supplies information about the events that will occur, along with reassurance, and (2) discusses coping mechanisms that the patient can use to handle stress and pain.

The anesthetist first needs to evaluate the level of the patient's desire for information. Care must be taken to avoid overbriefing. Some patients want only a minimal-to-moderate amount of simple, factual information; some want no information at all; and some do not want to know "too much." A simple explanation of the preoperative holding room, intravenous lines, and anesthesia induction will usually suffice. The patient may then lead the interviewer to answer specific questions. If questions are asked about diagnosis and surgical treatment, the anesthetist must be careful that answers do not conflict with those provided by others.

Preoperative information allows the patient to mentally "rehearse," to develop realistic expectations and plans for coping with the perioperative experience. As well as providing information, the anesthetist can counsel the patient about coping mechanisms. The anesthetist can provide active emotional support by fostering the patient's sense of control over destiny, e.g., by teaching the technique of coughing and deep-breathing, with a return demonstration by the patient, and at the same time explaining how this technique helps prevent atelactasis and maintain optimum lung function. In addition, reassurance can be given that postoperative analgesics will be available and the patient shown how to splint the incision. The anesthetist can also review the techniques for deep-breathing and relaxation as a method for coping with stress and postoperative pain.

SECURING INFORMED CONSENT

Securing informed consent for anesthesia services is a primary duty of the anesthetist making the preoperative visit. This responsibility can be difficult if the anesthesia care provider is not sure how much and how to inform the patient.

Most hospitals require patients to sign a blanket consent form agreeing to surgery and the necessary administration of anesthesia. Some departments of anesthesiology have developed a separate form that specifically describes the type of anesthesia proposed and requires the patient's signature.

Regardless of the type of form used, the quality and completeness of the anesthesia provider's explanation to the patient and the patient's genuine understanding of this information are required for a bona fide informed consent. An accurate explanation of the choices of anesthesia techniques available and their benefits is given to the patient. The anesthetist describes any discomforts or risks to the patient and identifies any technique or drug that is experimental. The anesthetist must also identify the other anesthesia care providers who will be involved in the anesthetic care. Any particular concerns of the patient should be documented in the chart.

Special problems with informed consent arise with a patient of limited intelligence or with a language barrier. The anesethetist must assess the degree of limitation and the patient's literacy before giving explanations or asking for written consent. If a language barrier exists, a neutral, objective translator must be located. The translator is instructed against interpreting or summarizing the information.

Even after informed consent is obtained, the anesthetist should offer to answer any questions about the planned anesthetic agent or technique. Legally the patient is free to withdraw consent at any time without future prejudice to care and treatment.

EVALUATION AND DOCUMENTATION OF ANESTHETIC RISK

One of the goals of the preoperative visit is to calculate the risk of anesthesia. A subjective evaluation of anesthetic risk has always been used to discriminate between very low and very high risk patients. The accurate estimate using subjective criteria is based on such factors as the anesthetist's previous experience with similar patients and operations, clinical history, physical examination, laboratory results, the skill of the surgeon, and the characteristics of the institution.

As awareness of preoperative complications increases, classification systems have been developed to objectively quantify the risks of anesthesia and surgery based on the patient's health status. The determination of risk is important because surgical indication itself is formulated on the basis of a risk:benefit ratio.

The American Society of Anesthesiologists (ASA) Classification of Physical Status, developed by Dripps, is one of the most commonly used systems to estimate patient risk. On the basis of preoperative assessment, the patient is assigned to a class. The categories of physical status are listed as follows:

Class I   The patient has no organic, physiologic, biochemical, or psychiatric disturbance. The pathologic process is localized and does not entail a systemic disturbance.
Class II   The patient has a mild to moderate systemic disturbance caused either by the conditions to be treated surgically or other pathophysiologic process. (Example: Controlled hypertension.)
Class III The patient has severe systemic disturbances that impact on activities of daily living. (Example: Brittle diabetic.)

Class IV   The patient has severe systemic disorders that are life-threatening and not necessarily correctable by surgical means. (Example: Widespread vascular disease and kidney failure.)

Class V   The moribund patient who is not expected to survive 24 hours. (Example: Head injury with stroke.)

Emergency   Any patient in one of the classes listed above who has surgery on an emergency basis.

Various indexes for estimated risk have been developed in addition to the Dripps system. A liver disease scoring system exists to predict patient outcome based on the presence of encephalopathy, bilirubinemia, increased prothrombin time, and decreased blood albumin. The Goldman Cardiac Operative Risk Index Scoring System (CRIS) is a multifactor index that has been used extensively for patients with cardiac disease to determine the risk and advisability of surgery (Table 11–4). The authors recommend that elective surgery not be performed on patients with total scores over 26 points, which is considered a Class IV risk. The preoperative interview should include identification of factors contributing to cardiac risk. Coronary artery disease should be suspected if predisposing factors are noted. The risk of developing coronary artery disease is doubled by smoking, increased four times by the combination of smoking and hypertension, and increased eight times in the presence of smoking, hypertension, and elevated serum cholesterol. Additional danger signals include obesity, glucose intolerance, occlusive vascular events, or a family history of heart disease.

Despite the many objective scoring systems devised to estimate patient risk, the Dripps system has prevailed as the standard in anesthesia practice. Other systems, such as CRIS, may be employed in special situations. The ASA classification is entered on the patient's record before anesthesia, thereby providing a baseline for later reference.

OPTIMIZATION OF PREOPERATIVE STATUS: REDUCTION OF PERIOPERATIVE MORBIDITY

One of the primary goals of the preoperative visit is to use the data obtained to plan and implement strategies that will optimize the patient's preoperative status. The preanesthetic evaluation that is done in sufficient time to allow further diagnostic tests and preparation of the patient may significantly reduce perioperative morbidity or mortality.

Frequently some facts come to light in the preoperative assessment that call for review of previous charts. Any suggestion that a personal or family history of anesthetic complications exists should be followed up. If the patient has previously had surgery at the same institution, old anesthesia records can be retrieved and studied. Any complications of postoperative jaundice should lead the anesthetist to review old charts; halothane should not be readministered to a patient with a history of halothane-associated hepatitis.

If the patient describes a history of prolonged apnea after a previous anesthetic, a thorough probe of possible causes is carried out; this may include a dibucaine number and a pseudocholinesterase level. Similarly, if the patient describes an episode that sounds like malignant hyperthermia, the patient can be further assessed with creatine phosphokinase levels or muscle biopsy with in vitro testing. Should the preoperative diagnosis of malignant hyperthermia be substantiated, strategies are undertaken to minimize the patient risk, including administration of preoperative dantrolene sodium and heavy sedation on the morning of surgery.

The nutritional status of the patient can be cause for preoperative intervention. Preoperative parenteral nutrition has been shown to decrease wound infections significantly in patients with low serum albumin.

The patient may relay information about earlier episodes of preoperative bleeding or a family history of coagulation disorder. In this case, routine preoperative laboratory evaluation includes prothrombin time, partial thromboplastin time, and a platelet count. Approximately 80 percent of unexpected bleeding complications during surgery are due to unappreciated aspirin use. Any patient who is taking aspirin or nonsteroidal anti-inflammatory drugs should be assessed for prolonged bleeding time. These findings should be taken into account when blood is ordered preoperatively.

If pulmonary dysfunction is suspected, an attempt is made to identify, treat, and reverse the pathologic condition as much as possible. It is well recognized that patients with pre-existing respiratory disease are at greater risk for development of postoperative pulmonary complications.

TABLE 11–4. GOLDMAN CARDIAC OPERATIVE RISK INDEX SCORING SYSTEM (CRIS)[a]

Factors	Points
1. History	
Age > 70 yr	5
Myocardial infarction within previous 6 months	10
Aortic stenosis	3
2. Physical examination	
Early diastolic gallop	11
JVD[b] or congestive heart failure	
3. ECG	
Nonsinus rhythm	7
>5 premature ventricular contractions/min	7
4. General information	
Pao_2 < 60 mm Hg	3
$Paco_2$ > 50 mm Hg	3
Potassium < 3 mEq/L	3
BUN > 50 mg/dl	3
Creatine > 3 mg/dl	3
Bedridden	3
5. Operation	
Emergency	4
Intrathoracic	
Intra-abdominal	3
Aortic surgery	3
Total	71

[a] Class I: 0–5 points.
    II: 6–12 points.
    III: 13–25 points.
    IV: 26 points or more.
[b] JVD = jugular venous distention.

Preparation for surgery in these patients is an important facet of preoperative evaluation. Modification of risk consists of correcting everything that is correctable and preparing the patient for the problems that remain.

A quality chest x-ray is necessary to search for effusions, atelectasis, edema, and pneumonia. Typical findings of chronic pulmonary disease include a low, flat diaphragm, hyperinflation, increased anterior-posterior diameter, and increased lung markings. Significant pulmonary dysfunction may be present despite a normal chest x-ray; therefore the anesthesia care giver still must rely on clinical signs when planning treatment.

An ECG is called for when pulmonary disease is suspected. Increased pulmonary vascular resistance is manifested on the ECG by signs of right ventricular hypertrophy, such as tall, peaked P-waves and right-axis deviation.

Spirometry provides useful quantification of pulmonary function. Investigators have outlined laboratory abnormalities, including pulmonary function test findings, that can be used as a basis for decision about elective surgery (Table 11–5). Special procedures may be indicated if thoracic surgery is planned. Radionuclide lung scanning is useful for comparing ventilation with perfusion. Spirometry may be done after selective occlusion of bronchi to determine the expected postoperative pulmonary status.

Arterial blood gases may be analyzed in the event of abnormal pulmonary function tests or if the physical assessment or health history indicates. Analysis of arterial blood gas results provides information about the adequacy of ventilation, oxygenation, and acid-base status. It has been shown that patients with abnormal spirometric values but normal arterial blood gases have few postoperative pulmonary complications. The combination of abnormal spirometric values, hypoxemia, and hypercarbia indicates that postoperative ventilation is likely to be necessary, and the patient should be informed of this possibility.

Preoperative measures can be instituted to minimize risk in the patient with pulmonary disease. The patient is taught the use of incentive spirometry and the importance of coughing and deep breathing. At this time the anesthetist explains the adverse effects of anesthesia, postoperative medication, dressings, and immobilization in the supine position on respiratory function. The patient is encouraged to quit smoking, recognizing that although carboxyhemoglobin levels will decrease immediately on cessation of smoking, improvement in pulmonary function requires several weeks. Administration of antibiotics, bronchodilators, steroids, or sympathomimetics may reverse bronchospasm. Mobilization of secretions should be attempted by hydration, aerosol therapy, expectorants, and chest physiotherapy.

General guidelines have been developed for the scheduling of anesthesia and surgery on the patient with pulmonary disease. Surgery is scheduled late in the day if the patient has chronic bronchitis, to allow for morning mobilization of sputum. A 2-week interval between the occurrence of upper respiratory tract infection and elective surgery is advisable to minimize the chance of pulmonary complications. Hyperirritability of the airways is present for several weeks after acute asthma attacks; therefore, it is recommended that the disease symptoms be pharmacologically controlled before surgery and anesthesia.

With the recent advances in pharmacology, it is common to find patients taking a number of prescription and over-the-counter drugs. This is especially true in patients over 55 years of age. Preoperative management of pharmacotherapeutic agents is specific to the individual drugs. Guidelines for preoperative preparation are found in Table 11–6.

SELECTION OF PREMEDICATION

After the preoperative assessment, a choice of preoperative medication is made. The primary factor in this decision is the individual patient's psychological need for pharmacologic anxiety relief or pain control. The patient's physical status and the planned surgery are also considerations. Some patients, such as the emergency room patient in shock, may require no preoperative medication. In contrast, the patient presenting for chemonucleolysis will require a series of premedication drugs according to protocol.

There is a multitude of drugs used for premedication purposes (Table 11–7). It is preferred that the drugs chosen have a synergistic effect with the planned anesthetic. A narcotic-tranquilizer combination may be an excellent preanesthestic medication when a balanced anesthetic technique is planned. Anticholinergics are avoided when regional anesthesia will be used. Preoperative medications are further discussed in Chapter 18. A preoperative holding area is the ideal setting for administration of preanesthetic medication for most patients. In this setting the anesthetist can safely administer intravenous medications, thus sparing the patient an additional intramuscular injection. Close nursing supervision of the patient is available in the preoperative holding area, allowing for optimum titration of the drugs.

FORMULATION OF ANESTHETIC CARE PLAN

The primary purpose of preoperative evaluation and preparation of the surgical patient is to allow for the generation of an anesthetic care plan that will provide maximum safety to the patient. The choice of anesthetic technique and agent is based on many factors, including patient condition and preference, type and duration of surgery, skill and prefer-

TABLE 11–5. LABORATORY ABNORMALITIES THAT CORRELATE WITH HIGH RISK CAUSED BY PULMONARY DYSFUNCTION

Function	Value
Maximum voluntary ventilation (MVV)	<50% predicted or <50 L/min
$Paco_2$	>45 torr
Forced expiratory volume (FEV$_1$)	<0.5 L
Forced expiratory flow (FEF)	25–75% <0.6 L
Forced viral capacity (FVC)	<1 L
Electrocardiogram (ECG)	Abnormal
Pao_2	<55
Maximum expiratory flow rate (MEFR)	<100 L/min

TABLE 11–6. DRUG MANAGEMENT AND PREOPERATIVE PREPARATION

Drug	Preoperative Preparation	Potential Intraoperative Problems
Antianginal medications	Sublingual tablets can be continued until induction with IV nitroglycerin or paste administered intraoperatively. Methemoglobin levels of heavy nitrate users should be monitored.	Potentiate hypotensive effects of some anesthetic agents, particularly in hypovolemic patients.
Antiarrhythmics	Continue to day of surgery.	Potentiate neuromuscular blockers.
Antibiotics	Avoid aminoglycosides (i.e., neomycin).	Aminoglycosides potentiate neuromuscular blockers and anesthetics that provide muscular relaxation.
Anticoagulants	Replace oral anticoagulants with subcutaneous heparin to ensure prompt reversal, if necessary, with IV protamine sulfate.	Oral anticoagulants are not reversed by protamine sulfate and it takes 24–48 hours for IV vitamin K_1 (phytonadione [AquaMEPHYTON]) to return prothrombin time to normal.
Antidiabetics	Measure preoperative blood sugar. Discontinue chlorpropamide 48 hours before surgery and continue all other oral hypoglycemics until the evening before surgery. Begin glucose/insulin infusion before surgery if indicated.	Intraoperative fluctuations in blood sugar.
Antihypertensives	Continue methyldopa, reserpine, and guanethidine to day of surgery. Continue clonidine parenterally to avoid severe rebound hypertension.	Unstable blood pressure with wide fluctuations.
Antiparkinson medications	Continue levodopa until night before surgery. If antiemetic is needed, antihistamine type (diphenhydramine) preferred over phenothiazine.	Phenothiazines nullify antiparkinson effects of levodopa. Aminoglycosides may interact to cause neuromuscular blockade.
Antiseizure medications	Phenytoin augments nondepolarizing neuromuscular blockade.	Continue phenytoin and phenobarbital to day of surgery.
Beta blockers	Continue to day of surgery. May be given IV if oral route contraindicated.	Potentiate cardiac depressant effects of some anesthetics.
Cardiac glycosides	Continue to day of surgery. Assess patient for signs of digitalis toxicity or potassium depletion and correct if present.	Potentiate nondepolarizing muscle relaxants.
Corticosteroids	Continue to day of surgery. Administer 100 mg hydrocortisone 1 hour before surgery.	Patients who are on corticosteroid therapy (7.5 mg daily prednisone or equivalent) for at least 2 months preceding surgery require intraoperative and postoperative supplementation.
Psychotropes	Monoamine oxidase (MAO) inhibitors should be discontinued 2 weeks before surgery. Continue tricyclic antidepressants, lithium, and phenothiazine antipsychotics to day of surgery.	MAO inhibitors interact with narcotic analgesics, (i.e., meperidine [Demerol]), local anesthetic/epinephrine combinations, and other vasopressors. Lithium prolongs the effect of depolarizing muscle relaxants.

TABLE 11–7. PREANESTHESIA MEDICATION

Classification	Drug	Adult Dosage (mg)
Narcotics	Butorphanol tartrate	2.0
	Fentanyl	0.05–.015
	Meperidine	50.0–100.0
	Morphine	5.0–15.0
Anticholinergics	Atropine	0.4–0.6
	Glycopyrrolate	0.2–0.3
	Scopolamine	0.3–0.5
Tranquilizers/ sedatives	Diazepam	5.0–10.0
	Droperidol	2.5–5.0
	Hydroxyzine	50.0–150.0
	Lorazepam	1.0–4.0
	Midazolam	4.0–5.0
	Promethazine	25.0–50.0

ence of the anesthetist, and characteristics of the surgeon and institution.

The anesthetist must first decide whether the anesthetic technique should be general, regional, or local. Once this decision is made, there is a multitude of choices, including the agents to be selected and the approach to be employed, i.e., spinal versus epidural, or endotracheal versus mask airway management. Once the anesthetic technique and drugs are selected then the appropriate monitoring modalities are chosen.

The formulation of the anesthetic care plan requires creativity on the part of the anesthetist, who must individualize the plan of care for every patient. It is at this point that the art and science of the practice of anesthesiology are merged.

BIBLIOGRAPHY

Bates B: A Guide to Physical Examination. 3rd ed. Philadelphia, Lippincott, 1983.

Bonebrake CR, Noller KL, Muhm JR, Fish CR: Routine chest roentgenography in pregnancy, JAMA 240:2747–2748, 1978.

Brechner VL: Unusual problems in the management of airways: I. Flexion-extension mobility of the cervical vertebrae. Anesth Analg 47:363, 1968.

Davies DW, Steward DJ: Unexpected excessive bleeding during operation: Role of acetylsalicylic acid. Can Anaesth Soc J 24:452–458, 1977.

Dripps RD, Lamont A, Eckenhoff JE: The role of anesthesia in surgical mortality. JAMA 178:261–266, 1961.

Elliot D, Linz DH, Kane JA: Medical evaluation before operation. The West J Med 137:351–358, 1982.

Goldman L, Caldera DL: Multifactorial index of cardiac risk in non-cardiac surgical procedures. N Engl J Med 297:845–850, 1977.

Hodgkin JE, Dines DE, Didier EP: Preoperative evaluation of the patient with pulmonary disease. Mayo Clin Proc 48:114–118, 1973.

Schellinger RR: The length of the airway to the bifurcation of the trachea. Anesthesiology 25:169, 1964.

Williams J, Jones JR, Workhoven MN: The psychological control of preoperative anxiety. Psychophysiology 12:50–54, 1975.

12

Intubation and Airway Management

Christine S. Zambricki

*A*irway management, including the placement of various pharyngeal or endotracheal airway devices, is recognized as an area in which the certified registered nurse anesthetist (CRNA) possesses skill and proficiency. In the operating room, the CRNA routinely assesses and manages airway problems ranging from simple to complex with the aid of neuromuscular blockers and sophisticated equipment. The CRNA also functions as a resource person outside of the operating room, providing airway management during cardiopulmonary resuscitation and situations of respiratory failure or insufficiency throughout the clinical site.

The physical placement of an endotracheal tube is a technical skill that can only improve with opportunity and practice. Good airway management is more than mechanical skill, however. It is an art requiring (1) sound clinical judgment based on knowledge of airway anatomy and physiology and a thorough history and physical assessment; (2) familiarity with state-of-the art equipment and techniques; and (3) an understanding of the risks related to instrumentation and placement of artificial airways.

This chapter provides the reader with a thorough review of the science of airway management as well as the technical aspects of instrumentation. The discussion will cover the anatomy and physiology of the respiratory passages, assessment of the respiratory passages, equipment, techniques used, and complications of artificial airways.

ANATOMY AND PHYSIOLOGY OF THE RESPIRATORY PASSAGES

This discussion will highlight only those anatomic structures pertinent to the placement of an artificial airway. An anatomic atlas should be consulted as an adjunct to this text.

The respiratory passages provide a mechanism for the exchange of air between a person and the environment. These passages have been divided into two areas in series: the upper airway and the lower airway (Fig. 12–1).

The Upper Airway

The term "upper airway" designates those portions of the respiratory passages superior to and including the larynx and comprises such structures as the nose, nasopharynx, oral cavity, laryngopharynx, and the larynx.

The nasal cavity is divided into two channels by the nasal septum, which is covered by vascular mucous membranes and supported by both bone and cartilage. Curving bony projections, called turbinates (superior, middle, and inferior), protrude into the nasal cavity from the lateral wall. The turbinates are covered by a mucous membrane well supplied with blood, which provides additional surface area for the cleansing, humidification, and warming of inspired air. The rich blood supply of the nasal passages presents a hazard when trauma is incurred during nasal intubation. Pharmacologic agents such as cocaine may be used to constrict the nasal vasculature, thereby expanding the size of the nasal inlet and facilitating passage of a nasopharyngeal airway or nasoendotracheal tube.

The nasopharynx extends from the sphenoid and occipital bones superiorly along the posterior nasopharyngeal wall to the level of the soft palate where it joins the oropharynx. The nasopharynx is of clinical significance because it houses the lymphoid tissue called the pharyngeal tonsils or adenoids. This tissue may swell and cause nasal obstruction in children—an important consideration when attempting to ventilate a child with a mask. In these cases, the anesthetist must take care to keep the mouth open with an oropharyngeal airway or by maneuvering of the mandible to achieve effective ventilation. The nasopharynx is connected to the middle by the eustachian tube.

The oropharynx is continuous with the nasopharynx, extending to the epiglottis inferiorly. The oropharynx can be seen through the oral cavity. The paired palatine tonsils can be seen in the fossae between the anterior and posterior pillars and may impede visualization of the larynx if enlarged. The vallecula is the space lying between the base of the tongue and the epiglottis. The tip of a curved laryngoscope blade is placed in the vallecula.

The oral cavity is bounded by the palate, oropharynx, tongue, and cheeks. Significant anatomic landmarks for the endoscopist include the uvula, soft palate, and the pos-

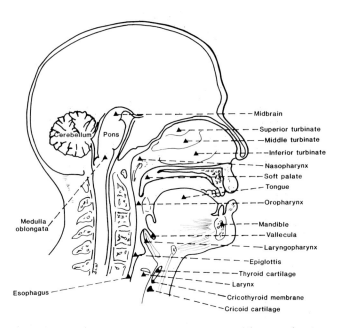

Figure 12–1. Sagittal section illustrating upper airway and superior portion of lower airway.

terior wall of the oropharynx. The tongue can be compressed and deflected, thereby enlarging the size of the oral cavity and improving visualization of anatomic structures.

The quality and quantity of the patient's dentition are factors of major importance to the anesthetist. The eruption of deciduous teeth generally begins by the age of 6 months and is complete by the age of 2½ years. Beginning at approximately 5 years of age and continuing until the 12th year, deciduous teeth are being replaced by permanent ones and are therefore loosely attached. The exposed incisors and canine teeth are most easily dislodged, being secured to the alveolar parts of the maxilla and mandible by only one root. The adult patient may have loose or diseased teeth, which are susceptible to accidental extraction.

The laryngopharynx extends from the epiglottis superiorly to the esophagus inferiorly. The laryngeal inlet lies anterior to the laryngopharynx at the level of C-4 to C-6. Important landmarks of endotracheal intubation, such as the epiglottis, aryepiglottic folds, and the mucous membrane covered arytenoid cartilages, are located within the laryngopharynx. The primary function of the pharyngeal musculature is to coordinate the act of swallowing with motor innervation via the vagus nerve (cranial nerve X). Sensory supply to the pharynx is by the glossopharyngeal nerve (cranial nerve IX).

Transition between the upper and lower airways occurs at the larynx. The opening to the larynx is called the rima glottidis. The predominant single cartilages forming the laryngeal skeleton are the thyroid, cricoid, and epiglottis. The cricoid cartilage is the narrowest point in a child's airway, a fact of clinical significance because its size cannot be estimated by direct visualization. The cricoid cartilage is the only complete tracheal ring. There is no room to accommodate swelling without increasing airway resistance. Because the cricothyroid membrane is below the level of the vocal cords, it is the site commonly used for emer-

gency entry into the trachea. The three sets of paired cartilages (arytenoid, corniculate, and cuneiform) articulate to effect vocal cord functioning.

The epiglottis, a flexible cartilage that lies superior to the vocal cords and attaches to the thyroid cartilage, provides an important anatomic landmark for endotracheal intubation. Its function is to occlude the glottic opening during swallowing.

The vocal cords are composed of muscle, ligament, submucosal soft tissue, and laryngeal mucosa. No cilia are present in the larynx. The vocal cords insert into the thyroid cartilage anteriorly and to the arytenoid cartilages posteriorly. Reinke's space, located just beneath the mucous membrane covering the vocal cords, is a space of potentially poor lymphatic drainage where fluid may accumulate and occlude the laryngeal inlet. Even slight swelling in this area will cause a tremendous amount of airway resistance, particularly in children.

The laryngeal ventricles lie above the true vocal cords. The false vocal cords, or vestibular folds, are located immediately superior to them. The false vocal cords function sphincterally to prevent aspiration of foreign material.

The larynx functions primarily as: (1) a gas-conducting conduit between the laryngopharynx and the trachea; (2) a sphincter to protect the lower airway from foreign substances; (3) a site of reflex origination, generating the cough reflex as well as cardiovascular and pulmonary changes; and (4) a speech generator, by modifying expired air in voice production.

The sensory and motor innervation to structures of the larynx is of clinical significance to the anesthetist. Sensory innervation to the superior surface of the epiglottis is via the glossopharyngeal nerve (IX), whereas the superior laryngeal nerve (a branch of X) provides the sensory pathway from the inferior aspect of the epiglottis to the vocal cords. Some clinicians cite this anatomic relationship as an advantage of intubation with a curved laryngoscope blade. The recurrent laryngeal nerve (a branch of X) is the primary motor supply to all muscles of the larynx except the cricothyroid, which is supplied by an external branch of superior laryngeal nerve. Injury to the recurrent laryngeal nerve will result in vocal cord dysfunction; the recurrent laryngeal nerve function can be checked in the nonparalyzed patient by direct laryngoscopy.

The Lower Airway

The lower airway extends from the tracheobronchial tree to the lung parenchyma. The function of the tracheobronchial tree is to conduct, humidify, and heat inspired air. The alveolocapillary membrane exchange occurs distal to the terminal bronchioles.

The trachea extends from the cricoid cartilage of the larynx to its bifurcation at the level of T-5. The trachea is approximately 14 cm in length and branches into two main bronchi at the carina. External landmarks for the tracheal bifurcation are the sternal angle anteriorly and the fourth thoracic spinous process posteriorly. The walls of the trachea are formed by a series of 16 to 20 C-shaped cartilages, whose open ends face posteriorly. The trachea is separated from the esophagus posteriorly by a muscle layer. A portion of the thyroid gland lies in front of the trachea at the second, third, and fourth tracheal cartilages. The trachea is near several large vessels of the neck, including the anterior and internal jugular veins, the inferior thyroid veins, and the innominate and carotid arteries. The vascular relationships are of paramount significance in the performance of tracheostomy or cricothyroidotomy.

The trachea bifurcates into a right and left mainstem bronchus with a 25-degree angle to the right and a 50-degree angle to the left. In the infarct, both mainstem bronchi form angles of approximately 55 degrees, making it possible for the endotracheal tube to slip into either mainstem bronchus. Because pediatric tubes are cuffless, it is very easy for unintentional endobronchial intubation to occur.

The mainstem bronchi are in series with the lobar bronchi, which then divide into segmental and subsegmental bronchi. Cartilage begins to disappear in the bronchioles; by the time the airway ends in the terminal bronchioles, the tissue is composed of simple epithelial cells. Distal to the terminal bronchioles are the alveoli, where the diffusion of gas occurs.

ASSESSMENT OF THE RESPIRATORY PASSAGES

Evaluation of the patient's airway is of primary concern to the anesthetist during the preoperative visit (see Chapter 11). This assessment begins with a review of the chart, watching for any suspicious findings such as altered arterial blood gases or abnormal pulmonary function studies. A lateral neck film may show a soft-tissue mass impinging on the trachea. A cervical film may demonstrate severe arthritic changes of the cervical spine. Whenever the anticipated surgery is related to the upper or lower respiratory passages, the chart is scrutinized for information about previous diagnostic or surgical procedures. Multiple attempts at intubation serve as warnings for airway difficulties.

The overwhelming importance of the airway to the anesthetic care of the patient makes a thorough history and physical examination imperative. The patient interview should include questions about the presence of dyspnea, orthopnea, exercise tolerance, previous surgery or pathology involving the airway, and smoking history. The physical examination should routinely include inspection of the nose, nares, nasal septum, temporomandibular joint, dentition, oropharynx, and structures contained therein. The chest should be auscultated. The neck should be observed for symmetry and size, and the thorax should be examined for signs of chronic lung disease. The anterior neck should be palpated for masses and the orientation of the trachea to midline. At the same time, an enlarged thyroid gland can be detected. Maneuvers such as flexion/extension of the head and opening of the mouth should be requested of every patient. Lateral roentgenograms or indirect laryngoscopy may be useful diagnostic adjuncts.

OBSTRUCTION

Upper Airway Obstruction

Upper airway obstruction is the most common type of obstruction encountered in the anesthetist's practice. The causes of upper airway obstruction are varied, and efforts must be made to distinguish the source of the problem so as to be able to relieve the obstruction.

Soft-tissue obstruction is encountered frequently both in patient units and in the operating room. One common cause of soft-tissue obstruction is the loss of muscle tone, caused either by pathologic conditions of the central nervous system (CNS), or by the effect of anesthetic agents, resulting in relaxation of the voluntary pharyngeal-laryngeal muscles. In a patient in the supine position, the tongue has a tendency to fall back to the pharynx, obstructing the laryngeal inlet. Soft-tissue obstruction is exaggerated in the edentulous patient, who may have resorption of alveolar bone.

Foreign material such as food, vomitus, chewing tobacco, gum, or dentures may lead to upper airway obstruction. Retching or vomiting during induction or emergence may be the result of opioid premedication, suction, airway insertion, movement of the patient, or distension of the abdomen with air. Esophageal reflux may occur secondary to the use of muscle relaxants or in patients with bowel obstruction or ascites or who have recently eaten. Excessive manipulation of the airway to gain visual exposure may cause edema, hematoma, or bleeding, precipitating complete obstruction. Occasionally, the cause of upper airway obstruction may be direct injury to the pharynx or larynx. If a patient passes through an excitement phase during induction, the jaw may clench tightly and the neck flex, resulting in obstruction.

The accumulation of secretions during the induction phase of general anesthesia may potentiate upper airway obstruction. This condition is aggravated by repeated injections of succinylcholine, which tend to have a parasympathomimetic effect. Concomitant hypercarbia and hypoxemia potentiate the effect of respiratory distress and lead to additional problems in airway management.

Respiratory obstruction in the anesthetized patient is recognized by the sound of snoring or the feel of vibrations when the mask is being held. The reservoir bag may or may not continue to move, but the characteristics of the movement will be different from that in the unobstructed state. Direct inspection of the patient to determine the quality of respirations is the best method for detection of airway obstruction. Indications of an obstructed airway are (1) the use of accessory muscles or presence of retractions; (2) a jerking, downward movement of the trachea known as "tracheal tug"; or (3) a "rocking boat" respiratory pattern characterized by chest restriction and abdominal motion as the diaphragm descends. These clinical signs indicate the need for immediate clinical intervention.

Laryngeal obstruction is commonly encountered during anesthesia. Laryngeal obstruction may be due to injury or pathologic conditions of the larynx or the presence of foreign material, edema, or hematoma at the laryngeal inlet. Laryngospasm may also cause laryngeal obstruction. Partial or total laryngospasm occurs when the airway is heavily manipulated during the light planes of anesthesia or in response to visceral stimulation via autonomic pathways.

The cause of upper airway obstruction dictates the strategy to be employed to deal with it. The anesthetist proceeds from simple corrective measures to more complex maneuvers involving instrumentation. Initially, an attempt is made to extend the neck, thereby positioning the tongue and soft tissue away from the posterior pharyngeal wall. A useful technique known as "angling the jaw" is employed next. The mandible is displaced forward with the anesthetist holding the angles of the patient's jaw slightly below and in front of each ear with bent forefingers. The thumbs assist in holding the mouth open. The mandible is pulled forward and maintained in this position. This strategy should only be employed for a short period of time because it may result in tenderness or swelling. This technique manually moves the tongue upward and may stimulate vigorous respirations to occur. Should mechanical positioning not relieve soft-tissue obstruction, an oropharyngeal or nasopharyngeal airway may be employed. If the obstruction persists, an endotracheal tube is placed. As a last resort, cricothyroidotomy or tracheostomy may be undertaken.

Treatment of laryngospasm requires different strategies from those used to relieve soft-tissue obstruction. Laryngospasm is heralded by a high-pitched crowing sound (partial laryngospasm) or the absence of sound and the inability to ventilate (complete laryngospasm). Dealing with laryngospasm requires distinguishing between partial and complete laryngospasm. The partial laryngospasm often occurs during light planes of anesthesia in response to surgical or pharyngeal stimulation. Attempts should be made to deepen anesthesia without additional provocation. The anesthetist relaxes his or her grip on the mandible and mask and observes the reservoir bag for excursion, providing gentle assistance to respiration if needed. Pharmacologic deepening of anesthesia must take place before further stimulation is continued. Partial laryngospasm can progress to complete laryngospasm with closure of the glottic opening.

Sustained, moderate pressure of approximately 20 cm H_2O applied to the reservoir bag is the first strategy employed to overcome complete laryngospasm. This maneuver is particularly successful in children. Continual assessment is essential while the patient is in spasm, because no air exchange and ventilation is taking place. Succinylcholine (20 to 40 mg) is used to relieve total laryngospasm in cases refractory to positive pressure.

Lower Airway Obstruction

Lower airway obstruction may be caused by a foreign body, lesions, excessive secretions, or bronchospasm. Pediatric patients are often found to have lower airway obstructions such as coins, food, and toys when they are brought to the operating room for bronchoscopy and removal of the foreign object. Adult patients may present with a pathologic lesion of the lower airway. This can be bypassed by a flexible wire-reinforced endotracheal tube. Depending on the level of the lesion, tracheostomy or cardiopulmonary bypass may be necessary for resection. Excessive tenacious secretions may be sufficient to obstruct the bronchial lumen totally, and removal may be required.

Bronchospasm is a form of lower airway obstruction manifested by bronchial smooth muscle contraction. The hallmark of bronchospasm is the patient's unexpected, total inability to ventilate in the absence of upper airway obstruction. Wheezes on both inspiration and expiration may precede bronchospasm; however, bronchospasm does not always follow wheezing. Intraoperatively, bronchospasm is treated by the administration of bronchodilating pharmacologic agents such as halothane, aminophylline, or terbutaline. In addition, endotracheal intubation may be necessary to ensure adequate oxygenation and ventilation.

AIRWAY MANAGEMENT: EQUIPMENT, TECHNIQUES, AND COMPLICATIONS

The anesthetist must rely on the use of a variety of respiratory equipment in the administration of anesthesia or at times when manual techniques fail to relieve airway obstruction. Anesthesia apparatus and airway equipment can be lifesaving in skilled hands but can be the cause of iatrogenic complications when used by the inexperienced.

The Use of a Face Mask

Fitting a mask and providing assisted or controlled ventilation via that mask is a primary responsibility of the anesthetist. Masks may be disposable or nondisposable (Fig. 12–2). A clear plastic mask allows detection of cyanosis or vomitus while the patient is wearing it; however, many anesthetists prefer the standard black masks, which are available in several shapes. A rubber mask may be surrounded by a pad that conforms to the shape of the patient's face. Some clear masks have a preinflated cushion designed for a tight seal. The preformed mask has no padding but is contoured to fit the patient's face and has minimal dead space. This is of particular importance in the pediatric patient.

A mask should be selected to provide the best fit for a given patient. It should be pliant enough to be adjusted to the shape of a patient's face, but it should be rigid enough not to dent when held tightly. A mask with a metal or plastic ring and hooks for head strap attachment allows easier airway management.

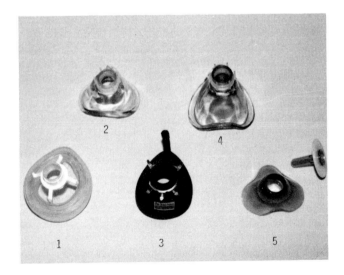

Figure 12–2. 1. Cushion-Flex single use face mask by Life Design Systems. 2. Transparent preformed single-use pediatric face mask by Dryden Corporation. 3. Multiple-use rubber face mask by Ohio Medical Products. 4. Transparent preformed single-use adult face mask by Dryden Corporation. 5. Pediatric anesthesia mask (PAM), scented with pacifier, by Plasmedics.

Selection of the proper size mask is of prime importance. After inspection of the patient's facial characteristics, the mask can be molded or manually shaped to approximate the patient's facial contours. A good fit can be obtained by spreading the bottom of the mask and placing it on the patient's chin before positioning the remainder of the mask (Fig. 12–3). The mask is held in place with the left hand, using the thumb to hold the top of the mask down and the little finger to hold the mandible cephalad. If the mask fit is good (Fig. 12–4), the anesthetist will not experience excessive fatigue or hand tremors. In some difficult or prolonged mask cases, the anesthetist may position his or her left elbow on the operating table to provide additional strength; however, this is not usually necessary. Anesthesia can be induced and maintained with a mask alone in many patients having minor surgery. Mask management is not appropriate for patients in the prone, sitting, or true lateral position.

Complications. Caution must be exercised when applying manual pressure on the mask to achieve a better airway. Excessive pressure will not correct the problem of respiratory obstruction and may damage the facial nerve. Once the mask is properly positioned and the airway secured, head straps may be applied to help stabilize the mask. The patient's ears must not be pinched or bent by the head strap, nor should the head strap apply undue pressure to the sides of the face or the eyes.

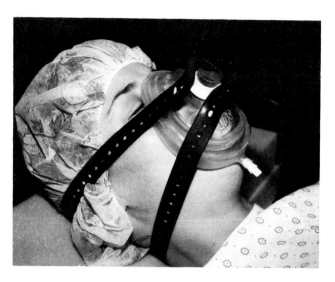

Figure 12–4. Proper mask fit with head strap attached.

Eye care is particularly important for the patient having general anesthesia by mask. The mask must not apply pressure to the eyes. Eyes should be lubricated and taped closed with eye patches applied if necessary. The danger of inadvertent damage by the anesthetist's fingers or the mask is compounded by the drying effect of gases that may blow on the eyes from small leaks at the bridge of the mask.

The Use of Pharyngeal Airways

Pharyngeal airways are employed when respiratory obstruction is refractory to manual corrective measures. Two types of pharyngeal airways are in use: oropharyngeal and nasopharyngeal (Fig. 12–5).

Oropharyngeal Airways. The oropharyngeal airway is inserted along the tongue and separates the posterior orophar-

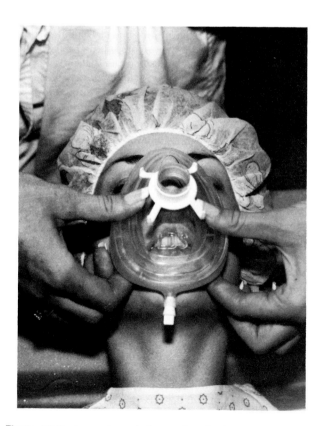

Figure 12–3. A good mask fit can be obtained by spreading the bottom of the mask and placing it on the patient's chin before positioning the remainder of the mask.

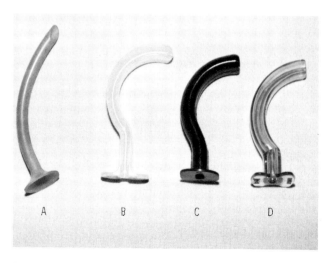

Figure 12–5. Pharyngeal airways. **A.** Robertazzi nasopharyngeal airway; **B.** Berman plastic oropharyngeal airway; **C.** Guedel rubber oropharyngeal airway; **D.** Guedel plastic oropharyngeal airway.

ynx and the base of the tongue. There are two basic styles of oropharyngeal airway, the Berman and the Guedel. Oropharyngeal airways are very stimulating to the awake or lightly anesthetized patient and may cause retching, vomiting, or laryngospasm. Care must be taken to select the proper size of oropharyngeal airway. Too large an airway may traumatize the oropharynx and mouth, whereas too small an airway may push the back of the tongue against the posterior pharyngeal wall, thus potentiating obstruction. In cases where obstruction to lymphatic drainage of the head is expected, one size smaller airway may be selected because macroglossia can occur. Such situations include head and neck surgery or sitting cervical laminectomy.

The oropharyngeal airway should be placed quickly and carefully to avoid injury to the lips, teeth, or gingiva. Using the left hand, a tongue blade is placed toward the posterior aspect of the tongue and the tongue drawn forward. The airway is inserted with the right hand. Under no circumstances should the airway be twisted into place or forced between the clenched teeth of a lightly anesthetized patient. Occasionally the condition of the tongue or teeth precludes the use of an oral airway. After airway insertion, the teeth and gums should be inspected for pressure or trauma. A suction catheter can be passed along the side of the oral airway as required.

Nasopharyngeal Airway. The nasopharyngeal, or Robertazzi, airway is a soft rubber tube designed to be inserted through the naris, passing along the curvature of the nasopharynx and oropharynx. When positioned correctly, this airway rests between the base of the tongue and the posterior pharyngeal wall. Because insertion of a nasopharyngeal airway is less stimulating than that of an oropharyngeal airway, it can be used in the awake or lightly anesthetized patient who develops airway obstruction and may not tolerate an oropharyngeal airway.

Nasopharyngeal airways come in different sizes ranging from pediatric to adult. To minimize trauma and bleeding, this airway should be lubricated with a local anesthetic lubricant before insertion. It use should be avoided in patients with nasal septal deformity, leakage of cerebrospinal fluid from the nose, or coagulopathy.

The nasopharyngeal airway should be inserted gently with the right hand. The left hand can be used to deflect the tip of the nose upward. The airway should be angled toward the occiput, following the natural contours of the nasal cavity, rather than superiorly. If resistance is encountered, the other naris should be tried.

The nasopharyngeal airway is an underestimated piece of anesthesia equipment. It may be inserted easily, requiring little skill, and it may be used for patients who are unable or unwilling to open their mouths. A suction catheter can be passed through the middle of the airway if necessary. Clinicians have reported circumstances in which airway obstruction was unrelieved by oropharyngeal airway insertion but was responsive to nasopharyngeal airway insertion. Regardless of whether an oropharyngeal or nasopharyngeal airway is selected, the anesthetist must develop the skill to insert the airway quickly and atraumatically.

Endotracheal Intubation

Cannulation of the trachea via the oral or nasal route is not a new procedure. As early as 1841, T. Spencer Wells provided instructions for nasotracheal intubation. In 1880, flexible orotracheal tubes were used and described by Macawen. Although technology has made tremendous strides in the manufacture of endotracheal tubes, the advantages of endotracheal intubation are the same as they were in the 19th century. First and foremost, the patency of the airway is maintained with a high degree of reliability if the endotracheal tube is in position and unobstructed. The endotracheal tube allows positive-pressure ventilation and at the same time minimizes intragastric air. In addition, a cuffed endotracheal tube provides marked protection against aspiration of regurgitant in contrast to pharyngeal airways, which provide no protection. Respirations can be maintained artificially by the anesthetist despite the position of the patient or the distance from the patient to the anesthetist. The tracheobronchial tree can be suctioned with relative ease. A further benefit is that the endotracheal tube reduces dead space by one-half. Thus, it is clear that the placement of an endotracheal tube, when indicated, will allow the anesthetist a degree of security not present when oro- or nasopharyngeal airways are used.

The numerous indications for endotracheal intubation can be classified in two broad categories: those mandated by patient characteristics and those mandated by surgical procedure. Airway problems may arise unexpectedly, and the anesthetist must learn to look for them even when they do not fall into one of these categories.

Indications for Endotracheal Intubation

Patient Characteristics. The features that mandate endotracheal intubation can often be assessed during the preanesthetic evaluation. The patient may possess anatomic traits that augur difficulty with a mask fit, such as protruding teeth or longstanding lack of teeth with concomitant resorption of alveolar bone, micrognathia or a malformed jaw, or facial features such as a prominant or broad, flat nose. The patient having a short, fat, or thick neck should be elevated carefully. Beards or facial burns can also make mask management difficult. The presence of a nasogastric tube makes an airtight seal with a mask difficult to achieve. The anesthetist may elect to perform endotracheal intubations for any such patient, even for a short surgical procedure, to optimize ventilation.

Certain skeletal malformations such as kyphoscoliosis, cervical arthritis, or severe pectus excavatum predispose the patient to difficulties with ventilation. Traumatic injuries resulting in fractured ribs and an unstable chest wall require immediate intubation.

Respiratory failure or insufficiency is an indication for endotracheal intubation. Severe respiratory dysfunction should be regarded as an indication for immediate intubation. The cause of respiratory distress must be determined to anticipate the possibility of prolonged postoperative intubation and ventilation.

The patient's general physical condition may be so poor that endotracheal intubation must be planned, even for the simplest procedure. For example, severe cardiac dysfunction, cachexia, or kidney failure render a patient a poor risk; thus, the anesthetist must plan to have two hands available for case management. Although the critically ill patient can be managed with mask ventilation, the anesthetist must also plan for the postoperative period when the patient will most likely require mechanical ventilation with an endotracheal tube.

For general anesthesia, intubation is required for any patient with known or suspected gastric contents. This includes the intoxicated patient as well as the patient with pyloric stenosis, bowel obstruction, ascites, or who is pregnant. Although the cuff on the endotracheal tube does not provide a waterproof barrier to aspiration, it is the safest technique available for airway management when general anesthesia is necessary.

Surgical Procedure. The position of the patient during surgery can preclude the use of a mask as the primary mechanism for ventilation. Patients assuming the prone or sitting position require endotracheal intubation. The true lateral position is an indication for placement of an endotracheal tube; however, mask management for patients in a modified lateral position has been reported. Although the lithotomy position does not require endotracheal intubation, the exaggerated lithotomy position makes mask management very difficult, especially when coupled with steep Trendelenburg.

Surgical procedures that involve the oral cavity, pharynx, or the neck will require that the patient be intubated. In this case, the surgeon and anesthetist will be sharing the airway; thus the only way to ensure ventilation is through endotracheal intubation.

Surgical procedures of the head and neck, such as neurosurgery, tympanomastoidectomy, or cleft-palate repair, will usually necessitate positioning the anesthetist distant from the patient's airway and from the surgical site. In this case, the anesthetist is able to maintain the patient's gas exchange with endotracheal intubation, whereas mask management would not be possible.

Intrathoracic surgery clearly indicates endotracheal or endobronchial intubation. First of all, the majority of patients undergoing thoracic surgery have lung disease and require careful monitoring of their respiratory status intraoperatively. General anesthesia coupled with thoracic surgery profoundly affects the ventilation-perfusion ratio, thereby potentiating existing problems. If pneumothorax is induced on incision into the thorax, the patient must receive controlled positive-pressure ventilation via the endotracheal tube to prevent paradoxical respiration and mediastinal shift.

Neurosurgical procedures also require endotracheal intubation because of the distance between the anesthetist and patient. In addition, controlled positive-pressure ventilation is needed for accurate maintenance of Pa_{CO_2} and Pa_{O_2} intraoperatively to avoid intracranial pressure increases.

Intubation is planned for intraabdominal procedures for several reasons. Surgical retractors in the abdomen push abdominal contents up against the diaphragm, making

mask ventilation difficult. Unintentional introduction of air into the stomach with mask ventilation hinders the surgeon's work and prolongs the duration of anesthesia. Patients undergoing abdominal surgery often have delayed gastric emptying time, enhancing the risk of aspiration. Relaxation of the abdominal muscles must be adequate to allow the surgeon to explore the area unhindered. Once paralyzed, the intubated patient can be mechanically ventilated with ease.

Although practice varies, it is generally agreed that any surgical procedure lasting longer than 2 hours justifies endotracheal intubation. Longer procedures frequently require massive fluid and blood replacement, multiple anesthetic agents, and adjunct drugs. Endotracheal intubation allows the anesthetist freedom to respond to the demands of major surgery. If the surgical procedure is long but not major, such as multiple tendon repairs of the hand, the anesthetist will elect to intubate as a matter of convenience when administering a general anesthetic.

In addition to these indications, other circumstances may dictate the choice of endotracheal intubation. Rather than following a memorized list of indications, the anesthetist applies the principles of sound airway management to the needs of the individual patient in the particular surgical situation. Sound clinical judgment and skilled technique are necessary to prevent mishaps caused by inappropriate airway management.

Equipment for Endotracheal Intubation. The basic equipment for intubation includes a laryngoscope, endotracheal tube, and assorted connectors, adaptors, forceps, and stylets.

Laryngoscopes may be divided into two broad categories: those with straight blades and those with curved blades (Fig. 12–6). The straight laryngoscope blade is designed to allow the tip of the blade to reach below the epiglottis and lift the epiglottis (Fig. 12–7). Because the underside of the epiglottis is innervated by the vagal nerve (X), some clinicians believe that this approach is more likely to lead to cardiac dysrhythmias. Nevertheless, the glottic structures are visualized in their entirety more frequently with the straight blade because of its direct lifting action. A Harlan lock may be fitted between the blade and the laryngoscope handle to alter the laryngoscope configuration and help expose anatomic structures.

The curved blade conforms to the curvature of the tongue, with the tip of the blade being placed at the vallecula (Fig. 12–8). As the laryngoscope is lifted forward and upward, the glottis is pulled anteriorly and the underlying cords are exposed. The blade tip is said to stimulate the glossopharyngeal nerve (IX) with less risk of vagus-induced cardiopulmonary changes. The curved blade allows more room for maneuvering the endotracheal tube in the mouth and for this reason may be more appropriate for use in the obese patient.

Curved and straight-blade laryngoscopes have several features in common. The blades are interchangeable and are connected to the laryngoscope handle by means of a hook-and-bar mechanism. Contact is made between the blade, which contains a bulb, and the battery-containing

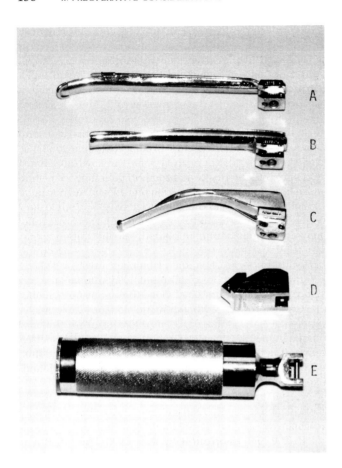

Figure 12–6. Laryngoscopes: **A.** Miller blade (straight); **B.** Wis-Foreggar blade (straight); **C.** MacIntosh blade (curved); **D.** Harlan lock; **E.** laryngoscopy handle with bar latch; batteries are inside cylinder, which is entered by unscrewing the bottom of the handle.

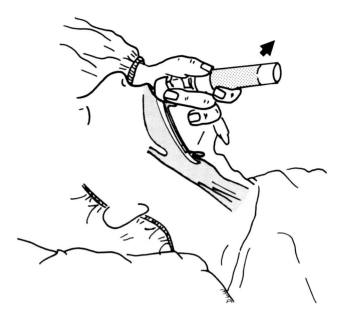

Figure 12–7. Proper placement of the straight blade on the inferior side of the epiglottis.

handle when the laryngoscope is open and ready for use. Batteries can be replaced by unscrewing the base of the handle. Blades are manufactured in sizes ranging from 0 to 4. The handle of the laryngoscope comes in different diameters and may be constructed of aluminum or steel.

Nontraditional laryngoscopes have been developed in recent years for specific functions. Plastic laryngoscopes, designed for one-time use, are now available. Fiberoptic laryngoscopes have a brighter, whiter light than traditional laryngoscopes, without the electrical problems caused by wires and bulbs in the blade. The cost of a plastic laryngoscope is less than an ordinary laryngoscope, but the plastic can be used only once. A fiberoptic laryngoscope costs about twice as much as a traditional laryngoscope.

Because the traditional-design laryngoscope has few working parts, troubleshooting in the event of malfunction is simple. The laryngoscope is checked before use by attaching the handle securely and opening it so that blade and handle are at 90-degree angles. The hook-and-bar latch must be securely in place or the equipment will not work. If the light does not go on, the bulb is checked to make sure it is screwed in properly. A new bulb may be substituted. The base of the handle can be unscrewed and the batteries

checked. Rarely, if the laryngoscope has been damaged, the wire connection between the bulb and the proximal portion of the blade may be broken and the blade will not work. The laryngoscope should always be cleaned after use by disconnecting the blade from the handle, scrubbing the handle and blade, and immersing the blade in a disinfectant solution before the next use.

Most endotracheal tubes in use today are disposable and made of polyvinylchloride (PVC) (Fig. 12–9). The tube wall is generally marked with radiopaque lines for checking tube placement by x-ray. Some hospitals still use tubes of natural or synthetic rubber. Rubber substances have been

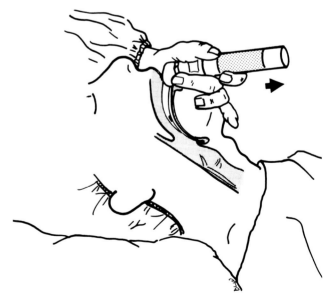

Figure 12–8. Proper placement of the curved blade with blade tip in the vallecula.

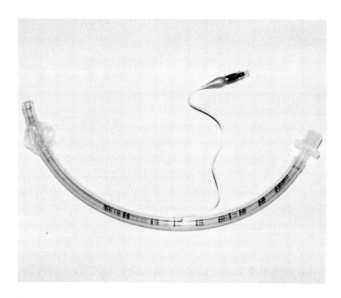

Figure 12–9. Disposable endotracheal tube with cuff and pilot balloon with valve.

found to be rigid, difficult to clean, and more irritating to tissue than the plastic substances available. PVC has gained popularity for artificial airways because it usually does not cause tissue reactions and is flexible within the airway. The PVC tube must be watched for kinking, especially when it is long and there are weighty rubber or metal corrugated tubes attached to it. Kinking may take place inside the mouth or nose.

Endotracheal tube sizes reflect the internal diameter in millimeters, ranging from 2.0 to 10.0 mm in 0.5-mm increments (Table 12–1). The internal diameter of the tube is the most critical factor in determining airflow resistance. According to the laws of physics, resistance varies inversely with the fourth power of the radius of the tube. Tube selection for oral intubation is generally determined by the age and size of the patient, a size 8.0 for the average female and a size 9.0 for the average male. A size 8.0 nasal endotracheal tube is the largest size used for female or male patients.

TABLE 12–1. ENDOTRACHEAL TUBE SIZES FOR AVERAGE PATIENTS BASED ON AGE AND SEX

Age/Sex	Internal Diameter (mm)
Premature	2.0–2.5
Newborn	2.5
6 months	3.5
1 year	4.5
2 years	5.0
4 years	5.5
6 years	6.0
8 years	6.5
10 years	7.0
12 years	7.5
14 years	8.0
Adult	
Female	8.0–8.5
Male	9.0–9.5

Pediatric oral endotracheal tube sizes can be estimated by the following formula, which takes into account conversion from the French number: age + 18/4 = size of tube. A tube that is one size larger and one that is one size smaller than the one selected should be immediately available at the intubating location. The tube used should be the largest one that can pass without force. The thickness of the tube may vary from 1 to 2 mm; therefore, a thin-walled tube will be easier to pass for a given size.

The tube length ranges from 11 to 28 cm and is designated on the tube, beginning at the distal end. Oral endotracheal tubes may require cutting before use if they are not precut by the manufacturer. The length required can be estimated by placing the endotracheal tube along the patient's face and measuring from the level of the mouth to the angle of Louis, which is assumed to be the level of the carina. The tube should be of the proper length to position the cuff in the upper portion of the trachea and extend slightly out of the nose or mouth to allow attachment of ventilatory equipment to the endotracheal tube connector.

Manufacturers have designed variations of endotracheal tubes suited for the particular needs of the patient and anesthetist (Fig. 12–10). The anode, or armored, tube has a coiled wire within the wall of the tube, which prevents collapse or kinking. Because the wire support is not continuous to the proximal end of the tube, kinking may still take place between the connector and the wire. Noncollapsible tubes are preferred in procedures such as a radical neck surgery, where the surgeon may be manipulating the tube to a sharp angle. The anode tube is also used in instances of tracheal stenosis or when tumor compression of the trachea is present. Some clinicians prefer this type of tube whenever the head will be sharply flexed intraoperatively.

The oral or nasal Rae tubes were developed with a natural curvature in the tube to eliminate the need for additional curved connectors or adaptors during special procedures. The oral Rae tube is useful when the anesthetist will be positioned to the side of the patient, whereas the

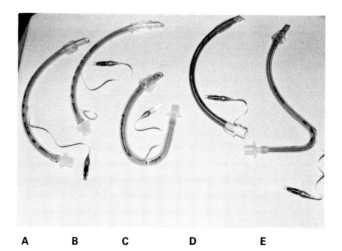

A   B   C   D   E

Figure 12–10. Variations of endotracheal tubes: **A.** traditional endotracheal tube; **B.** Endotrol by National Catheter, with plastic ring for deflecting tip of endotracheal tube; **C.** Rae tube for oral use; **D.** disposable armored tube; **E.** Rae tube for nasal use.

nasal Rae can be used in oral surgery when the tube and ventilating hoses must be directed toward the anesthetist at the head of the table.

Double-lumen endobronchial tubes such as the Carlens, White, or Robertshaw have been developed to provide preferential ventilation of one lung during anesthesia (Fig. 12–11). These tubes are also used to isolate one lung in the event of massive hemorrhage or infection. These endobronchial tubes are constructed differently from endotracheal tubes: there is a double lumen through the length of the tube and both a tracheal and bronchial cuff to allow for distribution of ventilation.

Federal standards have been developed for artificial airways and are designated on the endotracheal tube. I.T. stands for "implantation tested," meaning that rabbits have been injected with the material and have not reacted to it. The Z-79 on the side of the tube refers to the Z-79 Committe for Anesthesia Equipment for the American National Institute and indicates that the manufacturer has tested for substance toxicity and tissue irritation by using a cell culture technique. As Z-79 standards expire, they will be reviewed and revised by the American Society for Testing and Materials (ASTM) Committee F-29.

The tracheal tube cuff is generally built into the distal portion of the adult endotracheal tube and may be either "high residual volume" (low pressure) or "low residual volume" (high pressure). Pediatric tubes do not have a cuff because of the small diameter of the pediatric airway. The purpose of the cuff is to form a seal against the tracheal wall, thereby facilitating positive-pressure ventilation while at the same time discouraging aspiration of foreign material. Capillary blood flow in the area contacted by the cuff must be maintained.

The intra-arterial pressure of the tracheal wall has been estimated at 30 torr, whereas the venous end of the capillary bed has a pressure of 20 torr. Lymphatic flow in the tracheal

area operates at a pressure of 5 torr. Sensitive devices implanted into the anterior tracheal wall have shown that pressures exerted by the cuff during endotracheal intubation may exceed 100 torr. Studies have demonstrated that maintaining intracuff pressure in high-residual-volume, thin-walled cuffs between 17 to 23 torr during spontaneous or controlled ventilation forms an effective seal and allows adequate capillary mucosal blood flow.

In recent years, a significant number of studies have looked at the characteristics of tracheal tube cuffs and the complications resulting from their use. Various types of cuffs have been developed, including prestretched cuffs, cuffs filled with foam, and cuffs with pressure-regulating systems. The goal in developing these cuffs is to present the clinician with a high-residual-volume cuff that produces less tracheal wall pressure than the narrow, low-residual-volume cuff. Tracheal wall changes reported with the high-pressure cuff follow a distinct pattern. Mucosal inflammation and ciliary denudation occur under the cuff site within 2 hours. Within 24 hours mucosal edema is evident. Necrotic areas over the cartilaginous rings of the anterior tracheal wall will follow. Secondary infection may set in, and with continued cuff inflation, tracheal rings may soften. Further pressure can lead to posterior erosion into the esophagus or anterior erosion into the innominate artery. The changes are explained by the physical principles of cuff inflation within a closed space. As air is introduced, elastic forces within the cuff cause expansion until the cuff touches the walls of the trachea. As more air is added to the cuff, the trachea is further compressed. High-residual-volume cuffs have the advantage of conforming to the shape of the trachea with minimal increase in cuff or mucosal pressure. Although data suggest that endotracheal tubes with compliant cuffs should be chosen over those with stiff cuffs, certain precautions still must be observed. The compliant cuffs are easy to overinflate because little resistance is felt. Although inadvertent overinflation of the cuff is less likely to produce damaging pressure on the trachea, the cuff can occlude the beveled end of the endotracheal tube, obstructing the airway.

Nitrous oxide and other gases diffuse into air-inflated tracheal tube cuffs and increase volume and pressure in all cuffs. Intraluminal pressure may also increase as the air in the cuff is warmed to body temperature. Cuff volume increases will vary with exposure time, cuff thickness, partial pressure of nitrous oxide, and cuff composition. The anesthetist must assume that there is nitrous oxide diffusion into a cuff inflated with air and must deflate the cuff to the minimal occluding volume approximately every 30 minutes. The anesthetist can fill the cuff with the anesthetic gas mixture to prevent diffusion. A device that monitors the intraluminal pressure of the cuff is available. Cuff pressure can then be adjusted with a syringe to allow sufficient tracheal capillary blood flow.

Desirable cuff characterisics include (1) a thin wall, (2) a large diameter and high compliance, (3) a large enough residual volume to allow for positive endotracheal pressure, and (4) tear resistance. Cuff thickness determines the size of folds on channels formed when the cuff is inflated in the trachea. Thin folds decrease the channeling of liquids and offer better protection against aspiration. Although

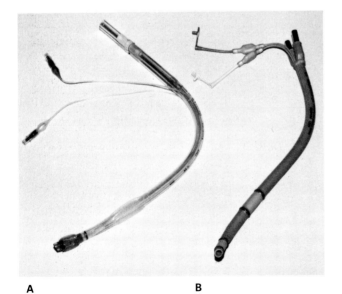

A   **B**

Figure 12–11. Endobronchial tubes: **A.** Robertshaw tube; **B.** Carlens tube.

thick cuffs slow the diffusion of nitrous oxide, eventually the same volume of nitrous oxide will diffuse.

The anesthetist's armamentarium for airway management includes other equipment (Fig. 12–12). Endotracheal tubes are supplied with straight 15-mm connectors, but curved connectors or plastic or metal may be substituted for convenience of positioning. Straight or curved adaptors can be used to link the connector with corrugated tubing or other ventilatory equipment. A specialized connector has been developed for use with a fiberoptic bronchoscope, allowing ventilation via the endotracheal tube during the procedure.

A stylet is a malleable probe used to give shape and form to the endotracheal tube. Stylets are constructed of copper or aluminum and may be plastic coated. The stylet is inserted into the endotracheal tube with its tip approximately ½ inch from the beveled end of the tube. The stylet should never extend into or beyond the bevel because tracheal perforation or vocal cord damage may result. The stylet is bent once, away from the operator at the tube connector, to prevent it from inadvertently going too far down into the tube.

McGill forceps are long-necked forceps that are commonly used to direct the tip of the tube anteriorly during nasoendotracheal intubation. These forceps grasp the tube immediately superior to the cuff. They may be helpful in guiding an oral endotracheal tube or nasogastric tube as well. Caution must be used to keep the forceps from inadvertently grabbing mucosal tissue or the uvula with their serrated tips. This complication may result in hemorrhage requiring surgical intervention.

A tonsil suction has an advantage over the traditional flexible suction catheter in that it can be manipulated with one hand during laryngoscopy. One disadvantage of the tonsil suction is that it cannot be used through an endotracheal tube.

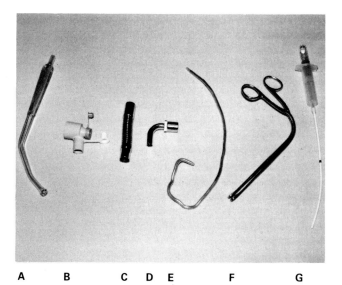

Figure 12–12. Additional airway equipment: **A.** tonsil suction; **B.** connector for use with fiberoptic bronchoscope; **C.** metal flex connector; **D.** metal curved connector; **E.** stylet; **F.** McGill forceps; **G.** laryngeal-tracheal anesthesia kit.

The laryngeal tracheal anesthesia kit contains local anesthetic for topical application to the lower pharynx, larynx, and trachea. The anesthesia requires laryngoscopy and is applied before placement of the endotracheal tube.

Technique for Endotracheal Intubation. The trachea can be cannulated using either the oral or nasal route. Many of the principles are the same regardless of the route employed. Before beginning the procedure, the patient must be positioned on a stationary table or bed with the head at the level of anesthetist's xiphoid process. The anesthetist should be positioned behind the patient's head. A 4-inch pad or pillow should be positioned under the patient's head to provide optimum alignment of the oral, pharyngeal, and laryngeal axes. Good lighting is essential to allow continual assessment of the patient's mucosa and integument for cyanosis. A tonsil suction is set up for use before the actual insertion of the endotracheal tube, and a suction catheter is available for deep tracheal suctioning afterward.

A resuscitation bag and mask of the appropriate size are necessary, not only for checking placement of the endotracheal tube but in the event that the anesthetist is unable to intubate a patient experiencing airway distress. The reservoir bag that is part of the anesthesia circuit may be used for the same purpose.

Oral Intubation. All required equipment should be assembled before beginning the procedure. For oral endotracheal intubation, the following equipment is necessary: local anesthetic lubricant, oral airway, tongue blade, laryngoscope, oral endotracheal tube with 15-mm connector, stylet, 10-ml syringe, and suction and positive-pressure ventilation apparatus.

The technique for oral endotracheal intubation is best learned through study of the following sequence and practice. Initial attempts at intubation should concentrate on maintaining good technique rather than focusing on the success of the placement. Common errors and difficulties of the novice are:

1. inserting laryngoscope blade too far;
2. excessive hyperextension of the head;
3. loss of control of the tongue;
4. blade not midline;
5. prying on the teeth.

Immediately before intubation, the patient's head must be properly positioned to maximize visualization. There are two head positions commonly used for endotracheal intubation (Fig. 12–13A, B). The "sniffing" or "amended" position has been shown to improve alignment of the axis of the oral cavity, the pharynx, and trachea (Fig. 12–13A). This position is achieved by placing a 4 inch pad or pillow under the patient's occiput, without elevating the shoulders. Extreme hyperextension of the head is not required; gentle extension of the atlanto-occipital junction will facilitate intubation. Although this position improves visualization, it does require the pad or pillow, which may not be readily available in the emergency situation. The sniffing position is contraindicated in patients with known or suspected injury of the cervical spine.

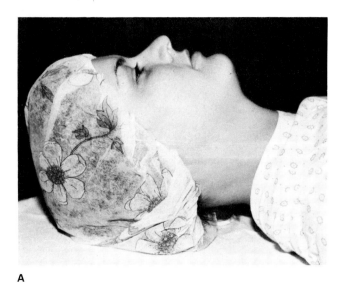
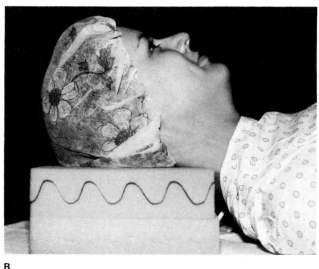

A   B

Figure 12–13. Positioning the head for endotracheal intubation: **A.** sniffing or amended position; **B.** classic or "jacksonian" position.

In contrast to the sniffing position, the classic or "jacksonian" position is one in which the patient's shoulders and head remain on the bed or table (Figure 12–13B). The disadvantage of this position is that the lip-to-glottis distance is elongated and the larynx rotated anteriorly. Gentle hyperextension of the head with the right hand at the occipit will stabilize the head during intubation (Fig. 12–14).

Oral Endotracheal Intubation Technique

Step 1:   Obtain good lighting. Position the patient on a nonmoving surface in sniffing position with the head at the level of the anesthetist's xiphoid process.

Step 2:   Open the mouth with the right hand by gently depressing the mandible. It is not usually neces-

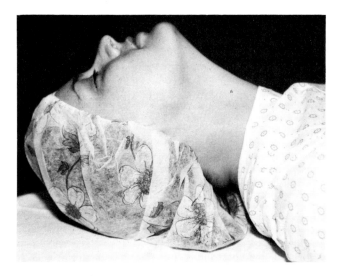

Figure 12–14. Classic or jacksonian position with gentle hyperextension.

sary to put the fingers in the mouth; on rare occasions, if the anesthetist's fingers are placed in the patient's mouth, gloves should be worn.

Step 3:   Using the left hand, place the laryngoscope blade in the right side of the mouth. Move the laryngoscope to the midline, deflecting the tongue to the left. The blade should be perpendicular to the patient's body.

Step 4:   Maintaining a midline orientation, continue to direct the laryngoscope blade down the pharynx. The anatomic landmarks seen will be the uvula, oropharyngeal wall, and the epiglottis.

Step 5A: If a straight laryngoscope blade is used, advance the blade approximately 1 cm beyond the epiglottis. At this point, the blade tip lifts up the epiglottis as the anesthetist lifts the laryngoscope forward and upward, and the glottis is exposed (direct exposure).

Step 5B: If a curved laryngoscope blade is used, advance the blade and place the tip in the vallecula. The laryngoscope is lifted upward and forward, thereby exposing the glottis (indirect exposure).

Step 6:   Using the right hand, direct the endotracheal tube into the right side of the oral cavity, pharynx, and through the vocal cords. If a stylet is used, it is withdrawn as the tube passes through the vocal cords. The anesthetist must watch the cuff pass through the cords.

Step 7:   Connect the apparatus for positive-pressure ventilation to the endotracheal tube. Listen to breath sounds bilaterally in all quadrants and auscultate the stomach. Inflate the cuff of the endotracheal tube by injecting air into the pilot balloon until there is no leak.

Step 8:   Insert an oral airway and secure the tube.

When learning the technique of laryngoscopy, it is helpful to memorize the anatomic landmarks in sequence (Table

TABLE 12–2. ANATOMIC LANDMARKS USED IN INTUBATION

Mouth
Uvula
Posterior pharynx
Epiglottis
Glottis

12–2). These can be used as checkpoints while performing laryngoscopy to ensure successful visualization.

Nasal Intubation. Certain situations indicate the need for a nasal approach to tracheal cannulation. A nasal tube is necessary for patients who are unable to open their mouth or hyperextend their neck, making laryngoscopy and ventilation impossible. It is desirable for oral surgical cases where the surgeon will be doing extensive work in the mouth or on the jaws. Nasoendotracheal intubation is a good choice for patients who will require long-term ventilation postoperatively because the tube is easier to stabilize and more comfortable for the patient. Patient oral hygiene is more readily maintained without an oral endotracheal tube in the mouth.

Contraindications to the nasal approach do exist. Patients with coagulopathies are not good candidates for nasoendotracheal intubation because of the vascularity of the nasal mucosa. This technique should be avoided in patients suffering from a dural tear presenting with cerebrospinal fluid draining from the nose, and those with a nasal injury, acute sinusitis, or mastoiditis. If the patient has an extremely deviated septum or difficulty breathing through the nose, nasal intubation should be avoided if possible.

All equipment for nasoendotracheal intubation must be assembled before beginning the procedure. Equipment necessary includes: vasoconstricting nose drops, laryngoscope, soft nasal airway, local anesthetic lubricant, nasal endotracheal tubes with 15-mm connector, oral tubes, 10-ml syringe, McGill forceps, and suction and postive-pressure ventilation apparatus. A stylet is never used for nasal intubation.

Immediately before intubation, the patient is properly positioned in the sniffing position. If the procedure is to be carried out on an awake patient experiencing respiratory distress, the patient may remain in a semi-Fowler's position. Oral endotracheal tubes are available for use in the event of difficulty with the nasal approach. Before attempting nasal intubation, the anesthetist should identify which naris is more patent by asking the patient which side of the nose he or she can breathe through better. If there is no surgical or patient-based indication to use the left naris, the right naris is preferred for mechanical convenience to the anesthetist. The anesthetist may also measure the length of the nasotracheal tube using anatomic landmarks (Fig. 12–15). The tube should be cut at the level of the naris and the connector reinserted to prevent kinking.

Technique for Nasal Endotracheal Intubation in the Anesthetized Patient

Step 1: Position the patient, apply the vasoconstricting drops to both nares. Anesthetize the patient.

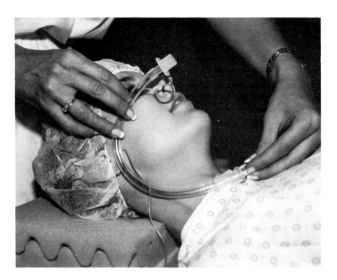

Figure 12–15. Measuring the length of a nasotracheal tube using external landmarks: suprasternal notch, earlobe, and naris.

Step 2: Insert a well-lubricated soft nasal airway in the naris to be used for intubation to ascertain nasal patency. Ventilate.

Step 3: Remove the nasopharyngeal airway. Using the left hand to gently push up on the tip of the nose, insert the lubricated nasal endotracheal tube, following the contours of the vestibule of the nose, going up from the nostril and backward and down into the nasopharynx. With steady pressure, advance the tube until loss of resistance occurs.

Step 4: Using the right hand, open the mouth by depressing the mandible and insert the laryngoscope blade into the right side of the mouth using the left hand.

Step 5: As the laryngscope is moved midline, the tip of the nasal tube should be seen in the pharynx. If it is not, the anesthetist advances the tube further until the tip is identified.

Step 6: The endotracheal tube and laryngoscope are advanced simultaneously. Exposure of the glottis is obtained and the tube inserted. The cuff of the tube should pass below the vocal cords.

Step 7: The laryngoscope is removed and the endotracheal tube connection attached to the breathing circuit. Listen to breath sounds bilaterally in all quadrants and ausculate the stomach. Positive pressure is applied, and the tube placement is checked by auscultating the chest bilaterally. The cuff is inflated until no leak is present and the nasal tube is secure.

Intubation via the nasal route has some disadvantages. It is not uncommon for the pressure of the tube to cause necrosis in the area of the ala nasi in patients requiring long-term intubation. Once in place, the nasal tube can totally obstruct sinus drainage, leading to acute sinusitis. It may also block the eustacian tube in the nasopharynx, resulting in otitis media. The nasal tube may kink within the nose, leading to acute airway obstruction. This most commonly occurs as the tube warms to body temperature.

Intubation of the Awake Patient. There are situations in which awake intubation is indicated, either in the operating room before surgery or in the patient's room. The nasal route is preferred for awake intubation unless contraindications to this approach exist. The nasal tube can often be placed "blindly," that is without laryngoscopy and visualization of the glottis. There is currently available a nasal tube that has at the proximal end a ring that is connected via the tube wall to the tip of the tube. Pulling up on the ring curves the tip of the tube upward so that it can pass through the vocal cords more easily. Blind nasal intubation can be facilitated by changing the position of the patient's head from side to side or from flexion to extension. The anesthetist listens to breath sounds from the endotracheal tube and advances the tube toward them. Loss of breath sounds is cause to withdraw the tube slightly and redirect it or reposition the patient. When the breath sounds become very audible or the patient coughs, the tube should be firmly advanced. Cessation of breath sounds, lack of humidity appearing on the tube, or regurgitant material in the tube are evidence of failure to pass the tube through the glottis. At times the tube may appear as a bulge on the outside of the neck. It should then be withdrawn slightly and redirected.

It is not possible to intubate every patient using the blind technique. If there have been several attempts, it is best to open the patient's mouth and proceed with direct laryngoscopy. McGill forceps may be necessary to direct the tube into the trachea. The patient in respiratory distress is a poor candidate for multiple intubation attempts; if the tube cannot be passed easily by the blind technique it is best to move quickly to direct laryngoscopy.

Oral endotracheal intubation can also be performed in the awake patient, although it is not usually attempted without using laryngoscopy. Awake oral intubation is chosen for the patient suspected of impending respiratory or cardiac arrest and for patients with nasal injuries requiring general anesthesia if the ability to ventilate the patient is in question. Awake intubation is the safest technique for a patient who has a full stomach and requires general anesthesia.

Awake intubation using either the nasal or oral approach is not without risk. The procedure is extremely stimulating and uncomfortable for the patient. Laryngoscopy can elicit violent cough and gag reflexes in the awake patient. This reaction is of particular danger to the patient with suspected cervical injury, increased intracranial pressure, or increased intraocular pressure. Complications may be induced in the patient with coronary artery disease, hypertension, or asthma. For these patients, awake intubation should be avoided if at all possible.

Before beginning awake intubation, the anesthetist should prepare the patient so as to minimize discomfort and maximize cooperation. The proposed procedure should be explained in simple terms, along with the reason why this approach is desirable. Whenever possible, time should be taken to provide maximum analgesia and amnesia for the procedure.

The patient can receive titrated doses of sedatives with an amnesic effect such as diazepam or lorazepam. Small doses of short-acting narcotics, such as fentanyl, can be given incrementally to minimize discomfort. The use of a fentanyl citrate and droperidol (Innovar) drip has also been reported for sedation. Caution must be taken to avoid respiratory depression lest the patient develop the airway problems that awake intubation is meant to avoid.

If nasal intubation is planned, vasoconstrictive drops should be applied at least 1 minute before beginning. A well-lubricated nasopharyngeal airway should first be passed to provide local anesthesia to the mucosal surface of the nose. Cocaine can be applied to the mucosa with either pledgets or cotton swabs, to minimize bleeding and achieve local anesthesia.

If laryngoscopy is necessary, the laryngoscope should be rinsed with warm water and the local anesthetic lubricant applied to the blade. A local anesthetic spray can be applied in stages to the oral cavity and pharynx. Once the tongue is anesthetized, it can be displaced forward with a tongue blade and the lower portion of the pharynx sprayed. The patient, if cooperative, can gargle with viscous lidocaine for additional anesthesia. A recurrent laryngeal or superior laryngeal nerve block may also be performed.

Complications with an Endotracheal Tube in Place. An endotracheal tube in place interferes with the normal functions of the airway, such as coughing, humidification, and speech. Because the patient cannot mobilize secretions with a cough, the anesthetist must suction the tracheobronchial tree via the endotracheal tube. Most patients will require suctioning periodically during lengthy surgery and at the end of the procedure; patients with copious secretions may require suctioning more frequently.

Serious complications may result from improper suctioning and therefore it is most important to incorporate sound procedure into the anesthetic care plan. Sterile technique, using a sterile glove for the hand holding the catheter, must be used whenever possible. The suction catheter should never pass from the oropharynx to the endotracheal tube. The suction catheter is inserted without vacuum, and intermittent suction is applied during removal. Suctioning during the surgical procedure is best performed during periods of maximal relaxation. The patient should be well oxygenated before and after tracheal suctioning. The suction catheter should remain in the airway no longer than 15 seconds.

Various humidified circuits are now available for use on anesthesia machines. These devices are particularly helpful for patients undergoing prolonged surgery or for pediatric patients receiving anesthesia via a nonrebreathing system.

When intubation is expected to continue in the recovery room, the patient should be instructed preoperatively about ways to communicate while the tube is in place. A pencil and pad of paper can be available at the bedside. All attempts at talking with the tube in place should be discouraged, because trauma to the vocal cords can occur.

Despite the many advantages of endotracheal intubation, the procedure is not without risk. Intubation may cause chipped or broken teeth and damage to the lips, tongue, or mucous membranes of the oral cavity and pharynx. Epistaxis and hemorrhage are possible.

Airway emergencies can still occur once the endotracheal tube is inserted. Tube obstruction may result from a variety of causes. The cuff can slip or overinflate, occluding the end of the tube. This can be relieved by deflating the cuff. The tube may kink or collapse. This can be corrected by manipulating the tube or the patient's head. Secretions or a foreign body may occlude the tube. Under normal circumstances, suction will remove the obstructing material; however, in certain situations the tube will have to be replaced. The bevel of the tube may lodge against the tracheal wall. This problem can be remedied by the tube manipulation.

Cuff leaks are not only bothersome but dangerous, and ventilation must be maintained with increased tidal volume while the cause of the problem is diagnosed. In the case of nasal intubation, cuff leakage is assumed to be due to damage to a cuff during insertion. Sudden air leakage and failure to maintain a closed system require performance of a direct laryngoscopy. Often the problem is that the cuff is superior to the cords. Passage of a nasogastric tube into the trachea resulting in a large air leak, has been reported. If tube replacement is necessary because of a damaged cuff, the new tube is inserted along the existing tube while the larynx is visualized. The malfunctioning tube is then removed and a new tube inserted under direct visualization.

Malpositioning of the tube is another airway problem that can occur after the anesthetist has completed the intubation procedure. The tube may slip down into the bronchial tree, resulting in ventilation-perfusion inequality. Sometimes it is difficult to hear breath sounds over the lung fields; in other instances auscultation of the chest produces the sound of air although the tube is positioned in the esophagus. When any doubt exists, the anesthetist should quickly auscultate over the stomach. If doubt lingers, laryngoscopy should be performed and the tube position verified. Observation of chest excursion and auscultation of breath sounds should always be repeated after the patient's position is changed intraoperatively.

The tube may become dislodged and unintentional extubation occur. This is an airway emergency that can have dire consequences if the patient is in the sitting or prone position. Prevention requires that the tube always be secured properly from the start. Continuous monitoring of lung sounds via a precordial stethoscope allows the anesthetist to detect intraoperatively extubation immediately. In the event of accidental extubation, the surgeon should be informed and the patient ventilated with 100 percent oxygen. Reintubation should take place as soon as possible.

Airway emergencies also occur when the tube is patent and properly positioned but there is a break in the ventilating circuit. This circumstance is characterized by complete loss of the patient's breath sounds and chest excursion. Systematic checking of the entire circuit, from patient to gas machine, will usually reveal the cause. If the cause is difficult to diagnose, the patient must be ventilated meanwhile, either by ambu bag or mouth-to-tube ventilation.

Intubation during light planes of anesthesia can result in breath holding, prolonged cough, and spasm of the chest wall or bronchi. Deepening of the anesthetic usually relieves the difficulty. Additional measures, such as the administration of succinylcholine or aminophylline, may be required.

Extubation. At the end of the surgical procedure, the patient is extubated if there are no indications for continued endotracheal intubation. One criterion for extubation is whether or not a muscle relaxant has been administered.

If no muscle relaxant has been used, the patient may be extubated either at a deep plane of anesthesia or when reflexes have returned. Extubation during light planes of anesthesia can result in breath holding and laryngospasm. Deep extubation takes place when spontaneous respirations are present but the patient has not begun to cough on the tube or move. The procedure for carrying out deep extubation is as follows:

When spontaneous respirations are present, the nitrous oxide is turned off and the anesthetic deepened by increasing the inhalation agent. Spontaneous respiration must be maintained. Suctioning may take place at this time. (Reflex response to suctioning occurs when the patient is at too light a plane of anesthesia.) If the patient is assessed to be in a sufficiently deep plane, the cuff is deflated and the tube removed while positive-pressure ventilation is applied. Extubation on inspiration is less likely to cause laryngospasm. If laryngospasm should occur, the lungs are full of oxygen so that passive diffusion may take place during the temporary lapse in ventilation.

Once the tube is removed, 100 percent oxygen is administered via mask and the patient is allowed to awaken. Miscalculation in timing of deep extubation may result in complications such as breath holding or laryngospasm.

Deep extubation is indicated when the patient's condition demands the absence of coughing or bucking on the endotracheal tube (e.g., with increased intraocular or intracranial pressure, asthma, or cardiovascular disease). Deep extubation is contraindicated in patients with a full stomach or airway difficulties.

Administration of muscle relaxant intraoperatively adds another dimension to the question of when to extubate. In this instance, the anesthetist is not only concerned that the patient be awake and reflexic but that an adequate number of skeletal muscle receptors be unoccupied.

There are several methods for assessing adequacy of muscle-relaxant reversal. The patient who can demonstrate a "train of four" in response to peripheral nerve stimulation has few occupied receptors. This tool is useful for assessment in the operating room but less suitable for the emerging or awake patient because the stimulus is painful.

Sustained antigravity movement, such as lifting the head on request, is a better alternative. The patient must begin in a supine position and deliberately raise his or her head without the use of handrails. The movement should be purposeful and sustained for 5 seconds. Jerking, coughing movements of the head in response to tracheal stimulus does not qualify the patient for extubation.

Grip strength is an indicator of receptor occupancy. Bilateral grip strength can be compared with preoperative norms. This measure, although difficult to qualify, is useful for patients who were unable to lift their heads preoperatively.

Measurement of the negative inspiratory pressure is a useful indicator of muscle power and the patient's ability to generate an effective cough. The equipment required is relatively inexpensive and simple to use. A manometer is connected via plastic tubing to a three-way adaptor, which is connected to the endotracheal tube. While the anesthetist occludes the port, the patient is instructed to breathe. Thus, the pressure measured on the manometer reflects the negative "pulling power" of the lungs and diaphragm. A negative inspiratory pressure (NIP) of -20 cm H_2O correlates with a vital capacity of 15 ml/kg or greater and compares well with the train of four for assessment of muscle-relaxant reversal.

The patient's ability to self-extubate is never considered an appropriate measure of muscle-relaxant reversal. The patient is receiving a strong airway stimulus from the indwelling endotracheal tube and possibly an oropharyngeal airway. The patient may muster all possible strength to remove the endotracheal tube, only to lapse into respiratory depression once the tube is out. Self-extubation does not guarantee that the patient has adequate muscle power to generate an effective cough or handle secretions. Damage to the vocal cords can result from self-extubation with the cuff inflated.

Once the decision has been made to extubate, the procedure should be explained to the patient in simple terms if the patient is alert enough to understand. The trachea, pharynx, and oral cavity should be suctioned. Oxygen is delivered after tracheal suctioning, before extubation. The cuff on the endotracheal tube is deflated and the tube removed on inspiration. The awake patient should be instructed to open his or her mouth and take a deep breath to facilitate a quick, safe extubation. Oxygen is administered after extubation and the patient is carefully observed for signs of obstruction or laryngospasm. The period immediately after extubation is a critical one because of the many complications that can follow extubation.

Postextubation Complications. Laryngospasm may occur when the patient is in a light plane of anesthesia and has been extubated. Laryngospasm may be caused by retained secretions that are at the vocal cords postextubation. Treatment of laryngospasm includes the administration of oxygen using positive-pressure apparatus and possibly succinylcholine.

Tracheal collapse after extubation has been reported in patients with prolonged intubation, which weakens the cartilaginous rings of the trachea. Thyroid disease or large cervical or mediastinal tumors may also result in tracheal collapse. Immediate reintubation is clearly indicated in this event.

Extubation is contraindicated in any patient suffering from respiratory distress. Poor arterial blood gas values should warn of the danger of proceeding with a planned extubation. Under no circumstances should a patient be extubated without the presence of someone who can ventilate the patient and replace the airway if necessary.

Many complications of endotracheal intubation manifest themselves only after extubation. Predisposing factors are varied and, in many cases, avoidable. Clinicians report that complications are more frequent in elderly, debilitated patients, with women affected more often than men. Factors that contribute to complications include excessive movement of the tube while in place, too large a tube for the

patient's larynx, traumatic intubation or multiple attempts at intubation, and poor sterile technique.

The most common complaint expressed by patients postextubation is sore throat and laryngitis because during the process of intubation the epithelial layer of the mucous membrane lining the respiratory tract is traumatized. This condition spontaneously clears up within 2 to 3 days with adequate hydration.

Glottic and subglottic edema may occur as a result of traumatic intubation of a tight-fitting tube. Rarely, a patient may develop edema in response to the PVC tube. Ventilatory obstruction results from subepithelial edema of the epiglottis, vocal cords, and subglottic area. High-pitched, progressive inspiratory stridor is a key indicator of subglottic or glottic edema. This condition is treated by reassurance, topical decongestant via aerosol, and possibly steroids. The patient must be carefully observed and intubation equipment kept immediately available in case reintubation is necessary.

Ulceration of the tracheal mucosa may occur at the cuff site or the anterior wall where the tip of the tube has denuded the epithelium. Infection may occur as a secondary complication.

Vocal cord injury or paralysis after endotracheal intubation has been reported. Ulceration, granuloma, or polyps on the vocal cords are suspected when hoarseness persists for several days. The absolute diagnosis is made via laryngoscopy. Trauma, excessive movement, allergic reaction to PVC, and tight-fitting tubes are possible causes of these complications. Surgery of the head and neck or mediastinum may lead to inadvertant ligation of the recurrent laryngeal nerve, resulting in vocal cord paralysis.

Tracheal stenosis or malacia are complications most often seen in patients undergoing long-term endotracheal intubation and ventilation. The development of tracheal stenosis or tracheal malacia is a result of several factors such as cuff pressure, duration of intubation, mean arterial blood pressure, and sensitivity to endotracheal tube materials. These complications rarely occur in patients undergoing short-term intubation for general anesthesia.

BIBLIOGRAPHY

Bernard AV, Cottrell JE, et al: Adjustment of intracuff pressure to prevent aspiration. Anesthesiology 50:363, 1979.

Bernhard WN, Yost LC, et al: Physical characteristics of the rates of N20 diffusion into tracheal tube cuffs. Anesthesiology 48:413–417, 1978.

Burtner D, Goodman M: Anesthetic and operative management of potential upper airway obstruction. Arch Otolaryngol 104: Nov., 657–661, 1978.

Cooper JD, Grillo HC: Analysis of problems related to cuffs on endotracheal tubes. Chest 62:2115, 1972.

Herrin T, Bruzustowics R, et al: Anesthetic management of neck trauma. South Med J 72:1102–1106, 1979.

Klainer AS, Turndorf H, et al: Surface alterations due to endotracheal intubation. Am J Med 58:674, 1975.

Knowlson GTC, Bassett HFM: The pressures exerted on the trachea by endotracheal inflatable cuffs. J Anaesthesiol 42:824, 1970.

Stanley TH: Effects of anesthetic gases on endotracheal tube cuff gas volumes. Anesth Analg 53:480, 1974.

Stauffer JL, Olson DE, et al: Complications and consequences of endotracheal intubation and trachestomy. Am J Med 70:65–76, 1981.

Part III

APPLIED PHARMACOLOGY

13

Principles of Drug Uptake and Distribution

Robert C. Reynolds

*A*nesthetists have a benefit not afforded to other medical specialists in that they work with short-acting drugs that have a very rapid onset of action. Careful observation of the response (or lack of response) of a patient to these drugs allows the anesthetist to follow one of the most important dictums of medical practice: "Each patient should determine the extent of his or her own therapy."

To take advantage of this important medical principle, it is absolutely essential that anyone administering a drug to a patient should have a thorough understanding of the physiologic, pharmacologic, and pathologic factors that influence the uptake, distribution, and action of that drug. Armed with this information, an anesthetist can practice more effectively, safely, and enjoyably his or her craft. By understanding the nature of a patient's pulmonary disease, an anesthetist can anticipate problems with the uptake of an inhalation drug. The observation that a patient has a delayed response to the injection of succinylcholine may suggest that one is dealing with a patient with a lowered cardiac output or diminished circulatory blood volume.

Many discussions of drug uptake and distribution use the presentation of mathematical models of pharmacokinetics. This extensive use of formulae, equations, and diagrammatic models often confuses and discourages a neophyte clinician. An attempt will be made in this chapter to minimize the use of mathematical equations. It is hoped the reader will be stimulated to study the subject more extensively.

BASIC MECHANISMS OF DRUG ACTION

The majority of drugs produce their effects on an organism by interacting with cellular receptors. These receptors appear to be macromolecular proteins, often influencing or participating in enzymatic activities of the cell. The interaction of drug and receptor is chemical in nature and can be represented by:

$$D + R \rightleftharpoons D\text{–}R \rightsquigarrow \text{effect}$$

Where D is the drug, R is the receptor, and D–R is the drug–receptor complex.

Drug receptor theory maintains that the magnitude of a drug effect is proportional to the number of drug–receptor complexes formed. This is the usual explanation of a dose–response curve. In most situations the number of available receptors remains constant, and so the number of drug–receptor combinations depends on the concentration of drug available at the receptor sites of the effector cell. For example, if muscle cholinesterase can be considered a receptor to react with the drug, neostigmine (a cholinesterase inhibitor), the greater the number of molecules of neostigmine available to interact with the cellular cholinesterase molecule, the greater will be the resultant cholinergic effect.

Not all drugs administered by an anesthetist react with specific receptors. The osmotic diuretics (e.g., mannitol) change the osmolality of fluids, producing secondary shifts of body water. The inhalational anesthetics are thought to have a nonspecific interaction with cellular membranes, resulting in a depression of cellular excitability. In either case, the same general principles of distribution of an appropriate amount of drug to the desired site of action apply to these drugs as well as to the drugs that depend on specific receptor combinations for their effect.

The routes by which drugs can be administered to a patient include parenteral (injection), inhalational, enterel (oral), and topical. The use of topical drugs is discussed in Chapter 16.

PARENTERAL UPTAKE AND DISTRIBUTION

The most reliable technique for introducing a drug directly into a patient's plasma is the intravenous (IV) route. Venous blood passing the injection site carries the drug directly to the cardiopulmonary circulation and to arterial blood going directly to effector organs. IV injection is the most precise form of drug administration (with the possible exception of intracardiac injections used as emergency procedures during cardiac arrest).

Factors that can interfere with IV uptake must not be ignored. Frequently a drug is injected into IV tubing that is carrying saline or other fluids. Obviously, if a drug leaks out of the administering equipment, it will have no effect on the patient. Keeping this possibility in mind has led to the discovery of disconnections of IV sets under surgical draperies when a patient did not respond to an injection of a muscle relaxant.

Pain is a factor in the use of parenteral medications. Most drug injections into a well-placed, free-flowing IV line are not painful. If a patient complains of pain after the injection of a test dose of 1 or 2 ml of a 2.5 percent solution of thiopental, this should serve as a warning to the anesthetist that the injection may not have gone entirely into the vein. Perhaps some of the very alkaline drug may have extravasated into the perivascular tissue, producing pain or, eventually, tissue destruction. The injection site should be examined before any further injection is made. Some drugs can be expected to produce pain when injected into an adequate IV perfusion. Concentrated solutions of potassium chloride produce pain along the vessel into which they are being injected. This pain can usually be relieved by slowing the rate of infusion. Drugs, such as diazepam, are irritating to vessels. An anesthetist can relieve a lot of anxiety by warning a patient in advance of the injection that he or she may "feel some burning at the injection site, but this will go away, and as it disappears you will feel yourself becoming more and more relaxed." This type of reassurance often adds to the desired pharmacologic sedation to be produced by the drug.

Premedicant drugs are often ordered to be given intramuscularly (IM) in a patient's room an hour or so before the patient is to be brought to the operating room. Since the medications are usually given by someone other than the anesthetist, the pain associated with injection is often ignored by everyone except the patient, and it can often counteract the desired sedative effect. Pain could be the result of the volume of the injection (100 mg of pentobarbital represents 2 ml of injected fluid) or of other materials injected with the medications (glycols are frequently used as drug solvents), or some drugs (phenothiazines) are naturally irritating. Pain at an injection site is a significant factor in drug uptake because it can cause local vasoconstriction, inhibiting blood flow to the area. Studies have shown that serum concentrations of diazepam rise more slowly after IM injections than after oral ingestion of the same dosage of the drug.

After a drug has passed through the cardiopulmonary circulation, its organ distribution will depend on tissue blood profusion. Such organs as the brain and heart receive a preferential blood supply even in the event of diminished cardiac output. In such situations the major portion of a single bolus of drug could be delivered to these organs and produce a profound effect. In contrast to a healthy patient, a patient with a low cardiac output or decreased blood volume might become unconscious or hypotensive after an injection of even a very small amount of thiopental.

Other organs that receive a high percentage of the cardiac output are the kidneys, liver, and viscera. Lean tissues, such as muscle, skin, and bone, receive a smaller allotment of the cardiac output, and fat receives the least percentage of circulatory volume. Therefore, after a single injection of a rapid-acting barbiturate, a patient may be rendered unconscious and, if there are any serious cardiovascular problems, hypotension may develop in the duration of one circulatory time. With continued circulation after a single injection, the drug will be redistributed from high-flow organs to lean tissues and finally to fat. In fact, the major factor in terminating the action of the short-acting barbiturates is not metabolism or excretion of the drug but the agent's redistribution to less responsive tissues. Total body stores of repeated injections of barbiturate probably play a role in the residual hangover effects of the drug.

Organ blood flow plays an important role in distribution with all forms of drug administration but probably is demonstrated most graphically by the response of a patient after a single IV injection of a rapid-acting agent.

PASSAGE OF DRUGS ACROSS BIOLOGICAL MEMBRANES

After a drug has been delivered to an effector organ, it must pass through one or more biological membranes before combining with an appropriate cellular receptor. The rapidity with which a drug passes through biological membranes depends on the physical and chemical characteristics of both drug and cellular barriers.

Biological barriers can be divided into three categories: capillary membranes, cellular membranes, and specialized membranes. Capillary membranes are generally the loosest and most easily penetrated of biological barriers. Small molecules can diffuse through numerous aqueous pores or channels of capillary walls, and larger lipid-soluble molecules can associate and diffuse through lipoprotein matrices of cell walls. Drug diffusion by either of these mechanisms is a passive process depending primarily on concentration gradients. A compound will pass from an area of high concentration to one of low concentration. Only large molecules, the size of proteins, are not able to diffuse across intact capillary membranes. This becomes a significant factor in considering drugs that are bound to plasma proteins.

Cellular membranes differ from capillary membranes primarily in the decreased number of aqueous channels available for transport of compounds into the cell. Lipoprotein dissolution and diffusion are much more important factors in the transport of drugs into and out of cells than across capillaries. Certain cell membranes, particularly in excitable tissues, have the ability to actively transport molecules into and out of cells, but this has not been shown to be a significant factor in the intercellular movement of drugs.

Not all drugs need to enter a cell to be effective. Many drug receptors are closely associated with cell membranes on the surface of effector cells. The catecholamines interact with receptors on the surface of heart, vascular, and muscle membranes, triggering a series of enzymatic reactions to produce their adrenergic effects. The neuromuscular blocking agents are highly charged, nonlipid, soluble molecules that combine with receptors on the muscular side of a neuromuscular junction to block the receptors for acetylcholine discharged from motor neurons. The rapid action of both types of drugs can be attributed to the supposition that neither drug needs to penetrate a cell wall to be effective.

A discussion of specialized biological membranes

should include the blood–brain barrier. The blood–brain barrier is probably not a single anatomic or functional feature that prohibits the passage of molecules from the cerebral circulation into the central nervous system (CNS). It is most likely a specialized version of other cellular membranes that allows only highly lipid-soluble compounds to pass into the CNS. Drugs that are not lipid soluble, for example, high molecular weight, ionized, or bound molecules, are barred entry into the CNS.

The placenta presents a somewhat different type of barrier to the passage of compounds from the maternal circulation to the fetus. As with other cell membranes, lipid-soluble drugs pass very easily through the placenta. However, the actual amount of drug that reaches the fetus is dependent more on the duration of the drug in the mother's circulation than on a single exposure to the drug. For example, the thiobarbiturates (thiopental) and the narcotic analgesics (morphine or meperidine) are very lipid-soluble CNS depressants, and since they freely pass the placenta, they present a potential threat of respiratory depression to a newborn infant. If a mother in labor is given an injection of morphine, a significant concentration of the analgesic will remain in her circulation for a long time, allowing a potentially harmful amount of the drug to pass from the mother to the baby. In contrast, if a mother is given a single IV injection of thiopental during delivery, the barbiturate will remain in her circulation for a relatively brief time, which limits the amount of the drug passing to the baby.

An example of the role of lipid solubility and drug activity can be observed in contrasting the effects of single IV injections of two commonly used tranquilizers. Diazepam and lorazepam are benzodiazepine derivatives that are used as premedicants to relieve anxiety and produce amnesia. The most obvious difference in the effect of these drugs is that diazepam produces evidence of CNS depression within 1 to 1½ minutes after injection, whereas the onset of lorazepam activity is not apparent for 15 to 20 minutes. The best explanation for the difference in activity is that diazepam is much more lipid soluble than lorazepam and is therefore able to pass the blood–brain barrier much more rapidly. Ease of membrane passage may also explain the difference in duration of effect of the two drugs. Diazepam-induced CNS depression is fairly short-lived after a single injection, whereas there is evidence of drug-induced amnesia lasting up to 24 hours after a single administration of lorazepam.

Many drugs exist as the salts of weak acids or bases. This means that in solution they are in two different forms: ionized molecules (with positive or negative electrolytic charges) and nonionized (neutral) molecules. The role of ionization and drug activity becomes meaningful when the clinician realizes that the ionized form of a drug may have a very different effect on an organism than has the neutral form of the same molecule.

Most neutral molecules are lipid soluble, whereas ionized forms of the same compound are repelled or absorbed by the protein portion of cell membranes and are unable to enter the cell. The degree of ionization of a molecule depends on only two factors: the pH of the solution, or the milieu surrounding the substance, and the pKa of the substance. The pKa is a physiochemical characteristic of the compound and is defined as the pH at which 50 percent

of the chemical will be in the charged form and the other half will be neutral. The actual charge on the molecule (positive or negative) depends on whether the compound ionizes as a base (positive) or as an acid (negative). A weak base (e.g., procaine, with a pKa of 8.5) will become ionized and less effective as the pH of the solution is lowered or becomes more acidic. Topical local anesthetic preparations are rendered more effective by slightly alkalinizing the solution; however, in most clinical situations an injected solution is quickly brought to extracellular pH by natural tissue buffers.

The local anesthetics are markedly affected by changes in pH because most of the agents have pKas just a bit higher than the physiological pH. If the pH of a solution is 1 unit below the pKa of the basic compound, the ratio of anion : unionized molecule will shift from 5:50 percent to 90:10 percent, and another shift of pH to 2 units below the pKa results in a ratio of 99:1 percent. This 10-fold shift in ionization is the result of the pH and pKa scales being logarithmic (Henderson–Hasselbalch equation).

Barbituric acid derivatives are another series of compounds with pKas very close to physiologic pH (thiopental, 7.4) whose activity may be changed by relatively small changes in pH. In contrast to local anesthetics, the barbiturates ionize as acids. Therefore, an increase in pH with hyperventilation or the infusion of bicarbonate increases the amount of negatively charged cation and decreases the amount of neutral lipid-soluble molecule, reducing the effectiveness of the drug.

Not all drugs are affected by changes of pH and ionization. The muscle relaxants with quaternary ammonium ions have pKas so distant from the normal biological pH that any possible shift in physiologic pH does not significantly change the ionization of these compounds. They are always ionized. Many biologically active drugs do not ionize at all, and so they are unaffected by changes in pH. Inhalational anesthetic agents and alcohols are examples of this latter category of drugs.

INHALATIONAL ANESTHETIC TECHNIQUES

The inhalational anesthetic agents are unique in the way they use the respiratory system for their uptake and, to a great extent, elimination from the body. Anesthetic gases or vapors are delivered to the lung, where they freely pass the alveolar membranes into the pulmonary circulation and are delivered to the brain and other body tissues.

Even though the exact mechanism of anesthetic action is not understood, it is generally agreed that the effect of an agent is directly proportional to the concentration, or more precisely, the partial pressure* of the anesthetic in

---

* The partial pressure of a gas is the pressure produced by the bombardment of molecules of a gas against a unit area of a wall of the container holding the gas. An increase in the density or concentration of molecules in the container will increase the number of bombardments and thereby increase the partial pressure of the gas. Partial pressure is usually expressed as millimeters of mercury or torr. The terms partial pressure and tension are used interchangeably. If more than one gas is present in a container, the tension of each gas is independent of the movements of the molecules of the other contained gases (Dalton's law). The total pressure is the sum of the pressure of each independent gas in the mixture.

the brain. By understanding the principles of anesthetic uptake and distribution, a skillful anesthetist is able to alter subtly the anesthetic tensions in a patient's brain and thereby vary the depth of anesthesia from moment to moment to suit the requirements of a surgical procedure.

The course of an inhalation anesthetic can be divided into three different phases:

1. Induction. The primary movement of the anesthetic agent is from the patient's lungs to the blood distributed to the brain.
2. Maintenance. This is the period during which the partial pressure of the anesthetic in the blood and brain is nearly equal to the partial pressure of the agent in the alveoli. In this phase, the movement of the anesthetic from the alveoli to the blood is closely matched with the amount of gas moving from the blood back into the alveoli. This stage is also referred to as *equilibrium* because of the nearly equal movements of gas in both directions.
3. Emergence. This is a stage at which the anesthetist purposely (or sometimes unwittingly) decreases the pressure of the anesthetic in the alveoli, and the movement of the gas is from a higher pressure gradient from the tissue (brain) to blood and into the lung.

Normal alveolar membranes provide no barrier to the movement of anesthetic gases in either direction. Gas movement between alveoli and blood is dependent on the dynamic interaction of three variables:

1. The concentration or partial pressure of the gas in the alveoli
2. The solubility of the gas in blood
3. The status of the blood in the pulmonary circulation

Alveolar Partial Pressure

The concentration of an anesthetic gas in the alveoli is the algebraic sum of the number of dynamic factors that affect the delivery and removal of the gas from the alveoli. An obvious way to increase alveolar gas concentration is to increase the inspired concentration of the anesthetic. However, only in a state of true equilibrium does the alveolar gas concentration approach that of the concentration of the inspired gas. An anesthetist must be aware that many factors can alter the concentration of an inspired gas as it approaches the alveoli. This is particularly true during the induction phase of anesthesia.

During the first breaths of an induction, the partial pressure of an inspired anesthetic is decreased most dramatically by the volume of exhaled inert gas (mostly nitrogen) moving from a patient's lungs and pulmonary circulation. This dilutional effect is exaggerated in patients who have a significant degree of obstructive lung disease because mixing of old and newly inspired concentrations can be delayed markedly in abnormal lungs. Anesthetic dilution can be somewhat overcome by preoxygenating, or more appropriately denitrogenating, a patient before the induction of an inhalational anesthetic. By having a patient breathe 100 percent oxygen before induction, much of the nitrogen will be removed from the patient's lung, enhancing induction with a greater movement of the gas toward the alveoli and the pulmonary circulation. It is important to remember that with a single inspiration of room air after a period of preoxygenation, the effort of several minutes of removing nitrogen from a patient's respiratory tree will be reversed.

Another effective way of overcoming the dilutional effects of residual lung contents is to markedly increase the volume of inspired gas delivered to a patient. A large volume of gas will wash the inert gas from the patient's lungs more rapidly than will a smaller delivered quantity of gas.

In the induction phase of an anesthetic, it is important to think in terms of not just the concentration of the anesthetic but also the actual volume of gas being delivered to the patient's pulmonary circulation. An anesthesiologist describing a routine IV induction would not say "the patient was given 2.5 percent thiopental"; more likely he or she would say "250 mg of thiopental was injected intravenously." The same type of thinking about the actual amount of agent being delivered to a patient should be considered when thinking about an inhalation induction.

The concentration of an anesthetic in the inspired gas can always be increased. This maneuver, however, may not necessarily increase the alveolar concentration of the agent. If the gas is irritating to the airway a sudden increase in concentration may provoke coughing, secretions, breath-holding, laryngospasm, and other unpleasant respiratory reflexes, leading to decreased minute ventilation. Gradual incremental increases in concentration of an anesthetic in the inspired gas mixture allow the airway to accommodate to these irritant effects. This is very important with such agents as ether and isoflurane but less significant with nonirritating nitrous oxide (N_2O) and halothane.

Respiratory depression is another factor that can markedly decrease the rate of delivery of an inspired gas to the alveoli. Decreased minute ventilation can be the result of a disease process or, more likely, the pharmacologic depression produced by preoperative medications (narcotic analgesics) or the anesthetic agents themselves. In the past, respiratory depression was overcome by allowing the patient's arterial P_{CO_2} to rise, stimulating ventilation. At present, respiratory depression is usually treated by mechanical assistance or control of ventilation.

Finally, alveolar anesthetic tension can be decreased by uptake of the agent into the pulmonary circulation. A high pressure gradient between alveolar gas and pulmonary venous blood enhances a movement of gas from the alveolus, thereby reducing alveolar tension. This movement is exaggerated during induction with increased cardiac output and high blood gas solubility.

Solubility of Anesthetic in Blood

The solubility of the anesthetic in blood is expressed as blood/gas partition coefficient, or Ostwald number (Table 13–1). This number represents the ratio of the concentration of an anesthetic in blood to the concentration in the gas phase at equilibrium. Blood/gas coefficients are simply de-

TABLE 13–1. PARTITION COEFFICIENTS (OSTWALD) OF WELL-KNOWN ANESTHETIC AGENTS

Anesthetic	Blood/Gas	Brain/Blood	Fat/Blood
Cyclopropane	0.46	1.3	21
Nitrous oxide	0.47	1.1	3
Isoflurane	1.4	3.7	45
Enflurane	1.8	2.6	105
Halothane	2.3	2.6	60
Ether	12.1	1.1	5
Methoxyflurane	13.0	2.0	63

termined by exposing a quantity of anesthetic gas to a volume of blood in a closed container. Initially, the gas will be dissolved into the blood, but at equilibrium, the number of molecules entering the blood will equal the number of molecules leaving to rejoin the gas. In other words, the partial pressure of the agent in the blood will equal that of the gas phase. At this point the concentration of anesthetic in each phase is measured, and the ratio of the concentration is the blood/gas coefficient.

The solubility of an anesthetic in blood plays an important role in the uptake and delivery of an agent to the brain. Blood acts not only as a carrier of an anesthetic but also as a reservoir. During induction with a very insoluble anesthetic agent, for example, N_2O or cyclopropane (blood/gas coefficient less than 0.5), the storage role of blood is minimal. Very little of the agent needs to be dissolved in the circulation before the partial pressure of the gas in arterial blood is high enough to permit the agent to be passed on to the brain. On the other hand, very soluble agents, such as ether and methoxyflurane (blood/gas coefficients greater than 12), may be as rapidly dissolved in blood, but a concentration of approximately 25 times greater than that of the insoluble agents is required before the gas reaches a partial pressure sufficient to pass the agent from the blood reservoir to tissue. In other words, a greater amount of soluble anesthetic must pass alveolar membranes to produce the same partial pressure in the circulation as that of an insoluble agent. Therefore, the tension in blood of a less soluble agent rises more quickly, and the onset of anesthesia is more rapid.

The transfer of gas from blood to tissue is dependent on three factors, very similar to those responsible for the transfer of gas to blood in the lungs:

1. The concentration or partial pressure of gas in arterial blood
2. The rate of delivery of the gas to tissue (or organ blood flow)
3. The relative solubility of the gas in tissue (blood/tissue solubility coefficient)

The same factors regulating delivery of an injected drug apply to the inhalational anesthetics. Vessel-rich tissues (heart, brain, and viscera) receive preferential blood flow over lean, fatty tissues. Anesthetic solubility in brain gray matter and other lean tissues plays a very minor role in

the relative rate of anesthetic induction.* In contrast to the variety of blood/gas solubilities of different anesthetic agents, brain/blood coefficients vary little more than unity (Table 13–1).

An example of the role properties of anesthetic agents play in the course of an induction is a contrast of the effects of ether and cyclopropane. Ether is a very soluble agent that is also extremely irritating to the airway. The inspired concentration must be gradually increased to allow the airway to adjust to its pungency. Because it is extremely soluble in blood, a great deal of the agent must be dissolved before the partial pressure of ether at the blood–brain barrier begins to approach that of the alveolus. An induction with ether may last from 7 to 30 minutes depending on the physical condition of the patient and the skill of the anesthetist. In contrast, cyclopropane is not very irritating and is insoluble in blood. Even though cyclopropane is a less potent anesthetic (minimum alveolar concentration [MAC] = 9.2 volumes percent) than ether (MAC = 1.9 volumes percent), a single breath of 50 percent cyclopropane can render a patient unconscious in the duration of one circulation time. The physical properties of the newer halogenated hydrocarbon anesthetics, halothane, enflurane, and isoflurane, fall between the extremes of cyclopropane and ether (Table 13–1), as do their pharmacologic properties.

SPECIAL CONSIDERATIONS ASSOCIATED WITH UPTAKE AND DISTRIBUTION OF NITROUS OXIDE

Even though N_2O is a benign and easily managed inhalational anesthetic, it has physical characteristics that call for special attention by a practicing anesthetist. The agent is very insoluble in blood (blood/gas partition coefficient = 0.47). N_2O is also a very weak anesthetic (MAC = 101 percent) and is usually given in 50 to 75 percent concentrations with oxygen. It may be combined with narcotics and other IV agents, or it is frequently used as a carrier gas for more potent volatile anesthetics.

During the induction of an anesthetic with high concentrations of N_2O, this very insoluble agent is rapidly absorbed by the pulmonary circulation from the alveolar gas, producing virtually a partial vacuum and pulling additional gas into the respiratory tree, thereby augmenting any mechanical ventilation. This supplementation of gas movement into the alveoli and alveolar circulation has been called the *concentration effect*.

When a high concentration of N_2O is used as a carrier gas with a much lower concentration of a potent inhalation agent (e.g., halothane), a phenomenon closely related to the concentration effect, known as the *second-gas effect*, occurs. The rapid movement of N_2O from the gas mixture in the alveoli increases the concentration or tension of the halothane in the alveoli and produces a more rapid passage

---

* *In contrast to lean organs, the solubility of anesthetics in fatty tissue varies considerably from agent to agent (Table 13–1). Since these organs receive a low percentage of cardiac output, their role in anesthetic uptake during induction is less important. Fat tissue plays a more relevant role in prolonged anesthetic uptake and subsequent emergence.*

of this second gas into the pulmonary circulation, resulting in an increase in the rate of induction of anesthesia.

The low solubility of N_2O in blood is usually viewed as an advantage of the agent. However, in some circumstances it can be a potential hazard. If blood saturated with N_2O contacts a compartment of gas in the body that does not contain N_2O, the N_2O in the blood will diffuse from the blood to reach an equilibrium with the gas in the enclosed space. This movement of N_2O from the circulation causes an increase in volume or pressure if the gas is tightly contained. If such a build-up of N_2O should occur during the placement of a graft during a tympanoplasty, the increase of pressure in the middle ear can interfere with the surgical procedure. The development of this same phenomenon during a pneumoencephalogram, or in the presence of a pneumothorax, or an air embolism could be devastating.

At the termination of N_2O anesthesia, the rapid movement of insoluble N_2O from the circulation into the pulmonary tree can produce a significant dilution of O_2 entering the lungs, resulting in a phenomenon known as *diffusion hypoxia*. This transient dilution of inspired O_2 should not be a problem in a patient with healthy lungs, but the hypoxia could be prolonged seriously in a patient with impaired ventilatory mixing. Diffusion hypoxia can be overcome easily by giving a patient supplemental O_2 in the first few minutes after the termination of N_2O anesthesia.

ENTERIC DRUG ADMINISTRATION

The most widely patient-accepted method of medication administration, the oral route, is probably the least used by anesthetists. With the exception of the occasional sedative prescribed to be given with water some time before an operation, anesthesia personnel are not happy with oral medication for several reasons.

First, anesthetists have a well-grounded fear of any possible cause for regurgitation and respiratory aspiration by an anesthetized patient. There is a tendency to take the nothing orally dictum almost too literally. Careful use of oral premedications does have a place in anesthesia practice and should not be ignored.

Second, and perhaps more important, is the problem of not being certain that everything taken orally by a patient will be absorbed by the gastrointestinal tract. Oral medication is relatively imprecise when compared to parenteral

or inhalational techniques. The problem was dramatically illustrated when a child who was thought to be susceptible to malignant hyperthermia was given a prophylactic treatment of oral dantrolene. Despite an appropriate 2-day regimen of dantrolene, the child experienced classic signs of malignant hyperthermia after a careful induction of anesthesia. It was speculated that the gastric irritation often produced by dantrolene inhibited the absorption of the medication. Fortunately, the child responded to subsequent IV administration of the drug.

A final problem associated with the oral administration of medication is related to drug metabolism. Some drugs (e.g., insulin) are denatured by gastric acidity or destroyed by digestive enzymes. Furthermore, the major portion of nutrients and medication absorbed from the gastrointestinal tract goes into the splanchnic circulation and passes through the liver before entering the systemic circulation. Drugs that are rapidly destroyed or inactivated by hepatic enzymes (e.g., most of the narcotic analgesics) are metabolized before they reach the peripheral circulation.

One form of enteric medication that has had varying degrees of acceptance by pediatric anesthetists is rectal hypnotics and sedatives. Intermediate-duration barbiturates (pentobarbital and secobarbital), available as rectal suppositories, can be used as premedication in children. Ultrashort-acting barbiturates (thiopental and methohexital) can be given rectally as a suspension or solution for the induction of anesthesia. The major problem with the use of rectal medications is that the absorption of the drug is very unpredictable because of expulsion or fecal obstruction. These factors can affect the onset and duration of drug activity.

BIBLIOGRAPHY

Albert A: Ionization, pH, and biological activity. Pharmacol Rev 4:136–167, 1952.

Eger EI: Anesthetic Uptake and Action. Baltimore, Williams & Wilkins, 1974.

Fitzgibbons DC: Malignant hyperthermia following preoperative administration of dantrolene. Anesthesiology 54:73–75, 1981.

Goodman LS, Gilman A: The Pharmacological Basis of Therapeutics, 7th ed. New York, Macmillan, 1985.

Hug CC: Pharmacokinetics of drugs administered intravenously. Anesth Analg 57:704–723, 1978.

Ketty SS: The theory and applications of the exchange of inert gas at the lungs and tissues. Pharmacol Rev 3:1–41, 1951.

14

Pharmacology of Inhalational Anesthetics

Jerrold H. Levy and John J. Savarese

*I*nhalational agents must be thought of as potent drugs with distinct pharmacologic and physiologic effects. The unique characteristics of each anesthetic agent must be considered before its use. Pharmocologic and physiochemical properties of the inhalational anesthetics and their effects on organ function are discussed in this chapter. Because, for example, one anesthetic agent may be better suited for use in neurosurgery than in cardiac or hepatic surgery, a major problem arises in patients with underlying multisystemic disease who require one operation with one anesthetic. A detailed knowledge of the inhalational agents and understanding of their organ effects are important in making a rational choice of agents in a clinical practice.

The original anesthetic agents, ether and cyclopropane, have been replaced by an entirely new class of pharmacologically active halogenated drugs. At present, nitrous oxide, halothane, enflurane, and isoflurane are the most commonly used inhalational anesthetics and are discussed in depth. Methoxyflurane, ether, and cyclopropane are mentioned briefly, although they are rarely used.

MINIMUM ALVEOLAR ANESTHETIC CONCENTRATION

The concept of anesthesia is to provide amnesia (transient loss of memory), analgesia (loss of pain), and muscle relaxation for an operation. The inhalational anesthetic agents all provide these prerequisites. Early in the development of the newer anesthetics, attempts were made to assess anesthetic potency. In the 1960s, Merkel and Eger established the concept of the minimal alveolar anesthetic concentration (MAC) required to abolish movement in response to a noxious stimulus. The noxious stimulus, as we clinically apply it, is the surgical manipulation, whether it is a skin incision, bone manipulation, or electrocautery of tissues. The concept as it was developed by Eger was the anesthetic partial pressure in the alveolus at equilibrium where 50 percent of the human subjects did not react to a skin incision by any "gross purposeful muscular movement." MAC is expressed in terms of percent of 1 atm.

The original studies by Eger et al involved exposing a human being or animal to a predetermined end-tidal (end-expiratory) anesthetic concentration of drug. This was held constant for approximately 15 minutes to achieve equilibrium among the alveolus, blood, and, most important, the brain. The stimulus was then applied. The concept of MAC is useful clinically as a standard of anesthetic potency, as a guide to clinical dosage, and as a means of comparing anesthetics during studies that require equipotent dosages.

Other considerations that are important in understanding the concept of MAC include the concomitant use of more than one drug. Although various medications may affect MAC, drugs that have specific analgesic or anesthetic effects will have additive effects when given together. For example, narcotics will decrease the MAC of any inhalational anesthetic agent. In sufficient quantities, narcotics can serve as the sole pharmacologic agent use for anesthesia. The use of narcotic premedicants will decrease the amount of inhalational agent required for an operation. Furthermore, MAC values are additive: 0.5 MAC of nitrous oxide (50 percent) and 0.5 MAC of halothane (0.37 percent) equals 1 MAC of anesthetic.

PHYSIOCHEMICAL PROPERTIES

Nitrous Oxide

Nitrous oxide is the most commonly used of all the inhalational agents, whether as an adjuvant to a more potent inhalational agent or as a primary anesthetic. It was introduced in the early 1840s when a chemist (Horace Wells) traveled the country giving public demonstrations of the effects of nitrous oxide for an admission charge of 25 cents.

Nitrous oxide is an odorless, colorless gas, which is stored in cylinders in a liquid form at 50 atm of pressure. The blood/gas partition coefficient at 37C is 0.47. The MAC of nitrous oxide is 100 percent, an obviously anoxic mixture. In 40 to 70 percent inspired concentrations it is used to supplement other anesthetic agents. Its other physiochemical properties are listed in Table 14–1.

TABLE 14–1. PROPERTIES OF INHALED ANESTHETICS

	Isoflurane (Forane)	Euflurane (Ethrane)	Halothane (Fluothane)	Methoxyflurane (Penthrane)	Nitrous Oxide
	$HC-O-CHCF_3$ (with F above and F, Cl below)	$CH-O-C-CH$ (with F above and F, F, Cl below)	$F-C-CH$ (with F, Br above and F, Cl below)	$H_3C-O-C-CH$ (with F, Cl above and F, Cl below)	$N{\equiv}N{=}O$
Molecular weight (g)	184.0	184.5	197.4	165.0	44.0
Boiling point (at 760 torr)	48.5C	56.5C	50.2C	104.7C	—
Specific gravity	1.50	1.52 (24C)	1.86 (22C)	1.41 (25C)	—
Vapor pressure (torr)	250.0	175.0 (20C)	243.0 (20C)	25.0 (20C)	—
		356.0 (37C)	480.0 (37C)	56.0 (37C)	—
Odor	Pleasant, pungent	Pleasant, ethereal	Pleasant, sweet	Pleasant, fruity	Pleasant, sweet
Preservative	Not necessary	Not necessary	Necessary	Necessary	Not necessary
Stability to					
Metal	Nonreactive	Nonreactive	May react	May react	Nonreactive
Alkali	Stable	Stable	Slight decomposition	Decomposes	Stable
Ultraviolet light	Stable	Stable	Decomposes	Decomposes	Stable
Explosiveness	None	None	None	None	None
Partition coefficients					
Blood/gas	1.4	1.9	2.3	13.0	0.47
Brain/gas	3.65	2.6	4.1	22.1	0.50
Fat/gas	94.5	105.0	185.0	890.0	1.22
Liver/gas	3.50	3.8	7.2	24.8	0.38
Muscle/gas	5.6	3.0	6.0	20.0	0.54
Oil/gas	97.8	98.5	224.0	930.0	1.4
Water/gas	0.61	0.8	0.7	4.5	0.47
Rubber/gas (at 23 C)	0.62	74.0	120.0	630.0	1.2
Minimum alveolar concentration (MAC) for humans (aged 19–30) at 1 atm % in					
100% Oxygen	1.3	1.7	0.75	0.16	110
70% N_2O	0.56	0.57	0.29	0.07	—
% recovered as metabolites (approx.)	0.2	2.4	15–20	50	—

From Wade JG, Stevens WC: Anesth Analg 60:666, 1981.

Halothane

Halothane is a volatile anesthetic agent. It is a liquid at room temperature and is readily vaporized by passing a carrier gas, such as oxygen, through the liquid. It was originally introduced by the British Medical Research Council after they had established a committee to investigate the use of nonexplosive agents. It is nonflammable and nonexplosive.

Halothane is a halogenated hydrocarbon with the structure shown in Table 14–1. It differs from diethyl ether, isoflurane, and enflurane because it does not contain the ether (—C—O—C—) configuration. Halothane has a molecular weight of 197, and its vapor pressure at 20C is 243 torr. The blood/gas partition coefficient at 37C is 2.3, and the MAC in humans is 0.75 percent. Other physiochemical properties are listed in Table 14–1.

Enflurane

Enflurane is a nonflammable, volatile liquid anesthetic. Its molecular weight is 184, and its vapor pressure is 171 torr at 20C. Enflurane has an odor similar to ether's. The MAC in humans is 1.68 percent in oxygen, and the blood/gas partition coefficient at 37C is 1.91. Its structural formula and additional physiochemical properties are listed in Table 14–1. Enflurane is readily vaporized by passing a carrier gas, such as oxygen, through the liquid.

Isoflurane

Isoflurane, an isomer of enflurane, is a clear, colorless volatile liquid with a pungent, musty odor. Its molecular weight is 184, and its vapor pressure is 238 torr at 20C. The blood/gas partition coefficient at 37C is 1.43. Isoflurane is the newest of the halogenated ethers to be introduced into clinical practice. The structural formula and additional physiochemical properties are listed in Table 14–1.

Methoxyflurane

Methoxyflurane is a clear, colorless liquid with a sweet, fruity odor. The vapor pressure at 20C is 25 torr. It is the most potent of all of the inhalational agents, with a MAC of 0.16 percent. Induction time is very slow because of its high blood/gas partition coefficient of 13 and high oil/gas coefficient of 900. Other physiochemical properites are listed in Table 14–1.

Cyclopropane

Cyclopropane is a colorless gas with an odor resembling that of petroleum ether. Its blood/gas partition coefficient at 37C is 0.46. It is explosive in concentrations as low as 2.4 percent. The MAC for cyclopropane is 9.2.

Diethyl Ether

Diethy ether was one of the first anesthetics to be used. It was first introduced in the mid-19th century by William T. G. Morton, a dentist at the Massachusetts General Hospital. It is still in common use in some parts of the world today. Ether is a volatile liquid with a boiling point of 36.5C. At 20C, it has a vapor pressure of 450 torr. The MAC for either is 1.9 percent, and it is explosive.

RESPIRATORY EFFECTS

Although all of the inhalational anesthetics may affect ventilation to some degree, these changes, as measured by carbon dioxide retention, can be further augmented by narcotics. Narcotics in general decrease the responsiveness of the brainstem, which normally regulates ventilation, to carbon dioxide. In view of the common use of narcotic premedicants, patients who are allowed to breathe spontaneously may have further respiratory depression in addition to the general respiratory depressant effects of the inhalational anesthetics.

Nitrous Oxide

Nitrous oxide causes minimal respiratory depression, even when delivered at 1 MAC in a pressure chamber (Fig. 14–1). When used in combination with other anesthetics, the

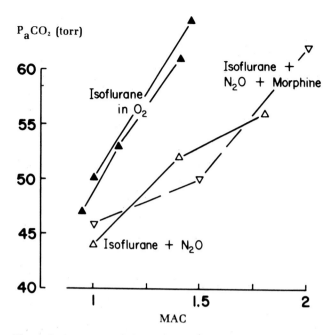

Figure 14–2. Values for $Paco_2$ versus MAC in unstimulated patients given isoflurane in oxygen, 70 percent nitrous oxide, and 70 percent nitrous oxide with 0.15 mg/kg morphine (*From Eger EI II: Isoflurane (Forane): A Compendium and Reference,* 2nd ed. Madison, WI, Anaquest, BOC, 1985.)

replacement of the more potent inhalational agents by nitrous oxide may decrease the respiratory depression (Fig. 14–2).

Halothane

Halothane decrease the ventilatory response to arterial carbon dioxide in normal patients but is less potent than either enflurane or isoflurane in this regard (Figs. 14–1, 14–3). Halothane will also decrease the ventilatory response to hypoxia. This is evident even at 0.1 MAC, whereas no response to hypoxemia is seen with any inhalational agent at 1.1 MAC (Fig. 14–4). Surgical stimulation will increase minute ventilation and decreases $Paco_2$ by increasing both tidal volume and respiratory rate (Figs. 14–5, 14–6), but this response can be ablated by increasing the depth of anesthesia. Minute ventilation may remain constant with increases in halothane concentrations from 1 to 2 MAC, but $Paco_2$ may rise (Figs. 14–6, 14–7). This is due to changes in the dead space:tidal volume ratios with less efficient ventilation (i.e., a rapid respiratory rate and shallow tidal volume) (Fig. 14–7).

Halothane is a potent bronchodilator and may be the agent of choice for use in asthmatics. The effects may be related to its ability to suppress airway reflexes. Because halothane is so potent in suppressing airway reflexes, it is useful in the management of patients with difficult airways (e.g., tracheal stenosis, croup, epiglottitis, or laryngeal tumors) and is used with 100 percent oxygen. It is still the agent of choice among many anesthetists for patients with irritable airways (e.g., chronic obstructive pulmonary disease, asthma, or bronchitis).

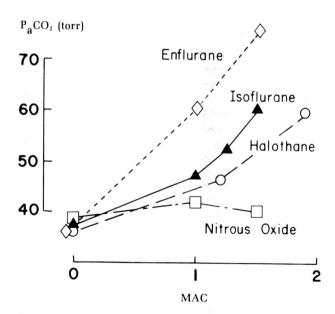

Figure 14–1. Arterial Pco_2 during spontaneous ventilation in unstimulated volunteers awake and during anesthesia. Nitrous oxide was administered in a pressure chamber. (*From Eger EI II: Isoflurane (Forane): A Compendium and Reference,* 2nd ed. Madison, WI, Anaquest, BOC, 1985.)

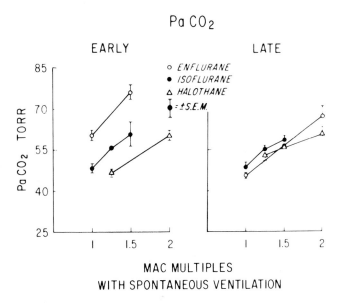

PaCO₂

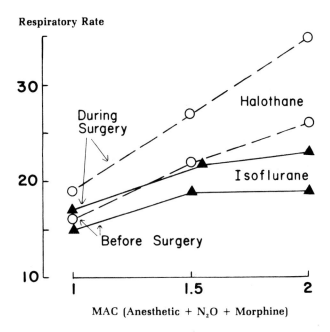

Respiratory Rate

Figure 14–3. Arterial P_{CO_2} changes produced during spontaneous ventilation during the first hour of halothane and isoflurane administration, during the second hour of enflurane administration, and later during the fifth hour of anesthesia. (*From Calverley RK, Smith NT, et al.: Anesth Analg 57:610, 1978*).

Figure 14–5. Increases in respiratory rate caused by the stimulus of surgery. (*From Eger El II: Isoflurane (Forane): A Compendium and Reference, 2nd ed. Madison, WI, Anaquest, BOC, 1985.*)

Enflurane

Enflurane is the most potent respiratory depressant anesthetic vapor used in humans. In unstimulated patients the Pa_{CO_2} at 1 MAC is 60 torr and increases as anesthesia is deepened (Figs. 14–1, 14–3). This Pa_{CO_2} increase may trend back toward normal to some extent over time (Fig. 14–3). Enflurane produces profound respiratory depression (Fig. 14–4) with little response to hypoxia. It has an ether-type odor that sometimes produces coughing and breath holding. This is seen more often if the anesthetic concentration is increased too rapidly. The effects on respiration are similar to those produced by isoflurane.

Isoflurane

Isoflurane is a potent respiratory depressant. In unstimulated patients during spontaneous ventilation, the Pa_{CO_2} at 1 MAC and 1.5 MAC is approximately 50 torr and 65 torr, respectively (Figs. 14–1, 14–3). Deepening anesthesia with isoflurane causes decreases in tidal volume but not in respiratory rate (Fig. 14–7). Isoflurane, when adminis-

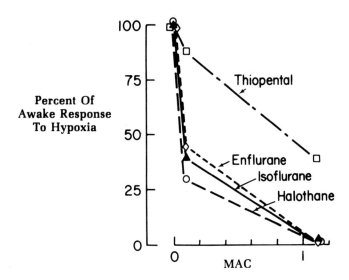

Figure 14–4. Ventilatory response to imposed decreases in Pa_{O_2} in humans. (*From Eger El II: Isoflurane (Forane): A Compendium and Reference, 2nd ed. Madison, WI, Anaquest, BOC, 1985.*)

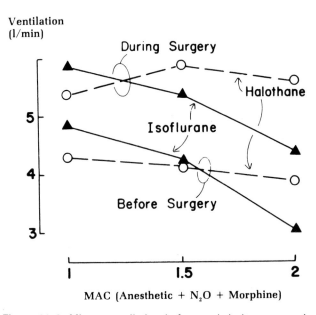

Figure 14–6. Minute ventilation before and during surgery in healthy patients. Morphine, 0.15 mg/kg, was administered 15 minutes before induction, and halothane or isoflurane was administered in 70 percent nitrous oxide. (*From Eger El II: Isoflurane (Forane): A Compendium and Reference, 2nd ed. Madison, WI, Anaquest, BOC, 1985.*)

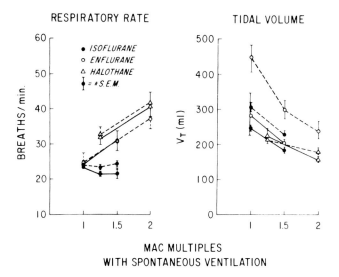

RESPIRATORY RATE   TIDAL VOLUME

• ISOFLURANE
○ ENFLURANE
△ HALOTHANE
= ± S.E.M.

MAC MULTIPLES
WITH SPONTANEOUS VENTILATION

Figure 14–7. Respiratory rate and tidal volume during spontaneous ventilation in patients during the first hour of isoflurane and halothane anesthesia, during the second hour of enflurane anesthesia (solid line), during the fifth hour of halothane and isoflurane anesthsia, and during the seventh hour of enflurane anesthesia (broken line).

tered with nitrous oxide, causes less hypercapnia at equivalent levels of anesthesia than those agents depicted (Fig. 14–2). Surgical stimulation will decrease arterial Pa_{CO_2} by 5 to 13 torr by increasing minute ventilation (Fig. 14–6).

As do the other agents, isoflurane produces profound reductions in the normal ventilatory responses to hypoxia (Fig. 14–4). Pulmonary airway resistance increases during isoflurane anesthesia. Isoflurane has a musty, pungent odor that may irritate airways and induce breath holding and coughing during induction, especially without barbiturates or narcotics as adjuvants. Isoflurane may cause pulmonary vasodilation and reverse hypoxic pulmonary vasoconstriction, which may produce changes in intrapulmonary shunts. However, this is usually not a problem.

Methoxyflurane

Methoxyflurane is a potent respiratory depressant that causes decreasing tidal volume but does not change respiratory rate. It is nonirritating to the airways, has a pleasant odor, and does not stimulate tracheobronchial secretions.

Cyclopropane

Cyclopropane is a respiratory depressant that decreases the ventilatory response to inspired Pa_{CO_2}. Respiratory rate increases and tidal volume decreases as the depth of anesthesia is increased. Cyclopropane is not irritating to the tracheobronchial tree.

Diethyl Ether

Diethyl ether increases the respiratory rate and minute ventilation and maintains normal Pa_{CO_2} levels during anesthesia, up to 2 MAC. With increasing concentrations, the sensi-

tivity of the respiratory response is reduced. Diethyl ether is a direct bronchodilator and stimulates tracheobronchial secretions.

CARDIOVASCULAR EFFECTS

Nitrous Oxide

Nitrous oxide is a relatively weak myocardial depressant that decreases both cardiac contractility and heart rate. Systemic vascular resistance can increase approximately 20 percent with the use of nitrous oxide because of sympathetic stimulation. The net effect of these changes in healthy people is a small increase in arterial pressure (Fig. 14–8). Although there are fewer myocardial depressant effects with nitrous oxide than with other more potent inhalational agents, as reflected by changes in stroke volume (Fig. 14–9), nitrous oxide must nevertheless be used with some caution in people with poor ventricular function. Nitrous oxide will also increase pulmonary vascular resistance and must be used with caution in patients with pulmonary hypertension.

Halothane

Halothane produces cardiovascular depression by a direct effect on the heart and sympathetic nervous system. This dose-dependent depression of left ventricular function can produce profound hypotension (Fig. 14–8) in patients with compromised ventricular function (e.g., congestive heart failure or coronary arterial disease with prior myocardial infarction). Depression of the medullary vasomotor center (part of the sympathetic central nervous system) by halo-

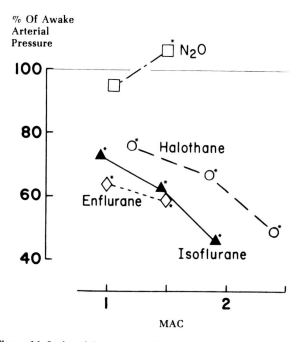

% Of Awake
Arterial
Pressure

N_2O

Halothane

Enflurane

Isoflurane

MAC

Figure 14–8. Arterial pressure with controlled ventilation during nitrous oxide, halothane, isoflurane, and enflurane in oxygen anesthesia. Values are expressed as percentage of awake arterial pressure. (*From Eger El II: Isoflurane (Forane): A Compendium and Reference, 2nd ed. Madison, WI, Anaquest, BOC, 1985.*)

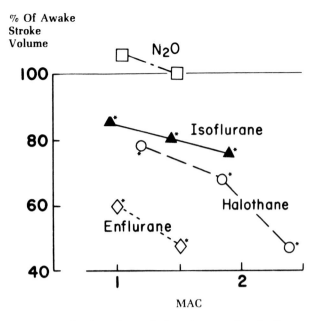

% Of Awake
Stroke
Volume

Figure 14–9. Stroke volume during nitrous oxide, isoflurane, halothane, and enflurane in oxygen anesthesia. Values are expressed as percentage of awake stroke volume. Asterisks indicate significant changes from values during the awake state. (*From Eger El II: Isoflurane (Forane): A Compendium and Reference, 2nd ed. Madison, WI, Anaquest, BOC, 1985.*)

thane or other inhalational anesthetics can result in profound hypotension in volume-depleted patients. Use of any potent gas or vapor anesthetic for patients in shock from any cause (hemorrhagic, cardiogenic, anaphylactic, septic, or neurogenic) can cause further depression of cardiovascular function and inhibition of compensatory reflexes and result in the need for cardiopulmonary support. The cardiovascular depression is due to interference with calcium—protein binding in sarcoplasmic reticulum. Healthy patients, however, tolerate the cardiovascular depression produced by halothane and other agents with minimal difficulty. Halothane produces decreases in cardiac output and arterial pressure and an elevation of left ventricular filling pressures, as measured by left ventricular end diastolic pressure (Figs. 14–8, 14–10, 14–11).

Halothane has profound effects on heart rhythm and rate, in addition to its effects on hemodynamic function. It sensitizes the myocardium to the effects of both endogenous and exogenous catecholamines, producing premature ventricular contractions and other ventricular arrhythmias, particularly if hypercarbia caused by hypoventilation is present. If epinephrine is to be used with halothane anesthesia, the dose of epinephrine should be limited to 1 to 1.5 µg/kg per 10 minutes, not to exceed 4 µg/kg per hour. Halothane can decrease conduction time in both the His-Purkinje and atrioventricular (AV) nodal pathways. This mechanism may produce clinical nodal rhythm with loss of the atrial contraction component for ventricular filling. Atrial filling of the ventricle normally contributes 15 to 25 percent of the left ventricular volume before ejection. This may increase to as high as 50 percent in patients with poor left ventricular function or with valvular obstruction to ven-

tricular filling in mitral stenosis. Halothane should be used cautiously in these patients because the development of nodal rhythm may seriously impair cardiac output and maintenance of adequate systemic pressures.

Enflurane

Enflurane produces a dose-related cardiovascular depression. In healthy patients, the initial changes are a dose-related depression of stroke volume and cardiac output with a decrease in arterial pressure (Figs. 14–8, 14–12). Tachycardia may occur to some extent in spontaneously breathing patients, but this may be related to increases in Pa_{CO_2}. During prolonged enflurane anesthesia at light levels, some recovery in cardiac output may occur (Fig. 14–12). Hypotension is a consistent sign of excessive enflurane concentration.

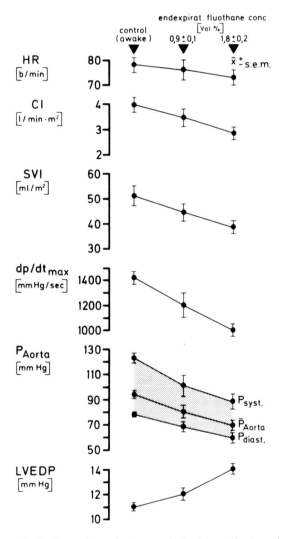

Figure 14–10. Hemodynamic changes in healthy patients undergoing halothane in oxygen anesthesia. CI = cardiac index; dp/dt max = change in pressure/change in time maximum; HR = heart rate; LVEDP = left ventricular end-diastolic pressure; P aorta = aortic pressure; SVI = stroke volume index. (*From Sonntag H, Donath U, et al: Anesthesiology 48:320, 1978.*)

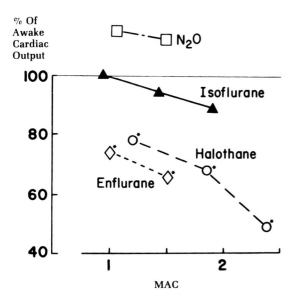

Figure 14–11. Cardiac output during nitrous oxide, isoflurane, halothane, and enflurane in oxygen anesthesia. Values are expressed as percentage of awake cardiac output. (*From Eger EI II: Isoflurane (Forane): A Compendium and Reference, 2nd ed. Madison, WI, Anaquest, BOC, 1985.*)

The mechanism of cardiovascular depression is thought to be interference with calcium–protein binding in the sarcoplasmic reticulum, as well as in the tropomyosin of cardiac myofibrils. Although it was initially reported that enflurane depressed myocardial contractility more than did halothane in equianalgesic concentrations, clinically this may not be noticeable because of enflurane's ability to produce vasodilation. Because blood pressure is a function of cardiac output and peripheral vascular resistance, less cardiovascular depression may be seen when peripheral resistance is also lowered.

Enflurane does not sensitize the myocardium to catecholamines. It does, however, increase induction time in the His-Purkinje and AV node conduction pathways of the heart, producing AV nodal rhythm.

Isoflurane

Isoflurane, like other halogenated hydrocarbons, decreases myocardial contractility, producing a decrease in stroke volume and arterial pressure (Figs. 14–9, 14–10). At equipotent doses in vitro, these effects are comparable to those of halothane and methoxyflurane but are greater than the effects of diethyl ether or enflurane. In contrast to studies in the isolated heart, studies in humans suggest that isoflurane produces less depression of cardiac output than does halothane or enflurane at concentrations from 1 to 2 MAC (Fig. 14–11). Cardiac output is maintained by an increase in heart rate and decrease in vascular resistance, which occurs in these dose ranges. The use of nitrous oxide with isoflurane produces less hypotension than does isoflurane–oxygen at equivalent doses. This may be due to nitrous oxide produc-

ing an increase in sympathetic tone and increases in peripheral vascular resistance with lower concentrations of isoflurane.

Isoflurane does not sensitize the myocardium to catecholamines. Approximately three times the injected dose of epinephrine that causes arrhythmias under halothane is tolerated without producing arrhythmias under isoflurane. Isoflurane has little effect on the His-Purkinje or AV node conduction time and produces a stable cardiac rhythm. Isoflurane may have a stimulating effect on heart rate, producing tachycardia during induction. In patients who require slow heart rates (e.g., valvular stenosis or coronary arterial disease), it may not be the inhalational agent of choice.

Methoxyflurane

The effects of methoxyflurane on the cardiovascular system are very similar to those of halothane. It is a myocardial depressant and decreases cardiac output and blood pressure. Deeper levels of anesthesia can produce an AV nodal rhythm.

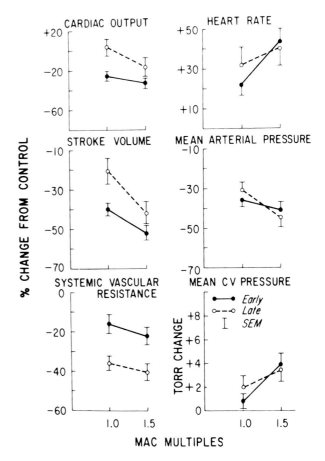

Figure 14–12. Percent changes from control values in some cardiovascular variables during continuous enflurane anesthesia in the first hour (solid line) and in the sixth hour (broken line) of anesthesia. (*From Calverley RK, Smith NT, et al: Anesth Analg 57:619, 1978.*)

Cyclopropane

There are minimal cardiovascular changes associated with the use of cyclopropane at concentrations required for general anesthesia. Cyclopropane produces an increase in sympathetic nervous system activity, which maintains both cardiac output and peripheral vascular resistance, and was once the agent of choice for the patient in shock for this reason. However, it markedly sensitizes the myocardium to both endogenous and exogenous catecholamines.

Diethyl Ether

Diethyl ether is a myocardial depressant but also produces an increase in sympathetic tone. Clinically, ether produces relative circulatory stability at levels required for surgical anesthesia. It does not sensitize the myocardium to catecholamines.

CENTRAL NERVOUS SYSTEM

Nitrous Oxide

Nitrous oxide, when used alone, causes a 20 to 200 percent increase in cerebral blood flow and an increase in cerebral metabolic rate (Fig. 14–13). These effects are easily modified by the concomitant use of other drugs and, particularly, prior administration of barbiturates (Fig. 14–13). In patients with head trauma, concentrations of 50 percent nitrous oxide can cause clinically significant increases in intracranial pressure. Nitrous oxide may have variable effects on the EEG, ranging from no changes to a loss of alpha rhythm and the appearance of theta waves.

Halothane

Halothane is the most potent cerebral vasodilator of all the halogenated inhalational anesthetic agents. The greatest increase in cerebral blood flow occurs at from 0.6 to 1.6 MAC, with an almost 200 percent increase in flow at 1.6 MAC (Figs. 14–13, 14–14). Halothane, however, decreases cerebral metabolic rate (Fig. 14–13). The brain normally autoregulates cerebral blood flow over a range of mean arterial pressures from 50 to 150 torr (Fig. 14–15). The normal flow in humans in a resting state is 50 ml/minute per 100 g of tissue. The arterial $Paco_2$ is also important in regulating

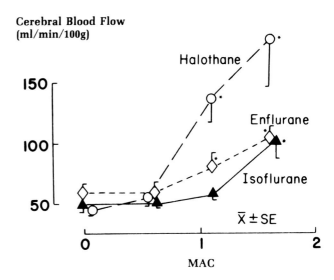

Cerebral Blood Flow
(ml/min/100g)

Figure 14–14. Cerebral blood flow in volunteers during halothane, enflurane, and isoflurane in oxygen anesthesia. Systemic blood pressure and $Paco_2$ were kept at normal levels. (*From Eger El II: Isoflurane (Forane): A Compendium and Reference, 2nd ed. Madison, WI, Anaquest, BOC, 1985.*)

blood flow, since carbon dioxide is a cerebral vasodilator (Fig. 14–15). At low concentrations, the volatile agents have minimal effects on autoregulation of cerebral blood flow. As the inspired concentration is increased, halothane increases flow until systemic hypotension reduces cerebral perfusion pressure (cerebral perfusion pressure equals mean arterial pressure minus intracranial pressure). The concomitant use of barbiturates with the inhalational agents decreases cerebral blood flow.

Enflurane

Enflurane causes an increase in cerebral blood flow and a decrease in cerebral metabolic rate (Fig. 14–13). At 1.1 MAC in humans, enflurane increases cerebral blood flow 38 percent and is less of a cerebral vasodilator than halothane (Fig. 14–14). Enflurane is unique in its ability to affect the electroencephalogram (EEG). At doses greater than 1.5 MAC, enflurane acts as a central nervous system irritant, producing spike wave activity on the EEG. When this oc-

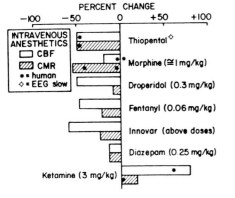

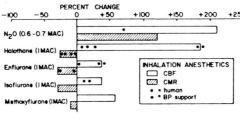

Figure 14–13. Overall effects of commonly used anesthetic agents on cerebral blood flow and metabolism. CBF = cerebral blood flow; CMR = cerebral metabolic rate; EEG = electroencephalogram. (*From Shapiro HM: Neuroanesthesia: Physiologic and pharmacologic principles. American Society of Anesthesiologists. Refresher Course Lectures, 1980.*)

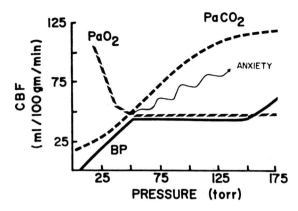

Figure 14–15. Overall cerebral blood flow responses to common physiologic stimuli.

curs, auditory stimuli can produce generalized seizure activity. The potential of any inhalational agent to cause seizures is related to the number of substituted halogenated groups. Hypocapnia with enflurane anesthesia may potentiate the epileptogenic effects of this agent.

Isoflurane

Isoflurane decreases cerebral metabolic rate but increases cerebral blood flow (Fig. 14–13). At a concentration of 1.1 MAC, cerebral blood flow increases 18 percent (Fig. 14–14). Although structurally similar to enflurane (its isomer), it does not induce spike activity on the EEG or cause electroencephalographic convulsive activity. Although isoflurane is the newest of the currently inhaled agents in clinical practice, it may ultimately prove to be the most useful of the inhalational anesthetics for neurosurgical procedures.

METABOLISM OF INHALATION ANESTHETICS

Originally, the inhalational agents were thought to be inert materials that did not undergo metabolic activity within the body, in contrast to the relatively high degree of metabolic activity of intravenous agents. Today we know this is not the case, and some inhalation agents may be metabolized to a considerable extent. Metabolism of these drugs, in general, may produce a product that is inert or possibly more toxic than the unmetabolized form. The liver is the primary site of metabolism of all inhalation agents. The smooth endoplasmic reticulum contains the enzyme system (the cytochrome P450 oxidizing system) responsible for metabolism of anesthetic agents. The kidney, as an excretory organ, eliminates the products of metabolism, which are usually more water-soluble than is the parent compound. Therefore, both the liver and the kidney may be target organs of toxic metabolites.

Nitrous Oxide

There is no evidence in humans that nitrous oxide is metabolized. Nitrous oxide can inactivate methionine synthetase and might ultimately affect DNA synthesis, although this has not been proven conclusively.

Halothane

Halothane undergoes significant metabolism in humans. Trifluoroacetic acid, its major metabolite, and, to a lesser degree, chloride and bromide ions are eliminated in the urine. Patients who are taking certain drugs that are known to induce hepatic microsomal enzymes (phenobarbital or phenytoin) may have increased halothane metabolism, although this has not been proven. Approximately 10 to 20 percent of absorbed halothane is metabolized and recovered as urinary metabolites in humans. The pathway of halothane metabolism and its implications in halothane hepatitis are discussed separately.

Enflurane

Enflurane is only slightly metabolized in humans, and pretreatment with enzyme inducers only slightly increases its metabolism. Approximately 2.5 percent of absorbed enflurane undergoes metabolic change, with only 0.5 to 1 percent of the dose metabolized releasing fluoride ions.

Isoflurane

Isoflurane undergoes an extremely low degree of metabolism in humans, being the least metabolized of all the halogenated agents currently used. Less than 0.25 percent of an absorbed dose of isoflurane is metabolized. Approximately 0.17 percent of the uptake is recovered as urinary metabolites in humans.

Methoxyflurane

Although methoxyflurane is not often used, it is of historical interest as the most extensively metabolized inhalation anesthetic agent. The major metabolites in humans are fluoride ions and dichloroacetic acid. The metabolism of methoxyflurane is increased after treatment with phenobarbital and phenytoin. Approximately 50 percent of the uptake of methoxyflurane is recovered as urinary metabolites in humans.

HEPATIC EFFECTS

Although abnormal liver function test results occur commonly after surgery (more frequently after abdominal surgery), the clinical importance of these findings is not clear. Sodium sulfobromophthalein (Bromsulphalein, BSP) excretion tests are sensitive indicators of hepatocellular dysfunction. BSP retention may occur in the absence of liver enzyme elevation, with alterations in hepatic flow, and postoperatively. Halothane, enflurane, and isoflurane all produce BSP retention in patients without any known clinical sequelae.

It is believed that the halogenated inhalational agents are not hepatotoxic, but their metabolic products or formed intermediate compounds may be. Three mechanisms were proposed by Brown to explain hepatic damage after the reactive metabolite formation of inhalational agents through reductive (nonoxygen-dependent) pathways.

1. Lipoperoxidation. Free radicals, formed as intermediate compounds of metabolism, remove hydrogen and incorporate oxygen into long-chain fatty acids of cellular membranes and organelles. This event causes the breakdown of structural, synthetic, and metabolic processes within the cell, with ensuing cellular destruction.
2. Antioxidant depletion. Reactive intermediate compounds deplete the levels of antioxidants intracellularly and intensify free radical reactions (i.e., lipoperoxidation). Normally, glutathione and alphatocopherol inhibit free radical reactions.
3. Covalent binding. Reactive intermediates bind to lipids and proteins and alter their structure and function. This causes a loss of cellular homeostasis and cellular death. There are certain conditions that favor the formation of reductive intermediates in experimental animals. Both hypoxia and hypotension favor the formation of metabolic products through reductive pathways.

Halothane

Halothane causes a 30 percent reduction in hepatic blood flow at 1.5 to 2 MAC. This agent has been implicated as possibly causing liver damage, especially upon reexposure at short intervals. The diagnosis is made on the clinical findings of unexplained fever, eosinophilia, rashes, and abnormal liver function tests within 2 weeks postoperatively, especially after a repeat exposure. It is postulated to be caused by a hypersensitivity-type reaction to a metabolite of halothane. The syndrome is more common in older and obese patients and has not been seen in pediatric populations. Although the National Halothane Study showed that halothane is a safe agent with a low incidence of hepatic necrosis, it may be best to avoid its use in patients with previous liver disease and to repeat exposures within short time intervals.

PHARMACOLOGIC PROPERTIES—RENAL

All of the known inhalational agents can affect renal function. The halogenated agents produce dose-dependent decreases in renal blood flow and glomerular filtration rate (GFR) (Figs. 14–16, 14–17), thus impairing the autoregulation that normally occurs in the kidney. In normovolemic patients this may not be important. In patients who are volume-depleted, these changes may result in further reductions in urine output and potentially affect postoperative renal function. These alterations may be a result of changes in the sympathetic nervous system, stress hormones, or a direct effect of the halogenated agents or their metabolic products. Urine output must be monitored in patients undergoing major surgery, extended surgery, or patients with impaired renal function. The clinical use of enflurane and methoxyflurane is considered separately, because they are able to release free fluoride ions, which can cause renal toxicity.

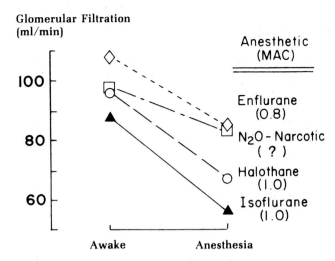

Figure 14–16. Renal blood flow as determined by para-aminohippuric acid (PAH) clearance in patients during enflurane, halothane, nitrous oxide–narcotic, and isoflurane anesthesia. (*From Eger El II: Isoflurane (Forane): A Compendium and Reference, 2nd ed. Madison, WI, Anaquest, BOC, 1985.*)

Enflurane

Enflurane has been shown to liberate fluoride ions during clinical use. If 1 MAC anesthesia is maintained for several hours, the serum level of fluoride is clinically insignificant. A 1.5 MAC level of enflurane for 6 and 10 hours of anesthesia will produce serum fluoride levels of 30 and 50 μM, respectively. At fluoride levels of 50 μM, transient renal dysfunction may occur, producing an inability to concentrate the urine. Because enflurane has a low potential for producing tubular dysfunction under such conditions, it should be

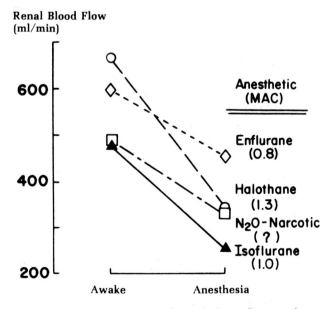

Figure 14–17. Urine flow in patients during enflurane, nitrous oxide–narcotic, halothane, and isoflurane anesthesia. (*From Eger El II: Isoflurane (Forane): A Compendium and Reference, 2nd ed. Madison, WI, Anaquest, BOC, 1985.*)

used cautiously in patients with preexisting renal disease or in those undergoing renal transplantation.

Methoxyflurane

Methoxyflurane undergoes substantial metabolism and can rapidly produce clinically significant serum fluoride levels. At 2.5 and 5 MAC hours, serum fluoride levels reach 50 to 60 μM and 90 to 120 μM, respectively. As serum fluoride levels increase greater than 50 μM, inability to reabsorb water in the tubules occurs. Methoxyflurane, therefore, produces a vasopressin-resistant polyuria characterized by serum hyperosmolarity, hypernatremia, polyuria, and urine hypo-osmolarity. For these reasons, methoxyflurane has only limited clinical use.

NEUROMUSCULAR EFFECTS

Halothane, enflurane, and isoflurane potentiate the effects of the nondepolarizing agents on neuromuscular blockade. This varies with equipotent doses of different inhalational agents. The degree of potentiation increases with anesthetic depth. At 1.25 MAC levels of enflurane and isoflurane, only approximately 30 percent as much D-tubocurarine is required to produce equal blockade as is required with nitrous oxide–narcotic. At the same MAC level of halothane, only 50 percent as much D-tubocurarine is required. The halogenated anesthetics produce slight augmentation of blockade when used with the depolarizing agent, succinylcholine.

UTERINE EFFECTS

Halothane, enflurane, and isoflurane all produce a dose-related depression of uterine contractility and frequency of contractions. All three agents increase uterine bleeding after abortion and cesarean section and should be used cautiously. In studies of the effects of halothane and isoflurane in pregnant ewes, both agents caused similar decreases in maternal blood pressure and uterine blood flow at MAC levels from 1 to 2.

Uterine tone is relatively well maintained with ether and cyclopropane. Although ether does not depress myometrial contractions at concentrations needed for delivery, it causes profound nausea and vomiting and was an unpopular and dangerous agent. It is no longer used in obstetric centers.

STRESS RESPONSES

Stress during anesthesia is assessed by the levels of catecholamines, cortisol, antidiuretic hormone, insulin, growth hormone, and other hormones that are part of the human physiologic systems that maintain homeostasis. Whether or not the blocking of the stress hormonal responses to a surgical stimulus is important in humans still remains to be documented. After surgical stimulation, significant increases in antidiuretic hormone, cortisol, and aldosterone occurred in patients receiving halothane but did not occur in patients receiving high-dose fentanyl. The increase in

stress response hormones in patients receiving halothane was associated with a decrease in creatinine clearance (a measure of renal blood flow and GFR). There were no differences in the clinical outcome in the two groups. The failure of the inhalational anesthetic agents to inhibit the release of stress hormones may explain the transient decreases in renal function associated with halothane, enflurane, and isoflurane use. Fentanyl, in contrast, has been shown to prevent increases in antidiuretic hormone associated with surgery.

SPECIAL CONSIDERATIONS

Nitrous oxide is far more soluble in blood than is nitrogen. This physiochemical characteristic in combination with increased alveolar partial pressures causes it to diffuse readily into the hollow structures of the body and expand these air-filled spaces. A pneumothorax can rapidly increase in volume if nitrous oxide is used. Other instances in which nitrous oxide should be discontinued include sudden air emboli during hepatic surgery or neurosurgery and placement of a graft on the tympanic membrane or on any other closed air pockets. During prolonged gastrointestinal surgery with an open abdomen, nitrous oxide may cause respiratory compromise and difficulty with wound closure from bowel distention. Gas may be trapped in endotracheal tube cuffs, with resultant increases in cuff pressure. During long procedures, this may produce ichemia of the tracheal mucosa. It is therefore prudent to routinely check cuff pressures when nitrous oxide is used.

After nitrous oxide is discontinued, 100 percent oxygen should be administered for 5 to 10 minutes, assuming normal ventilation. Just as large volumes of nitrous oxide are taken up initially during induction of anesthesia, upon discontinuing its administration, nitrous oxide readily diffuses out of the plasma and back into the lung. The rapid outpouring of nitrous oxide into the alveolar space may displace oxygen and cause hypoxia if additional oxygen in high concentration is not administered. Alveolar carbon dioxide also may be diluted and may initially depress respiratory drive. This may be of greater concern in patients with preexisting lung disease with ventilation and perfusion imbalances or in patients recovering from anesthesia, since these people may still be hypoventilating.

BIBLIOGRAPHY

Calverley RK, Smith NT, et al: Ventilatory and cardiovascular effects of enflurane anesthesia during spontaneous ventilation in man. Anesth Analg 57:610, 1978
Calverley RK, Smith NT, et al: Cardiovascular effects of enflurane anesthesia during controlled ventilation in man. Anesth Analg 57:619, 1978.
Cousins MJ, Greenstein LR, et al: Metabolism and renal effects of enflurane in man. Anesthesiology 44:44, 1976.
Deutsch S, Goldberg M, et al: Effects of halothane anesthesia on renal function in normal men. Anesthesiology 27:793, 1966.
Eger EI II: Isoflurane (Forane): A Compendium and Reference, 2nd ed. Madison, WI, Ohio Medical Products, 1985.
Eger EI II, Smith NT, et al: Cardiovascular effects of halothane in man. Anesthesiology 32:396, 1970.

Eisele JH, Smith NT: Cardiovascular effects of 40 percent nitrous oxide in man. Anesth Analg 51:956, 1972.

Fogdall RP, Miller RD: Neuromuscular effects of enflurane alone and in combination with D-tubocurarine, pancuronium, and succinylcholine in man. Anesthesiology 42:173, 1975.

Johnson RR, Eger EI II, et al: A comparative interaction of epinephrine with enflurane, isoflurane, and halothane in man. Anesth Analg 55:709, 1976.

Knill RL, Gelb AW: Ventilatory responses to hypoxia and hypercapnia during halothane sedation and anesthesia in man. Anesthesiology 49:244, 1978.

Mathers J, Benumof JL, et al: General anesthetics and regional hypoxic pulmonary vasoconstriction. Anesthesiology 46:111, 1977.

Neigh JL, Garman JK, et al: The electroencephalographic pattern during anesthesia with Ethrane: Effects of depth of anesthesia, Pa_{CO_2} and nitrous oxide. Anesthesiology 35:482, 1971.

Shapiro HM: Neuroanesthesia: Physiologic and Pharmacologic Principles. American Society of Anesthesiologists Refresher Course Lectures, 1980.

Sharp JH, Trudell JR, et al: Volatile metabolites and decomposition products of halothane in man. Anesthesiology 50:2, 1979.

Smith NT, Calverley RK, et al: Impact of nitrous oxide on the circulation during enflurane anesthesia in man. Anesthesiology 48:345, 1978.

Sonntag H, Donath U, et al: Left ventricular function in conscious man and during halothane anesthesia. Anesthesiology 48:320, 1978.

Stevens WC, Cromwell TH, et al: The cardiovascular effects of a new inhalation anesthetic, Forane, in human volunteers at constant arterial carbon dioxide tension. Anesthesiology 35:8, 1971.

Theye RA, Michenfelder JD: Whole-body and organ V_{O_2} changes with enflurane, isoflurane and halothane. Br J Anaesth 47:252, 1975.

Vitez TS, Miller RD, et al: An in vitro comparison of halothane and isoflurane potentiation of neuromuscular blockade. Anesthesiology 41:53, 1974.

Wade JG, Stevens WC: Isoflurane: An anesthetic for the eighties? Anesth Analg 60:666, 1981.

Waude BE: Decrease in dose requirement of D-tubocurarine by volatile anesthetics. Anesthesiology 41:298, 1979.

Weil JV, McCullough RE, et al: Diminished ventilatory response to hypoxia and hypercapnia after morphine. N Engl J Med 292:1103, 1975.

15

Intravenous Anesthetics

Doris J. Tanaka

PHARMACOKINETICS OF INTRAVENOUSLY ADMINISTERED DRUGS

The most efficient and commonly used methods of administration of anesthetics are by inhalation or intravenous routes. The following is a review of the pharmacokinetics and pharmacology involved in the actions of intravenously administered drugs. Pharmacokinetics describes the fate of drugs in the body, including the process of absorption from sites, distribution to body tissues and fluids, biotransformation, and excretion from the body. The knowledge of pharmacokinetics can be used to control the intensity and duration of drug actions and to understand the variable responses of individuals to anesthetic drugs.

Absorption

An intravenously administered drug bypasses the absorption phase and therefore has an onset and intensity of action that is more rapid and more predictable.

Distribution

After intravenous injection, there is first a dilution that occurs because of the mixing of the drug with the blood volume. An injected drug is mixed within 30 seconds and is distributed almost immediately. The blood plasma is the medium in which drugs are distributed and removed to their sites of action. The concentration of the drug delivered to these sites is therefore proportional to its concentration in the plasma.

The rate of tissue uptake of the intravenously administered drugs is determined by the rate of drug delivery to the tissue (cardiac output or blood flow) as well as the ability of the drug to enter the tissue (permeability). For those drugs that are able to pass rapidly through cell membranes, permeability can be the rate-limiting factor.

Variables that affect drug permeability are (1) lipid solubility, (2) ionization, (3) molecular size, and (4) protein binding. Lipid solubility is probably the most important property. The greater the lipid solubility, the more quickly a drug will penetrate the biologic membranes. Ionization of a drug will limit permeability by reducing its lipid solubility and also by causing it to be repelled by similarly charged parts of the membrane or attracted and bound by oppositely charged portions of the membrane. Ionization affects entry into cell membranes but does not seem to affect diffusion across capillary membranes. Molecular size affects penetration of the membrane via pores. Most intravenously administered anesthetic drugs are small enough to pass through the pores of vascular capillary membranes but are too large for penetration of pores in cellular membranes.

Protein-bound drugs cannot cross capillary or cellular membranes because of the nature of the protein, which has a large molecular size, is ionized, and has a low lipid solubility. Protein binding also reduces tissue uptake by reducing the concentration of the diffusable, free drug in the plasma. Only the unbound, free drug is able to reach the site of action.

Changes occurring in blood volume, cardiac output, and distribution of blood flow will alter the distribution and concentration of the drug. A decrease in blood volume will decrease dilution and result in an increased blood concentration of the drug. A lowered blood volume will also alter distribution of blood flow, decreasing blood flow to skin and muscle while preserving perfusion to the vital organs. Consequently, a greater portion of the administered drug will reach the brain and heart, which may cause an increase in both central nervous system and cardiac depression. A febrile state, apprehension, and sympathetic stimulation will result in an increased cardiac output and subsequently increased skin and muscle blood flow, which divert the drug from the brain and may result in a lighter-than-expected level of anesthesia.

Organs receiving a higher percentage of the cardiac output will initially receive the bulk of the active drug. The normal distribution of blood flow to various organs is shown in Table 15–1. Each group is differentiated from the others on the basis of the volume of blood flow to the tissues and on the tissue:blood partition coefficient. The rate at which each tissue equilibrates with the drug depends on the capacity of the tissue for the drug (volume of tissue times the tissue:blood partition coefficient) relative to the tissue perfusion.

TABLE 15-1. THE DISTRIBUTION OF BLOOD VOLUME TO VARIOUS ORGANS AND TISSUES

Organs and Tissues	Body Weight (%)	Cardiac Output (%)
Vessel-rich group (70–75% of cardiac output)		
Brain	2.0	14
Heart	0.5	5
Liver	4.0	28
Kidney	0.5	23
Total	7.0	70
Intermediate group		
Skeletal muscle	49	15
Skin	6	8
Total	55	23
Fat	19	6
Vessel-poor group (ligaments, tendons, bone)	19	1

Because of its high blood flow, the vessel-rich group initially receives the major portion of the drug. As the drug penetrates the vessel-rich group, the plasma concentration of the drug declines, and the partial pressure of the drug in the vessel-rich group exceeds that in the plasma now coming to it. The drug then reenters the blood and accumulates in fat and muscle at a rate dependent on solubility, tissue volume, and blood flow.

Biotransformation

Biotransformation of a drug to its metabolites will usually terminate its actions; however, this is not always true. Drug metabolites may be "active" or "inactive." The active metabolites may be more or less potent than the parent drug, and it is also possible for the metabolite to possess similar or dissimilar actions. The rate of biotransformation of most drugs is determined by the concentrations of the drug at the site of metabolism. This is dependent on the concentration in the plasma as well as the volume of blood flow to the liver. Biotransformation of some drugs can occur to a small extent in the brain, kidneys, and other tissues as

well. Other factors that also determine the rate of biotransformation are the numerous variables that affect enzyme activity, the particular chemical means by which the enzymes metabolize the individual drug, and the genetic, nutritional, physiologic, and pharmacologic state of the body.

Elimination

The kidneys and gastrointestinal tract are the major routes of drug excretion for intravenously administered drugs. Drugs may be excreted either in the unchanged form or after biotransformation. The rate of renal excretion of drugs is determined by glomerular filtration, tubular reabsorption, and tubular secretion.

The glomerular filtration depends on molecular weight, the plasma concentration of the unbound drug, and volume of glomerular filtrate.

Tubular secretion involves a selective active transport mechanism that removes drugs from the renal tubular plasma. The process is selective for certain drugs and metabolites and can affect free as well as protein-bound forms of the drugs.

Tubular reabsorption removes from the renal tubules drugs that entered by glomerular filtration and tubular secretion. The ability of a drug to be reabsorbed is determined by its ability to penetrate cellular membranes. Some drugs are reabsorbed very easily and therefore only small amounts of the unchanged drugs are lost in the urine. Biotransformation frequently produces more polar metabolites, which have less ability to penetrate the cell membranes, and therefore results in less tubular reabsorption and greater excretion in the urine. The rate of reabsorption may be altered by the degree of ionization, rate of tubular urine flow, and pH of the urine.

Intestinal excretion of drugs usually occurs to a much lesser extent than renal excretion. The biliary system acts as a transport mechanism for the intestinal excretion of drugs. The same factors that determine drugs' rate of absorption and ability to be absorbed from the gastrointestinal tract also affect the elimination of drugs and their metabolites via the biliary system. Specialized transport mechanisms resemble those of the renal system.

Barbiturates

Barbiturates are the most popular anesthetic induction agents in use today. Historically the first successful and extensively used intravenous anesthetic was a barbiturate known as hexobarbital introduced in 1932. Hexobarbital remained popular until the introduction of thiopental in 1934. Thiopental still remains the most widely used of all intravenous anesthetics. Intravenous methohexital, introduced in 1956, has been the only serious rival to thiopental. Thiamylal has limited popularity in the United States but

has not been a serious challenge to thiopental. Clinically, thiopental and thiamylal are very similar in action and the effects are almost indistinguishable. Methohexital is two to three times more potent than thiopental but has a shorter duration of action and rate of metabolism.

Thiopental and methohexital are probably the two most commonly used intravenous agents in anesthesia practice. Both drugs have been traditionally classified among the "ultra-short-acting" barbiturates. The classic grouping of barbiturates into long-, intermediate-, short-, and ultra-short-acting drugs is misleading. It is now known that the elimination half-lives do not coincide with the apparent duration of action. However, a more accurate classification has not yet been universally adopted.

Chemistry

The term *barbiturates* refers to any derivative of barbituric acid. Barbituric acid is formed by the condensation of malonic acid with urea and is 2,4,6-trioxohexahydropyrimidine. Barbituric acid itself lacks central depressant activity. Barbiturates are formed by certain substitutions made on the parent molecule of barbituric acid.

There are three chemical groups of barbiturates that have clinical use: oxybarbiturates, thiobarbiturates, and methylbarbiturates. Oxybarbiturates, such as pentobarbital, are used commonly as hypnotics for sleep or intramuscularly as anesthetic premedication. Oxybarbiturates are not routinely used for intravenous anesthesia, but the N-methylated oxybarbiturates, such as methohexital, are popular anesthetic induction agents for outpatients. Thiobarbiturates, such as thiopental and thiamylal, are used as anesthetic induction agents (Fig. 15–1).

Substitutions at the 5 carbon position R_1 or R_2 affect the potency. Both positions must be occupied by alkyl, straight saturated or unsaturated, branched or cycled, or aromatic groups to produce a sedative-hypnotic effect. An increase in length of one of these side chains will progressively increase the potency and decrease duration. There are normally no more than eight or less than four carbon atoms in the two chains. One side chain must remain short and simple, and together the two side chains should not number more than eight. The potency reaches a maximum when there are seven or eight carbon atoms. Beyond

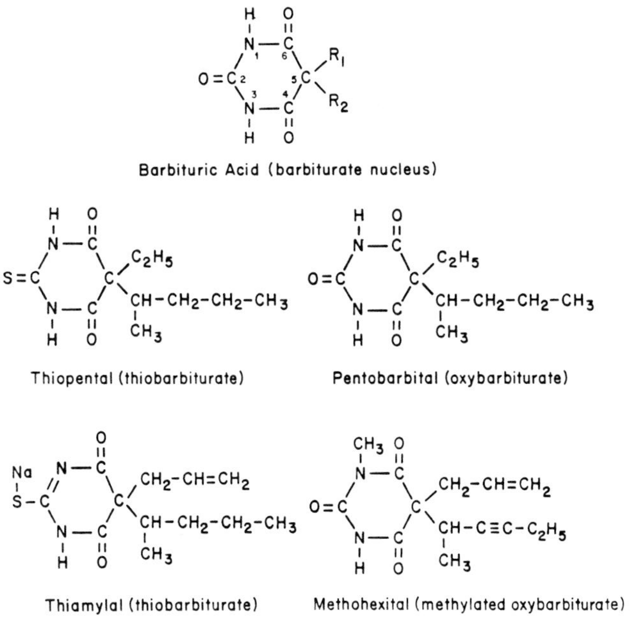

Figure 15–1. The barbiturate nucleus and four different barbiturates resulting from various substitutions.

TABLE 15–2. SUBSTITUTIONS ON THE BARBITURIC ACID MOLECULE THAT DISTINGUISH THE THREE MAJOR BARBITURATE GROUPS

Groups	Substitutions	
	Position 1	*Position 2*
Oxybarbiturate	H	0
Methylbarbiturate	CH_3	0
Thiobarbiturate	H	S

this, toxicity increases more rapidly than potency. Branching or unsaturated chains also tend to increase potency and provide greater hypnotic activity. An aromatic nucleus in an alkyl group that is directly attached to the 5 carbon position produces a compound with convulsant properties; however, direct substitution with a phenyl group confers anticonvulsant properties.

In position 1, a methyl (CH_3) or ethyl (C_2H5) group will often result in a compound with a more rapid onset and recovery but that will also produce a high incidence of excitatory phenomena such as tremor, hypertonus, or spontaneous involuntary muscle movements.

When position 2 is occupied by an oxygen atom, the oxybarbiturates are formed. A sulfur atom in this position forms the thiobarbiturate group, which is highly fat-soluble and is responsible for rapid onset of action and a very short duration of action. The thiobarbiturates also increase vagal activity (Table 15–2).

Physical Properties

Barbiturates that are supplied for clinical use are in the form of sodium salts. Barbituric acid derivatives do not readily dissolve in water, but the sodium salts of barbiturates will dissolve in water, forming an alkaline and unstable solution.

Thiopental is supplied for clinical use as thiopental sodium for injection, U.S.P. Each gram of thiopental sodium contains 60 mg of anhydrous sodium carbonate. The mixture is strongly alkaline (pH 11). Once in the circulation, the sodium carbonate becomes neutralized and the thiopental is converted to its acidic, nonionized form. Approximately 80 percent of the drug is bound to plasma proteins, mainly albumin, in an inactive form. The alkaline pH makes the solution bacteriostatic but also makes it incompatible with acid solutions. Unused solutions of thiopental should be discarded after 24 hours. Thiopental should be administered separately from other drugs to prevent precipitation in the intravenous lines.

Clinical concentrations used for intravenous administration vary between 2.0 percent and 5.0 percent. The 2.0 or 2.5 percent solutions are most commonly used. Concentrations greater than 2.5 percent are more likely to cause serious problems if inadvertent extravasation or intraarterial injection should occur. A 3.4 percent concentration in sterile water for injection is isotonic. Concentrations less than 2.0 percent in sterile water may cause hemolysis.

Methohexital, U.S.P., is supplied for use as methohexital sodium for injection. Each 500-mg ampule of methohexital contains 30 mg of anhydrous sodium carbonate. Sterile water for injection is the preferred diluent; however D$_5$W or 0.9 percent sodium chloride injection may be used. Methohexital sodium is *not* compatible with lactated Ringer's injection. The pH of the aqueous solution is 11. A 1 percent solution is recommended for induction of anesthesia and maintenance by intermittent injection.

Thiamylal is supplied as thiamylal sodium for injection, U.S.P. The pH of its aqueous solution is 11. The recommended diluents are sterile water, D$_5$W, or 0.9 percent sodium chloride for injection. A 2.5 percent solution is the recommended concentration for induction of anesthesia and maintenance by intermittent injection.

Pharmacokinetics

Distribution. Physical redistribution plays a crucial role in the termination of action in the ultra-short-acting, highly lipid-soluble barbiturates. The role of redistribution of the drugs from brain to other tissues has been studied most thoroughly using thiopental. The same principles apply to thiamylal and methohexital.

An intravenous injection of barbiturates is initially distributed to the central blood volume of the body. Dilution of the drug by the blood establishes an initial concentration, which is then further decreased by distribution to the tissues. Plasma levels of intravenous thiopental, 400 mg were studied by Collins (1976). He demonstrated an initial rapid decline within the first 5 minutes, representing drug distribution and establishment of plasma-tissue equilibrium. Within 15 minutes the plasma levels were less than one-half the initial concentration and the patient regained consciousness. A slower rate of decline in the plasma thiopental level occurs during the next 20 minutes and an even slower decline after 30 minutes until a plateau is reached at 120 minutes. The peak concentration in the muscles occurs within 20 to 30 minutes; the fat and vessel-poor groups may take up to 6 hours before reaching peak-concentration level. Intravenous barbiturates are highly lipid-soluble, but they are absorbed more slowly by fat because of the lower blood supply to these tissues (Fig. 15–2).

Clinical effects can be seen as the barbiturates undergo a rapid, flow-limited uptake into the most vascular areas of the central nervous system. Unconsciousness occurs in one arm-to-brain-circulation time (10 to 20 seconds) after a single intravenous anesthetic dose. The depth of anesthesia may increase for up to 40 seconds and then progressively decrease. Excessive or prolonged administration will lead to drug accumulation in all tissue compartments and may cause excessive drowsiness or unconsciousness in the postoperative period. The fact that thiopental remains in the body after it ceases to be active is the reason for cumulative effects of repeated doses. The rate of equilibration is determined not only by blood flow and cardiac output but also by the ability of the active drug to penetrate cell membranes. The three important factors governing the ability of barbiturates to cross cellular membranes are (1) lipid solubility, (2) degree of ionization, and (3) plasma protein binding:

1. The greater the lipid solubility, the more rapid is the redistribution and equilibration process. The less

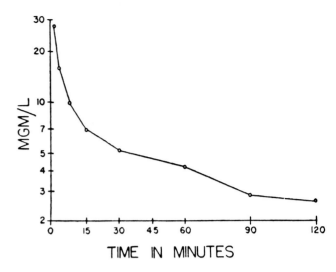

Figure 15–2. Thiopental levels after a single intravenous dose of 400 mg. Note that patients regain consciousness in a few minutes while blood levels are still high. (*From Brodie BB, Mark LC, et al: The fate of thiopental in man and a method of estimation in biological material. J Pharmacol Exp Ther 98:, 1950.*)

lipid-soluble oxybarbiturates equilibrate much more slowly than the thiobarbiturates because uptake is limited more by the drug's cell-membrane permeability than by blood flow.

2. The extent of dissociation of the intravenous barbiturates into an ionized form depends largely on the pH of the blood and tissues. There is greater ionization with alkalosis and less with acidosis. The nonionized active form crosses membranes more rapidly than the ionized form.

3. Barbiturates are bound to plasma proteins, mostly albumin. Approximately 75 to 80 percent of the injected barbiturate will bind with proteins. The unbound active form of the drug is available to penetrate cell membranes.

Keeping all of these variables in mind, the anesthetist can make sound judgments regarding dose, duration, and effect of the barbiturates. A patient who presents in an acidotic state with low plasma protein and blood volume can be expected to respond more dramatically to the usual doses of barbiturates. The patient's physiologic state can alter the normal kinetics of the drug.

Metabolism. The biotransformation of barbiturates is mediated by the microsomal enzyme systems, located primarily in the liver. The thiobarbiturates are also transformed to a small extent in the brain and kidneys. Methohexital is metabolized only by the liver.

Barbiturates are transformed by three main routes: (1) oxidation of radicals at carbon 5, (2) nitrogen dealkylation (methohexital undergoes N-demethylation to a very slight extent, but the rate of oxidation of the carbon 5 substitutes is so rapid that N-demethylation products make up only a minute fraction of the metabolites) and (3) desulfuration of thiobarbiturates.

The ultra-short-acting barbiturates are almost completely transformed in the body to an inactive form. The rate of transformation of thiopental is slow—approximately 10 to 15 percent per hour; 3 percent of the original dose may remain after 24 hours. Metabolism of methohexital is slightly more rapid and accounts for the more rapid recovery. Methohexital has been found to have a short half-life of 75 to 125 minutes.

The duration of action of intravenous barbiturate anesthesia is short and patients will regain consciousness fairly quickly. However, the duration of action of intravenous barbiturates has no correlation with the rate of biotransformation of the drugs. Patients awaken with a large amount of unmetabolized drug in the body. Although they may behave and speak normally, patients who have received intravenous barbiturates, especially outpatients, should be advised against taking alcohol or other drugs on the same day. Their effects may be enhanced by the subclinical levels of barbiturate still present in the body. This caution also applies to methohexital, although it is metabolized slightly more rapidly than thiopental.

Excretion. The transformed products of the intravenous barbiturates are excreted primarily by the kidneys; however, a small fraction may appear in the feces by way of the biliary system. Only minute traces (0.3 percent) of these drugs are excreted unchanged in the urine.

Pharmacologic Effects

Central Nervous System. The intravenous barbiturates rapidly cross the blood-brain barrier to produce a progressive central nervous system depression ranging from mild sedation to coma, depending on the dose injected and the rate of injection. The depth of anesthesia produced depends on the plasma concentration of the barbiturate but can be evaluated in terms of the initial dose and rate of administration. If very large initial doses are administered, the patient may awaken when the brain and plasma levels are significantly higher. This has been termed "acute tolerance"; a larger dose establishes a higher critical level. This fact has been accounted for on the basis of the "slug administration theory." The rapid entry of large doses into and out of the central nervous system causes a distortion of drug distribution between the brain and peripheral circulation that does not occur with slower rates of administration and can result in return of consciousness with higher-than-normal plasma concentrations.

General anesthesia with thiopental is believed to result from the supression of the reticular activating system. However, some researchers believe that there are certain cells in the cortex that have a high sensitivity to barbiturates, and it has been suggested that the anesthetic action may be due to a blocking of polysynaptic neuronal systems that exist not only in the brainstem but also in the cortex.

Central nervous system depression occurs in the same pattern as with inhalation anesthetics but the clinical state may not bear a precise relationship because the anesthetic state is reached more rapidly with intravenous agents. A patient given an intravenous barbiturate will go through the classical "stages of anesthesia," but at a much faster rate so that each stage may not be clearly appreciated by the observer. Stage I, consciousness, is lost first. The patient falls asleep suddenly. If there is conversation during induction, the patient's words may suddenly become jumbled and slurred, and he or she may take a few deep breaths or yawn before the eyelids close. There is loss of consciousness. Stage II, the excitement stage, is passed so quickly that it is usually not seen. Stage III is achieved very quickly: superficial and deep reflexes are diminished and will disappear. Pupils are constricted and the eyes are fixed at midline. The eyelid reflex is lost and there is profound relaxation of the pharyngeal and masseter muscles. This relaxation is most profound in the first minutes of anesthesia and is transient. Planes III and IV of this stage can only be obtained when extremely large, toxic doses are administered.

As with the inhalational anesthetics, the cerebral cortex is depressed first, followed by the subcortex (in stage II and III–plane I), and then the midbrain in the latter planes of stage III. Stage IV is reached when brain-stem depression or failure occurs.

The intravenous barbiturates, in doses insufficient to cause unconsciousness, can cause amnesia for events occurring during the time of sedation. This effect correlates well with the plasma levels of the drug.

The lower doses of barbiturates are also capable of increasing the sensitivity to painful stimuli. Barbiturates have little or no direct effect on pain relief. Subhypnotic doses increase the sensitivity to deep somatic pain, and especially visceral pain, while decreasing the sensitivity to pain from mild, superficial skin stimulation. The latter phenomenon is explained as a result of diminished apprehension and fear, not an analgesic effect. The hyperalgesia to deep somatic and visceral pain appears to be from depression of the inhibitory system in the ascending reticular activating system, which then permits facilitation of secondary slow pain impulses.

Clinically, small doses of thiopental can antagonize the analgesic actions of nitrous oxide or narcotic. Even large doses of thiopental appear to be lacking analgesic effects. The clinical level of anesthesia is related to the intensity of surgical stimulus. A patient may appear to be in a surgical plane of anesthesia and may even be apneic, but with surgical stimulation, he or she may reflexly initiate movement and respirations. Doses of thiopental sufficient to produce surgical anesthesia in the presence of strong stimulation may cause prolonged respiratory depression and unconsciousness when the stimulation ceases.

Cerebral blood flow and oxygen utilization are reduced with thiopental and the other barbiturates. This decrease in cerebral blood flow decreases intracranial pressure and this effect is frequently utilized in anesthesia for neurosurgery.

Thiopental and thiamylal produce a rapid, smooth, and quiet induction of anesthesia. Methohexital induction is followed by an appreciable incidence of excitatory phenomena such as tremor, hypertonus, and spontaneous involuntary muscle movements. The methyl group added to position 1 on the oxybarbiturate molecule is believed to be responsible for the excitatory phenomena. This incidence is reduced by narcotic premedication but increased by preoperative phenothiazines or anticholinergics. Methohexital is more likely to induce seizures in susceptible patients than the other intravenous induction agents.

Cardiovascular System. Clinical doses of thiopental, thiamylal, or methohexital will generally depress myocardial function. (Hemodynamic changes are usually fewer with methohexital than with the thiobarbiturates). The medullary vasomotor center is depressed as well as the hypothalamic centers, which regulate the force of myocardial contraction. A transient fall in the mean arterial pressure can be noted. There is a redistribution of the blood volume, with approximately 60 percent pooling in the systemic capacitance vessels. This shift causes a decreased venous return and a reduction in left ventricular diastolic filling pressure, leading to a reduced stroke volume and cardiac output. An increase in total calculated peripheral resistance occurs over a period of time and is believed to be compensatory to decreased cardiac output; however, a cause of central origin cannot be ruled out. The heart rate is usually slightly increased or unchanged. Arrythmias are uncommon, and there is no evidence of myocardial sensitization to catecholamines. Barbiturates selectively depress transmission in the sympathetic ganglia. This may partly account for the fall in blood pressure produced by these drugs.

The recommended induction doses of the ultra-short-acting barbiturates given to healthy individuals will cause only a minor and transient change in blood pressure and heart rate. However, the same "normal" dose given to hypovolemic, septic, hypertensive, or debilitated patients or to those with an already compromised hemodynamic state can produce an exaggerated effect. Severe and prolonged hypotension or cardiovascular collapse may result. Even very small doses of intravenous barbiturates have been known to produce hypotension in these patients and should be used with caution. Cardiovascular depression resulting from barbiturate administration in healthy individuals is usually the result of a rapid injection of very large doses (Table 15–3).

The redistribution of blood increases blood flow to the muscles and extremities while decreasing blood flow to the brain, renal, and splanchnic bed. A decrease in renal plasma flow and glomerular filtration occurs even in small doses. The release of antidiuretic hormone (ADH) by the barbiturates produces an antidiuretic effect.

There is some histamine release with the intravenous barbiturates, especially thiopental, but it does not appear to be significant in altering hemodynamics.

TABLE 15–3. HEMODYNAMIC EFFECTS OF INTRAVENOUS BARBITURATES

Stroke volume	Decreased
Cardiac output	Decreased
Mean arterial pressure	Decreased
Total peripheral resistance	Increased
Cerebral vascular resistance	Increased
Cerebral blood flow	Decreased
Cerebral oxygen consumption	Decreased
Renal and splanchnic blood flow	Decreased

Respiratory System. The ultra-short-acting barbiturates depress respirations by direct action on the medullary and pontine centers. The pulmonary stretch receptors, afferent and efferent nerves, and the neuromuscular junction are not affected to any significant degree. The aortic and carotid chemoreceptors are able to maintain their functions until deeper levels of anesthesia are reached.

The extent of respiratory depression depends on dose, rate of administration, and narcotic premedication. Small doses in patients without premedication will cause only a transient and minimal decrease in minute ventilation, primarily affecting the tidal volume. Arterial P_{CO_2} is minimally elevated. A larger dose will depress minute ventilation to an even greater extent and can transiently produce apnea. The period of apnea is brief and is attributed to the rapid rate of redistribution of the drug out of the central nervous system. After narcotic premedication, respiratory depression is more marked at all levels of barbiturate anesthesia.

The usual sequence of events after slow administration of thiopental in recommended doses is a few deep breaths or yawning, followed by reduction in ventilation or transient apnea. Surgical stimulus can stimulate respiration and offset the respiratory depression to a certain degree. A patient may breathe adequately during surgical manipulation but become apneic or subside into shallow respirations when the stimulus is removed. The respiratory depression and apnea produced by methohexital are usually not as prolonged as with the thiobarbiturates.

Laryngeal and pharyngeal protective reflexes are not completely obtunded by barbiturates until deep levels of anesthesia are reached. Laryngospasm can occur during barbiturate anesthesia, caused by surgical stimulation and by stimulation of the vagal nerve-endings in the larynx by mucus, blood, secretions, etc. A light level of anesthesia combined with any one or more of the various stimuli can produce a laryngospasm.

Coughing, sneezing, and hiccoughing can occur with any of the intravenous barbiturates but seem to occur more frequently with methohexital. These side effects can be minimized by the use of a small total dose and slow injection. Premedication with narcotics and anticholinergics have been noted to be helpful in this respect.

Intravenous thiobarbiturates appear to have a parasympathomimetic effect, which has been implicated in the bronchoconstriction and bronchospasms that are sometimes seen. Although bronchospasms after administration of thiopental are infrequent, clinical use of this drug in asthmatics or patients with increased bronchiolar tone is often avoided.

Indications and Contraindications

The induction of anesthesia using a barbiturate is simple, rapid, and not unpleasant for the patient. The majority of the general anesthetics administered are induced with an intravenous barbiturate regardless of the agent to be used for maintenance. However, the clinical use of intravenous barbiturates is not suitable for all patients.

When the adequacy of an airway is in doubt, intravenous barbiturates should not be used. Patients with head and neck tumors, gross anatomic abnormalities, or other patients who may lose a patent airway with loss of consciousness should not be induced with the barbiturates until an airway is secured.

Patients in hypovolemic shock, impending shock, a state of dehydration, or debilitation will not react normally to barbiturates, and thus these drugs should be used with extreme caution. Caution must be exercised with severe asthmatics and patients with other bronchospastic disorders.

Patients with acute intermittent porphyria may experience exacerbation of symptoms after barbiturate administration. This can sometimes be fatal; therefore barbiturates are definitely contraindicated for these patients.

Complications

Laryngospasm is not an uncommon problem during barbiturate anesthesia. Secretions or blood in the pharynx, stimulation of the pharynx with an airway, or peripheral stimulation during a light plane of anesthesia will induce a laryngospasm. The precipitating factor should be removed, anesthesia deepened, and the spasm relieved by application of constant, positive airway pressure with 100 percent oxygen. If the laryngospasm persists and cyanosis or arrythmias appear, a small dose of succinylcholine can be administered. Coughing, sneezing, and hiccoughing can also occur with barbiturate anesthesia. This occurs most frequently with methohexital.

Barbiturate solutions are very alkaline and therefore irritating to the tissues. If large amounts of the drug are placed extravascularly, necrosis of the subcutaneous tissue can result. The higher the concentration of the solution, the greater the danger of a serious problem. Methohexital is usually used in a 1 percent solution and carries a low risk of tissue damage with extravasation. Thiopental and thiamylal in a 2.5 percent solution are also unlikely to cause serious damage, and no permanent sequelae have been reported after use of this concentration. Extravasation of the 5.0 percent solutions of thiopental has been reported to cause serious damage.

Intraarterial injections of barbiturates have been reported when the antecubital site has been selected for the intravenous injection. Intraarterial injection in the awake patient will always result in severe pain described as hot or scalding. Arterial spasm occurs and a chemical endarteritis destroys the endothelial and subendothelial layers of the vessels. Muscle layers may also be involved and thrombosis can occur. The degree of damage depends on the amount and concentration of the solution injected.

Arterial spasms are believed to be due to the local release of norepinephrine. Necrosis and gangrene are believed to be the result of thrombosis and crystallization of the drug, causing vascular occlusion. Studies have shown that the necrotizing effect is a property of the drug and is not related to the alkalinity.

Treatment of intraarterial injection must be instituted immediately. The aim of therapy is to dilute the injected drug, overcome the arterial spasm, and prevent thrombosis. General anesthesia with an inhalation agent to promote vasodilation may be indicated if the patient is in much pain and is unable to cooperate for proper treatment; 10 ml of 1 percent procaine should be injected into the same needle or catheter used for the barbiturate injection. Local heparinization and injection of an alpha blocker such as phentolamine may be indicated. A stellate ganglion block or brachial plexus block can be performed to ensure vascular dilation. If arterial thrombosis occurs, operative removal of the clot may be required and should be undertaken within 6 hours of the initial injury. If necrosis and gangrene occur, amputation may be necessary.

Clinical Uses

There are a number of clinical uses of the intravenous barbiturates. The most popular use is for the induction of anesthesia. A bolus of the barbiturate is administered to supply sufficient depth of anesthesia, time for endotracheal intubation, and introduction of an inhalation agent or narcotic for maintenance. The induction dose is preceded by a 50 mg test dose to determine the pharmacologic effect before the bolus of the barbiturate is administered. There should be adequate time allowed for the test dose to exert an effect, if any, before proceeding with the induction. A blood pressure measurement should be made about 1 minute after the test dose and an assessment of the patient's consciousness should also be made at this time. Patients who are hemodynamically unstable may show an exaggerated fall in blood pressure in response to the test dose, whereas patients who are less tolerant of the effects of hypnotics may become very sedate and drowsy. Pain on injection may indicate extravasation, and the intravenous site should be checked before proceeding with the injection.

The induction dose of the barbiturates must be tailored to the individual patient. An assessment of the patient's size, premedication and its effect, and physical status (i.e., state of hydration and nutrition, metabolic and acid-base status, previous drug therapy, etc.) must be made when determining a proper dose. The amount of barbiturate given for induction may also vary with the technique or method of anesthesia to be employed. The following are the usual required doses for induction of anesthesia for *healthy* patients:

Induction Dose

Thiopental	3 to 4 mg/kg body weight
Methohexital	1 mg/kg body weight
Thiamylal	2 to 3 mg/kg body weight

Thiopental is the most widely used induction agent for all types of procedures. However, methohexital, because of its more rapid rate of metabolism and recovery, has challenged the use of thiopental for dental and other outpatient procedures of shorter duration. Methohexital also appears to be less toxic to the cardiovascular system and has found popularity for use in cardioversions and electroconvulsive therapy.

Barbiturates have been used as a sole anesthetic agent for short surgical procedures by either intermittent bolus injections or a continuous drip. These techniques can be used in conjunction with nitrous oxide or an intravenous narcotic premedication. A barbiturate alone is usually not sufficient for most surgical procedures, even with the addition of nitrous oxide, but can be used successfully for very short procedures that do not require relaxation. When doses greater than 500 to 1000 mg are required, or if the procedure lasts longer than 45 minutes to 1 hour, another anesthetic technique should be considered. These techniques should always be performed with supplemental oxygen, and resuscitative equipment should be available. The technique is usually as follows: Intermittent bolus injections of 25 to 75 mg are administered after a sleep dose of the barbiturate given according to clinical signs of anesthetic depth. An attempt is made to correlate dose and time of administration to the degree of surgical stimulus. Hypoventilation or apnea can occur at any time, and therefore the anesthetist must always be prepared to ventilate the patient. These procedures are frequently done as "mask" cases. Narcotic premedication will usually decrease the amount of barbiturate required to produce the desired effects and the respiratory depressant effects can be expected to be greater. For very brief procedures such as a closed reduction of a fracture or dislocation, one bolus injection of the barbiturate may be all that is required. Continuous barbiturate infusion is rarely used for anesthesia today and, when used, is usually limited to procedures of short duration. A dilute concentration should be mixed. A 0.1 percent concentration in D_5W with no more than 500 mg in the solution is a fairly safe mixture. Barbiturate drip anesthesia carries a risk of overdosage and prolonged depression, but the use of a dilute solution and a fixed amount of the drug will afford some protection. If it appears that the entire amount is required, an alternative method should be considered.

The barbiturate drip is started after a small sleep dose of the barbiturate. The infusion is used to maintain the patient in a consistent plane of anesthesia. This method usually requires nitrous oxide supplementation, and premedication is very helpful in maintaining a smooth course. The infusion rate can be increased, decreased, or stopped during the procedure according to the surgical stimulus and clinical signs of the depth of anesthesia. As always, when an intravenous barbiturate is used, resuscitative equipment should be available.

Eugenols

Eugenols are nonbarbiturate intravenous anesthetic agents derived from the oil of cloves. Propanidid is a synthetic eugenol derivative synthesized by Hietmann and introduced for clinical investigation in 1961. The chemical structure is shown in Figure 15–3.

Physical Properties

Propanidid is supplied in a 5 percent aqueous solution in 20 percent polyoxyethylated castor oil or Cremophor EL as a solvent. It is a yellow oil, poorly soluble in water, with a pH of 5.15. The solution is highly viscous but can be diluted with an equal volume of normal saline for easier administration. The mixture should always be freshly prepared. The usual dosage is from 5 to 10 mg/kg for adults.

Distribution, Metabolism, and Excretion

Fifty percent of the injected drug is immediately bound to plasma proteins and thus inactivated. The unbound drug is rapidly metabolized by plasma cholinesterases in both the blood and liver. There is an enzymatic splitting of the ester bond, which results in an inactive acid metabolite with no anesthetic properties. The metabolites are then excreted in the urine. Hydrolysis is fairly rapid, and the drug is usually not detected in the plasma 30 minutes after injection. Redistribution of the drug is normally unimportant unless there is a deficiency in plasma proteins or serum cholinesterases.

Pharmacologic Effects

Central Nervous System. The main characteristic of eugenol anesthetics is their truly ultra-short duration and the completeness of recovery. The duration of action is a result of detoxification rather than redistribution. After an injection of propanidid, consciousness is lost in one arm-to-brain-circulation time. Anesthesia lasts for approximately 3 to 6 minutes with complete recovery by about 10 minutes. During the brief period of anesthesia, pupillary, corneal, laryngeal, and pharyngeal reflexes are absent; there is a moderate degree of muscular relaxation.

General recovery and mental clarity after propanidid anesthesia is much more rapid and complete than with other intravenous anesthetics. After barbiturate anesthesia, there is a tendency toward periods of sleep during the

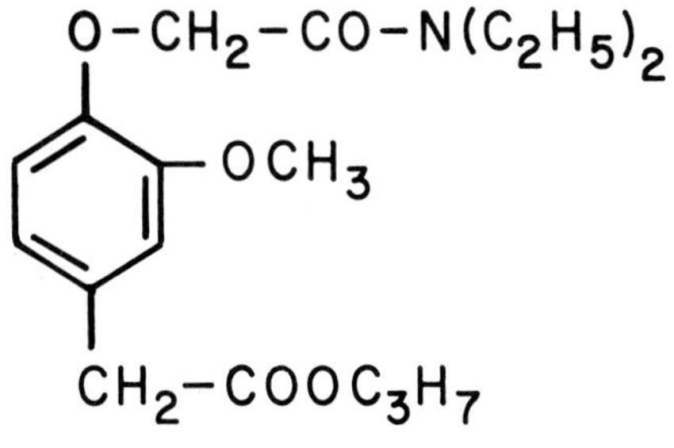

Figure 15–3. Chemical structure of the eugenol propanidid (Eptonol).

subsequent 12 to 24 hours after anesthesia but with propanidid this is less likely. The effects of alcohol ingestion after propanidid anesthesia were mild compared with methohexital or thiopental.

Large doses of propanidid seem to increase the excitatory phenomena. Doses greater than 8 mg/kg produce an incidence twice that of an equivalent dose of thiopental. The likelihood of coughing and hiccoughing on induction is also increased with increasing dose. Narcotic premedication tends to reduce these side effects, but phenothiazines and anticholinergics seem to increase the incidence.

This drug is not contraindicated in patients with seizure disorders.

The hyperalgesia caused by the barbiturates is not found with the eugenol anesthetics.

Postoperative nausea and vomiting after propanidid anesthesia is more frequent than after barbiturate anesthesia.

Cardiovascular System. Propanidid causes a fall in mean arterial pressure and a rise in heart rate. A 4 mg/kg dose of propanidid produces the same degree of hypotension as an equivalent dose of intravenous barbiturate. However, with larger doses (8 mg/kg) the incidence and degree of hypotension increases to greater extent than that seen with the barbiturates. The decrease in cardiac output and stroke volume is attributable to myocardial depression and peripheral vasodilation. The blood pressure normally returns to baseline levels within 3 to 4 minutes and the tachycardia subsides within 10 minutes after a single bolus injection.

Respiratory System. Respiratory stimulation is a characteristic of eugenol anesthetic administration. Hyperventilation immediately follows injection and can last up to 30 seconds. This is followed by a period of hypoventilation or apnea. The duration of hypoventilation is similar to the hyperventilation phase. Minute ventilation then returns to normal within a few minutes. Hypoventilation and apnea appears to be of greater magnitude in patients receiving narcotic premedication whereas the hyperventilation phase is less marked. Apnea requiring ventilatory assistance is less likely with propanidid than with equivalent doses of barbiturates.

Because plasma cholinesterase plays an important role in the inactivation of both propanidid and succinylcholine, competitive inhibition results when the two drugs are used for induction and intubation. Apnea after 50 mg of succinylcholine is significantly longer when propanidid is used for induction rather than a barbiturate.

Clinical Uses

Propanidid is a useful anesthetic for brief, minor surgical procedures because of its short duration of action. It is used most frequently for dental anesthesia in European countries. Patients are able to leave the surgical area much faster after propanidid anesthesia than after methohexital.

Propanidid can be used safely in patients with porphyria. Propanidid is not recommended for use with succinylcholine if nitrous oxide or other agents are not used for supplementation of anesthesia. There have been many instances of patients recovering from propanidid while still being paralyzed from the effects of succinylcholine.

Toxic reactions to eugenols such as hypotension and excitation are usually due to excessive doses. A unique phenomenon of propanidid is that the blood levels decrease more rapidly after a rapid injection than after a slow injection because a greater concentration of substrate becomes available for enzymatic hydrolysis. Increasing the dose of propanidid does not increase the duration of sleep but only increases the toxicity of the drug.

Propanidid can be used in the same manner as barbiturates: as an induction agent or as a sole agent for brief procedures.

Complications

Intraarterial injections of propanidid in humans have not shown significant histologic changes or damage, but they may produce irreversible damage, depending on the concentration and dose injected.

Propanidid does cause histamine release, but it is usually not of clinical significance. Hypersensitivity reactions reported were the result of overdosage or too rapid injection. Anaphylactic reactions to propanidid have also been reported. It has been suggested that Cremophor EL may be the initiating or sensitizing factor in anaphylactoid reactions.

At this time the eugenols are not approved for anesthetic use in the United States.

Althesin

Chemistry and Physical Properties

Althesin is an intravenous anesthetic that is a mixture of two steroids, alphaxalone and alphadolone acetate. Alphaxalone is the main anesthetic agent. Alphadolone contributes slightly toward the sedative effect but also helps increase the solubility of the two steroids in 20 percent Cremophor El and sodium chloride. Althesin is a clear isotonic solution of neutral pH. Each milliliter contains 9 mg of alphaxalone and 3 mg of alphadolone for a total of 12 mg/ml. The solution is viscid and insoluble in water but can be diluted with normal saline (Fig. 15–4).

Distribution, Metabolism, and Excretion

Intravenous injections will produce unconsciousness in one arm-to-brain-circulation time with a duration of 5 to 10 minutes. Large doses produce a slightly longer duration of

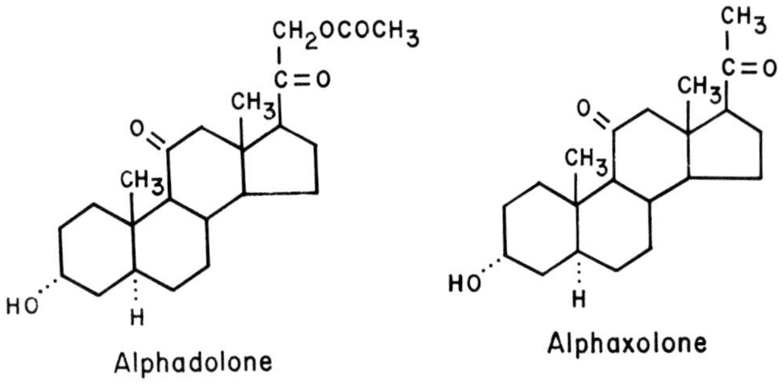

Figure 15–4. Chemical structure of the steroid compound althesin and its two components.

anesthesia, although the length of action even with a larger dose is still brief. The optimum induction dose is 50 to 100 μl/kg. There is a more rapid onset and recovery of unconsciousness than with thiopental.

The drug is approximately 30 to 40 percent bound to plasma proteins. The half-life is about 6 to 8 minutes. The rapid return of consciousness is due primarily to redistribution of the drug. Termination of action of the drug occurs in the liver by enzymatic reduction. The metabolites are excreted in the bile; approximately 70 percent appear in the feces, but because of enterohepatic recirculation, the remainder is excreted in the urine. Liver dysfunction or nephrectomy does not greatly prolong the duration of action.

Pharmacologic Effects

Central Nervous System. The exact mechanism of action of the steroid drugs in producing anesthesia is unknown but is believed to be through an action on cerebral function. Cerebral oxygen uptake, cerebral glucose utilization, and cerebral blood flow are reduced significantly.

There is a high incidence of excitatory phenomena with large doses, but this occurs less frequently than with methohexital. The incidence is reduced by narcotic premedication.

Althesin has been reported to produce some retrograde amnesia. There is good muscle relaxation after the onset of unconsciousness. Recovery is usually rapid and complete by 30 minutes. Nausea and vomiting are uncommon. There is no hyperalgesia as a result of althesin administration.

Cardiovascular System. After intravenous injection, there is a decrease in total peripheral resistance, which results in a 10 to 20 percent drop in the mean arterial pressure. The central venous pressure is also lowered but the cardiac output is usually maintained or increased, depending on the degree of tachycardia, which also occurs on injection

of althesin. The cardiovascular changes usually return to normal within 2 to 3 minutes. The onset of the cardiovascular changes correlate well with the changes seen in the respiratory pattern, suggesting a central effect of althesin.

Respiratory System. The ventilatory pattern is affected after induction. There is usually a brief period of apnea, which is followed by shallow and rapid respirations. A 2 to 3 mm Hg rise in P_{CO_2} can be seen. Coughing, hiccoughing, and laryngospasm can occur as a result of stimulation under light anesthesia, but these are rare.

Endocrine System. No significant hormonal effects of the steroid configuration have been noted.

Clinical Uses

Althesin is used for induction of anesthesia, particularly for outpatient procedures because of its rapid metabolism. Althesin has also been used as a sole anesthetic agent as a continuous infusion or intermittent injection for brief procedures. It appears to possess more analgesic properties and is less cumulative than the barbiturates. Althesin offers an advantage for use in neurologic procedures because of its ability to decrease cerebral blood flow and metabolism. It has been used as a continuous infusion in intensive care units to maintain reduced intracranial pressures and is an appropriate agent for patients with head injuries.

Precautions

There is a significantly greater incidence of hypersensitivity reactions after althesin administration. They have been classified as (1) histaminoid: vasodilation, edema, profound drop in mean arterial pressure; (2) bronchospasm: sometimes preceded by coughing and occurring before tracheal intubation; and (3) cardiovascular collapse: profound hypotension not accompanied by histamine reactions or bronchospasm. These reactions usually occurred immediately after intravenous injection, but histaminoid reactions occurring 12 to 80 minutes after injection have also been reported. Dosages were not a factor, since most reactions occurred after very small doses. The incidence of hypersensitivity to althesin is 10 to 20 times greater than that for thiopental. The problem of hypersensitivity has greatly decreased the use of althesin.

Althesin in patients with porphyria is believed to affect enzymes in a manner similar to the barbiturates and is contraindicated in these patients.

Althesin is not currently approved for use in anesthesia in the United States.

Etomidate

Etomidate is a relatively new hypnotic induction agent approved for clinical use in the United States in the 1980s. It was first synthesized in 1965 in the laboratories of Janssen Pharmaceutica at Beerse, Belgium.

Chemistry and Physical Properties

Etomidate, (R)−(+)-ethyl-1-(1-phenylethyl)-1*H*-imidazole-5-carboxylate sulphate is a carboxylated imidazole (Fig. 15–5). It is available as a water-soluble compound in 35 percent

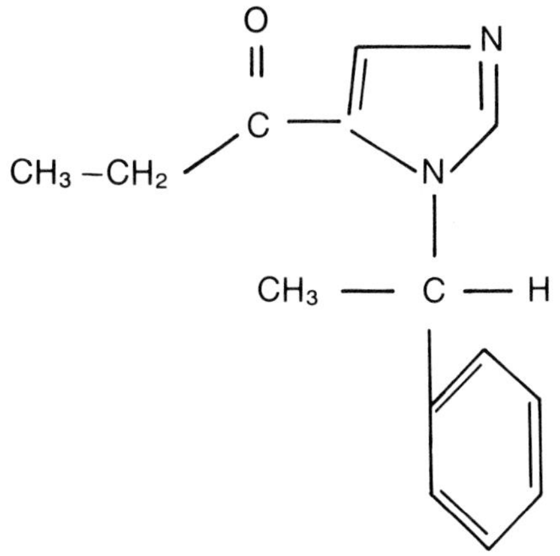

Figure 15–5. Chemical structure of etomidate (Amidate).

propylene glycol, with a pH of 5.6. Only the dextroisomer is anesthetically active. Etomidate is available in a 0.2 percent solution. This solution is very stable, and it can be left at room temperature for more than 2 years.

On a milligram per milligram basis, etomidate is approximately 25 times more potent than thiopental and approximately 6 times more potent than methohexital. It has a wider margin of safety than thiopental or methohexital. Its therapeutic index (LD_{50}/ED_{50}) is 26.0, whereas that of thiopental is 4.6.

Distribution, Metabolism, and Excretion

Intravenous injections of etomidate 0.3 mg/kg will produce unconsciousness in one arm-to-brain-circulation time. Etomidate is highly lipid-soluble and has a pKa of 4.2. Recovery from a single dose of etomidate is very rapid—approximately 3 to 5 minutes for responsiveness. It both enters and leaves the brain quickly because of rapid redistribution. The distribution half-life is just over 2 minutes. Much of the drug is distributed to fat and muscle. The duration of action is dose-dependent, usually about 3 minutes for a 0.3 mg/kg dose, and the duration is doubled when the dose is doubled. Etomidate is approximately 78 percent protein bound.

Metabolism of etomidate is through hydrolysis by esterases in both the liver and plasma. The compound is metabolized into pharmacologically inactive forms. Plasma levels of etomidate decrease rapidly during the first 30 minutes and less rapidly over the following 3 to 6 hours. Detectable amounts of etomidate can be found in the plasma for at least 6 hours. The elimination half-life is approximately 3 hours. Eighty-seven percent of the administered drug is excreted in the urine, 3 percent in an unchanged form. The remaining 13 percent is excreted in the bile. Eighty percent of the drug is excreted in 24 hours.

Pharmacologic Effects

Central Nervous System. Etomidate is a hypnotic agent and does not provide analgesic effects. The central depressant actions appear to be on the brainstem reticular forma-

tion by a gamma-aminobutyric acid (GABA) mimetic mechanism.

Electroencephalographic (EEG) changes noted after etomidate administration are similar to those of other intravenous anesthetics. Etomidate has effects on cerebral blood flow and cerebral metabolism similar to those of barbiturate anesthetics. Studies indicate that both cerebral blood flow and cerebral oxygen use are reduced.

A major problem associated with etomidate administration is myoclonic movements. These movements are involuntary, irregular contractions of individual or groups of skeletal muscles and are usually seen during anesthesia induction with etomidate. EEG patterns during these movements have not been indicative of seizure activity. The incidence of myoclonus has been reported to be between 10 and 60 percent. Premedication with fentanyl or diazepam appears to reduce the incidence of these movements.

Cardiovascular System. One of the major advantages of etomidate use is that it appears to have minimal effects on the cardiovascular system. Arrhythmias are not usually seen when this drug is used. When compared with other intravenous induction agents, etomidate produces fewer and milder consequences to the cardiovascular system.

In patients without cardiopulmonary disease, a dose of 0.3 mg/kg of etomidate does not produce significant alterations in the cardiovascular parameters. Heart rate and cardiac output are not significantly affected. The mean arterial pressure decreases slightly, as does the peripheral vascular resistance and myocardial oxygen consumption. Similar findings have been published with regard to patients with significant cardiovascular disease.

In contrast to some other drugs used in anesthesia, etomidate does not have histamine-releasing properties.

Respiratory System. Etomidate has minimal effects on blood gases and pulmonary function. Tidal volume and minute ventilation are reduced, whereas respiratory rate is increased. Transient apnea has been reported with 0.3 mg/kg doses, especially in the debilitated or geriatric population of patients. The incidence of apnea varies with premedications, but it is considerably less when compared with thiopental.

Endocrine System. The primary effect of etomidate on the endocrine system is its ability to block the effects of adrenocorticotropic hormone (ACTH) on the adrenal cortex. The resultant effect is a low plasma cortisol level. Studies have indicated that the reduction in plasma cortisol levels in patients who received etomidate was due to a lack of response to ACTH by the adrenal cortex and indicates a suppression at the glandular level.

Clinical Uses

Etomidate has been used in many clinical situations by various techniques. It is probably most commonly used as an induction agent for outpatient surgery, short diagnostic procedures, in the elderly, or in patients with some cardiovascular compromise. Because of the short duration of action and also the relatively hangover-free effect, it is suitable for outpatient use. Etomidate is used in the elderly and in those who may not tolerate other agents because of its minimal effect on the cardiovascular system. In such patients, the induction dose should be administered slowly and cautiously to avoid undesirable cardiovascular changes. Because etomidate does not appear to release histamine, it has been used in patients who are inclined to asthma and other forms of bronchospastic disorders. Etomidate may be useful in neurosurgical and ophthalmic procedures because of its ability to reduce cerebral blood flow, cerebral metabolism, and intraocular pressure. The administration of etomidate to patients with increased intracranial pressure (ICP) or open eye injuries for induction or maintenance may be very useful.

The use of etomidate in a continuous infusion for anesthetic maintenance is gaining popularity, especially when it is administered with intermittent injections of fentanyl. An infusion solution of 0.4 mg/ml may be used with an approximate infusion rate of 1.6 mg/minute.

The drug has also been used for sedation in patients receiving postoperative intermittent positive-pressure ventilation and for short oral surgery cases. In these instances etomidate was administered in small incremental doses of 0.1 mg/kg along with either fentanyl or diazepam in very small doses.

Undesired Effects and Side Effects

Pain on injection is a distinct side effect of etomidate. The average incidence of pain upon injection appears to be approximately 20 to 30 percent, although reported incidences vary from 30 to 80 percent. The incidence and severity of pain can be reduced by premedication or pretreatment of a vein with fentanyl or lidocaine or by using a larger vein. Pain occurs most frequently from injections given into small veins in the wrist or dorsum of the hand and when no premedication was given. Thrombophlebitis has been reported as a side effect of etomidate injection, although there is no conclusive evidence that the incidence is any higher with etomidate than with thiopental. An injection of etomidate instilled within 30 seconds apparently produces less pain than does an injection over a period of 60 seconds. It was once thought that the phenomenon of pain on injection was due to the acidity of the aqueous solution (pH = 3.2) and the carrier was changed to propylene glycol solution (pH = 6.0). Unfortunately, even the propylene glycol solution carries an undesirable incidence of pain.

Another major disadvantage of etomidate is the myoclonic movements produced on induction. As mentioned earlier, the incidence ranges from 10 to 60 percent and can sometimes be severe. The myoclonic movements are reduced when premedication with diazepam or fentanyl has been given. A second injection of etomidate may precipitate new myoclonic movements; external stimuli have also been implicated in causing these movements.

Nausea and vomiting can occur postoperatively after the administration of etomidate. The incidence is greater when etomidate is used for both induction and maintenance.

Precautions

Etomidate probably should be avoided in patients with a history of seizure disorder or in patients who require higher levels of cortisol and aldosterone during anesthesia and in the postoperative period.

Ketamine

Ketamine was introduced into clinical anesthesia by Corssen and Domino in 1966. It was first approved for human use in 1970.

Chemistry and Physical Properties

Ketamine hydrochloride is a phencyclidine derivative used to produce a state of "dissociative" anesthesia. It is sometimes referred to as a cyclohexylamine (Fig 15–6).

Ketamine is a water-soluble solution and can be administered intravenously or intramuscularly. The pH of ketamine is acidic, between 3.5 and 5.5, and it is available in 10, 50, or 100 mg/ml solutions. Benzethonium chloride (Phemerol) 1:10,000 is added as a preservative. Ketamine is nonirritant on injection. It is recommended that the higher concentrations of ketamine be diluted and administered slowly over 60 seconds.

An intravenous administration of 1 to 2 mg/kg will produce surgical anesthesia in one circulation time, lasting about 5 to 10 minutes. Repeated doses may be given for a prolonged effect without significant cumulative effects.

Intramuscular doses of 5 to 10 mg/kg of the 10 percent solution produces surgical anesthesia within 3 to 4 minutes and lasting approximately 15 to 30 minutes.

Metabolism and Excretion

Ketamine undergoes N-demethylation and hydroxylation of the cyclohexane ring, resulting in the formation of conjugates, which are then excreted through the kidneys. Ninety-three percent of the metabolites can be found in the urine and approximately 3% in the feces. The metabolites have very weak anesthetic potency. Adverse effects on the hepatic or renal systems have not been reported.

Pharmacologic Effects

Central Nervous System. Ketamine produces unconsciousness, analgesia, and amnesia; however, the patient does not appear to be anesthetized but is "dissociated" from his environment. Dissociative anesthesia, as it is

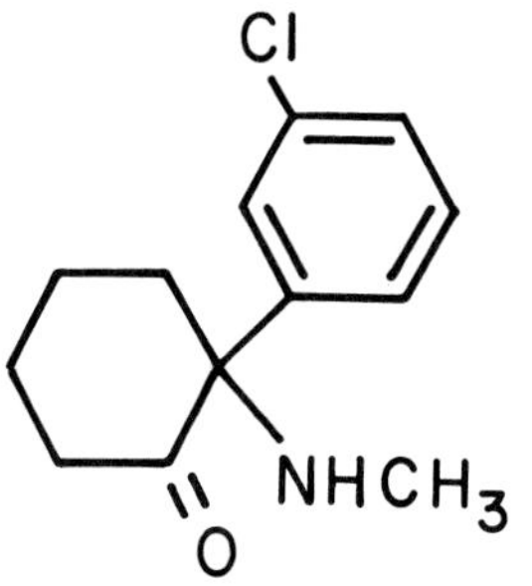

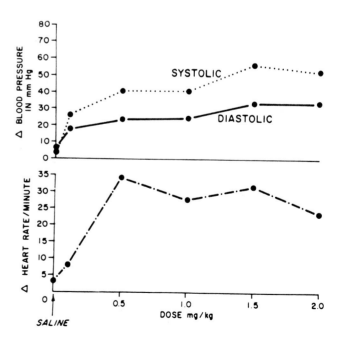

Figure 15–6. Chemical structure of the phencyclidine, ketamine hydrochloride (Ketalar).

termed, is characterized by catalepsy, catatonia, and hypertonus. The dissociative actions of ketamine produce surgical anesthesia that is very different from that produced by other anesthetics. When entering the dissociative state, the patient's eyes may remain open. Nystagmus occurs. A deep anesthetic level may be reached even though the eyes remain open.

Ketamine does not provide visceral analgesia and is not recommended for use as a sole anesthetic agent for abdominal or thoracic procedures.

Ketamine is believed to exert its effects by depressing the neocorticothalamic system, especially the association areas and the sensory and motor cortex; at the same time it stimulates areas of the limbic system. It has very little effect on the reticular activating system and the thalamic sensory nuclei, which is a distinguishing feature from most other anesthetics. Studies have shown that both visual and somatosensory impulses travel unimpaired from the periphery to the primary sensory cortex, but under the effects of ketamine the cortex is unable to interpet the afferent impulses and make appropriate responses.

Ketamine greatly increases the cerebral blood flow and cerebral metabolic rate and is not recommended for use in patients with cerebral vascular disease or space-occupying lesions. Ketamine also increases intraocular pressure and is contraindicated in open globe eye injuries.

Cardiovascular System. Unlike most other anesthetic agents, ketamine produces cardiovascular stimulation that affects both blood pressure and heart rate. Cardiac output is increased because of the rise in heart rate rather than because of an increase in stroke volume. In unpremedicated patients, the rise in blood pressure after an intravenous dose of 1 to 2 mg/kg is in the range of 20 to 40 mm Hg, with a slightly lower rise in the diastolic pressure. The rise in blood pressure occurs over the first 3 to 5 minutes and declines to normal values within 10 to 20 minutes. A rise in heart rate of approximately 15 beats per minute occurs immediately after intravenous injection. These changes in blood pressure and heart rate can be blocked or prevented by concomitant administration of halothane (Fig. 15–7).

After ketamine administration there is a rise in the circulating norepinephrine level. The hypertension and tachycardia are probably due to sympathetic stimulation, increased norepinephrine levels, and depression of barore-

ceptors. An effect similar to that seen with cocaine occurs: the reuptake of norepinephrine at the adrenergic nerve terminals is prevented.

There is wide individual variation in the blood pressure response to ketamine. There is very little evidence of a dose-related hypertensive effect and the rate of injection does not appear to affect the degree of hypertension. Premedication will decrease the rise in blood pressure, as will tubocurarine. Ketamine and pancuronium together will produce a rise in blood pressure and heart rate that is greater than that seen with ketamine alone.

Ketamine also appears to be an antiarrythmic agent. It blocks the oculocardiac reflex and, in small doses, has been noted to produce cardioversion.

Respiratory System. After intravenous injection, ketamine can produce a transient period of apnea. Slight respiratory depression without apnea may also occur and this is usually most pronounced 1 to 2 minutes after injection. The tidal volume is affected more than the respiratory rate. The initial period of apnea or respiratory depression is dose-dependent; larger doses appear to produce greater respiratory depression. Within a few minutes after induction, respiration is restored to normal or on many occasions, mildly stimulated.

The protective reflexes usually remain intact. Coughing, gagging, and swallowing can be seen with stimulation. Because both the pharyngeal and laryngeal reflexes remain intact, ketamine was at one time used for anesthetizing patients with full stomachs. It is now known that despite the presence of protective reflexes, aspiration can and has occurred. The incidence of aspiration is increased by narcotic premedication or preoperative sedation. Diazepam, droper-

Figure 15–7. Cardiovascular changes in response to ketamine administration. (*From Zsigmond, Domino. In Aldrete JA, Stanley TH (eds): Trends in Intravenous Anesthesia, 1980. Courtesy of the authors.*)

idol, and narcotics all depress laryngeal reflexes. Ketamine should be used with the same precautions as with any other general anesthetic agents.

In patients with bronchospastic disorders, including asthma, ketamine appears to offer protection and even reduce symptoms of an acute attack. The mechanism of action is believed to be due to the sympathetic stimulation (and consequent increased plasma catecholamine levels).

Ketamine produces an increase in salivation and tracheal mucus formation. An anticholinergic agent should be administered prior to the use of ketamine. Laryngospasm can occur with stimulation of the larynx by saliva or mucus, especially since the reflex activity remains intact.

Clinical Uses

Ketamine can be used as a sole anesthetic agent for minor procedures or as an induction agent. Indications for use as a sole agent are: (1) relatively short procedures that do not require muscle relaxation, such as minor orthopedic surgery (closed reductions of fractures), gynecologic procedures, neurologic diagnostic procedures (pneumoencephalograms, ventriculograms), ophthalmic examinations, or radiotherapy in small children; (2) mass casualty situations; (3) procedures where there is difficulty maintaining an airway, especially for burns and trauma that affect the face, neck, or upper airway; and (4) dressing changes in severely burned patients. Because this drug does not provide relief from visceral pain, it should not be used alone for abdominal and thoracic procedures.

Ketamine can be used as an induction agent before general anesthesia followed by conventional anesthetic techniques. Because of its effects on blood pressure, it is frequently used for poor-risk patients, such as patients suffering from shock or hypovolemia or any patient who might be a risk for severe hypotension should a barbiturate be used. Anesthetic induction in the asthmatic patient can be managed with ketamine if thiopental is to be avoided. Patients with porphyria who cannot receive barbiturate induction agents do well with ketamine.

Intramuscular ketamine is often very useful in young children who are unmanageable. Administered intramuscularly 5 to 10 mg/kg or less of ketamine will produce a mangeable child within 5 minutes. Nystagmus will occur as the child enters the dissociative state. The anesthetist can then apply monitors, place an intravenous line, and continue the anesthetic with another technique or continue on with intravenous doses of ketamine.

Undesired Effects and Complications

A commonly reported feature of ketamine anesthesia is the occurrence of an "emergence delirium" consisting of vivid, unpleasant dreams and bizarre hallucinations. Emergence delirium or excitement usually occurs in the immediate postoperative period and is characterized by restlessness, agitation, disorientation, moaning, or crying. The incidence of hallucinations in adults receiving ketamine anesthesia has been reported to be as high as 50 to 77 percent. It has occurred in approximately 50 percent of unpremedicated patients. Females appear to have a higher incidence of hallucinations than do men or children. Shorter procedures (5 to 10 min) seem to produce fewer problems with hallucinations than longer procedures (30 to 40 min) but is uncommon in prolonged procedures. It has also been suggested that emergence disturbances may be caused by stimulation during the arousal or emergence period.

Dreams and hallucinations can occur up to 24 hours after administration of ketamine. Amnesia persists for about an hour after the apparent recovery from anesthesia and the emergence delirium and excitement are usually not remembered. The dreams and hallucinations, however, are upsetting to the patient.

Medication with sedatives and narcotics or intravenous droperidol near the end of surgery appears to be effective in reducing the incidence of emergence delirium but not the dreams and hallucinations. Intravenous diazepam appears to decrease the incidence of unpleasant dreams, although it has little effect on emergence delirium. Physostigmine has been used for the emergence delirium with success.

Precautions and Contraindications

Ketamine is contraindicated in patients with coronary artery disease or angina. The increase in heart rate and blood pressure caused by this agent may increase myocardial oxygen demand while decreasing supply. Patients with a history of hypertension or cerebrovascular accident and patients at risk from increased intracranial or intraocular pressure should not be given this drug. A severe, sustained hypertensive episode has been reported in a patient on thyroid therapy; this can conceivably occur with the concomitant use of ergot derivatives and therefore should be avoided. Patients having a history of or suffering from neuropsychiatric disturbance should not be given this drug.

The major disadvantages of ketamine has been the postoperative hallucinations, dreams, and delirium seen even in patients without psychiatric disturbances. Another disadvantage of this agent is the slow recovery. Patients are usually in full control of their reflexes but it is often very difficult to determine the exact moment of emergence from the dissociative state. Patients should be left in an environment without a great deal of sensory stimulation to avoid emergence delirium and excitement. To prevent unpleasant reactions, the anesthetist should take care to select appropriate patients, order adequate premedication, be certain that the procedure is short, and avoid use of high doses.

Benzodiazepines

DIAZEPAM

Benzodiazepines were first synthesized in 1933. Chlordiazepoxide was the first compound introduced for clinical use. At present, there are a number of benzodiazepines available and they are used primarily as antianxiety agents and central-acting muscle relaxants. Of the benzodiazepines, diazepam is probably the most widely used and accepted. The new benzodiazepine, lorazepam, and diazepam are both used in anesthesia for a number of purposes, which will be discussed later in this section. Diazepam is considered the prototype drug for the benzodiazepines (Fig. 15–8).

Chemistry and Physical Properties

Diazepam is a benzodiazepine derivative; it is a colorless crystalline compound that is insoluble in water. It contains propylene glycol, ethyl alcohol, 5 percent sodium benzoate, and benzoic acid as buffers and benzyl alcohol as a preservative. Each milliliter contains 5 mg of diazepam. The pH of the solution ranges between 6.4 to 6.9. A transient cloudiness occurs when diazepam is diluted with water or saline, but this does not affect the potency. The manufacturer does not recommend dilution because it produces an emulsion of small, particulate matter. Diazepam should not be mixed with other drugs.

Metabolism and Excretion

After intravenous administration, redistribution is rapid and follows kinetics similar to highly lipid-soluble agents. Diazepam is 80 to 90 percent bound to plasma proteins. After distribution is complete, elimination proceeds at a slow rate because of a relatively long half-life.

In humans, the major metabolic pathway involves N-demethylation by hepatic microsomal enzymes. This process yields a pharmacologically active product, N-desmethyldiazepam, which is only slightly less potent than the parent compound. There is a constant rise in N-desmethyldiazepam levels over the first 24 hours, which is mirrored by the steady decline in diazepam levels. After 24 hours, both the metabolite and diazepam levels decline at approximately the same rate. There is an increase in plasma diazepam levels 6 to 8 hours after administration and then a second smaller rise at approximately 10 to 12 hours. This is believed to be due to enterohepatic recirculation but this has not been substantiated. The rise in plasma levels at 6 to 8 hours is of clinical significance because patients may become sedate and sleepy again at this time. Oxazepam is another active metabolite of diazepam and reaches a peak plasma concentration in 4 hours and is excreted as the glucuronide conjugate in the urine.

Approximately 70 percent of the drug is excreted in the urine as glucuronide and other inactive metabolites. The elimination half-life of diazepam is approximately 1 to 3 days. To date, there has been no evidence of impairment of liver or renal function in patients receiving diazepam.

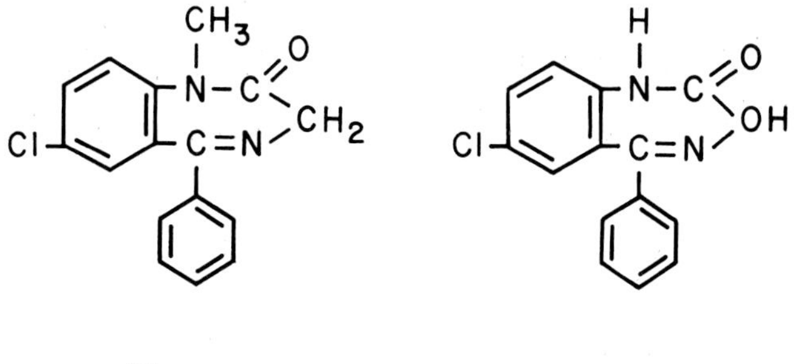

Pharmacologic Effects

Central Nervous System. The effects of benzodiazepines can vary from tranquility to sedation and, with larger doses, sleep. Diazepam also produces relaxation of striated muscles by a central action. Intravenous administration produces anterograde amnesia, but not retrograde amnesia.

Diazepam produces tranquility and sedation by its action on the limbic system, specifically the amygdala and the hippocampus. The mode of action of the benzodiazepines may be a competitive antagonism with norepinephrine. Another possibility is that these drugs act as agonists for gamma-aminobutyric acid (GABA), which is an inhibitory neurotransmitter.

When diazepam is administered intravenously, there is a delay of approximately 60 to 90 seconds before maximum depression occurs; however, there is a great deal of individual variation in response to diazepam.

The amnesic action is rare after oral or intramuscular administration but after intravenous injection of 10 mg diazepam, the peak effect occurs in approximately 2 minutes and will persist for about 5 minutes, declining over the next 30 to 40 minutes. The amnesic actions of benzodiazepines are most marked when sedation is produced. Patients may respond appropriately to questions or commands but recall for these events are suppressed (Fig. 15–9).

Diazepam is frequently used in anesthesia for purposes of sedation, reduction of anxiety, and amnesia. The level of sedation achieved is dose-related. Most patients will become heavily sedated with 20 to 40 mg. Thickened, slurred speech and nystagmus often precede the onset of sleep. Narcotics administered concomitantly will often reduce the required amount of diazepam to produce the desired effect as will alcohol ingestion, shock, or debilitation.

Diazepam   **Lorazepam**

Figure 15–8. Chemical structures of the two commonly used benzodiazepines: diazepam and lorazepam.

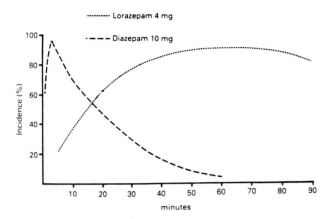

Figure 15–9. Comparison of the amnesic actions of diazepam and lorazepam. (Percentage incidence of patients who could not recall being shown objects at various times after the intravenous administration of diazepam and lorazepam.) (*Adapted from Dundee JN: In Feldman HS, Scurr E (eds): Current Topics in Anesthesia: Intravenous Anesthetics Agents. 1979.*)

Benzodiazepines are not analgesic and do not enhance the action of narcotics. The antianxiety effect combined with the soporific action may sometimes appear to produce analgesia.

Diazepam possesses anticonvulsant properties that can promptly control seizure activity by abolishing seizure discharge on the EEG within a few seconds of injection. It is often used as the drug of choice in status epilepticus. The anticonvulsant properties and the elevation of the seizure threshold by diazepam may be of clinical importance in patients who are to receive large doses of local anesthetics. Diazepam can be administered intramuscularly or intravenously for seizure control. Intravenous diazepam will control seizures within 20 seconds of intravenous injection and intramuscular injection within a few minutes.

In experimental models, the benzodiazepines suppress the spread of seizure activity in the cortex, thalamus, and limbic structures but do not appear to alter the discharge from the epileptogenic focus. Benzodiazepines also suppress polysynaptic activity in the spinal cord and decrease neuronal activity in the reticular system. It has also been suggested that benzodiazepines may mimic the effects of the inhibitory neurotransmitter glycine at strychnine-sensitive synapses.

Benzodiazepines have a centrally mediated muscle relaxant property, which is effective in the treatment of muscle spasms of varying etiology. This effect is believed to be due to the action of these drugs on the polysynaptic pathways within the spinal cord or on supraspinal structures. Diazepam has been used successfully for control of rigidity and muscle spasms caused by tetanus. Although diazepam produces a significant amount of relaxation of muscle rigidity and spasm, it does not produce adequate muscle relaxation for abdominal surgical procedures.

Cardiovascular System. The cardiovascular changes occurring with diazepam injection appear to be minimal. Intravenous injections of up to 0.8 mg/kg of diazepam by

one group of investigators produced no significant effects on cardiac output or blood pressure. The fall in systolic pressure did not exceed 20 mm Hg. Tachycardia has been reported after 0.2 mg/kg injection of diazepam but without changes in blood pressure or cardiac output. Other reports have demonstrated only a slight decrease in blood pressure and left ventricular stroke work with an increase in heart rate. It should be remembered that diazepam is not entirely devoid of cardiovascular depressant action. With large doses (60 mg), cardiovascular collapse has been reported after intravenous diazepam injection. The cardiovascular depressant effects of diazepam appear to be minimal in most patients, but the drug must be used with caution in patients with hypovolemic shock, advanced age, or in a debilitated state of health. Wide variations in the response to diazepam should always be kept in mind.

Diazepam has been used for cardioversions in poor-risk and emergency situations. When compared with thiopental, diazepam produces a significantly lower incidence of ventricular arrhythmias and hypotension with this procedure.

Respiratory System. Clinical doses of diazepam will cause a slight degree of respiratory depression. A significant rise in V_D/V_T and $Paco_2$ and decrease in tidal volume have been noted after doses of 0.14 mg/kg. Even small doses of diazepam administered intravenously have been reported to cause a transient period of apnea, especially if given with a narcotic. The ventilatory response to carbon dioxide is depressed.

Large doses of diazepam should be given with caution in patients with respiratory impairment, those receiving other central nervous system depressants such as barbiturates, or those who may have recently ingested alcohol. All these factors can lead to respiratory compromise or an exaggerated response.

Clinical Uses

Clinical uses of intravenous diazepam include the following:

1. Preoperative medication
2. Induction agent
3. Sedation and amnesia for local or regional anesthesia
4. Cardioversion
5. Long-term sedation and amnesia for intensive care patients
6. Control of seizures, tetanus
7. Treatment of severe delirium tremens

In anesthesia, diazepam is used most often for the first three of these purposes.

Diazepam is an excellent premedicant because of its efficacy in relieving anxiety and at the same time, producing sedation and amnesia. Intravenous diazepam can be administered in doses of 2.5 to 10 mg with or without a narcotic. If both narcotic and benzodiazepines are to be given, the doses should be adjusted accordingly. Oral diazepam is also very effective as a premedicant in doses of 5 to 10 mg. Gastrointestinal absorption of diazepam is rapid and complete, with plasma levels peaking shortly after administration. Intramuscular injections of diazepam are not as reliable in terms of absorption and distribution. The oral and intramuscular routes do not produce amnesia. If amnesia is to be a desired effect of premedication, diazepam must be injected intravenously.

Intravenous diazepam in doses of 0.2 to 0.6 mg/kg (in 5-to-10-mg increments at 1-to-2-minute intervals) may be required to induce general anesthesia. The dose may vary according to the degree of preoperative sedation. The onset of sleep after diazepam injection is 1 to 3 minutes. Diazepam induction is an alternative to the use of barbiturates in patients with porphyria, asthma, or bronchospastic disorders, and in poor-risk patients.

When patients induced with diazepam were compared with patients induced with thiopental, the following results were noted: Patients induced with diazepam had a longer duration of amnesia postoperatively, muscle relaxant requirements were approximately 8 to 10 percent lower in the patients induced with diazepam, hemodynamic parameters were essentially unchanged with diazepam, and the respiratory rate increased and tidal volume decreased, resulting in a 20 to 30 percent decrease in minute ventilation with diazepam. Postoperative nausea and vomiting occurred with the same frequency in diazepam and thiopental groups.

Because of the long half-life and the active metabolites present, patients may be sleepier after the large doses of diazepam used for induction.

Intravenous diazepam is used extensively for sedation for endoscopic procedures under local anesthesia and other minor surgical procedures carried out with local anesthesia, such as dental procedures or plastic surgery. Diazepam is also used in conjunction with a regional anesthetic technique to relieve anxiety and provide sedation and amnesia. Because diazepam does not provide analgesia, it can be given together with a narcotic to achieve a desired effect. Both the narcotic and the diazepam should be titrated carefully to avoid loss of consciousness or loss of airway because of upper airway obstruction. It must be remembered that under local anesthesia, with "sedation," the patient should be arousable, cooperative, and comfortable.

Contraindications and Complications

Injectable diazepam is contraindicated in patients with acute narrow-angle glaucoma and open-angle glaucoma unless patients are receiving appropriate therapy.

When administered intravenously, diazepam must be injected slowly to reduce the possibility of venous thrombosis, phlebitis, local irritation, and swelling. In a study conducted to investigate venous sequelae after diazepam and lorazepam injection, it was found that there was a significantly higher incidence of sequelae after intravenous diazepam than after lorazepam. Both thrombosis and phlebitis were found on the second and third days after injection, with an incidence of 23 percent for diazepam and 8 percent for lorazepam. Painless thrombosis that extended to the upper arm and axilla was noted at 7 to 10 days. Very long thrombosed segments of vein were found more often after diazepam; there was an incidence of 39 percent with di-

TABLE 15–4. INCIDENCE OF VENOUS SEQUELAE AFTER ADMINISTRATION OF INTRAVENOUS BENZODIAZEPINES

Drug	Dose (mg)	No.	Total Venous Sequelae (%)	
			2–3 days	7–10 days
Diazepam	10	44	23	39
Lorazepam	4	40	8	15

From Dundee JN: In Feldman HS, Scurr E (eds): Current Topics in Anesthesia: Intravenous Anesthetic Agents, 1979. Courtesy of the author.

azepam and 15 percent with lorazepam at 7 to 10 days (Table 15–4).

The complications occur most frequently when smaller vessels are selected for use. Venous thrombosis after diazepam is related to age. The incidence increases with age and increases sharply after age 60. Patients who are 70 years or older have almost a 100 percent chance of a venous thrombosis sequelae (Fig. 15–10).

Hypotension and apnea are always possible complications of intravenously administered central nervous system depressants. Resuscitative equipment should be available when moderate-to-large doses are administered. Diazepam must be administered with caution to patients in shock, taking barbiturates, phenothiazines, narcotics, MAO inhibitors, or alcohol, and elderly or debilitated patients.

LORAZEPAM

Chemistry and Physical Properties

Lorazepam is a new benzodiazepine derivative with actions very similar to diazepam. It is a white powder that is insoluble in water. Each milliliter contains polyethylene glycol in propylene glycol with benzyl alcohol as a preservative.

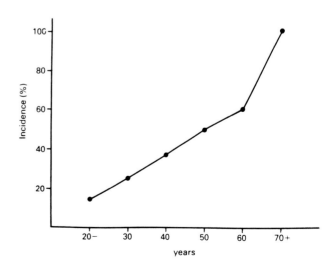

Figure 15–10. The incident of venous thrombosis after intravenous administration of 10 mg diazepam, related to the age of patients. (*From Dundee JN: In Feldman HS, Scurr E (eds): Current Topics in Anesthesia; Intravenous Anesthetic Agents, 1979. Courtesy of the author.*)

Absorption, Metabolism, and Excretion

Lorazepam is rapidly and virtually completely absorbed by the intramuscular route. Peak plasma concentrations are reached in 60 to 90 minutes. Maximum depressant effects after intravenous lorazepam do not occur for 10 to 20 minutes. After oral administration, peak plasma levels are reached within 2 hours. Absorption from the gastrointestinal tract is essentially complete. The mean half-life for intravenous or intramuscular lorazepam is approximately 16 hours. It is 80 percent bound to plasma proteins.

Lorazepam is conjugated in the liver into its major metabolite, lorazepam glucuronide. The metabolite is inactive and is excreted in the urine. The extent of drug accumulation with multiple-dose therapy is considerably less than that seen with diazepam.

Dilution of lorazepam with an equal volume of compatible solution is recommended before intravenous use.

Pharmacologic Effects

Lorazepam and diazepam have basically very similar effects on the central nervous, cardiovascular, and respiratory systems. The differences are discussed below.

Lorazepam has a much slower onset of action and a longer amnesic action. If lorazepam is to be given for sedation or relief of preoperative anxiety, it must be given earlier. The effects of a clinical dose of lorazepam usually last for 6 to 8 hours. The amnesic action peaks at 15 to 30 minutes intravenously and 2 hours intramuscularly and can continue for 4 to 8 hours. The degree of sedative and anxiety-relieving effects are similar for both diazepam and lorazepam. The amnesic effects occur more rapidly and also subside more rapidly with diazepam. Lorazepam is indicated when a longer period of sedation and amnesia are desired.

Lorazepam can be diluted with sterile water or sodium chloride for injection as well as D₅W injection. The drug should be administered slowly. The incidence of venous sequelae is much lower than with diazepam, probably because of the lower concentration of propylene glycol contained in the lorazepam.

Clinical Uses

Premedication and sedation for local or regional procedures can be accomplished quite nicely with lorazepam. However, inducing anesthesia with lorazepam is not recommended because of the slow onset of action. Other situations indicating benzodiazepines and requiring rapid onset of action would best be handled with diazepam. On the other hand, sedation and amnesia for intensive care patients on a respirator may be best accomplished with lorazepam.

Suggested doses for lorazepam are: intramuscular premedication 0.05 mg/kg up to 4 mg. For optimum amnesic effects, intramuscular lorazepam should be administered 2 hours before the anticipated procedure. For intravenous sedation and relief of anxiety, 0.04 mg/kg up to 2 mg total dose may be given. If optimum amnesic effects are required and would be beneficial, 0.05 mg/kg up to 4 mg may be administered intravenously.

TABLE 15–5. COMPARISON OF DIAZEPAM AND LORAZEPAM

	Diazepam	Lorazepam
1. Equivalent dose	10 mg	2.0–2.5 mg
2. Intravenous administration		
Peak effect	2–5 min	30–40 min
Duration of sedation	30 min–1 hr	3–6 hr
Duration of amnesia	3–30 min	30 min–4 hr
3. Active metabolites	Desmethyldiazepam 3-Hydroxydiazepam Oxazepam	None
4. Half-life	36 hr (20–50)	12 hr
5. Half-life of active metabolites	Desmethyldiazepam: 48–96 hr 3-Hydroxydiazepam: 15–20 hr Oxazepam: 6–8 hr	— — —

Precautions

As with diazepam, caution must be exercised when administering intravenous lorazepam. The same precautions should be taken regarding drug interactions, selection of patients, and availability of resuscitative equipment.

The manufacturer does not recommend the use of lorazepam in persons under 18 years of age.

Table 15–5 compares diazepam and lorazepam.

MIDAZOLAM

Midazolam is a relatively new benzodiazepine with actions very similar to those of diazepam. The principal differences between the two drugs are (1) the shorter duration of action, (2) the rapid metabolism, and (3) the water-solubility. Midazolam is approximately three times more potent than diazepam.

Chemistry and Physical Properties

Midazolam is the imidazole-1,4-benzodiazepine (Fig. 15–11) that is water-soluble in an acidic aqueous medium (pH < 4.0). At physiologic pH, midazolam becomes highly lipid-soluble and is one of the most lipid-soluble of the benzodiazepines. The high lipid solubility promotes rapid entry of the drug into the brain tissue. Studies have indicated that in an acid medium, the benzodiazepine ring opens and creates the desired water-soluble solution. At pHs close to 7.4 the ring closes, and the drug becomes lipid-soluble and readily crosses the blood–brain barrier. The therapeutic index (LD₅₀/ED₅₀) is 200.

Distribution, Metabolism, and Excretion

Intravenous administration of midazolam at physiologic pH produces a rapid onset of activity. Entry into brain tissue and clinical activity occur within 30 to 90 seconds. Midazolam's high lipid solubility and its rapid distribution and metabolism contribute to the drug's short duration of action. Midazolam is the shortest-acting benzodiazepine available.

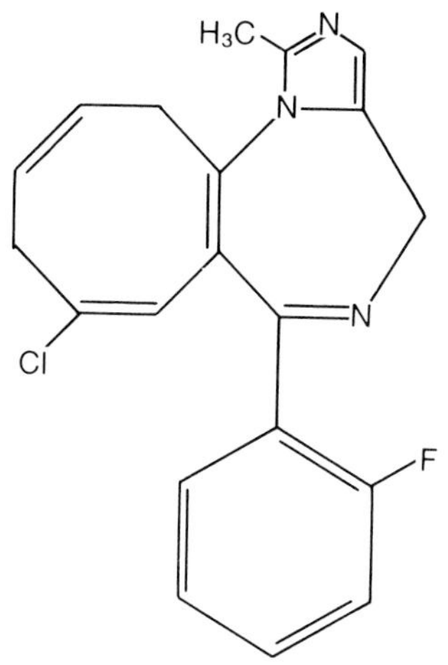

Figure 15–11. Chemical structure of midazolam.

The initial phase of drug disappearance is a result of drug distribution. This is followed by the less-rapid phase, which is attributed mainly to biotransformation. After distribution and equilibration, midazolam is rapidly eliminated. The half-life ranges from 1 to 4 hours.

Midazolam is approximately 96 to 97 percent protein-bound. The biotransformation involves hydroxylation by hepatic microsomal enzymes. The major metabolite is 1-hydroxymidazolam. There are two other metabolites formed in very small amounts, 4-hydroxymidazolam and 1,4-dehydroxymidazolam. The metabolites are excreted in the urine in the form of glucuronide conjugates. Both the 1- and 4-hydroxymetabolites possess pharmacologic activity, that is much less than that of the parent compound and is not believed to be a significant factor in the overall clinical effects.

Pharmacologic Effects

Central Nervous System. Once midazolam has crossed the blood–brain barrier, it works at the level of the central nervous system benzodiazepine receptors. Midazolam appears to have twice the affinity for these receptors as has diazepam. The actions are mediated by the potentiation of the gamma-aminobutyric acid (GABA) inhibitory effect, and GABA reuptake is inhibited.

Midazolam has similar clinical effects to diazepam. Premedicated patients will usually lose consciousness after intravenous doses of 0.2 mg/kg. Unpremedicated patients may require 0.3 mg/kg or more. Midazolam is an excellent hypnotic, anxiolytic, and amnesic. Anterograde amnesia can be obtained from both the intravenous and intramuscular routes of administration. The duration of amnesia is dose-related. Midazolam 0.15 mg/kg produced amnesia for approximately 40 minutes, whereas a dose of 0.3 to 0.35 mg/kg produced amnesia that lasted for 1 to 2 hours. Sedation and reduction in the level of anxiety are significantly obtained by intravenous doses of approximately 5 mg. Intramuscular doses for adequate sedation range from 0.07 to 0.08 mg/kg.

Midazolam possesses anticonvulsant actions similar to those of diazepam, but it appears to be more potent. The EEG changes produced by midazolam are also similar to those observed with diazepam. Cerebral blood flow and cerebral oxygen consumption are reduced much more effectively by midazolam than by diazepam. Intraocular pressures are reduced to a degree similar to the degree achieved with diazepam. Studies indicate that physostigmine is effective in reversing midazolam-induced sedation.

Cardiovascular System. Midazolam's cardiovascular actions are very similar to those of diazepam, although midazolam was found to produce a greater decrease in blood pressure. The decrease in blood pressure occurs by several mechanisms: (1) systemic vascular resistance is reduced, (2) venous return is therefore reduced, (3) contractility is decreased, and consequently (4) cardiac output is reduced. When these events occur, compensatory mechanisms respond immediately by mobilizing splanchnic blood flow to the central circulation and by a baroreceptor-mediated rise in heart rate and contractility, which returns cardiac output to normal levels. In general, blood pressures usually will decrease by 10 to 20 percent and heart rate will increase by about 15 percent.

When pulmonary artery occlusion pressures are initially high, midazolam has been shown to reduce them. Midazolam appears to maintain hemodynamic values in patients with ischemic heart disease. Samuelson et al reported a small increase in heart rate; small decreases in blood pressure, pulmonary artery pressure, and pulmonary artery occlusion pressure; and no change in cardiac output after induction with 0.5 mg/kg of midazolam. Cardiac arrhythmias have not been reported to be a problem.

Older patients and other poor-risk patients are more sensitive to midazolam. Volume-depleted patients may respond to midazolam with serious decreases in blood pressure; therefore, it would be wise to reduce the dose and to use caution. Although midazolam appears to produce only minimal cardiovascular depression, it has not been proven to be a safe agent for induction in hemodynamically unstable patients.

Respiratory System. Intravenous induction doses of midazolam will cause a transient respiratory depression (tidal volume reduction), apnea or both. The incidence of apnea varies between 18 and 78 percent, and the apneic period may last approximately 20 to 40 seconds. The respiratory depression and apnea appear to occur most frequently in patients premedicated with narcotics. Recovery from this depression corresponds with recovery from unconsciousness.

In patients with chronic obstructive pulmonary disease, there is a more profound and persistent depression of ventilation. This probably is true for the elderly and poor-risk patients, who are more sensitive to drugs. Sedation and respiratory depression can be reversed with physostigmine. Coughing, breath holding, and laryngospasms occur less frequently with midazolam than with thiopental.

Sedative doses of midazolam given intravenously may in some patients cause transient respiratory depression, and therefore patients should be observed closely whenever intravenous midazolam is used.

Renal System. Midazolam induction produces a reduction in renal blood flow and glomerular filtration rate (GFR), while increasing renal vascular resistance. These results are comparable to those observed with thiopental, with the exception of GFR reduction, which was less in patients who received midazolam.

Patients with chronic renal failure had shorter induction times and longer recovery times. These findings can be related to the lower degree of binding of midazolam to albumin and the greater availability of the active, unbound drug in these patients, who also showed a reduction of free drug clearance when compared with normal subjects.

Clinical Uses

Intravenous midazolam can be used for many of the same indications as diazepam: (1) as induction agent, (2) as maintenance agent, (3) as sedation for local anesthesia or regional techniques, and (4) as premedication.

Induction doses for midazolam range from 0.2 mg/kg to 0.5 mg/kg. The dose is influenced by premedication, age, physical status, speed of injection, and serum albumin concentration. Narcotic premedication appears to decrease the required dose of midazolam and shortens the induction time. Sedatives and hypnotic premedications do not have the same ability to reduce dosage or induction times.

Induction times vary from 30 seconds to almost 5 minutes depending on the speed of injection. When compared with thiopental, midazolam induction and emergence are considerably slower. Patients regained consciousness after midazolam in approximately 15 minutes. Although this is prolonged compared with thiopental, patients were considered street fit in 3 to 4 hours after induction with either midazolam or thiopental induction. It should be remembered that induction and emergence times may be abnormal in patients with chronic renal failure.

Midazolam offers no advantage over thiopental for speed of induction and is not more effective in maintaining cardiovascular dynamics than etomidate. The advantages of midazolam as an induction agent are its increased reliability, speed of induction, and duration of action when compared with diazepam.

Midazolam can be used during anesthetic maintenance in the same manner as diazepam. Midazolam lacks analgesic properties, so it must be used in combination with narcotics in a balanced technique or as an adjunct to an inhalation anesthetic. For short procedures, midazolam may be used in a similar manner to thiopental by giving small intermittent doses after induction, supplemented by nitrous oxide and a narcotic premedication.

To supplement a regional or local anesthetic, small doses of intravenous midazolam in combination with small doses of narcotics will produce hypnosis, sedation, and amnesia. Both midazolam and narcotics should be carefully titrated to obtain the desired effect. Close observation of blood pressure and respirations is crucial when any intravenous agent is administered for sedation.

Premedication with midazolam can be accomplished intravenously, intramuscularly, or orally. Intravenous premedication may supplement previously administered oral or intramuscular drugs or may be used for acute sedation in an unpremedicated patient. When used for sedation, intravenous midazolam should be titrated to obtain the desired effect. Intramuscular premedication with midazolam produces much of the same effects as are obtained by the intravenous route, namely, hypnosis, amnesia, and anxiolysis. The recommended intramuscular dose is 0.07 to 0.08 mg/kg approximately 1 hour before surgery. Oral midazolam is rapidly absorbed from the gastrointestinal tract. Peak plasma concentrations and clinical effects are noted within 1 hour. After oral administration, only 40 to 50 percent of the dose will be available in the systematic circulation in the intact form. This is due to extensive first-pass hepatic extraction and necessitates doses approximately twice the intravenous dose to achieve the same effect. The elimination half-lives of oral and intravenous midazolam are similar and are independent of the route of administration.

Advantages over Diazepam

Midazolam causes minimal local irritation and pain after intravenous or intramuscular administration. Intravenous midazolam has not been associated with the venous sequelae common with diazepam. Another advantage is the rapid onset of action and the rapid metabolism and half-life. Midazolam has superiority over diazepam in outpatient use and in short surgical or diagnostic procedures requiring sedation and amnesia.

Neuroleptanalgesia

Neurolepsis is a term coined by Delay and his colleagues in 1959 to describe a drug-induced behavioral syndrome consisting of diminished aggression, indifference to surroundings, and somnolence with easy arousability to full rational attention. Neuroleptic is the term used to describe drugs that produce neurolepsis or a neuroleptic state and is synonymous with the term "major tranquilizer."

In the same year that Delay defined neurolepsis, De-Castro and Mundeleer introduced neuroleptanalgesia at the French Anesthesia Congress in Lyon. Neuroleptanalgesia has since then become an extremely popular and useful anesthetic technique. As the name suggests, it is a state produced by combining a potent neuroleptic drug with a potent narcotic. DeCastro and Mundeleer emphasized the uniqueness of this technique from "balanced" techniques in that the patients were neither asleep nor awake but in a state of profound analgesia and psychomotor sedation. DeCastro and Mundeleer originally used haloperidol, with a narcotic, muscle relaxant, and oxygen. With the introduction of the potent narcotic fentanyl and the neuroleptic droperidol in 1963, the previously used drugs were discontinued and Innovar, a mixture of these two drugs, became the frequently used combination.

The effects produced by Innovar are the result of each component exerting its own pharmacologic effect independently of the other. The combination of fentanyl to droperidol is in a fixed ratio of 1:50; each milliliter of Innovar contains fentanyl 0.05 mg and droperidol 2.5 mg.

State of Neuroleptanalgesia

Neuroleptanalgesia has been described as a state of tranquilization and intense analgesia with little or no hypnosis. The technique affects the subcortical areas of the brain, the thalamus, hypothalamus, and reticular system to provide analgesia and sedation while leaving cortical functions intact. Central nervous system characteristics of this state include somnolence without loss of consciousness, psychological detachment from the environment, inhibition of learned behavioral activity and reflexes, and analgesia.

From an anesthetic viewpoint, neuroleptanalgesia offers several advantageous features: (1) mental withdrawal from the immediate situation with an ability to respond and cooperate when the need arises, (2) a disinclination to move, (3) potent antiemetic effects, (4) analgesia, and (5) cardiovascular stability. When undisturbed, the patient remains in a state of calm detachment. The technique has been especially useful for diagnostic or surgical procedures requiring consciousness and cooperation of the patient. If an anesthetic agent is added to produce unconsciousness and amnesia, the technique is termed "neuroleptanesthesia." A muscle relaxant can be added if required, and this technique then becomes very similar to balanced anesthesia.

The following discussion will treat the pharmacology of droperidol and fentanyl separately and then the clinical uses of the combined solution, Innovar.

DROPERIDOL

Droperidol is a neuroleptic derived from the butyrophenone series of drugs (Fig. 15–12).

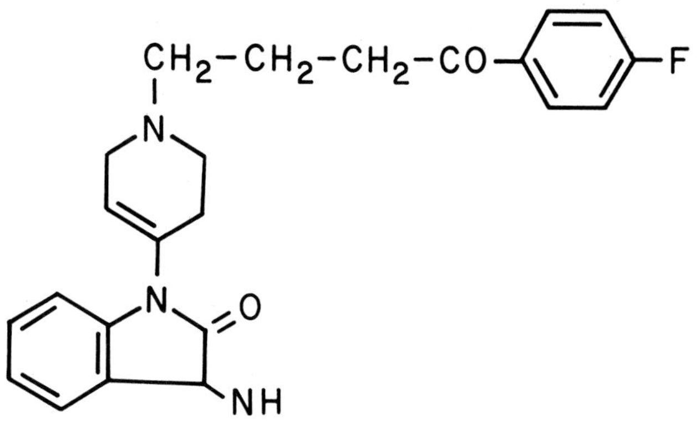

Droperidol is available alone in 2-, 5-, or 10-ml vials or in combination with fentanyl as Innovar. Whether alone or in combination with fentanyl, droperidol 2.5 mg is contained in each milliliter. The pH of the clear, colorless solution is adjusted to 3.5. The 10-ml vial contains methylparaben and propylparaben as preservatives. The onset of action after intravenous injection is 3 to 5 minutes. The full effect may not be apparent for 30 minutes. The duration of action is generally 2 to 4 hours, but the effects of the drug may be noted for up to 12 hours.

Metabolism and Excretion

Droperidol is metabolized in the liver. Excretion of the drug occurs by way of urine and feces with the majority of the metabolites being excreted within 24 hours. Approximately

Figure 15–12. Chemical structure of the butyrophenone droperidol (Inapsine).

10 percent of the drug is excreted intact through the kidneys.

No untoward effects on the liver or kidneys have been noted.

Pharmacologic Effects

Central Nervous System. The droperidol component of Innovar contributes most to the state of neurolepsis. Droperidol produces marked tranquilization and inhibits operant (learned) behavior. The butyrophenones are able to induce cataleptic immobility, in which patients appear tranquil and dissociated from the environment but are readily accessible when spoken to. Neuroleptics also inhibit symptoms of delusions, hallucinations, paranoia, and mania.

The outward tranquility induced by droperidol often masks a state of marked mental restlessness, agitation, apprehension, and fear. Numerous reports from patients indicate that although they appeared tranquil and calm, they felt extremely anxious and ill at ease. Droperidol alone has not been found to have a high degree of patient acceptance. Patients report an increase in their level of anxiety after receiving droperidol and an inability to express their anxiety while under the influence of the drug.

The ability of the neuroleptics to exert these effects on the central nervous system result from their ability to competitively antagonize the dopamine-mediated synapses in the brain. The action is on the postsynaptic neuron, where dopamine is the neurotransmitter. At certain synapses, gamma-aminobutyric acid (GABA) is the inhibitory transmitter and dopamine the stimulatory transmitter. It is believed that neuroleptics compete for the dopaminergic receptors to decrease transmission.

Neuroleptics have a predilection for areas in the brain that are high in dopaminergic receptors, including the chemoreceptor trigger zone (CTZ) and nigrostriatum. The marked antiemetic activity of droperidol is due to its action on the CTZ in the medulla. Droperidol does not antagonize motion sickness originating in the labyrinth. Extrapyramidal systems sometime occur as a result of dopamine blockade at the extrapyramidal nigrostriatum, and pseudoparkinsonian effects can be noted, though they may sometimes be delayed for up to 24 hours. This is usually associated with high doses but has also been reported with low doses administered intramuscularly. These effects respond to anticholinergics or antiparkinson therapy. Extrapyramidal side effects occur in approximately 1 percent of the patients who are given the drug.

Droperidol can potentiate the effects of other central-nervous-system depressants such as thiopental, other tranquilizers, narcotics, and general anesthetics. Dosage adjustments should be made accordingly.

Cardiovascular System. Droperidol has little or no effect on the myocardium, heart rate, or cardiac output. The systemic blood pressure falls slightly (in a normovolemic patient) because of the alpha-adrenergic blocking activity. This action is usually very mild, but hypotension can occur in a hypovolemic patient. There is also a small decrease in pulmonary vascular pressures caused by decreased resistance. In general, the cardiovascular hemodynamics are well maintained. There has been some evidence that droperidol may reduce the incidence of epinephrine-induced arrhythmias, but it does not appear to prevent other cardiac arrhythmias.

Body oxygen consumption is reduced slightly after droperidol administration.

Respiratory System. Droperidol has not been found to produce any significant degree of respiratory depression. Alterations in arterial blood gases have not been reported after doses of 10 mg of droperidol administered intravenously.

The respiratory depression occurring with the administration of Innovar is due to the narcotic component, fentanyl.

FENTANYL

Fentanyl is the narcotic component in Innovar. It is a synthetic narcotic that is structurally related to meperidine. Fentanyl is approximately 100 times more potent than morphine and 1,000 times more potent than meperidine. Fentanyl 0.1 mg is roughly equal to 10 mg of morphine or 75 mg of meperidine (Fig. 15–13).

Fentanyl is available alone or in combination with droperidol as Innovar. Each milliliter contains 0.05 mg of fentanyl. The pH is adjusted to 4.0 to 7.5 with sodium hydroxide. Ten percent of fentanyl is excreted unchanged; the remainder is degraded in the liver.

Liver function tests and renal function are unaltered by fentanyl.

Pharmacologic Effects

Central Nervous System. Fentanyl is a powerful and potent analgesic. After intravenous administration, there is an immediate onset of action, with its peak effect occurring at about 4 to 5 minutes. The analgesic effect lasts for 30 to 60 minutes after a single dose.

Pain from both somatic and visceral sources is relieved. The primary site of action appears to be the thalamus, hypothalamus, reticular system, and the gamma neurons. At the cortical level, an indifference to pain is noted. Fentanyl alone has very little hypnotic or sedative action. Fentanyl also possesses typical narcotic features, such as stimulation

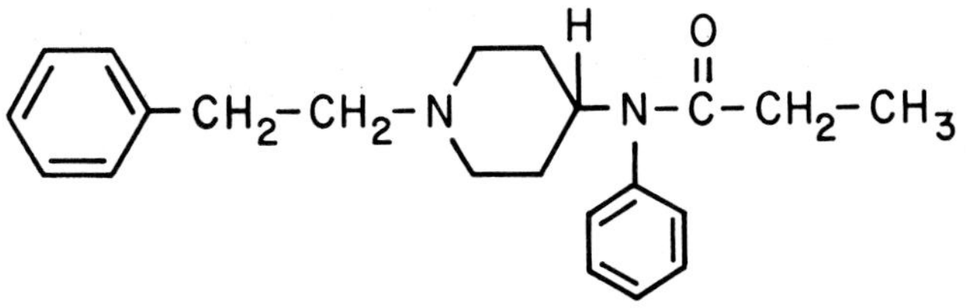

Figure 15–13. Chemical structure of the narcotic fentanyl (Sublimaze).

of miosis, euphoria, and depression of the ventilatory control centers.

Fentanyl appears to have less emetic activity than the other narcotic analgesics.

Cardiovascular System. Fentanyl has minor effects on the cardiovascular system. Cardiac output usually remains unchanged. Myocardial function is not depressed nor is the vascular system affected. A slight decrease in systemic blood pressure is sometimes seen. This is consistent with the effects of sedation and analgesia. Bradycardia may occur because of fentanyl's central vagotonic effect. This is easily reversed by anticholinergics.

Respiratory System. Fentanyl is a potent respiratory depressant; the degree of depression is directly related to dosage. Respiratory frequency and tidal volume are both affected. There is a lowered sensitivity of the ventilatory control centers to carbon dioxide levels. Larger doses may produce total apnea. The peak respiratory depressant effect of a single intravenous dose of fentanyl appears between 5 and 10 minutes after injection. The ventilatory status is usually returned to normal by approximately 30 minutes; however, altered responses to carbon dioxide have been noted for up to 4 hours after a single dose. This depression of carbon dioxide sensitivity may persist longer than the depression of respiratory rate or the analgesic effect.

Histamine release rarely occurs with fentanyl, but the possibility of bronchoconstriction caused by histamine is always a possibility.

Occasionally, there is difficulty ventilating a patient who has been given intravenous fentanyl. This is usually a result of muscle rigidity of the thorax and abdomen. The severity seems to be related to the dose and speed of injection and is believed to be the result of a direct excitatory effect on the spinal reflexes. This phenomenon has been referred to as the "stiff chest" syndrome and can be overcome with a small dose of succinylcholine. Slow intravenous injections will usually prevent this occurrence.

CLINICAL USES OF INNOVAR

Innovar has been used clinically for many procedures with great success and effectiveness. It has been especially useful when a sedated but cooperative patient is required. Patients undergoing diagnostic procedures, such as angiography, esophagoscopy, or bronchoscopy, who are given Innovar with local anesthesia appear to tolerate it well. The drug is also useful in providing sedation for surgical procedures under local or regional anesthesia.

An awake intubation is usually well tolerated by patients under neuroleptanalgesia, especially when cooperation is essential, as in an awake blind nasal intubation.

Innovar has been used for cardiopulmonary bypass surgery to avoid the depressant effects of volatile agents. It has also been used in neurosurgical procedures, such as stereotactic surgery, where conscious cooperation is required, and for craniotomies in combination with nitrous oxide and muscle relaxant. An advantage of neurolept-anesthesia using Innovar for neurosurgical procedures is that it reduces both cerebral blood flow and cerebral oxygen consumption.

Innovar has also been used for premedication, but there have been reports of the drug increasing the level of anxiety and apprehension to the point where patients have refused to have their surgery. It should also be kept in mind that the narcotic component is very potent and may lead to significant ventilatory depression in patients who are not closely watched.

Nitrous-narcotic techniques using fentanyl and nitrous oxide (with or without muscle relaxant) can be supplemented with Innovar or droperidol for tranquilizing effects.

Contraindications and Precautions

Innovar is contraindicated in patients with Parkinson's disease. The droperidol component can cause an increase in the symptoms caused by action on the dopaminergic synapses. Innovar is not recommended for use in outpatients because of the prolonged duration of action of droperidol. The safety of Innovar in children under 2 years of age and in pregnancy has not been established.

Innovar must be used with caution in elderly, debilitated, or hypovolemic individuals. Dosages should be titrated slowly. Caution must be exercised when administering this drug to patients who have compromised ventilatory reserve. The narcotic component may additionally reduce respiratory drive and increase airway resistance. The doses of other central nervous system depressants must be adjusted for patients who have received Innovar.

The advantages of neuroleptanalgesia are many and include (1) lowered incidence of nausea and vomiting, (2) profound sedation with easy arousability, (3) profound analgesia, and (4) cardiovascular stability. There are, however, certain disadvantages that must be considered as well when selecting an anesthetic technique. It must be remembered that Innovar can cause extrapyramidal side effects. The effects of droperidol will outlast the analgesic effects and may be prolonged, and the respiratory depressant effects often far outlast the analgesic effects. These facts must all be kept in mind when selecting an appropriate technique for each patient.

Narcotics

MORPHINE, MEPERIDINE, AND FENTANYL

Opium is a Greek word meaning *juice,* which describes the drugs obtained from the milky exudate of the incised unripe seed capsules of the poppy plant, *Papaver somniferum,* which is indigenous to Asia Minor. The term opioid refers to any natural or synthetic drug with pharmacologic properties similar to morphine. The term is synonymous with narcotic analgesics.

Opium has been used as a narcotic since the earliest time. Greek history contains records of opium use that date back to 300 B.C. It has been used throughout history for various purposes including pain relief and control of dysenteries. When opium was first used in connection with surgery is difficult to determine. The earliest known soporific sponge dates back to the ninth century. Soporific sponges were sponges filled with opium, *Mandragora, Cicuta,* and hyoscyamus and were used to relieve pain during operations in the 14th century. The first attempt to administer opiates intravenously for anesthesia was made by Elscholtz in 1665. In 1778, Boerhaave used opium for anesthesia as a vapor by inhalation and as a powder. The extreme variability of the opium in terms of doses and absorption rate often resulted in inadequate analgesia or coma and death. Pravaz in 1853 invented the syringe, and Alexander Wood developed the hollow needle in the same year. It was not until this time that accurate means of administering opiods became feasible.

In 1805, Serturner described a pure alkaloid base isolated from opium. In 1817, he published this report and called the compound morphine after the Greek god of dreams, Morpheus.

Opium, in the form of dried powder, contains a number of alkaloids. About 25 different alkaloids have been identified and have been placed into two groups. The phenanthrene group of alkaloids possess narcotic properties. Of this group, morphine and codeine are the two clinically significant opioids. The benzylisoquinoline group yields drugs such as papaverine, noscapine, and other related substances, which lack narcotic activity but are used as antitussives and smooth muscle relaxants.

Morphine constitutes approximately 10 percent of the opium powder and is the oldest narcotic in use at present. It is also the standard to which all other narcotics are compared.

Because morphine is the prototype for narcotics, the following information about this class of drugs will pertain to morphine as well as the others unless otherwise specified. The three narcotics to be discussed are morphine, meperidine, and fentanyl (Fig. 15–14).

Morphine and the other analgesic alkaloids are phenanthrene derivatives, so called because of the tricyclic system they contain. Meperidine is chemically dissimilar to morphine and is a phenylpiperidine derivative (Fig. 15–15).

The piperidine ring has a unique configuration and is common to morphine, meperidine, and benzomorphan derivatives. The analgesic activity of opiates is highly stereospecific in that the levo-isomer possesses most of the potency. A tertiary nitrogen, a quaternary carbon separated from the nitrogen by an ethane chain, and an electrophilic

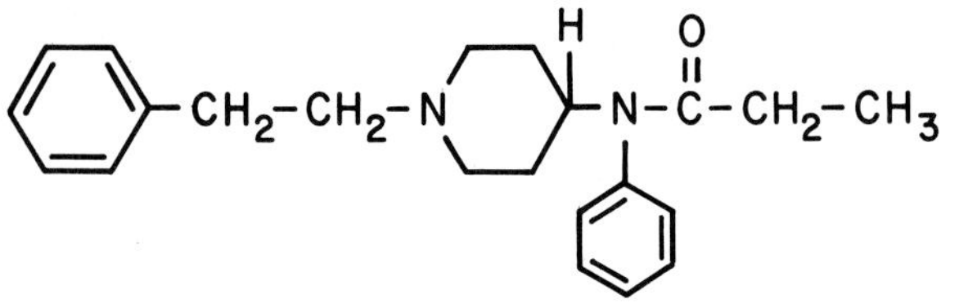

Fentanyl (Sublimaze)

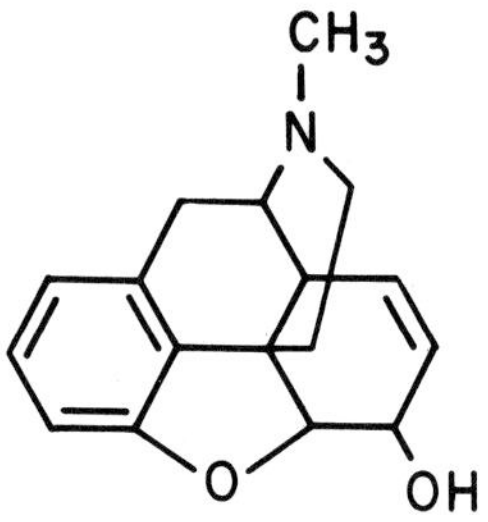

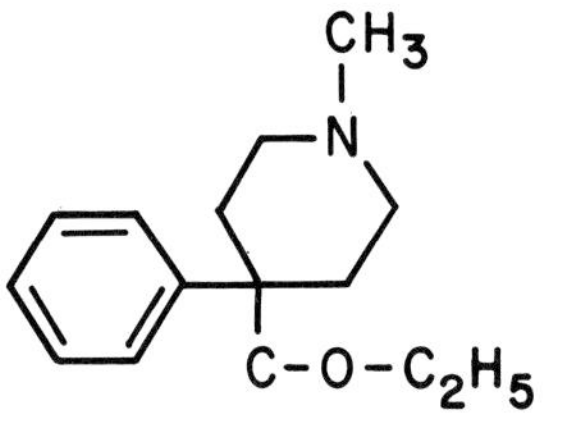

Morphine   **Meperidine (Demerol)**

Figure 15–14. Chemical structure of narcotics: morphine, meperidine, and fentanyl.

carbon that attaches a phenylic or ketone group appear to be common structural characteristics.

Meperidine is a totally synthetic opiate introduced in 1939 by Eisleb and Schaumann in Germany. It was originally studied because of its atropine-like effect and the similarity of its chemical structure to atropine. Initial tests demonstrated a narcotic analgesic property and subsequent studies verified this effect. Today, meperidine is one of the most widely used narcotic analgesics.

Like meperidine, fentanyl is a synthetic piperidine derivative. It was introduced in 1963 by Janssen as the narcotic component of Innovar.

Absorption, Metabolism, and Excretion

Narcotics are absorbed completely from all routes of administration. Those used for anesthesia are usually adminis-

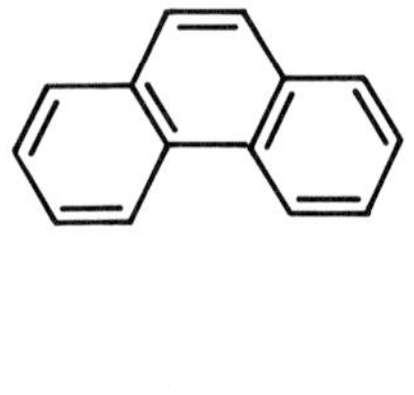

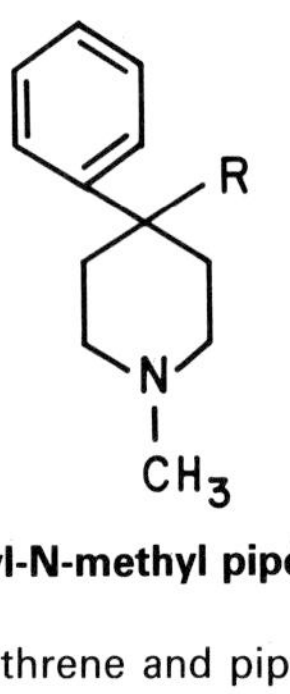

Phenanthrene   **α-Phenyl-N-methyl piperidine**

Figure 15–15. Structures of phenanthrene and piperidine. The phenanthene rings are evident in the structure of morphine; the piperidine structure is contained in meperidine.

tered by intravenous injection and therefore the pharmacokinetics of absorption are not a major consideration.

The tissue uptake and distribution of narcotics follow the same pharmacokinetic principles as other drugs injected intravenously. The plasma levels of narcotics fall rapidly after injection, and only a small percentage of the injected drug actually reaches the central nervous system tissues. Plasma concentrations of narcotics have been noted to be greater in older individuals and may possibly relate to cardiac output, but there is no available data that would confirm or refute this idea.

All three narcotics are metabolized in the liver and their primary route of excretion is the kidneys. Approximately 5 percent of morphine is N-demethylated and almost all of this is excreted as normorphine in the urine. Only about 5 to 10 percent of free morphine or any of its metabolites can be detected in the feces. Respiratory depression after morphine anesthesia has been found to be inversely related to urinary flow rate and excretion of morphine. Patients with low urine outputs have been shown to have a longer period of respiratory depression after high-dose morphine anesthesia.

Meperidine is N-demethylated to normeperidine and hydrolyzed to meperidinic acid. N-demethylation of the meperidinic acid occurs and normeperidinic acid is formed. The liver conjugates these metabolites with glucuronide before they are excreted in the urine.

A hydrolytic reaction in the liver metabolizes 80 to 90 percent of fentanyl and produces 4-n-(N-propronyl-anilino)-piperidine and proprionic acid. An oxidative reaction also occurs but to a much smaller extent. Only about 10 percent of fentanyl is excreted unchanged. Approximately 70 percent of the administration drug is excreted in 4 days with the greatest concentration detected between 8 and 24 hours after administration. The brevity of action of fentanyl is due primarily to rapid redistribution rather than to a rapid metabolism and excretion.

Pharmacologic Effects

Central Nervous System. Narcotic effects on the central nervous system include analgesia, drowsiness, mood changes, and mental clouding.

Analgesia is the main feature of narcotics. The analgesic action can usually be produced without disturbing other Central Nervous System functions. For a given degree of analgesia, the drowsiness or mental clouding produced by the narcotics is less pronounced and of a different character than, e.g., nitrous oxide, alcohol, or barbiturate intoxication.

The site and mechanism of analgesic action remains uncertain at the present time but is believed to be a result of stimulation of the pain-inhibiting system. The receptors of this system are excited by narcotics, endorphins, enkephalins, and electrical stimulation and are located around the third ventricle, cerebral aqueduct, and the rostral areas of the fourth ventricle. Stimulation of this system is believed to cause descending inhibition of transmission of nociceptive information through the spinal cord. Narcotics also induce an alteration in the limbic system response to painful stimuli without significant alteration of the sensory pathways. The narcotics do not alter the threshold or responsiveness of the nerve endings to painful stimuli, nor do they affect peripheral nerve conduction. The subjective perception and interpretation of the noxious stimulus are altered by the effects of narcotics on the cortical perception areas of the brain.

Clinically, pain threshold is raised and the perception of response to pain is blunted. The painful stimulus may be noted but not perceived as painful. Patients often report that the pain is present but tolerable.

Dull, continuous pain can be relieved more effectively than sharp intermittent pain but most types of pain can be relieved by narcotics if sufficient doses are adminstered. Analgesia usually occurs without loss of consciousness but sedation, drowsiness, and mental clouding become more prominent as the dose is increased. Therapeutic doses will usually produce minimal sedative effects, but increasingly larger doses produce effects that can range from sedation to coma.

When an appropriate amount of narcotic is administered to a patient with pain, discomfort, fear, anxiety, or tension, patients report that they are less distressed. Drowsiness, euphoria, or sleep may ensue. The onset of sedation is slower than that of the analgesic effect but its duration is greater. Narcotics given to patients who are without pain may cause dysphoria rather than euphoria and cause unnecessary anxiety or fear.

Although narcotics provide excellent analgesia, they do not always provide amnesia when used alone. Amnesia may be associated with loss of consciousness after large doses of narcotics. Narcotics combined with nitrous oxide will produce amnesia during general anesthesia but narcotic-with-oxygen techniques should not be relied upon to produce amnesia.

Nausea and vomiting are primarily due to the ability of narcotics to directly stimulate the CTZ located in the medulla. A vestibular component may be involved as well, because there appears to be a greater incidence of emesis in ambulatory patients. Other causes for nausea and vomiting after narcotic administration include a delayed time of emptying gastrointestinal contents, increased tone of smooth muscle and sphincters, and an increased volume of pancreatic and biliary secretions. Hypotension and inadequate cerebral perfusion may also stimulate the CTZ. Very large doses of narcotics may depress it. The emetic effect of morphine is counteracted by narcotic antagonists, phenothiazines, droperidol, and drugs used for motion sickness.

Cardiovascular System.
Myocardial depression is not a feature of intravenously administered morphine or fentanyl in intact humans and animals. Morphine has a positive inotropic effect on dogs that is dependent on the release of endogenous catecholamines. This effect can be blocked by beta blockers. Plasma and urine catecholamine levels are usually elevated after morphine administration. Whereas morphine and fentanyl are both benign with respect to myocardial function, meperidine has been found to cause significant depression.

Morphine and fentanyl are capable of producing vagal stimulation and bradycardia. There is also some evidence that morphine depresses intraatrial and AV nodal conduction. Intravenous administration of meperidine often causes a significant increase in heart rate as a result of a vagolytic effect.

All three drugs produce a certain degree of arterial and venodilating effects. Morphine is believed to possess an alpha-blocking property, and its effects on the capacitance vessels are much more profound and prolonged than on the arterial system. The venodilating effects appear to be dose-dependent and usually are not significant at lower doses. Histamine release also plays a role in vasodilation after morphine or meperidine administration. This effect is rarely seen with fentanyl.

Hypotension after narcotic injection is related to rate of injection and is a more frequent occurrence in the hypovolemic or hypertensive individual. Fluid administration and slight Trendelenburg position will usually correct the hypotensive episode. Hypotension after administration of fentanyl is usually due to bradycardia and is usually responsive to atropine administration.

Intravenous narcotics combined with nitrous oxide will produce cardiovascular effects that are quite different from the effects of the narcotic alone. The meperidine-nitrous oxide combination will produce a reduction in the arterial pressure and a significant lowering of cardiac output and stroke volume with an increase in peripheral vascular resistance. Nitrous oxide in combination with morphine or fentanyl produces a similar effect, though the increase in peripheral vascular resistance is not as pronounced. The reduction in cardiac output is usually greater than the reduction of the mean arterial pressure. Morphine reduces pulmonary blood volume and increases pulmonary artery pressure.

Cerebral blood flow is not directly affected by narcotics. Respiratory depression and carbon dioxide retention caused by large doses of narcotics will produce cerebral vasodilation and an increase in intracranial and cerebral-spinal fluid pressure. Artificial ventilation that maintains $Paco_2$ at normal levels will maintain a normal cerebral blood flow despite large doses of narcotics. Cerebral metabolic rate is reduced.

Respiratory System.
Therapeutic doses of narcotics will produce respiratory depression which can be detected without other apparent signs of central nervous system depression. The respiratory depression is dose-related and can proceed to apnea with large doses.

The mechanism of respiratory depression involves direct depression of the medullary centers involved in ventilatory control. There is a reduction in the response of the central chemoreceptors to carbon dioxide levels as well as a decrease in response of the carotid and aortic chemoreceptors to hypoxia. The carbon dioxide threshold is elevated and the Pco_2-alveolar ventilation curve is shifted to the right. The pontine and medullary centers involved in ventilatory rhythmicity are also depressed, which may result in irregular and periodic breathing. Often, the inspiratory phase is prolonged and expiratory phase is delayed.

Respiratory rate, minute volume, and tidal volume are all depressed. Small doses of narcotics will decrease the respiratory rate without significantly affecting tidal exchange, whereas anesthetic doses may terminate involuntary respirations. Voluntary mechanisms for ventilation remain intact and the patients are able to respond to commands to breathe. The respiratory rate is greatly depressed but at this stage the tidal volume is markedly increased to compensate. Narcotic overdoses and deaths result from profound respiratory depression and respiratory arrest.

Other effects of narcotics on respiration include depression of ciliary action within the bronchial tree, inhibition of the cough reflex caused by action on the cough center located in the medulla, and increased bronchial tone. It is not clear whether the latter effect is mainly a direct effect on smooth muscle or an indirect action caused by histamine liberation or by an elevation of the Pa_{CO_2}.

Miscellaneous Effects. Opiates will decrease gastric and intestinal secretions and motility and increase sphincter tone. There is a delay in gastric emptying and the passage of bowel contents. Because of the delay, water is more completely absorbed. This is believed to contribute to the constipating effects of narcotics. Propulsive contractions of the bowel are virtually abolished, and the tone may be increased to the point of spasm. Atropine will partially antagonize the spasmogenic action but has little effect on the decreased propulsive activity.

Because opiates tend to stimulate smooth muscle of the gastrointestinal and genitourinary tracts, the resulting spasms can create an increased pressure within these tracts to produce pain or rupture of smooth muscle that is weakened by surgery or disease. Biliary colic and spasm are intensified by morphine. Meperidine and fentanyl can also precipitate biliary colic but to a lesser degree than morphine. It has been noted that patients who are already suffering from colic can obtain relief of their pain from opiates even though these do increase the intensity of the spasm.

The opiates cause pupillary constriction, which occurs even in total darkness. The exact mechanism by which narcotics induce miosis is uncertain but is believed to be due to a central effect via the Edinger-Westphal nucleus of the oculomotor nerve rather than to an effect on the pupillary sphincter. Anticholinergics can counteract the opioid-induced miosis. Tolerance to the miotic effect is not usually seen, and miosis can be detected even in heroin addicts.

Renal System. It was previously thought that the antidiuretic effect of morphine was due to the release of ADH. It has recently been confirmed that this is not the case in humans. The decrease in urine output noted with use of morphine anesthesia is believed to be related to renal hemodynamics. Studies conducted on volunteers given morphine slowly in conjunction with fluid replacement necessary to maintain a stable cardiovascular status showed no significant changes in GFR or urine output. However, rapid administration of the drug and the addition of nitrous oxide decreased hemodynamic function enough that the GFR and urine output were markedly diminished. Fentanyl is believed to cause only minimal changes in renal function.

Uncatheterized patients may have a decreased urine output caused by the increased detrusor tone and contraction of muscles and urethral sphincters, which makes urination difficult. The central effects of the drugs may render the patient inattentive to the stimuli arising in the bladder.

SUFENTANIL

Chemistry and Physical Properties

The chemistry of sufentanil was first described in 1976. It is a thienyl derivative of fentanyl (Fig. 15–16). Its molecular weight is 578.68, and it is a white crystalline powder that is very soluble in water and organic solvents. Each milliliter of sufentanil citrate contains 50 µg of the drug. The drug is supplied in 1-, 2-, and 5-ml ampules. The solution has a pH range of 3.5 to 7.5.

Pharmacokinetics

Sufentanil is a highly lipophilic compound that is rapidly distributed to all tissues. Tissue levels studied in rats showed a peak level in the vessel-rich group in 2 minutes and in fat by 30 minutes. The major sites for sufentanil biotransformation are the liver and small bowel. Sufentanil in animals is metabolized by N-dealkylation and O-demethylation. The metabolites are essentially inactive except for one metabolite, which has approximately 10 percent of the activity of the parent drug. The exact mechanisms of metabolism in humans have not yet been determined. Approximately 80 percent of the drug is excreted in the urine and feces within 24 hours. Approximately 20 percent of the drug is excreted unchanged.

The therapeutic index of sufentanil has been determined to be much greater than all other currently available opioids. (Table 15–6). The drug is about 93 percent proteinbound. When compared to fentanyl, sufentanil is more rapid in onset and has a shorter elimination half-life. There is also less tendency for drug accumulation after repeated doses. When used as an agent in balanced techniques, the potency of sufentanil has been reported to be as much as 10 times greater than fentanyl.

Pharmacologic Effects

Sufentanil is a pure opioid agonist and, as such, has effects similar to those of other opioids in regard to respiratory depression, gastrointestinal spasm, and intrabiliary pressures. It is most similar to fentanyl and alfentanil in its cardiovascular stability. High doses of fentanyl and sufentanil have been used for high-risk cardiac surgical procedures with hemodynamic stability. Large doses of these drugs (fentanyl 50 to 100 µg/kg, sufentanil 5 µg/kg) produce loss of consciousness, analgesia, and prevention of normal endocrine and metabolic responses to surgery. Amnesia may not always be complete. Lorazepam or other reliable amnesics should be used when narcotic–oxygen techniques are employed.

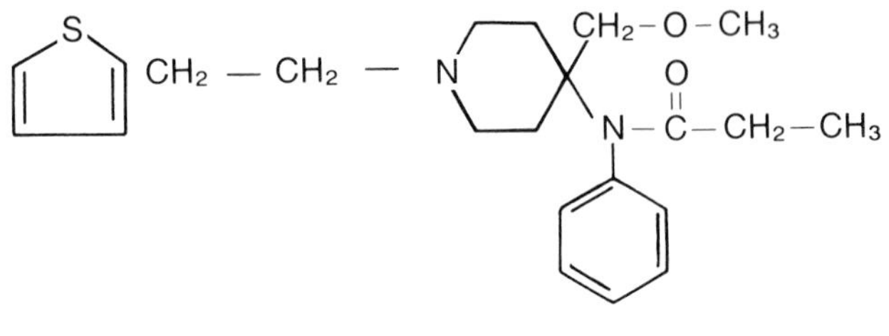

Figure 15–16. Chemical structure of sufentanil (Sufenta).

TABLE 15–6. COMPARISON OF FENTANYL, SUFENTANIL, ALFENTANIL, AND MORPHINE

	Fentanyl	Sufentanil	Alfentanil	Morphine
Potency	130	1,250	30	1
Therapeutic index	277	26,000	1,080	70
Elimination				
Half-life (min)	219	164	94	180
Volume of distribution (L/kg)	4	3	1	3
Clearance (L/kg/min)	13.0	12.7	5.0	14.7

Sufentanil is the most potent opioid available for clinical use. It is used in anesthesia as an opioid agent for balanced techniques and as the sole anesthetic agent for narcotic-oxygen techniques. Depending on the length and technique of anesthesia, doses of less than 1 μg/kg to 20 μg/kg have been used. The recommended dosage for procedures with a duration of 1 to 2 hours using nitrous oxide and oxygen is 1 to 1.5 μg/kg, followed by maintenance doses of 10 to 25 μg (0.2 to 0.5 ml) as needed. The total dose should not exceed 2 μg/kg. For surgical procedures of longer than 2-hours' duration, the recommended loading dose is 1 to 5 μg/kg administered with nitrous oxide and oxygen. Total dose should not exceed 8 μg/kg. For cardiovascular surgery using a narcotic–oxygen technique, 10 to 20 μg/kg is recommended. As with other drugs, doses must be adjusted appropriately for elderly and debilitated patients.

The side effects of sufentanil are similar to those of fentanyl. The advantages of sufentanil over fentanyl include (1) faster onset of action, (2) shorter duration of action, (3) greater effectiveness in reducing hormonal responses to surgical stress, and (4) higher potency and greater affinity for opiate receptors.

ALFENTANIL

Chemistry and Physical Properties

Alfentanil (R 39209) is the latest of the opioid drugs currently under clinical trials in the United States (Fig. 15–17). In 1987 alfentanil should be available to all anesthesia practitioners. Alfentanil and sufentanil are chemical analogs of fentanyl with very similar effects. The molecular weight of alfentanil is 416. It is readily soluble in water and is currently available in isotonic saline solutions.

Pharmacokinetics

Alfentanil is classified as an ultra-short-acting narcotic (as opposed to fentanyl and sufentanyl, which are short-acting). Alfentanil has a duration of action that is approximately one-third that of fentanyl. The shorter duration of action of alfentanil reflects its kinetic profile. Alfentanil is less lipid-soluble than are sufentanil and fentanyl. Its volume of distribution and clearance are lower, and its elimination half-life is much shorter. The lower volume of distribution results in greater access of the drug to clearing organs and a shorter elimination half-life despite the low clearance. In contrast to fentanyl, the clinical duration may be more dependent on metabolism than redistribution. There is less of a cumulative effect when compared with fentanyl.

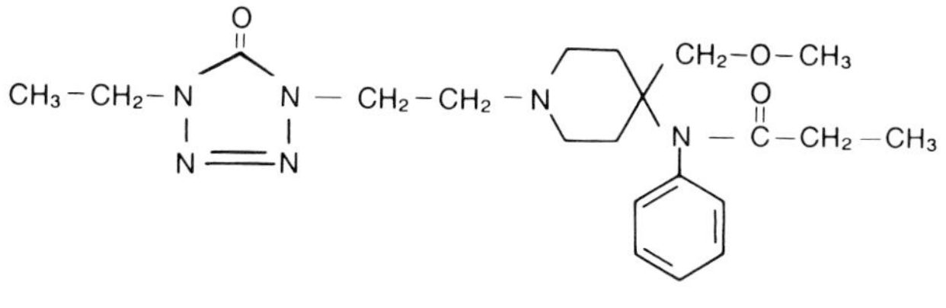

Pharmacologic Effects

Alfentanil produces all of the physiologic effects characteristic of opioids. It is unique in that it has the fastest onset and shortest duration of any opioid available. Its therapeutic ratio is high, but side effects of alfentanil are similar to those of other opioid compounds.

The potency and duration of action that are characteristic of alfentanil will find wide use in anesthesia practice. Alfentanil will be used extensively in procedures of short duration, because it allows rapid recovery of consciousness with less respiratory depressant effect. This should be an appropriate drug for outpatient procedures. Use of alfentanil as an induction agent will very likely become popular. Alfentanil 10 to 30 μg/kg with nitrous oxide-oxygen in unpremedicated patients produced good operating conditions and rapid recovery. This dose was sufficient for a 15- to 20-minute procedure. Induction doses of alfentanil used in preliminary studies range from 120 to 250 μg/kg.

Although induction using alfentanil has been found to be slower than that using thiopental, the hemodynamic stability during laryngoscopy and intubation was greater with alfentanil. There are some reports of hypotension and myocardial depression after induction in high-risk patients. It has not been determined in all cases whether this is due to interactions with the premedication, too rapid a rate of injection, differing cardiovascular effects in higher-risk patients, or any number of other factors. Alfentanil also has been studied in a continuous infusion form. There appear to be adequate surgical conditions with rapid recovery when the infusion is discontinued.

Caution should be exercised when administering an induction bolus of alfentanil to critically ill and debilitated patients. Because of the rapid onset of alfentanil, pretreatment with a nondepolarizing muscle relaxant may be indicated to reduce the occurrence of chest wall rigidity.

CLINICAL USES

In anesthesia, narcotics are often used (1) for premedication, (2) as adjuncts to regional or local anesthesia, (3) for postoperative analgesia, and (4) as anesthetic agents.

Figure 15–17. Chemical structure of alfentanil.

Premedication. Narcotic premedications should not be used routinely but are usually reserved for the patient with pain or patients who may require some analgesia before the induction of anesthesia. There are also those who believe that narcotic premedications lower the anesthetic requirements during general anesthesia and that certain narcotics in themselves will provide tranquilizing effects. Most anesthetists ordering a narcotic premedication will order a combination with a benzodiazepine, phenothiazine, barbiturate, or other major tranquilizer. This combination is often used for patients about to undergo surgery with regional or local anesthesia or narcotic-nitrous general anesthesia. Narcotic premedication can often provide some postoperative analgesia after inhalation anesthesia for a short surgical procedure.

Narcotic premedication should be avoided in patients who cannot tolerate even mild respiratory depression (e.g., those at risk of increasing intracranial pressure or with severe pulmonary compromise). Although histamine release from premedicant doses of narcotics is rarely a problem, this should be kept in mind when ordering morphine or meperidine for asthmatics. Administration of morphine to patients with biliary colic or some history of significant biliary tract disease is contraindicated.

Adjunct to Regional or Local Anesthesia. For this purpose, intravenous narcotics are used in conjunction with tranquilizers such as diazepam, lorazepam, or droperidol to provide sedation and analgesia. Some patients receiving a regional or local anesthetic are very anxious and will request sedation and or amnesia. Both the narcotic and tranquilizer must be titrated to achieve the desired effect. The desired effect is usually a calm, sedate but responsive and cooperative patient. Care should be taken not to oversedate and render the patient apneic or unresponsive.

Immediate Postoperative Analgesia. Anesthetists often administer analgesics in the recovery room for postoperative pain. The intravenous route is the route of choice because immediate effects can be seen and the uncertainty of the rate of absorption is not a problem. The drug must be titrated, starting with small doses. It must be remembered that the postoperative patient is frequently still depressed from the anesthetic agents received during the surgery. These patients usually require very small doses of narcotics to obtain analgesia. The respiratory rate should be monitored closely in patients receiving intravenous analgesics in the recovery room.

Narcotic Anesthesia. Narcotics are often used with nitrous oxide, oxygen, and a muscle relaxant for a technique known as balanced anesthesia. The narcotic provides analgesia while the nitrous oxide supplements the analgesic effect and provides amnesia. At least 60 to 70 percent nitrous oxide is required to provide adequate depth and amnesia for most patients. Muscle relaxation can be achieved by any nondepolarizing relaxant or a succinylcholine drip.

The aim of balanced anesthesia is to maintain a consistent level of narcosis during the anesthetic. This can be accomplished by titrating the narcotic so that the patient's respiratory rate is lowered to 5 to 8 per minute just before

induction. The patient will be sedate but responsive. The respiratory rate and the level of narcosis seem to correlate well. After induction, the respiratory rate can be used as a guide to the depth of anesthesia if muscle relaxants are not used. By this time, the nitrous oxide is also exerting an effect to supplement the narcotic agent. If muscle relaxants are to be used, clinical signs as well as the basic pharmacology (i.e., peak effect, duration of action) of the narcotic must be used to determine when additional doses of narcotics may be required.

If an adequate loading dose of morphine is given before induction, additional doses (2 to 5 mg) are rarely needed for the next 1 to 1½ hours. The blood pressure and heart rate may increase slightly after the start of surgery but will usually become stable and maintain a fairly consistent level. It is important to achieve adequate levels of morphine before stimulation because it is difficult to lower the blood pressure during morphine anesthesia once it has become elevated. At this point, additional doses of morphine will not usually lower the blood pressure. Adjunct drugs or a low concentration of a volatile anesthetic may be required for blood pressure control, if elevation occurs. The blood pressure may remain elevated despite adequate levels of anesthesia. The rise in blood pressure can be attenuated by the use of curare, rather than pancuronium.

Meperidine and fentanyl can be used in the same manner. The clinical signs of the anesthetic depth, such as blood pressure and heart rate, can be used with greater reliability with these agents. A rise in blood pressure will usually respond to additional doses of meperidine or fentanyl. Additional doses of meperidine (5 to 20 mg) are usually required every 20 to 30 minutes and fentanyl (25 to 50 µg) every 10 to 20 minutes to maintain a consistent level. Narcotics should be withheld for the last 20 minutes to 1 hour before the end of anesthesia. Patients anesthetized with this technique are usually able to tolerate wound closure well even at lighter levels of anesthesia.

Morphine and fentanyl do not alter cardiovascular dynamics to a great extent; however it should be remembered that with the addition of nitrous oxide, cardiovascular depression may occur.

Advantages of the Narcotic-Nitrous Technique. The advantages of the narcotic-nitrous techniques are that it (1) produces very little alteration in cardiovascular dynamics, (2) decreases laryngeal, tracheal, and cough reflexes, (3) produces no myocardial sensitization to catecholamines, (4) permits a smooth emergence, (5) provides postoperative analgesia, and (6) decreases metabolic rate.

Disadvantages. The technique does, however, have disadvantages, including (1) possible cardiovascular depression in the susceptible patient, especially if nitrous oxide is added, (2) chest wall rigidity with rapid administration, (3) no muscle relaxation, (4) requirement of at least 50 percent nitrous oxide (thus it may not be a wise choice for middle ear surgery or bowel obstruction), (5) possible renarcotization after reversal, and (6) decreased cough reflex postoperatively.

BIBLIOGRAPHY

Aldrete JA, Stanley TH: Trends in Intravenous Anesthesia. Chicago, Year Book Med Pub, 1980, pp. 173–187.

Barron DW: Methohexital. Int Anesthesiol Clin 7(1):33–42, 1969.

Blitt CD, Petty WC, et al: Clinical evaluation of injectable lorazepam as a premedicant: The effect on recall. Anesth Analg: 55:522–525, 1976.

Bovill JG, Sebel PS, et al: The pharmacokinetics of alfentanil (R 39209): A new opioid analgesic. Anesthesiology 57:439–443, 1982.

Bovill JG, Sebel PS, et al: Kinetics of alfentanil and sufentanil: A comparison. Anesthesiology 55:A–174, 1981.

Breimer DD: Pharmacokinetics of methohexitone following intravenous infusion in humans. Br J Anaesth: 48:643–649, 1976.

Brown AS: Neuroleptanalgesia. Int Anesthesiol Clin 7(1):159–175, 1969.

Bullingham RES: Clinics in Anaesthesiology. Opiate Analgesia. London, Saunders, 1983, Vol 1, No. 1.

Carson IW, Graham J, et al: Clinical studies of induction agents XLIII: Recovery from althesin—a comparative study with thiopentone and methohexitone. Br J Anaesth 47:358, 1975.

Clark N, Liu W-S, et al: Sufentanil versus fentanyl as a supplement to N_2O anesthesia during general surgery. Anesth Analg 63:198, 1984.

Clark RSJ: The eugenols—propanidid. Int Anesthesiol Clin 7(1):43–63, 1969.

Clark RS, Dundee JW, et al: Adverse reactions to intravenous anaesthetics. Br J Anaesth: 47:575–585, 1975.

Collins VJ: Principles of Anesthesiology, 2nd ed. Philadelphia, Lea & Febiger, 1976, Chaps. 21–23.

Conahan TJ: New intravenous anesthetics. Surg Clin North Am 55:851–859, 1975.

de Lange S, Stanley TH, et al: Catecholamine and cortisol responses to sufentanil-O_2 and alfentanil-O_2 anesthesia during coronary artery surgery. Can Anaesth Soc J 30:248–254, 1983.

DiPalma JR: Drills Pharmacology in Medicine, 4th ed. New York, McGraw-Hill, 1971.

Dundee JW: In Feldman HS, Scurr E (eds): Intravenous Anesthetic Agents: Current Topics In Anesthesia. Chicago, Year Book Med Pub, 1979.

Dundee JW: Comparative analysis of intravenous anesthetics. Anesthesiology: 35:137–148, 1971.

Dundee JW: Current views on the clinical pharmacology of the barbiturates. Int Anesthesiol Clin 7(1):3–25, 1969.

Dundee JW, Keilhy SR: Diazepam. Int Anesthesiol Clin (1):91–116, 1969.

Estafanous FG: Opioids in Anesthesia. Boston, Butterworth, 1984.

Fisher DM: Are the pharmacokinetics of alfentanil really predictable? Anesthesiology 59:256–257, 1983.

Foldes FF, Shiffman HP, et al: The use of fentanyl, meperidine or alphaprodine for neuroleptanesthesia. Anesthesiology 33:35–42, 1970.

Fragen RJ, Reves JG: Clinical perceptions of midazolam. Anesthesiol Rev 12:3S, 1985.

Garfield JM, Garfield FB, et al: A comparison of psychological responses to ketamine and thiopental-nitrous oxide-halothane anesthesia. Anesthesiology 36:329, 1972.

Ghoneim MM, Dhanaraj J, et al: Comparison of four opioid analgesics as supplements to nitrous oxide anesthesia. Anesth Analg 63:405–412, 1984.

Ghoneim MM, Korttila K: Pharmacokinetics of intravenous anesthetics: Implications for clinical use. Clin Pharmacokinet 2:344–372, 1977.

Greenblatt DJ, Shader RI: Pharmacologic understanding of antianxiety drug therapy. South Med J 71:2, 1978.

Hall GM, Whitwam JG, et al: Some respiratory effects of althesin. Br J Anesth 45:629–632, 1973.

Harvey SC: Hypnotics and sedatives. In Goodman A, Gilman L (eds): The Pharmacological Basis of Therapeutics, 6th ed. New York, Macmillan, 1980.

Heinanen J, Orko R, et al: Anaesthesia for cardioversion: A comparison of althesin and thiopentone. Br J Anaesth 45:49–54, 1973.

Heisterkamp DV, Cohen PJ: The effect of intravenous premedication with lorazepam (Ativan), pentobarbitone or diazepam on recall. Br J Anaesth 47:79–81, 1975.

Herr GP, Conner JT, et al: Diazepam and droperidol as IV premedicants. Br J Anaesth 51:537, 1979.

Howells TH, Harnek E, et al: Propanidid and methohexitone: Their comparative potency and narcotic action. Br J Anaesth 39:31, 1967.

Howie MB, Reitz J, et al: Does sufentanil's shorter half-life have any clinical significance? Anesthesiology 59:A146, 1983.

Hudson RJ, Stanski DR; Metabolism versus redistribution of fentanyl and alfentanil. Anesthesiology 59(3):A243, 1983.

Hug CC, Jr: What Is the Role of Narcotic Analgesics in Anesthesia? American Society of Anesthesiologists Annual Refresher Course Lectures, 1980.

Hug CC, Jr: Pharmacokinetics of Anesthetics: Intravenous Drugs. American Society of Anesthesiologists Annual Refresher Course Lectures, 1978.

Hug CC, Jr: Pharmacokinetics of drug administered intravenously. Anesth Analg 57:704–723, 1978.

Hug CC, Jr, Stanski DR: Reply to correspondence. Anesthesiology 59:257, 1983.

Hull CJ: The pharmacokinetics of alfentanil in man. Br J Anesth 55:157S–164S, 1983.

Hunter AR: Twenty years ago—pentothal sodium anaesthesia. Anaesthesia 23:450, 1968.

Jaffe J, Martin W: Opioid analgesics and antagonists. In Goodman A, Gilman (eds): The Pharmacological Basis of Therapeutics, 7th ed. New York, Macmillan, 1985.

Lamalle D: Cardiovascular effects of various anesthetics in man. Four short-acting intravenous anesthetics: althesin, etomidate, methohexital and propanidid. Acta Anaesthesiol Belg 27:208–224, 1976.

Ledingham IM, Findlay WE, et al: Etomidate and adrenocortical function. Lancet 1:1434, 1983.

Lorenz W, Doenicke A, et al: Histamine release in man by propanidid and thiopentone: Pharmacological effects and clinical consequences. Br J Anaesth 44:355, 1972.

Lowenstein E, Hallowell P, et al: Cardiovascular response to large doses of intravenous morphine in man. Eng J Med 281:1389, 1969.

Marshall B, Wollman H: General Anesthetics. In Goodman, A, Gilman L (eds): The Pharmacological Basis of Therapeutics, 6th ed. New York, Macmillan 1980.

Monheim LM: Pharmacology of intravenous anesthetic agents. Anesth Prog 17:195–200, 1969.

Morrison JD: Drugs used in neuroleptanalgesia. Anesthesiol Clin 7(1):141–154, 1969.

Murphy PJ: Biotransformation of methohexital. Int Anesth Clin 12:139–143, 1974..

Radnay PA: Epontol (propanidid) an ultrashort-acting intravenous anesthetic agent. Int Surg 52:163–172, 1969.

Rolly G, Kay B et al: A double blind comparison of high dose fentanyl and sufentanil in men: Influence on cardiovascular, respiratory and metabolic parameters. Acta Anaesthesiol Belg 30:247–254, 1979.

Roscow C: Sufentanil citrate: A new opioid analgesic for use in anesthesia. Pharmacotherapy 4:1, 1984.

Samuelson PN, Reves JG, et al: Hemodynamic responses to anesthetic induction with midazolam or diazepam in patients with ischemic heart disease. Anesth Analg 60:802, 1981.

Saidman LJ: Distribution and Metabolism Of Intravenous Anesthetics. American Society of Anestheologists Annual Refresher Course Lectures, 1978.

Saidman LJ: Uptake and Distribution of Intravenous Agents: The Thiopental Model. American Society of Anestheologists Refresher Courses in Anesthesiology, 1975. Vol. 3.

Sebel PS, Bovill JG, et al: EEG effects of high dose alfentanil anesthesia: Correlation with plasma concentration. 8th World Congress of Anesthesiologists, Manila, Philippines, Jan 22–27, 1984. Book of Abstracts II:A378.

Siker ES: Pros and Cons of Balanced Versus Inhalation Anesthesia. American Society of Anesthesiologists Annual Refresher Course Lectures, 1979.

Stanley TH: Pharmacology of Intravenous Non-Narcotic Anesthetics (Excluding Ketamine). American Society of Anesthesiologists Annual Refresher Course Lectures, 1980.

Stanley TH: Pitfalls and problems in using narcotics for anesthesia. Anesthetist Update Series, 1978, no. 1.

Stanley TH, Bidwai AV, et al: Cardiovascular effects of nitrous oxide during meperidine infusion in the dog. Anesth Analg 56:836, 1977.

Stanley TH, Liu W: Cardiovascular effects of meperidine-N$_2$O anesthesia before and after pancuronium. Anesth Analg 36:669, 1977.

Stanski DR: Narcotic pharmacokinetics. Can Anaesth Soc J 30:257–258, 1983.

Stanski DR, Hug CC, Jr: Alfentanil: A kinetically predictable narcotic analgesic. Anesthesiology 57:435–438, 1982.

Stovner J, Endresen R: Intravenous anesthesia with diazepam. Acta Anaesthesiol Scand 24:223, 1966.

Takahashi T, Takasaki M, et al: Effects of althesin on cerebrospinal fluid pressure. Br J Anaesth 45:179–184, 1973.

Tammisto T, Takki S, et al: A comparison of althesin and thiopentone in induction of anaesthesia. Br J Anaesth 45:100–107, 1973.

Tanaka DJ: The Effects of Diazepam on succinylcholine-induced Serum Potassium Changes. Master of science thesis, University of Claifornia, Los Angeles, 1981.

Thornton JA: Methohexitone and its application in dental anaesthesia. Br J Anaesth 42:255–261, 1970.

Thornton JA: Dixon RA, et al: Intermittent methohexitone. Br Med J, 691, 1969.

Trevor SJ: How Do Narcotics-Analgesics and Benzodiazepines Act? American Society of Anesthesiologists Annual Refresher Course Lectures, 1980.

Turner JM, Coroneos NJ, et al: The effect of althesin on intracranial pressure in man. Br J Anaesth 45:168–172, 1973.

Way WL: Ketamine: What Is Fact or Fantasy? American Society of Anesthesiologists Annual Refresher Course Lectures, 1980.

Wilson RD: Current States of Ketamine. In Hershey SG (ed): Regional Refresher Courses in Anesthesiology, 1973.

16

Pharmacology of Local Anesthesia

Michael Stanton-Hicks

Local anesthetics are chemical substances that can, by definition, cause the temporary loss of sensation in a circumscribed area of the body. This loss of sensation, or anesthesia, results from a reversible depression of the process of nervous conduction. Though such a state can be produced in nervous tissues by many physical and chemical agents, this discussion will be confined to those compounds that temporarily interrupt nerve conduction by preventing the process of depolarization (omitting those neurolytic substances that act in a different manner and are more commonly used in the treatment of intractable pain). Historically, local anesthesia began with the isolation of cocaine from the Erythroxylon coca bush, a plant indigenous to Peru, by Niemann in 1860, but any clinical application had to await the revelation by Koller, a pupil of Freud, of its use as a topical anesthetic for surgery on the eye. Soon after this discovery, cocaine was used for spinal anesthesia by Bier in Germany and within a year, in 1898, by Halstead in the United States for blocks of the brachial plexes. After its chemical identification as an ester of benzoic acid, many similar compounds were synthesized, among them the topical anesthetic benzocaine. Unfortunately, because of its addictive qualities, cocaine was very quickly relegated to the historical shelf, although because of its unique propensity among local anesthetics to produce vasoconstriction, it still has a limited but specific use to this day as a topical anesthetic for mucous membranes. While benzocaine was poorly soluble in water, procaine, another ester of para-aminobenzoic acid, synthesized by Einhorn and Braun in 1905, proved to be sufficiently water-soluble and have such a satisfactory margin of safety that its clinical use as an injectable agent was ensured. Of the many hundreds of ester local anesthetics synthesized in the ensuing half century, tetracaine, discovered in 1930, and chloroprocaine, in 1952, have remained clinically important. More of these ester-type local anesthetics would have been developed but for the fact that they are associated with the production of endogenous hypersensitivity.

A major departure from this class occurred when, in 1943, Löfgren synthesized lidocaine. This became the forerunner of a completely new type of chemical compound, the amino-amides. Fortunately, the amino-amides seem to be practically free from any tendency to produce allergic reactions and, in addition, possess other kinds of local anesthetic action that are an improvement over the esters. Most recently interest has centered around a group of biologically related substances called guanidines, which are extremely potent inhibitors of nerve function. At this time, however, these are still experimental curiosities; this account will concern itself with a description of the two main classes of local anesthetics already mentioned, the amino-esters and the amino-amides.

PHYSIOLOGY OF NERVE CONDUCTION

To understand the principles of local anesthetic pharmacology a description of neural anatomy and physiology is necessary.

Anatomy

All peripheral nerves contain a mixture of sensory and motor elements, whose size and histology vary with their particular function. The principal element, or axon, is surrounded by a connective tissue sheath called the endoneurium; groups of axons are bound together by more connective tissue forming an external sheath known as the perineurium. The perineurium then binds these groups of axons into what is seen as a peripheral nerve fiber (Fig. 16–1). The axon itself is encased in myelin and, depending on whether the myelin is in a single or multiple layers, the axon is referred to as unmyelinated (C fiber) or myelinated (A and B fibers) nerve, respectively. The myelin is produced by Schwann cells; the nuclei of these cells can be seen in histologic sections (Fig. 16–2). Although it consists primarily of lipid, the myelin sheath does contain some protein, which, when added to the cell membrane (axolemma), functionally alters the characteristics of the nerve fiber. Conceptually, the cell membrane consists of a bilaminar lipoprotein matrix with the lipoid and protein arranged in a heterogenous fashion as shown in Figure 16–3. The physicochemical properties of local anesthetics (i.e., water-solubility, lipid solubility, and protein-binding properties) not only determine the manner in which they interact with the cell membrane but also dictate the particular characteristics of the resulting nerve block.

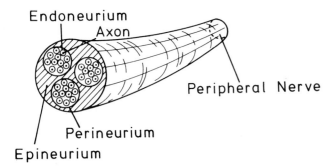

Figure 16–1. Schematic drawing of a peripheral nerve fiber in which the principal structures are illustrated.

Nerve Conduction

The nerve membrane behaves like a semipermeable structure that separates an electrolyte solution high in potassium concentration on the inside of the cell from one that is high in sodium on the outside. This lipoprotein membrane has small channels, or "pores," that under certain conditions allow the passage of ions in either direction (although the potassium ion, which is smaller than sodium, can move freely even when the cell is at rest). The selective permeability of this membrane is under the influence of tiny electrical fields. The analogy of small "gates" that control the transit of ions through these channels has been suggested.

Because of the ionic asymmetry across the membrane, an electrochemical potential is created that, at rest, is about −70 mV in mammalian nerves, the inside being negative in respect to the outside of the cell (Fig. 16–4). During this resting state the cell is said to be polarized, the opposite of which is depolarization. The electrochemical process of depolarization that results from the increase in ionic permeability occurs only when the nerve has been excited by a stimulus sufficient to achieve what is termed the depolarization threshold.

During the process of depolarization, the influx of sodium ions into the cell through the so-called sodium channels is so great that not only is the original electrical potential neutralized, but there is also a slight overshoot as can be seen in Figure 16–5. The "gates" close at this point and potassium ions now move out of the cell. The electrical disturbance created by depolarization spreads along the cell axon initiating a "wave" of depolarization that travels along the length of the fiber. Repolarization commences in each segment of a nerve immediately after the impulse or wave has been propagated along the complete length

of the nerve. This process is initiated by closure of the sodium gates, thereby preventing any further influx of sodium. Potassium, which has until now leaked outside of the membrane, commences its return into the cell, under the influence of both a concentration gradient and the pull of electrostatic forces within the cell. The ionic imbalance caused by sodium influx is now restored by an active metabolic process termed the "sodium pump," which continuously transports these ions out of the cell to satisfy the previous resting ionic equilibrium. Without such a mechanism requiring metabolic activity, the nerve cell would ultimately become exhausted and cease to develop the ionic gradients necessary for the creation of the electrochemical potential across the membrane.

The foregoing description of impulse propagation along a nerve by the creation of an electrochemical disturbance across its membrane applies only to unmyelinated nerves, which have a thin unilaminar covering of myelin. Propagation in myelinated nerves is different. Here, the electrical impulse jumps from node to node instead of propagating slowly and continuously along the membrane (Fig. 16–6). This saltatory (jumping) action is possible because the nerve membrane at each node of Ranvier is in direct contact with the extracellular fluid and consequently is more excitable than a membrane covered thinly but continuously with myelin. The speed of conduction in such nerves is about 100 m/second whereas in the smallest unmyelinated nerves (C fibers) the conduction speed is between 1 and 2 m/second.

MECHANISM OF LOCAL ANESTHETIC ACTION

Almost all of the commercially available local anesthetics are prepared as the hydrochloride (acid) salt of a basic amine. In this form the cation, which is positively charged, is in dissociation equilibrium with the uncharged local anesthetic base, which can be expressed in the following way:

$$pH = pKa - \log [BH^+]/[B],$$

where pH is the hydrogen ion concentration, pKa is a dissociation constant, $[BH^+]$ is the concentration of positively charged cation, and [B] is the concentration of uncharged base.

The pKa is a physical constant of any specific local anesthetic, but it is the pH of the solution (or surrounding tissues) that will determine the relative concentration of free base and cation that are present.

If the pH of the solution or environment decreases, which means the hydrogen ion concentration has increased

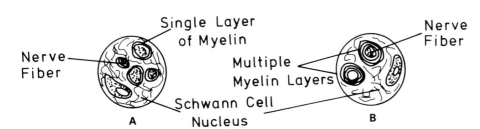

Figure 16–2. Cross-sections of a peripheral nerve showing the basic differences between **(A)** unmyelinated and **(B)** myelinated nerves. Schwann cell nuclei, from which myelin is produced, can also be seen.

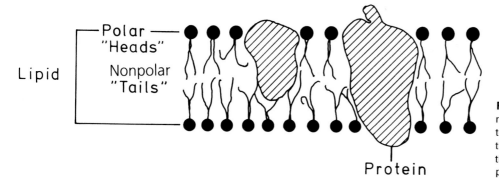

Figure 16–3. Conceptual nerve cell membrane as a bilaminar lipoprotein matrix is illustrated. Note that the protein molecules can "bridge" the entire membrane thickness in places.

(more acidic), the equilibrium in the relative concentrations of cation and base shifts so that more local anesthetic will exist in the cationic form. The converse would be true if the pH of the solution were to increase, in which case the equilibrium shifts so that more local anesthetic will occur as the base. This expression is another way of using the principle embodied in the Henderson-Hasselbalch equation, which can be written

$$pKa = pH + \log \frac{(cation)}{(base)}.$$

Present theory of local anesthetic action proposes that it is the cationic moiety that is ultimately responsible for producing neural blockade. However, in order for a local anesthetic to reach its site of action, the base must be present in sufficient concentration to facilitate its passage across (charged) membranes.

The events outlined in Figure 16–7 illustrate the passage of the local anesthetic from its site of deposition outside a nerve into the axon, where its site of action is believed to be. In fact, the description of local anesthetic dissociation is the basis for adding carbon dioxide to local anesthetic solutions to increase the concentration of cation as a result of the lower pH generated by the carbon dioxide inside the nerve membrane (Bromage et al, 1967). The actual site (receptor) where local anesthetics produce their block is probably at the internal end of the sodium channel. It is believed that displacement of calcium ions from their lipoprotein receptors by local anesthetic cations ultimately blocks the sodium channel, decreasing sodium permeability—thereby inhibiting membrane depolarization. In practice, the local anesthetic moves by diffusion along a concentration gradient from its site of deposition through the tissues and into the nerve. This diffusion continuously decreases the amount of local anesthetic present by dilution and absorption through lymphatic and vascular channels.

Because of an affinity for protein and lipid structures, much of the local anesthetic is also lost to the nerve by binding and dissolution in these structures. One means of achieving a higher concentration of local anesthetic to block the nerve is to add a vasoconstrictor, such as epineph-

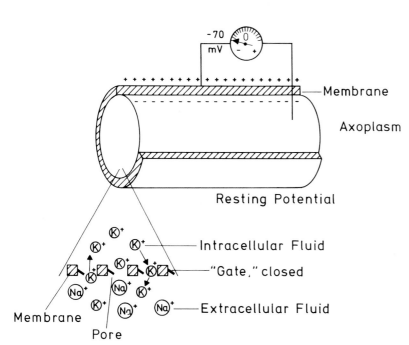

Figure 16–4. Diagram of an unmyelinated nerve fiber at rest. Note the resting potential of −70 mV, the inside of the cell being negative to the outside. The magnified section of the nerve membrane illustrates the ionic relationships during this resting phase. Note that ionic passage through the pores is controlled by "gates," which when closed allow free passage to potassium ions (K^+) but prevent the ingress of sodium ions (Na^+).

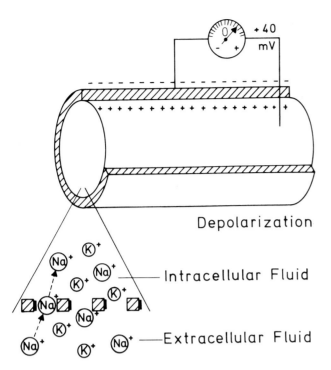

Figure 16–5. Diagram of an unmyelinated nerve fiber during depolarization. Note, in comparison with Figure 16–4, that the "gates" are now open, allowing sodium ions to pass into the cell. The electric potential is momentarily 40 mV, the outside of the cell now being negative to the inside.

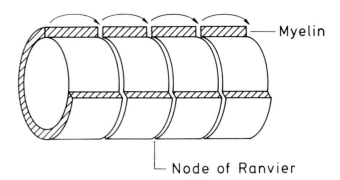

Figure 16–6. Diagram of depolarization in a myelinated nerve fiber, showing propagation of the electrical impulse from node to node. Voltage changes similar to those described for unmyelinated nerve fibers occur.

rine, which will decrease its rate of absorption into vascular channels. The size of the fiber also determines the quality of neural blockade. In a mixed nerve fibers are classified as A, B, and C fibers, representing the different modalities that are subserved by the nerve. These are of different sizes and in microscopic cross section appear to occur in a random distribution, although in reality there is a certain order. Fibers subserving proximal structures are situated concentrically on the outer aspect, or mantle, of the nerve, and those fibers that subserve more distal structures occupy the core of the nerve. Attention has been drawn to this order by de Jong. Its practical application is that during the onset of neural blockade, proximal structures will be blocked first and then, as the local anesthetic diffuses into the center of the nerve bundle, those last to be blocked will be the innermost or core fibers.

Because the small C fibers appear to be more easily blocked than large fibers, one might expect that it would be possible to block modalities served by these fibers by means of a given concentration of local anesthetic, thus sparing the function of thicker A fibers; this does indeed occur clinically and is responsible for what is referred to as a "differential block." However, recent experimental evi-

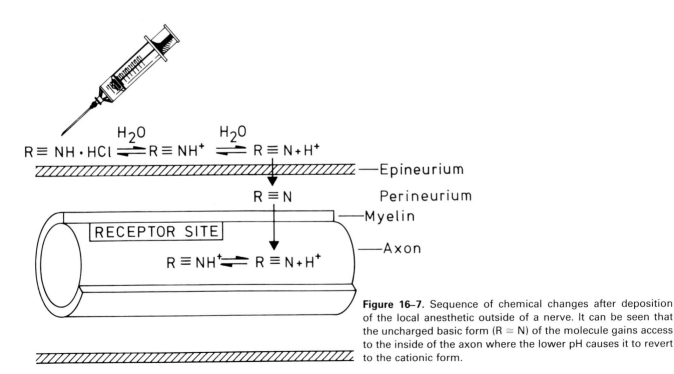

Figure 16–7. Sequence of chemical changes after deposition of the local anesthetic outside of a nerve. It can be seen that the uncharged basic form ($R \equiv N$) of the molecule gains access to the inside of the axon where the lower pH causes it to revert to the cationic form.

dence does not support this view; in fact, what appears to be a greater sensitivity to local anesthetic action by the small C fibers is in reality an artifact, caused by diffusion barriers, and is not a function of fiber size (Gissen et al, 1980; Sprotte, 1985). Therefore, to overcome these diffusion barriers, particularly when muscle relaxation is required in the region for which a nerve block is given, the concentration of the solution must be great enough to block the A fibers responsible for motor activity. A useful concept when considering local anesthetic action has been defined by de Jong as the minimum blocking concentration (C_M). This can be considered analogous to the minimum alveolar concentration (MAC) of a volatile anesthetic that is necessary to provide surgical anesthesia and implies that it is that concentration that will block all elements in a nerve.

One more factor that has a bearing on the effects of local anesthetic block is the frequency with which neural impulses travel along nerve fibers. For example, an isolated axon is much more sensitive to a local anesthetic when the frequency of neural traffic is increased than when fewer impulses are being transmitted. To look at it another way, a weaker local anesthetic solution may produce only partial blockade in a given axon under the influence of a low-frequency stimulus, but the same axon will become completely blocked when subjected to higher frequencies of stimulation. This effect is called "frequency-dependent conduction block" and is shared by all the clinically used local anesthetics, particularly those agents like bupivacaine and etidocaine that are highly lipid soluble (Courtney 1977).

Duration and recovery from nerve block are, again, dependent on the kinetics of local anesthetic action, which are regulated by laws of diffusion (along concentration gradients) and an affinity for lipoprotein structures, which assist in removing local anesthetic and will be discussed in more detail later. However, it is sufficient to say here that during recovery the diffusion gradient is reversed. The outer concentric layer of the nerve loses its local anesthetic to the extracellular fluid first and the core of the nerve somewhat later. The clinical implication of this sequence is that in blocks of the limbs, the proximal region tends to lose its anesthesia before the more distal regions, one of the reasons for early onset of tourniquet pain.

LOCAL ANESTHETIC POTENCY

A standard method of determining the C_M of local anesthetics is the 50 percent reduction of the action potential spike height in a sheathed frog sciatic nerve within 5 minutes, when the nerve is stimulated at a frequency of 30 impulses per second, in a solution having a pH of 7.2 to 7.4. Under such conditions, the potency of the commonly used anesthetics can be classified as shown in Table 16–1. From this table it can be seen that there is a strong correlation between the lipid solubility and potency where procaine (the least lipid soluble) is given a relative potency of 1 and etidocaine (the most lipid soluble) has a relative potency of 16. This means that local anesthetics with a high potency will produce their effects at lower concentrations than will agents of intermediate or low potency. It also means that in a mixed nerve, agents of high potency are more likely to block all neural components, i.e., the A, B, and C fibers, unless only dilute solutions are used. Latency of onset of local anesthesia and the duration of neural block are the two most important characteristics clinically. In a manner similar to that used to establish C_M, latency is determined by the concentration of a local anesthetic that will depress the action potential in the frog sciatic nerve by 50 percent in 10 minutes. Latency has no relation to potency, but is particularly dependent on the site of injection; there is also a correlation with the pKa and its lipid solubility concentration and therefore local anesthetic gradient is also important. By doubling the anesthetic concentration, there is a reduction in latency of roughly one third. Etidocaine, which is highly soluble and has the lowest pKa of all the clinically used local anesthetics, also has the shortest latency (Table 16–2). The duration of neural block is also related to lipid and protein affinity. Most agents can be separated into three groups, those of short, those of intermediate, and those of long duration. The local anesthetics in the latter group have not only the greatest affinity for lipids but are also highly bound to tissue and plasma proteins. While these in vitro models are important for the establishment of standard pharmacologic criteria, there will invariably be some differences between those data obtained from in vitro and in vivo animal studies and those data obtained from

TABLE 16–1. RELATIONSHIP OF ANESTHETIC POTENCY TO IN VIVO $C_M{}^a$ OF DIFFERENT AGENTS

Drug	Potency	C_M Rat Sciatic Nerve	Cat Sciatic Nerve
Procaine	1	1.000	4.0
Mepivacaine	2	0.500	2.0
Prilocaine	3	0.500	2.0
Chlorprocaine	4	1.000	2.0
Lidocaine	4	0.500	2.0
Tetracaine	16	0.125	0.5
Bupivacaine	16	0.125	0.5
Etidocaine	16	0.125	0.5

^{a} C_M = minimum anesthetic concentration to produce 50% block.
From Covino BG, Vassallo HG: Local Anesthetics: Mechanisms of Action and Clinical Use, 1976. Courtesy of Grune & Stratton.

TABLE 16-2. IN VITRO PHYSICAL AND BLOCK CHARACTERISTICS OF DIFFERENT AGENTS

Drug	Potency	Lipid Solubility	Latency	Duration
Procaine	1	0.6	1.0	1.00
Mepivacaine	2	1.0	1.0	1.50
Prilocaine	3	0.8	1.0	1.50
Chlororprocaine	4	—	0.8	0.75
Lidocaine	4	2.9	0.8	1.50
Tetracaine	16	80.0	2.0	8.00
Bupivacaine	16	28.0	0.6	8.00
Etidocaine	16	141.0	0.4	8.00

From Covino BG, Vassallo HG: Local Anesthetics: Mechanisms of Action and Clinical Use, 1976. Courtesy of Grune & Stratton.

patients. Most discrepancies, when they do occur, can result from such factors as species differences, different tissue sites, vascularity of the tissues, and the state of vascular tone in the respective tissues. Quite apart from these factors is the intrinsic pharmacologic activity of the different local anesthetics on blood vessels and the effects of vasoconstrictors when added to local anesthetic solutions.

Apart from potency, the most useful clinical criteria are a knowledge of the onset (latency) and duration that can be expected from a given local anesthetic.

CLINICAL PHARMACOLOGY AND LOCAL ANESTHETICS

The clinical features of local anesthetics, as well as those factors that govern their uptake, distribution, and metabolism, will now be considered.

Uptake and Distribution

Factors governing the uptake of local anesthetic by neural structures have already been discussed. The following discussion focuses on what happens to the portion of a dose of local anesthetic that does not reach the nerve and also the portion that has reached its target, performed its block, and then left the nerve. Factors that primarily affect the absorption of local anesthetics are

1. the site of injection (vascularity and type of immediate tissue, i.e., predominantly fat, muscle, connective, etc.);
2. pharmacology of the particular drug;
3. dose of drug; and
4. addition of vasoconstrictor.

For example, the highest blood levels of any local anesthetic are obtained after multiple intercostal blocks. The lowest levels are obtained after subcutaneous infiltration—given that equal volumes and concentrations of local anesthetic are used in each instance. The reasons for the differences are many; not the least important are the greater surface area, greater vascularity, and lower proportion of adipose tissue in the case of intercostal blockade.

The pharmacologic differences between the different

amide local anesthetics have been well studied; however, because of the rapid hydrolysis (metabolism) by pseudocholinesterase in body tissues, the majority of the ester local anesthetics have lacked similar studies. Using epidural anesthesia as a model, the amide local anesthetics have been classified according to the blood concentrations that were obtained after equipotent doses and, as can be seen in Table 16-3, etidocaine achieved the lowest blood concentrations and mepivacaine the highest. The possible explanation for these differences is the greater rate of tissue redistribution of etidocaine (giving lower blood concentrations). Mepivacaine has less lipid solubility and more vasodilator activity than etidocaine. In the case of prilocaine, which has about the same lipid affinity as mepivacaine, its high clearance (metabolism and excretion) results in low blood concentrations. All the local anesthetics, esters included, except cocaine produce vasodilation in the vicinity of the block site and, as a rule, those agents that produce the greatest degree of vasodilation are the ones that achieve the greatest benefit from added epinephrine. It is for this reason that epinephrine is added to many commercial preparations of local anesthetics. The vasoconstrictor actions are twofold: first, to increase the duration of action, and second, to reduce the potential toxicity from the absorbed local anesthetic. The dose of epinephrine most commonly used is 1:200,000 or 5 μg/ml. Higher concentration of epinephrine (except perhaps in oral mucous membranes where solutions may be used containing epinephrine in a dose of 1:80,000) may attain durations that are only marginally longer. As already mentioned, little advantage in duration, in spite of the reduction in blood concentration, results from the addition of a vasoconstrictor to the two long-acting agents, bupivacaine and etidocaine. Probably the high affinity for lipid structures and greater vasodilator activity of these agents are responsible. It is the local absorption of local anesthetic by protein in the surrounding tissues (as well as in the nerves) that provides a depot and concentration gradient in favor of the nerves, thereby providing a long duration. This effect offsets the high lipid solubility that favors vascular uptake. Also, epinephrine has only a relatively short duration of effect. The process of absorption of a local anesthetic from its site of deposition will be mirrored in the blood, producing a profile that will rise and fall at rates that are dependent on the rate of distribution from the vascular compartment to other tissue compart-

TABLE 16–3. INFLUENCE OF LIPID SOLUBILITY AND VASODILATOR ACTIVITY ON MAXIMUM BLOOD LOCAL ANESTHETIC CONCENTRATION DURING EPIDURAL BLOCK

Equipotent Dose (mg)		Lipid Solubility	Relative Vasoactivity	Blood Level µg/ml
Lidocaine	300	2.9	1.0	1.4
Prilocaine	300	1.0	0.5	0.9
Mepivacaine	300	0.3	0.8	1.5
Bupivacaine	150	28.0	2.5	1.0
Etidocaine	150	141.0	2.5	0.5

From Covino BG, Vassallo HG: Local Anesthetics: Mechanisms of Action and Clinical Use, 1976. Courtesy of Grune & Stratton.

ments and the elimination by metabolism and excretion. The circulatory concentration of local anesthetics may be expressed either as whole-blood or plasma concentrations, and these values may differ because of different uptake into blood cells. This knowledge is used by pharmacokineticists, who are able to calculate the relative distribution of these drugs to different tissues. Generally speaking, those tissues receiving a higher proportion of the circulation, such as the lungs and kidneys, will also contain higher concentrations of local anesthetics than poorly perfused organs. The rate of tissue redistributon is related in part to the protein-binding and lipid affinity of each agent. Therefore agents like prilocaine, which is poorly bound in plasma, and etidocaine, which is very fat-soluble, will rapidly equilibrate between the blood and tissue compartments. Such drugs tend to have much lower relative toxicities because the peak blood concentration from the same dose is always much lower than those obtained with other agents that are not so rapidly distributed.

Metabolism and Excretion

Local anesthetics are metabolized along one of two pathways, depending on whether they contain an ester or an amide linkage. Procaine, the forerunner of the ester class, chloroprocaine, and tetracaine are all hydrolyzed in the plasma by pseudocholinesterase to para-aminobenzoic acid derivatives. The rate of hydrolysis of chloroprocaine in plasma is extremely fast so that it is almost undetectable in blood after neural blockade. Procaine is hydrolyzed 4 times slower and tetracaine is 16 times slower again. However, the rates of metabolism of all esters are much faster than any of the amides. Unfortunately, para-aminobenzoic acid can form a hapten with antibodies in certain individuals and in such instances is responsible for allergic phenomena.

The metabolism of amide compounds is quite different from and much more complex than that of the esters. For these compounds the liver is the primary site of metabolism. The rate of metabolism does vary slightly from one agent to another with prilocaine clearly undergoing the most rapid degradation, followed by etidocaine, lidocaine, mepivacaine, and bupivacaine in that order. The metabolites differ with each drug and may themselves have clinically important actions. Normally, one would not expect these substances to have any untoward or toxic effects but, in renal failure and cardiac failure, these metabolites may accumu-

late and, added to their parent substances, generate increased potential for toxic side effects.

Liver disease with severe impairment of normal function can be the cause of toxic sequelae from the accumulation of unmetabolized local anesthetics in the circulation. Consideration of the use of regional anesthesia in such patients must take this factor into account, particularly if the regional anesthetic procedure calls for amounts of local anesthetic that are in the upper range of normal doses.

Impairment of metabolism will affect the clearance of these drugs from the body. Generally, greater than 90 percent of all local anesthetics are excreted as metabolites of their parent compounds. In humans, the kidney is the primary excretory organ. As is the case in impaired liver function, severe renal disease will directly affect the clearance and ultimate excretion of local anesthetic metabolites.

Renal disease can also contribute to toxic side effects from systemically absorbed local anesthetic agent when the local anesthetic is displaced from plasma protein by uremic products.

LOCAL ANESTHETICS AND THEIR USES

Esters

The following agents in this family of compounds will be discussed: cocaine, procaine, chloroprocaine, tetracaine, and benzocaine.

Cocaine. Cocaine is the historical prototype of this group and is supplied as a hydrochloride. The pKa is 8.6, and it is available in 1 percent to 20 percent solutions. The most common strength, used in otolaryngology, is 5 percent, which, when applied topically to mucous membranes, will provide anesthesia for about 60 minutes. It is sometimes used in conjunction with epinephrine, but as has already been mentioned, this is usually unnecessary because the drug provides its own vasoconstriction by preventing the reuptake of catecholamines that are released from vasomotor nerve endings.

The maximum safe dose is now considered to be 200 mg. Because of its stimulatory effects on the sympathetic nervous system, toxic side effects on the central nervous and cardiovascular systems can be expected if high blood levels of the agent occur. Therefore, extreme excitement, convulsions, tachycardia, and hypertension will all precede the depressant effects, which can be fatal when the myocardium is affected. Cocaine is metabolized by the liver and in red blood cells. Accumulation of uremic products in the blood can lead to exaggerated drug responses because the products may displace bound drug molecules from plasma proteins. Therefore, there is the potential for toxic side effects of this local anesthetic in patients with renal disease, although such effects have not been demonstrated experimentally.

Procaine (Novocain). This derivative of para-aminobenzoic acid is prepared as the hydrochloride with pKa of 9.

Concentrations and Uses. It is available in 1 percent, 2 percent and 5 percent solutions, the first two strengths being roughly equivalent in potency to similar concentrations of lidocaine when used for infiltration anesthesia. However, the latency and duration are inferior to those of lidocaine. The 5 percent solution can be used with D_5W to provide satisfactory spinal anesthesia with a duration of 30 to 45 minutes. Although it is not used very often today, it has been supplied as an alternative to the amide agents to provide anesthesia in patients known to be susceptible to malignant hyperthermia. There is, however, no definite proof that amide agents can precipitate this syndrome.

The maximum safe dose is 500 mg for plain solutions and 750 mg when epinephrine is added.

The drug is primarily hydrolyzed by pseudocholinesterase in the blood and by enzymes in the liver before being excreted in the urine.

Chloroprocaine (Nesacaine). Chloroprocaine shares many of the properties of procaine, the big exception being its greater affinity for lipid (approximately seven times more lipid soluble). This property is responsible for its superior anesthetic quality. The pKa is 8.7. Because it is the most rapidly hydrolyzed local anesthetic, chloroprocaine achieves very low plasma concentrations and is, therefore, the least toxic local anesthetic. Unfortunately, this quality also results in very short durations, the shortest being about 30 minutes seen in epidural anesthesia, although the addition of epinephrine will increase the duration by about 100 percent.

Concentration and Uses. Chloroprocaine is available in 1 percent, 2 percent, and 3 percent solutions. The 1 percent solution is used for infiltration anesthesia or peripheral nerve block and is quite useful for outpatient procedures requiring short durations. Durations of 45 to 90 minutes can be realized, depending on whether epinephrine 1:200,000 is used or not.

The most popular use of this drug has been in obstetric conduction anesthesia, either epidural or caudal. The rapid onset time, poor motor block, and low toxicity all contribute to its popularity in this group of patients. A 2 percent solution is generally adequate, although a 3 percent solution will shorten the latency and improve neural blockade. For this reason, the 3 percent solution is commonly used for emergency caesarian section.

The maximum safe dose is 600 mg for plain solutions, and 800 mg for epinephrine-containing solutions. Like procaine, it is hydrolyzed by pseudocholinesterase in the blood and is excreted by the kidney.

Tetracaine (Pontocaine). This is also an ester of para-aminobenzoic acid. Its pKa is 8.5, and it is much more lipid-soluble than chloroprocaine. It is readily bound to protein. Tetracaine is available as a solution or as crystals, the latter being more stable to heat sterilization.

Concentrations and Uses. Because of its potency, very low concentrations of tetracaine are used for infiltration and peripheral nerve blocks. A 0.1 percent to 0.2 percent solution is generally adequate for such blocks, but when larger volumes of solutions are required, as would be the case for multiple intercostal blocks, it is advisable to add epinephrine 1:200,000 to reduce the systemic uptake of drug. The latency is long, and complete block may take 45 minutes to develop fully.

Before the introduction of the long-acting agents, bupivacaine and etidocaine, it was common to add lidocaine to reduce its latency and also improve the quality of sensory block. For epidural or caudal anesthesia, a solution of 0.25 percent is required, and for spinal anesthesia, now its most useful application, a 1 percent solution is used. The 1 percent solution (or crystals of tetracaine) is mixed with distilled water or 10 percent dextrose, depending on whether hypobaric or hyperbaric anesthesia is required. These plain solutions will achieve excellent anesthesia for 60 to 90 minutes. The addition of epinephrine, 0.2 mg (0.2 ml of 1:1000) will prolong the block by about 60 percent. Phenylephrine 5 mg (0.5 ml of 1% solution) will prolong the block by 100 percent to 150 percent.

Unlike the prolonged latency that occurs when tetracaine is used for peripheral nerve block or epidural block, the onset of anesthesia after subarachnoid administration is rapid, taking only 5 to 10 minutes.

The maximum dose of 100 mg should not be exceeded unless a vasoconstrictor is added, in which case up to 150 mg can be used. The metabolism of tetracaine by pseudocholinesterase, subsequent breakdown by the liver, and excretion are much slower than for the other esters. Therefore, tetracaine is potentially much more toxic than procaine or chloroprocaine.

Benzocaine. This is a relatively insoluble drug in water; it has, however, found considerable use as a topical anesthetic. For this reason it is not available in an injectable form, although it has been incorporated with dextran as a 2 percent solution for the provision of anesthesia lasting many hours, such as for the pain from fractured ribs.

Uses. Benzocaine is used as a spray or incorporated into ointments and gels for the anesthesia of mucous membranes and the skin.

Amides

Most of the amides, with lidocaine as the parent congener, are anilides. Only one, dibucaine, is a quinoline derivative. The following agents will be discussed: lidocaine, prilocaine, mepivacaine, bupivacaine, etidocaine, and dibucaine.

Lidocaine (Xylocaine). Lidocaine is generally dispensed in aqueous solutions as the hydrochloride salt. It has a pKa of 7.9, is moderately lipid-soluble, and has a plasma-protein binding of about 67 percent. In some countries, lidocaine is marketed as a carbonated salt that is buffered to a pH of 6.5. This permits a high proportion of the drug to assist as the "lipid-soluble base" that facilitates its penetration through lipid membranes. As the carbon dioxide is given off (prepared under a pressure of 2 atmospheres), the pH rises to 7.5, again improving conditions for transportation of the uncharged base through lipid barriers. The diffusing carbon dioxide rapidly penetrates the membrane, where the pH falls, thus "trapping" the local anesthetic in the active cationic form.

As a consequence of this activity, the latency is shortened and the quality of anesthesia is improved, although there is little effect on duration.

Concentrations and Uses. Lidocaine is available in 0.5 percent, 1 percent, 2 percent, 4 percent, and 5 percent solutions, to which epinephrine may be added as a vasoconstrictor. Because of the large volumes that may be required, only 0.5 percent solutions are use to provide satisfactory infiltration anesthesia. The duration of the 0.5 percent solution may be increased from 75 minutes to about 240 minutes with 1:200,000 epinephrine. A 1 percent solution will provide about 120 minutes of anesthesia, or 400 minutes with added epinephrine. Only in dental anesthesia, because of the highly vascular tissue and the small volumes necessary, is a 2 percent solution with epinephrine 1:80,000 used. The duration that can be expected is about 150 minutes.

A 0.5 percent lidocaine solution will provide excellent intravenous analgesia in the upper limbs. Higher concentrations are unnecessary and increase the risk of toxicity. Most peripheral nerve blocks and plexus anesthesia require a 1 percent solution, but satisfactory digital nerve block can be provided by a 0.5 percent solution.

The latency for individual nerve blocks is short, about 5 minutes, and about 20 minutes for plexus anesthesia. Durations of 60 minutes can be increased up to 130 percent by the addition of epinephrine. Epidural and caudal anesthesia require either a 1 percent or 2 percent solution, depending on whether less or more motor block is required. The addition of epinephrine 1:200,000 reduces the latency, improves motor block, increases duration, and when large volumes are used, reduces the potential for toxic side effects. Duration of surgical anesthesia is increased from 60 minutes to 100 minutes when epinephrine is added.

Spinal anesthesia of 45 to 60 minutes' duration can be provided by a plain 5 percent solution of lidocaine in 7.5 percent dextrose. The duration is increased by up to 50 percent with 0.2 mg of epinephrine. The solution has a specific gravity of 1.035 at body temperature, which causes it to spread rapidly, and therefore, the onset of anesthesia is almost immediate.

A 4 percent solution of lidocaine is available for topical anesthesia and in some countries, a 10 percent spray is available for the same purposes. The maximum recommended dose of lidocaine is 400 mg, or 500 mg when epinephrine is added.

Lidocaine is metabolized by the liver. Less than 4 percent is excreted unmetabolized in the urine.

Prilocaine (Citanest). The pKa of prilocaine is 7.9; it has a lower lipid solubility than lidocaine and is approximately 55 percent bound to plasma protein. Unlike the other amides, which are tertiary amines, prilocaine is a secondary amine and is a toluidide (i.e., derivative of ortho-toluidine or 2 methylaniline) rather than a 2, 6 dimethyl aniline like the direct descendents of lidocaine.

Concentrations and Uses. Prilocaine is available in 0.5 percent, 1 percent, 2 percent, and 3 percent solutions. All solutions may be incorporated with a vasoconstrictor.

Like lidocaine, prilocaine 0.5 percent to 1 percent will provide satisfactory infiltration anesthesia lasting from 75 to 280 minutes, depending on whether epinephrine is added or not.

Prilocaine 0.5 percent solution is probably the anesthetic agent of choice for intravenous regional anesthesia because it is the least toxic of the amide local anesthetics and, therefore, the least likely to produce toxic sequelae during sudden deflation of the tourniquet. In peripheral nerve block, 0.5 percent to 1.5 percent solutions will provide conditions similar to those seen with lidocaine, although in plexus anesthesia, prilocaine will generally provide durations that are 50 percent longer. In this respect prilocaine is more useful than lidocaine when anesthesia of moderate duration is desired for patients in whom epinephrine is contraindicated.

Although not commonly employed for epidural and caudal anesthesia, prilocaine is used in either a 2 percent or 3 percent solution. There is little difference in the quality of anesthesia compared with lidocaine, although when the 2 percent solution is used without a vasoconstrictor, excellent anesthesia with minimal motor block and low toxicity make this a very suitable agent for outpatient surgery.

The maximum dose of prilocaine is 400 mg, or 600 mg when epinephrine is added. If a dose of 600 mg is exceeded, the development of clinical methemoglobinemia is possible. This is manifested by cyanosis, which can be treated by the administration of methylene blue in a dose of 1 mg/kg. While methemoglobin has little effect on the oxygen-carrying capacity of hemoglobin, except in the presence of severe anemia below 5000 mg/100 ml, it is aesthetically displeasing and also masks the normal clinical observation of hypoxia in patients. For this reason, prilocaine should probably not be used in obstetrics. However, it should be emphasized that because prilocaine is four times less cardiotoxic and neurotoxic, it is probably the safest short-acting amide local anesthetic available. Prilocaine is partially metabolized in the liver to *o*-toluidine, and a metabolite of this is probably responsible for the production of methemoglobinemia. This metabolic reaction cannot occur with the direct descendents of lidocaine. The metabolites are excreted by the kidneys.

Mepivacaine (Carbocaine). This substance has a pKa of 7.6 and a similar lipid solubility to lidocaine. However, it is more plasma-protein-bound than either of these two agents, having a range of 68 to 84 percent.

Concentrations and Uses. Mepivacaine is equipotent with lidocaine and is, therefore, available in the same range of concentrations with the exception of topical solutions.

The drug has the same indications as lidocaine, except that it is probably not the drug of choice for obstetrics as neonatal metabolism may be slower than is the case with lidocaine; in addition the placental transfer of mepivacaine is greater.

The maximum safe dose of mepivacaine is 400 mg, and 500 mg with epinephrine. Most of the animal studies indicate that mepivacaine is slightly more toxic than lidocaine, and epinephrine is not quite as effective in either increasing the duration of block or in lowering the blood concentrations when added to mepivacaine. Like lidocaine, metabolism of mepivacaine takes place in the liver with most of the drug being then eliminated as metabolites by the kidneys.

Bupivacaine (Marcain). Bupivacaine belongs to the same group of anilides as mepivacaine, having been synthesized at the same time, although prepared commercially some years later. A butyl group replaces the methyl group in the piperidine ring, and it is this alteration of the molecule that is responsible for its being much more lipid soluble than mepivacaine.

The pKa is 8.01, it is 88 percent plasma-protein-bound and highly lipid-soluble. This high lipid affinity accounts for its high potency and also its greater toxicity.

Concentrations and Uses. Solutions of 0.25 percent, 0.5 percent, and 0.75 percent are available. No solution is available for topical anesthesia. A 0.125 to 0.25 percent solution with or without epinephrine is satisfactory for infiltration anesthesia. Latency is short and durations of 200 minutes or 400 minutes are achieved with added epinephrine.

For peripheral nerve block, solutions of 0.25 to 0.5 percent, with or without epinephrine, are satisfactory. However, latencies are long, particularly in the case of plexus anesthesia, which may require 30 minutes to achieve complete block. The 0.5 percent solution will provide good motor block and the quality of sensory anesthesia is better than that obtained with the 0.25 percent solution. There is extreme variability in the duration of anesthesia, which may range from 400 minutes to 24 hours. Epinephrine has an unreliable effect on the duration but does reduce the uptake of the drug (and hence its toxicity). In epidural and caudal anesthesia, the most commonly used concentrations are 0.5 and 0.75 percent, depending on whether a more profound motor block is desired. No alteration in duration is achieved by the addition of epinephrine, but the ensuing blood concentrations are lower. Obstetrics is a special situation for which motor block is not required, and bupivicaine in concentrations as low as 0.125 percent, or more commonly 0.25 percent, will provide very satisfactory analgesia in this group of patients. The only disadvantage of these weaker solutions is the shorter duration that results.

Bupivacaine is now available in the United States as either a 0.5 percent isobaric or hyperbaric solution for spinal anesthesia. The duration is very similar to tetracaine, the main difference being a superior sensory analgesia but poorer motor block. The maximum safe dose is 150 mg for plain solutions and 200 mg with epinephrine.

Bupivacaine is about four to five times more toxic than lidocaine. The liver is responsible for its metabolism, and the metabolites are excreted via the kidneys.

Etidocaine (Duranest). This drug, also developed from lidocaine, has a pKa of 7.74. Etidocaine has the highest lipid solubility of all clinical local anesthetics, and a plasma binding of 94 percent. It is not equipotent with bupivacaine and is less toxic. It does, however, provide similar durations and a more profound motor block than bupivacaine when twice the concentration is used.

Concentrations and Uses. Etidocaine is available in 0.5 percent, 1 percent, and 1.5 percent solutions. It is not available as a topical anesthetic, but its ability to penetrate lipid barriers would make it a very effective agent. The 0.5 percent solution without epinephrine will provide infiltration anesthesia rapidly with durations similar to those seen with bupivacaine.

When etidocaine is used for peripheral nerve block, the onset is much quicker than with bupivacaine and there is little difference in the durations. A 0.5 percent solution, with or without epinephrine, is used and when large volumes are required, it is safer than bupivacaine because of its lower toxicity.

Epidural and caudal anesthesia are provided by 1 to 1.5 percent solutions, depending on the degree of motor block desired. Even a 1 percent solution of etidocaine will provide a motor block superior to 0.5 percent bupivacaine, which is equally potent. In fact, because of this ability to affect motor function while providing only partial analgesia, this drug is not satisfactory for obstetric use.

The latency when a 1.5 percent solution is used is extremely short, and complete anesthesia may take place within 20 minutes. Epinephrine has no effect on duration, a marginal effect on blood concentrations, but does intensify motor block. Because of the degree of motor block, etidocaine is well suited for operations requiring profound relaxation. The maximum dose is 300 mg and 400 mg with epinephrine.

Etidocaine is metabolized in the liver with less than 1 percent being excreted in the urine unchanged.

Dibucaine (Nupercaine). This is a quinoline derivative having an amide link in the intermediate chain.

It has a pKa of 8.5, is very lipid-soluble, and is very potent.

Concentration and Use. The most common solution now available is 0.5 percent in 6 percent dextrose, having a specific gravity of 1.025, which is used for hyperbaric spinal anesthesia. A hypobaric solution is also available. The latency is greater than that for tetracaine, 5 to 10 minutes, and it has a duration of 3 hours. If epinephrine 0.2 mg is added, this can be increased to 4 hours. Even longer durations up to 130 percent can be achieved when phenylephrine 5 mg is added. The range of dose used varies between 5 to 15 mg. The maximum dose is 50 mg.

Dibucaine is metabolized in the liver, but little is known of its metabolites.

Vasoconstrictors

Although a number of vasoconstrictors have been synthesized, epinephrine, introduced by Braun (1903) is still the most widely used and most reliable adjunct for this purpose today. Vasoconstrictors are added to local anesthetic solutions to retard the absorption of the local anesthetic, thereby improving its uptake by nerves, increasing the duration of action, and reducing systemic toxicity.

Epinephrine. While epinephrine has both alpha- and beta-adrenoceptor effects, it is only for the alpha effects that epinephrine is incorporated with local anesthetic. It is quite rapidly oxidized, and for this reason it is probably better to add it to the local anesthetic solution immediately prior to its use. Commercially prepared epinephrine-containing solutions, usually in a concentration of 1:200,000 (5 μg/ml), have a low pH (3 to 4.5) and contain an antioxidant, sodium metabisulphite. They can be autoclaved once without materially affecting the potency of the vasoconstrictor. The total dose of epinephrine should be kept below 200 μg. Toxic side effects are mainly caused by the beta-adrenergic stimulatory effects (tachycardia, bradycardia, and cardiac arrythmias), but high doses will also result in the stimulation of alpha-adrenergic receptors causing hypertension.

Epinephrine should be avoided in patients with thyrotoxicosis and hypertension.

Phenylephrine. This is the only other vasoconstrictor that has been used with local anesthetics that is presently available in the United States. It is a synthetic drug with predominantly alpha agonist effects. It is usually used in a concentration of 1:20,000 (20 μg/ml) and has been very popular as an adjunct for spinal anesthesia, where durations are prolonged by 100 to 150 percent. It is not widely used as a vasoconstrictor for other regional anesthetic procedures because of the widespread systemic effects, but it can be used as an alternative to epinephrine in those cases where epinephrine is contraindicated.

TOXIC EFFECTS OF LOCAL ANESTHETICS

Because of their ability to influence excitable membranes, local anesthetics can be expected to have far-reaching effects on the central nervous and cardiovascular systems should large amounts enter the systemic circulation (Scott and Cousins, 1980).

Central Nervous System

When the local anesthetic level in the blood increases, a recognizable series of reactions are seen in the central nervous system (CNS). Among toxic manifestations are excitatory subjective phenomena such as light-headedness, dizziness, tinnitus, and difficulty in focusing. Objective signs are slurred speech, shivering, muscular twitching, and tremors. As the blood concentration increases, generalized convulsions will ensue. These effects are thought to be an initial action on the inhibitory systems in the CNS, which may be more sensitive to local anesthetic action than are the facilitatory systems, which therefore tend to exert their circulatory effects unopposed. If local anesthetic blood concentrations continue to rise, generalized CNS depression will occur and, if allowed to continue unchecked, will lead ultimately to respiratory arrest. Local anesthetic toxicity is enhanced by elevated hydrogen ion (pH) and carbon dioxide (P_{CO_2}) concentrations in the patient. A number of mechanisms may be involved. These include the increased cardiac output associated with a respiratory or metabolic acidosis, the resulting increased cerebral blood flow and vasodilation, which delivers a high local anesthetic dose to the brain, and finally a reduction in intraneural pH, which causes more local anesthetic to exist in the cationic, or active, form. Convulsive activity can be terminated by the administration of an ultra-short-acting barbiturate such as thiopental in a dose of at least 4 mg/kg, or diazepam in a dose of 0.1 mg/kg. de Jong has suggested that diazepam can be given prophylactically, although there are other data that contradict this suggestion. Although excitatory effects can result from local anesthetic overdose, it is not generally realized that all local anesthetics have anticonvulsive activity. However, the doses associated with these effects are much lower than those that cause seizure activity.

Cardiovascular System

Local anesthetics are described as having biphasic effects on cardiac and vascular muscle. This means that at low concentrations stimulatory effects are seen and at high concentrations depressant effects are manifested. Since the introduction of procaine and, later, lidocaine, these cardiac and vascular actions have been studied extensively. In fact, the margin of safety from cardiovascular toxicity with local anesthetics is very large; blood concentrations of short-acting local anesthetics must be some ten times greater than those necessary to cause toxic effects on the CNS, those of the long-acting agents four times greater. Lidocaine, of course, is used extensively as an antiarrythmic agent and induces its activity at concentrations that are well below those that will cause toxic effects. High blood concentrations of local anesthetic, however, result in depression of both the myocardium and the vascular tissue.

As the local anesthetic concentration in the blood rises, a predictable series of changes is seen in the heart. There is a prolongation of conduction time in most regions of the heart, an increased PR interval, increased QRS duration, bradycardia, and finally cardiac arrest in asystole. These electrophysiologic changes are identical to the effects that have already been described in relation to the effects of local anesthetics on nerve membranes.

On vascular tissue, both in vitro and in vivo studies have demonstrated similar effects, with vasoconstriction occurring at low local anesthetic concentrations and vasodilation with increasing concentrations. However, the effect that predominates at a given local anesthetic concentration depends on such factors as the background vascular tone and the particular vascular bed concerned. For example, intra-arterial administration of mepivacaine to human volunteers caused a decrease in forearm blood flow, but when the concentration was increased, the resistance fell and flows increased. As already discussed, the only local anesthetic that consistently causes vasoconstriction is cocaine;

therefore, the toxic vascular effects that can be expected with this agent are profound, widespread vasoconstriction causing hypertension.

High doses of all other local anesthetics will cause cardiovascular collapse secondary to cardiac depression and vasodilation (Reiz and Nath, 1986). The vascular bed that seems to react differentially is the pulmonary vasculature, which responds with vasoconstriction to high concentrations of most local anesthetics.

Indirect Effects of Local Anesthetics

Because of the interference with the sympathetic nervous outflow, major conduction anesthesia, which includes spinal and epidural anesthesia, is responsible for profound physiologic changes. The degree of the disturbance is dependent on a number of factors. These include hypovolemia from whatever cause, the concurrent administration of CNS-depressant drugs, the presence or absence of a vasoconstrictor (in the case of epidural anesthesia), and the physiologic status of the patient.

Basically, one can expect an increasing tendency toward hypotension to develop because of vasodilation in the blocked areas and a decrease in venous return caused by pooling in the capacitance system of the skin and muscles. Many of these changes are compensated by vasoconstriction in the unblocked parts of the body. When an increasing number of segments are blocked (above T-5), one can expect an increasing inability for compensatory adjustments to cope with the loss of vasomotor control. The speed with which hypotension occurs during spinal anesthesia is much faster than is the case during epidural anesthesia, although in most surgical patients with blocks extending to T-5 (which is adequate for most abdominal operations), the ultimate level to which the blood pressure falls in either case is about 15 percent of the control pressure. Therefore, use of either of these two techniques in the presence of uncorrected hypovolemia is contraindicated. When epinephrine-containing solutions are used for epidural anesthesia, there may be an increased tendency for hypotension to develop even in normovolemic subjects because of the widespread beta-adrenergic effects that oppose any compensatory vasoconstriction in the unblocked areas, e.g., upper limbs and torso (Bonica et al, 1971). One must also expect additional depressant effects on the cardiovascular system when CNS-depressant drugs, such as those that have been administered for premedication or sedation, are used in conjunction with the conduction anesthetic. These drugs may increase the tendency for hypotension and must be taken into consideration to maintain homeostasis at the desired level.

Finally, although spinal or epidural anesthesia may be selected over general anesthesia for the debilitated patient, it should be remembered that any concurrent circulatory disturbances in such patients also require close observation because of the additional potential for hypotension associated with such anesthetic techniques.

The only other toxic effects that are attributable to local anesthetics are allergy, which can, as has been mentioned, attend the use of the ester local anesthetics, and histotoxic effects when local anesthetics are repeatedly applied to striated muscle. However, these histotoxic effects are not permanent and regeneration is usually complete within 2 weeks' cessation of the last application of the particular local anesthetic. Recently, the histotoxic effects that had been attributed to the accidental injection of chloroprocaine into the subarachnoid space, causing partial and permanent neurologic lesions, have been shown to have resulted from the antioxidant used to preserve these solutions. Chloroprocaine has been remanufactured with a greatly reduced concentration of the antioxidant, sodium bisulfite, from 0.2 percent to 0.07 percent. In vivo and in vitro experiments appear to have reestablished the safety of using this drug as it is now formulated.

REFERENCES

Bonica JJ, Akamatsu TJ, et al: Circulatory effects of peridural block: II. Effects of epinephrine. Anesthesiology 34:514, 1971.

Braun H: Über den Einfluss der Vitalität der Gewebe auf die örtlichen und allgemeinen Giftwirkungen localanaesthesirender Mittel und über die Bedeutung des Adrenalins fur die local Anaesthesie. Arch Klin Chir 69:541, 1903.

Bromage PR, Burfoot MF, et al: Quality of epidural blockade: III. Carbonated local anesthetic solutions. Br J Anaesth 39:197, 1967.

Courtney KR: Mechanism of frequency-dependent inhibition of sodium currents in frog myelinated nerve by lidocaine derivative GEA 968. J. Pharmacol Exp Ther 195:225–236, 1977.

de Jong RH: Physiology and Pharmacology of Local Anesthesia, 2nd ed. Springfield, Ill., Chas. C Thomas 1977.

Gissen AJ, Covino BG, et al: Differential sensitivities of mammalian nerve fibers to local anesthetic agents. Anesthesiology 53:467, 1980.

Reiz S, Nath S: Cardiotoxicity of local anesthetic agents. Br J Anaesth 58:736–746, 1986.

Scott DB, Cousins MJ: Clinical pharmacology of local anesthetic agents. In Bridenbaugh PO, Cousins MJ (eds): Neural Blockade: In Clinical Anesthesia and Management of Pain. Philadelphia, Lippincott, 1980, pp.86–121.

Sprotte, G. Thermographic investigations into the physiological basis of regional anaesthesia. Anaesthesiology and intensive care medicine, 159. Berlin, Heidelberg, New York, Tokyo, Springer-Verlag, 1985.

17

Muscle Relaxants

Leah E. Katz and Ronald L. Katz

PHYSIOLOGY OF NEUROMUSCULAR TRANSMISSION

Skeletal muscles receive somatic efferent innervation from fast-conducting group A axons, which have cell bodies located in the midbrain or anterior horn of the gray matter of the spinal cord. As an axon approaches muscle, repeated divisions occur according to the function of the innervated muscle; larger muscles are supplied by axons with few divisions, and muscles controlling fine function are densely innervated and are supplied by axons with many divisions.

As the terminal branch of the axon reaches the muscle, it loses its myelin sheath and forms multiprocessed endings. These endings lie in grooves in the postjunctional membrane of the muscle cell, a specialized part of the muscle membrane that consists of folds serving to increase the surface area opposite the nerve terminal (Fig. 17–1). These folds are the site of acetylcholine receptors. Acetylcholinesterase, an enzyme that rapidly ends the action of acetylcholine, is located in the folds. The gap between the nerve and muscle membrane is approximately 200 to 300 Å wide and is continuous with the extracellular space. When a nerve is stimulated, the nerve impulse causes the release of acetylcholine, which diffuses across the gap and reacts with the receptors on the postjunctional membrane, initiating the process of excitation in the muscle. The acetylcholine molecule, because of its quaternary nitrogen group, is attracted to anionic receptors on the endplate (Fig. 17–2). After the acetylcholine reacts with the receptor, channels open that alter sodium and potassium conductance. Sodium ions enter the cell and potassium ions exit, causing a depolarization, the endplate potential (EPP).

The normal resting membrane potential of skeletal muscle is -85 to -95 mV, with the area inside the muscle cell being negative in respect to the outside. As the membrane potential becomes less negative during the EPP and when the threshold level of approximately -45 mV is reached, conductance is altered in the nearby muscle membrane, causing propagation of the muscle action potential. This action potential causes calcium to be released from the sarcoplasmic reticulum that subsequently is able to bind with troponin. The binding of calcium and troponin permits actin and myosin to combine, and muscle contraction occurs. Adequate adenosine triphospate (ATP) is necessary for this process.

Acetylcholinesterase, which is readily available in the area of the postjunctional membrane, rapidly hydrolyzes acetylcholine to acetate and choline. Following the muscle action potential, the resting membrane potential is reestablished as sodium ions again are extruded to the extracellular space and potassium ions return to their intracellular location. (A very small amount of acetylcholine is not broken down but diffuses away from the area of the neuromuscular junction, also contributing to termination of action.) Since the sequence of events occurring at the neuromuscular junction takes only a few milliseconds under normal conditions, rapid repetitive synaptic transmission is possible.

ACETYLCHOLINE SYNTHESIS, STORAGE, AND RELEASE

Acetylcholine is synthesized in the motor nerve endings by acetyl coenzyme A and choline acetyltransferase. Energy for this reaction is supplied by ATP. After formation, acetylcholine passes by a carrier system into vesicles located within the nerve endings. When acetylcholine is stored in the vesicle, it is available for release into the synaptic cleft in uniform amounts called "quanta."

When a nerve impulse reaches the nerve ending, calcium gates located in the terminal axon membrane are opened and there is an influx of calcium. Calcium causes the vesicles containing acetylcholine to attach and fuse with the membrane of the axon. An all-or-none discharge of the acetylcholine (exocytosis) into the synaptic cleft follows. It is postulated that 100 to 200 quanta of acetylcholine may be released simultaneously; each vesicle or quanta is thought to contain at least 1000 molecules of acetylcholine.

Under normal resting conditions, miniature endplate potentials (MEPP) occur continuously without motor nerve stimulation. The MEPPs are caused by spontaneous release of acetylcholine quanta and have an amplitude of 1 to 2 mV. They are not of sufficient amplitude to cause depolarization. An EPP generated by nerve stimulation results in the synchronous release of 100 to 200 quanta of acetylcho-

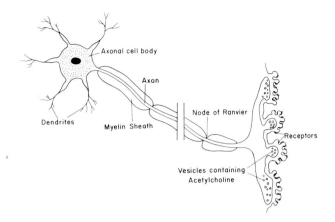

Figure 17–1. Anatomy of a neuron, indicating the neuromuscular junction, vesicles containing acetylcholine, and the acetylcholine receptors on the postjunctional membranes.

line. If the EPP is sufficiently large (40 to 45 mV) a propagated muscle action potential will be triggered.

One may think of acetylcholine as stored in nerve endings in three compartments:

1. Vesicular stores. Release from the vesicles depends on the presence of adequate calcium and adequate frequency of stimulation.
2. Mobilization stores. Acetylcholine passes from mobilization stores to the vesicles at a rate slower than the rate of vesicular release; therefore, it is theoretically possible for the vesicles to become depleted after frequent stimulation.
3. Synthesis and reserve sites. Acetylcholine synthesis is thought to occur in the cytoplasm. After synthesis, acetylcholine is carried to the mobilization stores and then on to the vesicles for release. As the immediately available acetylcholine located in the vesicles is used, the mobilization stores replenish acetylcholine stored in the vesicles.

The amount of acetylcholine released after a stimulus is directly related to the amount immediately available in vesicular stores. As this supply is decreased, the number of quanta released during stimulation is decreased, and fade in contraction may occur. Fade will continue until the vesicular stores of acetylcholine are replenished. Although fade does not usually occur in the normal situation, it does occur with nondepolarizing relaxants because of the prejunctional effects, which inhibit release of acetylcholine.

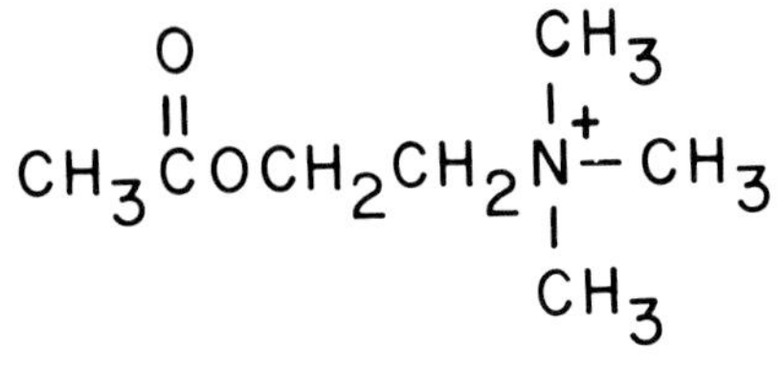

$$CH_3\overset{\overset{\displaystyle O}{\|}}{C}OCH_2CH_2\overset{\overset{\displaystyle CH_3}{|}}{\underset{\underset{\displaystyle CH_3}{|}}{N}}{}^{+}\!-CH_3$$

Figure 17–2. Structure of acetylcholine.

Neuromuscular transmission may be modified by muscle relaxants in several ways. Nondepolarizing relaxants block postjunctional acetylcholine receptors. In addition, it is thought that these drugs block the ionic channels through which, during depolarization, sodium and potassium ions are interchanged. Therefore, depolarization is prevented by both receptor block and channel block (Fig. 17–3). Postjunctional block occurs when acetylcholine is released but depolarization does not take place. This may be due to receptor occupation by a nondepolarizing agent (competitive inhibition), or the receptors may already be depolarized (i.e., by succinylcholine or decamethonium). The latter is referred to as a "depolarization block." Another possibility is that the receptors may be incapable of responding to depolarizing agents (desensitization block). This may be seen after prolonged depolarization and may be due to a modification in the sodium channels causing sodium to enter the cell at a less than normal rate.

Presynaptic receptors may be stimulated by depolarizing relaxants, allowing greater mobilization of acetylcholine to the vesicles. Nondepolarizing relaxants may block prejunctional receptors and inhibit the mobilization of acetylcholine. The relative effect on prejunctional receptors varies with different nondepolarizing muscle relaxants. Table 17-1 illustrates modification in events leading to muscle contraction.

PHARMACOLOGY OF NEUROMUSCULAR BLOCKING AGENTS

Neuromuscular blocking drugs contain at least one and usually two quarternary groups on each molecule. It was formerly believed that two quaternary nitrogens were required for neuromuscular blocking action, but it is now known that one is sufficient. The quaternary nitrogen acts on the cholinergic receptors in place of acetylcholine by either activating receptors, as in the case of succinylcholine or decamethonium, or inhibiting receptors, as in the case of *d*-tubocurarine, pancuronium, dimethyl tubocurarine, and gallamine. The molecules of drugs that activate receptors (depolarizing agents) are flexible, long molecules of relatively low molecular weight that structurally resemble acetylcholine. The nondepolarizing agents that inhibit the receptors of the endplate are, in contrast, bulky, more rigid molecules of a relatively high molecular weight that join with the receptors, thus preventing acetylcholine from doing so. Therefore, they prevent development of changes within the receptor that normally initiate depolarization.

Because of the similarity of the molecular structure of the neuromuscular blocking agents to that of acetylcholine, the neuromuscular blocking drugs are able to act as agonists or antagonists (i.e., stimulate or block) at any receptor site that normally is affected by acetylcholine. These cholinoceptive receptor sites are (1) nicotinic sites and (2) muscarinic sites. Nicotinic receptors are located at the neuromuscular junction and at autonomic ganglia. In contrast, muscarinic receptors are located at postganglionic parasympathetic sites. Some of these clinically important sites are the salivary glands, stomach, bowel, bladder, bronchi, and sinoatrial node of the heart. Depolarizing agents, acting in a manner similar to acetylcholine, usually stimulate cholinoceptive

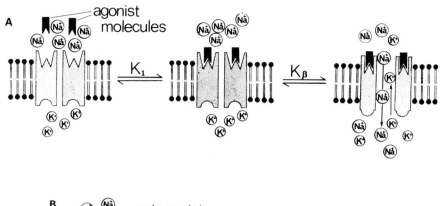
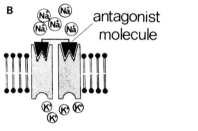
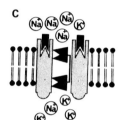

Figure 17–3. Diagrammatic representation of the interaction of acetylcholine and *d*-tubocurarine with endplate cholinoceptors. **A.** Acetylcholine molecules combine with the recognition sites of the receptor and induce a conformational change in the ion conductance modulator protein. Ion channels open, allowing diffusion of Na^+ and K^+ ions down their concentration gradients. **B.** *d*-Tubocurarine has combined with the recognition sites of the closed channel form of the receptors. No conformational change is induced. **C.** *d*-Tubocurarine molecules have entered and plugged the open channel form of the receptor, the ion channel having been opened by acetylcholine molecules. Such an effect might contribute to tetanic fade. (*From Bowman WC: Anesth Analg 59(12), 942, 1980.*)

TABLE 17–1. THE PHYSIOLOGIC EVENTS LEADING TO MUSCLE CONTRACTION CORRELATED WITH POSSIBLE MODIFIERS OF EACH EVENT

Physiologic Effect	Modifiers of Normal Effect
Nerve action potential	Block by local anesthetics
↓	↓
Depolarization of nerve terminal	—
↓	↓
Acetylcholine release (calcium ion required)	Blocked by hemicholinium, botulinum toxin, procaine, magnesium ion, lack of calcium ion, beta-bungarotoxin, small block of nondepolarizing relaxants, decreased synthesis and storage of acetylcholine
↓	↓
Acetylcholine diffusion into synaptic cleft	—
↓	↓
Acetylcholine combination with postjunctional membrane receptor and receptor activation	Blocked by nondepolarizing relaxants. Activation terminated by hydrolysis of acetylcholine by acetylcholinesterase, reuptake of acetylcholine into the vesicles, diffusion of acetylcholine away from receptors
↓	↓
Increase in permeability of postjunctional membrane to sodium and potassium	Modified by acid–base balance, calcium ion, nondepolarizing muscle relaxants
↓	↓
Depolarization of postjunctional membrane	Excitation enhanced by succinylcholine, decamethonium, and neostigmine, blocked by potassium ion
↓	↓
Propagation of muscle action potential	Excitation enhanced by calcium ion and veratrum alkaloids; blocked by quinine
↓	↓
Excitation–contraction coupling	Blocked by lack of calcium ion
↓	↓
Muscle contraction	Blocked by lack of calcium ion, procaine, dantrolene, acidosis

sites, whereas nondepolarizing agents block these sites. Effects of the relaxants other than at the neuromuscular junction may usually be attributed to the effects of the drugs at cholinoceptive sites. Pancuronium is thought to be cardioselective in its antimuscarinic action.

Recent studies have shown that relaxants may have a channel blocking effect that inhibits ionic movement and, therefore, muscle function and recovery. This effect provides an additional mechanism of action of neuromuscular blocking agents. However, for the relaxants currently available, the predominant effects are at the receptor. It is important to remember that channel block is not competitive and that cholinesterase inhibitors will not antagonize a channel block.

CHARACTERISTICS OF DEPOLARIZING BLOCK

Depolarizing block occurs after the administration of such agents as succinylcholine and decamethonium. The motor endplate is depolarized, as occurs with acetylcholine, but depolarization is more prolonged. Repolarization is inhibited, preventing impulse transmission, which would normally occur in response to the release of acetylcholine.

After injection of succinylcholine, fasciculation of body muscle groups is commonly seen, due to depolarization. When a peripheral nerve stimulator is used, the response to tetanic stimulation (50 to 100 Hz) is usually well sustained, and posttetanic facilitation is not noted. However, depending on the degree of block, the anesthetic technique used, and the muscle studied, tetanus may not consistently be 100 percent sustained. Drugs, such as neostigmine or pyridostigmine, increase a depolarizing block.

CHARACTERISTICS OF NONDEPOLARIZING BLOCK

When receptors are occupied by nondepolarizing agents, such as *d*-tubocurarine or pancuronium, a nondepolarizing block occurs. Since the muscle cells have not been depolarized, no fasciculation is seen. When using a peripheral nerve stimulator, one will see a decreased twitch response. During tetanic stimulation there will be fade, which is seen mechanically as a decrease in muscle tension despite continued stimulation.

If the muscle response is electromyographically recorded, fade will be seen as follows. The first action potential during tetanic stimulation will be the largest, followed by smaller action potentials. The first four to eight action potentials will show diminishing height, and then a stable level will be reached. Whether recorded mechanically or electromyographically, when tetanic stimulation is decontinued and single stimuli (twitches) are again applied, the first twitch is larger than the last one administered before tetanus (posttetanic facilitation). This is followed by a subsequent decrease in twitch height on continued stimulation, and a new stable level of twitch height is attained. Depending on the circumstances, this new level may be equal to or somewhat larger than the level seen before tetanic stimulation (posttetanic decurarization). Drugs, such as neostig-

mine, pyridostigmine, and edrophonium, counteract the nondepolarizing type of block.

DESENSITIZATION BLOCK (PHASE II BLOCK, DUAL BLOCK)

After prolonged depolarization induced by the continuing administration of a depolarizing agent, such as succinylcholine or decamethonium, a change occurs in the postsynaptic membrane. The membrane becomes partially repolarized but is in a state of desensitization (i.e., unresponsive to acetylcholine). Characteristics noted with this block include poorly sustained tetanus and posttetanic facilitation. These characteristics of the desensitization block are similar to those seen with a nondepolarizing block. However, despite this superficial similarity, the nondepolarizing and desensitizing blocks are different entities.

When desensitization block occurs, one initially may note tachyphylaxis (the need for an increasing dose of the depolarizing drug to cause the same effect) in approximately 50 percent of patients. The postjunctional membrane then becomes less and less sensitive to acetylcholine or succinylcholine. The occurrence of desensitization block usually depends on the dose and duration of time over which a depolarizing relaxant has been administered. The longer the time of drug administration and the larger the dose, the more likely is the appearance of a desensitization block.

Although it is commonly stated that a block is initially depolarizing and abruptly changes to desensitizing, this is not necessarily true. After the first dose of succinylcholine, a few muscle fibers are probably in the desensitized state. With additional time and administration, more fibers convert to the desensitized state until the majority of the muscle fibers are desensitized. Thus, there is a varying balance of fibers in the depolarized and desensitized states, with more being depolarized initially and later more being desensitized. The dose of succinylcholine required for desensitization block varies with both the patient and the anesthetic technique used. Administration of 4 to 5 mg/kg of succinylcholine in combination with halothane anesthesia has been noted to cause desensitization block, but when the nitrous oxide–oxygen–narcotic technique is used, desensitization block has required 7 to 8 mg/kg of succinylcholine. In patients with atypical plasma cholinesterase, desensitization block has been described immediately after the first dose of 1 mg/kg of succinylcholine.

MONITORING OF NEUROMUSCULAR FUNCTION

As the anesthetist gains experience, the effect of relaxants is often assessed by the feel of the anesthetic reservoir bag. In the normal patient this may be an excellent guide, but in patients with respiratory obstruction or bronchopulmonary disease, when the surgeon has placed a number of packs in the chest or upper abdomen, or when the assistant is leaning on the chest, such assessment becomes more difficult. Observation of airway pressures in both the manually and artificially ventilated patient provides another adjunct to assessment of the relaxant effect. This again may be misleading in respiratory obstruction or in the presence of anesthetic agents that modify respiration. The opinions of the surgeon and the anesthetist are valuable in assessing relaxation but may be affected by anesthetic agents, bowel distention, patient pathophysiology, or surgical technique. In the conscious patient, the hand squeeze or head lift held for 5 seconds or more may be helpful in assessing recovery. Inspiratory force measurement, noting negative pressure against an occluded airway, may also be used.

Because agents other than muscle relaxants may influence all these factors it was thought necessary to develop a method of monitoring the effects of muscle relaxants that was more specific to the effects of the drugs used. This is done with the aid of a peripheral nerve stimulator. The muscle response evoked by nerve stimulation can be visually observed or measured with a transducer. The spontaneous electrical muscle activity can also be measured, but this is not a suitable method for routine clinical use. Therefore, the most effective monitoring technique currently available is to measure the effects of muscle relaxants with a nerve stimulator. This technique does not require patient cooperation and may be used at any point before, during, and after the anesthetic. The ulnar nerve is usually stimulated at the elbow or wrist with surface or needle electrodes, and the effects of the stimulus may be observed visually or measured mechanically or electrically. The mechanical method of evaluating muscle response involves the application of a force transducer that measures the adduction force of the adductor pollicis muscle or other hand muscles after stimulation of the ulnar nerve. The muscle response may be measured electrically by recording the compound action potential of the adductor pollicis or other muscle. In clinical practice, the most common monitoring method is the visual observation of contraction of the hand muscles in response to ulnar nerve stimulation.

Electrical stimulation of the ulnar nerve may vary from one stimulus every 5 to 10 seconds to tetanic stimulation at a rate of 50 to 100 Hz. Normally, tetanus can be maintained in the adult for at least 20 seconds at 50 Hz. After this, the first signs of fatigue become apparent from depletion of the readily available stores of acetylcholine.

In addition to measuring changes in single twitch height and tetanic response, the train of four technique has recently been used for clinical monitoring. The major advantages of this technique are that a control response is not necessary before administration of anesthetic agents and that it is less painful than tetanic stimulation. The train of four technique involves stimulating a nerve at 2 Hz for 2 seconds, thus evoking four responses. The ratio of the fourth to the first response is used to assess the degree of block. With a nondepolarizing agent, the second, third, and fourth responses are progressively less than the first response. This is really an example of fade. The smaller the train of four ratio, the greater the block. With depolarizing agents, there is no fade of train of four until desensitization block occurs.

The presence of a normal twitch height does not indicate that all of the muscle fibers are functioning normally. It has been shown that approximately 75 to 80 percent of receptors must be occluded before neuromuscular transmission is interrupted at slow rates of stimulation (twitch). High-frequency tetanic stimulation may be a more sensitive measure of residual curarization than the single twitch. It has been shown that 50 percent of the receptors must be available to sustain a tetanic stimulation at 100 Hz.

The greater number of receptors blocked would yield a greater degree of muscle relaxation, at least in theory, and conversely, restoration of normal neuromuscular function would indicate that few receptors are blocked by residual muscle relaxant drug effects. Adequate surgical relaxation may be best assessed by measuring the train-of-four response. Ninety to ninety-five percent twitch suppression indicates a dose of nondepolarizing muscle relaxant appropriate to achieve surgical relaxation during nitrous oxide anesthesia. If potent inhaled agents are administered, adequate surgical relaxation may be achieved at 75 percent twitch depression.

Observation of the level of neuromuscular blockage during general anesthesia must include correlation of evoked responses with clinical signs. Endoscopy and endotracheal intubation may be performed when twitch suppression is 95 percent or more. Abdominal muscle relaxation may appear to be surgically inadequate at 25 percent twitch suppression. However, the patient may not be able to lift his/her head until the twitch height is at a minimum of 90 percent of the premuscle relaxant control. Recovery from neuromuscular blockade must also be evaluated utilizing both clinical signs such as adequacy of ventilation and muscle strength. These clinical signs can be correlated with evoked responses. The assessment of a train-of-four response which is 75 percent or higher should ensure adequate ventilation and muscle control has been restored.

DEPOLARIZING MUSCLE RELAXANTS

Succinylcholine (Anectine)

Succinylcholine was first prepared in 1906 by Hunt and Taveau. In 1949 and 1950 respectively, Bovet and colleagues and Castillo and de Beer described the paralyzing action of the bis-choline esters of succinic acid, and showed that succinylcholine was hydrolyzed by cholinesterase and that this hydrolysis could be reduced by cholinesterase inhibitors. The clinical use of succinylcholine was described in Europe in 1951 by Thesleff, Brock et al, Mayerhaufer and Hassfurther, and Scurr. In 1952 Foldes described the clinical use of succinylcholine in anesthesia in the United States.

Physical and Chemical Properties. Succinylcholine is a bisquaternary ammonium compound (Fig. 17–4) that appears as white crystals with a melting point of 150C. In solution, it is relatively unstable and should be kept cool during storage, otherwise potency may be decreased over time. Plasma cholinesterase (pseudocholinesterase) hydrolyzes the drug to succinylmonocholine and choline. Succinylmonocholine, which is much less active than succinylcholine, is slowly broken down by plasma cholinesterase to succinic acid and choline.

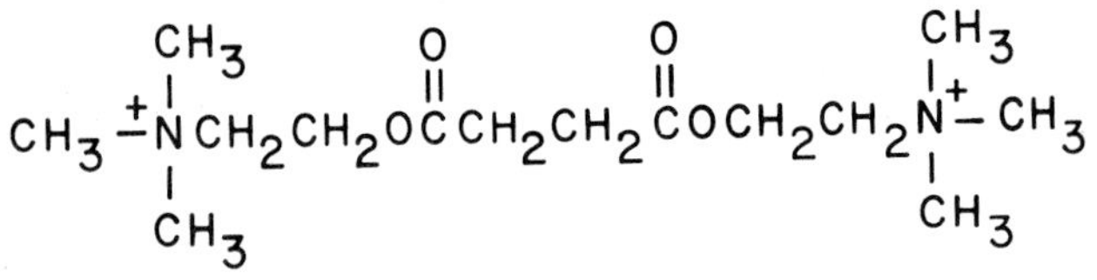

$$CH_3 \overset{\overset{CH_3}{|}}{\underset{\underset{CH_3}{|}}{N^+}} CH_2 CH_2 O \overset{O}{\overset{||}{C}} CH_2 CH_2 \overset{O}{\overset{||}{C}} OCH_2 CH_2 \overset{\overset{CH_3}{|}}{\underset{\underset{CH_3}{|}}{N^+}} CH_3$$

Figure 17–4. Structure of succinylcholine.

Drug Action. Succinylcholine causes muscle relaxation within 1 minute. It is therefore frequently used for endotracheal intubation. The usual dose required to produce satisfactory conditions for intubation is 0.5 to 1 mg/kg. In normal patients relaxation persists for approximately 3 to 5 minutes, but complete recovery may require up to 20 minutes. When a prolonged effect is desired, succinylcholine has been instilled by continuous infusion. Ninety percent twitch depression may be maintained with approximately 1.5 to 15 mg/kg per hour. Because of the variable effects of succinylcholine, a peripheral nerve stimulator is particularly helpful during the administration of a continuous infusion. Recovery from 1 hour of succinylcholine infusion has been found to require from 3 to 21 minutes. After 2 hours of continuous infusion, recovery was found in some patients to be markedly prolonged, and it was therefore recommended that succinylcholine continuous infusion be used only in procedures lasting 1 hour or less. It is possible to use succinylcholine infusion safely by intermittent rather than continuous infusion, but the availability of other, better agents for this purpose (nondepolarizers) has diminished the use of succinylcholine for procedures lasting more than 1 hour.

Uptake, Distribution, and Elimination. Normal plasma half-life of succinylcholine is 1 to 2 minutes. Succinylcholine and its breakdown products, succinylmonocholine and choline, are normally completely excreted within 3 hours. Although succinylcholine is bound to plasma protein (approximately 30 percent during a 3-hour period), no clinical effect should be noted after a single dose because of rapid breakdown and elimination. With continuous infusion, protein binding may be clinically significant.

In patients with abnormal pseudocholinesterase, elimination occurs primarily by redistribution and renal excretion. Because these effects are much slower than normal breakdown, it may be necessary to ventilate patients artificially with abnormal pseudocholinesterase. The duration of artificial ventilation depends on the amount of drug given. With the use of a peripheral nerve stimulator, the diagnosis of abnormal pseudocholinesterase can be made after the first dose of 0.5 to 1 mg/kg is given, and only a few hours of ventilation are required.

Pseudocholinesterase. Pseudocholinesterase (plasma cholinesterase), necessary for the rapid hydrolysis of succinylcholine, is synthesized in the liver and found in the plasma, kidney, liver, brain, intestine, and pancreas. True cholinesterase, or red cell cholinesterase, differs from pseudocholinesterase. True cholinesterase is present at the myoneural junction and in the red blood cells. It hydrolyzes acetylcholine but not succinylcholine. Because of rapid hydrolysis by pseudocholinesterase, only a small fraction of injected succinylcholine reaches the endplate of the neuromuscular junction. Low pseudocholinesterase levels may be found in pregnancy, liver disease, or malnutrition. A prolonged response may occur in patients with low pseudocholinesterase, and the prolongation of a dose of 1 mg/kg may be from a normal of 20 minutes to 30 to 60 minutes.

A much greater prolongation of the activity of succinylcholine is seen in patients with an atypical enzyme that is minimally effective in hydrolyzing succinylcholine. Patients may have one (heterozygotes) or two (homozygotes) abnormal genes for pseudocholinesterase. The presence of atypical pseudocholinesterase can be found by determination of the dibucaine number. Dibucaine normally inhibits the hydrolysis of benzylcholine, a substrate of pseudocholinesterase. The dibucaine number is the percent inhibition by dibucaine of the hydrolysis of benzylcholine by pseudocholinesterase. Patients with two normal genes for pseudocholinesterase have a dibucaine number of 70 or greater. In patients with atypical pseudocholinesterase (homozygotes with two abnormal genes), the dibucaine number is 30 or less. Heterozygotes have a dibucaine number between 30 and 70 (Table 17–2).

The concentration of pseudocholinesterase is not reflected in the dibucaine number. This number reflects only the activity of the pseudocholinesterase that is present. A patient with liver disease may have a reduced amount of pseudocholinesterase but a normal dibucaine number. If succinylcholine is required in the clinical care of patients suspected of having atypical pseudocholinesterase, a small test dose of 0.1 mg/kg of succinylcholine is recommended. A patient with atypical pseudocholinesterase (homozygote) will become completely paralyzed and apneic with this dose; however, complete recovery should occur within 45 to 60 minutes. If the patient with atypical pseudocholinesterase is instead given the normal dose of 1 mg/kg, recovery may take 2 to 4 hours. With heterozygotes the response is variable. Some will respond normally to succinylcholine, whereas others may have prolonged response, but the prolonged response will not be as great as that of a homozygote with two abnormal genes.

The frequency of occurrence of atypical pseudocholinesterase is approximately 1 in 25 patients for heterozygotes and 1 in 2500 patients for homozygotes with two abnormal genes. The fluoride number and succinylcholine number have been used to study atypical pseudocholinesterase, but not as commonly as the dibucaine number. Another genetic abnormality affecting pseudocholinesterase is the silent gene. Homozygotes with two silent genes have little or no pseudocholinesterase activity.

The C_5 Variant gene is a rare variety of gene affecting plasma cholinesterase. In contrast to the previously presented abnormalities, a very rapid hydrolysis of succinylcholine is seen in patients with this gene. Thus, these patients are relatively resistant to succinylcholine.

Management of Patients with Abnormal Pseudocholinesterase. Monitoring of patients with a peripheral nerve stimulator will help diagnose as well as treat patients with atypical pseudocholinesterase. The patient should be

TABLE 17–2. HEREDITARY VARIANTS OF PSEUDOCHOLINESTERASE RESULTING FROM FOUR ALLELIC GENES

Genotype	Frequency in a British Population	Response to Succinylcholine	Typical Dibucaine Number	Typical Fluoride Number
N–N	Normal population	Normal	80	60
D–D	1 in 2,800	Greatly prolonged	20	20
F–F	?1 in 300,000	Moderately prolonged	70	30
S–S	?1 in 140,000	Greatly prolonged	—	—
N–D	1 in 26	Slightly prolonged	60	45
N–F	?1 in 280	Slightly prolonged	75	50
N–S	?1 in 190	Slightly prolonged	80	60
D–F	?1 in 29,000	Greatly prolonged	45	35
D–S	?1 in 20,000	Greatly prolonged	20	20
F–S	?1 in 200,000	Moderately prolonged	65	35

N = Gene for normal pseudocholinesterase; D = Gene for dibucaine-resistant variant; F = Gene for fluoride-resistant variant; S = Gene for absence of enzyme activity (silent gene).
(*From Lehman H, Liddell J: Br J Anaesth 41:235, 1969.*)

allowed to recover fully from the initial dose of succinylcholine before administration of further depolarizing or nondepolarizing relaxants. Failure to do so has resulted in missing a diagnosis of atypical pseudocholinesterase. If one encounters a patient with a prolonged response to succinylcholine, it is thought best to sedate and ventilate the patient until the patient recovers from the block. The administration of anticholinesterase agents is not always successful and may serve only to confuse the diagnosis.

Effects of Succinylcholine Other Than on the Neuromuscular Junction. Succinylcholine acts on nicotinic and muscurinic sites where acetylcholine is normally the transmitter. Thus, it exhibits many of the same effects as are seen with acetylcholine.

Cardiovascular Effects. Succinylcholine has been shown to produce bradycardia in infants and children after an initial dose. Reports of bradycardia and brief periods of cardiac standstill have, to a lesser extent, been reported in adults. However, these have occurred most frequently after a second dose. The time interval between the first and second dose of succinylcholine is significant, with bradycardia being seen most commonly with a time period of 5 minutes between the first and second doses. The cause of bradycardia or asystole has not been definitively determined, and current theories include (1) baroreceptor stimulation, (2) reflex bradycardia, (3) sensitization of the heart by succinylmonocholine to subsequent doses of succinylcholine, and (4) direct acetylcholine-like effect on the heart. The cardiovascular effects are dose related and are blocked by atropine or the prior injection of a nondepolarizing agent.

Cardiac arrhythmias, ranging from occasional premature ventricular contractions to ventricular fibrillation and cardiac arrest, may occur when succinylcholine is given to patients after trauma, burns, tetanus, hemiplegia, spinal cord transection, cerebral vascular accidents, neuromuscular disorders with muscle wasting, and long-term immobilization. The arrhythmias are due to a plasma potassium increase from normal (3.5 to 4.5 mEq/L) to levels as high as 12 to 14 mEq/L. In the normal patient, serum potassium increases only 0.5 mEq/L after the administration of succinylcholine. The profound increase noted in patients with neuromuscular disorders, trauma, or burns is thought to be due to a supersensitivity phenomenon resulting in the entire muscle membrane becoming permeable to sodium and potassium.

The time of susceptibility to succinylcholine-induced hyperkalemia varies with the cause. After burns, the patient is most likely to demonstrate significant potassium increase from the 20th day to the 60th day, although many exceptions have been noted. Patients with massive trauma may demonstrate significant succinylcholine-induced potassium levels immediately following trauma until the lesion is covered by skin. After spinal cord injury or lower motor neuron damage, the danger period may last 6 months or more. These ranges are simply reported times of release of high levels of potassium. Individual patients may demonstrate high levels of potassium release after succinylcholine administration at times other than those listed. In cases of progressive neuromuscular disease and atrophy, the danger period may last indefinitely. It is extremely important that succinylcholine be avoided or given with care in patients with potential large serum potassium increase.

Pretreatment with nondepolarizing muscle relaxants or diazepam has been studied to determine the effect on potassium rise. Although there is partial protection in some cases, these techniques do not assure total protection. Therefore, it appears to be far safer to avoid the use of succinylcholine in any high-risk patient.

Often, concern is expressed about the use of succinylcholine in patients with renal failure. Studies have demonstrated that the increase in serum potassium in renal patients is similar to that seen in normal patients (0.5 mEq/L). There is no increase in extrusion of intracellular potassium as is seen with burns, trauma, or neuromuscular disorders. One should be cautious, however, in giving succinylcholine to renal patients, since a 0.5 mEq increase in serum potassium might be dangerous in a patient with a previously increased serum potassium level.

A less well known effect of succinylcholine is hypertension due to succinylcholine per se. Endotracheal intubation may cause hypertension, but it is possible to demonstrate a rise in arterial pressure after succinylcholine, followed by an additional rise in arterial pressure after intubation. The mechanism of succinylcholine hypertension appears to be stimulation of sympathetic ganglia (a nicotinic effect), resulting in the release of catecholamines. Caution should be used in administering this drug to patients with cerebral aneurysms, dissecting aortic aneurysms, or other vascular conditions where hypertension may cause complications.

It should be remembered when considering the cardiovascular effects of any drug that the response of an individual patient depends on the state of balance of the autonomic nervous system, the anesthetic agents the patient receives, and the conditions surrounding the administration. Succinylcholine has many different actions and may induce effects on any of the nicotinic or muscarinic receptors of the autonomic nervous system. Therefore, the results may be variable in individual patients, and the drug should be used in each individual after considering the patient's condition and the need for this mode of muscle relaxation.

Effect on the Eye. Succinylcholine causes contraction of both the extraocular muscles and the intraorbital smooth muscle of the eye. The extraocular muscles are unusual in that two types of muscle fibers are present, a twitch system and a tonic system. The twitch system is the muscle system found in other skeletal muscles of humans. The tonic system has been found in humans only in the extraocular muscle. The effect of succinylcholine on the twitch system is depression. In contrast, the tonic system responds with contracture. This contracture of the extraocular muscles, plus the contraction of intraorbital smooth muscle can lead to a marked increase in intraocular pressure. In a patient with an open eye, this increase may be sufficient to cause extrusion of the vitreous and subsequent blindness.

An additional cause of increased intraocular pressure has been related to a rise in systemic BP. This is less important than the effect on the extraocular muscles, since there is only approximately 1 mm of intraocular pressure rise for every 10 mm rise in systemic pressure. The administration of a nondepolarizing relaxant before administration of succinylcholine depresses the effect on both the twitch and tonic eye muscle groups and on the intraorbital smooth muscle. However, the degree of depression varies and depends on the dose of nondepolarizer and the dose of succinylcholine. It should be remembered that if pretreatment with a nondepolarizing agent, such as *d*-tubocurarine (3 to 6 mg) or gallamine (20 to 40 mg), is carried out, a larger dose of succinylcholine is required for intubation. With pancuronium pretreatment (0.5 to 1 mg), a larger dose of succinylcholine is not required, since the pseudocholinesterase-inhibiting action of pancuronium balances the antagonism of the depolarizing action of succinylcholine by the nondepolarizing agent. Hexafluorenium has also been used as pretreatment to prevent the increase in intraocular pressure found with succinylcholine. The effects of this drug are discussed in a later section.

Gastrointestinal System. Succinylcholine has been found to cause increased intragastric pressure, which may result in increased susceptibility to vomiting or silent regurgita-

tion. The pressure required to open the cardioesophageal sphincter varies depending on the circumstances and the patient. In most patients, the rise in intragastric pressure after succinylcholine administration is not sufficient to cause problems, but it is not always possible to predict in which few patients a potential problem exists. The intragastric pressure increase may be prevented by administration of a nondepolarizing relaxant 3 to 5 minutes before administration of succinylcholine. Atropine 0.6 mg has been found to increase the gastric opening pressure to a pressure higher than is generated in most circumstances by the administration of succinylcholine. Sellick's maneuver (pressure on the cricoid cartilage to compress the esophagus against the cervical spine) and awake intubation have been used to prevent regurgitation and aspiration in susceptible patients. There is a great deal of debate at present about which of these techniques or combinations is best to prevent regurgitation and aspiration. Our preference is for awake intubation whenever possible.

Effects on the Uterus and Placenta. Succinylcholine may be used safely in the obstetric patient without effects on the newborn. With IV doses under 200 mg, succinylcholine has not been found in the umbilical venous blood of newborn infants. In larger doses, 300 to 500 mg, small amounts can be found in the blood of the umbilical vein, but effects on the newborn have not been noted.

Obstetric patients often have lower than normal levels of pseudocholinesterase, and, therefore, smaller doses of succinylcholine may achieve effects equal to those seen in nonpregnant patients. In addition, normally safe doses of succinylcholine may cause problems in the fetus of a mother with atypical pseudocholinesterase.

Succinylcholine has no effect on uterine smooth muscle contraction.

Histamine Release. Histamine release after administration of succinylcholine is thought to be approximately 1/100 of that seen after the administration of *d*-tubocurarine, although intradermal injection of small doses of succinylcholine may cause a wheal and a flare. There are occasional case reports noting anaphylaxis, bronchospasm, hypotension, and pharyngeal and facial edema, but these are rare.

Muscle Pain. Muscle pain and stiffness are frequently seen following the use of succinylcholine. This effect usually occurs within 12 to 14 hours after succinylcholine administration but may be seen earlier or later. The duration is usually 2 days but may be as long as 5 or 6 days. Possible sites of pain are the neck and shoulders, abdomen, chest, back, jaw, and limbs. Patients frequently describe the discomfort as similar to that noted after strenuous exercise. The reported incidence of pain has been quite variable, ranging from a low of 0.7 percent to a high of 89 percent. Differences in the types of patients studied, the definition of muscle pain, and the circumstances surrounding the study may account for the difference in results.

Muscle pain is reported more frequently in females than males, more often in the 20 to 50 year age group than at other ages, and, most important, more commonly in patients undergoing minor operative procedures who ambulate immediately after surgery. The following mechanisms have been considered as causes of muscle pain: (1) mechanical damage to the muscle cell, (2) potassium release, (3) lactic acid release, and (4) the effect of succinylcholine on the muscle cells. The exact mechanism of muscle pain has not yet been determined. Pain has not been related to the release of potassium or to the observation of fasciculation.

The injection of hexafluorenium before succinylcholine administration has been demonstrated to prevent muscle pain. The administration of thiopental immediately before the administration of succinylcholine may decrease the incidence of muscle pain, as may the prior administration of a small dose of nondepolarizing relaxant (3 to 6 mg of *d*-tubocurarine, 20 to 40 mg of gallamine, or 0.5 to 1 mg of pancuronium). The prior administration of diazepam in as small a dose as 0.05 mg/kg has been reported to prevent succinylcholine muscle pain. Since diazepam does not modify the neuromuscular effects of succinylcholine and the muscle relaxants do, this drug appears to be the most logical method of preventing muscle pain.

Myoglobinemia and Myoglobinuria.

Myoglobinuria has been seen after injection of succinylcholine, although renal failure has not necessarily followed. The incidence appears to be far less in adults than in children, and effects are frequently noted when halothane is used for induction. It has been shown that the administration of thiopental immediately before succinylcholine administration will prevent this effect.

Abnormal Response.

Rarely, succinylcholine may produce contraction rather than relaxation. This has been noted in patients with muscle disease, particularly myotonia congenita and myotonia dystrophica. Myoglobinuria may then result. It is best to avoid the use of succinylcholine in patients with myotonia, since contractions may be so severe that the patients cannot be ventilated. There have been cases in which administration of a nondepolarizing relaxant has relieved the contraction, but because of the nature of the disease, this effect is not assured.

Decamethonium

History.

The depolarizing effects of decamethonium (Syncurine) were described in 1948 by Barlow and Ing and by Patton and Zaimis. In 1949, Organe et al reported the use of this drug in clinical anesthesia. Decamethonium is not widely used in anesthesia today.

Physical and Chemical Properties.

Decamethonium is a water-soluble crystalline powder that is relatively stable (Fig. 17–5). It is not irritating to tissues and is not destroyed by acetylcholinesterase.

Clinical Effects.

Decamethonium is a depolarizing agent with effects similar to those of succinylcholine. It differs, however, in that its duration of action is longer and it more readily causes tachyphylaxis upon repeated injection. The duration of action is approximately 20 to 30 minutes after

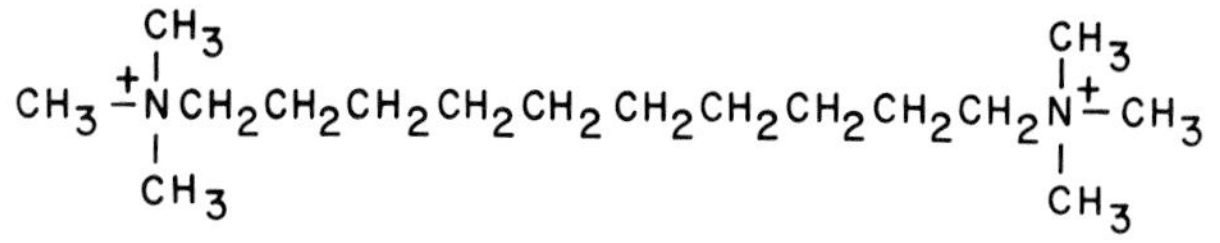

$$CH_3 \overset{+}{N} CH_2 CH_2 CH_2 CH_2 CH_2 CH_2 CH_2 CH_2 CH_2 CH_2 \overset{+}{N} CH_3$$

Figure 17–5. Structure of decamethonium.

a dose of 4 mg used to facilitate intubation. Termination of action is due to redistribution and renal elimination. This drug is not thought to undergo significant breakdown in vivo. Eighty to ninety percent of the total dose has been recovered unchanged in the urine over a 24-hour period. Therefore, this drug should not be used in patients with impaired kidney function.

Decamethonium may cause fasciculation and muscle pain but apparently does so to a lesser extent than succinylcholine. Histamine is released in amounts less than after *d*-tubocurarine administration but more than after succinylcholine administration. Serum potassium is increased in amounts equal to that seen with succinylcholine.

Four to six milligrams of decamethonium is required for endotracheal intubation, and satisfactory conditions are noted within 2 to 3 minutes. Two to four milligrams provides satisfactory abdominal relaxation in the previously intubated patient. The size of repetitive doses should be dependent on the degree of tachyphylaxis.

NONDEPOLARIZING RELAXANTS

d-Tubocurarine

History.

The South American Indians originally used *d*-tubocurarine (curare) as an arrow poison. In 1850, Sir Benjamin Brodie administered curare to a donkey and kept the animal alive through artificial ventilation. The animal completely recovered. In 1850, Claude Bernard noted that curare caused paralysis of the skeletal muscle of a frog, yet the muscle still responded to direct stimulation. He, therefore, concluded that the effect of the drug was between the nerve and the muscle. Kuhne, in 1862, noted that the effect of curare was at the neuromuscular junction. In 1935, the pure alkaloid of *d*-tubocurarine was isolated from the plant *Chondodendron tomentosum*. Bennett et al., in 1940, described the first administration of *d*-tubocurarine in humans to diminish skeletal muscle movements during electroconvulsive therapy. Griffith and Johnson, in 1942, first used curare in anesthesia.

Physical and Chemical Properties.

The original formula of *d*-tubocurarine chloride has recently been found to be incorrect. Chemical analysis of this particular drug is very difficult. The formula reported by Everett et al. in 1970 demonstrates that *d*-tubocurarine has only one stable quaternary ammonium group (Fig. 17–6). This finding elucidated the fact that it is not required that a neuromuscular blocker be a bisquaternary ammonium compound.

Pharmacologic Action.

d-Tubocurarine was the first of the neuromuscular blocking drugs and is used as the prototype of all nondepolarizing neuromuscular blocking agents. It

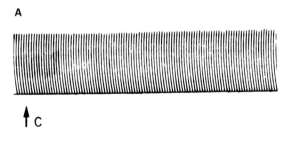

Figure 17–6. Structure of *d*-tubocurarine.

binds with receptors used normally by acetylcholine and prevents its binding. It is also thought to block depolarization by blocking the sodium–potassium interchange channels.

The clinical characteristics of nondepolarizing neuromuscular blockers have been discussed previously and can be summarized as (1) the presence of fade during tetanic stimulation of the nerve, (2) posttetanic facilitation on return to a twitch rate of stimulation, and (3) antagonism by anticholinesterase drugs. The individual response to *d*-tubocurarine varies markedly, as shown in Figure 17–7.

The dose of *d*-tubocurarine required for endotracheal intubation varies from 0.4 to 0.7 mg/kg. The dose required for satisfactory abdominal relaxation varies from 0.1 to 0.4 mg/kg. The duration of action of *d*-tubocurarine depends on the degree of block produced by the dose given, the pH level of the blood, the degree of surgical stimulation, and the degree of basal anesthesia. Repeat doses of the drug rarely exceed one fifth of the original amount given

due to residual receptor occupancy. Because of the extreme variability in patient response, it is important that the patients be monitored by a nerve stimulator and the dose of relaxant titrated until the desired effect is noted (Fig. 17–8).

The effects of *d*-tubocurarine may be antagonized by the administration of edrophonium, neostigmine, or pyridostigmine. These drugs are discussed later in this chapter. The interaction between *d*-tubocurarine and various general anesthetic agents is listed in Table 17–3.

Uptake, Distribution, and Elimination. *d*-Tubocurarine is approximately 40 to 50 percent protein bound, although this amount varies among normal individuals. This may account in part for the variation in patient response to similar doses of *d*-tubocurarine.

d-Tubocurarine demonstrates a widespread distribution throughout the body at active and inactive tissue sites. The predominant locations other than at the neuromuscular junction are the kidneys, liver, and spleen.

The initial termination of effects of this drug occurs because the plasma concentration falls below the critical threshold level required for neuromuscular block. This effect is due primarily to redistribution rather than to urinary or biliary elimination.

In contrast to earlier data, *d*-tubocurarine is now thought to be excreted largely unchanged in the urine, but the biliary system does offer an alternative pathway. In patients with renal failure, the excretion of drugs through the biliary tract is increased.

Recurarization. Although recurarization has been reported, it is likely that most, if not all, of these cases were due to lack of full recovery that was not initially appreciated but later was noted and thought to be recurarization. This has been clearly demonstrated with the use of a peripheral nerve stimulator.

Cardiovascular System. It is well known that *d*-tubocurarine produces hypotension, which was thought to be due to a negative inotropic effect of the drug. However, this effect was subsequently found to be due to preservatives in solution with *d*-tubocurarine. Hypotension after the administration of large doses of *d*-tubocurarine is due mainly to the effects of histamine release and some ganglionic blockade (Fig. 17–9).

The fall in blood pressure has been used by some to assist in the production of controlled hypotension, especially during halothane anesthesia. If not desired, the fall in blood pressure may usually be eliminated by the administration of small doses of *d*-tubocurarine rather than the administration of the total required dose in one bolus.

d-Tubocurarine may inhibit acetylcholine at the cardiac ganglia as it does at the neuromuscular junction. An effect on the vagal afferents has been suggested that may contribute to prevention of succinylcholine-induced bradycardia and arrhythmias when *d*-tubocurarine is used as pretreatment. There is substantial uptake of *d*-tubocurarine by the cardiac muscle, an additional response indicating that it is not unlikely that cardiovascular effects may occur.

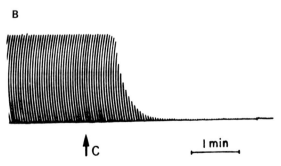

Figure 17–7. Effect of *d*-tubocurarine. **A.** *d*-Tubocurarine (0.1 mg/kg) given at ↑ c did not depress twitch height. **B.** *d*-Tubocurarine (0.1 mg/kg) given at ↑ c abolished the twitch response. (*From Katz RL: Anesthesiology 28:237, 1967.*)

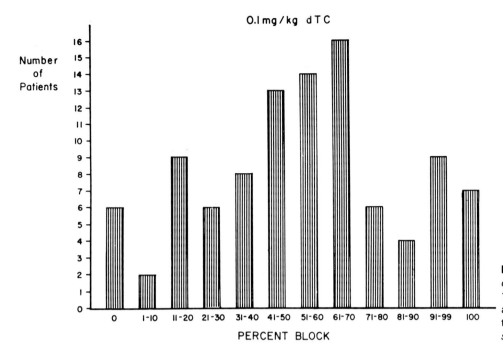

Figure 17–8. Effect of 0.1 mg/kg of *d*-tubocurarine on twitch height in 100 patients. Note the marked variation in percent block produced by this dose. (*From Katz RL: Anesthesiology 28:237, 1967.*)

Central Nervous System Effects. Although there are many conflicting reports of the effects of *d*-tubocurarine on the central nervous system, it is currently thought that normally there is no passage of *d*-tubocurarine across the blood–brain barrier. The barrier may be altered, however, under such conditions as dehydration, pH change, and anesthesia, and small amounts may traverse from the blood to the brain.

An indirect effect of *d*-tubocurarine on the state of consciousness may sometimes be seen due to a decrease in afferent impulses from joints and muscle. This may produce a decrease in central nervous system activity and a decrease in the amount of anesthetic agents needed.

A notable experiment regarding the effects of *d*-tubocurarine on the central nervous system was performed by Dr. Scott Smith, an anesthesiologist, who himself received approximately 1 mg/kg of *d*-tubocurarine IV. Following this, he was ventilated until recovery and afterward reported no analgesia, loss of consciousness, clouding of sensorium, or memory impairment.

Skeletal Muscles. Skeletal muscle relaxation after administration of *d*-tubocurarine is first noted in the eye muscles and subsequently spreads to the face, limbs, and abdominal muscles. The diaphragm is the last to be paralyzed. Since the abdominal muscles are paralyzed, the function of the respiratory muscles is seriously impaired to the point that assistance is required.

Uterus and Placenta. In the normal pH range, *d*-tubocurarine is ionized and therefore is relatively insoluble in lipids. It does not cross the placenta in amounts significant to affect the fetus. Because of the small doses of *d*-tubocurarine normally used in obstetric anesthesia and the relative impermeability of the placenta, this drug has been used successfully and safely in large numbers of obstetric patients

TABLE 17–3. INTERACTION BETWEEN *d*-TUBOCURARINE AND GENERAL ANESTHETIC AGENTS

Anesthesia	No. of Patients	Mean Age (yr)	Mean Dose (mg)	10 Percent Recovery Time[a] (min)	Mean Percent Twitch Depression	Percent Patients with Total Paralysis
Diethyl ether-nitrous oxide-oxygen	20	87	13.5	30 ± 11	98	65
Methoxyflurane-nitrous oxide-oxygen	20	36	13.7	29 ± 11	94	80
Cyclopropane-oxygen	20	38	13.4	23 ± 9	98	65
Halothane-oxygen	20	34	14.7	21 ± 8	98	70
Halothane-nitrous oxide-oxygen	85	42	13.5	20 ± 9	94	48
Trichloroethylene-nitrous oxide-oxygen	20	39	14.1	18 ± 9	91	20
Meperidine-nitrous oxide-oxygen	20	42	13.8	17 ± 11	85	30
Innovar-nitrous oxide-oxygen	20	37	13.7	15 ± 6	93	25

[a] Mean and S.D.
(*Reproduced with permission from Walts LF, Dillon JB: Anesth Analg 49:18, 1970.*)

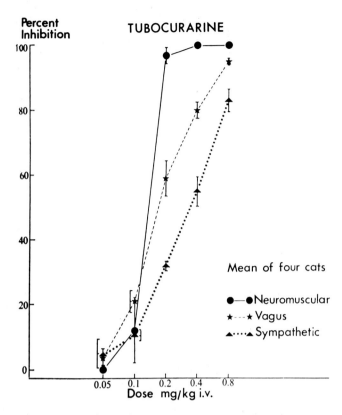

Figure 17–9. Dose–response curve showing blockade of neuromuscular and autonomic mechanisms by IV tubocurarine in cats anesthetized with chloralose. Each point represents the mean of four observations. (*From Hughes R, Chapple DJ: Br J Anaesth 48:59, 1976.*)

and has shown no clinical effect in the newborn. The administration of *d*-tubocurarine has no effect on the uterine smooth muscle and does not depress uterine contraction.

Histamine Release. It has been well documented that histamine release occurs following injection of *d*-tubocurarine. However, the clinical significance of this effect may be minimal. In the administration of doses of 0.1 to 0.3 mg/kg, evidence of histamine release is unusual except in extremely sensitive individuals. In these individuals, flushing, hypotension, urticaria, wheals, laryngeal and pharyngeal edema and increasing respiratory resistance may be noted. When doses of 0.6 to 0.7 mg/kg are used for endotracheal intubation, the effects of histamine release are more common.

Pancuronium Bromide

History. In 1964, Hewitt and Savage noted that when two acetylcholine moieties were incorporated into an androstane nucleus, neuromuscular blocking agents were formed. Pancuronium bromide (Pavulon) is an effective neuromuscular blocking agent that shows no evidence of steroid activity. This drug was introduced into clinical anesthesia by Baird and Reed in 1977.

Physical and Chemical Properties. Pancuronium, a bis-quaternary amino steroid (Fig. 17–10), induces a neuromuscular block of the nondepolarizing type. It is a white, crystalline powder melting at 215C and is a relatively stable agent.

Pharmacologic Action. Pancuronium acts at the neuromuscular junction as a nondepolarizer. The response to pancuronium varies markedly among patients in a manner similar to that seen with *d*-tubocurarine. At lower dose levels, 0.02 mg/kg pancuronium is thought to be five times as potent as *d*-tubocurarine. However, the dose–response curves of the two drugs are not parallel, and 0.08 mg/kg of pancuronium is approximately equal to 0.67 mg/kg of *d*-tubocurarine, a ratio of approximately 8:1. Pancuronium 0.04 mg/kg is thought to provide adequate muscle relaxation for abdominal surgery in the average patient; 0.08 mg/kg has provided relaxation satisfactory for endotracheal intubation, although the range used clinically has been 0.06 to 0.15 mg/kg. Conditions satisfactory for rapid intubation (within 1 to 1.5 minutes) were found with 0.15 mg/kg, thus avoiding the need for administration of a depolarizing agent in patients with a full stomach. Three minutes are usually required to achieve the desired level of relaxation for intubation with a dose of 0.08 mg/kg. The duration of action of pancuronium varies in different patients, as it does *d*-tubocurarine, although it roughly correlates with the amount of block present. Two patients with the same degree of neuromuscular block may, however, have widely differing durations of action. The duration of action of the ED_{95} dose of pancuronium is shorter than that of the ED_{95} doses of *d*-tubocurarine, metocurine, and gallamine.

Pancuronium may be antagonized by the administration of neostigmine, (0.04 to 0.08 mg/kg), pyridostigmine (1.6 to 3.2 mg/kg), or edrophonium (0.5 to 1 mg/kg).

Uptake, Distribution, and Elimination. Pancuronium has not been shown to be significantly bound to plasma proteins. The distribution in the body is thought to be similar to that of *d*-tubocurarine, and as with other relaxants, the kidney is relied on as the main route of elimination. Since a small amount of pancuronium is deacetylated in the liver and subsequently excreted in the bile, this route can be an alternative pathway in the presence of kidney disease.

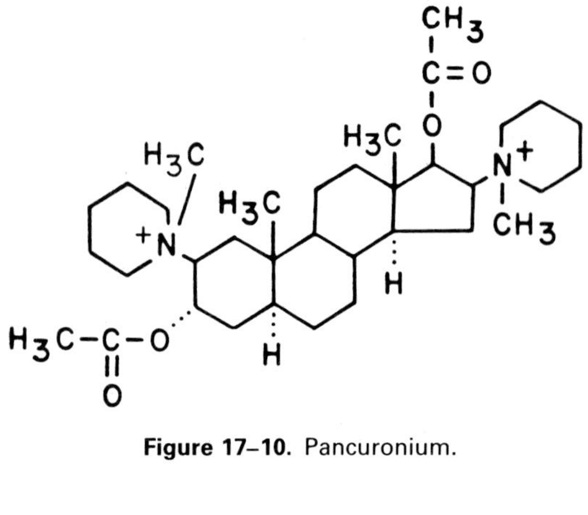

Figure 17–10. Pancuronium.

Cardiovascular System. In clinical doses, pancuronium does not appear to have a significant ganglionic blocking effect in humans. At doses below 0.06 mg/kg, little change in pulse rate is seen, although some vagolytic activity may occur with higher doses (Fig. 17–11). It has been shown that cardiac effects are greater in the patient anesthetized with the balanced technique than in those anesthetized by inhalation agents. Tachycardia noted following pancuronium is both dose related and cumulative and is probably related to muscarinic receptor blockade. The increase in heart rate and arterial pressure is much more profound if the patient is unpremedicated and has not received a belladonna drug. In patients with a higher basal heart rate or who are well anesthetized, little cardiovascular effect is seen (Fig. 17–12). Pancuronium may also prevent reuptake of catecholamines by the sympathetic nerve endings. These effects may contribute to increases in mean arterial pressure and cardiac output.

Central Nervous System Effects. Because pancuronium bromide is a charged ion with little lipid solubility, it is not believed to cross the blood–brain barrier. There is no evidence to indicate that it has any effect on the central nervous system.

Uterus and Placenta. Pancuronium has been used widely for cesarean section without apparent effect on the newborn. In clinical doses, little drug crosses the placenta. Although pancuronium has been noted in the urine of infants whose mothers received the drug, the infants did not exhibit clinical effects.

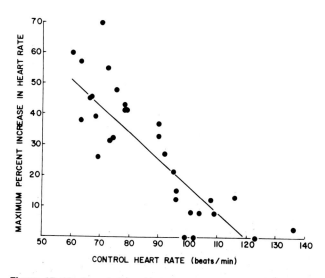

Figure 17–12. Correlation of heart rate before pancuronium administration (control heart rate) with maximum percentage increase in heart rate after pancuronium administration. The line represents analysis of linear regression ($r = 0.85$). (*From Miller RL, Eger EI, Stevens WC, et al: Anesthesiology 42:354, 1975.*)

Histamine. Allergic reactions have been recorded following administration of the drug, but there is no evidence to suggest that significant histamine release occurs. This is thought to be an important contribution to the lack of hypotension and bronchospasm noted after pancuronium is administered.

Duration of Action and Antagonism. Paralysis after an ED_{90} dose of pancuronium lasts for approximately 30 to 40 minutes, and as with curare, a dose approximately one fifth of the original dose may be used to maintain relaxation. Pancuronium is easily reversed by neostigmine, pyridostigmine, or edrophonium in doses similar to those used with *d*-tubocurarine.

Pancuronium is a weak inhibitor of plasma cholinesterase. This effect is clinically significant in that pancuronium 0.5 to 1 mg given before succinylcholine increases the action of succinylcholine, whereas *d*-tubocurarine 3 to 6 mg or gallamine 20 to 40 mg given before succinylcholine decrease the action of succinylcholine. Thus, when pancuronium is given before succinylcholine, the dose of succinylcholine does not have to be increased as it must with *d*-tubocurarine or gallamine.

Metocurine

History. In 1935, King first described metocurine (Metubine) as a methylated derivative of *d*-tubocurarine. In 1950, Collier described its pharmacologic action in animals, and its clinical use was described in the same year by Wilson.

Chemical and Physical Properties. Metocurine (Fig. 17–13) is available as a chloride or iodized salt with a melting point of 236C. It is approximately twice as potent as *d*-tubocurarine and is longer acting. The block may be

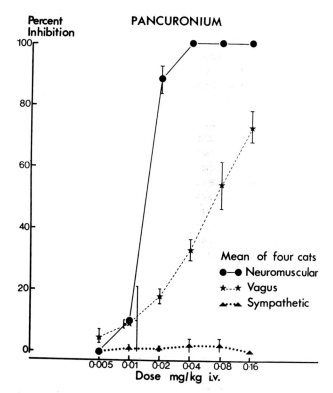

Figure 17–11. Dose–response relationship for pancuronium given IV. (*From Hughes R, Chapple DJ: Br J Anaesth 48:59, 1976.*)

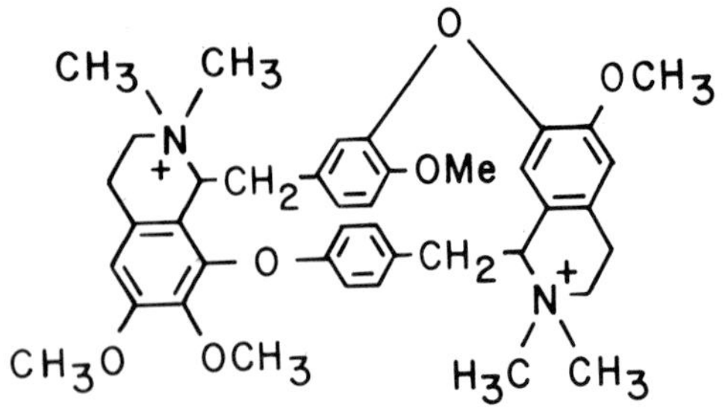

Figure 17-13. Metocurine.

antagonized by neostigmine, pyridostigmine, or edrophonium.

Because of difficulty of synthesis, metocurine initially was not widely accepted. In addition, until recently, it was thought to be three times as potent as *d*-tubocurarine rather than twice as potent. It has lately become increasingly popular because of its comparatively minimal cardiovascular effects when compared with *d*-tubocurarine and pancuronium.

Cardiovascular Effects and Histamine Release. Metocurine has no vagolytic effect at neuromuscular blocking doses. This drug may be particularly useful in patients in whom tachycardia, hypertension, and hypotension are to be avoided, such as in patients suffering from coronary arterial disease (Fig. 17-14).

In doses less than 0.4 mg/kg, histamine release should not be significant. However, if doses exceeding this amount are given as a bolus, hypotension secondary to histamine release may be seen. No evidence of bronchospasm has been reported.

The excretion of metocurine is carried out entirely through the kidneys. Its use should, therefore, be avoided in patients with renal disease.

Gallamine

History. Gallamine (Flaxedil) was found in response to the search for a synthetic agent with an action similar to that of *d*-tubocurarine. Bovet et al described the relaxant properties of this drug in 1947, and the clinical effects in humans were first described in France by Huguenard and Boue in 1948, and in 1949 in England by Mushin et al. Gallamine is safely used clinically today.

Physical and Chemical Properties. The white amorphous powder of gallamine has a melting point of 145 to 150C (Fig. 17-15). It is synthetically prepared and is relatively stable in solution.

Pharmacologic Action. Gallamine acts at the neuromuscular junction as a nondepolarizing muscle relaxant. It is approximately one-sixth to one-seventh as potent as *d*-tubocurarine. The duration of action of gallamine was originally thought to be between 20 and 35 minutes and therefore slightly shorter than that of *d*-tubocurarine. However, it has been shown that gallamine is longer acting than pancuronium, *d*-tubocurarine, and metocurine.

Uptake, Distribution, and Excretion. Gallamine is thought to be significantly protein bound in a manner similar to *d*-tubocurarine. It is excreted almost totally through the kidneys, and, therefore, its use is usually avoided in patients with renal impairment, since there is no significant alternate pathway of elimination.

Cardiovascular Effects. Gallamine does not seem to have a direct action on the myocardium, although there is a very marked vagal blocking effect of the drug. The vagal blocking effect occurs at a lower dose than that required for neuromuscular block, thus assuring that the heart rate will increase if adequate neuromuscular relaxation has been achieved (Fig. 17-16). Tachycardia is also enhanced due to norepinephrine release at cardiac postganglionic adrenergic neurons. Since atropine given after the administration of gallamine has produced an even further increase in heart

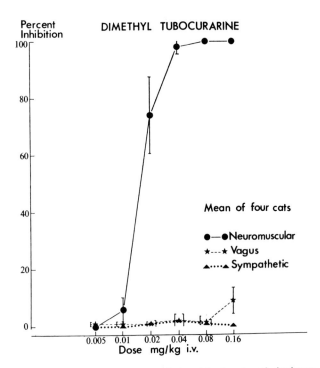

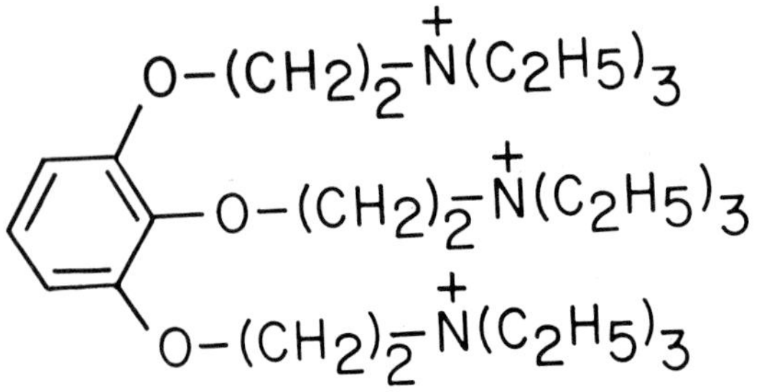

Figure 17-14. Dose–response relationships for dimethyl tubocurarine given IV. (*From Hughes R, Chapple DJ; Br J Anaesth 48:59, 1976.*)

Figure 17-15. Gallamine.

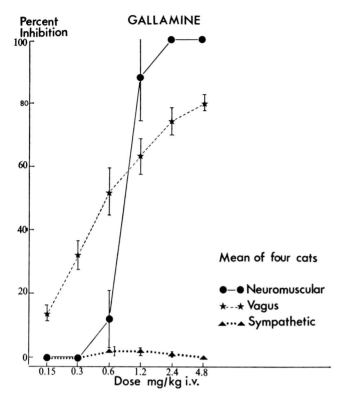

Figure 17–16. Dose–response relationships of gallamine given IV. (*From Hughes R, Chapple DJ: Br J Anaesth 48:59, 1976.*)

rate, either the vagal block is incomplete or the drug action may be at a different receptor site in the heart from that of atropine. Arterial pressure after administration of gallamine increases from 10 to 15 percent, cardiac output increases 20 to 50 percent, and heart rate increases 20 to 100 percent. These changes may be noted within 1 to 2 minutes after the IV administration of the drug. Figure 17–17 shows a comparison of the commonly used relaxants in relation to cardiovascular parameters.

Central Nervous System. When injected IV there is no evidence that gallamine crosses the blood–brain barrier in amounts significant to exert an effect. If injected intrathecally, convulsions have been noted.

Uterus and Placenta. In contrast to other frequently used nondepolarizing muscle relaxants, gallamine has been shown to cross the placenta in amounts sufficient to be noted in the fetus. These infants, however, showed no evidence of muscle weakness. Because of the apparent increase in placental transfer of gallamine when compared to other nondepolarizing and depolarizing relaxants, its use in obstetric patients is not recommended.

Histamine. Gallamine is much less capable of releasing histamine than *d*-tubocurarine, but histamine release has been noted.

Antagonism. Gallamine is effectively antagonized by neostigmine, edrophonium, and pyridostigmine, although an-

tagonism may require larger doses than necessary for equivalent doses of *d*-tubocurarine or pancuronium.

Vecuronium

Physical and Chemical Properties. Vecuronium (Norcuron) is a monoquaternary amino steroid (Fig. 17–18). It differs structurally from pancuronium only in that the nitrogen on the A-ring of the steroid nucleus is a tertiary rather than a quaternary amine. Changing from a quaternary to a tertiary amine profoundly affects the action of the drug in two ways: (1) the vagal blocking action is eliminated in the dosage range that produces neuromuscular block, and (2) the potency of the drug is increased over that of pancuronium by approximately 20 percent, and the duration of action is decreased by approximately 30 percent.

Drug Action and Effects. Because different investigators have used different measurement techniques, the reported ED_{90} of vecuronium varies from 0.023 to 0.044 mg/kg. The time from administration to peak effect varies from 4 to 8 minutes for doses eliciting less than 100 percent depression of twitch height. When doses three to four times the ED_{95}

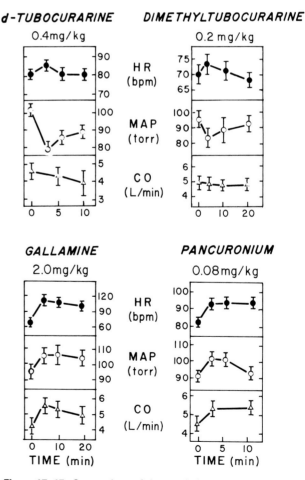

Figure 17–17. Comparison of changes in heart rate, mean arterial pressure, and cardiac output after administration of nondepolarizing neuromuscular blocking agents. (*Courtesy of RK Stoelting: Anesthesiology 36:613, 1972.*)

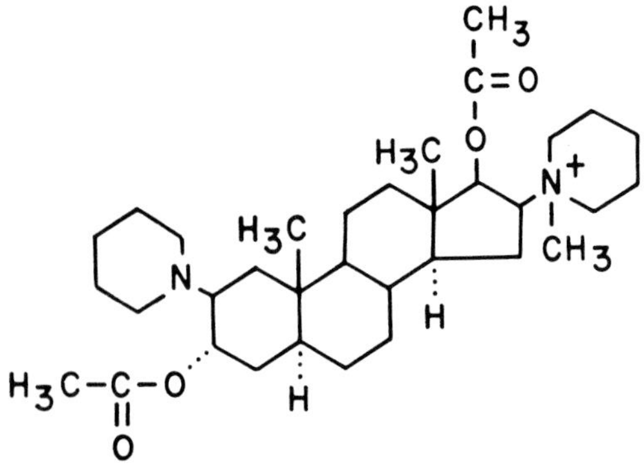

Figure 17–18. Vecuronium.

are given, time from administration to complete abolition of the twitch is 1.3 minutes.

Duration of action (time from injection to 90 percent recovery) varies from 30 to 45 minutes after administration of the ED_{95} dose and is approximately 60 minutes when twice the ED_{95} dose is given. Recovery time (time from 25 percent to 75 percent recovery of twitch height) varies from 9 to 12 minutes.

After an initial dose of vecuronium is given and recovery to 25 percent of control is achieved, a dose can be selected that repeatedly produces the same degree of depression and recovery over several hours. Because of this, it has been said that vecuronium has no cumulative effect. Strictly speaking, this is incorrect. Vecuronium does have a cumulative effect, but it is possible to choose doses and times of administration so that the consistent effect described previously is seen and no cumulative effect is clinically apparent. This allows the same dose to be administered repeatedly and produce the same duration of action.

An important advantage of vecuronium is its lack of side effects in doses as large as 0.28 mg/kg. There is no evidence of histamine release or ganglionic or vagal blockade. Thus, even at this large dose, no cardiovascular effects are seen.

Interaction with Other Drugs. The neuromuscular blocking activity of vecuronium is affected by inhalation agents but to a lesser degree than is seen with pancuronium or *d*-tubocurarine. The prior administration of succinylcholine increases the neuromuscular blocking activity of vecuronium. Antibiotics may also increase the neuromuscular blocking action.

Elimination. The major route of elimination of vecuronium is the bile. Therefore, as expected, in the few studies carried out, the effect of vecuronium is prolonged in patients with liver disease.

Only 10 to 25 percent of vecuronium is excreted in the urine. In animals whose kidneys were eliminated as a source of excretion, the duration of action was similar to that in normal animals. Although there are only a limited number of studies, it appears that the action of vecuronium is not significantly prolonged in patients with renal failure.

The metabolites of vecuronium are (1) 3-hydroxy, (2) 17-hydroxy, and (3) 3- and 17-hydroxy metabolites that are believed to have little activity. The percentage of metabolities recovered, however, has been small, and the largest percentage of drug recovered in the urine and bile is vecuronium itself.

Clinical Use. Vecuronium may be used for both facilitation of intubation and maintenance of relaxation or for maintenance only after intubation facilitated by succinylcholine. If succinylcholine is contraindicated, vecuronium is an effective alternative. The recommended intubation facilitating dose of vecuronium is 0.1 mg/kg, and the recommended initial dose after succinylcholine is 0.05 mg/kg.

Whether vecuronium can safely be used to facilitate intubation in a patient with a full stomach is still being debated. Those advocating its use have followed two basic approaches. The first, which is based on the priming principle, involves the injection of 15 to 20 μg/kg of vecuronium, followed in 3 to 6 minutes by injection of 80 to 85 μg/kg along with an appropriate induction agent, usually thiopental. Most clinicians find that they are then able to satisfactorily intubate the trachea in 1 minute or less. A potential undesired effect of this technique is that some patients may become weak after the initial dose. However, if this possibility is explained to the patient preoperatively, there is usually no problem.

A second approach is to use a very large dose, such as 0.25 mg/kg, as a single bolus along with the induction agent. With this dose it is possible to intubate within 1 minute. There is insufficient research to date to establish which of the two techniques is better or whether either of these techniques will be used routinely.

After the initial dose of vecuronium, depending on the clinical circumstances and effect seen while monitoring with a peripheral nerve stimulator, relaxation is usually satisfactorily maintained with 10 to 20 μg/kg of vecuronium given every 15 to 30 minutes.

The rate of twitch height recovery after vecuronium use is much faster than after the use of either pancuronium or *d*-tubocurarine. A peripheral nerve stimulator is therefore an extremely helpful aid to indicate the need for additional muscle relaxant before the surgeon realizes this or the patient makes gross movements.

Vecuronium neuromuscular block is usually easily antagonized by 0.5 to 1 mg/kg of edrophonium. Recovery of twitch height to control level is seen within 5 to 10 minutes. It is difficult to be specific about the details of antagonism, since the speed of recovery depends on the degree of block at the time of antagonism as well as on the dose and antagonist given.

Atracurium

Physical and Chemical Properties. Atracurium (Tracrium), a quaternary ammonium compound (Fig. 17–19), differs from other neuromuscular blocking agents because it breaks down by either Hoffman elimination or ester hydrolysis. It was originally reported that Hoffman elimination was the major route, but at present this is controversial and the precise amount of breakdown due to each of the two pathways is uncertain. Regardless of the final portion-

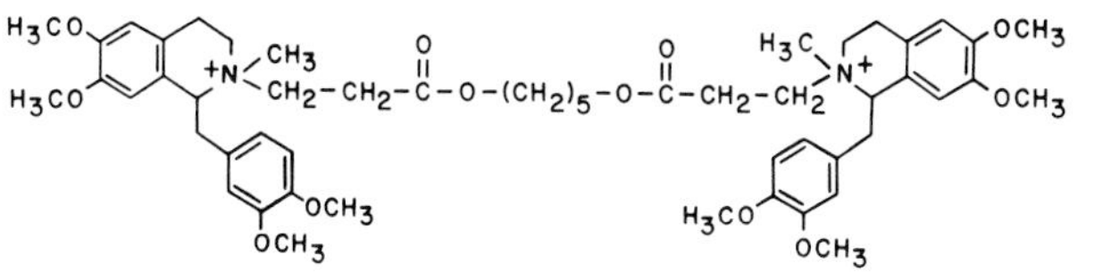

Figure 17–19. Atracurium.

ing, it appears that Hoffman elimination and ester hydrolysis are significant methods of atracurium degradation.

Drug Action and Effects. The ED_{90} of atracurium ranges from 0.1 mg/kg to 0.25 mg/kg, and the onset time is 4 to 8 minutes. This onset time is similar to that of vecuronium. After three times the ED_{95} is given, the onset time is approximately 1.3 minutes. When the ED_{95} is given, recovery to 90 percent of control twitch height occurs in approximately 30 to 45 minutes; when twice the ED_{95} dose is given, approximately 60 minutes is required for recovery.

Atracurium has not been found to have a clinical cumulative effect, probably because recovery is primarily due to breakdown as opposed to redistribution. However, as with vecuronium, it may be possible to experimentally show a small cumulative effect, depending on the study design.

Since atracurium is metabolized, one would not expect to find significant amounts in the bile or urine. Neither renal failure nor hepatic failure increases the duration of neuromuscular block because of the mode of elimination. The major breakdown products are laudanosine and monoacrylates. With clinical doses of atracurium, laudanosine levels probably will not result in cardiovascular or neurologic effects, although studies of this possibility are not yet complete.

It was initially reported that atracurium had no cardiovascular effects. More recently, it was observed that atracurium does release histamine; it has one third to one fourth of the histamine-releasing potential of *d*-tubocurarine when equivalent doses are given. As with *d*-tubocurarine, histamine release is modified by the speed of injection—the slower the rate of injection the less histamine release. When atracurium doses are limited to 0.5 mg/kg (maximum recommended by manufacturer) few or no cardiovascular changes are seen. If the dose is increased to 1.5 mg/kg, histamine release and hypotension occur in approximately 20 percent of patients, and tachycardia occurs in approximately 10 to 15 percent of patients.

It is clear that cardiovascular effects can be seen if the atracurium dose exceeds the amount recommended by the manufacturer. It is also clear, however, that the cardiovascular changes noted usually do not pose a significant clinical problem. Further experience with the drug is needed to determine whether this is correct.

Clinical Use. As with vecuronium, atracurium may follow the use of succinylcholine to facilitate intubation or may be used as the sole relaxant. After recovery from 1 mg/kg of succinylcholine, 0.3 mg/kg of atracurium is given to initially produce relaxation. If succinylcholine is not used, 0.4 to 0.5 mg/kg of atracurium may be used to facilitate intubation. With either of these techniques, subsequent doses of 50 to 100 μg/kg every 15 to 30 minutes are usually appropriate, depending on clinical conditions and the effect observed using a peripheral nerve stimulator.

Debate continues about whether atracurium should be used to facilitate intubation in patients with full stomachs. Those who use it for rapid sequence induction follow either of two techniques. Based on the priming principal, an initial dose of 0.08 to 0.1 mg/kg may be given, followed in 3 to 7 minutes by an additional 0.4 mg/kg. It is then usually possible to intubate the trachea within 1 minute. Alternatively, 1.2 to 1.5 mg/kg may be given in a single bolus with intubation following in 1 minute. Whether either or both of these techniques will stand the test of time is not yet known. As with vecuronium, a peripheral nerve stimulator is very useful when using atracurium because of the rapid recovery time.

Summary of Intermediate Acting Nondepolarizing Muscle Relaxants

Both vecuronium and atracurium have some advantages over other available nondepolarizing relaxants. Although the two drugs are quite similar, there are pharmacologic differences. However, because these differences seem minor, other factors, such as marketing, price, or the need for refrigeration or mixing, may determine the relaxant selected. An important practical difference is that atracurium must be stored in the refrigerator, whereas vecuronium must be mixed by adding fluid to powder.

It is our belief that these drugs are a way station on the route to even better neuromuscular blocking agents. The manufacturers of both drugs are currently evaluating new compounds that promise to be even better than the drugs now available. These new compounds may replace both agents in the future.

Hexafluorenium

Chemical and Physical Properties. Hexafluorenium (Mylaxin), an inhibitor of pseudocholinesterase, also has a mild competitive neuromuscular blocking property and an inhibiting action on true cholinesterase (Fig. 17–20). Because of the inhibiting action of pseudocholinesterase (its main effect), the neuromuscular blocking action of succinylcholine is significantly prolonged in both magnitude and duration of action. Administration of hexafluorenium before succinylcholine diminishes fasciculation, prevents muscle pain, and prevents the increase in intraocular pressure induced by succinylcholine.

The usual method of administration is an initial IV dose of hexafluorenium of approximately 0.4 mg/kg followed by a dose of succinylcholine of 0.4 mg/kg. This will cause muscle relaxation within 30 to 60 seconds, which will last approximately 20 to 30 minutes. Subsequent similar doses of succinylcholine will have a briefer action as the effect of hexafluorenium wears off. After 1 to 1.5 hours, additional doses of hexafluorenium will be required if succinylcholine potentiation is sought.

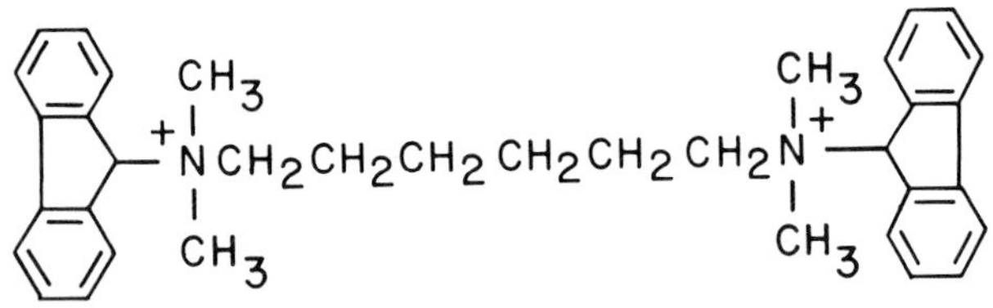

Figure 17–20. Hexafluorenium.

Reversal of Hexafluorenium. One of the disadvantages of the hexafluorenium–succinylcholine combination is that there is no antagonist available. Once the succinylcholine block becomes desensitizing in nature, edrophonium often will successfully antagonize the block. However, because antagonism of a nondepolarizer is more certain, the hexafluorenium–succinylcholine combination never achieved widespread popularity. In addition, misuse of the combination may lead to severe bronchospasm and cardiac arrhythmias.

FACTORS AFFECTING ADMINISTRATION OF MUSCLE RELAXANTS

Pharmacokinetics

Figure 17–21 shows the distribution of muscle relaxants. When a drug is administered IV, the concentration in the bloodstream is determined by (1) bolus size of the dose injected, (2) dose of the drug injected, and (3) rate of injection. Dispersion and delivery of the drug to the site of action are dependent on the cardiac output and circulation time. The cell membrane of the red blood cell, because of its lipophilic nature, presents a barrier to muscle relaxants. Entry into red blood cells is, therefore, relatively insignificant for the period of action of these drugs.

Loss of Active Drug

Intravascular degradation of drug is significant in the case of succinylcholine, which has a half-life of 1 to 2 minutes. With succinylcholine, because of intravascular degradation, a considerable amount of drug is lost before it reaches the muscle capillary beds.

Relaxants are readily filtered by the renal glomerulus, and because they are highly ionized reabsorption back into the circulation is prevented. Relaxants are, therefore, readily eliminated by the kidney, the main route of elimination for all except succinylcholine and atracurium. Pancuronium is eliminated through the kidney to a larger extent than is *d*-tubocurarine and, therefore, may potentially cause a more prolonged block than *d*-tubocurarine in patients with renal failure. This, however, has not been clinically observed.

Hepatic metabolism and biliary excretion is the alternative pathway of elimination for *d*-tubocurarine and, to a lesser extent, pancuronium. It is also the most important route of elimination for vecuronium. The hepatic metabolism of gallamine, decamethonium, metacurine, and atracurium is negligible.

Biliary obstruction and cirrhosis can alter the pharmacokinetics of the drugs by increasing the volume of distribution of the relaxants, thereby decreasing the concentration at the active tissue sites and prolonging the elimination phase. Theoretically, more relaxant would be necessary to produce a satisfactory level of block in patients with larger blood volume. However, since the elimination of the drug is decreased, the duration of action is increased.

Because many factors may influence the pharmacologic effect of drugs in patients with hepatic insufficiency, it is important to use a peripheral nerve stimulator and give individualized amounts of relaxant for each patient. If the drug is titrated, prolonged recovery should rarely occur.

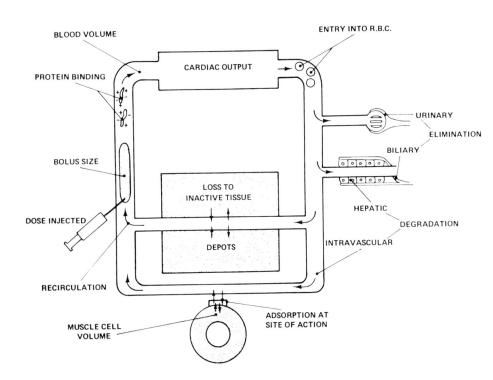

Figure 17–21. Diagram showing the main factors that influence the amount of unbound muscle relaxant in the bloodstream. (*From Crankshaw DP, Cohen EN: Uptake, distribution, and elimination of skeletal muscle relaxants. In RL Katz (ed): Muscle Relaxants. New York, American Elsevier, 1975, p 127.*)

Protein Binding

d-Tubocurarine binds approximately 16 percent with albumin and approximately 24 percent with gamma globulin. With pancuronium, comparable figures are 34 percent albumin binding and 58 percent gamma globulin binding. With metocurine, 35 percent binds to a plasma protein fraction.

Theoretically, the more a drug binds to plasma protein, the less free drug is available to act at the neuromuscular junction. In contrast, if fewer plasma proteins are available, more drug would be free to bind at the active sites.

Any disease, such as hepatitis or infection that increases plasma protein concentration, would then increase the dose needed to produce neuromuscular block, and less would be needed in disease states where less proteins are available for binding. This is modified, however, by the fact that volume of distribution is increased in these patients and, therefore, the drug is diluted to a larger extent. Because of these opposite effects it is often difficult to predict the net result.

Blood Flow and Temperature

It is believed that the onset and duration of block are related to the blood flow. With increased circulation time, the onset of block is more rapid and the duration of action is shortened. With decreased circulation time, the onset of block is slower and the duration is lengthened.

The effects of temperature are complicated. Temperature reduction may reduce the onset of paralysis but prolong the drug effect due to diminished perfusion, diminished metabolism, and diminished excretion. The rate of breakdown of atracurium is reduced when temperature is reduced.

The pharmacodynamics of the plasma concentration of drugs are altered during hypothermia, and the effect is not identical for all relaxants. For example, for a given amount of paralysis, the plasma concentration of *d*-tubocurarine is greater at lower temperatures, whereas the plasma concentration of pancuronium is less. The rate of breakdown of atracurium is reduced when temperature is reduced.

In addition to the altered pharmacologic effects of relaxants during hypothermia, lowered temperatures may have a direct mechanical effect on the muscle, which slows both contraction and relaxation. This in itself enhances neuromuscular blockade. In general, one may conclude that neuromuscular blockade is prolonged during hypothermia and that the time of onset of block may be increased. One should wait approximately twice the normal time to observe the effect in hypothermic patients so that one does not initially overdose with muscle relaxant. The peripheral nerve stimulator should act as a guide to determine the appropriate dose.

Acid–Base Balance

Acid–base balance influences different relaxants in varying ways. In general, respiratory acidosis tends to augment neuromuscular block and oppose antagonism by neostigmine. Respiratory alkalosis tends to decrease the action of *d*-tubocurarine and pancuronium, but it increases the block produced by gallamine.

Clinically, one notes that with hyperventilation, muscle relaxation is enhanced. This is due to an effect of the hyperventilation itself on abdominal muscle tone (diminishing it) rather than an effect of the relaxants.

Electrolytes

The ratio of intracellular to extracellular concentration of potassium and sodium determines the transmembrane potential. In hypokalemia or hypernatremia, transmembrane potential is increased, threshold for depolarization is increased, and the action of nondepolarizing agents is prolonged. This situation also increases the release of transmitter, which tends to decrease the action of nondepolarizing relaxants. The net effect appears to be that hypokalemia decreases the amount of *d*-tubocurarine and pancuronium needed to produce a given degree of block and increases the amount of neostigmine required to antagonize a nondepolarizing neuromuscular block.

Calcium has various actions in muscle function. It is necessary for the release of transmitter from the nerve terminal, it decreases the sensitivity of the postjunctional membrane to a transmitter, and it is required for the excitation–contraction coupling of the muscle. Because of the increase in acetylcholine release facilitated by calcium, this ion has been reported to antagonize some types of neuromuscular blocks. This is not, however, a reliable effect.

Effects of magnesium are essentially opposite to those of calcium. This ion decreases the release of acetylcholine from the nerve terminal and also reduces the sensitivity of the postjunctional membrane to the transmitter. Both of these effects increase the action of nondepolarizing relaxants. The amount of neuromuscular blocker used for patients who have received magnesium sulfate (such as obstetric patients who are toxemic) should be reduced, and these patients should be monitored with a nerve stimulator.

DRUG INTERACTION

Mixing of Muscle Relaxants

One might think it unwise, in theory, to use two drugs of differing actions on the neuromuscular junction in the same patient during the same anesthetic episode. However, succinylcholine is used commonly to produce adequate relaxation for intubation and is followed by a nondepolarizing relaxant. The use of a single dose of succinylcholine after a nondepolarizing block is more of a problem. The response to succinylcholine under these conditions depends on the prior dose of nondepolarizer and the dose of succinylcholine. The clinical effect may be either to antagonize or to enhance the underlying nondepolarizing block. Since it is impossible to determine the effect exactly and since there usually are alternative satisfactory solutions, we do not recommend the routine use of succinylcholine after a nondepolarizer.

Pseudocholinesterase Inhibitors

The effect of hexafluorenium as a pseudocholinesterase inhibitor has been discussed. Other drugs that lower pseudocholinesterase levels and increase the action of succinylcholine include echothiophate (Phospholine) eyedrops and certain antitumor drugs that alkylate the active site of pseudocholinesterase. Pregnant patients and patients with liver disease may have low levels of pseudocholinesterase, which may prolong their response to succinylcholine.

Antibiotics

Patients are often given antibiotics IV, intraperitoneally, or intrapleurally during anesthesia administration. These antibiotics may increase the action of both nondepolarizing relaxants and depolarizing relaxants.

Antibiotics have both prejunctional and postjunctional effects on the neuromuscular junction. For example, one effect of neomycin is a decrease in endplate potential and membrane sensitivity to acetylcholine. Although the neuromuscular blocking actions of all antibiotics are not identical, one factor responsible for prolongation of the effects of muscle relaxants is a presynaptic factor related to decreased transmitter release. It is thought that the block produced by erythromycin, clindamycin, polymyxin, and tetracycline is related to a direct effect on muscle contractility, in contrast to other antibiotics that produce a presynaptic block.

Antibiotics that can cause or prolong neuromuscular block include neomycin, streptomycin, kanamycin, colistin, polymyxin, bacitracin, tetracycline, clindamycin, gentamicin, and lincomycin. Penicillin G, cephradine, and cephaloridine are antibiotics that are known to be without neuromuscular effects.

Attempts at antagonism of antibiotic blocks have been carried out with neostigmine and calcium. These attempts may sometimes be successful, but there is no way to predict the outcome. In general, it is worthwhile to attempt antagonism of the mixed muscle relaxant–antibiotic block with neostigmine or pyridostigmine, but if this fails, artificial ventilation is the next choice. Although calcium has sometimes been effective, it is unreliable and may even increase the block. In addition, calcium has significant cardiovascular effects that may be unwanted. Finally, calcium may counteract the antibacterial action of some antibiotics. For all of these reasons, we prefer to ventilate the patient if neostigmine or pyridostigmine is not effective.

Local Anesthetics

Local anesthetics may enhance the action of both nondepolarizing and depolarizing muscle relaxants. Local anesthetics that may produce or enhance neuromuscular block include procaine, lidocaine, prilocaine, mepivacaine, and bupivacaine.

Anesthetic Agents

Inhalation anesthetics produce muscle relaxation in and of themselves and, in addition, may increase the action of neuromuscular blocking agents, primarily the nondepolarizers. Inhalation agents cause their relaxant effect mainly by depressing synaptic transmission at the level of the spinal cord. Inhalation agents also have a weak depressant action at the neuromuscular junction and on the muscle itself.

These latter actions account for potentiation of the action of muscle relaxants.

When using a peripheral nerve stimulator with potent inhalation agents, muscle relaxation may be greater than would be expected by observing twitch height. This is because the major mechanism by which inhalation agents produce muscle relaxation is at the level of the spinal cord. The effect is not observed on response to nerve stimulation, since this test only assesses the block peripheral to the site of stimulation.

The inhalation agents that most enhance the action of the nondepolarizing neuromuscular blockers are diethyl ether, methoxyflurane, enflurane, and isoflurane. When these agents are used with nondepolarizing relaxants, the dose required may be only one-third to one-half that required with balanced anesthesia. A lesser effect is seen with halothane, but even this agent produces significant enhancement of the block, and only one-half to two-thirds the dose of muscle relaxant is necessary compared with balanced anesthesia.

COUNTRY OF PRACTICE

It has been observed that patients in the United Kingdom require larger doses of d-tubocurarine to produce a given effect than do patients in the United States. Higher levels of cholinesterase inhibitors have been found in animal tissue in the United States than in animals in the United Kingdom, and this in part may explain the difference.

USE OF MUSCLE RELAXANTS IN OBSTETRICS

Muscle relaxants may be used in obstetric patients for reasons similar to their use during surgery. It should be noted, however, that skeletal muscle tone is markedly decreased with pregnancy, and, therefore, a lesser degree of block is usually required during obstetric procedures. Smooth muscle of the uterus is not affected by skeletal muscle relaxants, and therefore, relaxants will not decrease contraction nor will they assist in extraction of the baby during cesarean section. One should use care when using relaxants in patients who have been given magnesium sulfate. This drug may increase the effects of both succinylcholine and nondepolarizing relaxants.

Prolonged apnea has been noted after the administration of succinylcholine in pregnant patients who have not received magnesium. This has been attributed to a decline in the pseudocholinesterase level that occurs in the first trimester of pregnancy and persists until the early postpartum period.

USE OF MUSCLE RELAXANTS IN PEDIATRICS

Studies documenting the effect of muscle relaxants in children have had differing results, perhaps due to the variety of study techniques. When doses were calculated on a milligram per kilogram basis, results differed from those obtained when body surface area was used to calculate doses. In children, the ratio of body surface area to body weight is greater than in adults. Using weight as a criterion, newborns were more resistant to succinylcholine. When comparing dose to body surface area, it was found that neonates were more sensitive to *d*-tubocurarine than were adults. In contrast to the results found with *d*-tubocurarine, the requirement for pancuronium is greater in the child than in the adult, and the child recovers more quickly from a similar level of block.

Because of the conflicting reports about the effect of muscle relaxants in children and the extreme variability among children, it is important to monitor the effect of the block. Commonly, 0.5 to 1 mg/kg of succinylcholine is used to facilitate endotracheal intubation. If using nondepolarizing relaxants, a test dose of 0.1 mg/kg of *d*-tubocurarine or 0.02 mg/kg of pancuronium is widely used. Subsequent doses are then selected on the basis of response to the test dose and the clinical circumstances.

In children, antagonism of nondepolarizing relaxants may be carried out with 0.4 to 0.8 mg/kg of neostigmine or 0.16 to 3.2 mg/kg of pyridostigmine. Atropine 0.02 to 0.04 mg/kg or glycopyrrolate 0.01 to 0.02 mg/kg is given before neostigmine or pyridostigmine.

USE OF MUSCLE RELAXANTS OUTSIDE THE OPERATING ROOM

Relaxants may be used in the intensive care unit for intubation or for facilitation of prolonged ventilation. Nondepolarizing relaxants are usually used for long-term ventilation and are administered either by dilute infusion or by intermittent bolus. It must be emphasized that the block should be monitored and only the amount necessary to achieve the desired effect should be given. If possible, the patient should be sedated so that the unpleasant effects of paralysis without sedation are avoided.

Muscle relaxants are often used during electroconvulsive therapy to prevent injury from vigorous muscle contractions. Because of its short duration and rapid recovery, succinylcholine is usually the relaxant of choice. If a tourniquet is used to prevent the intravenously given succinylcholine from reaching the hand, it is possible to monitor the motor effects of the therapy while eliminating gross total body movements that may cause injury.

CHOLINESTERASES AND ANTICHOLINESTERASES

The two enzymes that hydrolyze esters of choline are acetylcholinesterase, which is found in the red cells, nerve, and muscle, and pseudocholinesterase or plasma cholinesterase, which is synthesized in the liver and found in the plasma, liver, brain, kidney, intestine, and pancreas. Pseudocholinesterase is not found at the myoneural junction. It has no known physiologic function but is important in anesthesia because it hydrolyzes succinylcholine.

Acetylcholinesterase, which is capable of hydrolyzing acetylcholine, cannot hydrolyze succinylcholine. Normally, acetylcholinesterase will hydrolyze acetylcholine within milliseconds, and the endplate is then able to be repolarized rapidly.

Acetylcholinesterase has two active sites: (1) an anionic site, which binds the positively charged end of the acetylcholine molecule and orients it so that the molecule can

be hydrolyzed, and (2) the esteratic site, which acts as the cleavage site. The esteratic site contains an electronegative group that contributes a pair of electrons that bond with the acetate portion of acetylcholine. This bonding terminates the action of the acetylcholine and produces free choline and an intermediate product, the acetylated enzyme. This enzyme combines with water to regenerate acetic acid and additional free enzyme (Fig. 17–22).

Anticholinesterases are drugs that inhibit the action of the cholinesterases. Usually, both pseudocholinesterase and acetylcholinesterase are affected by the anticholinesterases. However, a drug may be more effective against one enzyme than the other.

The anticholinesterase drugs may react with the anionic site (prosthetic inhibitors) or affect both the anionic and the esteratic sites (oxadiaphoric or acid-transferring inhibitors). Anticholinesterases affecting only the anionic site compete with acetylcholine for that site. When the anticholinesterase molecules diffuse away from the site, acetylcholine can again be broken down. The effect of this type of inhibitor is short. Edrophonium is the most common example of this type of drug.

Inhibitors affecting the esteratic and anionic sites include two groups of anticholinesterase agents: (1) the organophosphates (echothiophate, insecticides, and nerve gases) and (2) the carbamates (neostigmine, pyridostigmine, and physostigmine). The organophosphates bind to form a very stable compound. The anticholinesterase enzyme is permanently inactivated, and acetylcholine is hydrolyzed

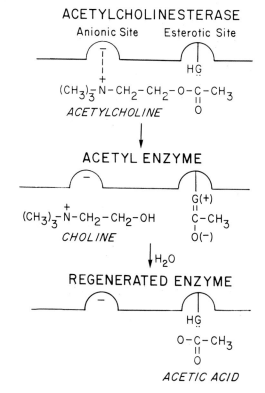

Figure 17–22. Hydrolysis of acetylcholine. (*Adapted from Koelle, 1970; from Pantuck EJ, Pantuck CB: Cholinesterases and anticholinesterases. In RL Katz (ed): Muscle Relaxants. New York, American Elsevier, 1975, p 144.*)

again only after synthesis of a new enzyme. This takes a period of 2 to 4 weeks. The carbamates are esters of carbamic acid and bind to both the esteratic site and the anionic site in a manner similar to the binding of acetylcholine. A carbamyl ester bond is hydrolyzed very slowly when compared with acetylcholine (Fig. 17–23).

In summary, the half-life of the acetyl enzyme (resulting from binding of acetylcholine and acetylcholinesterase) is measured in microseconds, the half-life of the carbamylated enzyme (resulting from binding of neostigmine, pyridostigmine, and acetylcholinesterase) is measured in minutes, and the half-life of the phosphoryl enzyme (resulting from binding of echothiophate or insecticides and acetylcholinesterase) is measured in weeks.

Mechanism of Action

It is thought that the antagonism of nondepolarizing neuromuscular block occurs because acetylcholine is allowed to build up. The most commonly known cause of this buildup of acetylcholine is the inhibition of breakdown of acetylcholine by acetylcholinesterase, as discussed previously. Other important actions of anticholinesterases, however, have been well documented. These include (1) repetitive firing of the motor nerve terminals due to the increased concentrations of acetylcholine, which cause brief tetanic contractions and increase the overall strength of contraction, and (2) direct depolarization of the motor nerve terminal and endplate. It is not possible at this time to state with certainty the precise role of the cholinesterase-inhibiting action and the presynaptic mechanisms. Cholinesterase inhibition is important, but the presynaptic actions unrelated to cholinesterase inhibition are also important.

Pharmacologic Properties

Anticholinesterase drugs can produce muscarinic and nicotinic actions at the autonomic effector organs. The effect of a given drug on nicotinic and muscarinic structures depends on the balance between the ganglionic and peripheral components of the drug action and the nature of the cho-

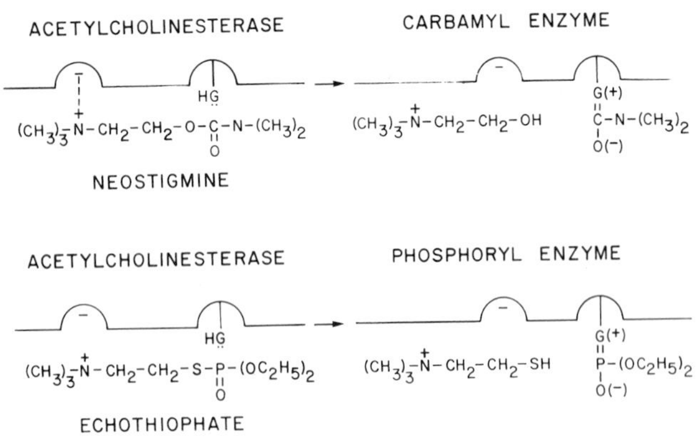

Figure 17–23. Inhibition of acetylcholinesterase. (*Adapted from Koelle, 1970; From Pantuck EJ, Pantuck CB: Cholinesteraseses and anticholinesterases. In RL Katz (ed): Muscle Relaxants. New York, American Elsevier, 1975, p 145.*)

linergic impulses on the effector organs. Atropine blocks the actions of neostigmine, pyridostigmine, and edrophonium on the autonomic effector cells. Thus, bradycardia, salivation, and bronchoconstriction are prevented. A dose of atropine of 0.15 to 0.2 mg/kg is commonly used before or at the same time as the cholinesterase inhibitor. Glycopyrrolate has been used as an alternative to atropine and is given in a dose one-half that of atropine. It has the advantage of not crossing the blood–brain barrier.

At one time it was thought that the use of neostigmine in patients who had undergone bowel anastomoses might result in disruption of suture lines. This is now known to be false, and neostigmine is not contraindicated in patients who have undergone bowel surgery.

Edrophonium

Edrophonium (Tensilon), an antagonist, has not commonly been used because of its presumed short duration of action. Recently, it has been suggested that increased doses may result in action similar to that of neostigmine. The former recommended dose was 0.15 mg/kg, but the increased dose recommended for more sustained response is 0.5 to 1 mg/kg. When used in this large dose, there is a faster onset of action than with neostigmine and pyridostigmine. Atropine is injected before injection of edrophonium.

Neostigmine

Neostigmine (Prostigmin) is probably the most commonly used of the anticholinesterase drugs. It must be preceded by atropine to block its muscarinic effects. The usual dose is 0.15 mg/kg of atropine given before 0.04 mg/kg of neostigmine. These doses may be repeated once if necessary. If a satisfactory response is not obtained after the second dose, it is recommended that the patient be ventilated until adequate recovery is seen.

Pyridostigmine

Pyridostigmine (Regonol) was originally used for myasthenic patients because the duration of action permitted a longer time between doses than did neostigmine. The usual dose for antagonism of nondepolarizing neuromuscular blockers is 0.15 to 2.0 mg/kg preceded by 0.015 mg/kg of atropine. The dose of both drugs may be repeated if necessary. However, if adequate antagonism does not occur after a second dose of pyridostigmine, the patient should be artificially ventilated. The advantage of pyridostigmine over neostigmine is that pyridostigmine causes fewer muscarinic side effects and a lower incidence of cardiac arrhythmias in elderly patients.

The criteria for adequate antagonism of the neuromuscular block include (1) a return of twitch height to control level, (2) a train of four ratio of 0.7 to 1.0, and (3) well-sustained tetanus of 50 to 100 Hz for 5 seconds. In addition, an inspiratory force of −20 or greater, sustained head lift for 5 seconds, and a grip strength similar to control should be achieved.

BIBLIOGRAPHY

Ali HH, Wilson RS, Savarese JJ: The effect of tubocurarine on indirectly elicited train-of-four muscle response and respiratory measurements in humans. Br J Anaesth 47:570–574, 1975.

Bowman WC: Prejunctional and post-junctional cholinoreceptors at the neuromuscular junction. Anesth Analg 59:935–943, 1980.

Bush GH, Stead AL: The use of *d*-tubocurarine in neonatal anaesthesia. Br J Anaesth 34:721–728, 1962.

Chang CC: Use of alpha and beta bungarotoxins for the study of neuromuscular transmission. Anesthesiology 48:309–310, 1978.

Cook D: Clinical use of muscle relaxants in infants and children. 28th Anesthesiology Review Course Lecture Notes. Society of Air Force Anesthesiologists, 1981.

Cooperman LH: Succinylcholine-induced hyperkalemia in neuromuscular disease. JAMA 213:1867–1871, 1970.

Feldman SA: Muscle Relaxants. London, Saunders, 1973.

Foldes FF: Muscle Relaxants. Philadelphia, FA Davis, 1966.

Ham J: Factors affecting administration of non-depolarizing neuromuscular blocking agents. ASA Refresher Course in Anesthesiology. Hershey SG (ed). 1980.

Hughes R, Chapple D: Effects of non-depolarizing neuromuscular blocking agents on peripheral autonomic mechanisms in cats. Br J Anaesth 48:59–68, 1976.

Katz RL: Clinical considerations of muscle relaxants. 28th Anesthesiology Review Course Lecture Notes, Society of Air Force Anesthesiologists, 1981.

Katz RL (ed): Muscle Relaxants. New York, American Elsevier, 1975.

Katz RL: Monitoring of muscle relaxation and neuromuscular transmission. In Crul JF, Payne JP (eds): Patient Monitoring. Amsterdam, Excerpta Medica, 1970, pp 125–142.

Katz RL: Neuromuscular effects of *d*-tubocurarine, edrophonium and neostigmine in man. Anesthesiology 28:327–336, 1967.

Katz RL: A nerve stimulator for the continuous monitoring of muscle relaxant action. Anesthesiology 26:832, 1965.

Lebowitz R, Savarese JJ: Cardiovascular and autonomic effects of neuromuscular blockers. ASA Refresher Course in Anesthesiology. Hershey SG (ed). 1980, Vol 8.

Lee C, Chen O, Katz RL: Characteristics of non-depolarizing block: Post-junctional block by alpha bungarotoxin. Can Anaesth Soc J 24:212–219, 1977.

Lehman H, Liddell J: Human cholinesterase: Genetic variants and recognition. Br J Anaesth 41:235–244, 1969.

Mark LC, Papper EM: Advances in Anesthesiology Muscle Relaxants. New York, Harper & Row, Hoeber Medical Division, 1967.

Miller RD: Reversal of neuromuscular blockade. 28th Anesthesiology Refresher Course Lecture Notes. Society of Air Force Anesthesiologists, 1981.

Miller RD, Savarese JJ: Pharmacology of muscle relaxants: Their antagonists and monitoring of neuromuscular function. In Miller RD (ed): Anesthesia. New York, Churchill Livingstone, 1986, pp 871–888.

Miller RD, Eger EI, Stevens WC, et al: Pancuronium-induced tachycardia in relation to alveolar halothane dose of pancuronium and prior atropine. Anesthesiology 42:352–355, 1975.

Miller RD, Way WL, et al: The dependence of pancuronium and *d*-tubocurarine-induced neuromuscular blockade on alveolar concentrations of halothane and forane. Anesthesiology 37:573, 1972.

Savarese JJ: Pharmacology of present and future neuromuscular blocking drugs. 28th Anesthesiology Refresher Course Lecture Notes. Society of Air Force Anesthesiologists, 1981.

Savarese JJ, Kitz RJ: The search for a short acting non-depolarizing neuromuscular blocking agent. Acta Anaesth Scand [Suppl] 53:43, 1973.

Standaert FG, Dretchen KL: Cyclic nucleotides in neuromuscular transmission. Anesth Analg 60:91–99, 1981.

Stoelting RK: Hemodynamic effects of pancuronium and *d*-tubocurarine in anesthetized patients. Anesthesiology 36:612–615, 1972.

Walts LF, Dillon JB: The influence of the anesthetic agent on the action of curare in man. Anesth Analg 49:17–21, 1970.

Walts LF, Dillon JB: Clinical studies of the interaction between *d*-tubocurarine and succinylcholine. Anesthesiology 31:35–38, 1969.

18

Pharmacologic Adjuncts to Anesthesia

Vasoactive Adjuncts

Roy Aston

Cardiovascular adjuncts in anesthesia are those parenterally administered agents that are employed to treat hypotensive or hypertensive emergencies, or to selectively alter cardiac preload or afterload in the treatment of ischemic heart disease, severe congestive failure, or acute myocardial infarction.

Such adjuncts include, among others, the adrenotropic pressor amines, and the direct-acting vasodilators. The latter may or may not exhibit specificity for resistance or for capacitance vessels.

A consideration of the pharmacology of adrenotropic and some cardiovascular drugs requires some review of the functions of the autonomic nervous system and of the processes of adrenergic neurotransmission. Direct-acting vasodepressors appear to act by a number of indirect mechanisms that ultimately reduce the availability of free calcium ion within vascular smooth muscle cells. The mechanisms by which this is accomplished are discussed under the individual vasodilators.

ADRENOTROPIC PRESSOR AMINES

The Autonomic Nervous System

Anatomic Overview. Adrenotropic agents are those that influence noradrenergic (norepinephrine) neurotransmission or adrenergic (epinephrine) responses in the body. The noradrenergic nervous system is largely equivalent to the anatomic sympathetic nervous system, the classic exception being the sympathetic nerves to the sweat glands, which are cholinergic fibers.

The sympathetic and parasympathetic divisions of the autonomic nervous system together comprise the efferent control mechanism for the smooth muscle and glands of the body. Teleologically, these organs represent the hardware, provided by evolution, for the sustenance and safety of the brain, which may be assumed to represent the physical substratum of our conscious "selves." Whenever this

internal hardware begins to malfunction, producing a potential threat to our well-being, or whenever external threats appear, the brain immediately provides chemical messages to this peripheral hardware to readjust its functional level to meet the threat. These chemical messages may be relayed to the whole body in a diffuse fashion by way of hormones secreted into the bloodstream, e.g., adrenal medullary epinephrine secretion. Alternatively, these messages may be delivered in a discrete point-to-point fashion by means of nerves, which function to deliver localized chemical messages to specific pieces of our peripheral hardware. This latter function is subserved by the autonomic nervous system.

The autonomic efferent system is a bineuronal output that originates in cell bodies within the central nervous system. These cells give rise to nerve fibers (preganglionic) that synapse with postganglionic neurons in peripheral ganglia. Postganglionic fibers distribute to the internal organs and glands. The two divisions of the autonomic system are anatomically differentiated by the relative length of pre- and postganglionic fibers. The parasympathetic system possesses very long preganglionic fibers with ganglia located within the tissue of the innervated organ, giving rise to very short postganglionic fibers. The reverse is generally true of the sympathetic system.

The parasympathetic or craniosacral division arises from cell bodies within the midbrain or medulla and from the second to fourth sacral segments of the spinal cord. The nerve supplying parasympathetic innervation to the organs of the thorax and abdomen is the vagus nerve.

The sympathetic or thoracolumbar division of the autonomic system arises in the first thoracic through the third lumbar spinal segments. The majority of these preganglionic fibers are short and synapse in the paravertebral ganglia, with the postganglionic fibers being distributed to peripheral organs along with their arterial blood supply. Some preganglionic fibers, however, fail to synapse in their respective segmental ganglia. Some of these fibers pass upward or downward in the chain to synapse in more superior or inferior ganglia. Others pass through their segmental ganglion and synapse in the more peripheral celiac or mesenteric ganglia. Certain of the preganglionic sympathetic fibers pass uninterrupted through both the paravertebral and the celiac ganglia to synapse with adrenal medullary cells, eliciting the release of hormonal epinephrine.

Autonomic Functions. Most organs of the body receive both parasympathetic and sympathetic innervation, and in most cases the two divisions produce opposite effects on the innervated organ. Thus, autonomic innervation is described as dual and reciprocal. The parasympathetic division provides discrete innervation of individual organs. Thus, an increase in heart rate will prompt a reflex parasympathetic bradycardia without producing alterations in the secretion of hydrochloric acid by the stomach. Sympathetic output, on the other hand, elicits a diffuse, whole-body response both because its anatomic distribution is diffuse and because the all-or-none sympathetic response includes adrenal epinephrine release.

Responses to stimulation of the two autonomic divisions are listed in Table 18–1, in which the sympathetic responses are further qualified as being α_1, α_2, β_1, or β_2 responses, depending upon the nature of the specific receptor areas on effector organs that respond to epinephrine. These receptors are discussed later in this section. Parasympathetic responses are concerned with sustenance, and function to produce and conserve energy. This involves stimulation of the digestive process from which we ultimately derive all body energy and inhibition of other body functions that would deplete energy body stores. Therefore, parasympathetic stimulation promotes increased peristalsis and gastrointestinal secretions together with relaxation of sphincters, while heart rate declines. Airways constrict to reduce oxygen intake, which, in turn, serves to restrict metabolism of glucose reserves. Pupils constrict to reduce the visual stimulation that could result in increased energy-dissipating activity. The urinary tract responds in the same way as the gastrointestinal tract. The parasympathetic system predominates during eating and sleeping.

Sympathetic responses, listed in Table 18–1, are concerned with safety, and function to mobilize energy and expend it in skeletal muscle activity in response to an acute stress situation (the so-called fight-or-flight reaction). The sympathetic system fires off as a single unit, eliciting whole-body mobilization of energy stores. Both hepatic and skeletal muscle glycogen stores are released as glucose into the bloodstream. Oxygen supply is enhanced through airway dilation. The increased glucose and oxygen supply is preferentially channeled into skeletal muscle by dilation of blood vessels in the skeletal muscle mass, and constriction of vessels in other nonessential areas such as skin, mucosa, and gastrointestinal tract. The heart is stimulated chronotropically and inotropically to drive more blood into the dilated vascular bed of skeletal muscle. Mydriasis occurs, enhancing our ability to visualize environmental threats. Sweating is enhanced, thus allowing the dissipation of excess body heat derived from increased metabolic and skeletal muscle activity.

Although autonomic innervation is dual and reciprocal, relative autonomic tone differs in most organs. Thus, sympathetic tone predominates in peripheral vasculature and in the airways. Parasympathetic tone predominates in the heart and the gastrointestinal and urinary tracts. In addition, autonomic tone varies with age. Parasympathetic tone is relatively low in both the infant and the elderly.

Autonomic Neurotransmitters. In all autonomic ganglia, acetylcholine functions as the excitatory transmitter substance, being released by all autonomic preganglionic fibers. Acetylcholine causes depolarization of both postganglionic autonomic neurons and adrenal medullary cells; the latter respond by secreting epinephrine. Autonomic ganglia also possess dopamine-secreting interneurons. Dopamine exerts a modulatory inhibition on ganglionic transmission by producing hyperpolarization of the postsynaptic neuron through an action upon specific dopamine receptors.

TABLE 18–1. RESPONSES TO AUTONOMIC NERVE STIMULATION

Effector	Parasympathetic	Sympathetic	Receptor
Heart			
SA node	↓ Rate	↑ Rate	β_1
AV node	↓ Conduction rate	↑ Conduction rate	β_1
Ventricles	—	↑ Contractility	β_1
	—	↑ Automaticity	β_1
Blood Vessels			
Skin and mucosa	—	Constriction	α
Salivary glands	Dilation	Constriction	α
Abdominal viscera	—	Constriction	α
Renal	—	Constriction	α
Skeletal muscle	—	Dilation	β_2
Other Smooth Muscle			
Bronchial	Contraction	Relaxation	β_2
GI muscle	↑ Tone, ↑ motility	↓ Tone, ↓ motility	α, β_1
GI sphincters	Relaxation	Contraction	α
Metabolic			
Adipose tissue	—	Lipolysis	β_1
Liver	Glycogen deposition	Glycogenolysis	β_2
Skeletal muscle	Glycogen deposition	Glycogenolysis	β_2

Postganglionic parasympathetic fibers produce their effects upon effector organs by the release of acetylcholine. The postganglionic sympathetic transmitter is norepinephrine. Somatic nerves also convey their excitatory impulses to skeletal muscle by release of acetylcholine.

Nerves employing acetylcholine or norepinephrine as transmitters are referred to as cholinergic and adrenergic (or more specifically as noradrenergic) nerves, respectively. Cholinergic sites within autmonic ganglia and at the somatic neuromuscular junction are collectively referred to as nicotinic. Postganglionic cholinergic sites are referred to as muscarinic.

Autonomic Receptors. The effects of neurotransmitters upon effector cells are mediated via specific proteins, embedded in the phospholipid membranes of tissue cells, termed receptors. Each receptor possesses a relatively fixed topology and will interact only with endogenous or exogenous substances possessing complementary surface configurations. A high correlation between chemical structure among such receptor-active agents and pharmacologic effect is evident.

Adrenoceptors, i.e., those receptors interacting with epinephrine, are subdivided into four types: α_1, α_2, β_1, and β_2. Of these, α_1 and β_1 receptors are located postsynaptically at noradrenergic nerve endings and respond preferentially to the neurotransmitter, norepinephrine. The α_2 and β_2 receptors are located both presynaptically and at extrajunctional sites on peripheral tissues. These latter receptors respond preferentially to the sympathetic hormone, epinephrine, and to exogenous catecholamines. Mixtures of these receptors occur in most adrenergically innervated tissues, the tissue response to epinephrine being dictated by the relative preponderance of one or another receptor type.

The α_1 receptors mediate excitatory responses, resulting in the contraction of smooth muscle cells. These responses include constriction of blood vessels in which α_1 receptors predominate, i.e., arterioles in skin, mucosa, abdominal viscera, and lungs. This is true also of all veins. The α_1-mediated contraction of the radial pupillary dilator muscle of the iris results in mydriasis.

Presynaptic α_2 receptors seem to be exclusively concerned with inhibition of exocytotic norepinephrine release from nerve endings. Postsynaptic α_2 receptors, on vascular smooth muscle at sites remote from the noradrenergic neuroeffector junction, mediate muscle contraction and vessel constriction. The α_2 receptors predominate in larger veins and the α_1 receptors in larger arteries, while a significantly mixed α population occurs in most arterioles.

The β_1 receptors mediate cardiac stimulation and lipolysis. Thus β_1 activation results in increased cardiac nodal rate, cardiac contractility, atriovenous (AV) conduction rate, and stimulated fatty acid mobilization from adipose tissue.

Presynaptic junctional β_2 receptors are reported to facilitate neuronal norepinephrine release. Postsynaptic extrajunctional β_2 receptors are primarily associated with smooth muscle relaxation, mediating bronchodilation, and vasodilation in skeletal muscle, heart, and lung. These receptors also appear to promote glycogenolysis in skeletal muscle.

At the present time, the clinical significance of postsynaptic α_2 and presynaptic β_2 receptors is largely speculative.

Receptors that mediate the effects of acetylcholine in the body are referred to as cholinoceptors and are divided into muscarinic and nicotinic types. Unlike the adrenoceptors, where mixed receptor populations exist in the same tissue, the cholinoceptors are distributed in a clear-cut fashion at one or another tissue site. Muscarinic receptors are found at all postsynaptic postganglionic parasympathetic sites. Thus, all responses of the body to parasympathetic stimulation are mediated by muscarinic cholinoceptors. Those cardiac muscarinic receptors of the sinoatrial (SA) node, however, appear to represent a distinct subgroup among the muscarinic receptors, inasmuch as some drugs, such as gallamine, can block nodal muscarinic receptors without affecting muscarinic responses elsewhere in the body.

The nicotinic cholinoceptors, though sharing an affinity for many drugs such as nicotine, do exhibit two differential drug response spectra, implying the existence of two subpopulations of nicotinic receptors. The first of these is by nicotinic receptors located postsynaptically in all autonomic ganglia and responsible for rapid ganglionic stimulatory transmission. The second class of nicotinic receptors are those located upon the muscle endplate of skeletal muscle fibers, which are responsible for the contractile response to acetylcholine liberated by efferent motor neurons.

All these receptors, except the very rapidly acting nicotinic receptors, appear to produce their effects on cells by increasing the formation of cyclic nucleotides, which, in turn, ultimately control the level of activity of many cellular enzymes responsible for energy production, transmembrane ion flux, and so on. Thus, β adrenoceptors and dopamine receptors directly activate specific membrane-bound adenylate cyclases, which are responsible for the conversion of cellular adenosine triphosphate (ATP) to a cyclized form of adenosine monophosphate [3',5'-cyclic adenosine monophosphate (cAMP)]. The α adrenoceptors and muscarinic receptors appear to act indirectly by causing an influx of calcium ions into cells. This influx of calcium ions into cells may act as a common trigger that precipitates biologic events ranging in effect from events as gross as muscular contractions, through hormone secretions, to as singular an event as activation of a single enzyme guanylate cyclase. The elevated intracellular calcium activates cytoplasmic guanylate cyclase, which converts guanosine triphosphate (GTP) to cyclized guanosine monophosphate [3',5'-cyclic guanosine monophosphate (cGMP)]. These cyclic nucleotides, cAMP and cGMP, activate specific protein kinases, which activate, through phosphorylation, specific regulator proteins. One such regulator protein, phosphoglucomutase, is involved in the conversion of glycogen to glucose in skeletal muscle in response to β_2 adrenoceptor activation. Both cAMP and cGMP are subsequently hydrolyzed by phosphodiesterases to their respective inactive 5' - nucleotides, AMP and GMP.

Adrenergic Neurotransmission

The process of postganglionic adrenergic neurotransmission involves both presynaptic and postsynaptic events. The presynaptic event includes the synthesis, storage, release, and inactivation of norepinephrine. The postsynaptic event includes the interaction of the transmitter with the various adrenoceptors on effector cells. Adrenotropic cardiovascular agents may act at any point in these transmittitory processes. The overall process of adrenergic neurotransmission, together with the sites of action of several of these agents, is illustrated in Figure 18–1. Each of the four presynaptic processes and the postsynaptic receptor interactions are considered separately below.

Norepinephrine Synthesis. Enzymes responsible for the formation of norepinephrine in adrenergic nerve endings are synthesized in the neuron cell body and conveyed to the nerve terminals by axonal cytoplasmic flow. The primary substrate for the synthesis of norepinephrine is the dietary amino acid tyrosine. The conversion of tyrosine to norepinephrine is accomplished by the sequential actions of three enzymes which convert the amino acid substrate to the catecholamine structure of the transmitter.

Tyrosine Hydroxylase. Tyrosine is a phenolic amino acid that is converted, by 3-hydroxylation of the benzene ring, into a catecholamino acid, dihydroxyphenylalanine (DOPA). The enzyme catalyzing this conversion, tyrosine

hydroxylase, requires tetrahydropteridine as a cofactor. Tyrosine hydroxylase activity is inhibited by cytoplasmic norepinephrine, which competes with the enzyme for the pteridine cofactor. This negative feedback mechanism is responsible for reducing norepinephrine synthesis in the nerve ending when excess amounts of the transmitter accumulate.

α-Methyltyrosine (Metytosine) inhibits tyrosine hydroxylase activity by competing with tyrosine for active sites on the enzyme, thus blocking the conversion of tyrosine to DOPA. This results in a 50 to 80 percent decrease in catecholamine tissue stores, including the adrenal medulla. The drug is indicated for the management of hypertensive episodes in patients with inoperable pheochromocytoma, as well as for preoperative treatment for surgical removal of the tumor. The recommended oral dosage is 250 mg q.i.d. initially, and then titrating the patient with daily increases in dosage of 250 to 500 mg up to a maximum of 4 g/day. The peak effect of the drug is evident in 2 to 3 days. A return to pretreatment plasma catecholamine levels is seen 3 to 4 days after the drug is stopped. In the case of surgery, it is recommended that the optimal dose be established and continued for 5 to 7 days preoperatively.

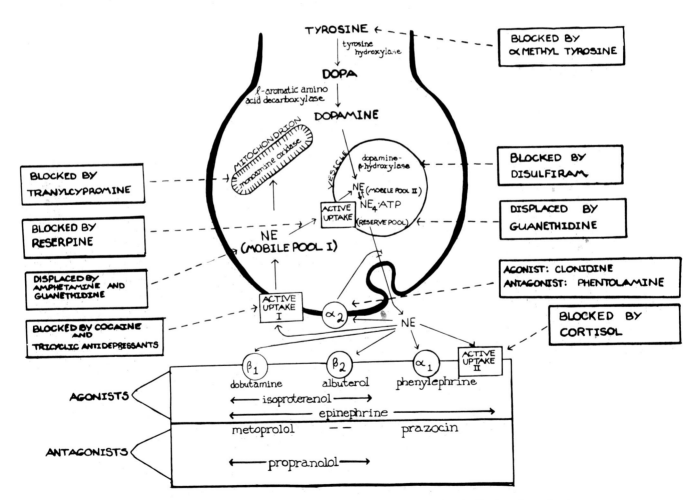

Figure 18–1. Processes involved in noradrenergic neurotransmission, indicating sites of action of presynaptic and postsynaptic adrenergic agonist and antagonist agents. Processes and drug effects are discussed in the text.

It is necessary to maintain a fluid intake of at least 2 L/day to avoid crystalluria. Sedation, anxiety, tremor, and diarrhea may be observed. The drug potentiates the extrapyramidal side effects of phenothiazines and similar drugs.

L-Aromatic Amino Acid Decarboxylase. The catechol-amino acid, DOPA, which is slowly formed from tyrosine, is rapidly decarboxylated in adrenergic tissues to form the catecholamine, dopamine. The enzyme catalyzing this step is L-aromatic acid decarboxylase, which requires pyridoxal phosphate (vitamin B_6) as cofactor. Dopamine is the first of a sequence of catecholamines that may be synthesized in tissues. Certain neurons lack the enzyme necessary for conversion of dopamine to norepinephrine. In such dopaminergic cells, dopamine functions as a neurotransmitter.

Dopamine-β-Hydroxylase (DBH). Dopamine that is formed in adrenergic nerves and adrenal medullary tissue is taken up and stored in granules or vesicles within the cytoplasm. In these vesicles, dopamine is converted to norepinephrine by β-hydroxylation. This step is catalyzed by dopamine-β-hydroxylase (DBH), a copper-containing enzyme requiring ascorbic acid as cofactor. DBH is found both in the membrane wall and in the contents of the adrenergic vesicle.

Disulfiram (Antabuse), although not employed as a cardiovascular agent, may produce cardiovascular complications during anesthesia. Chronic disulfiram use leads to inhibition of DBH, and can produce partial depletion of norepinephrine from adrenergic tissues. Under these circumstances, patients undergoing stimulation during anesthesia may exhibit a sudden fall in blood pressure by as much as 50 percent.

Phenylethanolamine-N-Methyl Transferase (PNMT). The phenylethanolamine is not present in adrenergic nerve endings and is, therefore, not illustrated in Figure 18–1. It is, however, present in the chromaffin cells of the adrenal medulla, where it functions to N-methylate norepinephrine, converting it to epinephrine. PNMT synthesis is stimulated by adrenocortical steroids. In pheochromocytoma, therefore, as the enlarging medullary tumor causes compression atrophy of the adrenal cortex, corticosteroid production is decreased, leading to reduced medullary PNMT synthesis. This results in reduced epinephrine production and accumulation of norepinephrine in the tumor.

Norepinephrine Storage. As indicated above, dopamine, which is formed in the cytoplasm of the nerve ending, is taken up by dense-core vesicles and converted within the vesicle to norepinephrine by the vesicular enzyme DBH.

Dopamine uptake into the vesicle is an active process requiring ATP and Mg^{2+} ion. Intravesicular dopamine is rapidly converted to norepinephrine. Free vesicular norepinephrine (mobile pool II norepinephrine) exists in an equilibrium state with norepinephrine bound to ATP in the ratio of four catecholamine molecules to each ATP molecule (reserve pool norepinephrine).

Total norepinephrine represents 21 percent of the dry weight of the vesicle. Proteins comprise the bulk of the remaining dry weight. Among these, DBH and the densely

staining chromogranin A make up the chromogranin content of the vesicle and account for 30 percent of the dry weight. Not only is newly synthesized norepinephrine found within the vesicle, but cytoplasmic catecholamine (mobile pool I norepinephrine) is also taken up by vesicles through an ATP-Mg^{2+}-dependent pump mechanism, where it contributes to mobile pool II and reserve pool catecholamine.

Reserpine interferes with vesicular catecholamine storage because it is avidly taken up by the vesicle (10,000 times more than norepinephrine) and displaces vesicular norepinephrine. Guanethidine (Ismelin) and certain of the indirect-acting amines, e.g., tyramine, also displace vesicular norepinephrine. Tyramine, however, releases only mobile pool II, whereas guanethidine displaces total vesicular norepinephrine. Of the norepinephrine released into the cytoplasm, some diffuses out of the nerve ending to activate adrenoceptors, while the remainder largely is metabolized by mitochondrial monoamine oxidase.

Norepinephrine Release. Release of norepinephrine from nerve endings can be produced by vesicular displacement, as with tyramine and guanethidine, and by displacement of cytoplasmic mobile pool I by drugs such as amphetamine. However, physiologic transmitter release is through exocytosis, a process by which the vesicle fuses with the presynaptic nerve membrane and evaginates to release its contents into the synaptic cleft.

The arrival of a nerve impulse at a nerve ending opens calcium channels in the presynaptic membrane. This results in a brief increase in intracellular calcium concentration, which, in an unknown fashion, triggers the exocytotic phenomenon. An integral facet of this process appears to be the activation of enzymes that methylate negatively charged carboxyl groups on the vesicular membrane surface. Since the presynaptic membrane also carries an excess negative charge, this methylation reduces the tendency of the vesicular and the neuronal membranes to repel each other, increasing the likelihood of random encounters between the two membranes. Vesicles that reach specific exocytotic sites on the presynaptic membrane become attached to these sites. The vesicular membrane then fuses with, and flows into, the presynaptic membrane, expelling the total contents of the vesicle into the synaptic cleft. Both norepinephrine and DBH are released from the nerve. Plasma levels of DBH correlate with adrenergic activity levels in the body. Plasma DBH levels are increased in torsion dystonia and reduced in familial dysautonomia.

Exocytotic release of catecholamines is negatively modulated by presynaptic $α_2$ adrenoceptors. Extracellular norepinephrine activates these receptors, which, in turn, inhibit further exocytosis. The $α_2$ adrenoceptors are also activated by epinephrine. The antihypertensive agent clonidine (Catapres) appears to exert its therapeutic effect by inhibiting central noradrenergic activity through this mechanism. Other drugs, notably the classic α adrenolytics, phentolamine (Regitine) and phenoxybenzamine (Dibenzyline), inhibit the activity of peripheral $α_1$ and $α_2$ adrenoceptors. This effect is most noticeable in the heart, where the resulting excess norepinephrine concentration accumulating at nerve endings is sufficient to produce an exaggerated $β_1$-

mediated cardioacceleration, even though the transmitter itself possesses only weak β_1 activity.

Inactivation of Norepinephrine. Inactivation of released monamines is accomplished through two processes, biotransformation and tissue uptake. The former process eliminates body stores of transmitters while the latter process conserves them.

Biotransformation of norepinephrine is governed by the enzymes monoamine oxidase (MAO) and catechol-O-methyl transferase (COMT). MAO is found associated with mitochondria within the noradrenergic nerve terminal and in many other body tissues, especially liver and kidney. The enzyme exists in two variants, MAO-A and MAO-B, which exhibit relative substrate specificities. The former variant has a high affinity for norepinephrine and dopamine and is the only form present in noradrenergic nerve endings. MAO-B has a high affinity for phenylethylamine. In the brain, it is selectively localized in astrocytes and serotineogic neurons. MAO functions primarily to deaminate intraneuronal catecholamines. COMT is a ubiquitous intracellular enzyme responsible for the O-methylation of catecholamines. Extraneuronal amines are directly O-methylated, while intraneuronal norepinephrine is initially deaminated. COMT is found only in nonneuronal elements in brain.

The sequence of metabolic disposition of endogenous norepinephrine is outlined in Figure 18–2.

MAO is responsible for the intraneuronal oxidative deamination of norepinephrine, cleaving the terminal amine group from the molecule by oxidation of the β carbon of the ethylamine side chain. This forms a short-lived aldehyde metabolite, which, in brain, is rapidly reduced to 3, 4-dihydroxyphenylethylene-glycol (DHPG). In the periphery the transient aldehyde is oxidized to form 3, 4-dihydroxymandelic acid (DHMA).

COMT functions to transfer a methyl radical to the meta-hydroxyl group of the catechol ring, converting norepinephrine to normetanephrine. Acting in concert, MAO and COMT produce the metabolite 3-methoxy-4-hydroxyphenylethylene glycol (MHPG). MHPG is the major norepinephrine metabolite found in brain tissue and cerebrospinal fluid. In the periphery, DHMA is similarly O-methylated by COMT, forming 3-methoxy-4-hydroxymandelic acid [vanillylmandelic acid (VMA)].

The central nervous system accounts for 15 to 20 percent of urinary norepinephrine metabolites, with the remainder arising from peripheral sites. Total urinary metabolites of endogenous norepinephrine consist about 60 percent VMA, 35 percent MHPG, and 5 percent normetanephrine. The total of urinary metabolites amounts to 30 to 35 μmol/day.

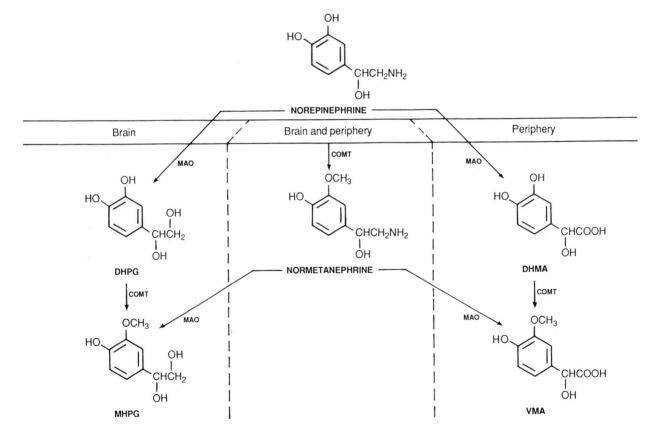

Figure 18–2. Biotransformation of norepinephrine. Enzymes involved are monoamine oxidase (MAO) and catechol-O-methyl transferase (COMT). Sequential metabolites in brain are 3,4-dihydroxyphenylethyleneglycol (DHPG) and 3-methoxy-4-hydroxyphenylethyleneglycol (MHPG). Sequential metabolites in the periphery are 3,4-dihydroxymandelic acid (DHMA) and 3-methoxy-4-hydroxymandelic acid (vanillylmandelic acid; VMA).

Tissue uptake mechanisms involve the transfer of released monoaminergic transmitters into cells through an energy-requiring amine pump mechanism that can concentrate norepinephrine inside cells against a concentration gradient. There are two such uptake pumps, as defined by substrate specificity and by location: the neuronal uptake mechanism (uptake 1) and the nonneuronal or effector tissue uptake mechanism (uptake 2). Among the endogenous monoaminergic transmitters, norepinephrine is taken up preferentially by uptake 1, and epinephrine by uptake 2.

Substances other than norepinephrine and epinephrine are taken up by these amine pumps. Dopamine is taken up by both uptake 1 and 2 mechanisms, metaraminol is avidly taken up by adrenergic neurons, displacing vesicular norepinephrine and producing adrenergic responses. It is less avidly taken up by extraneuronal tissues as well. Isoproterenol is not taken up by nerve endings but is subject to extraneuronal uptake. Certain indirect adrenergic agents, such as amphetamine and ephedrine, do not appear to enter neurons via uptake 1, and probably gain access to the interior of adrenergic nerve endings by simple diffusion.

A wide variety of substances are known that inhibit norepinephrine uptake processes. Most of these selectively inhibit neuronal uptake. Among the potent selective inhibitors of neuronal uptake are tricyclic antidepressants, neuroleptic phenothiazines, cocaine, metaraminol, dopamine, d-amphetamine, and α-methylnorepinephrine. Phenoxybenzamine blocks both neuronal and extraneuronal uptake. Hydrocortisone has been shown to be a selective inhibitor of the extraneuronal uptake process. This explains steroidal potentiation of the cardiovascular response to epinephrine, which is preferentially subject to uptake 2. Preferential inhibition of uptake 2 by hydrocortisone also explains the failure of the steroid to influence the 2-minute alpha half-life of norepinephrine in humans, since this initial pharmacokinetic phase is largely dependent on neuronal uptake.

Postsynaptic Receptor Interactions. As outlined above, smooth muscle, cardiac tissue, and glands throughout the body possess varying densities of adrenoceptors on their postsynaptic membranes. Responses to activation of the postsynaptic α_1, α_2, β_1, and β_2 adrenoceptors are outlined in Table 18–1 and summarized in Table 18–2, where the relative affinity of many adrenotropic agents for the various receptor types is indicated. The agonists listed in Table 18–2 represent drugs employed as pressor agents (epinephrine, norepinephrine, methoxamine, phenylephrine) or as cardiostimulants (isoproterenol, dobutamine). The antagonists in Table 18–2 represent vasodilators (phenoxybenzamine, phentolamine) or antidysrrhythmic agents (propranolol).

Adrenotropic Pressor Amines

Those amines most commonly employed to treat hypotensive episodes are listed in Table 18–3. They are classified according to their mode of action. Direct-acting amines are those that act upon postsynaptic adrenoceptors to produce their effects. The indirect-acting metaraminol produces its effects by presynaptic liberation of norepinephrine and, therefore, exhibits effects that largely parallel those of norepinephrine, except that its duration of action is more prolonged. The mixed-acting amines act both directly and indirectly. These drugs exhibit both α and β adrenergic activities, mimicking the actions of epinephrine. In this category, dopamine exhibits some unique characteristics inasmuch as its activation of vasodilatory dopaminergic receptors in mesenteric and renal beds results in a decline, rather than an increase, in mean arterial peripheral resistance.

Epinephrine (Adrenalin). Epinephrine, the hormone of the adrenal medulla, is an α,β-adrenotropic, direct-acting agent.

TABLE 18–2. RECEPTORS AND ADRENERGIC RESPONSES

Drug	Site: Postsynaptic $\alpha_1{}^a$	Presynaptic $\alpha_2{}^b$	Postsynaptic $\beta_1{}^c$	Postsynaptic $\beta_2{}^d$
Agonists				
Epinephrine (Adrenalin)	+	+	+ +	+ +
Norepinephrine (Levophed)	+ +	+ +	±	±
Methoxamine (Vasoxyl)	+ +	0	0	0
Phenylephrine (Neo-Synephrine)	+ +	0	0	0
Clonidine (Catapres)	0	+ +	0	0
Isoproterenol (Isuprel)	0	0	+ +	+ +
Dobutamine (Dobutrex)	0	0	+ +	±
Antagonists				
Prazosin (Minipress)	+ +	0	0	0
Phenoxybenzamine (Dibenzyline)	+ +	+	0	0
Phentolamine (Regitine)	+	+ +	0	0
Propranolol (Inderal)	0	0	+ +	+ +
Metoprolol (Lopressor)	0	0	+ +	±

^{a} Constriction of vessels in skin, mucosa, and abdominal viscera; mydriasis.
^{b} Inhibition of presynaptic norepinephrine release.
^{c} Increased cardiac rate, contractility, and atrioventricular conduction; lipolysis.
^{d} Dilation of vessels in skeletal muscle, heart, and lungs; relaxation of bronchial muscle; decreased gastrointestinal motility.

TABLE 18–3. CARDIOVASCULAR EFFECTS OF PRESSOR AMINES

| Mode of Action | Drug | Receptor Activity | | Effects upon[a] | | |
		Alpha	Beta	Heart Rate	Cardiac Output	Mean Peripheral Resistance
Direct	Epinephrine	+	+	↑	↑	↑ ↑
	Norepinephrine	+	±	Reflex ↓	0, ↑	↑ ↑
	Phenylephrine	+		Reflex ↓	↓	↑ ↑
	Methoxamine	+		Reflex ↓	0, ↓	↑ ↑
Mixed	Ephedrine	+	+	0, ↑	↑ ↑	↑ (Direct)
	Mephentermine	+	+	↓ ,0, ↑	↑	
	Dopamine[b]	+	+	0, ↑	↑ ↑	0, ↓
Indirect	Metaraminol	+		Reflex ↓	0, ↓	↑ ↑

[a] ↑ = increase, ↓ = decrease, 0 = no change.
[b] Although dopamine mimics epinephrine, its specific dopaminergic dilation of renal and mesenteric vessels dilutes its effect upon peripheral resistance.

Cardiac Effects. Cardiac β_1 receptors respond to epinephrine by increasing cellular cAMP levels. The increased cAMP has two effects: it enhances glycogenolysis, thus providing glucose as an energy source, and it enhances Ca^{2+} influx into cells through the slow calcium channels. These actions result in positive chronotropic and inotropic effects on the heart.

Heart rate is increased by enhancing the rate of calcium influx in SA nodal cells. This results in an increased rate of diastolic depolarization and an enhanced rate of SA discharge. Similar effects on the AV node and conducting tissue can lead to the production of multifocal ectopic pacemakers.

Epinephrine increases the force of ventricular contraction through its β_1 actions, resulting in an increased rate of rise of ventricular systolic pressure and a reduced ventricular residual volume. These positive inotropic ventricular effects are indirectly augmented through an increase in atrial contractility that causes an enhanced end-diastolic pressure in the ventricles. This stretches ventricular fibers and, in accordance with Starling's law, further augments ventricular contractions. Overall cardiac output is increased by epinephrine. Oxygen consumption, however, is enhanced to a degree proportionately greater than cardiac work, so that cardiac efficiency is reduced.

Vascular Effects. Epinephrine, through an action on β_2 receptors, elicits vasodilation in cerebral and coronary vessels and in the vasculature of skeletal muscle. Activation of α_1 adrenoceptors, which requires higher local concentrations of epinephrine than does β_2 activation, results in vasoconstriction. This response is observed in splanchnic, renal, cutaneous, and pulmonary vessels. Marked α-mediated venoconstriction occurs as well.

Blood Pressure Effects. A small intravenous (IV) dose of 1 µg epinephrine may produce a fall in mean arterial blood pressure (mABP) due to preferential β_2-mediated vasodilation. Doses of 10 to 15 µg epinephrine IV (1 to 5 ml of 1: 100,000 epinephrine) prompt significant β_1-mediated cardiac stimulation with an increase in cardiac output and systolic blood pressure. Reduced peripheral resistance and diastolic pressure due to β_2 effects offset the cardiac effect,

and mABP is generally unaltered while pulse pressure is markedly increased. Large doses of epinephrine, e.g., 0.5 mg IV, elicit marked α_1-mediated peripheral vasoconstriction. This widespread constriction overrides vasodilation in skeletal muscle beds and produces a rise in diastolic pressure that, together with the marked enhancement of cardiac output, results in an increase in mABP. Administration of such large doses of epinephrine to an individual who has received an α-blocking agent results in the unmasking of profound β_2-activated vasodilation, and a decline in mABP. This response is referred to as "epinephrine reversal." It occurs when epinephrine is mistakenly employed to correct hypotension due to such α-adrenolytic agents as phenoxybenzamine and chlorpromazine. On the other hand, propranolol, a β-blocker, will potentiate the pressor effects of epinephrine, particularly at high doses. In the face of significant β-blockade, large doses of epinephrine produce a pure α-mediated vasoconstriction and a marked rise in mABP. In these circumstances, 0.3 ml of 1:1000 epinephrine IV can lead to a fatal hypertensive crisis.

Other Effects. Epinephrine produces all the responses obtained by stimulation of the sympathetic nervous system. In the eye, mydriasis occurs due to α_1 contraction of the dilator pupillae muscle. This contraindicates the use of epinephrine, or any other α_1-adrenergic agents, in cases of narrow-angle glaucoma. Vasoconstriction in the iris, however, reduces the production of aqueous humor, and such drugs are indicated in the treatment of open-angle glaucoma.

Epinephrine causes marked relaxation of bronchial and bronchiolar smooth muscle through its β_2 actions. Dilation of the airways is accompanied by α_1-mediated mucosal vasoconstriction, which reduces the production of airway fluids and enhances the drug's antiasthmatic effect.

The increase in blood glucose observed after epinephrine administration has a mixed genesis. Pancreatic insulin release is subject to α_1 inhibition, while β_2 activity enhances insulin release. The latter effect is, however, of secondary importance. Concomitant β_2-mediated skeletal muscular glycogenolysis leads to elevated blood glucose levels. Epinephrine should be employed cautiously in the diabetic patient.

Uses, Side Effects, and Cautions. Intravenous epinephrine can produce transient feelings of anxiety or panic, fear, apprehension, restlessness, and dizziness. Palpitations, skin pallor, headache, and tremor may occur. Epinephrine must be employed judiciously in hypertensive patients. The recommended maximum dose in stabilized heart disease is 0.2 mg, while in patients without cardiovascular complications the maximum recommended dose is 1.0 mg. Epinephrine can cause severe hypertensive reactions in hyperthyroid patients, perhaps due to an increase in the number of cardiac β-receptors induced by thyroxine. Epinephrine may also precipitate anginal pain since it induces a relative oxygen deficit in stimulated cardiac muscle.

In treatment of hypotension, epinephrine, because of its arrhythmogenicity, has been superseded by other pressor amines. The main uses of epinephrine are as a bronchodilator, a localized vasoconstrictor, and in emergency treatment for anaphylactoid reactions.

Epinephrine as a 1:1000 solution may be employed as a topical hemostatic agent to control arteriolar or capillary bleeding. Epinephrine is employed as a vasoconstrictor in local anesthetic solutions, usually in a concentration of 1:100,000. Vasoconstrictors should not be employed for this purpose in appendages such as digits because intense ischemia may develop, leading to gangrene. Concentrations in excess of 1:100,000 should not be employed since extreme tissue ischemia and necrosis may occur.

Epinephrine must be used with caution in the diabetic and is contraindicated in narrow-angle glaucoma.

Acute bronchospastic episodes are terminated with 0.2 to 0.5 mg epinephrine subcutaneously or by inhalation of 1 percent (1:100) epinephrine.

Drug Interactions. It may be worthwhile to further examine the influence of drug interactions, once again using sympathominetics as the model system.

Most epinephrine drug interactions result in either hypertension or arrhythmias. Acute hypertensive episodes may occur if epinephrine is employed in combination with drugs that inhibit the catecholamine uptake process. This is true even of the low epinephrine concentrations employed in local anesthetic solutions. The amine is contraindicated in patients receiving tricyclic antidepressants and guanethidine for this reason. The risk is reduced in patients on monoamine oxidase inhibitors such as tranylcypromine (Parnate) for depression or pargyline (Eutonyl) for hypertension, although these situations should be treated as contraindications. Severe ventricular arrhythmias may develop if epinephrine is given in combination with sodium thyroxine or with certain inhalational anesthetics. The manufacturers' recommended arrhythmogenic limits for epinephrine are 10 ml of 1:100,000 solution per 50 kg body weight per 10 minutes for enflurane and 25 ml of 1:100,000 epinephrine for isoflurane anesthesia. It is suggested that epinephrine be used with caution, if at all, during halothane anesthesia.

Norepinephrine (Levophed).
Norepinephrine is primarily an agonist with weak β activity. It has a pKa of 8.6. Its elimination half-life is 2 minutes.

The main cardiovascular response to norepinephrine is peripheral vasoconstriction and a rise in diastolic blood pressure and mABP for 5 to 14 minutes. This is accompanied by a reflex vagal bradycardia and a reduced or unaltered cardiac output. These same responses are observed at all dose levels of the drug.

The drug is employed in hypotension by IV infusion of 2 to 4 μg/min of the base in a 4 μg/ml solution after initially titrating the patient's response to test rates. Norepinephrine is also employed as a vasoconstrictor in local anesthetic solutions in concentrations of 1:3000 to 1:2500.

The adverse effects of norepinephrine are similar to, but less intense than, those of epinephrine. The most common are anxiety, palpitation, and headache.

Due to lack of major β influences in the pressor response to norepinephrine, interactions with other adrenergic agents are minimal. Although α-blockers reduce the blood pressure rise due to norepinephrine, they do not produce a "reversal." Propranolol, which potentiates the pressor response to epinephrine, will slightly reduce the pressor effect of norepinephrine, probably by blocking its minor cardiac actions.

Norepinephrine causes severe hypertension with headache and vomiting in hyperthyroid patients. Patients on tricyclic antidepressants receiving 1:2500 norepinephrine as a vasoconstrictor adjunct to local anesthesia have developed fatal hypertensive crises. The drug should not be used in patients taking monoamine oxidase inhibitors. The β_1 cardiac effects of norepinephrine, though much less prominent than those of epinephrine, are sufficiently pronounced to precipitate severe ventricular arrhythmias and fibrillation when given together with halothane, enflurane, or isoflurane anesthesia.

Phenylephrine (Neo-Synephrine).
Phenylephrine is a noncatecholamine, α_1 adrenergic agonist with a pKa of 9.8. In the treatment of hypotensive episodes, the drug produces vasoconstriction, a marked increase in peripheral vascular resistance, and a profound reflex bradycardia with a decline in cardiac output. It produces no central stimulant effects.

Phenylephrine may be given, to treat hypotension, in a dose of 5 to 10 mg IM or 0.8 mg slow IV. The onset of pressor effect by the IM route is 10 to 15 minutes, with a duration of 1.0 to 1.5 hours. The drug may be employed by the IV route for treating paroxysmal atrial tachycardia. It is also used as a constrictor adjuvant with local anesthetics in a concentration of 1:2500.

Phenylephrine is contraindicated in patients on tricyclic antidepressants or monoamine oxidase inhibitors because of the likelihood of causing severe hypertension. It should be employed cautiously in the hyperthyroid or hypertensive patient, as well as in patients with cardiac failure. The lack of cardiac stimulant effects, however, means that phenylephrine is not arrhythmogenic and can be employed safely in combination with agents such as halothane.

Methoxamine (Vasoxyl).
Methoxamine is a direct α_1 agonist and produces effects similar to those of phenylephrine. It is usually administered intramuscularly in a dose of 10 to 20 mg. The pressor response, which is characterized by marked vasoconstriction and an absence of direct cardiac effects, lasts 60 to 90 minutes.

Ephedrine. Ephedrine is a mixed-acting amine. Its cardiovascular effects are largely indirect, but it has some direct actions, particularly upon β receptors. Although the drug is a weak inhibitor of uptake 1, it is not actively transported itself. It enters the noradrenergic nerve ending passively, displacing cytoplasmic norepinephrine. Repeated administration causes marked tachyphylaxis to its peripheral actions.

Ephedrine is an α_1, β agonist, and produces cardiovascular effects similar to those of epinephrine, but lasting from 0.5 to 0.75 hours. The drug augments cardiac output through an enhanced contractility, with heart rate unchanged or slightly increased. Peripheral vasoconstriction is a less important factor in the pressor response. Ephedrine produces mild central nervous system stimulation. Its primary pressor use is in hypotensive states due to spinal anesthesia or anaphylactic reactions. The usual dose is 15 to 50 mg subcutaneously or 20 mg IV. The drug is also used to treat nasal congestion, bronchial asthma, enuresis, and myasthenia gravis.

As is true with other indirectly acting amines, hypertensive crisis may result from its administration to patients being treated with monoamine oxidase inhibitors.

Mephentermine (Wyamine). Mephentermine is a mixed-acting amine with effects similar to those of ephedrine. It is used primarily in hypotensive states in a dose of 10 to 30 mg subcutaneously or intramuscularly, with pressor effects lasting 30 to 60 minutes and 4 hours, respectively. The drug lacks central stimulant effects in pressor doses.

Metaraminol (Aramine). Metaraminol is the most purely indirect acting of the pressor amines. It is taken up avidly by the uptake 1 mechanism, displaces vesicular norepinephrine, and produces noradrenergic effects. Marked vasoconstriction occurs with reflex bradycardia. Cardiac output is unchanged or slightly reduced. Both venous tone and pulmonary blood pressure increase, while cerebral blood flow is reduced. It lacks central stimulant activity.

Metaraminol is used almost exclusively to treat hypotension. Doses of 5 mg IM elevate blood pressure for 90 to 120 minutes.

The rise in blood pressure is attenuated in the presence of tricyclic antidepressants (which block uptake 1), but may be fatally potentiated in the presence of monoamine oxidase inhibitors.

With prolonged infusions, metaraminol is released by exocytosis, along with norepinephrine, and can produce profound hypotension.

Dopamine (Intropin). Dopamine mimics epinephrine in its effects upon α and β adrenoceptors, but, in addition, produces specific dopaminergic vasodilation in splanchnic and renal vascular beds. The receptor activity of dopamine appears to be, in decreasing order; dopamine receptors, β_1 receptors, β_2 receptors, and α_1 adrenoceptors.

Intravenous doses of 1 to 2 μg/kg/min dilate splanchnic and renal vessels, increasing glomerular filtration rate, sodium excretion, and urinary output. Doses of 2 to 10 μg/kg/min also produce β_1-mediated cardiac stimulation with an increased cardiac output, a reduced peripheral vascular resistance, but little change in heart rate or blood pressure. Doses of 10 to 20 μg/kg/min stimulate α_1 receptors, causing peripheral vasoconstriction and a rise in blood pressure. Such vasoconstriction, at doses above 20 μg/kg/min, may reverse the dopaminergic dilation of renal vessels. Overdosage, in the range of 750 to 1000 μg/kg/min, produces marked rises in systolic pressure, with little change in diastolic pressure, reflex bradycardia, and ventricular arrhythmias.

Dopamine is indicated in shock due to myocardial infarction, trauma, sepsis, open heart surgery, renal failure, and congestive heart failure.

Dopamine hydrochloride is supplied in 5-ml ampules containing 200 mg of the drug, which must be diluted in 250 or 500 ml of a neutral or acid (lactate) solution before use. A microdrip regulator is essential for infusion. In shock, hypovolemia must be initially corrected with blood or plasma expanders. IV infusion of dopamine is then begun, initially with 2 to 5 μg/kg/min and increasing as necessary, by increments of 5 to 10 μg/kg/min. Constant monitoring is required to maintain desired blood pressure and urine flow.

In the treatment of shock, 2 to 20 μg/kg/min dopamine causes a 30 to 40 percent increase in cardiac output, a 6 to 30 percent increase in mean arterial pressure, and a 200 to 500 percent increase in urine flow.

Nausea, vomiting, and ventricular ectopic beats are the most common adverse effects of dopamine. Its arrhythmigenicity is enhanced by halogenated anesthetics such as halothane. Monoamine oxidase inhibitors potentiate the effects of dopamine, and patients receiving such drugs should be given only one tenth the usual initial dose of dopamine. The drug is contraindicated in patients with pheochromocytoma, since higher doses of dopamine do exert an "indirect amine" effect.

Dobutamine (Dobutrex). Dobutamine is a chemical analogue of dopamine lacking significant vasoactive effects. It is a selective β_1 agonist, of short duration, producing enhancement of cardiac contractility and stroke volume, with little effect on heart rate. Employed in a dosage of 2.5 to 10μg/kg/min intravenously, it is useful for inotropic support in a variety of low output states, such as that occurring subsequent to cardiopulmonary bypass surgery.

DIRECT-ACTING VASODILATORS

Nitrate Venodilators

Nitrites and organic nitrates are general vasodilators, which exhibit more prominent effects upon capacitance than resistance vessels, and which dilate larger arteries more effectively than arterioles.

Amyl nitrite was advocated for the treatment of angina pectoris in 1867, twelve years before the introduction of nitroglycerin for the same condition. A number of organic nitrates have been synthesized, in an attempt to produce longer-acting agents for prophylactic use in ischemic heart disease. The clinical utility of nitroglycerin has expanded recently due to the introduction of novel formulations and drug delivery systems.

The more commonly used agents in this class are listed in Table 18–4, along with doses, routes of administration, and onset and duration of action.

Amyl nitrite (Vaporole) is a volatile liquid prepared in easily crushed ampules. The vapor is inhaled at the first sign of an anginal attack. The drug is inactive orally, due to rapid hydrolysis within the gastrointestinal tract.

Nitroglycerin is an explosive oily liquid which is safely compounded with mannitol in tablet form. Nitroglycerin tablets U.S.P. lose activity within 2 to 3 days if exposed to the atmosphere. Stored in a tightly sealed dark-colored glass container (without a cotton plug), the tablets have a shelf-life of about 6 months. Active tablets produce a burning sensation when placed under the tongue. A more stable tablet with a shelf-life of 2 years is available as Nitrostat. The drug is also available as a 2 percent ointment for cutaneous application, and in ampules in solution to be diluted for IV use. Accurate dose delivery of the drug by IV infusion has been limited in the past, by a 40 to 80 percent absorption of nitroglycerin by the polyvinylchloride tubing of common IV infusion sets. Special prepackaged infusion sets, employing nonabsorbing polyethylene tubing which allows accurate IV delivery of the drug, are now widely available.

Isosorbide dinitrate (e.g., Isordil, Sorbitrate) is available as sublingual, chewable, and oral tablets for prophylactic use in angina. Pentaerythritol tetranitrate (e.g., Peritrate, Pentritol) cannot be employed sublingually, because of its limited aqueous solubility.

In view of the widespread, and expanding, clinical role of nitroglycerin, the following discussion will be restricted to nitroglycerin, unless otherwise noted.

Administration and Uptake. Nitroglycerin is poorly absorbed by the oral route because of a high presystemic elimination rate, due to both hepatic and intestinal mucosal biotransformation. Large oral doses, however, saturate responsible enzyme systems, and long-lasting therapeutic blood levels (>5 to 10 ng/ml) can be achieved. Doses in the range of 2.5 to 6.5 mg of the drug, taken orally, can provide prophylactic antianginal activity for 4 to 6 hours.

The drug is well absorbed through skin and mucous membranes. Since only about 15 percent of total cardiac output is delivered to the liver, these sites of administration successfully circumvent the process of presystemic elimination.

The sublingual route is standard for the treatment of acute attacks of myocardial ischemia. A dose of 0.3 to 0.4 mg of nitroglycerin provides a peak plasma level of 1.4 ng/ml after 5 minutes, which declines to 0.7 ng/ml at 10 minutes. Doses of 0.3 to 0.6 mg nitroglycerin provide clinical relief within 2 to 5 minutes, which is maximal in 3 to 15 minutes, and lasts 20 to 30 minutes.

Cutaneous application of 2 percent nitroglycerin in an ointment base provides up to two times greater bioavailability than the oral route. Different areas of skin exhibit different absorption rates, with the forehead and ankle both possessing greater absorption rates than the skin of the chest. Usually ½ to 2 inches of ointment, as it is squeezed from the tube, is applied in a thin layer to the chest. An occlusive dressing hastens absorption. Onset of action is about 15 to 30 minutes by the percutaneous route, with a duration of 3 to 7 hours. Transdermal systems, consisting of a variable dose nitroglycerin reservoir with an adhesive ring, are also available. Steady-state nitroglycerin blood levels are achieved in 1 to 4 hours and are maintained for about 24 hours.

Intranasal administration of 0.8 mg of nitroglycerin in 1 ml of solution via a 16 gauge IV Teflon catheter produces peak levels, after 1 to 2 minutes, of 2.5 and 11.5 ng/ml in peripheral and central venous blood, respectively. This time course of absorption closely parallels that of IV bolus administration.

Bolus IV administration of 4 to 8 μg/kg of nitroglycerin produces hypotensive effects within 30 seconds, which peak at 1 to 2 minutes and last 3 to 5 minutes.

For intravenous infusion of drug, the recommended dosage is 5 μg/min, with incremental increases of 5 μg/min every 3 to 5 minutes, until a required response is obtained.

Following absorption, nitroglycerin is not significantly bound to plasma proteins. Based on peripheral venous

TABLE 18–4. ORGANIC NITRITES AND NITRATES USED IN ISCHEMIC HEART DISEASE

	Route	Usual Single Dose	Onset of Action	Duration of Action
Amyl nitrite	Inhalation	0.3 ml	30 sec	5 min
Glyceryl trinitrate (nitroglycerin)	Sublingual	0.6 mg	2–15 min	30 min
	Percutaneous	½–2 inches of 2% ointment	15–30 min	5 hr
	Oral	2.5–6.5 mg	Variable	5 hr
	Intranasal	0.8 mg	1–2 min	4 min
	Intravenous	0.5 mg	30 sec	4 min
Isosorbide dinitrate	Sublingual	5 mg	5 min	2 hr
	Oral	10–30 mg	30 min	5 hr
Pentaerythrityl tetranitrate	Oral	20 mg	30–60 min	5 hr

blood sampling, the V_d of the drug is about 4.2 L/kg, indicating significant extravascular sequestration.

Elimination. The elimination of nitroglycerin in humans can be described as a first-order monoexponential kinetic process with a $t_{1/2}$ of 2 to 6 minutes, and a clearance of about 500 ml/min/kg.

The first step in the biotransformation of nitroglycerin is a hepatic reductive denitration of either the 2- or 3- position of the drug molecule, catalyzed by the enzyme, organic nitrate ester reductase (ONER), coupled with reduced glutathione as cofactor. This results in the formation of both 1, 2- and 1,3-glycerol dinitrates, oxidized glutathione, and inorganic nitrite ion, which is subsequently oxidized to nitrate and excreted in the urine. This initial denitration is a rapid process, resulting in the brief $t_{1/2}$ of nitroglycerin.

The high intrinsic hepatic ONER activity is largely responsible for limiting the oral bioavailability of nitroglycerin to 40 percent. The system is saturable, however, presumably through depletion of glutathione cofactor. This accounts for the successful prophylactic use of large oral doses of nitroglycerin in angina.

The glycerol dinitrate metabolites are further denitrated by the ONER-glutathione system, forming 1- and 2-glycerol mononitrates. This proceeds at a rate that is only 2 to 5 percent of the initial denitration. The dinitrate metabolites reportedly have a V_d of 0.34 L/kg and an elimination clearance rate of 2.2 ml/min/kg. This provides a calculated $t_{1/2}$ of 108 minutes.

The primary metabolites in blood are 1,3-glycerol dinitrate and the two mononitrate derivatives. They have elimination $t_{1/2}$s to 2 to 4 hours but possess only limited pharmacologic activity. Urinary di- and mononitrates account for 80 percent of an administered dose of nitroglycerin. A portion of the dose is converted to carbon dioxide and eliminated through the lungs.

ONER activity is not restricted to the liver, but is found at significant levels in both kidney and intestinal mucosa, the latter likely contributing significantly to the presystemic elimination of oral doses of nitroglycerin.

Mechanism of Action. Organic nitrites and nitrates belong to the group of "nitric oxide vasodilators," which includes sodium nitroprusside and hydroxylamine (NH_2OH) as well as nitric oxide (NO) itself. These agents all appear to cause vasodilation by forming common intermediates, i.e., S-nitrosothiols.

Organic nitrates appear to act at sulfhydryl-containing receptor sites within vascular smooth muscle cells. The nitrates liberate nitroso groups (-NO) intracellularly. The nitroso group is very reactive and readily combines with two hydrogen atoms to form more stable compounds. Such available hydrogen atoms within the cell are found in reduced thiol compounds, specifically cysteine in the case of nitroglycerin. The resulting S-nitrosocysteine activates guanylate cyclase, resulting in measurable increases in intracellular cGMP levels, which in turn enhances intracellular calcium binding and causes relaxation of vascular smooth muscle.

In support of this theory are an observed dose-dependent arterial hypotension in cats produced by injection of S-nitrosocysteine, and a reported relaxation of isolated smooth muscle cells after microinjection of cGMP.

Cardiovascular Effects. The primary effect of nitroglycerin is differential relaxation of vascular smooth muscle. The predominant action is venodilation. Nitroglycerin causes a maximal reduction of tone in isolated arteries of only 50 percent, at concentrations that are ten times those producing complete inhibition of venous tone. The drug is, in turn, 10,000 times more potent in relaxing coronary, than femoral, isolated canine vascular rings that are in a state of monoamine-induced spasm.

The predominant venodilation causes a decrease in cardiac venous return and in left ventricular end diastolic volume (LVEDV) and pressure (LVEDP). The reduced LVEDP has two consequences. First, there is a decline in ventricular size and wall stress, with an accompanying reduction in myocardial oxygen consumption. Second, since endocardial vascular perfusion is greatly affected by pressure changes within the ventricles, the reduced LVEDP results in enhanced ventricular transmural blood flow and in a significant increase in endocardial/epicardial blood perfusion. A selective increase in subendocardial tissue P_{O_2} results. The reduced ventricular oxygen consumption together with the increase in endocardial blood flow and oxygenation are largely responsible for the salutary effects of nitroglycerin in myocardial ischemia.

The less pronounced arteriodilation caused by the drug results in two effects that contribute to its antianginal efficacy. First, the resulting decline in systemic arterial blood pressure reduces resistance to ventricular ejection, thus reducing cardiac workload and oxygen demand. There is an associated reduction in left ventricular systolic pressure, which, like the reduced LVEDP due to the decline in cardiac preload, contributes to a reduced compression of the endocardium and an increase in oxygen supply to this area. Second, coronary arteries dilate, larger vessels more so than smaller. This produces a decline in total coronary blood flow, but, at constant mean arterial blood pressure, there is an associated 18 percent increase in collateral blood flow to experimentally induced ischemic areas of canine myocardium.

In clinical studies of volunteer subjects, an intravenous bolus dose of 4 to 8 µg/kg nitroglycerin produces a 20 percent fall in mean arterial blood pressure, a 21 to 24 percent reflex rise in heart rate, and an 83 to 117 percent increase in cerebrospinal fluid pressure coupled with a 29 to 32 percent fall in mean cerebral perfusion pressure. Arterial P_{O_2}, P_{CO_2}, and pH are unchanged. Thiamylal–N_2O–O_2 anesthesia does not alter these responses significantly.

Other Effects. Organic nitrates are generalized smooth muscle relaxants with no significant actions on other systems. Nitroglycerin is clinically effective in relaxing the biliary tract, but other gastrointestinal spasm is unrelieved except by large doses of the drug, which causes significant hypotension.

Bronchial smooth muscle tone is reduced by nitrates, but nitroglycerin is only weakly antiasthmatic. An additional effect upon respiration is carotid chemoreceptor stimulation by inhaled amyl nitrite, resulting in a brief hyperpnea, followed by a compensatory hypopnea.

Adverse Effects. Transient throbbing headache, which may be severe, frequently results from nitroglycerin administration. It is due to a rise in cerebral blood flow and cerebrospinal fluid pressure. It has been observed in 2 of 15 conscious patients receiving 8 μg/kg of the drug IV. Tolerance to this effect occurs after several days of nitrate administration.

Postural hypotension, due to predominant venodilation, is not uncommon, especially in the erect patient. This is accompanied by weakness, vertigo, dizziness, and palpitation. The syndrome is more severe after higher doses of nitroglycerin ("nitrate syncope"), and the resulting tachycardia and enhanced myocardial contractility may, in itself, lead to exacerbation of anginal symptoms. Nitrate syncope is potentiated by ethyl alcohol. Severe hypotension in overdose results in hypokinetic anoxia due to peripheral pooling of blood in the extremities. Such reactions are effectively treated by placing the patient in the Trendelenburg position to increase venous return and cardiac output.

A severe idosyncratic hypotension (blood pressure of 65/40) with bradycardia (heart rate of 14 to 44 beats/min) has been reported in angina patients within 2 to 6 minutes of receiving nitroglycerin sublingually. The reaction is terminated by employing the Trendelenburg position and administering 0.5 to 2.0 mg atropine sulfate IM.

Nitroglycerin is believed to dilate retinal blood vessels and increase intraocular pressure. However, it appears to be completely safe for use in glaucomatous patients.

Cutaneous vasodilation may result in flushing in the head and neck region, although this is most usually observed only after amyl nitrite inhalation.

Methemoglobinemia is rapidly produced by the nitrite ion through oxidation of the iron atom in heme to the ferric state. Both amyl nitrite and sodium nitrite are effective in generating methemoglobin, and, for this reason, are employed in the treatment of cyanide poisoning. Cyanide ion is then innocuously bound as cyanomethemoglobin. Nitrates do not normally cause methemoglobinemia, but may do so in infants under 6 months of age, after being converted to nitrite by bacterial action in the gastrointestinal (GI) tract. These nitrate-reducing bacteria require a near neutral environment, and are able to thrive in the upper GI tract of infants, whose stomach contents are much less acid than the adult. In addition, the infant form of hemoglobin is more susceptible to oxidation than the adult form. Infantile erythrocytes are also deficient in methemoglobin-reducing enzyme. Cases of methemoglobinemia, with functional anemia, chocolate-colored blood, and cyanosis, are occasionally reported in infants in rural areas who drink well water that has been contaminated with nitrate-containing fertilizers.

Nitroglycerin blood levels of up to 45 ng/ml increase bleeding time by one third and reduce platelet aggregation, most probably by enhancing the synthesis of prostacyclin (PGI_2).

The intermittent use of nitrates in ischemic heart disease does not lead to tolerance to the effects of the drugs. However, persons involved in the manufacture of explosives, who are chronically exposed to nitrates, develop headache and dizziness to which they become tolerant after a few days. Symptoms reappear after a weekend away from the job ("Monday disease"). Complete tolerance to the vasodepressor effects of nitroglycerin has been produced both in intact rats and in isolated aorta. This tissue tolerance appears to be due to a nitrate receptor mechanism, inasmuch as exposure of the tolerant tissue to dithiothreitol, a disulfide-reducing agent, restores reactivity to nitroglycerin. Although nitrate tolerance has not been a clinical problem in the past, the increasing use of high-dose regimens may result in significant tolerance development.

A form of chronic nitrate dependence has been observed in munitions workers, characterized by coronary arteriospasm, with chest pain, myocardial infarction, and even death during temporary withdrawal from nitrate exposure. These symptoms of severe ischemic heart disease (IHD) are relieved by nitroglycerin. Although no firm evidence exists of nitrate dependence during therapeutic use of these drugs, patients with IHD or congestive failure should be warned not to discontinue their therapy abruptly.

Volatile organic nitrites, though nonaddictive, are frequently abused by inhalation to produce a transient euphoric experience. Amyl nitrite was long available as an over-the-counter drug for angina, but due to abuse, under street names such as "poppers" and "Amy Joy," was placed on prescription. Today, an analog, butyl nitrite, is widely available, ostensibly marketed as a "liquid incense" or a "room deodorizer" under such trade names as Locker Room, JacAroma, or Bullet. "Sniffing" this product produces a "rush," with a sense of being in slow motion, a feeling of warmth, hypotension with dizziness, rapid pulse, and flushed face for a few seconds to 1 minute. Deaths have occurred after oral ingestion of butyl nitrite, in one reported case in an amount of 8.6 g (about 9.5 ml of room deodorizer). In rats, butyl nitrite toxicity is manifested as cyanosis, dyspnea, ataxia, extensor spasm, and fasciculations.

Long-acting nitrates must be employed with caution in anginal patients with a history of cerebrovascular disease, especially those exhibiting residual paresis. In such cases, nitrates have caused transient cerebral ischemia with temporary exacerbation of paralysis.

Nitroglycerin is contraindicated in cases of severe anemia, increased intracranial pressure, constrictive pericarditis, or pericardial tamponade. Hypotension or uncompensated hypovolemia are contraindications because nitroglycerin can produce severe hypotension or shock under these conditions.

Uses. The main use of nitrite compounds is the treatment of cyanide poisoning resulting either from industrial use of cyanide or from nitroprusside overdose. Cyanide ion has a high affinity for ferric iron and, in vivo, complexes with the ferric form of cytochrome c reductase, inhibiting the enzyme. This interferes with oxygen utilization in tissues, producing rapid death due to cytotoxic anoxia. The immediate goal in treatment is to form an excess pool of oxidized iron to compete for cyanide ion. This is accomplished by producing large quantities of methemoglobin quickly. Amyl nitrite is administered by inhalation, for 30 seconds every minute, while a 3 percent solution of sodium nitrite is prepared. A dose of 15 mg/kg of the latter solution is administered slowly IV. The large amount of methemoglobin formed competes favorably for cyanide ion, and cytochrome c reductase activity is restored. The resulting cyanomethemoglobin complex is nontoxic. Elimination of cyanide from the body is accomplished by the IV administration of 150 mg/kg sodium thiosulfate given over a 15-minute period. Thiosulfate and cyanide are enzymatically converted, by the enzyme rhodanese, to thiocyanate ion, which is readily eliminated in the urine.

The primary clinical indication for organic nitrites and nitrates is IHD in its progressive manifestations as angina, congestive heart failure and myocardial infarction. Nitroglycerin is also employed to lower peripheral arterial blood pressure when indicated.

IHD, due to progressive coronary insufficiency, is usually a consequence of the formation of atherosclerotic plaques and intimal thickening in major coronary arteries. Slowly developing IHD is manifested as angina pectoris, which becomes more severe with age. Dysrhythmias occur if the conducting tissue of the heart becomes involved. Congestive heart failure may develop as the disease progresses. Sudden blockage of a major coronary vessel leads to myocardial infarction, with rapid death often resulting from ventricular fibrillation.

Angina pectoris is characterized as sudden severe suffocating precordial pain, which is often referred to the left shoulder and arm, and may radiate to the left side of the face, including the jaw, teeth, and throat. Angina is precipitated by a variety of factors, including anxiety, pain, fatigue, exercise, cold, or even partaking of a meal. In addition to the precordial pain, the patient suffers a feeling of choking and a fear of impending death. Frequent nocturnal attacks are seen, due to sympathetic stimulation during REM sleep.

Angina is produced by insufficient oxygen supply in the myocardium to meet oxygen demand. In angina, an atheromatous lesion in an epicardial coronary artery has two adverse consequences. First, diastolic pressure within the artery is reduced from the normal 80 mm Hg to as low as 25 mm Hg at a point distal to the lesion. Secondly, transmural arterioles, carrying blood to the subendocardial vascular plexus, and the endocardial vessels themselves, are maximally dilated at rest due to tissue hypoxia resulting from reduced tissue perfusion. (It is for this reason that a drug that is a pure coronary dilator is of no benefit in angina.) During exercise in an anginal patient, impaired myocardial blood flow may result in acute left ventricular failure characterized by an increase in LVEDP. Now subendocardial vascular perfusion pressure is the coronary artery diastolic pressure minus the LVEDP. In IHD, during exercise, the coronary artery diastolic pressure is reduced due to occlusion, and LVEDP is increased due to acute failure. The result is markedly reduced subendocardial perfusion pressure, blood flow, and oxygen supply, resulting in the pain of angina.

By reducing cardiac preload and LVEDP, nitroglycerin allows an increase in net subendocardial blood flow and reduces myocardial oxygen demand. In addition, a reduction in afterload reduces ventricular work, while dilation of coronary arteries increases collateral blood flow to areas distal to the site of coronary occlusion.

In chronic IHD, nitroglycerin is employed prophylactically by the oral or percutaneous route. The rapid onset of sublingual action makes this route useful for aborting or treating an acute anginal attack (Table 18–4). The IV route is indicated during surgery if ECG evidence of myocardial ischemic is observed.

Direct coronary artery dilation appears to be the principal action of nitroglycerin in the rapid alleviation of acute attacks in variant (Prinzmetal's) angina. This disease appears to be due to periodic α-adrenoceptive-mediated coronary artery vasospasm.

Nitrates can improve cardiac output and reduce pulmonary and peripheral edema in congestive heart failure, even in some patients who are unresponsive to digitalis treatment.

Nitroglycerin, given to normal individuals, causes a decline in cardiac output because of venodilation and reduced cardiac preload. In heart failure, on the other hand, because cardiac output is inadequate, there is a compensatory sympathetically induced increase in peripheral vascular resistance that helps to maintain arterial blood pressure. In this situation, nitroglycerin tends to cause an increase in cardiac output by reducing cardiac afterload. The ventricles empty more completely with less energy cost. Nitrates also produce a marked reduction in preload, resulting in a decrease in LVEDP, which reduces pulmonary congestion. Ventricular size is also reduced.

Patients most likely to respond are those in severe failure, with a high LVEDP, high systemic resistance, and low cardiac output. Benefits are seen with both short- and long-term nitrate therapy. Pentaerythritol tetranitrate, taken in doses of 80 mg orally provides relief in congestive failure for at least 5 hours. The drug produces a fall in mean systemic vascular resistance and arterial blood pressure, a decline in right atrial pressure and capillary pulmonary wedge pressure, and an increase in stroke volume and cardiac index. In digitalis-refractory heart failure, it is common to add oral hydralazine to the nitrate regimen. Hydralazine, a pure arteriolar dilator, maximizes the reduction in afterload and the increase in cardiac output, without producing marked alterations in blood pressure or heart rate in such patients.

Intravenous nitroglycerin is indicated in acute myocardial failure associated with myocardial infarction.

Chronic, as well as acute, pulmonary hypertension is ameliorated by nitroglycerin given IV at rates that avoid tachycardia. Intravenous infusion of 24 to 120 μg/min of the drug was reported to reduce pulmonary vascular resistance by 50 percent while increasing cardiac output by 61 percent due to the reduced right-side afterload. Mean arterial blood pressure declined by only 11.4 percent.

Intravenous infusions of nitroglycerin appear to be of value in the early treatment of acute myocardial infarction. The two main sequelae of acute myocardial infarction are acute heart failure leading to pulmonary hypertension and edema, and the formation of a residual infarct due to localized myocardial anoxia. The relief of acute heart failure and pulmonary congestion has been described above. Experimental clinical evidence indicates that nitroglycerin, by reducing myocardial oxygen demand, and redistributing blood flow to the infarcted area, may reduce both infarct size and the incidence of ventricular arrhythmias if it is administered early in the infarct episode.

Nitroglycerin IV is also indicated intraoperatively to produce controlled hypotension or to control systemic or pulmonary hypertension during surgery.

Sodium Nitroprusside (Nipride)

Sodium nitroprusside (SNP), $NaNOFeCN_5$, is a general vasodilator, of short onset and duration of action, which is used for the production of intentional hypotension or for the treatment of acute hypertensive crisis.

The drug is available in vials as 50 mg of a reddish-brown powder for dilution, immediately prior to use, with 500 ml of 5 percent dextrose, to provide a solution of 1.0 mg/ml for intravenous infusion.

Administration. Solutions of SNP must be fresh, and they should be discarded if more than 24 hours old. The drug is administered, by intravenous infusion with a microdrip regulator, at an initial rate of 0.5 to 1.5 μg/kg/min. The flow is rapidly titrated to the desired arterial blood pressure, and continued under constant monitoring to prevent severe hypotension. The mean adult infusion rate is 3 μg/kg/min, with a maximum of 10 μg/kg/min. The maximum allowable dose is 1.5 mg/kg, though in hypothermia this is reduced to 0.45 mg/kg. This latter dosage adjustment is necessary because low body temperatures reduce the activity of SNP detoxifying enzymes.

During administration, the infusion vessel and delivery tubing must be shielded from light, since light promotes the rapid chemical breakdown of SNP to inactive substances.

Elimination and Toxicity. The disposition of SNP is illustrated in Figure 18–3. The cardinal feature of SNP elimination is the production of toxic cyanide ion (CN^-) in the amount of five moles of CN^- per mole of SNP. This occurs

through a nonenzymic redox reaction with hemoglobin in which SNP oxidizes heme iron to form methemoglobin with the generation of CN^-. Since CN^- has a high affinity for ferric iron (Fe^{3+}), the formation of methemoglobin allows part of the cyanide ion to be bound in an inactive form as cyanomethemoglobin.

The remainder of the CN^- generated from SNP follows one of three pathways. Some binds firmly, but reversibly, to the Fe^{3+} of cytochrome c reductase, the terminal respiratory enzyme in tissues. Inhibition of this enzyme results in fatal cytotoxic anoxia. This process is accompanied by metabolic acidosis, due to the accumulation of blood lactic acid generated by anaerobic carbohydrate metabolism, and by a rise in venous P_{O_2}, due to the lack of tissue utilization of oxygen. The minimum lethal whole blood cyanide concentration is 340 μg/dl. Metabolic acidosis is consistently produced by erythrocytic CN^- levels greater than 0.75 μg/ml. However, 90 percent of whole blood CN^- is found in erythrocytes, presumably in an inactive form, so that erythrocytic CN^- levels probably represent an indirect estimate of free plasma CN^- concentrations. The human adult lethal CN^- plasma level is estimated to be 10 to 20 × 10^{-6} M.

Two thirds of the generated blood CN^- is converted to the less toxic metabolite, thiocyanate (SCN^-), by the transfer of a neutral sulfur atom from the endogenous donor, thiosulfate (SSO_3^-), to the nucleophilic acceptor cyanide ion. This reaction is catalyzed by the enzyme rhodanese (thiosulfate sulfur transferase), which is bound within the mitochondria of liver and kidney cells. Rhodanese requires vitamin B_{12} as a cofactor. The thiocyanate is excreted in the urine. Although oliguria or anuria do not enhance the risk of cyanide toxicity, renal insufficiency can lead to thiocyanate accumulation. Excessive blood thiocyanate levels may cause miosis, tinnitus, confusion, psychosis, and convulsions.

The third cyanide pathway involves combination of

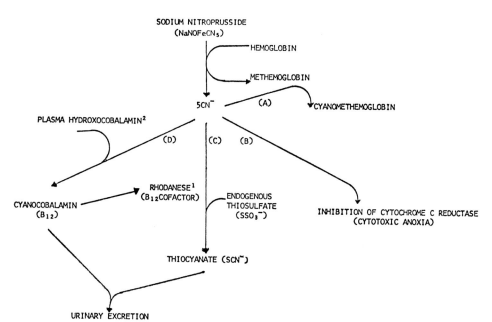

Figure 18–3. The in vivo disposition of sodium nitroprusside. Path B represents cyanide (CN^-) toxicity, with attendant metabolic acidosis and elevated plasma lactate and venous P_{O_2}. Paths A, C, and D represent routes of detoxification of CN^-. [1] Rhodanese (thiosulfate sulfur transferase) is a mitochondrial enzyme found in liver and kidney. [2] Plasma vitamin B_{12} includes cyano-, hydroxo-, methyl- and adenylcobalamins.

CN^- with plasma hydroxocobalamin to form cyanocobalamin, which, as indicated above, functions as a cofactor in the rhodanese-catalyzed detoxification of cyanide ion. Cyanocobalamin is poorly bound to plasma protein and is excreted in the urine.

Cyanide toxicity is reported to occur at SNP doses greater than 3.0 mg/kg, with death occurring at doses greater than 7.0 mg/kg. It may be noted that, in humans, infusion of 4.3 μg/kg/min for 3 hours (total dose of 0.89 mg/kg) increases whole blood cyanide from a control level of 3.6 up to 65.7 μg/dl.

Cyanide toxicity is treated by amyl nitrite inhalation (for 30 seconds each minute), coupled with slow IV administration of 15 mg/kg sodium nitrite, to promote the formation of methemoglobin to which CN^- binds. This is followed by slow IV introduction of 150 mg/kg sodium thiosulfate to provide substrate for the rhodanese-catalyzed conversion of CN^- to thiocyanate. It has also been suggested that hydroxocobalamin be administered along with SNP to reduce the likelihood of cyanide toxicity.

Mechanism of Action. SNP is one of the group of "nitric oxide vasodilators." It appears to act by generation of nitroso groups, forming intracellular S-nitrosothiols that, in turn, activate guanylate cyclase. This results in relaxation of vascular smooth muscle through the same mechanism as that of the organic nitrates. In the case of SNP, however, both resistance and capacitance vessels are dilated.

The drug also appears to stimulate cAMP production, as evidenced by SNP-induced increases in plasma levels of both cGMP and cAMP in humans.

Cardiovascular Effects. SNP causes an immediate dose-related decline in blood pressure, prompted by both venous and arterial vasodilation. This hypotensive response is associated with a reflex increase in heart rate of 15 to 50 percent. Cardiac output is slightly reduced, because of the decline in preload, although it may increase somewhat in the anesthetized individual. During controlled hypotension with SNP, carotid sinus blood flow is elevated and myocardial oxygen consumption is reduced. With excessive doses of the drug the blood pressure may disappear altogether.

Tachyphylaxis to the hypotensive effects of SNP has been noted, as has rebound hypertension following infusion of the drug. Tachyphylaxis may result from CN^- accumulation during prolonged infusions of SNP, since CN^- has been shown, in isolated smooth muscle, to antagonize both the vasodilation and the increase in cellular cGMP levels produced by SNP. Resistance of some patients to SNP vasodepression may be the result of impaired rhodanese function and rapid CN^- accumulation. The tendency to increase SNP infusion rates in such patients could lead to accelerated CN^- accumulation and toxic effects.

Rebound hypertension following infusion of SNP is related to the increased plasma levels of cAMP that are associated with increased norepinephrine and epinephrine plasma levels and with a rise in plasma renin activity. Both propranolol and captopril (3.0 mg/kg orally immediately before surgery) pretreatment prevents rebound hypertension, and both attenuate catecholamine release during SNP hypotension. Propranolol also reduces plasma renin activity, during controlled hypotension, whereas captopril, by inhibiting conversion of angiotensin I to angiotensin II, suppresses negative feedback and causes further renin release and a rise in plasma renin activity.

Uses. SNP is employed as a universal treatment for acute hypertensive crises. In this use, as in others, continuous monitoring of blood pressure, blood pH and lactate, and venous P_{O_2} is required to prevent excessive hypotension or cyanide toxicity. Because SNP is converted to thiocyanate, serum levels of the latter ion should be determined every other day if the infusion is maintained for longer than 72 hours. The infusion should be terminated if serum thiocyanate level exceeds 1.2 mg/dl, in order to avoid thiocyanate toxicity. SNP infusion should be particularly closely supervised in patients with cerebrovascular or coronary insufficiency, because the drug can produce rapid and precipitous declines in blood pressure.

The drug is frequently employed for controlled hypotension to produce a drier surgical field and to reduce surgical blood loss. SNP will enhance renal blood flow in postoperative cardiac surgery, provided that hypotension is prevented by intentional expansion of fluid volume.

SNP has been used to treat severe congestive heart failure through its actions in reducing both cardiac preload and afterload. The decline in afterload reduces end-systolic ventricular volume and promotes an increase in stroke volume and a reduction in heart size. The drug also enhances left ventricular function when given after acute myocardial infarction.

Hydralazine (Apresoline)

Hydralazine (1-hydrazinophthalazine) is an arterial vasodilator, employed parenterally in cases of acute hypertension and orally in the treatment of essential hypertension and of severe chronic congestive failure refractory to digitalis.

The drug is available as hydralazine hydrochloride (Apresoline) in 10-, 25-, 50-, and 100-mg tablets for oral use, and in 1.0-ml ampules containing 20 mg of drug for intravenous or intramuscular use.

Administration. The initial oral dose is 10 to 20 mg two to four times a day. This dose is increased until either a desired clinical response or toxicity is produced. Oral dosage should not exceed 400 mg/day for extended periods.

For the treatment of acute hypertensive episodes, 10 to 50 mg of the drug may be administered IM. For IV use, 10 to 20 mg of drug, in a volume of 20 ml, is administered, from a 20- to 50-ml syringe, at a rate not exceeding 0.5 ml/min. Blood pressure should be monitored continuously during administration, and the injection should be stopped frequently, when the blood pressure is dropping, to avoid hypotension. The injection of hydralazine from a syringe has advantages over the microdrip-regulated intravenous infusion because of the continual surveillance required for vasodilators like sodium nitroprusside or nitroglycerin.

In Vivo Disposition. Hydralazine is a base with a pKa of 7.1. Peak blood levels are achieved in 3 to 4 hours following oral administration. The drug is 90 percent bound to plasma protein and has a steady-state V_d of 2 to 6 L/kg. It appears to concentrate for long periods in the walls of muscular arteries, which may be the basis for its selective effect upon resistance vessels.

Elimination of intravenous hydralazine is reported as biphasic, with a distribution $t_{1/2}$ of 5 minutes and a terminal $t_{1/2}$ of 40 to 55 minutes. By the oral route, however, the terminal $t_{1/2}$ of the drug is about 25 minutes. The reason for this difference in $t_{1/2}$ by the two routes of administration is unclear. Mean total plasma clearance ranges from 4.4 to 8.3 L/kg/hr.

Hydralazine undergoes biotransformation both in liver and plasma. Hepatic metabolism involves both ring hydroxylation with glucuronide formation, and sequential acetylation and oxidation of the hydrazine side chain. The hydrazine side chain ($-NHNH_2$) on the phthalazine ring structure of the drug is acetylated to form N-acetylhydralazine. The acetylated hydrazine side chain undergoes rapid spontaneous cyclization to form 3-methyltriazolopthalazine (MTP), which is subsequently oxidized to form 3-hydroxymethyltriazolophthalazine (HMTP).

In the plasma, hydralazine is converted to acid-labile conjugates by interaction with carbonyl groups of endogenous aldehydes, ketones, and alpha-keto acids, to form hydrazones. This reaction proceeds even in blood samples "in vitro." One such derivative, hydrazine pyruvic acid hydrazone (HPH), makes up the major portion of such plasma conjugates. The elimination of $t_{1/2}$ of HPH is about 250 minutes. HPH plasma levels are usually 2.5 to 4 times those of hydralazine.

Hepatic acetylation of hydralazine is catalyzed by N-acetyl transferase. This is a polymorphic enzyme existing as a "slow" and a "fast" variant, distributed bimodally in the North American population. The population is thus divided equally between "fast" and "slow" acetylators. Fast and slow acetylator phenotypes are generally identified by measuring the acetylation of administered sulfamethazine. The fast and slow phenotypes acetylate about 60 and 15 percent of the drug, respectively, in 4 hours.

Acetylator phenotype does not influence intravenous hydralazine kinetics because extrahepatic clearance is much greater than hepatic clearance when the liver is bypassed using this route and because plasma conversion to hydrazone conjugates is not phenotype-dependent. Oral absorption of hydralazine, however, does correlate with acetylator phenotype, due to first-pass hepatic drug clearance. Oral hydralazine bioavailability is about 8 percent in fast, and 35 percent in slow, acetylators, providing peak drug plasma levels of 23 and 100 μM, respectively, following an oral dose of 1 mg/kg. The ratio of acetylated metabolites, such as MTP or HMTP, to HPH in 24-hour urine samples is ten times greater in fast than in slow acetylators.

Mechanism of Action. Hydralazine may cause vasodilation by inhibition of cyclic 3', 5'-nucleotide phosphodiesterase, resulting in an increase in intracellular cAMP, which stimulates calcium binding in smooth muscle cells, inducing relaxation of smooth muscle. This results in dilation of arterioles and arteries, with little effect on capacitance vessels, perhaps as a result of preferential distribution of the drug to arterial smooth muscle.

Cardiovascular Effects. The major pharmacologic effects of hydralazine are related to the cardiovascular system. Dilation of resistance vessels causes a decline in peripheral vascular resistance and mean arterial blood pressure, with diastolic pressure being more affected than systolic. Activation of the baroceptor reflex leads to tachycardia. The degree of tachycardia is unrelated to acetylator phenotype, but does correlate with a bimodal population distribution of sensitivity of baroceptor reflexes.

The positive chronotropic effect of hydralazine may have a central component, inasmuch as intracerebroventricular injection of small doses of the drug in animals causes tachycardia with no effect on blood pressure. The increased heart rate, together with the preferential decline in afterload, causes an increase in cardiac output, which is of benefit in congestive heart failure, but which may blunt the hypotensive response in acute hypertension.

Hydralazine enhances regional blood flow in coronary, cerebral, splanchnic, and, if blood pressure does not decline too severely, in renal vascular beds. Blood flow is generally unaffected in cutaneous and skeletal muscle vascular beds.

In clinical reports, the hypotensive response to intravenous hydralazine is dose related, with mean arterial pressure declining 8 percent and 17 percent at doses of 0.2 and 0.45 mg/kg, respectively. In initial clinical doses of 0.3 to 0.375 mg/kg intravenously, diastolic blood pressure declines by one third and mean arterial pressure by 12 to 13 percent, while heart rate increases by 40 percent. Onset of intravenous effect is 15 to 30 minutes.

By the oral route, 75- to 100-mg doses of hydralazine, in patients with refractory congestive failure, reduce systemic vascular resistance by 25 to 45 percent with minimal effects on mean arterial blood pressure and no influence on heart rate or right atrial pressure. As a result of reduced afterload, however, cardiac index, stroke volume index, and stroke work index all increase by 25 to 50 percent. In normal volunteers, 0.5 to 1.0 mg/kg orally reduces diastolic blood pressure by 25 percent, accompanied by a 27 percent increase in heart rate. Onset of action by the oral route is 45 to 75 minutes.

Hydralazine alters renal hemodynamics by enhancing renal blood flow, usually without affecting glomerular filtration rate or urine volume. Like many anti-hypertensives, however, the drug can cause sodium retention and a reduction in urine volume. This action may result in an increased plasma volume, leading to tolerance to the cardiovascular effects. This is prevented by coadministration of thiazide diuretics. When furosemide is given with hydralazine, the enhanced renal blood flow produced by the latter drug promotes a one-third increase in furosemide renal clearance (and an 18 percent decline in furosemide elimination $t_{1/2}$) by increasing proximal tubular secretion of the diuretic. Since furosemide acts at an intraluminal site in the ascending limb of the loop of Henle, its diuretic effect is enhanced by hydralazine.

Patients with heart failure respond to 75 to 100 mg oral hydralazine with a 32 percent decline in pulmonary vascular resistance and an 11 percent fall in mean pulmonary arterial pressure. Unlike other vasodilators, such as nitroglycerin and sodium nitroprusside, hydralazine does not inhibit pulmonary vasoconstriction in hypoxic areas of canine lung. Thus, shunting of blood from underventilated to ventilated alveolar areas is unimpaired by hydralazine, and the drug should not produce additional hypoxemia in patients with abnormal lungs, as do other vasodilators.

Adverse Effects. Intravenous hydralazine commonly causes facial flushing, vascular headache similar to that caused by nitroglycerin, and coldness of the extremities due to reflex vasoconstriction. The latter may cause paresthesias resembling Raynaud's disease. About one-third of treated patients vomit. Palpitations due to reflex tachycardia are often observed. Reflex myocardial stimulation may precipitate anginal attacks, or even myocardial infarction, in patients with IHD. The problem may be compounded by "coronary steal," i.e., dilation of patent coronary vessels diverting blood through collateral channels away from poorly perfused tissues supplied by obstructed coronary vessels. Among these side effects, beta-blocking agents significantly reduce the likelihood of palpitation, angina, facial flushing, and vascular headache.

Adverse effects of oral hydralazine are similar to those above, except that palpitations and angina are rare, and headache develops slowly over 2 to 6 hours only in slow acetylators. Vomiting is uncommon by the oral route.

A serious complication of longer-term oral hydralazine therapy is an apparent autoimmune reaction resulting in a syndrome resembling rheumatoid arthritis, which may progress to a state that mimics systemic lupus erythematosus (SLE). The arthritic picture develops in 10 percent of patients taking greater than 400 mg/day of the drug for more than 4 months, although the syndrome has developed in some patients receiving 100 mg/day for 3 weeks. The disease is phenotype dependent and is likely to occur in slow acetylators taking over 200 mg/day of the drug.

Drug-induced SLE differs from spontaneous SLE in that cardiovascular and renal involvement is rare, and men and women are almost equally affected. Symptoms include arthritis, myalgia, arthralgia, pleuritic pain and effusion, fever, weight loss, and hepatomegaly. Laboratory values show a consistent positive test for antinuclear antibody and for antibodies against single-stranded DNA. Elevated erythrocyte sedimentation rates and serum gamma-globulin levels are also common. Clinical signs of the disease resolve within a few months of drug withdrawal, but long-term corticosteroid therapy may be required. Serologic abnormalities may persist for several years. The SLE syndrome can be fatal if the drug is continued.

Uses. Hydralazine is of proven value in the treatment of mild to moderate essential hypertension, usually in conjunction with a thiazide diuretic and/or reserpine. It is also employed in patients with digitalis-refractory severe chronic cardiac failure where the drug produces a marked increase in cardiac output. Nitrates are also frequently coadministered to reduce cardiac preload and left ventricular filling pressure.

In hypertensive emergencies, hydralazine is particularly useful in those cases associated with acute glomerulonephritis or toxemia of pregnancy. In the latter situation, hydralazine, by relaxing uterine muscle and delaying labor, may prevent eclampsia-induced premature delivery. The drug is not consistently effective in controlling hypertensive encephalopathies associated with essential hypertension.

Diazoxide (Hyperstat IV)

Diazoxide is a direct-acting vasodilator with primary effects upon small arteries and arterioles, causing a prompt and profound reduction in blood pressure in hypertensive emergencies. It is chemically related to the thiazide diuretics but lacks diuretic activity.

The drug is available as Hyperstat IV in 20 ml ampules containing 300 mg diazoxide.

Administration. Diazoxide solutions are very alkaline and care must be taken to avoid extravasation. The intravenous dose is 5 mg/kg or 300 mg total. The drug must be administered rapidly in a single bolus dose from a syringe (within 15 seconds) to prevent inactivation by extensive plasma protein binding. In hypertensive patients with a mean control blood pressure of 230/130 mm Hg, 300 mg of diazoxide lowered blood pressure to 110/70 for 8 hours when injected in less than 10 seconds but only to 160/110 for 4 hours when the same dose was injected over a period of 4 minutes. Blood pressure declines in 3 to 5 minutes and remains reduced for 4 to 18 hours without wide fluctuations, largely obviating the need for close observation of the patient in an intensive care unit. Blood pressure rarely declines below the normal range, though postural hypotension may be severe for the initial half hour after injection.

In Vivo Disposition. Diazoxide is 90 percent bound to plasma albumin. The drug must, therefore, be administered rapidly since the concentration of free drug reaching vascular smooth muscle will be inadequate if time is allowed for equilibration with the binding protein.

Diazoxide exhibits biexponential elimination kinetics, with a distribution $t_{1/2}$ of about 10 minutes, and a terminal $t_{1/2}$ of 22 to 31 hours. Postdistributional plasma levels of about 20 μg/ml are achieved 10 to 15 minutes after a single intravenous dose of 300 mg. Steady-state V_d of diazoxide is 0.2 L/kg, and plasma clearance rate is 7 ml/min, with about one third due to renal clearance.

Cardiovascular Effects. Like hydralazine, diazoxide acts by blocking calcium-induced contraction of vascular smooth muscle by an undefined mechanism, resulting primarily in vasodilation of resistance vessels. Systolic and diastolic blood pressures promptly decline, eliciting sympathetically mediated reflex increases in heart rate, stroke volume, cardiac output, and plasma renin activity. All reflex responses are obtunded by beta-blocking agents.

Diazoxide-induced hypotension is generally so profound that cardiac workload and oxygen consumption are reduced, and the drug may safely be employed in patients with reduced myocardial reserve.

Pulmonary arterial pressure is usually unchanged, since pulmonary vasodilation offsets the increase in right ventricular output.

Adverse Effects. The major adverse effects of diazoxide relate to the cardiovascular and renal systems. Excessive hypotension, if induced, leads to cardiac stimulation, which may result in myocardial ischemia and infarction.

The renal effects of diazoxide are opposite to those of the thiazide diuretics, despite their chemical similarity. Diazoxide acts directly on the kidney to promote renal tubular sodium and water retention. This effect is exaggerated by a reduced glomerular filtration rate and renal blood flow when excessive hypotension is produced. The resulting expansion of fluid volume can cause frank edema in patients with myocardial inadequacy. This response is readily antagonized by coadministration of 40 mg furosemide intravenously.

In common with thiazide and loop diuretics, diazoxide inhibits proximal renal tubular secretion of uric acid, and may precipitate hyperuricemia.

Diazoxide also shares a hyperglycemic effect with thiazide diuretics. The mechanism appears to be inhibition of pancreatic insulin release (perhaps through an alpha-adrenergic mechanism), reduction of peripheral utilization of glucose, and release of endogenous catecholamines. The hyperglycemic response is enhanced by beta blockers, and attenuated by alpha-adrenergic blockade.

Chronic oral use of diazoxide in hypoglycemic patients has been associated with hypertrichosis, especially of the face.

Like hydralazine, diazoxide is a consistent relaxant of both the gravid and nongravid human uterus.

Uses. Diazoxide is useful in the treatment of crises associated with malignant hypertension, chronic or acute glomerulonephritis, eclampsia and hypertensive encephalopathy. The drug is not indicated in hypertension due to vascular abnormalities, or in cases involving excess catecholamine activity.

Diazoxide is available as Proglycem, in 50- and 100-mg oral tablets, for the control of hypoglycemia, including that due to insulin-secreting tumors of the pancreatic islet cells. A single dose increases blood glucose for up to 8 hours. The usual dosage is 3 to 8 mg/kg/day orally in divided doses for both adults and children.

Cardiovascular and Other Pharmacologic Adjuncts

Philip B. Hollander

ANTIARRHYTHMICS

*C*ardiac arrhythmias are initiated and defined by three conditions: (1) a disfunction or loss of impulse initiation in the sinoatrial (SA) node—the SA node is the normal site of electrical impulse formation; (2) a disturbance in impulse conduction; or (3) any combination of these two processes. If for any reason impulse formation occurs in cells other than those in the SA node then an arrhythmia is said to exist. If impulse conduction is altered thereby producing an altered, slower, or blocked impulse, then an arrhythmia is said to exist. Drugs used in the treatment of cardiac arrhythmias are selected to decrease the oxygen requirement, reduce automaticity and/or alter the reentry mode of the cardiac impulse. However, the administration of drugs may also result in a drug–drug interaction and establish the conditions which alter physiological function leading to a compromise in cardiac function. Cardiac arrhythmias occur in about 25% of the patients treated with digitalis, 50% of the patients undergoing anesthesia, and at least 80% of the patients presenting with an acute myocardial infarction. Cardiac arrhythmias have been redefined and explained in terms of the cellular mechanisms coincident with one or more phenomena associated with enhanced automaticity, abnormal excitability, and alteration in impulse conduction usually resulting in reentry. Delivery of a total or universally accepted antiarrhythmic drug therapy still awaits implementation. However, some useful antiarrhythmic drug therapy combinations are available to help prevent or abolish cardiac rhythm disorders that are present as slow (brady-), fast (tachy-), or other aberrant rhythms.

Electrophysiology

The preponderance of information defining the actions of antiarrhythmic agents is based upon microelectrode techniques used to develop theory (Hodgkins and Huxley, 1952a, b; Cole, 1968) applicable to nerve fibers. These techniques were extended to investigate the electrophysiology and electropharmacology of isolated cardiac tissues sections from different parts of the mammalian heart (McC. Brooks et al, 1955; Hollander and Webb, 1955; Webb and Hollander, 1956; Hollander and Webb, 1957; Hollander and Webb, 1967; Walsh et al, 1969; Ito et al, 1970; Hollander and Justus, 1971; Hollander and Moorman, 1974; Cranefield, 1975). Within the last 10 years some of these studies have been repeated and others undertaken using the patch clamp technique with an isolated approximate 0.3-μm diameter section of cell membrane (Sakmann and Nehr, 1983). This technique has been used to elaborate and define the various characteristics of the ion channels in cellular membranes (Flaim and Zelis, 1982). The patch clamp technique may be considered as an elegant modification of the microelectrode technique. In situ electrophysiological studies were also carried out using both animals and humans and it was found that the dog model mimicked the human very well. The cardiac action potential, obtained with microelectrodes inserted into isolated Purkinje fibers of the ventricle of dogs, has been defined by five phases. See Figure 18–4.

Phase 0 begins with a depolarization or upstroke of the action potential which is initiated when the resting membrane is stimulated to produce a voltage shift to its threshold of activation. In atrial and ventricular fibers this

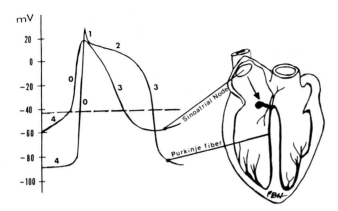

Figure 18–4. Diagrammatic representation of the heart and a normal action potential obtained from the sinoatrial node and Purkinje fibers. The horizontal dashed line represents the approximate threshold of activation for the sinoatrial node. The threshold of activation for the Purkinje fibers is in the range of −75 to −60 mV. The abscissa represents the time function; a full cycle of the normal action potential of the Purkinje fiber is approximately 1000 to 750 msec or 60 to 90 bpm.

is associated primarily with an immediate enormous increase in fast inward current carried primarily by an influx of sodium ions in designated channels. Some time later there is a slower inward current carried primarily by an influx of calcium ions in designated channels. When the level of membrane depolarization exceeds the threshold of activation, then depolarization becomes regenerative and further stimulation is not required.

Phase 1 is an early and transient voltage shift or repolarization most readily seen in Purkinje fibers. This repolarization may be associated with inward currents carried by an influx of chloride and calcium ions. Designated chloride channels have yet to be positively identified.

Phase 2 is seen as a momentary plateau with approximate zero or slowly moving to a negative membrane voltage. There is a balance between a slow inward current and a delayed rectifier current. Calcium ions are carried by the slow inward current and the delayed rectifier current is carried by potassium, or, simplistically, there is an increased inward current carried by an influx of calcium ions and decreased potassium and chloride flux.

Phase 3 is seen as the rapid repolarization of the membrane toward the resting membrane potential. There is an outward current associated with an increased efflux of potassium and inhibition of residual inward currents carried by sodium and calcium currents initiated during phases 0 through 2.

Phase 4, or diastole in cells other than nodal tissue, is the voltage–time sequence when the cell membrane potential is relatively constant and is in its unstimulated or resting state. During this phase of resting membrane potential there are slow changes in both potassium influx and sodium efflux which aid in restoring the intracellular milieu to its prestimulated state. This coupled exchange flux of potassium and sodium ions during phase 4 is under control of Na^+, K^+-ATPase, which participates in actively pumping these ions across the cell membrane.

Phase 4, or diastolic depolarization in nodal tissues, presents as a gradual decrease in outward potassium current that enables a small background inward current carried by sodium or calcium or outward chloride current to create the conditions essential for nodal activation. This condition is seen as a progressive decrease of the negativity of the membrane potential toward its threshold of excitation. When the progressive depolarizing membrane potential exceeds its threshold, then a regenerative depolarization is initiated. This is seen as a nodal action potential with voltage characteristics that however differ from nonnodal or normal "follower cells." All transmembrane potential voltages and their rates of change during an action potential cycle of nodal tissue are decreased in the range of 20% to 40% when compared to follower cells. It would appear that the inward current in nodal tissue is carried primarily by an influx of calcium ions, and response is usually seen in cells that have intrinsic rhythmicity. It also appears that there is a calcium channel which allows sodium entry. The paucity of sodium channels and lack thereof of a fast inward sodium current may explain the decreased conduction velocity in nodal tissues when compared to atrial or ventricular tissues.

Conduction velocities of all action potentials appear to be largely determined by the maximum velocity of the voltage change V_{max} of phase 0. The maximum in turn is dependent in part upon the polarity and magnitude of the membrane voltage at the beginning of phase 0. The more positive the resting membrane potential, the lower the depolarization and conduction rates. Thus there appears to be a direct relationship between the speed of depolarization or voltage change of phase 0 and the conduction velocity. The action potential depolarization and conduction rates of follower cells is 10 to 100 times higher than that observed in nodal tissues. A decreased conduction velocity may establish the conditions favorable for reentry of the conducted impulse into tissues and thereby induce an arrhythmia.

Pharmacology

Arrhythmias may be produced by different mechanisms and various arrhythmias respond to antiarrhythmic agents in a different manner (Miura and Rosen, 1983). Antiarrhythmic agents do not constitute a homogeneous chemical class and there are obvious differences in their pharmacology. All antiarrhythmic agents enumerated have the following general pharmacokinetic characteristics: Phenytoin appears to be the only drug that has zero-order pharmacokinetics; all other agents have first-order pharmacokinetics. Zero-order pharmacokinetics indicates that irrespective of the amount of drug in the body, only a constant amount will be metabolized or biotransformed in a given time. First-order pharmacokinetics indicates that a constant proportion of the drug contained in the body will be metabolized or biotransformed in a given time. With the exception of an unknown quantity for bretylium and less than 50% for lidocaine, oral absorption of all the indicated agents was between 75% and 90%. The volume of distribution, or tissue localization, for all agents was 0.5 (phenytoin) to more than 5 L/kg (amiodarone). Plasma protein binding is generally more than 60% to 95%, with the exception of procainamide

TABLE 18–5. ANTIARRHYTHMIC DRUGS (SUMMARY)

Drugs	Actions	Use
Bretylium	Increases action potential duration and inhibits the release of norepinephrine	Ventricular tachyarrhythmia
Cholinesterase inhibitors; e.g., neostigmine	Parasympathomimetic, blocks reentry	Paroxysmal supraventricular tachycardia (PST)
Digitalis	Increases AV conduction time, decreases atria and ventricle muscle refractory period	PST, atrial flutter and/or fibrillation
Lidocaine, phenytoin	Decreases automaticity and refractory period duration	Decrease ventricular arrhythmias
Propranolol, amiodarone	Slows nodal conduction time antiadrenergic action	Superventricular tachyarrhythmia
Quinidine, procainamide, disopyramide, encainide (phenytoin), mexiletine, tocainide	Decreases V_{max} and conduction rate and increases action potential refractory period	Suppress tachycardia and inhibits premature ventricular activities
Verapamil, nifedipine, diltiazem, aprinidine	Decreases calcium influx, depresses impulse formation, slows AV conduction, decreases contractile force	PST, superventricular tachyarrhythmias

and disopyramide which is less than 60%. Their half-life, $t_{1/2}$, or time to reduce the drug concentration to one-half the administered dose in the body, ranges from about 0.3 hours (lidocaine, tocainide and mexiletine) to 20 days (amiodarone). Lastly, all agents, with the exception of bretylium, are generally metabolized 35% to 95% by the liver; the kidney is the main route of excretion. Bretylium may be excreted unchanged. A summary of antiarrhythmic drugs is given in Table 18–5.

Many of the underlying factors that predispose cardiac muscle to arrhythmias appear operant primarily in ischemic tissue. These factors include an early significant shortening of the action potential duration and coincident refractory period, changes in threshold or excitability, automaticity changes in normal or induced ectopic foci, and conduction changes coincident with the depolarization rate of the cardiac action potential. Most antiarrhythmic agents may be ordered into four distinct groups: (1) local anesthetics, (2) antiadrenergic, (3) calcium channel blockers, and (4) other agents. This classification, based upon factors established by and associated with electrophysiology and pharmacology, enables a great deal of information to be readily presented and easily compared.

Group 1 drugs that block sodium channels and therefore demonstrate depressant or local anesthetic properties, include quinidine, procainamide, disopyramide, encainide, lidocaine, mexiletine, tocainide, aprindine and phenytoin. The electrophysiological effects usually demonstrated by quinidine are shared by procainamide, disopyramide, encainide, and somewhat by aprindine. Similarly, the effects attributed to lidocaine, seen later, are shared by mexiletine, tocainide, phenytoin, and somewhat by aprindine. Significant differences exist between the action of quinidine and lidocaine. For example, the effects of quinidine, dependent upon the heart rate because it binds more slowly and more progressively, appear to act both during depolarization, or V_{max}, and repolarization phases of the action potential. Quinidine is also anticholinergic. Lidocaine has a minimal

electrophysiological effect on normal tissues. Its action is dependent upon the initial state of the membrane depolarization voltage and appears to act primarily in the depolarization phase of the action potential. Lidocaine does not appear to alter the action potential plateau characteristics suggestive that there is no calcium channel involvement. Phenytoin seems to be the best drug available for digitalis intoxication. The local anesthetic properties assigned to drugs in this group also produce a decreased spontaneous rate due to (1) an elevation of the threshold of regenerative activation and (2) a depression of the spontaneous diastolic depolarization of cells in normal pacemaker or ectopic focal sites. There is also noted a depression in the conduction velocity which is related to a depression of V_{max} coincident with phase 0 or depolarization of the action potential. Lastly, there is an alteration, increase by quinidine or decrease by lidocaine, of the refractory period coincident with an inhibition of reentry.

Group 2 drugs, including propranolol, nadolol, timolol and amiodarone, alter catecholamine-induced effects because of their antisympathetic or sympatholytic actions. Generally, these agents decrease automaticity and oxygen demand of the heart by decreasing heart rate and contractile force. Amiodarone depresses the action potential V_{max}, prolongs the action potential duration, and significantly increases the force of cardiac contraction in compromised hearts. The depression of the V_{max} may be the cause for slowing the sinus rate and AV conduction, while the prolongation of the action potential duration would result in an increase of the refractory period inhibiting impulse reentry.

Group 3 consists of calcium-blocking drugs including verapamil, nifedipine, nicardipine, and diltiazem. These drugs may depress or inactivate the slow calcium channel without influencing the V_{max}. On the other hand, the effects of calcium blockers may be influenced by sodium channel responses. Impulse formation in the sinus and AV node, and subsequent conduction of the electrical response is in part associated with a slow inward calcium current especially when sodium current is inactivated. Verapamil reduces the rate of rise and phase 4 diastolic depolarization potential in the sinus node. Diltiazem is also used as a coronary and systemic vasodilator (Priebe and Skarvan, 1987). The pharmacological effects of the calcium blockers may be manipulated through the use of anesthetic agents. Halothane, enflurane, and/or isoflurane depress the sinus node rate of discharge and conduction. This action mimics calcium channel blocking activity, and seems to alter intracellular calcium kinetics as calcium blockers (Bosnjak and Kampine, 1983; Lynch, 1986; Lynch, et al, 1981; Lynch et al, 1982; Merin, 1987). Closed chest patients with reasonable ventricular function tolerate inhalation anesthetics and reasonable doses of calcium channel blockers. It was suggested that use of calcium channel blocking drugs during closed chest surgery may aid in the control of supraventricular tachycardia, hypertension, or coronary spasm. Bradyarrhythmias, if induced by calcium blockers, are readily treated with atropine or isoproterenol.

Group 4 drugs include bretylium and digitalis. Bretylium directly prolongs the action potential duration and refractory period of ventricle without altering V_{max}. This action would thus reverse the effects of ischemia, where the refractory period is shortened. Bretylium also markedly increases the stimulus required to initiate ventricular fibrillation. Lastly, bretylium also prevents the release of catecholamines. Digitalis is used in atrial flutter/fibrillation, and paroxysmal atrial or supraventricular tachycardia by increasing the refractory period and reducing conduction velocity in the AV-node. This action is induced by both parasympathomimetic and direct effects.

The clinical treatment, therapeutic guidelines, for management of arrhythmias can now be indicated. Treatment indicated starts with first line therapy and progresses through alternatives given in descending order.

1. Sinus bradycardia [<60 beats/min (bpm)] usually does not require treatment unless occurence is due to a secondary disease. Rates <40 bpm respond to IV or IM atropine.
2. Sinus tachycardia (100–160+ bpm) will respond to propranol TID or QID. Patient must be monitored due to negative inotropic effects of propranolol.
3. Acute atrial premature beats or paroxysmal supraventricular tachycardia or paroxysmal atrial tachycardia (PAT) (150–250 bpm) usually does not require treatment. Chronic atrial premature beats may be treated with quinidine, disopyramide, or procainamide.
4. Atrial flutter/fibrillation (245–350/350–600 bpm) are treated to reduce the ventricular rate by slowing the AV conduction and restoring normal rhythm. The choice of therapy depends in all cases on the state of the patient and the ventricular rate. Acute flutter/fibrillation treatment is based on DC-conversion, digitalis, verapamil, or propranolol. Chronic atrial fibrillation/flutter may be treated with digitalis, verapamil or amiodarone.
5. Acute paroxysmal premature beats may be treated with verapamil, digitalis and propranolol. Chronic paroxysmal premature beats may be treated with digitalis, verapamil, quinidine, or amiodarone.
6. Acute ventricular premature beats may be treated with lidocaine, procainamide, quinidine, or disopyramide. Chronic ventricular premature beats may be treated with quinidine, procainamide, disopyramide, or amiodarone.
7. Acute ventricular tachycardia (150–250 bpm) may be treated with DC-conversion, lidocaine, procainamide, disopyramide, quinidine, or bretylium. Chronic ventricular tachycardia may be treated with procainamide, disopyramide, quinidine, or amiodarone.
8. Wolff–Parkinson–White syndrome with or without PAT has a short PR interval and wide QRS complex may be treated with quinidine, procainamide, and propranolol.
9. Stokes–Adams disease is present as episodes of acute cerebral ischemia with impaired consciousness following sudden changes in cardiac rate, rhythm, or output. Treatment consists of sharp thumping on the precordium, IV infusion of isoproterenol or epinephrine, and temporary or permanent pacing.

Cardiac Glycosides (Digitalis)

In 1775, William Withering first published his classic description of his clinical experiences with purple foxglove, known today as digitalis, which was obtained from the plant *Digitalis purpurea*. Subsequent analysis has shown that he was so astute with his experimentation using the foxglove plant preparations that he produced a compound with a dose equivalent in activity to that used clinically today. One is now aware, due to the work of Johann Schmiedeberg, that the active ingredient in foxglove is digitoxin. Present-day economics dictate that digitoxin still be produced from the plant, rather than synthetically, using essentially the same techniques reported by Schmiedeberg more than 100 years ago.

Digitalis is today the fourth most prescribed drug in the United States and one of the most valuable cardiovascular active drugs in our armamentarium. It has, however, one of the lowest therapeutic indices of most drugs used (20 percent). Research to date has shown that digitalis glycoside is the only inotropic drug that also slows ventricular response in atrial flutter and fibrillation. This research also increased our comprehension of the mechanisms of cardiac contractility and has elaborated the possible iatrogenic causes of digitalis toxicity. Of all the 24 agents classified and tested for positive inotropic action, with the exception of calcium and digitalis, no reported agent investigated to date is a pure inotrope. However, all agents tested can exert positive inotropic and vasodilatory actions. It also has been demonstrated that one essential activity of digitalis is to specifically inhibit a membrane-bound Na–K-activated ATPase, which is instrumental in transmembrane transport of sodium and potassium. Recently it has been suggested that there appears to be a calcium entry regulatory mechanism that may augment the digitalis response producing a positive inotropy.

All cardiac glycosides do not have the same pharmacokinetic properties, resulting in differences of clinical effects. These consist of differences in uptake by the heart and the CNS, distribution, inotropic responses, and toxicities. The area postrema and surrounding sites in the CNS appear to be involved in toxic manifestations as well as regulation of systemic, peripheral, and coronary vascular resistance. Another significant factor in the toxicity of digoxin can be seen with the concurrent administration of quinidine. There appears to be a doubling of serum digoxin when quinidine is administered to patients who are receiving digoxin dosages to maintain their therapeutic plateau. Amiodarone, lorcainide, propafenone, and verapamil also have been shown to induce an increase in serum digoxin concentration. Most anesthetic agents tested, with the exception of cyclopropane, appear to protect against experimental dysrhythmia in dogs. Similarly, many antacids, barbiturates, lidocaine, and phenytoin may interact with digitalis and afford some protection against toxicities. Obviously there are different mechanisms of action to explain how the various agents listed above can afford some protection against digitalis toxicity. On the other hand, calcium, hypokalemia, many diuretics, large glucose infusion, insulin, liver disease, hypomagnesemia, quinidine, reserpine, and succinylcholine may all be contributing factors to digitalis toxicity.

Calcium (Antagonists) Blockers

In 1937, Heilbrunn was the leading proponent that calcium was the essential element within the cell that was critical for activity. The influx of calcium ions through calcium channels in eukaryotic cells is now accepted to be a second messenger, link, in the modulation and regulation of a host of physiologic functions, including contraction of skeletal, smooth, and cardiac muscles. All eukaryotic cells can alter their activity under the influence of appropriate stimuli by increasing the amounts of free cytoplasmic calcium. Calcium influx from the extracellular medium, primarily through calcium channels, is increased by membrane alteration or excitation. This enhanced calcium influx from the extracellular medium increases the amounts of free intracellular calcium, to the micromolar range, and is one of several determinants of muscle activity. The increase in free calcium is augmented also from calcium stores within the cell; intracellular increases of free calcium, converting bound to free calcium, are thought to occur during membrane activation as well as by translocation of calcium or sodium into the cell. Sodium is thought to occupy the same binding site as calcium and cause its competitive release into the cytoplasm. These increased free calcium ions are bound to calcium receptors. The chemical states of these receptors are altered and usually activated, thereby in turn enabling interaction with specific proteins producing enzymatic and corresponding physiologic activities. Obviously, association of calcium with a particular receptor will dictate the succeeding physiologic activity. Generally, calmodulin presently appears to be the only calcium-binding protein thought to be a universal regulator of the calcium messenger or signal, regulating more than 30 different proteins and enzymes in a calcium-modulated manner. To date publications have

shown that there are more than 26 calmodulin antagonists, including verapamil, diltiazem, haloperidol, and beta-endorphins. Specifically, binding of calcium to the protein, troponin C, found in skeletal and cardiac muscle, will thereafter initiate a contractile event. Calcium has been shown not only to be generally essential for automaticity and contractility in cardiac muscle, but also to play a significant role in linking excitation of smooth muscle membrane to contraction—the excitation–contraction coupling link (E-C link).

Based on the foregoing, judicious selective inhibition of calcium channels by calcium antagonists represents a major therapeutic breakthrough. At least 26 examples can be found for alleviation of disease states after treatment with calcium blockers. What Heilbrunn is to calcium and cellular function, Fleckenstein is to calcium blockers. He published 20 years ago that this new class of drugs, using verapamil as the model, would mimic the cardiac effects of simple calcium withdrawal. The inhibitory effects of verapamil would be promptly nullified through addition of calcium, cardiac glycosides, or beta-adrenergic catecholamines. These data would suggest that cardiac glycosides, beta-adrenergic catecholamines, or both modulate calcium in a different way than do calcium blockers. It is now generally accepted that the calcium blockers represent a drug group that is clearly different from beta-receptor blockade as represented by propranolol. Organic calcium-channel blockers may be divided into five distinct chemical groups: (1) papaverine derivatives like verapamil; (2) dihydropyridine derivatives like nifedipine; (3) benzothiazine derivatives like diltiazem; (4) piperazine derivatives like lidoflazine and flunarizine; and (5) others, like prenylamine, perhexiline, and terodiline, to mention just three. It is of some interest that the piperazine group of drugs also are potent antihistamines. The wide range of chemical structures, indicated above, suggests that there may be more than one mechanism by which this group of drugs acts at cellular membranes, if this is indeed the only site of their action. There may be three possible sites of action at the membrane for this group of drugs: the outer mouth of the calcium channels, with which agents such as dihydropyridines interact; the inner mouth of the calcium channels, with which agents such as verapamil interact; and another site of action, possibly in the "middle" of the calcium channels, with which agents such as diltiazem interact. It is also of some interest that flunarizine is more than 15 times more active on smooth muscle than on atrial muscle. All of the calcium blockers appear to increase coronary blood flow and redistribute the flow to favor subendocardial layers. Blood flow to the brain is also increased. Generally speaking, the half-life of these calcium-channel blockers ranges from 2 to 8 hours. It may be possible that the wide variation in effect and specificity of calcium-channel blockers can be explained by the way these drugs interact with the calcium channels and their dissimilarity in chemical structure, which would lead to wide variation in their pharmacokinetics. As more is learned about calcium-channel blockers and their mechanisms of action, it is likely that the knowledge gained will not only aid in the rational use of these drugs, but that more specific agents will be developed to modify and correct other physiologic or pathologic functions.

Drug–Drug Interactions

Current clinical anesthetic practice encompasses the actions and interactions to multiple drugs that act generally to induce hypnosis, skeletal muscle relaxation, analgesia, and blocking of reflexes as well as specifically to induce and obtund cardiovascular reflexes and offer cardiovascular protection. The use of adjuvant drugs, so-called since they assist in the control of the patient responses in the practice of clinical anesthesia, facilitates titration of the state of awareness of the patient currently unobtainable through the use of most inhalation volatile anesthetics. The time of the use of a single general anesthetic agent, to provide all of the requirements for anesthesia, may have been relegated to history.

A simple review of some basic pharmacologic principles and that of drug interaction seems warranted. Summation, or a dose–effect additive effect, is seen when the combined effect of two or more drugs acting simultaneously is the same as the arithmetic sum (S) of the effect of the individual drugs A + B in their selected doses (A + B = S). Synergism indicates that the simultaneous total effect of drug A + B will be greater than the effect of either drug A or B, provided that both drugs evoke a similar response (A + B > A or B). Potentiation, which may be considered a special case of synergism, is the augmentation of an effect of drug A by drug B even though drug B may not have any discernible effect on its own (A + B > A, B = 0). By definition, antagonism is that effect where the administration of drug A in the presence of drug B decreases the effectiveness of drug B (A + B < B).

Agonism would be the effect observed when an exogenously administered drug mimics the effects observed with endogenous drugs. Intrinsic activity is the ability of an exogenously administered drug to produce an effect usually seen with an endogenous substance. Drug allergy is due to an altered state of reaction to drugs produced from a prior sensitization. Idiosyncrasy is defined as an untoward or abnormal response to a drug. Tolerance will be noted when there is a decreased physiologic response with repeated drug administration of the same or chemically related drugs. Tachyphylaxis is that special case of tolerance that occurs rapidly with repeated frequent drug administration. Cumulation is seen when the body does not completely metabolize one dose of a drug prior to administration of the second dose. Drug dependence, preferred to the previous terminology of habituation and addiction, may be physical or psychic. Physical dependence refers to an altered physiologic state that produces enormous physical discomfort when the drug is withdrawn. Psychic dependence denotes the emotional reliance on drugs to maintain oneself and "function" in an acceptable fashion.

Drug interactions may be separated into three divisions. However, these divisions are strictly a didactic tool. Some drugs, like phenothiazines, show interactions that encompass all three of the divisions.

- *Division 1* includes pharmaceutical interactions that occur in vitro and/or in vivo. These drug–drug interactions may be due to chemical, physical, or physiologic influences. For example, penicillin G is incompatible with heparin when mixed together in a single tube or bag for administration; cholestyramine administration decreases digitalis availability for, and utilization by, the body; agents that alter gastric pH will influence the absorption of acetylsalicylic acid by the gut; opiate administration alters gastric motility and slows the drug absorption processes.

- *Division 2* includes pharmacokinetic factors that may be attributed to the physiologic state of the patient or the influence of other drugs. For example, the presence of lipids will slow the absorption of alcohol from the gut; alcohol or phenylbutazone will alter the plasma-protein binding of warfarin; kidney disease will prolong the duration of those drugs requiring the kidney for their route of elimination; the genetic lesion resulting in a decreased metabolism of succinylcholine is well known; propranolol administration will produce bronchoconstriction, increase airway resistance, and thereby decrease the ventilation–perfusion ratio in patients; sulfonamides inhibit and barbiturates stimulate the hepatic microsomal drug metabolizing enzyme system.

- *Division 3* includes pharmacodynamic interactions due to the ongoing effects of endogenous and/or exogenous drugs as associated with active or silent receptors. For example, halothane will produce cardiac arrhythmias when the catecholamines level is excessive; administration of a therapeutic concentration of potassium will modify the influence of digitalis on cardiac muscle; and neostigmine will alter the effects of succinylcholine.

Since drug effects can be strictly quantified only in a mathematical sense, one is constrained to deal with mean distribution for normal and abnormal responses. However, there are rarely sufficient data on hand to obtain these distributions and the anesthetist must be aware of and prepared to deal with possible untoward responses.

Preoperative Medications

Historically, preoperative medications have consisted of a combination of one or more of the following drugs: a narcotic, an antisialagogue/antimuscarinic, and a barbiturate/tranquilizer. With the increase in the number of surgeries being done on an outpatient basis, we have seen a concurrent decrease in the use of "traditional" preoperative medications. Also, there has been an increased use of oral medications versus intramuscular injections as the route of administration of these drugs. Narcotics, barbiturates, and tranquilizers are covered in other chapters so that pharmacology of those drugs will not be covered here.

Antisialagogue/Antimuscarinic Agents. Antisialagogues have long been employed as part of the preoperative regime to block the effects of parasympathetic autonomic discharge. The commonly employed drugs are atropine, scopolamine, and glycopyrrolate. The primary target areas for preanesthetic use of these drugs are the CNS, the cardiovascular system, the respiratory system, and the gastrointestinal (GI) system.

In doses usually administered clinically, the CNS responses to atropine and glycopyrrolate are minimal, although a mild stimulant effect on the medullary centers has been reported following atropine administration. However, scopolamine has a marked sedative effect, producing drowsiness and amnesia in some individuals. Under certain circumstances, administration of scopolamine followed by a painful stimulus has led to profound CNS stimulation and agitation in the patient.

Innervation of the atria of the heart and the sinoatrial node by parasympathetic (vagal) fibers accounts for the sensitivity of these fibers to muscarinic receptor blockade. Small preoperative doses of atropine, scopolamine, or glycopyrrolate may provide limited cardiac protection through vagal blockade.

Reduction of airway secretions is obtained even with preoperative doses of atropine, scopolamine, and glycopyrrolate. The upper and lower airway are innervated with parasympathetic fibers through the bronchial musculature and the salivary glands, allowing them to be particularly sensitive to the "drying" effects of these drugs. The relative value of this drug effect and its administration must be evaluated in individuals with respiratory diseases in whom more copious secretions may be beneficial, particularly in the postoperative period.

Blockade of muscarinic receptors reduces motility and secretions of the gastrointestinal tract. Therapeutic doses of glycopyrrolate appear to be effective in reducing the volume and amount of hydrochloric acid and mucin. However, relatively large doses of atropine must be administered to achieve this effect.

Antacids, H_2-Receptor Antagonists, Antiemetics. There has been an increased interest in anesthesia practice regarding the effects of gastric volume and pH on aspiration pneumonitis and in the use of antiemetics, particularly for outpatient surgery. Postoperative nausea and vomiting have long been associated with the effects of anesthetic agents, and recently considerable research has been conducted on prevention of nausea and vomiting in the postoperative period. Achievement of the goal to prevent postoperative nausea and vomiting begins with the administration of preventive drugs in the preoperative period.

Antacids are weak bases that react with gastric hydrochloric acid to form a salt and water. Their usefulness in the prevention of aspiration pneumonitis is to reduce gastric acidity by increasing gastric pH. Drugs such as aluminum hydroxide and magnesium hydroxide have been used to reduce gastric acidity. One of the disadvantages of these two drugs is that they both contain particulate matter that could cause pulmonary lesions if aspirated. Sodium citrate is a useful nonparticulate antacid that rapidly neutralizes gastric contents. A dose of 15 to 30 ml of a 0.3-M solution suffices to neutralize gastric acid in most cases.

H_2-receptor antagonists were introduced in the 1970s and their popularity has increased steadily. The most common preanesthetic agent of this type is cimetidine. This drug inhibits the action of histamine on the H_2 receptors of parietal cells, thereby reducing gastric acid output and concentration. The administration of cimetidine will lead to reduced volume and increased pH of gastric secretions.

The usual preoperative dose is 300 mg orally, but a patient can receive 300 mg four times a day if necessary. This drug may be administered intravenously as well.

A variety of other antiemetic drugs act centrally to block impulses in the chemoreceptor trigger zone. Metoclopramide is a potent central dopamine antagonist. This appears to be the principal effect responsible for its antiemetic properties. However, metoclopramide also has a stimulant effect in the gastrointestinal tract that accelerates gastric emptying. Metoclopramide appears to block the emetic effects of fentanyl and other narcotics. It can be given orally or intravenously in usual preoperative doses of 20 mg. Droperidol, a butyrophenone, has been shown to provide excellent protection against postoperative nausea and vomiting when administered preoperatively or early in the anesthetic process in doses of less than 2.5 mg administered intravenously. Numerous other agents may be used as antiemetics. Those mentioned here are simply the drugs that seem to be most commonly employed in clinical anesthesia practice today.

BIBLIOGRAPHY

Aaron H (ed): Dopamine for the treatment of shock. Med Lett 17:13–14, 1975.

Abrams J: Nitroglycerin and long-acting nitrates. N Engl J Med 302:1234–1237, 1980.

AMA Committee on Hypertension: The treatment of malignant hypertension and hypertensive emergencies. JAMA 228:1673–1679, 1974.

Andersson K-E: Calcium-entry blockers. A heterogenous family of compounds. Acta Med Scand 694 (Suppl):142–152, 1984.

Ariens EJ, Simonis AM: Physiological and pharmacological aspects of adrenergic receptor classification. Biochem Pharmacol 32:1539–1545, 1983.

Attia RR, Grogono AW, Domer FR (eds): Practical Anesthetic Pharmacology, 2nd ed. New York, Appleton & Lange, 1987.

Bowman WC, Rand MJ: Textbook of Pharmacology, 2nd ed. Oxford, Blackwell, 1980.

Bosnjak ZJ, Kampine JP: Effect of halothane, enflurane, and isoflurane on the SA node. Anesthesiology 58:314–321, 1983.

Cole KS: Membranes, Ions and Impulses. Los Angeles, University of California Press, 1968.

Cranefield P: The Conduction of the Cardiac Impulse. Mount Kisco, New York, Futura, 1975.

Dempsey PJ, Cooper T: Pharmacology of the coronary circulation. Annu Rev Pharmacol 12:99–110, 1972.

Diamond MJ: Anesthesia and emesis: Clinical usefulness of metoclopramide. Can Anaesth Soc J 32:198–204, 1985.

Faulks E, Jenkins LC: A comparative evaluation of cimetidine and sodium citrate to decrease gastric acidity; Effectiveness at the time of induction of anesthesia. Can Anaesth Soc J 28:29–32, 1981.

Flaim SF, and Zelis R: Calcium Blockers. Mechanisms of Action and Clinical Applications. Baltimore, Urban & Schwarzenberg, 1982.

Fleckenstein A: Verh Dtsch Ges Kreislaufforsch 34:15–34, 1968.

Goldberg LI: Cardiovascular and renal actions of dopamine: Potential clinical applications. Pharmacol Rev 24:1–29, 1972.

Janis EA, Triggle DJ: 1,4-Dihydropyridine Ca^{2+} channel antagonists and activators: A comparison of binding characteristics with pharmacology. Drug Dev Res, 4:257–274, 1984.

Johnson J, Mills JS: Calmodulin. Medical Research Reviews 6:341–363, 1986.

J Clin Pharmacol 25, 1985. The entire issue is dedicated to digitalis.

Hodgkin AL, Huxley AF: Currents carried by sodium and potassium ions through the membrane of the giant axon of loligo. J Physiol 116:449–472, 1952a.

Hodgkin AL, Huxley AF: A quantitative description of membrane current and its application to conduction and excitation in nerve. J. Physiol 117:500–544, 1952b.

Hollander, PB, Justus, JP: Electropharmacological control of cardiac myogenic activity in embryos. Comp and Gen Pharmacol 2:211, 1971.

Hollander PB, Moorman M: Direct determination of the electropharmacological factors modulating the refractory period of cell membranes of mammalian myocardium. Pharmacologist 16:268(442), 1974.

Hollander PB, Webb JL: Cellular membrane potentials and contractility of normal rat atrium and the effects of temperature, tension and stimulus frequency. Circ. Res. 3:604–612, 1955.

Hollander P, Webb JL: Effects of adenine nucleotides on the contractility and membrane potentials of rat atrium. Circ. Res. 5:349–353, 1957.

Hollander PB, Webb JL: Procedure to initiate a sustained aconitine-induced electrical arrhythmia in isolated intrinsically beating paired atria. Life Sciences 6:249–260, 1967.

Ito M, Hollander PB, Marks BH, Dutta S: The effects of six cardiac glycosides on the transmembrane potentials and contractile characteristics of right ventricle of guinea pig. J Pharmacol Exper Ther 172:188–195, 1970

Katz AM, Selwyn A: The Cardiac Arrhythmias. Sunderland, MA, Sinauer, 1983

Katzung BG: Basic and Clinical Pharmacology, 3rd ed. Los Altos, CA, Lange, 1987.

Kopin IJ: Catecholamine metabolism: Basic aspects and clinical significance. Pharmacol Rev 37:333–364, 1985.

Kruszyna H, Kruszyna R, Smith RP: Nitroprusside increases cyclic guanylate monophosphate concentrations during relaxation of rabbit aortic strips and both effects are antagonized by cyanide. Anesthesiology 57:303–307, 1982.

Lynch C: Differential depression of myocardial contractility by halothane and isoflurane in vitro. Anesthesiology 64:620–631, 1986.

Lynch C, Vogel M, Sperelakis N: Halothane depression of myocardial slow action potentials. Anesthesiology 55:360–368, 1981.

Lynch C, Vogel M, Pratila MD, Sperelakis N: Enflurane depression of myocardial slow action potentials. J Pharmacol Exp Ther 222:405–409, 1982.

Merin RG: Calcium channel blocking drugs and anesthetics: Is the drug interaction beneficial or detrimental? Anesthesiology 66:111–113, 1987.

McC.Brooks C, Hoffman B, Suckling EE, Orias O: Excitability of the heart. New York, Grune and Stratton, 1955.

Miura DS, Rosen MR: New directions in the development of antiarrhythmic drugs. J Clin Pharmacol 24:333–341 1983.

Myers MG, Harris L: Antiarrhythmic drugs. In H Kalant, WHE Roschlau, EM Sellers (eds): Principles of Medical Pharmacology, 4th ed. New York, Oxford University Press, 1985.

Priebe AJ, Skarvan K: Cardiovascular and electrophysiologic interactions between diltiazem and isofluorane in the dog. Anesthesiology 66:114–121, 1987.

Reece PA, Cozamanis I, Zacest R: Kinetics of hydralazine and its main metabolites in slow and fast acetylators. Clin Pharmacol Ther 28:769–778, 1980.

Sakmann B, Neher E: Single-Channel Recording. New York, Plenum Press, 1983.

Sellers EM, Koch-Weser J: Protein binding and vascular activity of diazoxide. N Engl J Med 281:1141–1145, 1969.

Shepherd A, Lin MS, McNay J, Ludden T, Musgrave G: Determinants of response to intravenous hydralazine in hypertension. Clin Pharmacol Ther 30:773–781, 1981.

Shlevin HH: Animal pharmacology of nitroglycerin. Life Sci 30:1233–1246, 1982.

Smith NY, Miller RD, Corbascio AN: Drug Instructions in Anesthesia. Philadelphia, Lea & Febiger, 1981.

Tinker JH, Michenfelder JD: Sodium nitroprusside: Pharmacology, toxicology, and therapeutics. Anesthesiology 45:340–354, 1976.

Vennesland B, Castric PA, et al: Cyanide metabolism. Fed Proc 41:2639–2648, 1982.

Walsh MJ, Hollander PB, Truitt EB Jr: Sympathomimetic effects of acetaldegyde on the electrical and contractile characteristics of isolated left atrium of guinea pigs. J Pharmacol Exper Ther 167:173–186, 1969.

Webb JL, Hollander PB: Metabolic aspects of the relationship between the contractility and membrane potential of the rat atrium. Circ Res 4:618–616, 1956.

Wester RC, Maibach HI, Guy RH, Noonan RC: Nitroglycerin pharmacodynamics monitored noninvasively by laser Doppler velocimetry. Clin Pharmacol Ther 33:263, 1983.

Wilson SL, Martina NR, Halverson JD: Effects of atropine, glycopyrrolate, and cimetidine on gastric secretions in morbidly obese patients. Anesth Analg, 60:37–40, 1981.

Part IV
APPLIED PHYSIOLOGY

19

Nervous System Physiology

Joseph T. Rando

The human nervous system is an extensive network of billions of interconnected neurons supported by glial cells. The complexity of this system presents an overwhelming number of details. It is therefore recommended that this chapter be read and reviewed in an effort to understand the role that the nervous system plays in the function of the entire human organism.

GROWTH AND DEVELOPMENT OF THE NERVOUS SYSTEM

Embryonic Formation

The embryonic formation of the human brain requires the production of 45,000 neurons per minute, assuming a typical human gestation period of 40 weeks. The neurons form by mitosis throughout gestation, their production ending shortly before parturition. Although all of the neurons are formed by the time of birth, noticeable changes occur thereafter. These will be elaborated in this chapter. It has been demonstrated that the human nervous system is functional by the end of the second month of gestation. Activity is manifested by the avoidance reflex, which the fetus expresses by moving the head when stimulated.

The brain develops from the ectodermal layer of the neural plate. As the ectoderm thickens along what will become the back, it begins to curl into a neural tube. The first part of the neural folds to fuse are in the cervical region. As the fusion continues caudally and cephalically, additional areas of ectoderm develop to form primordial structures of the sense organs—i.e., ears, nose, and eyes. The cephalic portion of the neural tube enlarges as it fuses and becomes the brain. The neural tube is completely fused by the 24th gestational day, leaving down its center a lumen that becomes the ventricular system of the brain and the central canal of the spinal cord.

As the neural tube continues to develop, the spinal cord portion differentiates into three distinct cell layers. The inner layer of cells lining the central canal is made up of columnar epithelial cells and is called the matrix. Through mitosis, it is the source of origin of the other

two layers. The middle layer of cells, called the mantle layer, is high in neuron content. It becomes the gray matter of the spinal cord. The outer layer of cells is also formed from the matrix, and these cells migrate to their final position, where they become the white matter of the spinal cord. These cells make up the marginal layer of the cord.

Sensory and motor neurons form from the matrix cells of the neural tube as the tube becomes grooved by the sulcus limitans, an indentation on the lateral aspect of the entire length of the spinal cord. The area posterior to the sulcus limitans, called the dorsal or alar plate, becomes the sensory nuclei associated with input from the peripheral, spinal, and cranial nerves. The alar plate also forms the telencephalon and diencephalon portions of the brain, which will be discussed later in this chapter. The area anterior to the sulcus limitans, known as the ventral or basal plate, becomes the motor nuclei. It is also associated with the functions of cranial and spinal nerves and forms the lobes of the brain known as the metencephalon, rhombencephalon, and myelencephalon. Recognizing this developmental anatomy aids in understanding the premise of the Bell–Magendie law, which states that sensory nerve fibers enter the posterior cells of the spinal cord and motor neurons exit the anterior spinal segments.

Until the third prenatal month, the spinal cord extends the entire length of the vertebral column and the nerves entering and leaving the cord exit the vertebral column at right angles. After the third gestational month, the vertebral column elongates faster than the spinal cord. At birth, the spinal cord ends at the level of the third lumbar vertebra. This disproportionate elongation of spinal cord and vertebral column results in the nerves leaving the lumbar, sacral, and coccygeal areas at an acute angle caudally. Additionally, the subarachnoid space below the first lumbar area is occupied by multiple nerves making up the cauda equina.

Adjacent to the neural tube as it develops are 31 pairs of somites arranged in sequence from the first cervical to the coccygeal level. Each of these pairs of somites differentiates into muscles, bone, and connective tissues and is innervated by one pair of spinal nerves. As these somite structures grow and develop, they take their innervation along. This is exemplified by the diaphragm, which originates at the cervical level and pulls the innervation from C3, C4, and C5 to its final location in the abdomen.

The brain is a three-vesicled organ prior to the second gestational month. It consists of a prosencephalon, mesencephalon, and rhombencephalon. At about the 36th day of gestation, the prosencephalon subdivides into the telencephalon and the diencephalon and the rhombencephalon subdivides into the metencephalon and the myelencephalon. After this, the brain continues to grow in size by becoming more contorted through the formation of flexures and enlarged areas. The surface area of the brain is increased by the formation of sulci and gyri, which are generally present by the seventh gestational month, are patterned individually, and continue to form unique individual patterns throughout life.

Postnatal Development

It is well recognized that the brain of the newborn is proportionately larger than that of the adult (10 percent of body weight and 2 percent of body weight, respectively). The newborn's brain continues to develop rapidly, and by the end of the second year of life the relative size and proportions of all parts of this organ are similar to those of the adult brain. From an average birth weight of 350 g, the brain grows to approximately 1000 g. By puberty, it has reached the adult size of 1450 g in the male and 1350 g in the female. We can determine from these figures that the newborn brain triples in size during the first year of life.

Among the documented functions of the nervous system is the avoidance reflex at 8 weeks of gestation. The fetus will withdraw the head in response to stimulation of the upper lip. There is also evidence of intercostal muscle activity by 13 weeks. Another sense that has been documented at birth is the sense of touch, which is well developed. Vision develops rapidly in the newborn, who can at first only distinguish light from dark. By 1 month of age, newborns can follow an object placed in front of their eyes, although newborns are usually farsighted. Hearing is rudimentary at birth, because the structures in the middle ear are not well developed. In addition, there is no air in the eustachian tube at birth. The senses of taste and smell are present at birth and become well developed in the first 2 months of life. Pain sensations are also present at birth, although the infant cannot localize pain. It is thought that infants have decreased sensitivity to pain, and it has been established that they certainly are easily distracted from painful stimuli by stronger reflexes such as sucking.

As we explore the changes that occur in the brain and nervous system with age, we note that the neurons are essentially formed and differentiated at birth. We see that the number of neurons decreases with age, because when neurons die they are not replaced by new ones. This loss is generally not noticeable for several years, since humans have an excess and the remaining neurons will compensate for slight losses. One estimate of the rate of neuron loss between 20 and 70 years of age places the loss at 100,000 neurons per day, or a 10 percent total loss over that half century of aging. Of course, a person can exaggerate that rate of destruction through abuse. Several changes have been documented to occur in neurons as they age. There

is an increase in pigmentation, especially up to the age of 40 years. This is the result of an accumulation of RNA within the neurons. By contrast, there is a decrease of Nissl substance, which has been identified as ribosomes. RNA decreases after about 60 years of age. There is a decrease in total brain weight with age. Cerebral blood flow decreases approximately 20 percent by age 75. There is a 66 percent decrease in taste buds and a 10 percent decrease in the velocity of impulse conduction in aged persons. In addition, there are meningeal calcification, increased ventricular size, and atrophic changes in the rhinencephalon, insula, and frontal and parietal lobes.

Developmental Abnormalities

A number of developmental abnormalities affect the nervous system. Noback and Demarest (1981) classified them into two categories—genetic and environmental. Among the developmental abnormalities of the nervous system associated with genetic origin is Down's syndrome. The occurrence of this abnormality is 1 in 800 births. More than 90 percent of these cases are due to the presence of extra material at chromosome 21. Another genetic abnormality is phenylketonuria, which results in an accumulation of phenylalanine hydroxylase. Environmental factors can also influence central nervous system formation. Some of these factors include German measles, syphilis, increased irradiation, birth trauma, or chemical exposure. Cytomegalovirus infection in the mother is most detrimental to the fetus in the second trimester of pregnancy. The incidence is 4 to 10 infected infants per 1000 live births, and manifestations include mental retardation, micrencephaly, and deafness. Maternal nutritional deficiencies may affect the infant. Infant or childhood nutritional deficiencies can manifest as marasmus or kwashiorkor, especially during the first 2 years of life. Cretinism may occur in the infant of a mother who had decreased thyroid function during the last trimester of pregnancy. Hypoxia during the last half of pregnancy or the first month of life may lead to cerebral palsy, mental retardation, cortical atrophy, or sclerosis of white matter. Finally, developmental abnormalities of the neural tube can lead to a number of central nervous system anomalies including anencephaly, spina bifida, and meningomyelocele. Their occurrence is more frequent in female infants, and the overall combined incidence is approximately 5 in 1000 live births.

NEURONS AND REFLEX ARCS

Classification, Structure, and Function of Neurons

The neuron is recognized as the basic structural and functional unit of the nervous system. Along with connective tissue, it makes up the totality of the nervous system. Neurons interconnect across synapses, which will be described in more detail later in this chapter.

The cell body is an important component of a neuron because it acts as a necessary part—without it the neuron would die. The cell body is also called the soma or the perikaryon, and most are visible with a light microscope. They are polymorphic and are surrounded by a cell membrane made up of the typical sugar-fat-protein configuration. Within the cell membrane of the cell body are several organelles. Along with the typical nucleus, nucleolus, and endoplasmic reticulum are also large numbers of mitochondria, especially at synapses and nodes of Ranvier, which will be described later. The cell bodies also contain structures called Nissl bodies, which are large granules of ribonucleoprotein such as is found in the ribosomes of other cells. They are located on the endoplasmic reticulum and are also freely distributed in the cytoplasm of the cell body. These Nissl bodies are critical to normal cell function, protein synthesis, and neuronal repair; increasing as these processes are carried out. There is very little chromatin (DNA), possibly reflecting the cell body's inability to regenerate. Neurofibrils made up of strands of protein can be seen throughout the cytoplasm, especially if neuronal regeneration is occurring. Golgi bodies and lyosomes typically exist in the cell body, conducting functions similar to those in other cells. The cell body varies in size from 0.1 to 13.5 millimicrons. Cell bodies are found in the gray matter of the brain and in the peripheral nervous system as autonomic nervous system ganglia and dorsal root ganglia, and as sensory ganglia of the cranial nerves.

The functions of the cell body are to receive nerve endings that convey excitatory or inhibitory stimuli generated in other nerve cells and to transmit them to the remainder of the neuron. It must also be kept in mind that the cell body contains the organelles essential for the overall functioning of the neuron as a viable unit.

Another component of the neuron is the dendrite. The dendrite is usually short, seldom extending more than 700 millimicrons from the cell body. Generally, there are many dendrites extending from the cell body, with as many as 4000 being identified from some neurons. This extensive arborization allows far-reaching relay of stimuli. In addition, the dendrites have small, spinelike projections called gemmules, which increase the surface area for contact. Dendrites lack a Golgi apparatus but do have Nissl bodies, mitochondria, and neurofibils. The function of a dendrite is to conduct excitatory or inhibitory impulses to the cell body.

A third component of the neuron is the axon. It originates from a broadened area of the cell body known as the hillock. Only one axon arises from a cell body, and it enlarges slightly in diameter beyond the first 100 μm of the hillock. This portion of the axon from the hillock to where the axon begins to enlarge is called the initial segment. The axon is longer and narrower than the dendrite and composes the bulk of the nervous system white matter. Axons have terminal branches that arborize, and each of these branches is known as a telodendron. The end of each telodendron has an enlarged knob called a bouton. It is these boutons that liberate a neurohumoral transmitter substance to aid in the transmission of a "message" from one neuron to another. Many of the axons are covered by a layer of fat and protein material known as myelin. It is arranged like a jelly roll around the axon and is avascular, thereby giving the axon a white appearance. The myelin is secreted by cells that surround all peripheral axons. Schwann's cells are present in the axon, and they originate from an outer layer covering the axon also known as neurilemma. In contrast to the myelin, the neurilemma is a thin,

delicate, nucleated, fatty substance. Axons with a diameter greater than 2 μm are usually myelinated and those smaller are not. The myelination of axons occurs in an intermittent fashion, and each portion of myelin sheath is 0.08 to 1 mm long. The gap between two adjacent Schwann's cells wrapped around the axon is called the node of Ranvier. It is from these gaps or nodes of Ranvier that collateral axons extend from the main axon, usually at a 90-degree angle.

The axon functions to conduct stimuli away from the cell body of its neuron. Because of the elaborate array of telodendrons and collateral axons, impulses can be conducted to (1) the dendrite of an adjacent neuron, in which case there is axondendritic conduction; (2) the cell body of an adjacent neuron, called axosomatic conduction; or (3) the axon of another neuron, called axoaxonal conduction.

Generally, no neuronal covering exists around the cell body or dendrites of a neuron; nor does it exist around the teledondrons or boutons. Axons may have various types of coverings. Peripheral axons are encircled by the neurilemma, consisting of a sheath of Schwann or Schwann's cells. Smaller-diameter axons (less than 2 μm) have only a single layer of covering and are therefore said to be unmyelinated. Larger axons of the peripheral nervous system have a thicker layer of myelin, as described earlier. This myelin is secreted by the neurilemma and lies inferior to it in a jelly-roll fashion. It accounts for the white appearance of nerves. The amount of myelinization of nerves differs, but all peripheral nerves contain this covering, with the exception of some postganglionic autonomic nerves and some afferent nerves transmitting pain sensation (slow pain fibers). The myelinization of nerves is incomplete at birth. Sensory fibers are almost completely myelinated, but motor nerves require 2 to 3 years for complete myelinization to occur. Myelinization serves several functions and provides certain advantages. Myelin covering prevents cross-talk or interference between impulse conduction among adjacent axons. Myelinated nerves are less susceptible to damage and have a faster rate of impulse conduction, in addition to requiring less ion flux, because they only depolarize at the node of Ranvier. This is further explained later in this chapter. In the central nervous system, myelin is secreted by connective tissue cells known as oligodendroglia since there is no neurilemma covering these axons. Myelin does cover those central nerves outside the gray matter, accounting for the white appearance of white matter of the brain and spinal cord.

In looking at the organization of nerves, we find that the axon is central to what is often called a nerve fiber. The axon is surrounded immediately by myelin, which is then covered by neurilemma. An additional covering known as endoneurium closely surrounds the neurilemma. Several fibers thus invested are surrounded by perineurium, a thicker connective tissue covering, collecting these fibers into fascicles. The fascicles in turn are joined together by a similar covering of connective tissue known as epineurium. Finally, nerves are often grouped together into fascial compartments separating them from muscles and blood vessels.

Neurons have typically been classified in three ways based on the number of processes, the diameter of the axon, or the length of the axon. Based on the number of processes, bipolar neurons have dendrites on one end and an axon on the other with a cell body interposed between. The unipolar neuron is called a modified bipolar neuron in that a common pathway is shared by the axon and dendrite connecting the cell body. A multipolar neuron has many short dendrites and one long axon, which may have collateral branches off the axon at a 90-degree angle near the cell body.

Classification of neurons based on the diameter is somewhat more complex, but it is commonly referred to by clinicians and academicians alike. The first group is referred to as A-type neurons. They are myelinated and have the largest-diameter axons, ranging from 2 to 22 μm. Since the velocity of neuron conduction varies directly with the diameter of the axon, it is obvious that this group has the greatest velocity of conduction, 12 to 120 m/second. A-type neurons are further subdivided into alpha, which conduct impulses of proprioception and somatic motor innervation; beta, which conduct impulses of touch and pressure; gamma, which innervate muscle spindles; and delta fibers, which conduct temperature and fast pain impulses. A second group of neurons classed according to axonal diameter is known as B type. They are also myelinated, have a diameter of 1 to 3 μm, have a conduction velocity of 3 to 14 m/second, and function as preganglianic autonomic fibers. The third type of neurons in this group is C type. They are usually unmyelinated or only lightly myelinated and have a diameter of 0.3 to 1.3 μm and a conduction velocity of 0.2 to 2 m/second. These fibers serve two functions—to conduct slow pain impulses and to make up the postganglionic autonomic fibers.

The third means of classifying neurons is according to axonal length. This is an older and less frequently used method. The Golgi I neurons have long axons and make up spinal and peripheral neurons. Golgi II have short axons and are found in the brain and the interneurons of the spinal cord.

Neuronal Degeneration and Regeneration

In the process of degeneration and regeneration, the entire neuron responds to the injury, which acts as a stimulus to the neuron. In the process of degeneration, the whole neuron irreversibly degenerates if there is no neurilemma or if the cell body is destroyed. If the axon is cut, the distal portion and the myelin covering degenerate and macrophages consume the debris. This is termed Wallerian degeneration of the neuron conducting sensory impulses. Sensation would be interrupted to the affected area. If the neuron conducted motor impulses, the muscle would undergo atrophic changes. The proximal segment of the axon may show retrograde degeneration stopping short of the cell body. If the cell body is involved, no regeneration will occur.

The process of regeneration depends on

1. the presence of neurilemma
2. no cell body injury or involvement in degeneration
3. a minimal gap between the proximal and distal segments of the axon.

Regeneration occurs if the proximal end of the axon grows toward the neurilemmal sheath or shell of the distal portion of injured neuron. The neurilemma does not secrete a new axon, however. As the axon grows, if the distal portion of the neurilemmal sheath has not shifted or become distorted in any way, the growing axon will recannulate the distal portion of the axon and functional integrity will be reestablished. There is no proven chemical attraction between the two ends of the injured axon. The axon will regenerate at a rate of approximately 3 to 4 mm/day.

Reflex Arcs

Functionally integrated neuronal units incorporate the principles of the Bell–Magendie law, which states that "in the spinal cord the dorsal roots are sensory and the ventral roots are motor." Reflexes are traditionally classified according to the components of the unit into three types. The monosynaptic reflex is the simplest and, as its name implies, has one synapse. It includes a sensory receptor and a sensory neuron, which conduct afferent impulses into the dorsal horn of the spinal cord. This apparatus synapses in the cord, with a motor neuron carrying efferent impulses to an effector unit, usually a skeletal muscle. In response to stretching of the sense organ in the muscle—namely, the muscle spindle intrafusal fibers lying parallel to the regular muscle contractile unit—activation causes the efferent limb of the reflex arc to produce motor activity. This is typified by the well-known knee jerk.

The disynaptic reflex arc has the same components mentioned above, plus one interneuron interposed in the spinal cord between the afferent and efferent neurons. This allows further nervous system integration, as exemplified by the reflex withdrawal from a noxious stimulus. Finally, the polysynaptic reflex arc is the most complex, having multiple interneurons all linked through collateral branches arranged in parallel chains. The branching is variable and causes prolonged responses. The complexity of this reflex system allows for coordinated flexion and extension of muscles supplying body parts to allow smoother reflex activity of the organism as a whole.

MEMBRANE EXCITATION AND IMPULSE TRANSMISSION

Characteristics of the Stable Membrane

Typically, the distribution of electrolytes inside and outside of the cell of the nervous system is similar to the makeup of other cells in the body. In the extracellular environment, there is 10 to 14 times more sodium than is found inside the cell. Extracellular sodium is also present in much greater concentrations than is extracellular potassium. The principal extracellular anion is the chloride ion. There is far more intracellular potassium—some 30 to 40 times more—than extracellular potassium. There is considerably less sodium within the cell in the resting state, and the intracellular anions consist of proteins, organic phosphates, and sulfates as well as bicarbonate.

Factors Maintaining the Polarized State

In the resting state, there exists a potential charge across the cell membrane. The charge is always measured on the inside and is negative relative to the outside. This is referred to as the transmembrane potential or the resting membrane potential. This actual value differs with the type of cell in which it is measured but for most neurons is −90 mV as measured on the inside of the cell. This transmembrane potential requires some basic conditions to maintain it. First, the cell membrane must be selectively permeable, allowing the more rapid diffusion of some ions over others. This allows a concentration gradient to be established for various anions and cations on either side of the cell membrane. The consequence of this is to provide the membrane with the potential to react—that is, to do whatever is characteristic of that tissue type—muscle tissue to contract, glandular tissue to secrete, and nervous tissue to conduct an impulse.

Because of the differences in concentration of the ions on either side of the cell membrane, there is a natural tendency for them to diffuse to equilibrium. Therefore, sodium ions enter the cell and potassium ions exit. This "leak" is thought to occur through pores or sodium channels. This selective permeability of the cell membrane is far less for sodium than it is for potassium. Perhaps 50 to 100 times more potassium leaks out of the cell than sodium leaks in. The rationale behind this is that the hydrated potassium ion is smaller than that of sodium and can therefore pass more freely through the cell pore. Only minimal amounts of chloride ions enter the cell, because there is a relatively small gradient on the two sides of the cell membrane for this anion. The intracellular anions are generally too large to diffuse out of the cell and are therefore said to be nondiffusible. In addition to the minimal permeability of the cell membrane to sodium and potassium ions, there is an adenosine triphosphate (ATP)-utilizing carrier system that keeps ahead of diffusion by carrying back out much of the sodium that diffuses into the cell and carrying the potassium into the intracellular cytoplasm.

Sequence of Depolarization Events

Before the activity of depolarization begins, the resting membrane potential must drop to −65 mV from −90 mV. This point of −65 mV is called threshold. When it is reached, selective permeability is lost, sodium ions rush into the cell causing the development of an action potential, and depolarization of the cell occurs. The cell thus performs its designated function as described above. With the development of an action potential, the intracellular electrical potential changes from −90 mV at rest to +45 mV during the initial period of depolarization. Stimuli can be of a chemical, mechanical, thermal, or electrical nature. Irrespective of the type of stimulus, the common result is a change in the membrane, making it much more permeable to sodium and later to potassium. It is postulated that the pores of the cell membrane are lined with calcium ions. This bound calcium alters the pore diameter and tends to decrease its permeability. The stimulus displaces the calcium from its membrane binding sites, thereby increasing the cell membrane permeability. Sodium ions rapidly diffuse into the

cell at a rate hundreds of times greater than during the resting state. This overpowers the active transport mechanism, which attempts to move excess sodium ions into the extracellular environment. Potassium ion flux changes very little. There also is some movement of chloride ions into the cell, but this is minimal and not instrumental in effecting depolarization of the cell. The net gain of intracellular cations causes the intracellular membrane potential to go from −90 mV to +45 mV. This is referred to as a reversal potential. As a consequence of this action potential and with the achievement of the reversal potential, cells are excited and perform their characteristic function by contracting, transmitting impulses, secreting their contents, and so on. This process of depolarization takes approximately 0.4 msec. The process is terminated by the diffusion of potassium out of the cell. This movement of potassium begins approximately 0.3 msec after stimulation of the cell and continues for another 0.4 msec, ending when the resting membrane potential reaches −94 mV. This state of hyperpolarization is due to the outpouring of potassium and the slight influx of chloride ions into the cell. The period of hyperpolarization lasts from 50 msec to seconds and is called a positive afterpotential, a confusing term since it is even more negative than the resting membrane potential.

Once a cell has depolarized, it is said to be refractory or resistant to subsequent stimuli while it reestablishes the ionic distribution that exists at rest. This refractory period is divided into an initial one-third of the repolarization period, in which the cell is completely resistant to further stimuli irrespective of strength or duration of the stimulus. This is referred to as the absolute refractory period. It is followed by the last two-thirds of the repolarization period, in which a stimulus of greater than normal magnitude or duration may cause subsequent depolarization of the cell. This is called the relative refractory period.

Several characteristics of the stimulus should be considered. As mentioned earlier, the stimulus can be chemical, mechanical, thermal, or electrical in nature. It must be of sufficient magnitude to cause depolarization of a cell. It is thus said to be of rheobase strength. The stimulus must also be applied for sufficient time to cause depolarization. This is known as utilization time. The term *chronaxie* applies to the length of time a stimulus of two rheobase intensity must be applied to produce depolarizing action of a cell.

SYNAPSE AND MUSCLE CONTRACTION
General Description and Location

A synapse is defined as a functional connection between neurons, neurons and receptors, or neurons and effector organs. There is considerable morphologic and physiologic variation between synapses. In general, all are involved in impulse transmission. Since the average axon terminates in 1000 synapses and since dendrites can receive synaptic contact from 100,000 axons, we can see that there is tremendous proliferation of synapses throughout the body.

Structural and Functional Characteristics

The most frequently studied synapse is that between the motor efferent neuron and the skeletal muscle effector. It is large, having the dendrites and cell body of the efferent neuron in the anterior horn of the spinal cord. The axon emerges from the anterior horn, forms a spinal nerve, and terminates by synapsing at the sarcolemma of a skeletal muscle fiber. The axonal ending forms a bouton or knoblike terminal at the telodendron. The end of the neuron is called the presynaptic terminal or end-plate; the membrane around these terminal ends of the neuron is the presynaptic membrane. There is a space separating the presynaptic membrane from the skeletal muscle. This space is known as the synaptic cleft or space, and it varies in synapses from 2 to 20 millimicrons. The membrane of skeletal muscle lying across from the presynaptic membrane is the postsynaptic membrane or sole plate. This postsynaptic membrane is specialized tissue differing from adjacent areas of skeletal muscle in that it is specifically adapted to receive and react to chemical substances released by the presynaptic terminal.

Mechanism of Impulse Transmission

Within the boutons of the telodendron, high concentrations of mitochondria produce a great deal of ATP, the source of considerable energy for the body. There are also several vesicles that contain the chemical neurohumoral transmitter substance specific for that neuron. In the specific effector neuron-skeletal muscle unit, that chemical is acetylcholine. Therefore, it is that transmitter that is described in detail here.

The depolarization wave passes down the axon to the terminal bouton and causes the vesicles adjacent to the synaptic cleft to rupture and exocytose their contents into the cleft. Approximately 2 to 300 such vesicles release their contents in this process. The exact mechanism by which the depolarization wave causes the vesicles to rupture is unclear, but it has been determined that the impulse causes an in-rushing of calcium ions through the terminal knob at the time of the action potential. The liberated acetylcholine transits the synaptic cleft and attaches to the specific receptor site on the postsynaptic membrane. It alters the permeability of the postsynaptic membrane, increasing the permeability to sodium and thereby causing depolarization of the sarcolemma. This depolarization next spreads in all directions to the skeletal muscle.

Before repolarization can occur and the muscle respond to another stimulus, the acetylcholine must be removed from the receptor sites. This occurs by two processes. A small amount is reabsorbed into the presynaptic terminal and back into vesicles, where it is in the inactive state. The predominant amount of acetylcholine is chemically inactivated by the enzyme acetylcholine esterase, which is present along the synaptic cleft. This enzyme is specific for the hydrolysis of acetylcholine. Another esterase found in brain, liver, and plasma is pseudocholinesterase, or nonspecific cholesterase, which is effective in hydrolyzing succinyldicholine into succinylmonocholine. Acetylcholinesterase breaks acetylcholine into choline and acetate, which is reabsorbed back into the presynaptic terminal, where it is acted on by cholineacetylase, an enzyme found in that terminal. Once synthesized, the newly formed acetylcholine is taken into vesicles and stored. These vesicles have been alternately called packets and quanta.

Synaptic Transmitter Substances

The postsynaptic membrane is specifically adapted to receive and react to the substance released by the presynaptic terminal. There are two general categories of neurohumoral transmitters. Some excite the postsynaptic membrane, causing depolarization, and these include acetylcholine, norepinephrine, and epinephrine. Others are limited to the central nervous system and include dopamine, serotonin, histamine, a number of hypothalamic-stimulating hormones, as well as enkephalins and endorphins. Inhibitory neurohumoral transmitters are also released at some synapses. These are said to stabilize or inhibit depolarization of the postsynaptic membrane. Examples of such inhibitory substances include glycine and gamma-aminobutyric acid. In addition, the excitatory neurohumoral transmitters can stimulate inhibitory fibers, which act to produce negative feedback inhibition of neurons.

Muscle Contraction and Relaxation

In considering the activity of muscle, we must first understand the makeup of a muscle fiber. The typical muscle fiber comprises hundreds of actin and myosin filaments attached end to end the entire length of the fiber. The actin filaments are thin, double-helical strands of protein extending on either side of a so-called Z band as fingers extend from a hand. Interdigitating with the actin are thicker protein molecules known as myosin. There are generally twice as many actin as myosin filaments in a myofibril. The Z band passes between myofibrils all along the muscle fiber. The part of the muscle lying between two successive parallel Z membranes including the projections of actin from each and the interdigitating myosin filaments is referred to as a sarcomere. The sarcomere is approximately 2 μm in length when completely relaxed. Thus, a myofibril if viewed in transverse cross section will appear as one myosin filament surrounded by six actin filaments in a regular hexagonal pattern. This pattern of actin and myosin filaments continues repeatedly up to approximately 3000 actin and 1500 myosin filaments over the entire length of each myofibril. As mentioned previously, hundreds to thousands of these myofibrils lie parallel to each other to form a muscle fiber, and many muscle fibers compose a muscle. The muscle fiber is distinguished by a surrounding cell membrane known as sarcolemma. Interweaving around the individual myofibrils is a lacelike structure of sarcoplasmic reticulum. This consists of complex channels that connect with a transverse tubular system running the length of the myofibril and connecting the sarcoplasmic reticulum with the extracellular environment. The T-tube system, as it is called, contains extracellular fluid. Several mitochondria are found between the myofibrils. The sarcoplasmic reticulum also has enlarged areas or terminal cisterns near the junction with the T-tube system. These terminal cisterns contain calcium ions.

The interdigitating makeup of actin and myosin molecules gives skeletal muscle its typical striated appearance. In addition to the Z bands, several other anatomic demarcations of the myofibril are evidenced. The portion of the sarcomere where the actin overlaps with myosin is termed the A band; where the actin does not overlap myosin, the I band; and finally the central portion of the myosin where there is no overlapping actin, the H band.

Arranged recessed in the cleft of the double-helical actin strand is a double strand of tropomyosin, which contains regularly spaced subunits of troponin. Both tropomyosin and troponin are proteins—the latter being made up of three differing subunits (I, T, and C). The tropomyosin/troposin complex prevents muscle contraction and is therefore known as an inhibitory complex. Tropomyosin covers the receptor sites on the action filament and prevents the interaction of actin and myosin.

With this background of the anatomy of the muscle unit, we can begin to consider the process of excitation-contraction coupling. When an action potential occurs in muscle, the impulse spreads throughout the muscle by way of the transverse tubular system. As the action potential moves past the terminal cisterns of the sarcoplasmic reticulum, calcium is released into the vicinity of the myofibril. This calcium binds with troponin C and moves the tropomyosin/troponin complex away from the receptor sites on the actin. This then sets the stage for muscle contraction. Excitation-contraction coupling occurs between the actin and myosin filaments. The myosin filament consists of a single strand of protein with shorter projections extending along the filament in much the same way that the feathers extend from the shaft of an arrow. These extensions are meromyosin cross-bridges protruding each 120 degrees around the myosin filament and spaced every few millimicrons apart for the entire length of the myosin filament. The meromyosin strands extend from the center of the myosin filament toward the ends in both directions. They characteristically are slender and have a bulbous head at the end opposite to that which attaches to the myosin filament. The meromyosin strands generally lie closely arranged around the myosin. There are two areas of the meromyosin strand that "hinge," allowing it to move further away from the myosin filament and the head portion to attach to the receptor sites of the action. The very center of the myosin filament has no meromyosin strands extending from it.

When the calcium released from the terminal cisterns moves the inhibitory proteins away from the receptor sites of the actin, the heads of the meromyosin attach to these sites and swivel in unison in a "cocking" motion, moving the two opposing actin filaments of the sarcomere closer to each other and interdigitating over a greater portion of the myosin. Once the meromyosin head has swiveled, moving the actin filament, the receptor site on the actin is exposed and the head detaches from the actin receptor site. ATP binds with the head, causing it to detach from the actin. Once the head becomes detached from the actin, an enzyme (ATPase) that is found in the meromyosin molecule causes the ATP to be split from the meromyosin head. This splitting causes the head to be recocked into position to once more reattach to a receptor site on the actin filament and move the actin again along the myosin filament. This process occurs repeatedly in a cogwheel fashion and is called the "ratchet theory" of muscle contraction.

Relaxation of the muscle occurs when the calcium ions are pumped back into the sarcoplasmic reticulum. This pro-cess occurs by active transport utilizing ATP. The inhibitory bonds are reestablished between the actin, troponin, and tropomyosin. Energy for the process of contraction and relaxation of muscle utilizes oxygen to supply ATP and phosphocreatine to supply anaerobic supplies of energy.

Comparison of Muscle Types

Skeletal muscle makes up about 40 percent of the body weight, smooth muscle and cardiac muscle another 10 percent. Although skeletal muscle has regularly occurring cross-striations as a result of organized, recurring actin and myosin filaments, the same characteristic is not evidenced by smooth muscle. This is because smooth muscle is arranged in an irregular pattern. There are two types of smooth muscle. The first, visceral smooth muscle, is found in the walls of hollow organs such as the intestines, ureters, urinary bladder, and uterus. This muscle type has a tightly connected border between cells, allowing inherent, rhythmic contractions without extraneous innervation. These cells have an unstable resting membrane potential because of a greater sodium and potassium leak than skeletal muscle has. There is therefore continuous depolarization, a summation of repetitive action, and a rippling of action potentials, resulting in tonic contractions lasting several seconds. The second type of smooth muscle is a multiunit type that consists of discrete muscle fibers with each fiber having a nerve ending and contracting only when directly stimulated. It is found in blood vessels and the iris of the eye.

Smooth muscle has a poorly developed sarcoplasmic reticulum and no transverse tubule system. It also differs from skeletal muscle in that it has autonomic nervous system innervation instead of spinal nerve innervation. The fibers of smooth muscle are smaller in diameter and shorter in length than those of skeletal muscle.

Cardiac muscle has some of the characteristics of both smooth and skeletal muscle. There are visible cross-striations and a well-developed sarcoplasmic reticulum. The T-tubule system opens at the Z lines rather than at the A-I band junction as occurs in skeletal muscle. The duration of action potentials in cardiac muscle is 15 to 30 times longer than in skeletal muscle, and it is also intrinsically self-excitable, as is smooth muscle, because of greater permeability to sodium ions. Cardiac muscle has intercalated disks, which are areas where the ends of muscle fibers abut each other through an extensive series of folds, forming a strong union. Because of the intercalated disks and tight cell junctions or borders, cardiac muscle cells contract when denervated, although they are generally innervated by the autonomic nervous system.

SPINAL CORD, MENINGES, AND CEREBROSPINAL FLUID

Spinal Cord Structure

The spinal cord is an elongated cylindrical structure approximately 1 cm in diameter and 42 to 45 cm long. The cranial end of the cord extends to the medulla oblongata at the upper border of the atlas, and the caudal end terminates at the body of the second lumbar vertebra in the adult.

The spinal cord tapers caudally to a blunt end, which is called the conus medullaris. It is suspended and supported laterally by the dentate ligament and is surrounded by meninges, which will be discussed later. The filum terminale is the delicate filament continuing down the vertebral canal from the conus medullaris to the first coccygeal vertebra. It is approximately 20 cm long, the first 15 cm being contained within the dura mater and surrounded by nerves of the cauda equina. This is called the filum terminale interum because it is invested by dura mater. The lower 5 cm has dura mater adherent to it and extends to the dorsal border of the first coccygeal vertebra, where it attaches to become the periosteum of the coccyx. This lower 5 cm is called the filum terminale externum. The blood supply to the spinal cord consists of spinal branches arising from the vertebral, deep cervical, intercostal, and lumbar arteries, with branches of the anterior and posterior spinal arteries. There is an extensive array of spinal vasculature. The venous drainage of the spinal cord collects into venous plexuses and empties into the vena cava. The external configuration of the cord shows it to be slightly flattened anteroposteriorly, with a cervical enlargement from the third cervical to the second thoracic vertebra corresponding to large nerves supplying the upper extremities. A similar enlargement corresponding to the nerves supplying the lower extremities is found in the lumbar region.

In cross-sectional view, the gross appearance of the spinal cord is a central area of gray matter immediately surrounding the central canal. The gray matter is made up primarily of dendrites, cell bodies, unmyelinated axons, and neuroglia arranged horizontally. The H-shaped distribution of gray matter varies with the amount of tissues innervated by the different segments. The thoracic segment of the cord has smaller proportions of gray matter; the cervical, lumbar, and sacral have proportionately a greater amount. The gray matter of the thoracic and upper lumbar areas shows small lateral projections (lateral horns) giving rise to the sympathetic preganglionic fibers. The horns of the gray matter are arranged so that they divide the gray matter into anterior, lateral, and posterior columns. Each of these columns is further subdivided, carrying nerve fibers to and from respective areas of the body. A transverse commissure of gray matter connects the right and left columns, forming a central gray isthmus. A hole can be seen in the middle of the gray commissure, and this extends from the fourth ventricle of the brain and travels the length of the spinal cord. It contains cerebrospinal fluid (CSF) and is called the central canal. The gray matter is the area of synapse of afferent, internuncial, and efferent neurons. The posterior horn is the point of synapse for most somatic afferent fibers and the anterior horn, the area where impulses are relayed for voluntary movement, as well as effector neurons of spinal reflex arcs.

The white matter of the spinal cord generally surrounds the gray. It consists primarily of myelinated afferent and efferent axons vertically arranged as projection tracts. The white matter in each half of the cord is divided into three columns of funiculi—namely, the anterior, lateral, and posterior. Each funiculus is subdivided into fascicles or tracts representing groups of axons carrying similar sensory or motor impulses. The specific tracts will be discussed elsewhere in this chapter.

Spinal Cord Coverings

The coverings of the brain and spinal cord are one and the same, with some differences evidenced in the two areas. They generally consist of nonneuronal connective tissue arranged in three separate but continuous layers around the brain and spinal cord. The meninges are innervated by somatic and visceral afferent fibers from spinal and autonomic nerves.

The outermost layer, the dura mater, is a tough, non-elastic, fibrous layer of connective tissues. Around the brain, the dura is composed of two layers. The outer, endosteal layer is the same as the periosteum of the skull and is adherent to the inner tablet. It sends many fine fibrous and vascular projections into the base, giving it a fuzzy appearance when peeled off from the bone. There is no real space between this outer layer and the skull; however, hemorrhage may occur in this area separating the outer dura from the skull. This extradural hemorrhage usually occurs from tearing of the middle meningeal artery, most commonly in the temperoparietal area.

The inner layer of dura is the meningeal layer, which is generally adherent to the outer layer, forming one membrane. The meningeal layer does separate from the endosteal layer and follows the large fissures between the cerebral hemispheres to form the falx cerebri, which extends down to the corpus callosum and from the crista galli anteriorly to the occipital tuberance posteriorly. The cerebral hemispheres are similarly separated by a fold of dura known as the falx cerebelli. In addition, the dura forms a tent separating the occipital lobe from the cerebellum and is called the tentorium cerebelli. The two layers of dura mater also separate to form large dural sinuses, which are venous channels draining blood from the brain into the internal jugular veins. These veins have no valves and are situated between the two layers of dura. There are two such groups of sinuses. The anterior-inferior group drains that portion; the posterior-superior group, including the largest, the superior sagittal sinus, drains the upper posterior brain. Below the inner layer of dura, there is a potential space that contains a few milliters of lubricating fluid in immediate contact with the dura. This subdural space exists around the brain but does not follow the fissures or sulci except as do the falx and tentorium.

Around the spinal cord we find the dura mater losing its double-layered configuration, which ends at the foramen magnum. The endosteal layer is represented below the foramen magnum as the periosteum of the vertebrae. The subdural space continues in the same way as it does around the brain. In addition, there is an epidural space around the spinal cord since the cord does not completely fill the vertebral canal. This space contains adipose and areolar tissue, blood vessels, and nerve roots. The dura continues caudally below the conus medullaris to form a sac called the lumbar cistern, extending to the second sacral vertebra. Below this the dura attaches to the coccygeal vertebrae, becoming the periosteum of the coccyx.

The arachnoid mater is a single-layered, avascular covering around the brain and spinal cord. It lies below the dura and dips into the fissures and sulci of the brain only, as do the falx and tentorium. It is separated from the dura mater by the subdural space and has a real space below the arachnoid mater known as the subarachnoid space. This space contains CSF and is continuous with the ventricular system.

As mentioned above, the arachnoid mater does not follow the contours of the brain but rather bridges over portions of the brain that do not fill the cranial vault. This bridging effect varies in different areas of the brain, with two being of greater interest—namely, the cisterna magna, lying below the cerebellum, and the lumbar cistern, lying below the conus medullaris at the caudal end of the spinal cord. These cisterns are filled with CSF.

The arachnoid mater has unusual thin, vertically arranged filaments that traverse the subarachnoid space attaching it to the underlying pia mater. There is no known function for these filaments, known as trabeculae, which give the arachnoid mater a weblike appearance. The arachnoid continues below the level of the conus medullaris to terminate at the level of the second sacral vertebra along with the dura after forming the lumbar cistern.

Arachnoid villi or granulations are extensions of the arachnoid membrane into the venous sinuses. They appear as berrylike tufts and are usually not found before the age of 3 years, but they increase in number and size with age. These granulations push against the dura mater and eventually cause the absorption of bone, leaving a depression in the inner table of the skull. These arachnoid villi are discussed further in the paragraphs that follow.

The pia mater is a thin, delicate layer of connective tissue adherent to the brain and spinal cord, following all fissures and sulci. It contains the blood supply of the brain and spinal cord, with the spinal portion being somewhat less vascular. The pia mater extends into the transverse cerebral fissure to contribute to the formation of the choroid plexus of the lateral, third, and fourth ventricles. The pia mater continues as a fibrous thread at the conus medullaris into the filum terminale. The pia also forms the denticulate ligament, which extends laterally on either side of the spinal cord and attaches to the vertebral bodies, providing support and stability to the spinal cord.

Cerebrospinal Fluid

A discussion of the formation, circulation, and absorption of CSF must be preceded by the anatomy of the cerebral ventricular system. The lateral ventricles lie within each cerebral hemisphere in the midbrain below the corpus callosum. The right and left lateral ventricles connect to a centrally located third ventricle by a foramen of Monro from each. The third ventricle is also located in the midbrain, above the area of the brain stem. The cerebral aqueduct, or aqueduct of Sylvius, connects the third with the fourth ventricle. The fourth ventricle is in the area of the brain stem anterior to the cerebellum. Its contents drain into the cisterna magna via three openings. One foramen of Magendie opens posteromedially, and two foramen of Luschka open laterally into the cisterna magna. From there the CSF normally circulates freely around the spinal cord and brain.

The formation of CSF occurs primarily with the action of the choroid plexus in each ventricle and to a much lesser extent by the same process in the perivascular spaces of the brain. The process begins with the secretion of sodium ions by the cuboidal cells of the choroid plexus. This devel-

ops a positive charge in the CSF. This in turn attracts chloride ions into the CSF. The excess of ions causes increased osmotic pressure in the ventricular fluid, exerting a pressure up to 160 torr greater than plasma osmotic pressure. Water and dissolved substances therefore move through the choroidal membrane into the CSF. The fluid circulates through the subarachnoid space around the brain and spinal cord by virtue of this CSF pressure.

The absorption of CSF occurs into large venous sinuses because of the pressure gradient within the subarachnoid space. When the pressure of the CSF is greater than venous sinus pressure, leaflike unidirectional valves in the arachnoid villi open, allowing CSF to drain into the dural sinuses. When the venous pressure is greater than the CSF pressure, the valves close and prevent a backflow of blood into the subarachnoid space.

Although different figures are quoted, the average adult male has a total of about 150 ml of CSF, approximately two-thirds of this in the ventricular system and one-third in the subarachnoid space. CSF is formed at a rate of 0.58 ml/minute, or 835 ml/day. Obviously, a similar amount must be absorbed into the venous sinuses each day as well. This formation of CSF produces a CSF pressure ranging from 6 to 18 cm H_2O with a mean pressure of 13 cm H_2O. The mean opening pressure for the arachnoid granulations is 6.8 cm H_2O. These figures can be converted to millimeters of mercury by dividing by 1.36.

Examining the chemistry of CSF shows a composition similar to plasma in many respects because of the intimate contact between CSF and plasma. Sodium concentration is 145 mEq/L, magnesium 2.3 mEq/L; chloride 113 mEq/L, potassium 2.85 mEq/L, and calcium 2.45 mEq/L. There is slightly less glucose in CSF than in plasma and considerably less protein. Few red and white cells are found in the CSF. When they are present, red cells indicate frank hemorrhage and white cells point to viral or bacterial infections. The specific gravity of CSF ranges from 1.003 to 1.009, and the pH is 7.32 to 7.35.

The overall functions of CSF are protective. The brain floats in CSF, decreasing its relative weight. The fluid also acts as a shock absorber, reducing trauma to the brain when rapid movement occurs. Finally, the CSF regulates the composition of neuronal environment within narrow limits that are required for normal functioning.

SPINAL NERVE ACTIVITY

General Diagram of Spinal Nerves

Each spinal nerve is composed of an afferent sensory component and an efferent motor component, with afferent neurons entering the spinal cord by the posterior horn and the efferent neurons exiting the anterior horn. The sensory and motor axons are termed rootlets. These rootlets meet at the point of exit from the vertebral column to form one spinal nerve. All of the sensory rootlets are axons entering into formation of one spinal nerve, termed the sensory roots of that nerve. The same makeup is seen in the motor roots of spinal nerves.

With the exception of the first cervical spinal nerve, which has only motor fibers, all spinal nerves have both sensory and motor components. The sensory and motor roots join to become one nerve from the vertebral column to the area of receptor and effector. The roots of the spinal nerve traverse the space between the cord and inner wall of the vertebral canal. The anterior and posterior roots unite in the area of the intervertebral foramen to form the common spinal nerve. The intervertebral foramen is a hole formed by the inferior vertebral notch located on the inferior surface of one vertebra and the superior vertebral notch of the vertebra below it. Most of the spinal nerves exit the vertebral column by way of the intervertebral foramen.

Prior to entering into formation of the common spinal nerve, each sensory neuron has its cell body. The cell body is located at a point just before the spinal roots become one common spinal nerve and leave the vertebral column. The cell body, which is within the bony framework of the vertebra, is known as a dorsal root ganglion.

The common spinal nerve runs for only a short distance before dividing into a larger and more important anterior primary ramus and a generally smaller, posterior primary ramus. Each ramus carries sensory and motor fibers. The anterior primary ramus sends off the lateral cutaneous and anterior cutaneous branches. The anterior primary ramus connects with the sympathetic paravertebral ganglia. The posterior primary ramus divides into a medial and a lateral branch. Before branching into primary rami, the spinal nerve sends off a meningeal branch carrying sensory and motor fibers back into the intervertebral foramen to supply the meningeal vessels.

The anterior primary rami leave the numbered spinal nerves, and some enter into plexus formation. The nerves exiting the plexuses are named for the specific area that they supply. These nerves supply sensory and motor innervation to the arms, legs, front and sides of the neck, thorax, and abdomen. The larger of these plexuses will be discussed later in this section. The posterior primary rami do not enter into plexus formations, do not extend into the extremities, but rather are limited to sensory and motor innervation to the muscles of the back and neck and the skin of the back and neck.

Origin and Nomenclature

The naming and number of spinal nerves occurs with the distribution of the 31 pairs into 8 cervical, 12 thoracic, 5 lumbar, 5 sacral, and 1 coccygeal. With the exception of the first pair of cervical spinal nerves, which are strictly motor, all have sensory and motor fibers. In general, spinal nerves are named for the vertebra above or below their point of exit through the intervertebral foramen. As we examine the human vertebral column, we note 7 cervical, 12 thoracic, 5 lumbar, 5 sacral, and 4 to 5 fused coccygeal vertebrae. The first pair of cervical spinal nerves exits between the first vertebra or atlas and the occiput. The second through seventh pairs exit through the intervertebral foramen and are named for the cervical vertebrae below their point of exit. The eighth pair of cervical spinal nerves exits below the seventh cervical vertebra. The thoracic, lumbar, and sacral spinal nerves are named for the vertebrae above their point of exit from the vertebral column.

Each pair of spinal nerves innervates a specific area of the body with its sensory, motor, and accompanying autonomic nerve components. The areas overlap considerably, and any specific area of the body is innervated by more than one pair of spinal nerves. Because the nerves below the thoracic level do not exit the intervertebral foramen corresponding to their level of origin off the spinal cord, the areas of the body that these nerves innervate are not transverse to the level from which the nerves originated. Named in reference to their point of origin, the cervical spinal nerves extend at a more or less right angle off the cord and exit the intervertebral foramen at about the same level. These nerves are the most horizontal of all spinal nerves. Beginning with the thoracic level, the nerves run down from the point of origin and exit the vertebral column approximately one vertebral body lower. Below the level of the second lumbar vertebrae, we find the spinal nerves extending below the end of the spinal cord and exiting the vertebral column much lower than their origin off the cord. This forms a network of loosely arranged spinal nerves referred to as the cauda equina because, like the horse's tail, the central mass ends much higher, with many fibers extending downward.

As the spinal nerve roots pass through the subarachnoid space surrounding the spinal cord, they first pierce the pia and arachnoid mater, which form a sleeve around the roots known as the perineurium. When these roots reach the outer dural membrane, an outer sleeve of dura mater surrounds the roots and common spinal nerve; this is known as the epineurium.

Functional Anatomy of the Brachial Plexus

The brachial plexus is repeatedly instrumented by the nurse anesthetist, and it is therefore imperative to have a thorough understanding of the anatomy of this plexus. The brachial plexus includes all nerve structures arising from the fifth cervical spinal nerve through and including the first thoracic spinal nerve. This plexus furnishes almost total somatic, autonomic, sensory, and motor innervation to the upper extremities. The anterior primary rami of the fifth, sixth, seventh, and eight cervical as well as first thoracic spinal nerves intertwine after exiting the intervertebral foramina, passing through the posterior triangle of the neck, which is formed by the trapezius and sternocleidomastoid muscle and the middle third of the clavicle between the anterior and middle scalene muscles. Roots from the fourth cervical and second thoracic spinal nerves occasionally contribute to the makeup of this plexus. The subclavian artery accompanies the roots as they pass between the scalene muscles. The roots of the above-mentioned spinal nerves collect while between the anterior and medial scalene muscles into three trunks named in reference to their position one to another. They are the superior trunk, made up of fibers from the fifth and sixth cervical spinal nerves; the middle, made up of fibers from the seventh cervical; and the inferior, made up of fibers from the eighth cervical and first thoracic spinal nerves. These three trunks exit from between the scalene muscles and run behind the clavicle to extend to the lateral aspect of the first rib, where they separate into six divisions, each trunk forming an anterior and posterior division at the lateral border of the first rib. These divisions lie behind the clavicle and subclavius muscle, descend into the axilla with the axillary artery, and collect into three cords.

The three cords are named in relation to their position around the axillary artery. The lateral cord is formed by the union of anterior divisions of the superior and middle trunks, and it carries fibers from the fifth, sixth, and seventh cervical spinal nerves. The medial cord arises from the anterior division of the inferior trunk; it carries fibers from the eighth cervical and first thoracic spinal nerves. The posterior cord is a combination of the posterior divisions of all three trunks and so has fibers from all five spinal nerves of this plexus.

The cord gives rise to several branches and terminal nerves. We shall discuss the origin and termination of six of the peripheral nerves of the brachial plexus. The musculo-cutaneous nerve is one of two nerves resulting from the bifurcation of the lateral cord. Motor fibers innervate the muscles that flex and adduct the upper and lower arm as well as supinate the hand. Sensory components innervate the skin over the radial half of the forearm from just above the antecubital fossa to the wrist, anteriorly and posteriorly.

The radial nerve originates as a continuation of the posterior cord. It supplies motor activity to the muscles flexing, extending, adducting, and abducting the arm. It also provides sensory innervation posteriorly, over the middle aspect of the forearm and to the dorsal surface of the hand to the lateral half of the ring finger excluding the tips of the thumb, index, middle, and ring fingers. Anteriorly, the radial nerve supplies the lateral margins of the thumb and hand.

The median nerve is made up of roots from the lateral and medial cords. Its motor fibers innervate muscles that serve to move the thumb and first two fingers and hand, giving them flexion, adduction, and abduction of the fingers and pronation of the hand. Sensory fibers extend to the anterior palmar surface from a line running through the ring finger to the wrist just short of the extreme lateral aspect of the thumb and palm. On the posterior aspect of the hand, the median nerve supplies the tips of the thumb and index and middle fingers, as well as the lateral aspect of the tip of the ring finger.

The ulnar nerve originates as a continuation of the medial cord after the cord makes its contribution to the median nerve. Motor fibers innervate all the intrinsic hand muscles, providing flexion, extension to the fingers, and extension and adduction of the hand. The sensory fibers innervate the medial aspect of the hand, anteriorly and posteriorly, from the middle of the ring finger, to and including the little finger.

The medial cutaneous nerve of the arm originates off the medial cord prior to the formation of the ulnar nerve. It terminates in sensory fibers only to the medial aspect of the upper arm from the axilla to the antecubital space.

Finally, the medial cutaneous nerve of the forearm originates off the medial cord and also has only sensory fibers, which in this case innervate the medial aspect of the forearm from the wrist to above the antecubital space and elbow both anteriorly and posteriorly.

SPINAL TRACTS AND SPECIAL RECEPTORS

Cross Section of the Spinal Cord

The reader is referred to the previous section of this chapter for a review of the anatomic divisions of the cross section of the spinal cord. The ascending and descending spinal tracts travel in the anterior, lateral, or posterior columns, bilaterally. Each of these columns or funiculi are further subdivided into fascicles or tracts that represent groups of axons carrying similar sensory or motor information to or from the brain. Detailed anatomy texts describe more than 20 spinal cord tracts transferring information to and from the brain. A lengthy discussion of each is beyond the scope of this text, but several of the more commonly understood are presented here.

Ascending Spinal Tracts

Sensory input to the central nervous system occurs by a series of three afferent neurons. The first-order neuron originates in receptors widely distributed in the periphery. Specific receptors will be discussed at length later in this section. This neuron commonly terminates in the posterior horn of the gray matter. There are exceptions that terminate in the medulla. Sensory neuron I, as it is referred to, synapses in the posterior horn with sensory neuron II. This second-order neuron ascends the spinal cord in a named tract of fibers located in the white matter to the thalmus. Some of the second-order sensory neurons travel up the cord in a tract on the same side as that entered by the first-order neuron. These fibers are said to be traveling in ipsilateral named tracts as we will see. Some of the second-order neurons cross the spinal cord in the anterior commissure or isthmus and ascend the cord in the contralateral spinal tract to the thalamus. In the thalamus, these neurons synapse with sensory neuron III, which has axons extending through the corona radiata and internal capsule, finally terminating in the sensory area of the postcentral gyrus of the parietal lobe.

Most of the sensory neurons form synapses with many other neurons located at various levels of the spinal cord and brain. This is referred to as the principle of divergence. The anesthetist should understand the major ascending pathways for the transmission of pain, temperature, touch, pressure, proprioception, and kinesthesia.

The lateral spinothalamic tract carries sensations of pain and temperature from the periphery to the brain. Sensory neuron I originates in the skin, muscles, tendons, and viscera and terminates in the posterior horn of the cord. Fibers making up sensory neuron II of this tract originate in the posterior horn, and the axons decussate before ascending in the lateral spinothalamic tract, terminating in the thalamus. Sensory neuron III originates in the ventrolateral nucleus of the thalamus, and the axons radiate to the cerebral cortex by way of the thalamocortical tract via the internal capsule.

The ventral spinothalamic tract functions to transmit sensations of touch and pressure from the periphery to the postcentral gyrus. Although the receptors are different from those for pain and temperature and the tracts in which the fibers of the second sensory neurons travel are different, the routes of each of the other fibers of this tract are similar to those traveled by fibers of the dorsal spinothalamic tract to the postcentral gyrus.

A third ascending tract is made up of fibers from the funiculus gracilis, which carries impulses from below the sixth thoracic spinal level and the funiculus cuneatus, carrying fibers above the sixth thoracic level. Together these fibers make up the medial lemniscal tract. This tract transmits sensations of conscious kinesthesia, vibration, stereognosis, deep touch, pressure, and two-point discrimination. Sensory neuron I for this tract originates at peripheral receptors, enters the posterior horn of the cord, decussates at the level of entry, and extends up the spinal cord to the nuclei of gracilis and cuneatus in the medulla instead of terminating in the posterior columns of the cord. Sensory neuron II originates in these nuclei of the medulla and extends through the midbrain to the thalamus. Sensory neuron III of this tract extends from the thalamus to the cerebral cortex, as have other radiating fibers.

The dorsal spinocerebellar tract carries sensations of unconscious kinesthesia from cord levels of the sixth cervical through the second lumbar regions. They originate in the Golgi apparatus and muscle spindles and travel to the posterior horns of gray matter. Sensory neuron II extends up the cord ipsilaterally as the dorsal spinocerebellar tract to the cerebellar cortex, which has a homunculus similar to that of the cerebrum. There are no third-order sensory neurons for the spinocerebellar tract.

The fibers of the ventral spinocerebellar tract carry unconscious kinesthetic sensations from below the second lumbar level into the cerebellum as uncrossed fibers. The second- and third-order sensory neurons originate and terminate in the same areas as those for the dorsal spinocerebellar tracts.

Descending Tracts

Four major descending tracts are presented here. They consist of fibers traveling in either pyramidal or extrapyramidal tracts. The pyramidal tracts are phylogenetically newer and are those whose fibers converge in the medulla to form pyramids. Their axons originate from cell bodies located in the cerebral cortex Betz's cells in the precentral gyrus of the frontal lobe. These tracts are necessary for skilled voluntary movements or coordination. Their fibers terminate at various levels of the cord in synapses with interneurons, which in turn synapse with anterior horn neurons. Approximately 80 percent of the fibers of the pyramidal tracts decussate in the medulla and extend down the cord in named tracts. Impulses traveling over these tracts stimulate individual muscles to contract.

Extrapyramidal tracts are phylogenetically older and more complex. They consist of all pathways between the motor cortex and the anterior horn cells except those of the pyramidal system, and they conduct impulses important to muscle tone, automatic movements, and facial expression. The extrapyramidal fibers originate from areas of the brain other than the cerebral cortex. Many of the fibers of the extrapyramidal tracts project directly from the motor cortex into several components of the basal ganglia.

Specific descending motor tracts include two pyramidal and two extrapyramidal tracts. The lateral corticospinal tract carries pyramidal crossed fibers. It controls voluntary movement, contraction of individual or small groups of muscles, particularly those moving hands, fingers, feet, and toes of the opposite side of the body. Dendrites and cell bodies of these neurons originate in areas one through six of the precentral gyrus. The axons descend through the cerebrum and brain stem, decussate in the medulla, and continue down the cord in the lateral corticospinal tract in the lateral white columns prior to terminating in the internuncial neurons of the gray matter. Roots go to the spinal nerves and terminate in somatic effectors such as skeletal muscles.

The ventral corticospinal tract is a direct pyramidal tract. Its functions are the same as those of the lateral corticospinal tracts except that it controls the muscles on the same side of the body. The dendrites, cell bodies, and axons are the same as those for the lateral corticospinal tract, except that the fibers descend uncrossed in the ventral corticospinal tract in the anterior white column and then into spinal nerves to somatic effectors.

The lateral reticulospinal tract is an extrapyramidal tract consisting of fibers facilitating flexor and inhibiting extensor activity. They influence motor neurons to skeletal muscles controlling posture and expression. Their neurons originate in the lateral reticular formation of the brain stem. They terminate in the internuncial neurons sending fibers to the spinal nerves supplying flexor and extensor muscles contralaterally.

Fibers of the medial reticulospinal tract facilitate extension and inhibit flexor activity of skeletal muscles. They originate in the reticular formation of the medulla and descend in the medial reticulospinal tract, controlling flexion and extension ipsilaterally.

Special Receptors

Special receptors are structures responsible for responding to stimuli. They are intermediate transducers between the stimulus and the sensory neuron. These receptors are modified sensory nerve endings or modified dendrites, and they are modified in two ways. First, the peripheral fiber loses both myelin and neurilemma near its end. The remaining free or naked nerve ending becomes the receptor. The second modification occurs where the peripheral portion of the dendrite loses its coverings as above and becomes encased in a special capsule or end organ. With this modification, it is said to have formed an accessory structure.

There are several systems for classifying special sensory receptors. The one used here is related to the nature of the stimulus and recognizes mechanoreceptors, thermoreceptors, chemoreceptors, and electromagnetic receptors.

The mechanoreceptors respond to stimuli that distort specific accessory organs or free nerve endings. Three receptors in this category respond to light touch. Meissner's corpuscles are definite accessory structures with widespread, uneven distribution under the epidermis. They are most numerous in hairless areas such as hands, feet, forearms, tongue, lips, and nipples. These receptors are useful in defining texture and movement of light objects over the skin as well as detecting low-frequency vibrations. Merkel's disks are a second type of touch receptor with distribution similar to Meissner's corpuscles, initially transmitting strong but adapting touch sensations of objects on the skin as occurs when one applies clothing. The last type of touch receptor is the free nerve ending, which is located around the base of hair follicles and serves to sense movement along the surface of the body. Pressure receptors respond to a mechanical force greater than touch. Known as Pacinian corpuscles, they are located deeper than touch receptors and are anatomically separate from other receptors. Pacinian corpuscles are found in mesentery, periosteum, subcutaneous, submucous, subserous connective tissue as well as in the palms, soles, and genitalia.

There are many varieties of stretch receptors in the body. Those known as proprioceptors provide information with regard to position or orientation of the body in space or body movement. They are stimulated as muscles become stretched preceding or during movement. There are muscle spindles attached in parallel to skeletal muscles, Golgi tendon organs that detect the stretching of tendons and free nerve endings located in joint capsules. Other stretch receptors termed baroreceptors are located in the bifurcation of the common and internal carotid. These are called carotid sinuses. In addition, there are similar stretch receptors in the arch of the aorta called aortic sinuses. These receptors respond to the stretch of vascular smooth muscle, as occurs with a change in blood volume, and help to maintain blood pressure. Hering–Breuer stretch receptors located in the smooth muscles of the bronchi and bronchioles respond to stretch of the airways during inflation of the lungs and help to prevent overinflation. Finally, stretch receptors located in the wall of the right atrium are stimulated by increased venous return to the right heart and cause an increase in heart rate. These are called Bainbridge receptors.

Another type of mechanoreceptor is found in the inner ear. The vestibule receptors function to maintain equilibrium and to provide knowledge of body position and movement. The stimulus is a fluid wave in the semicircular canals of the inner ear. Changes in this fluid level are sensed by the otoliths of that vestibular apparatus. Additionally, in the inner ear receptors known as organs of Corti perceive sound and are stimulated by fluid waves secondary to vibration of the tympanic membrane.

The last example of a mechanoreceptor is found in skin and deeper structures and responds to tissue damage whatever the cause. These free nerve endings transmit painful stimuli to the spinal cord and higher centers to provide basic protective responses for the organism.

A second category of receptors, according to our classification, is the thermoreceptors. They are specific accessory organs sparsely located in the skin and mucosa of the lips, tongue, and genitalia. Cold receptors are also called end bulbs of Krause. They respond to a negative quantity or lack of heat. They are typically stimulated at temperatures less than 25C to as low as about 15C. Below this level, end bulbs of Krause are nonfunctioning and pain receptors are stimulated. Interestingly, physiologists have found that these bulbs are again stimulated at approximately 45C, as are pain receptors. Ruffini's corpuscles are specific receptors stimulated between 25 and 45C. They are, therefore, respon-

sive to heat. The distribution of Ruffini's corpuscles is similar to that of cold receptors.

The next category of receptors, chemoreceptors, includes five types of receptors. Central receptors are diffusely located in the medulla, aiding in the regulation of respirations. They are stimulated by hydrogen ion and carbon dioxide concentrations in the arterial blood and CSF. Likewise, peripheral receptors located in the carotid bodies and aortic bodies respond to low arterial oxygen tensions and stimulate the respiratory center. Another type of chemoreceptor is located in the mucous membrane of the roof of the nasal cavity. Specific rods and cilia are responsive to inhaled vapors and initiate the sense of smell. Taste buds located in the tongue respond to salt, sour, bitter, and sweet stimuli, and osmoreceptors aid in the regulation of water balance by sensing changes in the osmolality of arterial blood. These receptors have not been specifically identified but are theorized to be located in the anterior hypothalamus.

The final category of receptors, electromagnetic receptors, are involved in visual perception. Light is the stimulus, and the receptors are the rods and cones of the retina. Light acts to decompose the chemical composition of opsins, in turn stimulating the specific receptors.

Stimuli are applied to receptors, and if they are of sufficient magnitude, they produce receptor depolarization. This is referred to as generator or receptor potential. The generator potential in turn acts as a stimulus to depolarize the peripheral sensory fiber. If encapsulated in a corpuscle, the peripheral fiber depolarizes at the first node of Ranvier, eliciting an action potential. Generator potentials differ from action potentials in that they do not become self-propagated. Instead, the magnitude of the receptor potential is determined by the magnitude of the stimulus. It does not follow the all-or-none law of the action potential.

Another characteristic of special sensory receptors is receptor specificity. A specific stimulus for which a receptor is adapted will most readily cause depolarization of that receptor. That is, threshold is lowest for the specific stimulus for which the receptor is adapted. Nonspecific stimuli can cause receptor depolarization but must be of greater intensity than the specific stimulus.

Modality specificity is another characteristic of sensory receptors. Sensations perceived will be those for which the receptor is adapted regardless of the type of stimulus or where along the neuron it is applied. We also see a phenomenon of these receptors dealing with adaptation. This can be defined as a decreased frequency of receptor response or depolarization in the presence of continued application of the stimulus. The degree of adaptivity varies with the receptors. For example, we see that pain receptors, muscle spindles, Golgi tendon apparatus, Hering–Breuer receptors, pressoreceptors, and chemoreceptors are poorly adaptive. Thermoreceptors are moderately adaptive, and touch and pressure receptors are readily adaptive.

AUTONOMIC NERVOUS SYSTEM
General Concepts

The autonomic nervous system has been referred to by many other names by various writers. It has been called the visceral nervous system since it innervates and regulates visceral function by innervating smooth muscle, cardiac muscle, and glands. It has been called the involuntary/automatic nervous system, since most responses and actions occur automatically on an unconscious level. It has been called the vegetative nervous system, referring to the influence of basic or primitive influences of the hypothalamus on its activities. Finally, it has been most often, and perhaps erroneously, called the autonomic nervous system. It was thought to function independently but to be influenced by other components of the nervous system. This is seen as fallacious if we try to imagine a "fight-or-flight response" without skeletal muscle integration as well as autonomic.

In the overall placement within the nervous system, the autonomic system is a subunit of the peripheral nervous system along with the spinal and cranial nerve components.

Sensory and Motor Components

There are no inherent sensory components of the autonomic nervous system per se; however, sensory input from the viscera occurs by way of neurons arising from sensors in the smooth muscles, cardiac muscles, or glands. The afferent fibers travel from these sensors back to the spinal cord with spinal nerve afferent fibers. These visceral afferent fibers, as the autonomics are sometimes called, have their cell body in the dorsal root ganglia as do spinal (somatic) afferent neurons. The visceral fibers terminate in the lateral horn of the gray matter of the spinal cord, where they synapse with the nuclei of visceral efferent neurons. These efferent autonomic fibers involve two efferent neurons and a synapse that occurs at a ganglion. The efferent fibers then terminate in smooth muscle, cardiac muscle, and glandular epithelium. The efferent fiber originating in the lateral horn of the spinal cord exits the anterior horn of the cord and travels a short distance with the spinal nerve roots and common spinal nerve. The function of the autonomic nervous system primarily involves monitoring, via visceral efferent fibers, the body's internal activities through coordinated efforts of the central nervous system.

Sympathetic Division

The autonomic nervous system is thought of as two divisions based on structural and functional differences. These differences become evidenced as we discuss the makeup of each.

Beginning with the anatomy of the sympathetic division, we find that the cell body and dendrites of the preganglionic efferent fibers originate in the lateral horn of the spinal cord from cord levels of the first thoracic spinal nerve through the second lumbar spinal nerve. It is therefore also referred to as the thoracolumbar division of the autonomic nervous system. The preganglionic sympathetic fibers are multipolar, B-type, lightly myelinated fibers.

As mentioned earlier, the preganglionic fiber exits the cord with the spinal nerve through the intervertebral foramina and follows the anterior primary ramus of the spinal nerve for a short distance. The sympathetic efferent fiber then leaves the common spinal nerve and enters a ganglion located approximately 1 inch lateral to the vertebral body, where it meets the dendrites and cell body of the postgan-

glionic sympathetic fiber. The portion of nerve fiber running from the common spinal nerve out to the paravertebral ganglion is known as a white ramus communicans. Although several routes or "fates" are evidenced by sympathetic postganglionic fibers, one very common route is back to the common spinal nerve from the paravertebral ganglion by a separate track called the gray ramus communicans. As we look at these loops, the white ramus occurs distal to the gray along the spinal nerve. The postganglionic fiber that travels with the anterior primary ramus of the spinal nerve leaves it at some point more distal to the innervation of its intended viscera.

An explanation of sympathetic paravertebral ganglia seems in order, since they are involved in all of the fates of the efferent fibers. The sympathetic paravertebral ganglion consists of a chain of 20 to 24 pairs of ganglia found 1 inch lateral to either side of the vertebral column and extending from a level of the second cervical vertebra to the coccygeal vertebra. At each vertebral level, we find 3 pairs of ganglia at the cervical level, 10 to 12 pairs at the thoracic level, 2 to 4 pairs at the lumbar level, 4 pairs at the sacral level, and 1 pair at the coccygeal level. The ganglia appear as polymorphic nodular beads strung on a chain, the string being represented by nerve fibers interconnecting one bead with the next. At the coccygeal end of the chain of ganglia, we find a single ganglion, the coccygeal impar joining together the right and left chain.

Some complexity is added to the sympathetic division because there are four distinctly different fates in addition to the one already described. A second fate of the preganglionic fiber is to enter the paravertebral ganglion but it does not synapse therein. Instead, it passes to a different ganglion up or down the chain and synapses at that level. The postganglionic fiber then travels back to the spinal nerve by way of the gray ramus communicans and travels with the anterior primary ramus of the spinal nerve. By this method, sympathetic nerve fibers can come off at one spinal cord level and innervate a higher or lower level of the body. It is by this method, for example, that structures above T1 and below L2 receive sympathetic innervation. A third fate of the preganglionic fiber is to enter the paravertebral ganglion at its level of origin from the cord, synapsing within the ganglion and then sending the postganglionic fiber not back to the spinal nerve but rather to exit the ganglion as a postganglionic fiber to an effector organ. Another fate of the preganglionic sympathetic fiber is to pass through the paravertebral fiber and travel to the periphery to synapse in a prevertebral ganglion. The fiber synapses within the prevertebral ganglion and sends a postganglionic fiber to the effector organ. Finally, there are preganglionic sympathetic fibers that pass through both the paravertebral and prevertebral ganglia and synapse right on the effector organ, namely the adrenal medulla, the adrenal being referred to as a postganglionic sympathetic fiber.

The Parasympathetic Division

The parasympathetic division of the autonomic nervous system has its origin from cranial and sacral outflow tracts. The nuclei of the cranial outflow lie near the nuclei of cranial nerves III, VII, IX, and X. Their fibers extend along with fibers of the respective cranial nerves to the effector. The cell body of the parasympathetic fibers traveling with the oculomotor nerve arise in the Edinger–Westphal nucleus near the aqueduct of Sylvius. As is characteristic of the preganglionic parasympathetic fibers, they are lightly myelinated, type C fibers approximately equal in length to the postganglionic parasympathetic fibers. The preganglionic fiber synapses just behind the globe of the eye in the ciliary ganglion, and the postganglionic fiber innervates the intrinsic eye muscles. The fibers traveling with the facial nerve originate in the upper medulla and synapse in the sphenopalatine ganglion near the lacrimal gland and in the submandibular ganglion near the parotid gland. The postganglionic parasympathetic fibers of this nerve innervate the nasal mucosa, lacrimal glands, and salivary glands. The nuclei of the parasympathetic preganglionic outflow traveling with the glossopharyngeal nerve originate in the upper medulla and synapse in the otic ganglion. The postganglionic fibers innervate the parotid glands. Finally, the vagus nerve has parasympathetic nuclei in the medulla and synapses in the thorax and abdomen, with the postganglionic fibers innervating the thoracic and abdominal viscera excluding the distal half of the large bowel.

The sacral portion of the parasympathetic division originates in the lateral horn of gray matter of spinal cord levels S2, S3, and S4. The preganglionic fibers exit with the spinal roots, follow the anterior primary rami to peripheral ganglia, and there synapse with postganglionic fibers that innervate the distal half of the colon, the rectum, bladder, musculature, sphincter, uterus, uterine tubes, and genitalia.

Transmitter Substances

The hallmark of the sympathetic division of the autonomic nervous system is diffuse, mass action effects on several organs and systems simultaneously. Several anatomic and physiologic parameters support this diffuse action. The paravertebral chain affords the sympathetic division a method of spreading influence to various levels above and below the actual point of origin off the cord. One preganglionic neuron can synapse with an average of thirty postganglionic neurons, and one postganglionic neuron synapses with several effector sites. Splanchnic nerves provide additional divergence to the sympathetic division. The adrenal medulla is directly innervated by splanchnic fibers that pass through the celiac plexus, causing the adrenal medulla to liberate epinephrine and to a lesser degree norepinephrine into the bloodstream. These sympathetic neurohumoral transmitters are inactivated more slowly than the parasympathetic transmitters. The sympathetic system is involved with the control of fight-or-flight mechanisms that bring about coordinated changes controlling the internal environment during stress states. These processes are catabolic in nature, requiring the breakdown of energy stores.

The parasympathetic division, by contrast, functions in a discrete manner controlling one organ or system. This system lacks chain ganglia or adrenal medulla. There is less divergence between the pre- and postganglionic parasympathetic neurons and between postganglionic neurons and effectors. The parasympathetic neurons liberate acetylcholine at the preganglionic fibers, just as occurs in the sympathetic preganglionic fibers, and acetylcholine is also the neurohumoral transmitter liberated by the postganglionic parasympathetic fibers. The predominant response due to parasympathetic stimulation results in anabolic responses building up body energy stores. The parasympathetic system dominates the control of visceral activities under basal conditions and is responsible for long-term, day-to-day regulation of visceral functions.

Muscarinic and Nicotinic Effects

Muscarine is a parasympathomimetic substance derived from a poisonous mushroom. This substance exhibits a cholinergic effect on smooth muscle, cardiac muscle, and glands but has essentially no effect at the ganglionic synapses or at the motor end-plates of skeletal muscles. Muscarinic responses occur by stimulating visceral effectors innervated by cholinergic postganglionic neurons.

The agents included in this category include acetylcholine, congeners of acetylcholine estrase. Diisopropyl fluorophosphate, organophosphates, and other anticholinesterases are examples of these substances. Atropine-like drugs block the muscarinic actions of acetylcholine by preventing it from acting at visceral effector organs.

Nicotine has a dual effect on autonomic ganglia and skeletal muscles but no direct effect on smooth muscle, cardiac muscle, or glands. It initially stimulates and then inhibits the excitation of postsynaptic neurons or muscles. The initial effect is to depolarize the postsynaptic membrane, resulting in postganglionic neuron depolarization. The subsequent effect is to maintain depolarization so the postsynaptic membrane cannot be further stimulated.

Actions of the Autonomic Nervous System

Before considering specific organ effects of autonomic stimulation, the reader should become familiar with the concept of alpha and beta receptor sites. This concept is only applicable to the sympathetic division and applies because it is untrue that sympathetic stimulation produces strictly excitatory responses. Researchers of physiologic processes found that the responses of effector organs when sympathetic fibers were stimulated could be excitory or inhibitory. On inspecting the effectors, they found that the postganglionic neurons were identical, each liberating epinephrine and norepinephrine. If the neurons and the neurohumoral transmitters were the same, then the difference in response must be due to some difference in the effector. Since the receptors could not be identified anatomically but could be separately identified by physiologic response to pharmacologic agents, Ahlquist in 1948 proposed that they be termed alpha and beta responses and that the receptors be referred to as alpha and beta receptors or cells located on the effector organ.

Generally speaking, one type of receptor is present on an effector. However, some have both alpha and beta receptors, with a balance being maintained between the two. In some effectors, one receptor type will predominate. It can be said that stimulation of alpha receptors causes effector excitation and that beta receptor stimulation causes inhibition. There are two exceptions to this concept that the reader must note. First, the myocardium is innervated by beta receptors but stimulation of these receptors causes positive chronotropic and positive inotropic activity. Second, the bowel has alpha receptors that when stimulated result in decreased peristalsis and tone.

An additional subdivision of the beta receptors exists as determined by the effects of certain drugs on some but not all of the beta receptors. These receptors are designated beta$_1$ and beta$_2$. Beta$_1$ receptors are found in the heart and beta$_2$ receptors in the coronary vessels, ciliary muscle of the eye, bronchi, urinary bladder, and uterus.

Two alpha-adrenergic receptor subtypes have been identified. According to Hoffman and Lefkowitz, presynaptic alpha receptors differ in pharmacologic properties from postsynaptic alpha receptors. They are designated alpha$_1$ and alpha$_2$ receptors and are sites on the cell membrane where pharmacologic substances are bound, leading to characteristic physiologic changes in the cell. Alpha$_1$ receptors include the postsynaptic receptors mediating smooth muscle contraction, and alpha$_2$ receptors are located in the presynaptic bulb and to a lesser extent in postsynaptic receptors. Stimulation of presynaptic alpha$_2$ receptors inhibits norepinephrine release. Alpha$_1$ stimulation will cause smooth-muscle contraction. The physiologic responses of alpha receptors are currently under extensive pharmacodynamic investigation, evaluating the agonist–antagonist responses of drugs through these receptors. A clearer understanding should soon be provided by either the physiology or pharmacology literature.

In considering the autonomic responses, it should be kept in mind that the preganglionic fibers, both sympathetic and parasympathetic, liberate acetylcholine and are known as cholinergic neurons. The postganglionic parasympathetics likewise release acetylcholine to the effector organ. The postganglionic sympathetic fibers, however, are adrenergic—that is, they liberate norepinephrine, which stimulates alpha receptors, and to a lesser extent epinephrine, which stimulates both alpha and beta receptors.

The organ effects of autonomic nervous system stimulation usually involve dual innervation. Few structures have only one division innervating an effector. Where there is dual innervation, both divisions exert tone, as is seen in blood vessels. Under basal conditions, the parasympathetic division usually predominates; during stress states, the sympathetic division usually dominates. The actions of the two autonomic divisions are synergistic.

Looking at specific organ responses, we find that stimulation of the sympathetic fibers supplying the iris of the eye causes contraction of the radial muscle, resulting in dilation of the pupil (mydriasis). Parasympathetic stimulation causes contraction of the sphincter muscle of the iris and constriction of the pupil (miosis). The lens of the eye is held in a flattened configuration by the tension on radial ligaments. Stimulation of the parasympathetic fibers causes the lens to become increasingly convex to accommodate for near vision. There is little or no sympathetic effect on the lens of the eye.

Sympathetic stimulation of the myocardium consists of beta$_1$ stimulation, but as an exception to the rule, the result is an increase in heart rate and contractile force leading, to increased cardiac output. Parasympathetic stimula-

tion causes negative inotropism and negative chronotropism. Sympathetic stimulation of blood vessels causes constriction of coronary, skin, cerebral, skeletal muscle, pulmonary, and abdominal vessels. Parasympathetic stimulation, by contrast, causes vasodilation.

Glandular secretions follow the expected pattern of autonomic responses. Sympathetic stimulation of sweat glands results in copious sweating; parasympathetic stimulation has no effect. Sympathetic stimulation causes inhibition of gastric secretions, and parasympathetic stimulation causes increased secretion. Nasal, lacrimal, and salivary glands produce sparse, thick secretions when stimulated by sympathetic fibers and produce profuse, watery secretions when stimulation of the parasympathetic fibers occurs.

Bronchial smooth muscle relaxes when its sympathetic innervation is stimulated. Parasympathetic stimulation causes bronchiolar constriction. The latter effect is due to vagal stimulation of the bronchiolar smooth muscle. The smooth muscle of the bowel is the second exception to the rule that alpha-receptor stimulation causes excitation, because, although alpha receptors predominate, sympathetic stimulation causes a decrease in intestinal tone and a decrease in peristaltic activity. Parasympathetic stimulation, on the other hand, causes increases in tone and peristalsis. The smooth muscle of the urinary bladder relaxes with sympathetic and contracts with parasympathetic stimulation. The action on the bladder sphincter is just the opposite, however. Sympathetic stimulation contracts the sphincter to prevent urination; parasympathetic stimulation relaxes it, allowing urination.

The autonomic influence on the liver results in glycogenolysis with sympathetic stimulation, thereby releasing more glucose for ready access as a source of energy to meet the additional demands during stressful circumstances. Pancreatic secretions are decreased and the gallbladder relaxes, preventing emptying. Parasympathetic stimulation produces the opposite effects, resulting in glycogen synthesis by the liver, secretion by the pancreas and gallbladder.

The response to autonomic stimulation of the kidneys is unique. Sympathetic stimulation causes a decrease in urinary output by decreasing renal blood flow. The mechanism by which this occurs is through increased renin secretion by the juxtaglomerular cells of the kidneys. Parasympathetic system stimulation results in no clinically significant effects on renal function.

THE BRAIN: GENERAL ORGANIZATION AND FUNCTIONS

Telencephalon

The cortex is the convoluted outer gray mantle of brain tissue made up of multiple layers of neuronal cell bodies. It ranges in thickness from 2 to 5 mm and represents a recent phylogenetic development. The cortex appears gray because of the dense concentration of unmyelinated cell bodies. The convoluted pattern is typical, providing a large surface area of approximately 2 square feet. Examination shows that two-thirds of the surface area lies within the convolutions and therefore is not grossly visible in the intact human brain. The cortex makes up about one-third of the brain's weight.

The white matter of the brain lies below the cortical layer and above the diencephalon. It consists of myelinated axons from sensory and motor fibers arranged as tracts interconnecting different areas of the brain with one another or with the spinal cord. Three pathways are commonly taken by these fibers. Projection tracts interconnect higher centers of the cortex with more caudal areas of the brain and cord. Commissural tracts interconnect the right and left hemispheres and association tracts, anterior portions with posterior portions of the brain.

The telencephalon (or forebrain) is the larger portion of the prosencephalon. It is divided into six lobes by fissures or sulci. The frontal lobe is the largest of these lobes and is located anterior to the central sulcus, above the lateral fissure and medially, anterior to the central sulcus and above the cingulate sulcus. In 1909, a German neurologist mapped out 47 areas of localized functions of the cortex. This has been referred to as Brodmann's cytoarchitectural graph. He found that several areas of specialization are ascribed to the frontal lobe. The area of the precentral gyrus just anterior to the central sulcus is termed the primary motor area. This area, numbered 4 and 6, extends from the lateral surface of the frontal lobe to the medial surface. Areas of the body have representation in a motor homunculus, a disporportioned human figure whose toes stand in the cingulate sulcus medially, hips extending to the top of the longitudinal fissure and then draped laterally, extending toward the lateral fissure. Areas more important in reacting or responding to the external environment such as the head, hands, and thumbs are represented by larger areas of distribution on the cortex of each hemisphere. This is also the area of origin of corticospinal tracts carrying motor impulses from the cortex to the spinal cord.

Broca's area, numbers 44 and 45, is the motor area controlling speech. It lies on the inferior, lateral aspect of the frontal lobe, bilaterally. It is dominant in the dominant hemisphere, and damage to or destruction of this area leads to the inability to articulate speech, thus motor aphasia.

There is also a secondary or associative motor area, number 8, located anterior to the primary motor strip and with a homunculus similar to that of the primary motor area. This secondary motor area has a higher response threshold, and the result is a less refined motor response.

The prefrontal area, numbers 9 through 12, is located anterior to areas 44, 45, and 46 and operates in the formulation of abstract thinking, in the ability to plan or predict, and in judgmental abilities. It is also involved in the appreciation of and reaction to pain. It was thought by previous investigators to be the seat of intellect, but present researchers have indicated that intellect is not isolated to the cortex of any single lobe but rather involves cortical activity of all the brain.

The parietal lobe of the telencephalon consists of the area of the brain posterior to the central sulcus and anterior to the parieto-occipital sulcus. Medially it is bounded by the longitudinal fissure down to the cingulate sulcus. The parietal lobe houses the primary sensory area, numbers 1, 2, and 3, known as the postcentral gyrus. The homunculus is the same as that of the primary motor area, again with the larger areas devoted to parts of the body that have greatest importance in interpreting stimuli. This sensory area is the point of termination of all third-order neurons, which carry sensory impulses from peripheral receptors to the cortex of the telencephalon.

The temporal lobe is located inferior to the lateral fissure and anterior to the parieto-occipital sulcus. It is responsible for audition, and the posterior portion is involved in the visual interpretation of lines, borders, and angles. Disease affecting this lobe may lead to the inability to identify objects and marked distractibility. Olfactory areas are also associated with temporal lobe control.

The occipital lobe extends posterior to the parieto-occipital sulcus and is the primary visual area, number 17. This is also a bilateral area, as are all the areas in the telencephalon. Part of the visual cortex is located within the calcarine fissure of the occipital lobe.

Another lobe of the telencephalon is the limbic lobe. It is central to the cingulate sulcus, forming a ring of cortical tissue visible on the medial surface only. This is the older name for the cingulate gyrus, parahippocampus, and uncus. This area of the brain controls functions associated with aggression, arousal, and primitive drives related to self-preservation including feeding behavior, sexual behavior, rage, fear, and motivation.

The insula lies within the lateral sulcus and cannot be seen from the lateral view of the telencephalon until the temporal lobe is retracted downward at the lateral sulcus and the tissue of the frontal and parietal lobes is retracted upward at the sulcus. The insula therefore lies medial to the temporal, frontal, and parietal lobes and lateral to the lentiform nucleus. Functions of the insula include the communication of sensory and motor impulses to and from the viscera. Stimulation of the cortex of the insula evokes epileptic-type motor activity and visceral sensations.

Diencephalon

The diencephalon, or interbrain, lies deep in the ventromedial aspect of the cerebrum, connecting the cerebrum with the midbrain. It lies above the mesencephalon and below the white matter surrounding the third ventricle. There are five principal divisions of gray matter making up the diencephalon.

The epithalamus, a narrow band of tissue at the roof of the diencephalon, houses the pineal gland. This was once considered a vestigial structure with a possible role in hypothalamic and endocrine functions in growth and development. More recently, the pineal gland has been identified as a neurosecretory structure analogous to the adrenal medullae and neurohypophysis. Sympathetic stimulation leads to secretion of melatonin, a hormone that acts on the ovaries to inhibit ovulation.

Another structure of the diencephalon is the subthalamus, which lies lateral and inferior to the thalamus. It contains some extrapyramidal fibers and has a stabilizing role in extrapyramidal motor activities because it receives fibers from the basal ganglia prior to the descent of these fibers into the spinal cord.

The thalamus consists of bilateral egg-shaped masses of gray matter lying one in each hemisphere beside the third ventricle. Each is 1 cm wide and 3 cm long. Fibers from numerous corticospinal tracts synapse in the thalamus, as do fibers from the basal ganglia. It also acts to relay impulses to and from the hypothalamus and various areas of the cerebral cortex. A number of functions are recognized as being mediated by the thalamus. As mentioned, it is a relay point for impulses traveling between the cortex and cord. The thalamus provides the first conscious awareness of sensory impulses. Interpretation is crude and localization is poor, however. It aids in arousal and alerting of the organism and is linked to the reticular activating and limbic system. Finally, the thalamus monitors and influences voluntary and involuntary motor activities.

The hypothalamus is an area lying below the thalamus on either side of the third ventricle, above the midbrain and optic chiasm. Four separate areas of the hypothalamus include the preoptic, supraoptic, tuberal, and mamillary areas. The hypothalamus receives input from almost every area of the nervous system. It acts as a moderator or clearing house for impulses coordinating critical vegetative functions. The hypothalamus regulates autonomic nervous system excitation or inhibition and controls the release of hormones from the pituitary gland.

The hypothalamus functions to influence heart rate, force of contraction, and vessel diameter through autonomic nervous system control. The hypothalamus monitors the temperature of the blood perfusing thermoreceptors; promotes heat loss through vasodilation and decreases in basal metabolic rate; or promotes heat gain by vasoconstriction, increases in metabolic rate, and shivering. It also secretes or controls secretions of the neurohypophysis and the adenohypophysis. The regulation of body water is controlled by the hypophysis, which monitors blood osmolality via osmoreceptors and adjusts thirst through the secretion of antidiuretic hormone by the posterior pituitary. Gastrointestinal activity and feeding action are stimulated through the monitoring of blood sugar by the hypothalamus.

The hypothalamus houses areas of rage, docility, pleasure, and punishment. Emotions of rage and docility are moderated and expressed by blushing, palpitations, tears, and so on. The lateral and medial hypothalamus house areas of pleasure and punishment, respectively. In addition, the hypothalamus integrates sleep and awake states, with input from the reticular activating system.

The final division of the diencephalon to be considered is the basal ganglia. It is made up of several small areas of gray matter. There are three major subdivisions. The corpus striatum is made up of the lentiform nucleus, the globus pallidus, putamen, and caudate nucleus. A second subdivision is termed the amygdala, and a third known as the claustrum. All of these areas of the basal ganglia are interconnected with one another and act to coordinate voluntary motor activity to prevent purposeless movements. Recent studies show that the basal ganglia appear to be involved in the planning and programming of voluntary movement. Disorders such as chorea, athetosis, and Parkinson's disease are seated in the basal ganglia.

Mesencephalon

The midbrain is located below the thalamus, above the metencephalon, and in front of the cerebellum. The mesencephalon interconnects these three areas with the higher centers. These fibers are made of myelinated tracts passing between the spinal cord and higher centers. There are also nuclei for the oculomotor, trochlear, and trigeminal nerves. The mesencephalon functions to interconnect the higher centers with the spinal cord and cerebellum. It is also the location of reflex centers for hearing and sight.

Metencephalon

The metencephalon is made up of the pons varolii and the cerebellum. Along with the myelencephalon, the metencephalon forms the rhombencephalon.

The pons is a bulbous enlargement on the anterior superior surface of the brain stem. It forms one continuous structure with the mesencephalon and the medulla. The nuclei for cranial nerves VI, VII, and VIII are located in the pons. Along with acting as an interconnecting pathway between the brain stem and higher centers, the pons also houses the pneumotaxic and apneustic centers, which influence respiratory activity.

The cerebellum is located posterior to the pons, the medulla oblongata, and the fourth ventricle. It lies in the posterior fossa of the occipital bone, connecting to the pons and midbrain by three stalks of white matter known as peduncles. The cerebellum consists of two hemispheres separated by the falx cerebelli. They have regularly spaced furrows and have a cortex and white matter similar to the telencephalon. The tentorium cerebelli is a fold of dura mater separating the cerebellum from the occipital lobe above. The cerebellum derives sensory input from spinocerebellar tracts and contributes to the control of auditory and visual responses, motion sickness, equilibrium, stretch reflexes, and adjustments for posture and movement. Cerebellar lesions lead to scanning speech, intention tremors, and inability to stop movement promptly.

Myelencephalon

The medulla oblongata is separated superiorly from the pons by a transverse sulcus. It is cone shaped, with the apex pointed toward the spinal cord. The inferior border is located above the highest rootlet of the first cervical spinal nerve. The medulla is slightly longer than two centimeters. The rootlets of cranial nerves IX, X, and XI emerge from the dorsolateral sulcus of the medulla, the rootlet of the hypoglossal nerve emerging from the ventrolateral sulcus. Internally the medulla is mixed white and gray matter.

The medulla oblongata has three major functions. First, it contains vital reflex centers for the control of heart action, blood vessel diameter, and respirations. It is also the control center for such nonvital reflexes as vomiting, sneezing, coughing, hiccuping, and swallowing. Finally, the medulla houses projection tracts interconnecting the brain with the spinal cord. Those fibers that decussate do so in the medulla.

CEREBRAL CIRCULATION

Vascular Circuits

The entire blood supply to the brain arises from the internal carotid and vertebral arteries. Venous drainage is completed by the superior sagittal sinus and sigmoid sinuses into the internal jugular veins.

The internal carotid arteries extend up the neck, entering the cranial vault by way of the posterior portion of the foramen lacerum and the petrous portion of the temporal bone. It enters in the area of the temporal bone without branching. It generally supplies the anterior portions of the brain, especially the cerebrum. After ascending to the area of the temporal lobe, it gives rise to three main branches. The first, the middle cerebral artery, is the largest of the three. It extends laterally along the lateral sulcus and continues posteriorly. The middle meningeal artery supplies portions of the temporal, parietal, and frontal lobes, including portions of the primary motor and sensory areas. The anterior cerebral artery branches from the internal carotid, entering the basal portion of the superior longitudinal fissure and extending medially and anteriorly. It supplies portions of the frontal and parietal lobes as well as the medial aspects of the primary sensory and motor gyri. The right and left anterior cerebral arteries are joined by the anterior communicating artery, which is approximately 4 mm long. The anterior cerebral artery ends in an anastomosis with the posterior cerebral artery, coming off from the vertebral artery circuitry. Finally, the third branch of the internal carotid artery forms the right and left posterior communicating arteries. These vessels pass posteriorly to supply portions of the thalamus, internal capsule, and the walls of the third ventricle. They terminate by joining with posterior cerebral arteries.

The vertebral artery network is somewhat less complex. The vertebral arteries also arise as bilateral structures from the brachiocephalic artery on the right and directly from the aorta on the left. The vertebral arteries ascend through the foramina of the transverse processes of the upper six cervical vertebrae. Before entering the cranium, the vertebral arteries give rise to the posterior inferior cerebellar arteries. Entering the cranial vault via the foramen magnum, the vertebral arteries next anastomose to form a single basilar artery. The basilar artery runs a short distance along the pons, giving off several small branches along its route. These supply the cerebellum, pons, and middle ear. It then divides into two main branches—namely, the right and left posterior cerebral arteries. These arteries supply the lateral portions of the temporal and occipital lobes and end by anastomosing with the posterior communicating arteries.

The network of anastomosing blood vessels at the base of the brain surrounding the optic chiasm allows for collateral circulation to the brain. It provides union of blood vessels supplying the brain by way of the carotid and vertebral arteries. This network of vessels, known as the circle of Willis, includes the anterior and posterior cerebral arteries and the anterior and posterior communicating arteries.

Physiology

Cerebral blood flow is maintained relatively constant at a rate of 45 to 50 ml/100 g of tissue weight per minute. The average adult male brain weighs 1450 g, the female 1350 g. Cerebral blood flow therefore is approximately 665 ml/minute, or 15 percent of the cardiac output. The regional distribution of cerebral blood flow results in the white matter receiving only 20 ml/100 g of tissue and the gray matter

40 ml/100 g. This obviously shows that gray matter receives a proportionately greater amount of blood flow owing to its greater metabolic rate. The overall oxygen consumption in the brain is 3.3 ml of oxygen per 100 g of tissue weight per minute. We see that the ratio of cerebral blood flow to cerebral metabolic rate of oxygen is approximately 15 to 1. In spite of this disproportionately high ratio, there is little basal oxygen reserve in the brain, and interruption of adequate blood flow for as little as 10 seconds can lead to loss of consciousness.

The constancy of cerebral blood flow is assured by maintaining a stable effective perfusion pressure to the brain. The perfusion pressure is the mean pressure difference between the veins and arteries. Venous pressure is relatively low and constant, typically being less than 10 mm Hg in the internal jugular veins. The mean arterial blood pressure therefore generally ranges between 90 and 95 mm Hg, keeping cerebral blood flow relatively constant. The cerebral vasculature is extremely sensitive to changes in tissue oxygen and carbon dioxide tensions. These vessels have the ability to constrict and dilate to autoregulate cerebral blood flow within certain limits of perfusion pressures, thereby helping to assure adequate cerebral perfusion. The limits spoken of above include mean arterial blood pressure between 60 and 180 mm Hg, which encompasses most normal fluxes of systemic blood pressures. Above mean arterial blood pressures of 180 mm Hg, the cerebral vasculature can no longer constrict to keep cerebral blood flow within normal limits and the flow increases. This results in increased intracranial pressure and may lead to intracranial hemorrhage. Below mean pressures of 60 mm Hg, cerebral vessels can dilate no more to keep blood flow constant and flow begins to decline. At this point, an additional mechanism ensures adequate cerebral tissue oxygenation. Below a mean pressure of 60 mm Hg to a pressure as low as 35 mm Hg, the cerebral tissue can extract more oxygen from hemoglobin to maintain adequate tissue oxygenation. Below arterial pressures of 35 mm Hg, signs of cerebral hypoxia are seen and irreversible brain damage may occur.

Other factors in addition to perfusion pressure maintain normal cerebral blood flow. There appears to be no evidence of direct action of autonomic nervous system influence on human cerebral blood flow. Carbon dioxide and oxygen do affect changes in blood flow by acting to dilate or constrict arterial diameter, however. Carbon dioxide is the most potent dilator and constrictor, exerting its effect directly on the vascular smooth muscle, resulting in a direct relationship between Pa_{CO_2} and cerebral blood flow and an inverse relation between Pa_{O_2} and cerebral blood flow. Between Pa_{CO_2} of 25 and 115 mm Hg, there is a 1 ml/100 g/minute change in cerebral blood flow. The range of influence seen with Pa_{O_2} on cerebral flow is narrower, in the range of 25 to 50 mm Hg. At a Pa_{O_2} of 50 mm Hg, there is a cerebral flow of approximately 50 ml/100 g/minute, and at a Pa_{O_2} of 25 mm Hg the cerebral blood flow is approximately 100 ml/100 g/minute. This gives a ratio of change of 2 ml increase in cerebral blood flow for each 1 mm Hg decrease in Pa_{O_2} between 25 and 50 mm Hg Pa_{O_2}.

It is important for the anesthetist to have some understanding of the effects of anesthetics on cerebral blood flow and cerebral metabolic rate. The following table summarizes these effects.

Agent	Cerebral Blood Flow	Cerebral Metabolic Rate
Halothane	+++	– –
Enflurane	0	– – –
Isoflurane	0	0
Ketamine	+++	– –
Thiobarbiturates	– – –	– – –
Fentanyl/droperidol	– –	–
Diazepam + N_2O	– – –	– – –

The agents listed above relate to either 1 minimum alveolar concentration (MAC) level of inhalation agents or levels of clinically effective levels of anesthesia. The + symbols represent increases and the – symbols decreases in the parameter reported.

Blood–Brain Barrier

The concept of a blood–brain barrier was developed in an attempt to explain the very different rate of permeability of most substances between the capillary bed and interstitial fluids of the brain compared with the more rapid equilibration between these two compartments as noted in other organ systems. It was noted that water, carbon dioxide, oxygen, and glucose move more readily from the blood into brain tissue. In general, the rapidity of the movement of all substances follows the specifics of Graham's law. Although many substances require longer time to equilibrate, very few if any substances are totally prohibited entry. The cerebral capillaries are more permeable in the newborn, and the blood–brain barrier develops in the first few years of life. This explains why in jaundiced infants bile pigments enter the nervous system and produce damage to the basal ganglia, resulting in kernicterus.

Some areas of the brain are more impregnable than others. The pineal gland, posterior pituitary, and areas surrounding the ventricular structures are more susceptible to substances circulating in the plasma. Such ions as Na^+, K^+, Mg^{++}, Cl^-, HCO_3^-, and $HPO_4^=$ equilibrate with CSF but may require up to 30 times longer than water. Bile salts, catecholamines, and proteins have very limited access to the adult brain. Acid substances and cations penetrate more slowly than bases and anions. Finally, there is a very high correlation between lipid solubility and penetrability.

The clinical implications associated with the permeability of the blood–brain barrier to drugs are that those anesthetics that have a high solubility coefficient generally cause unconsciousness more quickly. Drugs enter the brain at differing rates, with sulfadiazine and erythromycin entering readily, penicillin and chlortetracycline hydrochloride (Aureomycin) entering slowly. Atropine readily crosses the blood–brain barrier; glycopyrrolate does not. The clinician should also be aware that the blood–brain barrier breaks down as the result of irradiation and local infection and in areas of tumor growth.

CRANIAL NERVES

Categorization

The cranial nerves can be thought of as peripheral nerves arising from the brain. They consist of 12 pairs of nerves numbered in reference to their sequence coming off the brain stem from anterior to posterior or superiorly to inferiorly. The nerves are each named nerves and are also represented by Roman numerals. Cranial nerves enter or exit the brain by way of foramina in the base of the cranium. Because of the higher level of development of cephalic structures, the cranial nerves are more complex than spinal nerves. They are primarily involved in innervation of structures of the head and neck and are further differentiated on the basis of input or output to special senses. The cranial nerves consist of either sensory or motor fibers, with some nerves containing both types. Along with the commonly learned mnemonic representing the first letter of each named nerve, there is also one indicating whether the nerve is sensory, motor, or both. The mnemonic for learning the names is "On Old Olympus Towering Tops, A Finn and Visiting German Viewed Some Hops" and that designating function, "Some Say Marry Money But My Brothers Say Bad Business Marry Money." There are a number of variations that creative students have devised over the years, and the reader may have learned others.

Specific

Each of the cranial nerves will be presented in a format indicating the type and course of the nerve, its function and pathology.

    I. Olfactory
      A. Type—Sensory.
      B. Course—Receptors are modified, exposed dendrites located in the nasal cavity and sensitive to a variety of vapors. The cell bodies are embedded in respiratory mucosa covering the cribriform plate of the ethmoid bone. The axons terminate in the primary area for smell (area 36) in the temporal lobe.
      C. Function—Sense of smell is relatively poorly developed in humans compared to lower animals.
      D. Pathology—Usually local dysfunction due to respiratory mucosal inflammation leading to anosmia. May be due to intracranial tumors or head injuries, which can present as olfactory hallucinations or anosmia.
    II. Optic
      A. Type—Sensory.
      B. Course—The dendrites and cell bodies are in the retina and are not directly stimulated by light, but rather the stimulus causes a release of chemical transmitters, rhodopsin in the rods and iodopsin and photopsin in cones. From the retina, the optic nerve travels to the optic chiasm, where medial fibers from each eye decussate. Each tract from the optic chiasm to the visual cortex (area 17) of the occipital lobe carries fibers from both eyes. The visual cortex is necessary for conscious perception of an upright image. Collateral fibers of this nerve also extend to the cranial nerves involved in extraocular movement to coordinate globe movement with visual perception.

C. Function—Vision.

D. Pathology—Prechiasmic involvement produces ipsilateral blindness; chiasmic or postchiasmic pathology, varieties of hemianopsia.

III. Oculomotor

A. Type—Somatic and visceral motor.

B. Course—Somatic fibers originate in the Edinger–Westphal nucleus of the midbrain and synapse with all extraocular muscles except the superior oblique and lateral rectus muscles in addition to muscle elevating eyelids. Visceral fibers have the same origin, with the preganglionic fibers terminating in the ciliary muscle of the lens and the sphincter muscle of the iris.

C. Function—Somatic fibers innervate levator palpebrae, inferior oblique, inferior rectus, medial rectus, and superior rectus extraocular muscles to provide conjugate globe movement. The visceral nerves provide accommodation for far vision and for constriction of the iris.

D. Pathology—Disjunctive eye movements, ptosis, and loss of accommodation.

IV. Trochlear

A. Type—Somatic motor.

B. Course—Fibers originate in the midbrain at the floor of the cerebral aqueduct at the junction of the upper pons and cerebellar peduncles. These fibers terminate in the superior oblique extraocular muscle.

C. Function—Allows conjugate globe movement medially.

D. Pathology—Unable to turn eyes downward and outward, with vertical diplopia.

V. Trigeminal

A. Type—Sensory and somatic motor.

B. Course—Sensory receptors for touch, pressure, pain, and temperature originate in the anterior half of the head. The cell body is in the Gasserian ganglion, and fibers terminate in the pons. The somatic motor fibers originate in the pons and terminate in the muscles of mastication and the tympanic membrane.

C. Function—General sensation to the anterior half of the face, with three divisions. The ophthalmic division is sensory, the maxillary division sensory, and the mandibular division both sensory and motor. The motor components control mastication, swallowing, movement of the soft palate, and eardrum tension.

D. Pathology—Injury to the sensory root results in anesthesia to the anterior half of the face, dryness of nose, and loss of sense of taste. Motor root involvement results in loss of mastication and paralysis of facial muscles, as well as tic douloureux.

VI. Abducens

A. Type—Somatic motor.

B. Course—The multipolar neurons of this nerve originate in the pons and innervate the lateral rectus extraocular muscle.

C. Function—Operate conjugate globe movement temporally.

D. Pathology—Internal or convergent squint.

VII. Facial

A. Type—Sensory and somatic and visceral motor.

B. Course—Sensory unipolar neurons have their receptors in the taste buds of the anterior two-thirds of the tongue. Somatic motor fibers course from the pons to the facial muscles. Visceral fibers synapse in parasympathetic ganglia and terminate in salivary glands.

C. Function—Sensory (taste in the anterior two-thirds of the tongue); somatic motor (facial expression); visceral motor (salivary, nasal, lacrimal, oral secretions).

D. Pathology—Loss of sensation of taste in the anterior two-thirds of the tongue, Bell's palsy, and inability to grimace.

VIII. Vestibulocochlear

A. Type—Sensory.

B. Course—The vestibular portion has receptors and cell bodies in the otoliths and semicircular canal of the inner ear and terminates in the cerebellum. The dendrites of the cochlear portion of this nerve originate as dendrites in the organ of Corti of the inner ear and terminate in the primary auditory area (area 41) of the temporal lobe.

C. Function—The vestibular division ensures equilibrium, and the cochlear division, hearing.

D. Pathology—Results in vertigo and perceptive deafness.

IX. Glossopharyngeal

A. Type—Sensory and somatic and visceral motor.

B. Course—Sensory neurons originate from the taste buds in the posterior third of the tongue, chemoreceptors in the carotid bodies, and pressoreceptors in the carotid sinuses, as well as general sensory receptors in the oropharynx and hypopharynx and middle ear. They terminate in the medulla oblongata. Somatic and visceral motor fibers originate in the medulla, with somatic efferents innervating the pharyngeal constrictor muscles and the visceral efferent fibers terminating in the salivary glands.

C. Function—Taste, general sensation in the throat, swallowing, salivation; monitors blood pressure, Pa_{O_2} and Pa_{CO_2} levels.

D. Pathology—Loss of taste in the posterior third of the tongue, inability to swallow, loss of the gag reflex.

X. Vagus

A. Type—Visceral sensory and motor.

B. Course—Sensory fibers originate from abdominal and thoracic viscera, as well as chemo- and pressoreceptors. They terminate in the medulla. The motor fibers originate as preganglionic parasympathetic fibers in the medulla and after synapsing innervate smooth muscle, cardiac muscle, and glands.

C. Function—Sensory components provide general visceral afferent sensations and monitor blood pressure, Pao_2, $Paco_2$, left heart filling, and lung inflation. Motor components provide the characteristic parasympathetic autonomic excitatory effects.

D. Pathology—Sensory dysfunction ranges from anesthesia of the larynx to overdistension of the lungs. Motor dysfunction results in paralysis of laryngeal function, absence of bowel activities, and generalized decrease in daily anabolic functions.

XI. Spinal accessory

A. Type—Somatic motor.

B. Course—The cell bodies of this nerve originate in the medulla and the anterior horn gray matter of the first five cervical spinal cord segments. The cranial fibers terminate in pharyngeal and laryngeal muscles, whereas the spinal fibers innervate muscles of the neck and shoulders.

C. Function—The cranial segment aids in swallowing and phonation; the spinal segments in movement of the head and shoulders.

D. Pathology—Dysphagia, hoarseness, and weakness of head and shoulder muscles.

XII. Hypoglossal

A. Type—Somatic motor.

B. Course—The cell body of this neuron originates in the medulla and terminates in the tongue.

C. Function—Movement of the tongue.

D. Pathology—Inability to extend the tongue or weakness in movement of the tongue.

BIBLIOGRAPHY

Anthony CP, Thibodeau LC: Textbook of Anatomy and Physiology, 11th ed. St. Louis, Mosby, 1983.

Bates B: A Guide to Physical Examination, 3rd ed. Philadelphia, Lippincott, 1983.

Carpenter MB: Human Neuro-Anatomy, 8th ed. Baltimore, Williams & Wilkins, 1982.

Collins VJ: Principles of Anesthesiology, 2nd ed. Philadelphia, Lea & Febiger, 1976.

Cousins MJ, Bridenbaugh PO (eds): Neural Blockage in Clinical Anesthesia and Management of Pain. Philadelphia, Lippincott, 1980.

Crelin ES: Clinical Symposia: Development of the Nervous System. Ciba, Summit, 1974, Vol. 26, no. 2.

Eliasson SC, Prensky BH Jr: Neurological Pathophysiology, 2nd ed. New York, Oxford University Press, 1978.

Ellis H, McLarty M: Anatomy for Anesthestists, 2nd ed. Philadelphia, Davis, 1968.

Ericksson E: Illustrated Handbook in Local Anesthesia, 2nd ed. Philadelphia, Saunders, 1980.

Ganong WF: Review of Medical Physiology, 12th ed. Los Altos, Lange, 1985.

Goodman AG, Gilman A: The Pharmacological Basis of Therapeutics, 7th ed. New York, Macmillan, 1985.

Gray TC, Nunn JF, and Utting JE: General Anesthesia, 4th ed. London, Butterworth, 1980.

Guyton, AC: Textbook of Medical Physiology, 6th ed. Philadelphia, Saunders, 1981.

Hoffman BB, Lefkowitz RJ: Alpha-adrenergic receptor subtypes. N Engl J Med 302:1390, 1980.

Junqueirra LC, Carneiros J: Basic Histology, 4th ed. Los Altos, Lange, 1983.

Kandel ER, Schwartz JH: Principles of Neural Science, 2nd ed. New York, Elsevier/North-Holland, 1985.

Katz J, Benumof J, Kadis LB: Anesthesia and Uncommon Diseases, 2nd ed. Philadelphia, Saunders, 1981.

Merritt HH (ed): A Textbook of Neurology, 6th ed. Philadelphia, Lea & Febiger, 1979.

Miller RD (ed): Anesthesia, 2nd ed. New York, Churchill-Livingstone, 1986.

Mountcastle VB: Medical Physiology, 14th ed. St. Louis, Mosby, 1980.

Murray JM, Weber A: The cooperative action of muscle proteins. Sci Am 230:58–71, 1974.

Netter FH: The Ciba Collection of Medical Illustrations. Nervous System, Summit, Ciba, 1953, Vol. 1.

Noback CR, Demarest RJ: The Human Nervous System, Basic Principles of Neurobiology, 3rd ed. New York, McGraw-Hill, 1981.

Pansky B, Allen DJ: Review of Neuroscience. New York, Macmillan, 1980.

Rosenberg H: Skeletal Muscle Structure and Function, ASA Refresher Courses in Anesthesiology. Philadelphia, Lippincott, 1977, Vol. 5, Chapter 12.

Ruch TC, Patton HD: Physiology and Biophysics, 19th ed. Philadelphia, Saunders, 1974.

Shapiro HM: Physiologic and Pharmacologic Regulation of Cerebral Blood Flow, ASA Refresher Courses in Anesthesiology. Philadelphia, Lippincott, 1977, Vol. 5, Chapter 13.

Warwick R, Williams PL: Gray's Anatomy, 35th ed. Philadelphia, Saunders, 1973.

20

Integrated Circulatory Physiology

Dean H. Morrow and Lewis A. Coveler

The responsibilities of a teacher are to summarize pertinent information and to provide examples which make this information useful to the student. If the student is confused by the presentation or lost in detail the teacher has failed. It is our impression that many students are bewildered by cardiovascular physiology both by the presentation and detail to which they have been exposed. The intent of this presentation is to develop a concept of circulatory physiology which is conceptually accurate and yet simplistic enough to serve as a basis for informed problem solving during the conduct of anesthesia. Care has been taken to use common clinical situations to emphasize physiologic principles.

The primary purpose of the circulatory system is to provide blood flow consistent with the metabolic requirements of organs and tissues and, in special circumstances, with the needs of cell groups within an organ. On a moment-to-moment basis, blood flow is dependent on the interaction between pressure and resistance. This relationship is expressed by the blood flow equation: $Q = \Delta P/R$, where flow (Q) is in ml/min., the arterial-venous pressure difference (ΔP) is in mm Hg, and resistance (R) is in dyne-sec-cm^{-5}.

Although it is necessary to be familiar with the blood flow equation as a physiologic concept, it is more useful to express flow in terms of the intact circulation. Under this circumstance, flow in the systemic circulation becomes

$$\text{Left ventricular output} = \frac{\text{Mean arterial pressure} - \text{Mean right atrial pressure}}{\text{Systemic vascular resistance}}$$

and flow in the pulmonary system becomes

$$\text{Right ventricular output} = \frac{\text{Mean pulmonary artery pressure} - \text{Mean left atrial pressure}}{\text{Pulmonary vascular resistance}}$$

It is emphasized that although blood flow is the primary function of the circulation and although measurements of cardiac output (CO) and blood flow in selected arteries are becoming more common in some clinical environments, the measurement of blood flow in most organs or tissues

is quite difficult in the majority of patients. Since flow measurements are not yet practical on a routine basis, we must use other more easily measured, albeit less direct, variables to determine the status of the circulation in our patients. This reasoning, of course, is responsible for the emphasis placed on the monitoring and recording of blood pressure as an indirect indicator of systemic blood flow. Indeed, systemic arterial pressure (SAP) is quite useful in assessing the status of the circulation providing that the several variables that are physiologically integrated to produce and regulate the blood pressure are clearly understood.

Figure 20–1 illustrates the physiologic variables interacting moment-to-moment to determine SAP. We have found the schema illustrated in the diagram to be useful in problem-solving situations in the perioperative period.

The upper portion of Figure 20–1A, illustrates those physiologic variables related to the CO. The lower portion, B, illustrates variables influencing systemic vascular resistance. The center portion of the figure, C, illustrates the mechanism by which changes in blood pressure, acting via regulatory centers in the brain stem, adjust through the autonomic nervous system both CO and total peripheral resistance. To help understand the information summarized in Figure 20–1, it is useful to describe each of the three divisions independently.

VARIABLES RELATED TO THE CARDIAC OUTPUT

CO is the product of heart rate and stroke volume. The stroke volume is the difference between end-diastolic volume (EDV) and end-systolic volume (ESV). EDV may be modified by alterations in blood volume, heart rate, venous tone, and ventricular compliance. ESV is most closely correlated with the contractile state of the ventricle.

Heart Rate

Under normal circumstances, the heart rate is determined by the frequency of spontaneous discharge of automatic (pacemaker) cells in the sinoatrial (SA) node. Physiologic factors and drugs increasing the heart rate are categorized as producing a *positive* chronotropic response. Factors and

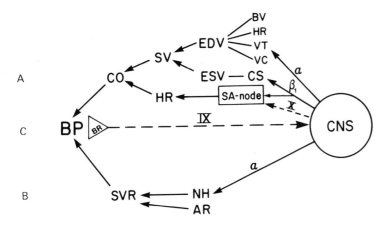

Figure 20–1. Schema of physiologic variables involved in systemic arterial pressure (BP). CO: cardiac output; SV: stroke volume; HR: heart rate; EDV: end-diastolic volume; ESV: end-systolic volume; BV: blood volume; VT: venous tone; VC: ventricular compliance; CS: ventricular contractile state; SVR: systemic vascular resistance; NH: neurohumoral; AR: autoregulation; BR: baroreceptors; α: alpha-mediated, efferent adrenergic response; β_1: beta-mediated, efferent adrenergic cardiac responses. (*Modified from Goldberg AH: Cardiovascular function and halothane. In Greene NM (ed): Halothane. Clinical Anesthesia. Philadelphia, Davis, 1968, pp. 23–60. Reproduced with permission.*)

drugs decreasing the heart rate are categorized as producing a *negative* chronotropic response. It is apparent from Figure 20–1A that an increase in heart rate will within limits permit a normal CO at a reduced stroke volume and that an increased stroke volume will within limits permit a normal CO at a reduced heart rate.

The physiologic mechanism altering the discharge rate of SA nodal pacemaker cells under usual circumstances is efferent vagal activity and the release of acetycholine. A decrease in efferent vagal activity—that is, fewer impulses from the vagal nuclei in the brain to the SA node—results in less acetycholine release and an *increase* in heart rate. Similarly, an increase in efferent vagal activity with more acetycholine release *decreases* heart rate. Thus, either an increase or decrease in heart rate can significantly modify CO if stroke volume remains constant.

Although the vagus is the primary determinant of heart rate under usual circumstances, it is well known that the pacemaker firing rate can be altered by efferent adrenergic (sympathetic) nerve activity and the release of norepinephrine. Importantly, many abnormalities in cardiac rhythm occurring during anesthesia and surgery can be attributed to increased adrenergic activity.

Physiologically, heart rate changes produced by efferent adrenergic discharge are categorized as β_1 responses. As is discussed in more detail below, drugs mimicking the activity of norepinephrine on the β_1 receptors and the antagonists of this action (e.g., propranolol) are of obvious importance in understanding drug-induced changes in physiologic responses. Adrenergic-related changes in heart rate and contractile state are β_1 responses, since these are the *only* adrenergic receptors in the heart.

End-Diastolic Volume

EDV is the volume of blood contained within the ventricle just prior to the onset of ventricular systole. Ventricular filling during diastole is due to both venous return, which is of course dependent on an adequate circulating blood volume, and to heart rate. Optimal EDV occurs with a physiologically normal or reduced heart rate, because there is adequate time for blood to flow into the heart. An increase in heart rate results in a shorter diastolic (filling) time and creates the potential for a decrease in EDV. Venous tone refers to the relative degree of contraction or relaxation of

smooth muscle contained in venous vessels. If tone is high, the capacitance or volume of the venous system is reduced. Theoretically, high venous tone and the resultant decrease in venous capacity would favor venous return to the heart by decreasing the quantity of blood in the total venous system. In contrast, low venous tone would favor decreased venous return. Although it is known that drugs such as norepinephrine and methoxamine (α-adrenergic agonists as in the section Neurohumoral Control) increase venous tone and that halothane decreases venous tone, the precise influence of these changes on EDV have yet to be completely elucidated in the intact patient. Additionally, reductions in ventricular compliance or a decrease in the relative distensibility of the ventricle may also reduce the EDV.

In the patient with hypovolemia secondary to blood loss, EDV may be reduced by both the inadequate circulating blood volume and compensatory increase in heart rate (shorter diastolic filling interval). Patients subjected to positive end-expiratory airway pressure (PEEP) have a decreased EDV through decreased venous return and diastolic filling. In patients with pericardial tamponade, ventricular compliance is mechanically decreased by external pressure. As a result, the EDV and, in turn, the stroke volume are usually decreased.

End-Systolic Volume

ESV is the volume of blood remaining in the ventricle after systole is complete. ESV is directly dependent on the contractile state of the ventricular musculature, as well as the resting fiber length of the ventricular muscle at the time systole begins. Since resting fiber length in the ventricle is established by the volume of blood in the ventricle at the onset of systole (EDV as described earlier), it is more correctly described as the end-diastolic ventricular fiber length (EDVFL).

Ventricular Contractility

Contractile state can be considered the end result of a series of biochemical and electromechanical events that produce shortening of the myofibrils composing the muscular syncytium of the ventricular wall. As a result of this shortening, the volume of the cardiac chamber decreases, intraventricular pressure rises, and a portion of the EDV is ejected into the aorta or pulmonary artery. The volume of blood ejected with each ventricular contraction is the stroke volume.

End-Diastolic Ventricular Fiber Length

The amount of tension in the ventricular muscle produced by the EDV determines the resting fiber length (EDVFL), from which ventricular mechanical systole begins. The relationship between the EDVFL and ventricular contractility is described by the Frank–Starling law, as illustrated in Figure 20–2.

The relationship between EDVFL and stroke volume (Fig. 20–2) is useful clinically to describe the contractile state as a function of work performed by the ventricle—that is, the stroke volume generated. Thus, ventricular contractility is related to both EDVFL and to the intrinsic biochemical-mechanical properties of the ventricle on a moment-to-moment basis. By convention, increased ventricular work, stroke volume from a given EDVFL (Fig. 20–2A), represents increased contractile state. Physiologic factors and drugs increasing ventricular contractility are said to produce a positive inotropic response. Decreased ventricular work from a given EDVFL (Fig. 20–2B) represents decreased contractile state. Factors and drugs that decrease the contractile state are said to produce a negative inotropic response. A unified hypothesis for explaining certain adrenergic physiologic responses and the action of inotropic drugs in either increased or decreased contractile state is, first, stimulation of β_1 cardiac receptors and, second, the increased release of ionized calcium within the sarcolemma of the myofibril. This calcium in turn regulates the physiochemical interaction between actin and myosin, which shortens the myofibrils, the major mechanical event of the systole. The source of the ionized calcium is currently understood to be the longitudinal tubular system of the sarcolemma. An increase in ionized calcium results in increased contractility (increased actin–myosin interaction); decreased ionized calcium results in a decrease in contractility (reduced actin–myosin interaction). Physiologic factors such as increased efferent sympathetic discharge to the heart and various drugs including cardiac glycosides and isoproterenol increase sarcolemmic ionized calcium. Decreased efferent sympathetic discharge to the heart and drugs such as nifedipine, a calcium antagonist, decrease sarcolemmic ionized calcium. Additionally, the negative inotropic action of halothane has also been ascribed to a drug-dependent decrease in ionized calcium within the sarcolemma. Although the hypothesis of calcium-dependent regulation has not yet been tested for all physiologic events and drugs known to alter the contractile state, it is the opinion of the authors that this relationship should be retained as an important principle on which future data can be interpreted.

The increase in SAP that usually occurs in the hypovolemic patient with the rapid intravenous infusion of fluids is the result of increased EDV, increased EDVFL, and improved contractile state. As a result, the stroke volume and CO increase and the product of CO and systemic vascular resistance (SVR), SAP, increases. As pointed out earlier, the magnitude of the CO increase may be even larger if there is a concomitant increase in heart rate. In contrast, rapid blood loss decreases the intravascular blood volume, decreases EDV, reduces EDVFL, decreases contractile state, decreases stroke volume, and decreases CO at the same SVR. In this circumstance, SAP will decrease when the product of the compensatory increase in heart rate and decreased SVR result in a decrease in CO. In either situation, the predicted physiologic response may be altered by the action of depressant drugs, which interfere with contractile state.

VARIABLES RELATING TO SYSTEMIC VASCULAR RESISTANCE

SVR is the sum of the resistances within the vascular system opposing ventricular systole and ejection of the blood. The product of SVR and CO is SAP. Functionally, resistance increases with decreasing vessel diameter so that resistance is least in the aorta and larger arteries and greatest in the precapillary arteries and capillary beds. It follows that blood flow will be highest in the large vessels close to the heart and least in the peripheral capillaries, where resistance is greatest. The reduced blood flow at the capillary level facilitates the metabolic exchange between blood and cell. Physiologically important is the fact that the amount of smooth muscle contained within the walls of the arterial division of the vascular system increases from the aorta to the periphery. The vessels designated as precapillary arterioles are most heavily invested with smooth muscle. Excitation of this smooth muscle reduces the internal diameter of the precapillary arteriole and results in a decrease in distal blood flow. Conversely, relaxation of the smooth muscle increases the internal diameter of the precapillary arteriole and results in increased distal blood flow. The relationship between blood flow and the diameter of the peripheral arterioles is described by Poiseuille's law. For any pressure, blood flow

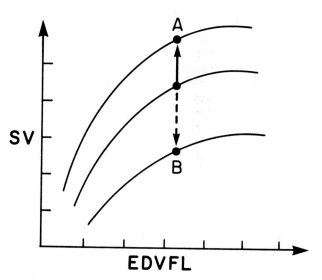

Figure 20–2. Family of ventricular function curves illustrating relationship of stroke volume (SV) and end-diastolic-ventricular-fiber-length (EDVFL). A: increased SV from same EDVFL (positive inotropic response). B: decreased SV from same EDVFL (negative inotropic response).

is proportional to the fourth power of the internal radius of the blood vessel. Thus, a decrease in arteriolar diameter from four units to two units results in a 16-fold ($4 - 2 = 2$; $2^4 = 16$) decrease in blood flow. On the other hand, an increase in vessel diameter from one unit to two units will increase flow 16 times at the same pressure. By virtue of the large amount of smooth muscle in the precapillary arteriolar vessels, the human organism has an exquisitely sensitive system for the regulation of local blood flow over a wide range of CO and SAP.

It is appropriate to consider the mechanism by which SVR is adjusted as required for meeting regional blood flow requirements. The modulating mechanisms are (1) neurohumoral control and (2) autoregulation.

Neurohumoral Control

Neurohumoral control is the physiologic mechanism responsible for *gross* adjustments in SVR. As implied by the term, neurohumoral control results from the release of endogenous vasoactive hormones from either the adrenal medulla or adrenergic nerve endings in the autonomic nervous system. Epinephrine is the primary chemical mediator released by the adrenal medulla, whereas norepinephrine is the mediator released from terminal adrenergic neuronal endings. The released epinephrine is carried in the blood to the physiologically active receptor areas within the circulation, including vascular smooth muscle. In contrast, norepinephrine is released in close proximity to the vascular receptors and is the final result of efferent adrenergic nerve discharge. Because most of the norepinephrine released locally is taken up again in the adrenergic neuronal nerve ending, it usually does not enter the blood in high concentrations. Physiologically, each of these chemical mediators is classified as an α-*adrenergic agonist* by virtue of the ability to produce contraction of arteriolar smooth muscle. Gross adjustments in SVR result from more or less adrenergic mediator release and the relative degree of vascular smooth muscle contraction. Since relatively more smooth muscle is present in the precapillary arteriole, the amount of contraction–relaxation response (more or less distal blood flow) is greatest at the level of the metabolically important capillary bed.

Smooth muscle contained within the venous segment of the circulatory system is similarly reactive to α-adrenergic agonists. Thus, the relative contraction or relaxation of venous smooth muscle is dependent on circulatory vasoactive hormones, as well as locally released norepinephrine (more or less efferent adrenergic nerve activity). As pointed out earlier, this adrenergic smooth muscle modulation is reflected in venous tone, the capacity of the venous circulation and venous return to the heart.

It is also known that there are vasodilator nerve fibers within skeletal muscle. Since the chemical mediator released by the fibers is acetycholine, they are classified as parasympathetic vasodilators. Although this parasympathetic influence on SVR is known, its importance in other than extreme stress such as marathon running remains hypothetical. Therefore, from a practical point of view, SVR can be considered to be a function of relative α-adrenergic stimulation on vascular smooth muscle.

The episodic hypertensive crisis in the patient with pheochromocytoma is a classic example of excess neurohumoral control. SVR is intermittently increased tremendously by the release of α-agonist from the "adrenal medulla-like tumor"; the SAP, in turn, is elevated (normal or reduced CO and an elevated SVR). On the other hand, the sudden relative decrease in adrenergic neuronal norepinephrine release accompanying "neurogenic shock" may result in a profound decrease in SAP (normal or elevated CO and a reduced SVR in both the arterial and venous systems). A clinically useful concentration of halothane may decrease the heart rate, reduce contractile state and in turn SV and CO, while concomitantly reducing SVR. Under this circumstance, SAP decreases. Similarly, the hypertensive patient under therapy with an α-receptor blocking drug (e.g., phenoxybenzamine) will have a lower SVR and a lower SAP for a given level of stroke volume and CO.

Autoregulation

Autoregulation is the physiologic phenomenon of constant blood flow occurring at different pressures. It is considered to be an intrinsic property of a vascular bed and is independent of nerve activity and circulating hormones. Although autoregulation has not been completely explained, it appears to be a property of most vascular beds, with significant variability depending on the circulatory area under consideration. Two explanations for autoregulation that seem to have the greatest clinical relevance are the myogenic hypothesis and the metabolic theory.

The *myogenic hypothesis* maintains that the smooth muscle of the vascular wall contracts and relaxes depending on pressure (tension) within the blood vessel. If pressure within the vessel increases, the smooth muscle contracts and the radius of the vessel is decreased. As explained before, flow under this circumstance would decrease by the fourth power of the change in radius. The opposite would be true for a decrease in pressure within the blood vessel. Importantly, the net effect of myogenic autoregulation is a more constant distal blood flow over a wide range of arterial pressure.

The *metabolic theory* is dependent on the concept that as pressure in a vessel decreases, flow decreases and oxygen supply to the vessel wall is also decreased. In response to the oxygen decrease, metabolites are released, and these produce vasodilatation and increased blood flow even at the lower pressure. At the present time, however, the specific metabolite responsible for vasodilatation under this circumstance has not been identified. The fact that decreased P_{O_2}, increased P_{CO_2}, or a decrease in pH is known to result in relaxation of vascular smooth muscle would appear particularly relevant to the anesthetized patient. For example, it is known that P_{CO_2} is the most important metabolic factor regulating flow in the cerebral circulation. A deficiency in the metabolic theory is that it does not appear to explain constant flow at *increased* perfusion pressures.

With respect to understanding those factors that integrate to produce the blood pressure (CO × SVR), it is emphasized that neurohumoral control and autoregulation are useful concepts for problem solving. Neurohumoral control is responsible for gross changes in SVR, whereas autoregulation either myogenically or metabolically adjusts regional blood flow to meet cellular metabolic requirements. Although there are some experimental data related to drug actions on local blood flow, the precise influence of many physiologic events important to the perioperative period, as well as the specific action of anesthetic drugs in patients, has yet to be clarified.

INTEGRATION OF CIRCULATORY EVENTS

The center portion of Figure 20–1C illustrates the physiologic mechanisms by which CO and total peripheral resistance are modulated to produce the spectrum of flow-resistance-pressure relationships required by various physiologic stresses including surgery and anesthesia. The baroreceptors (mechanoreceptors or pressoreceptors) are free nerve endings concentrated in the adventitia of the carotid sinus and the wall of the aortic arch. These nerve endings appear to be sensitive to the stretch of the vessel wall in which they are located. When pressure within the vessels containing these nerve endings increases or decreases, there is a resultant increase or decrease in afferent nerve impulses that are transmitted to the cardioregulatory centers in the brain stem. These afferent impulses travel over branches of the glossopharyngeal (cranial nerve IX). The control centers respond by physiologic readjustments decreasing or increasing both CO and total peripheral resistance. Thus, arterial pressure is physiologically lowered or raised. This sequence of events is referred to as the carotid sinus or baroreceptor reflex. When SAP is decreased, afferent impulses to the cardioregulatory centers decrease. As a result, efferent parasympathetic (vagal) discharge to the SA node decreases and heart rate is increased. Concomitantly, efferent adrenergic impulses to the heart, venous smooth muscle, and precapillary arterioles are increased (Fig. 20–3). As a result, the contractile state, venous tone, and SVR are increased. The increase in heart rate and contractile state, in combination with the increase in EDV and EDVFL produced by increased VT and venous return, increases stroke volume and CO. SAP increases since CO and SVR are increased. Conversely, an elevation in SAP decreases CO, decreases peripheral resistance, and decreases arterial pressure. Thus baroreceptor-related afferent nerve discharge and the resultant alterations in CO and SVR produced by the efferent parasympathetic and adrenergic autonomic responses is of primary importance in modulating blood flow.

The tachycardia frequently accompanying hypovolemia is the result of reduced baroreceptor stimulation, decreased afferent input to the cardioregulatory centers, and decreased efferent vagal discharge to the SA node. In a further effort to elevate SAP under this circumstance, contractile state, SVR, and venous return are increased by increased efferent adrenergic impulses. Thus, CO is increased (SV × heart rate) and SAP is elevated (CO × SVR).

Figure 20–1 also serves as a useful reference for the student in categorizing the anticipated physiologic effect of drugs with actions on the autonomic venous system. It is apparent that β-adrenergic agonists or antagonists (e.g., isoproterenol or propranolol) will exert their *primary* action

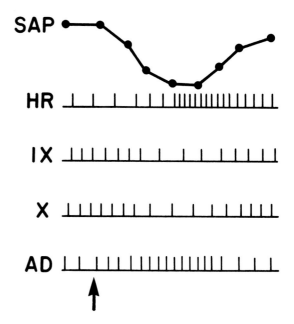

Figure 20–3. Schema illustrating integrated responses occurring with a decrease in systemic arterial pressure (SAP). HR: heart rate; IX: ninth cranial nerve afferent impulses; X: vagal efferent cholinergic impulses; AD: efferent adrenergic impulses; ↑ : onset of hypotension. Refer to text for details.

on contractile state with a secondary action on heart rate. Similarly, α-adrenergic agonists or antagonists (e.g., norepinephrine or phenoxybenzamine) will exert their primary action on SVR and venous tone. Similarly, the primary action of parasympathetic agonists or antagonists (e.g., neostigmine and atropine) will be on heart rate.

SUMMARY

The primary function of the circulation is to provide blood flow to meet cellular metabolic needs. Because blood flow measurements have limited application at the present time, indirect measurements are used to determine the status of the circulation. SAP is a useful index of circulatory status, if the related variables are clearly understood. An understanding of these variables, their interaction, and the mechanisms by which they are modulated is useful for problem solving during anesthesia and surgery.

SAP is the product of CO and total SVR. CO is the product of stroke volume and heart rate. Stroke volume is the difference between end-diastolic volume and end-systolic volume. End-diastolic volume is related to blood volume and venous return, venous tone, and ventricular compliance. End-systolic volume is most closely related to ventricular contractility. Ventricular contractility is an intrinsic property of ventricular actin–myosin interaction and is influenced by end-diastolic ventricular fiber length, relative efferent adrenergic discharge (β1 response), and ionized calcium release within the sarcolemma of the myofibril. Heart rate is primarily related to more or less efferent parasympathetic (vagal) discharge and secondarily to relative degrees of efferent adrenergic nerve discharge and β_1 receptor stimulation.

SVR is the sum of the forces opposing ejection of blood from the heart. Smooth muscle in the precapillary arteriole adjusts SVR and modifies distal blood flow to meet individual organ or capillary metabolic needs. Clinically, gross changes in SVR are the result of neurohumoral control. More discrete changes in vascular resistance are due to autoregulation. Neurohumoral control is produced by the release of vasoactive hormones and their reaction on α-adrenergic receptors in vascular smooth muscle (α response). Autoregulation may be due to intrinsic properties of smooth muscle or the local release of metabolites.

Pressoreceptors in the carotid sinus and aortic arch are responsive to changes in SAP. Afferent nerve impulses generated in response to pressure changes modulate CO and SVR. The afferent systemic pressure information is integrated in the cardioregulatory centers in the brain stem, modifying efferent parasympathetic and adrenergic discharge to the heart and peripheral vasculature as appropriate for adjustments in the physiologic status of the circulation.

BIBLIOGRAPHY

Guyton AC: An overall analysis of cardiovascular regulation. Anesth Analg 56:761–768, 1977.

Hoffman BF, Cranefield PF: The physiological basis of cardiac arrhythmias. Am J Med 37:670–684, 1964.

Morrow DH: Ventricular function during anesthesia. In Price HL, Cohen PJ (eds): Effects of anesthetics on the circulation. Springfield, IL, Chas C Thomas, 1964, pp. 122–134.

Morrow DH, Logic JR: Management of cardiac arrhythmias during anesthesia. Anesth Analg 48:748–754, 1969.

Morrow DH, Morrow AG: The effects of halothane on myocardial contractile force and vascular resistance: Direct observations in patients during cardiopulmonary bypass. Anesthesiology 22:537–541, 1961.

Morrow DH, Pierce GE: The effect of halothane on systemic venous reactivity. J Surg Res 8:115–121, 1968.

Opie LH: Calcium Antagonists and Cardiovascular Disease. Perspectives in Cardiovascular Research. New York, Raven Press, 1984, Vol. 9.

Rein J, Austen WG, Morrow DH: Effects of guanethidine and reserpine on the cardiac responses to halothane. Anesthesiology 24:672–675, 1963.

21

Hepatic and Excretory Systems

Sister Mary Arthur Schramm

The hepatic and excretory systems are similar in that both receive a large portion of the cardiac output and both function to control the excretion of chemicals and the maintenance of fluid, electrolyte, and other nutritional constituents. Each system has its own unique functions as well.

HEPATIC SYSTEM

A knowledge of this system is imperative for the anesthetist because of the malnutrition, environmental pollution, illicit drug use, and other predisposing factors to liver disease that are so common in our society.

Anatomy

The liver is the largest glandular organ in the body. It lies in the right upper quandrant of the abdomen, just below the diaphragm, at a level of ribs 5 through 11. Its location may vary slightly due to the specific body build of the individual person. The anterior linear projection in the mid-clavicular line is 15 ± 2 cm; in the midsternal line, it is 4 ± 1 cm. The nerve supply includes the sympathetic (thoracic 7 through 10), the parasympathetic (right and left vagus), and the right phrenic nerves. The autonomic control travels through the celiac ganglion to the hepatic vessels and bile ducts. Enlargement or tenderness of the liver locally produces a right-sided pain.

Physiology

The liver is composed of four discrete interrelated structures.

Circulatory–Lymphatic System. Two major vessels—the hepatic artery, which conveys oxygenated blood to the liver, and the portal vein, a combination of the mesenteric and splenic veins, which conveys blood with nutrients, metabolic substances, and toxins from the gastrointestinal tract—form a dual blood supply. The blood vessels are accompanied by lymphatics, nerve fibers, and biliary ducts. Both blood supplies empty into the sinusoids which surround all but one side of the hepatocyte. Once the blood is filtered and processed, it returns to the systemic circulation via the central vein, which leads into a system of hepatic venules and veins, finally emptying into the inferior vena cava by way of the hepatic vein just below the right atria.

The lymphatic vessels carry liver lymph with its high protein content from the organ into the general circulation and aid in the transport of substances from the splanchnic bed to the systemic circulation. The liver is the largest source of lymph in the body. The intrasinusoidal pressure, a combination of portal vein and hepatic artery pressures, is normally about 8 to 12 mm Hg. It is lowered by a decrease in entry of blood or a reduction in sinusoidal resistance. The pressure is raised by an increase in venous or arterial inflow or by obstruction of the hepatic venous outflow either within the liver or in the right atria. Subsequently, engorgement of the liver and of those vessels draining the stomach and the intestines will follow. The liver can store up to 400 ml of blood whenever there is a small hepatic venous pressure increase.

Biliary System. The bile canaliculi are formed by the plasma membrane of the hepatocytes. These canaliculi empty into bile ductiles that lead into an organized duct system and finally into the hepatic duct. The hepatic duct combines with the cystic duct to form the common duct. The bile empties either directly into the duodenum or is diverted to the gallbladder. The bile is composed of bile salts, bilirubin, cholesterol, lecithin, and electrolytes. The bile salts have two important actions: a detergent action on fat particles in foods so that the fat can be broken into smaller fractions; and the more important action of aiding in the absorption of fatty acids, monoglycerides, cholesterol, and other important lipids as well as the fat-soluble vitamins

A, D, E, and K. Vitamin K is required for the production of the blood coagulation factors prothrombin, VII, IX, and X. Most of the bile salts are reabsorbed by an active transport in the intestinal mucosa of the distal ileum back into the portal blood and returned to the liver. This recirculation process is termed enterohepatic circulation. It includes the reabsorption in varying quantities of other secreted chemicals and drugs such as *d*-tubocurarine, sulfonamides, penicillins, thyroxine, steroids, and calcium.

Reticuloendothelial Cells. Three different types of cells make up this system in the liver and comprises 60 percent of the body's reticuloendothelial system. One type of cell is the immunocytic sinusoidal cell that participates in humoral and cell-mediated immunity, the gamma-globulin synthesis, which in turn determines the body response to noxious agents. A second type is the stellate phagocytic cell, called Kupffer cell, that removes foreign substances, including infectious agents, and serves as a storage depot for iron, vitamins A, D, and B_{12}, and lipids. The third type of cell is the fiber-forming sinusoidal cell that leads to collagen deposition and a supernatant of hyperactive lymphocytes and is counterbalanced by enzyme degradation, a repair mechanism.

Hepatocytes. These liver cells are polyhedral in form and are surrounded on all sides but one by the sinusoids. These cells maintain a constant interchange with the vascular and biliary systems that border them. The liver cells around the terminal afferent vascular twigs receive more oxygen and nutrients than those around the venous outflow vasculature, and the former have more endoplasmic reticulum and enzyme activity. The hepatocytes are involved in the synthesis and degradation pathways of proteins, fats, carbohydrates, and nucleic acids. Malnutrition, toxic injury, and prolonged administration of drugs can alter the effectiveness of the endoplasmic reticulum. Hepatocytes have a vital function in protein metabolism by way of amino acid deamination in urea formation to decrease ammonia levels and in plasma protein synthesis, including albumin, the clotting factors V, VI, VII, IX, and X, and amino acid interconversions. Hepatocytes rapidly affect fat metabolism more than other cells in the formation of lipoproteins and cholesterol, the conversion of carbohydrates and proteins to fats, and in beta oxidation of fatty acids. The liver cells are very important in carbohydrate metabolism, especially the glucose-buffering power for the blood due to its metabolic processes of glycogenolysis, glycogenesis, and gluconeogenesis.

Pathology

Hepatic disease may affect a single unit of the liver initially, but ultimately all units are involved. The most common circulatory disturbance affecting the liver is congestion associated with heart failure. The characteristic findings include enlargement and tenderness of the liver, altered biochemical function tests, and, eventually, chronic passive congestion, in which the liver becomes small and firm. Similar changes result from shock when the lowered blood pressure produces stasis and accumulation of vasopressor substances.

Circulatory derangements lead to portal hypertension caused by portal or hepatic vein blockage, cirrhosis, fibrosis, neoplasms, and other less common factors which result in blood stasis, hypoxia, and ischemic necrosis. Diseases associated with the biliary passages (Table 21–1) include (1) jaundice, which may be classed as unconjugated hyperbilirubinemia, such as physiologic jaundice or Rh incompatibility in the newborn, conjugated, such as obstructive jaundice, or mixed, such as cholestasis due to infection, cholelithiasis, or neoplasms, (2) metabolic disorders, usually congenital, due to Tay–Sach's (involving lipidosis) or von Gierke's (involving glycogen storage or porphyria) diseases, which are latent until barbiturates are administered, (3) hepatitis due to infection, alcoholism, or drugs, (4) fibrosis and cirrhosis due to various forms of liver-cell necrosis and inflammation, and (5) neoplastic lesions, benign or malignant, the latter being either primary or due to secondary metastasis.

Assessment

Cirrhosis. In cirrhosis the symptoms may be vague—malaise, dyspepsia, weight loss, loss of libido, menstrual disturbances, skin changes, finger clubbing, spider nevi, high output state with flushed extremities, dilated veins, capillary pulsations, and collapsing pulse, enlarged or atrophied liver due to jaundice, edema, ascites, flapping tremor of the hands, and coma are noted. The major complications are encephalopathy, ascites, gastrointestinal hemorrhage, infection, jaundice, and vitamin deficiency.

Jaundice. Jaundice exists when the bilirubin serum level exceeds 1.5 mg/100 ml. In hemolytic jaundice, the increased plasma bilirubin results from the destruction of red blood cells with rapid release of bilirubin into the bloodstream. The indirect van den Bergh test for free bilirubin is positive. The other cause of jaundice is obstruction; in this instance the direct van den Bergh test for conjugated bilirubin is positive. Bilirubin excreted into the intestines is converted to urobilinogen, which is reabsorbed by the enterohepatic circulation and excreted by the kidneys. In total obstruction of bile flow the test for urine urobilinogen is negative. Lack of bile pigments in the intestinal tract also produces the clay-colored feces. A high aminotransferase (AMT) level and a moderate increase in alkaline phosphatase (APT) level indicate hepatocellular damage. A high APT and a small AMT indicate obstruction.

Viral Hepatitis. Hepatitis can cause liver dysfunction, ranging from a mild systemic illness, with or without jaundice, to acute liver failure. The patient may recover completely, with immunity, become a carrier of the virus, or progress

TABLE 21–1. DISEASES ASSOCIATED WITH BILIARY TRACT

1. Jaundice
2. Metabolic disorders
3. Hepatitis
4. Fibrosis and cirrhosis
5. Neoplasms

through various stages to reach chronic liver disease. Viral hepatitis is a potential risk to anesthesia. Immunologic tests for hepatitis A and B may aid in diagnosing patients who are incubating the virus. Care should be taken in the presence of persons who have acute or chronic liver disease, require dialysis, have undergone renal transplants or treatment by immunosuppressant drugs, have received transfusions from paid donors, or have visited abroad, stayed in countries with a high incidence of hepatitis, been tattooed, been drug addicts, prostitutes, or prison inmates, or stayed in psychiatric institutions.

Portal Hypertension. Ninety percent of the patients with portal hypertension have nutritional cirrhosis and alcoholism. The serious complication is bleeding from esophageal varices and this must be controlled. Nonoperative methods of control have met with little success; surgically, portacaval shunt has been somewhat helpful. The ascites is due to the increased hydrostatic pressure, lowered plasma colloidal osmotic pressure, increased plasma aldosterone concentration with sodium and water retention, and, possibly, an excessive lymph production. Treatment calls for low salt solutions, administration of vitamin K, glucose, and protein, and adequate available fresh blood to provide clotting factors, platelets, and prothrombin and to dilute the ammonium content of the blood. One must anticipate anemia due to hemolysis, iron deficiency, folic acid deficiency, or bleeding, along with thrombocytopenia and granulocytopenia, decreased renal function resulting from decreased blood flow due to decreased cardiac output, and cellular damage resulting from shock-producing agents excreted by the diseased liver, prolonged drug metabolism, endocrine changes in the presence of decreased conjugation by the liver, hypoglycemia, decreased magnesium and potassium with muscle weakness, decreased prothrombin time due to decreased absorption of vitamin K, and coma, which can be precipitated by surgery as well as by gastrointestinal bleeding, increased protein consumption, alkalosis, severe infection, sedation, diuretics, and hypokalemia.

Liver Function Tests. These are utilized to evaluate the following functions:

1. Carbohydrate, fat, and protein metabolism
2. Production of various substances
3. Destruction of breakdown products
4. Storage
5. Immunity
6. Bile formation
7. Detoxifiction of drugs

These liver function tests include:

1. *Serum levels of the following:*
   Sodium 130 to 145 nmol/L
   Potassium 3.5 to 5 nmol/L
   Bicarbonate 20 to 28 nmol/L
   Urea 3.3 to 6.7 nmol/L
   Creatinine 0.04 to 0.1 nmol/L
   Bilirubin 3 to 20 nmol/L
   Alkaline phosphatase (ALP) 30 to 85 IU/L
   Aspartate aminotransferase (AST) or (SGOT) 10 to 50 IU/L

   Lactic dehydrogenase (LDH$_5$) 90 to 300 IU/L
   Hydroxybutyrate dehydrogenase (HBD) 100 to 250 IU/L
   Gamma-glutamyl transpeptidase (GGT) <45 (M) to <35 (F) IU/L
   Globulin 25 to 30 g/L
   Albumin 35 to 50 g/L
   Total protein 60 to 80 g/L
   Glucose 80 to 120 mg/100 ml
   Prothrombin time 12 to 13 sec
   A/G ratio 1.5:1 to 2.5:1
2. *Dyes to evaluate bilirubin and blood flow:*
   Bromsulphalein (BSP) 67 to 100 percent recovered in 2 hours via bile
   Indocyamine Green (ICG) removed completely by the liver
   Rose Bengal I-131—excreted by the liver
3. *Glucose metabolism:* tolerance tests for glucose, fructose, galactose, and lactic acid.
4. *Storage:* levels of iron and B$_{12}$ in the serum.
5. *Liver cell degeneration:* levels of α-fetoprotein (AFP), which occurs especially in hematomas, but also in hepatitis and cirrhosis.
6. *Others:*
   Radiography—checks for blood flow and stones
   Angiography—checks portal pathway and drainage in the event of possible tumors
   Liver scan—checks for focal lesions such as deposits and abscesses
   Fiber optic endoscopy—checks esophagus, stomach, and duodenum for varices occurring with obstruction to blood flow
   Liver biopsy

History. In reviewing the patient's history in order to rule out liver disease, one must look for symptoms of discomfort of the nervous and gastrointestinal systems. It is important to document nausea, vomiting, anorexia, chronic indigestion, fatty food tolerance, food preference (especially fats, carbohydrates, protein, and sodium), clay-colored stools, melena, disturbed bowel habits, hemorrhoids, steatorrhea, dark yellow urine, site and type of pain if present, abdominal colic or tenderness, ascites, edema of limbs, jaundiced eyes or skin, skin or membrane disruptions, nose bleeds, bruises, use of drugs and alcohol, occupational history of hepatoxins, and other environmental factors such as exposure to hepatitis.

Physical Examination. A thorough examination is usually helpful and should include abdominal palpation for tenderness, liver size, presence of masses and consistency and size of the spleen, and a comprehensive inspection of the abdomen for ascites, venous collateral network common to cirrhosis, jaundice, purpura, hair loss, weight loss, enlarged breasts, spider angiomas, and reddened palms.

Anesthesia

The effect of anesthesia on the liver is one of decreased blood flow regardless of the agent or technique; therefore, one tries to choose an agent that will minimize the effect.

The fall may not be as significant with a patient with a healthy liver as with one who has a diseased liver (Table 21–2). The surgical manipulation is believed to have the more significant effect on liver blood flow. Spinal and epidural techniques are related to a decrease in mean arterial pressure; therefore, maintenance of blood pressure is important. Oxygen/nitrous oxide/air anesthesia with intermittent positive pressure breathing appears to have the least effect on blood flow. Both hyperventilation and hypoventilation can be harmful to flow and acid–base balance. Volatile agents such as halogenated agents need not be harmful; dosage correlates well with the alterations in blood flow and metabolism. Blood glucose levels increase with most agents; this is probably a stress response. Increased adrenaline levels and sympathetic activity during surgery may also decrease insulin release. Lipid-soluble agents are converted by the liver to water-soluble agents that have higher molecular weights and are more easily excreted. This is a function of the microsomal enzymes in the endoplasmic reticulum of the hepatocytes. There is usually severe disease before these enzymes are nonfunctional. Levels of microsomal enzymes and cytochromes such as P_{450} may rise, which may increase the drug metabolism in general. This action has occurred in hepatic porphyria in which barbiturates precipitate the increased production of enzymes that lead to acute porphyria. Oral anticonvulsants may affect calcium metabolism and folate deficiency may also occur. A number of drugs cause enzyme induction; these include ethanol and some phenothiazines, antihistamines, sedatives, corticoids, anticonvulsants, and volatile anesthetic agents such as methoxyflurane and possibly halothane. Some drugs such as disulfiram and SKF-525A will inhibit liver enzymes as well. One's concern rests on maintenance of blood pressure and avoidance of vasoconstrictors (Table 21–2). In liver disease, assessment is very important and selection of agents varies little with the type of pathology. All anesthetic drugs are protoplasmic poisons to some degree and lower splanchic blood flow, which is harmful because the liver is decompensated. Liver cells receive a lower oxygen saturation so they are the first to be damaged as saturation falls either due to shock or a fall in oxygen content.

The anesthetist strives to maintain normal P_{CO_2} levels, normotension, and adequate oxygenation. In most surgery, attention is given to treatment with vitamin K, premedication with meperidine hydrochloride (Demerol) or another preferred narcotic, and a tranquilizing agent, the use of hydrocortisone, mannitol, and antibiotics if they are indicated, an induction with a small amount of thiopental unless contraindicated as in porphyria (ketamine, etomidate, or another nonbarbituric agent may then be advisable), succinylcholine for a rapid intubation, pancuronium if it is a slower intubation, oxygen and nitrous oxide or air mixture with narcotic or halogenated agent, intermittent positive pressure ventilation to maintain normocapnia (regional anesthesia is also useful if prothrombin time is acceptable), monitoring of pulse, oxygen perfusion, blood pressure, electrocardiogram, central venous pressure or wedge pressure, fluids, and urinary outflow via a catheter and a volume device, the use of 5 percent dextrose by infusion, and the availability of blood via a warming apparatus, if indicated. A light level of anesthesia is maintained. The intermediate-acting muscle relaxants have much to offer. Some narcotics constrict the common duct.

Postoperatively, oxygen, and adequate ventilation should be maintained. Five to ten percent mannitol as indicated, and antibiotics and incentive spirometry to prevent lower lobe collapse should also be considered.

If cirrhosis is present, patients are graded (Table 21–3) on the basis of degree of encephalopathy (none, minimal, or coma), bilirubin level (under 25, 25 to 40, or over 40 nmol/L), albumin level (35, 28 to 35, or under 28 g/L), and prothrombin time (1 to 4, 4 to 6, or over 6 seconds). When levels are abnormal, surgery is delayed until the patient can be prepared. If portal hypertension surgery occurs, a thoracotomy for esophageal transection will require a double lumen endobronchial tube to facilitate the surgery. Large-bore infusion tubes for both 5 percent dextrose (D_5W) in water and for fresh blood are indicated. In all types of surgery involving patients with liver disease one must be conscious of the fact that the liver must metabolize all drugs administered for induction, relaxation, and analgesia.

In trauma, a hepatic resection may be indicated. If the patient has a noncirrhotic liver, the recovery is good. Because there is a great splanchnic bed sequestration large amounts of fluid are required, usually 10 percent dextrose and water pre- and postoperatively until oral intake is adequate. Albumin, vitamins A, D, and K, and high-caloric, high carbohydrate diets as well as fresh plasma and blood are indicated. The serum K and inorganic P levels are followed; antibiotics are necessary. The bilirubin levels will rise slightly but return to normal in approximately 1 to 3 weeks; 80 to 90 percent liver regeneration is estimated to occur over a 3-week period. Liver failure is a concern postoperatively, especially when the liver is already diseased. Prevention is aided by good hydration, mannitol or furosemide (Lasix) diuresis, invasive blood pressure monitoring, and urine outputs of greater than 50 ml/hr.

Acute liver failure occurs as a gradual deterioration, beginning with euphoria, mild confusion, and drowsiness

TABLE 21–2. MEANS OF REDUCING OXYGEN DELIVERY TO THE LIVER

1. Anesthesia
2. Decreased FIo_2
3. Hepatotoxins
4. Medication such as cimetidine
5. Obstruction
6. Portal hypertension
7. Positive end expiratory pressure (PEEP)
8. Pulmonary hypertension
9. Pyrexia
10. Reduced cardiac output

TABLE 21–3. GRADATIONS OF CIRRHOSIS

	I	II	III
1. Encephalopathy	none	minimal	coma
2. Bilirubin levels (nmol/L)	25	25–40	>40
3. Albumin levels (g/L)	35	28–35	<28
4. Prothrombin times (sec)	1–4	4–6	>6

and leading into a coma with electroencephalogram changes from normal to slowing to delta activity, then triphasics becoming flat due to increased protein metabolic disturbances, an increase in ammonia, variations in quantities of amino acids, increased blood insulin, increased fatty acid levels, progression to hypoxia, hypoglycemia, hypovolemia, and hypotension, convulsions ensuing with acid–base disturbances, hypocapnia, and respiratory alkalosis, which culminate in renal and hematologic disturbances.

Hepatorenal Syndrome

The hepatorenal syndrome is characterized by histologically normal kidneys, oliguria, azotemia, and high urine osmolality due to alteration in renal cortical perfusion and a reduction in effective renal blood flow. The etiology is not known but it is associated with hepatocellular failure.

EXCRETORY SYSTEM

The emphasis on renal physiology has increased in the past few decades due to renal and diabetic research, the longer life span and aging process, methoxyflurane toxicity, renal dialysis and transplants, and legislative support for treatment of renal failure.

Anatomy

Each kidney is located retroperitoneally in the lumbar area; the right one is slightly lower than the left, with its upper pole resting on the 12th rib. Each kidney weighs approximately 125 to 180 g. The functional unit is the nephron. Each kidney comprises approximately 1,200,000 nephrons. The upper pole of each kidney supports the adrenal gland. The renal vessels and ureter join the kidney at the hilum, wherein the ureter expands into the pelvis of the kidney. In a cross-sectional view, the kidney is composed of an outer cortical area and an inner medullary area. The latter also divides into an inner and outer region. The kidney is divided into segments by the blood supply. The sympathetic nerve supply arises from thoracic 11 through lumbar 2 via the celiac ganglia and the renal plexus and the parasympathetic travels through cranial nerve X, the vagus. There are adrenergic, dopaminergic, and cholinergic receptors. There is also an intrinsic autoregulation that maintains arteriole diameter and thus mean pressure to the glomerulus as long as the renal blood pressure is in the range of 80 to 180 mm Hg; this assures a constant pressure for glomerular filtration.

Physiology

The formation of urine is a secondary effect of the kidney; the primary function is to maintain body fluids and remove waste products of body metabolism. The renal blood supply arises directly from the abdominal aorta, providing a higher hydrostatic pressure than is common in most capillary beds in the glomerular capillary bed. The renal artery enters at the hilum, divides into interlobar arteries that traverse the medulla of the kidney between the segments, and forms the arciform arteries at the junction between the medulla

and the cortex where intralobular branches are given off as afferent arteries to the glomerulus. Approximately 90 percent of the blood is filtered; the other 10 percent provides nutrition to the renal structures. The glomerular capillary bed reforms into the efferent arteriole which flows into the peritubular capillary, except for 3 percent of the blood which flows through the vasa recta. The glomerular capillary bed maintains a mean pressure of approximately 70 mm Hg, which provides a pressure head for the movement of approximately 20 percent of the renal plasma as a filtrate into the blind pouch, Bowman's capsule, that surrounds the glomerulus. The efferent arterioles, due to vascular resistance, decrease the pressure to less than that in the tubular lumen by the time the blood enters the peritubular capillaries, which aids in the reabsorption of fluid from the tubule back into the blood stream.

The Function Unit. The nephron consists of three structures:

1. *The malpighian corpuscle* is composed of the glomerulus and Bowman's capsule wherein filtration over a 24-hour period reaches 170 to 180 L of fluid containing in milliequivalents 24,500 of sodium, 17,800 of chloride, 4,900 of bicarbonate, 700 of potassium, 780 of glucose, 870 of urea, 12 of creatinine, 50 of uric acid, and many other substances in smaller amounts.

2. *The tubules,* into which the capsule filtrate diffuses, are composed of three segments: (a) The proximal convoluted tubule, about 14 mm in length, located in the cortex, signified by the large number of mitochondria in each lumen cell and the villi projections that form a brush border on the luminal side to perform the large reabsorptive function reclaiming 65 to 80 percent of the filtrate sodium and water (obligatory), all of the glucose, potassium, and amino acids, and the greater portion of the bicarbonate, phosphate, and urea as well as the secretion of hydrogen ion and foreign substances, and yet, maintaining an isotonic filtrate. (b) The loop of Henle, which narrows as it dips into the medulla to form the descending and ascending limbs, widening as the tubule passes through the outer medullary zone back into the cortical region (12 percent of the nephrons have the long, well-developed loops for salt conservation termed juxtamedullary nephrons); the loop has the ability through the countercurrent mechanism to passively receive salts from the progressively hypertonic medullary interstitium into the lumen filtrate down the descending limb and to actively return sodium chloride through the ascending limb wall, which is impermeable to water, and thus to replenish those salts to the interstitium as the filtrate passes through the ascending limb, forming a hypotonic filtrate by the time the loop reaches the third segment, which is termed the distal convoluted tubule. (c) The distal convoluted tubule begins in the cortical zone at a point where the juxtaglomerular apparatus (a number of packed nuclei termed the *macula densa* lie between the afferent

arteriole and the distal tubule, which are associated with the sensing of the filtrate tonicity and secrete the renin involved in the renin–angiotensin–vasoconstrictor/aldosterone mechanism) has fewer villi and functions in the buffering of volume, and acid–base water (antidiuretic hormone required), secretion of potassium, hydrogen, urea and ammonium to yield a filtrate that is controlled in volume, pH, and concentrate (tonicity).

3. *The collecting duct,* which receives the filtrate from several tubules as it traverses the cortical zone through the medullary zone, secreting and reabsorbing sodium, potassium, hydrogen, and ammonia as well as absorbing water (antidiuretic hormone required) and ultimately emptying into the short papillary ducts of Bellini, which lead into the renal calyces and finally into the renal pelvis and the ureter.

Pathology

Parenchymal diseases of the kidney include those of transport, which are infrequent, such as renal tubular acidosis, renal glycosuria, renal hypophosphatemia, aminoaciduria, and nephrogenic diabetes insipidus and those of inflammatory and degenerative nature which the anesthetist may more often encounter in the chronic than in the acute stage. The functional impairment is directly proportional to the amount of nephron damage and can be a cause of postoperative oliguria.

Glomerulonephritis. The acute form is abrupt in onset, more common in children and young adults, and characterized by hypertension, and occurs after a recent upper respiratory or focal skin infection producing an antistreptococcus, group A, beta and other microbes. Although a few patients die from the disease, 90 percent will recover within 3 to 4 weeks, which leaves about 8% who will go on to develop the chronic stage characterized by hypertension and albuminuria. These patients may be on antihypertensive therapy, diurectics, digitalis, or corticosteroids.

Pyelonephritis. The acute form of this disease is sudden in onset, with chills, rise in body temperature to 102 to 105F, cystitis, and dull pain in the kidney region. In initial attacks, the patient completely recovers but the disease may develop into a chronic state with recurrent bacterial kidney infections. Symptoms of tubular impairment include excessive sodium and potassium loss, inability to secrete a strongly acid urine, inability to produce ammonia in response to acidosis and dehydration, and hypovolemia related to the loss of medullary salt-concentration mechanism.

Arteriolar Nephrosclerosis. This condition may affect one kidney more than the other, the benign form progressing with age. Other causes are occlusion of large vessels in the kidney due to sclerotic construction from various disease processes. The kidney is unable to develop collateral circulation and so in time the kidney becomes reduced in size and develops a nodular surface, diminishing its functional capacity.

Nephrotic Syndrome. This syndrome, due to increased glomerular permeability, is not a specific disease but a stage in renal disorders wherein proteininuria develops into hypoproteinemia and subsequent retention of sodium and water, leading to edema. These patients may be on diuretics, steroids, and antihypertensive medications and require albumin and potassium replacement prior to anesthesia.

Shock. This is an ischemic state due to severe circulatory shock, because of the strong sympathetic vasoconstriction caused by a lowered perfusing volume of fluid. The lack of nutrition destroys epithelial cells which slough and plug the tubules. Blood transfusions may cause reactions that may advance the disease process by hemolysis, with large amounts of hemoglobin released into the plasma to further plug the tubules. Hypovolemia can be a prerenal cause of postoperative oliguria.

Endocrine Gland Disorders. Examples of this group are diabetes mellitus, in which lesions occur in the glomeruli, tubules, and arterioles, the prevalence of acute pyelonephritis and the presence of proteinuria, leading later to symptoms of azotemia and hypertension, adrenal diseases such as Addison's and Conn's, which affect the levels of steriods, including the production of aldosterone, and pituitary disorders, which affect the release of antidiuretic hormone (ADH).

Renal disease can also be associated with gout, hypertension, rheumatoid arthritis (and large intake of analgesic drugs), systemic lupus erythematosus, and periarteritis nodosa.

Renal causes of oliguria usually result from ischemia or toxicity. Anoxia due to low ambient flows of oxygen or decreased perfusion of tissues and toxins such as those due to methoxyflurane, carbon tetrachloride, gold therapy, and other drugs are main causes of postoperative renal oliguria.

Renal Failure. Renal failure, the inability of the kidney to vary urine volume and content in response to homeostatic needs, is associated with circulatory problems impairing renal perfusion such as hypovolemia and disease. The overall changes associated with acute or chronic stages of renal failure will include:

1. Psychological dependence, depending upon the severity and length of the failure, due to the need for medication and dialysis, oversolicitous relatives and friends, fear of invalidism or death, and economic insecurity.
2. Physiologic abnormalities in fluids, electrolytes, and metabolism:
   a. Anemia, low platelet count, and clotting abnormalities due to reduction of erythropoietin from the kidney.
   b. Hypertension due to disorders of the renin–angiotensin–aldosterone/vasoconstrictor secretion.
   c. Metabolic acidosis due to the elevation of hydrogen ion concentration as well as rises in organic acids, sulfate, and phosphate.

d. Hyperkalemia excess of 0.3 to 3.0 mEq/L which may affect the neuromuscular blockage.
e. Hypoproteinemia with edema.
f. Axotemia due to rise in urea, uric acid, creatinine, amino acids, and polypeptides.
g. Total lipid, cholesterol, phosphorus, and neutral fat levels increased.
h. Heart failure and abnormalities in liver function that increase the edema and may cause pulmonary congestion.

3. Abnormalities caused by drug therapy, especially steroids, which increase susceptibility to infection, impaired wound healing, skeletal decalcification, bone and joint changes, suppressants that increase susceptibility to infection and decrease white cell and platelet counts, and drugs that aggravate renal failure due to toxicity such as antibiotics, isoniazid, procainamide, and hydrolazine.

Renal Function Tests

Laboratory tests useful in determining the presence and extent of renal disease include:

1. *Urinalysis.* A number of tests together can present a reliable picture of renal disease.
   a. Appearance and odor may indicate bleeding, infection, or systemic disease.
   b. pH may indicate the ability of the kidney to acidify urine or the presence of certain diseases.
   c. Specific gravity and osmolarity can indicate the ability of the kidney to concentrate urine, which will decrease much earlier in disease than the ability to dilute urine.
   d. Until negated by other tests, protein concentration is usually a sign of disease.
   e. Glucose presence usually means that an abnormally large load has been presented to the tubules and further check for systemic diseases is required.
   f. Microscopic findings of casts, bacteria, and blood are indicative of further study.
   g. Ketones may indicate various systemic metabolic disorders.
   h. Occult blood is indicative of further search for bleeding disorders.
   i. Sediment can indicate inflammation due to infection or systemic disease.
   j. Amount of urine in relationship to intake of fluid.
2. *Blood/Serum Levels.* The correlation of tests such as the blood urea nitrogen (BUN), nonprotein nitrogen (NPN), and creatinine levels to those in the urine may be significant. Serum electrolytes, pH, and blood gases, and a complete blood count may also aid in the determination of the extent of renal disease.
3. *Radiologic Exam.* This area would include chest and abdominal flat plates, intravenous pyelogram (IVP), retrograde pyelogram, and angionephrotomography for the presence or absence of the organ, tumors, structures, and function.

4. *Electrocardiogram (ECG).* The ECG will reflect electrolyte changes such as calcium and potassium levels, changes due to drugs such as digitalis and heart myopathies due to increased workload.
5. *Intake/Output Data.* The correlation between intake and output along with daily weights can be indicative of fluid accumulation.
6. *Urine Collection Tests.* These tests include glomerular clearance by use of urea, creatinine, or insulin, tubular concentration and dilution regimes, and renal blood flow (renal clearance) evaluation by the use of paraminohippuric acid (PAH), iodopyracet (Diodrast), or inulin (Iopax) secretion.

Physiologic Composition of Urine

1. 1500 ml daily output: 60 g solute and 90 percent water
2. Organic wastes—35 g
   a. Urea—30 g
   b. Creatinine—1 to 2 g
   c. Ammonia—1 to 2 g
   d. Uric acid—1 g
   e. Others—1 g
   Inorganic wastes—25 g
   a. Chloride
   b. Sulfate
   c. Phosphorus
   d. Sodium
   e. Potassium
   f. Magnesium
3. pH—acid (5.5 to 6.5)
4. Specific gravity (1.010 to 1.025)
5. Clear yellow color, ammonia odor
6. Negative for sugar, acetone and albumin
7. Clearance
   a. Urea—40 to 65 ml/min
   b. Creatinine—125 $\pm$ 15 ml/min
   c. Insulin—120 to 125 ml/min
8. Renal Blood Flow
   PAH/idopyracet—600 to 800 ml/min

Physiologic Composition of the Blood

1. Cardiac output—5000 ml/min
2. Organic substances (per 100 ml)
   a. Urea—33 to 67 nmol
   b. Creatinine—0.7 to 2.0 mg/4 to 10 nmol
   c. Uric acid
   d. Organic acid—0.5 mEq
   e. Protein—6 to 8 g
   f. BUN—10 to 20 mg
   g. NPN—15 to 35 mg
   h. Albumin—3.5 to 5.0 g
   Inorganic substances (mEq/L)
   a. Chloride—98 to 110
   b. Sulfate—1.0
   c. Phosphate—2.0
   d. Sodium—138 to 146
   e. Potassium—3.5 to 5.5
   f. Magnesium—1.5 to 2.5
   g. Calcium—5.0
   h. Bicarbonate—24 to 31
3. pH—7.35 to 7.45
4. Glucose—80 to 120 mg

TABLE 21–4. DIURETIC AGENTS EFFECTS ON KIDNEY FUNCTION

Drug	Site of Action	Indications	Side Effects	Potency
Mannitol	Osmotic, primarily proximal tubule, dilute Na concentration	Potentiates excretion of salicylates and phenobarbitone, reduces brain volume, prevents acute renal failure, protects against nephrotoxins	Ensure against extravascular linkage	Ineffective in azotemia
Urea	Osmotic, primarily proximal tubule	Similar to mannitol	Arrhythmias and increased blood pressure, hemolysis	Less effective than mannitol
Mercurials Mersalyl acid Merphyllin Salyrgan Thiomerin	Acts on several sites in proximal tubule primarily by inhibiting intracellular enzyme systems; thus Na^+ and Cl^- transport in all areas	Rarely used; other agents safer and more reliable	Increases blood levels, causes renal tubular damage, metabolic alkalosis due to Cl^- loss	Variable; more effective if acidosis present
Azetazolamide Diamox (a sulfonamide derivative)	Inhibits carbonic anhydrase in proximal and distal tubule, decreases H^+ and HCO_3 reabsorption, affects whole nephron	Used with organic mercurials in the treatment of edema associated with CHF and in glaucoma	Metabolic acidosis occurs with retention of Cl^-, K^+ is excreted in exchange for the Na required to absorb HCO_3 rather than H^+	Similar to mercurials
Metyrapone Metopirone	Inhibits production of aldosterone and cortisone, adrenal cortex	Diagnostic tool for adrenal ACTH disorders	Induction of acute adrenal insufficiency if patient has reduced adrenal secretory capacity already	Not utilized as diuretic
Ammonium chloride NH_4Cl	Acidifies, decreases urine pH, mainly in proximal tubule, converts NH_3 to urea by liver, urea and Cl^- act as osmotic diuretics, H^+ exchanges for Na^+	Used in pethidine, lead, and bromide intoxication and to enhance mersalyel, resupplies lost Cl.	Enhances metabolic acidosis. Dangerous in liver and renal failure	Mild diuresis until NH_3 production over 3–4 days, then ineffective
Spironolactone Aldactone	Competitive blocker of aldosterone at the distal tubule, primarily prevents reabsorption of Na^+ and excretion of K (K^+ sparing)	Edema of CHF, ascites, and nephrotic syndrome, in hypertension and myasthenia gravis, in secondary aldosteronism	Reabsorption of K^+	Powerful if used with other diuretics to conserve K^+
Triampterene Dyrenium Dytac (pteridine derivative)	Effect on distal tubule mainly, increases urine pH and HCO_3^- excretion, does not inhibit carbonic anhydrase (K^+ sparing)	Edema of CHF, cirrhosis, nephrotic syndrome, idiopathic and drug-induced edema, used with thiazides	Minor effects, some azotemia, slight increase in Na^+, Cl^-, and H^+ excretion but blunts K^+ excretion caused by diuretics given concurrently with them	Weaker natriuretic effect than thiazides, similar to Aldactone in K conservation but not aldosterone dependent
Amiloride	Similar to triampterene, works primarily on distal tubules, blocks Na^+–K^+ exchange directly	Similar to triampterene	Similar to triampterene	Similar to triampterene
Azolimine	Perhaps a combination of all K^+-sparing diuretics	Similar to other K^+-sparing diuretics	Similar to other K^+-sparing diuretics	Partially aldosterone dependent but active without, too.
Thiazides Chlorothiazide Diuril Bendroflumethiazide Naturetin (sulfonamide derivatives)	Works all along tubule, greatest effect on prevention of Na^+ reabsorption in distal loop of Henle and in the early part of distal tubule, weak inhibitor of carbonic anhydrase, increases HCO_3^- and K^+ excretion, decreases blood pressure, direct action on total peripheral resistance	Edema of chronic CHF, hepatic or renal disease, and in hypertensive disease	Hypokalemia, hyperuricemia, hyperglycemia, azotemia, hypocalcemia, and hyponatremia are possible	Effective diuretic, especially in cortical portion of ascending limb
Ethacrynic acid Edecrin (phenoxyactetide derivative)	Proximal convoluted tubule, ascending limb (Cl^-) of loop of Henle (medullary) and distal tubule, increases excretion of Na^+, K^+, H^+, and Cl^-	Acute pulmonary edema and other emergencies, in edema resistant to other diuretics	Hypokalemia, hypochloremic alkalosis and sudden fluid loss, dehydration, hyperuricemia, hyperglycemia, azotemia	Effective in azotemia and decreases GFR, 5× as powerful as the thiazides

TABLE 21–4. *Continued*

Drug	Site of Action	Indications	Side Effects	Potency
Furosemide Lasix (sulfonamide derivative)	Same as ethacrynic acid, also redistributes renal blood flow to cortical zone	Similar to ethacrynic acid; enhances the effect with spironolactone	Same as ethacrynic acid plus ototoxicity, hypercalcemia, and hyponatremia, photosensitivity, rashes, bone marrow depression	Effective in poor renal function and in pulmonary edema
Bumetamide	Loop diuretic Ascending limb	40× more potent than furosemide	Similar to above	Similar to above
Tienilic acid	Affects loop Ascending limb	Moderately saliuretic	Uricosuric	
MK-196	Loop diuretic Ascending limb	Long duration of action. Saliuretic	Antihypertensive mildly uricosuric	

Diuretics and Ion and Water Reabsorption

Diuretics have been a part of renal therapy since the early 1920s, when the organomercurials were introduced. The carbonic anhydrase inhibitors became available between 1940 and 1948, acetazolamide and *p*-carboxybenesulfonamide in 1954, chlorothiazide and spironolactone in 1957 and 1959, respectively, and triamterene, furosemide, and ethacrynic acid in the early 1960s. Our newest agents in the late 1970 era are bumetanide, tienilic acid, and MK-196.

The major indications for diuretics include:

1. Inappropriate water and electrolyte retention due to disease processes.
2. Anesthesia and surgery to prevent ischemic renal failure.

The basic concepts behind diuretic therapy are to change the renal blood flow and intrarenal distribution (mannitol and furosemide) and to increase sodium excretion (all diuretics) which is termed a natriuretic effect.

Table 21–4 offers a summary of the diuretics. The natriuretic diurectics cause one or more of the following:

1. Increase the glomerular filtration rate (GFR) either by raising the blood pressure or by dilating renal afferent arterioles.
2. Inhibit sodium reabsorption by increasing peritubular–capillary oncotic pressure (because of decreased filtration fraction).
3. Inhibit directly the active-transport system for sodium (block its energy supply or that of chloride in the loop).
4. Inhibit secretion of renin or aldosterone.
5. Block action of aldosterone.
6. Act as an osmotic diuretic by its osmotic contribution.
7. Inhibit active secretory system for hydrogen (block carbonic anhydrase).

Anesthesia in Renal Disease

The anesthetist should manage the patient with suspected renal disease and known renal failure in much the same manner.

Preoperative Preparation and Medication

The patient's history, laboratory findings, and symptoms must be taken into careful consideration. If the patient is on chronic hemodialysis, the patient may need to be dialyzed immediately prior to surgery if electrolyte shifts are rapid or the day prior to surgery if no emergency exists. Hypertension secondary to hypervolemia is corrected by ultrafiltration and a serum potassium level of 5.0 to 5.5 mEq/L or less is advocated. The potassium level may be buffered by chemical means such as adequate calcium ratios, increased uptake of potassium by the cell through the infusion of glucose solution and insulin administration, or the rectal instillation of resins to exchange potassium. Hemoglobin levels should be greater than 5 g/100 ml, and this may require packed erythrocytes, but levels above 9 to 10 g/100 ml are hard to achieve and these lower levels are usually satisfactory.

The primary objective of the premedication is to achieve adequate sedation without significant respiratory and circulatory depression. Many anesthetists suggest modest doses of diazepam, 60 to 90 minutes prior to surgery, but others advocate shorter-acting agents in this family of drugs, especially if there is central nervous system depression since diazepam has a half-life of 24 hours. Long-acting barbiturates are avoided since they are excreted unchanged by the kidney. Narcotics are metabolized prior to excretion by the kidney but one may wish to avoid them particularly in the debilitated patient in which their action is intensified; these drugs cause small reduction in glomerular filtration, urinary volume, and urinary solute excretion without an increase in urine concentration. If ADH is stimulated, this reduction is counterbalanced. Phenothiazines increase volume and dilution of urine, probably by suppressing ADH. Chloral hydrate has little effect on renal function. Of the anticholinergics, neither scopolamine nor atropine has an effect on renal function. Since patients may have dry mucous membranes already, one may wish to avoid all drying agents. Since droperidol may cause an unpredictable increase in apprehension, it may be avoided as a supplement or premedication for local and regional anesthesia.

One must measure hemoglobin, blood urea, and electrolyte levels and take all precautions for any patient with a full stomach if emergency surgery is necessary.

Monitoring. The usual monitoring devices—blood pressure cuff, precordial/esophageal stethoscope, temperature probe, oximeters, and electrocardiogram—are utilized. Intravenous routes, as indicated, are instituted for the administration of fluids and other components. An indwelling catheter aids in monitoring available urine output. Central venous pressure and pulmonary capillary wedge pressure are utilized to monitor fluid replacement if the patient's reserves are questionable. Cannulation of the dorsalis pedis artery can provide serial evaluation of serum electrolytes, blood gases, acid–base status, and direct arterial pressure during longer procedures. If the patient is being dialyzed, shunts and fistulas must be carefully protected; a Doppler sensor over the shunt or fistula provides continuous monitoring of patency.

Induction. Induction is associated with profound changes in renal hemodynamics and water and electrolyte excretion.

Anesthesia is usually induced by an ultrashort-acting barbiturate but sleep doses can cause severe cardiovascular depression. Thiopental sodium must be given carefully if uremia is present because there are lowered albumin levels to bind it and acidosis reduces ionized and bound portions, thus increasing the effect. Small doses of diazepam may be adequate; some anesthetists prefer etomidate, or the steroids propanidid or althesin; the latter is not available in the United States. Halothane may be indicated, using high flows, especially in children and adults whose veins do not yield easily to puncture or to insertion of a catheter. Controversy exists around the usage of succinylcholine to facilitate intubation if the patient is hyperkalemic or on immunosuppressant therapy since these drugs depress pseudocholinesterase. In chronic renal failure, patients with potassium serum levels of 3 to 4 mEq/L, no significant increase has been shown with the injection of succinylcholine, nor has metabolism of the drug been prolonged beyond what occurs in the general population. Hypertension preoperatively predisposes to hypotension during induction.

Maintenance. The main objective is to avoid hypotension, low cardiac output, and anoxia during the perioperative period. All inhalation agents depress renal function by reducing total renal blood flow (glomerular filtration to approximately one third of normal) electrolyte excretion and urinary flow. Neuroleptanalgesia apparently causes no depression of these parameters, probably due to the adrenergic blocker effect of agents like droperidol. Methoxyflurane (Penthrane) is definitely contraindicated in renal insufficiency because of the direct depression on tubular function, and one should evaluate enflurane closely because it metabolizes to some fluoride as well. Halothane is preferred by many anesthetists even though it has a direct effect on sodium transport and an indirect one on circulatory, endocrine, and sympathetic nervous systems, sensitizing the heart to catecholamines when the patient may already be hyperkalemic, hypocalcemic, and acidotic. Isoflurane may now be the agent of choice. Nitrous oxide should not exceed 50 percent if the patient is anemic. Due to elimination problems in renal insufficiency, volatile agents need not be metabolized and eliminated whereas intravenous agents do.

Other recommendations include spinal or epidural anesthesia at levels of T1–T2. Blockers of compensatory autonomic activity are poor choices because the delicate homeostatic balance is essential especially if the patient is fragile.

Muscle Relaxants. Decamethonium, gallamine, and succinylmonocholine, a breakdown product of succinylcholine, are excreted by the kidney and prolonged paralysis usually occurs; some advocate very small doses depending on the severity of the renal disease. If a patient is on dialysis, one can reverse the drug postoperatively by dialysis. Nondepolarizing neuromuscular blocking agents such as *d*-tubocurarine and pancuronium have been used with good results and these drugs do have an alternate pathway of excretion through liver metabolism and biliary excretion. The newer agents atracurium and vecuronium have been indicated because their elimination does not depend upon the kidney function. If there is a questionable renal dysfunction these drugs may be preferred.

It is important to remember that hyperkalemia, hypermagnesemia, hypercalcemia, and hypernatremia may alter neuromuscular blockage and induce arrhythmias.

Antagonists. These agents seem to have little effect upon the kidney but their efficiency may be altered due to electrolyte shifts and metabolism of the fixed drug that is to be reversed. If the patient is in renal failure, postoperative dialysis may be required to reverse the agent.

Fluid Therapy. If shock occurs, maintenance of cortical flow is most important to prevent renal ischemia, which correlates with time and severity of the shock. To maintain flow, careful replacement with fluids such as Ringer's lactate, saline, and blood are important; the use of adrenergic blockers, such as dopamine, that decrease arterial pressure but not resistance, and the use of diuretics, such as furosimide, that reroute the renal flow and thus increase cortical flow through the peritubilar capillaries (salt wasting zone) as well as decrease resistance, are of greatest importance. The avoidance of vasoconstrictors is crucial since their effect on renal flow is extensive.

If the patient has renal insufficiency, the restriction of fluids is essential and only insensible water loss is replaced. One must closely monitor "third space" water as well as water sequestered in traumatized tissue. Replacement methods utilize balanced salt solution for sequestered fluids and 5 percent dextrose in water for water loss. The cause of hypotension and hypovolemia must be ascertained so that appropriate fluids can be selected to expand blood volume. Postoperative hemodialysis can remove the excess fluid.

Other Anesthesia Problems. Patients receiving continuous positive pressure ventilation (CPPV) frequently have fluid retention and decreased urinary output. An increase in plasma ADH and decrease in renal cortical perfusion are believed responsible.

In hypertensive crisis, many anesthetists prefer trimethaphan (Arfonad) because it is metabolized by cholinesterase. If at all possible one should avoid preoperative digitalization in patients suspected of renal disease.

Postoperative Care. Signs and symptoms of acute renal failure are insidious. Diagnostic increases in levels of urea and creatinine occur only when more than 60 percent of the renal function is lost. At this stage there is still little change in electrolyte and water metabolism. Disease may have already existed preoperatively and aggressive fluid therapy or hypovolemia and anoxia during surgery may have aggravated the disease.

Postoperative renal failure is usually manifested by a urine output of less than 400 ml per 24 hours. It may be due to prerenal hypovolemia, renal acute tubular necrosis, either ischemic or nephrotoxic, or postrenal obstruction. Differentiation of treatment usually includes laboratory tests such as glomerular filtration rate, BUN or serum creatinine ratio, and mannitol or furosemide challenge.

SUMMARY

In order to prevent kidney disorders during surgery and to manage those that occur one must:

1. Assess the patient carefully for a history of hypertension, diabetes, or proteinuria.
2. Review and correlate the routine urinalysis findings to previous admission studies.
3. Interpret the BUN measurement in the light of the patient's metabolic state and adequacy of hydration.
4. Compare the serum creatinine value with past levels or that after the last dialysis.
5. Review electrolyte, hemoglobin, and cardiac output studies.
6. Assess the length of time and dosage of all drugs administered to the patient relative to depression or toxicity of the kidney, homeostasis, and interactions with each other.
7. Prevent periods of hypovolemia, overhydration, and anoxia during the surgical procedure.
8. Monitor urinary output and other parameters as indicated in the perioperative period.

BIBLIOGRAPHY

Appel GB, New HC: Nephrotoxicity of antimicrobial agents, Part I. N Engl J Med 296:663–670, 1977.

Bastrom RD, Perkins FM, Pyne JL: Autoregulation of renal blood flow during halothane anesthesia. Anesthesiology 46:142–144, 1977.

Bevan OR: Kidney and Anesthesia. In Scurr C, Feldman S (eds): Scientific Foundation of Anaesthesia, 3rd ed. London, Heinemann, 1982, pp 309–323.

Beyer KH: Diuretics in perspective. J Clin Pharmacol 17:618–625, 1977.

Brobeck JR (ed): Best and Taylor's Physiological Basis of Medical Practice, 11th ed. Baltimore, MD, Williams & Wilkins, 1985.

Brown R: Enzymes of biotransformation as related to anesthesia. ASA Refresher Courses in Anesthesiology 3:27–38, 1975.

Cawson RA, McGracken AW, Marcus PB: Pathological Mechanisms and Human Disease. St. Louis, Mosby, 1982, p 369.

Deutsch S: Effects of anesthetics on the kidney. Surg Clin North Am 55:775–786, 1975.

Gebman S, Fowler KC, Smith LR: Regional blood flow during isoflurane and halothane anesthesia. Anesth Analg 63:557, 1984.

Gifford RW: A guide to the practical use of diuretics. JAMA 235:1890–1893, 1976.

Goldberg LI: L-dopa effect on renal function (Letter). N Engl J Med 297:112–113, 1977.

Goodman LS and Gilman A (eds): Pharmacological Basis of Therapeutics, 7th ed. New York, Macmillan, 1985, pp 222–323.

Goth A: Medical Pharmacology. 11th ed. St. Louis, Mosby, 1984.

Gussin RZ: Potassium—sparing diuretics. J Clin Pharmacol 17:651–662, 1977.

Guyton AC: Textbook of Medical Physiology, 7th ed. Philadelphia, Saunders, 1986.

Harries JD: Evaluation of renal function. ASA Refresher Courses in Anesthesiology 4:39–50, 1976.

Holder J: Anesthesia for renal transplants. AANAJ 49:498–502, 1981.

Katz J, Benumof J, Kadis L: Anesthesia and Uncommon Diseases, 2nd ed. Philadelphia, Saunders, 1981.

Kessane JM (ed): Anderson's Pathology 8th ed., St. Louis, Mosby, 1985, pp 1147–1148.

Kimberly RP, Plotz PH: Aspirin—induced depression of renal function. N Engl J Med 296:418–424, 1977.

Leevy CM: Evaluation of Liver Function in Clinical Practice, 2nd ed. Indianapolis, IN, Lilly Research Laboratories, 1974.

Luckman J, Sorensen K: Medical-Surgical Nursing, 2nd ed. Philadelphia, Saunders, 1980.

Miller RD (ed): Anesthesia, 2nd ed, 3 vols., New York, Churchill Livingstone, 1986, pp 318–319, 898–903, 1199–1123, 2339–2340.

Nechay BR: Biochemical basis of diuretic action. J Clin Pharmacol 17:626–641, 1977.

Parker PO: Anesthetic management of the patient with hepatic dysfunction. Anesthesiol Rev, 12:9, 1985.

Pitts RF: Physiology of the Kidney and Body Fluids, 3rd ed. Chicago, Year Book Med Pub, 1974.

Powell B: Preoperative evaluation and physical assessment of the patient. AANAJ 49:613–624, 1981.

Radnay PA, Duncalf D, et al: Common bile duct pressure changes after fentanyl, morphine, meperidine, butorphanol, and naloxone. Anesth Analg 63:441, 1984.

Reece EL: Preoperative evaluation and physical assessment of the patient. AANAJ 49:516–522, 1981.

Schramm MA: Anatomy and physiology of the kidney. AANA J 43:39, 1975.

Stoelling RK: Estimation of hepatic function—Effects of the anesthetic experience. ASA Refresher Course in Anesthesiology 4:139–150, 1976.

Strunin L: The Liver and Anesthesia. Philadelphia, Saunders, 1975, Vol 3.

Strunin L: Liver and anesthesia. In Scurr C, Feldman S (eds): Scientific Foudation of Anaesthesia, 3rd ed. London, Heinemann, 1982, pp 323–329.

Sullivan L: Physiology of the Kidney. Philadelphia, Lea & Febiger, 1975.

Vander AJ: Renal Physiology. New York, McGraw-Hill, 1975.

Wood M, Wood AJJ (ed): Drugs and Anesthesia. Baltimore, Williams and Wilkins, 1982, p 323.

Zakin D, Boyer TD: Hepatology. Philadelphia, Saunders, 1982, pp 455–561.

Zauder HL: Anesthesia for patients who have terminal renal disease. ASA Refresher Course in Anesthesiology 4:163–173, 1976.

22

Respiratory Physiology

Susan Ward, Joseph Kanusky, and James Hunn

MECHANICS OF VENTILATION

The exchange of air between atmosphere and alveoli is defined as ventilation, and it requires the alternate expansion and contraction of the lungs. This requires the generation of force by the respiratory muscles, which, in turn, depends on delivery of oxygen to the sites of local energy expenditure. There are several factors that favor either lung inflation or collapse, apart from any action of the respiratory muscles.

Factors Favoring Lung Collapse

The lung has a natural tendency to collapse or recoil, because it is predominantly an elastic structure. In the absence of other forces, the lung will recoil down to a very small volume—the relaxation volume of the lung—at which the lung recoil force is zero. As the lungs are inflated progressively from this volume, the magnitude of the lung recoil force increases. This inherent recoil constitutes the principal force that must be overcome to expand the lung during a normal inspiratory movement.

A crucial factor tending to collapse the lung is the intra-alveolar surface tension. The inner surfaces of the alveoli are covered with a thin layer of liquid. The molecules in this liquid strongly attract one another and, like a drawstring, pull the alveoli down to a smaller volume. In accordance with Laplace's law, a much greater force is required to expand the alveoli, owing to their reduced radius.

Also, the nonelastic structures of the lung, such as bone, cartilage, vessels, nerves, and connective tissue, act as a dead weight that must be moved or displaced whenever the lung is inflated. In brief, these tissues are a hindrance to lung inflation, because of their intrinsic elastic character.

Factors Favoring Lung Expansion

There are two components on the other side of the balance that favor lung expansion and thus oppose collapse.

First, although the lung has a natural tendency to collapse, the thorax has a constant similar tendency to expand outward into a hyperinflated position because of the particular geometry created by the arrangement of elastic fibers, skeletal muscle, and ribs. This outward recoil is the main force resisting the lungs' tendency to collapse. In contrast to the lungs, the passive relaxation volume of the thorax is large (about two-thirds of the total lung volume) and is not normally encroached upon. Thus, the chest wall recoil force will increase as the lungs become smaller (c.f., the lungs).

Next, if the surface tension forces within the alveoli could be decreased, their tendency to retract would be less. Pulmonary surfactant, a complex phospholipid produced by specialized cells in the alveolar wall and secreted at the alveolar surface, acts to decrease the attraction that exists between the molecules of liquid and in this way decreases surface tension. Therefore, pulmonary surfactant is a favoring factor for lung expansion. The synthesis of pulmonary surfactant begins in utero. However, prior to about the 30th week of gestation, insufficient quantities are produced to permit normal lung inflation. Hence, premature births are frequently associated with neonatal respiratory distress syndrome, characterized by abnormally stiff lungs with varying degrees of alveolar collapse.

A Balance of Forces

At the end of a normal expiration, those forces tending to collapse the lung are effectively held in check by those forces favoring lung expansion; that is, the recoil forces of the lung and chest wall are balanced. If these forces did not counter one another, the thorax would flare outward into a position of hyperexpansion and the lung would collapse to a volume approaching zero. However, neither event normally occurs because the thorax and lung are closely apposed and thus move together, i.e., when the thorax expands, the lungs inflate, and when the lungs retract, the thorax follows. The factor that bonds these two structures together is the subatmospheric, or negative pressure, seal within the intrapleural space that exists between the thorax and the lung. This seal ensures that, under normal

The opinions and assertions contained herein are the private views of the authors and are not to be construed as official or as reflections of the Department of the Army or the Department of Defense.

circumstances and throughout the breathing cycle, the thorax is held in check and cannot freely recoil outward during inspiration or the lung freely collapse during expiration.

Each lung is surrounded by its own membrane, or pleura, composed of two layers. The outermost (superior) layer, the parietal pleura, is attached to the inner surface of the thorax, whereas the inner (inferior) layer, the visceral pleura, is bonded to the lung's surface. There is only a small volume (a few milliliters, at most) of lubricating serous fluid between the two layers and, although it is possible to introduce air or liquid between the two, they are normally in direct contact and thus the space is only potential.

Because the structures (thorax and lung) to which the two pleural layers are attached are pulling in opposite directions, the pressure within the potential intrapleural space is less than atmospheric (atmospheric pressure is normally about 760 mm Hg) or negative (for the same reason that the space within a syringe becomes negative if the outlet is blocked and the plunger and barrel are pulled in opposite directions). Thus, a balance exists between the thorax and lung: neither can obey its natural tendency to recoil completely if the pleural space remains closed to the atmosphere. As a result of the two opposing (though balanced) forces the pressure within the intrapleural space is slightly subatmospheric; a typical value at the end of a quiet expiration is -4 cm H_2O (Fig. 22–1).

Lung Compliance

Lung compliance is a measure of lung distensibility, or of how much air is moved into the lung per unit of "distending" pressure change (Fig. 22–2). The "distending" (or transpulmonary) pressure is the difference between the pressure immediately outside the lung (intrapleural) and the pressure within the lungs (intra-alveolar). A normal value for compliance is 200 ml/cm H_2O. If, for whatever reason, a given pressure differential moves less air than normal, the lungs are considered less distensible, i.e., compliance has decreased (e.g., fibrosis, neonatal respiratory distress syndrome). If more air is moved per unit of pressure differential, then the opposite is said to be true (e.g., emphysema).

It is important to recognize that the tidal volume is

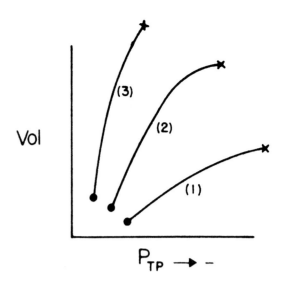

Figure 22–2. Compliance curves for normal lung (2), for lung with high recoil (e.g., fibrosis) (1), and for lung with low recoil (e.g., emphysema) (3). P_{TP} = transpulmonary pressure. (*From Whipp, 1982. Courtesy of Year Book Med Pub.*)

not distributed uniformly throughout the lung, even in healthy individuals with no evidence of pulmonary dysfunction. This reflects the effects of gravity on the lung tissue volume (which is made up largely of water). As a consequence, the intrapleural pressure at the base of the lung (i.e., in the dependent region) is more positive (or less negative) than at the apex; and the basal alveoli are thus smaller than are those at the apex. This is schematized in Figure 22–3, which shows that, at the end of a quiet expiration, the larger apical alveoli are located on the upper, flatter portion of the compliance curve (at ●, *a*), whereas the smaller basal alveoli lie on the lower, steeper portion of the curve (at ●, *b*). Both apical and basal units will expand during the subsequent inspiration in response to a given increment of intrapleural pressure (ΔP_{ip}), and to an extent dictated by the regional compliance. Thus, the basal alveoli—although smaller—will expand more than the apical alveoli. Hence, the alveolar ventilation is distributed preferentially to the dependent portions of the lungs.

Quiet Breathing

For air to enter the lungs, the muscles of inspiration must contract and thus expand the internal diameter of the thoracic cavity. In other words, the muscles of inspiration serve to shift the balance just described in favor of lung inflation.

The diaphragm is the principal muscle responsible for moving air during a quiet inspiration. This dome-shaped skeletal muscle is attached around its periphery to the sternum, costal cartilage, muscle, and vertebrae; it thus effectively separates the thoracic and abdominal cavities. It has orifices for the esophagus, aorta, vena cava, and nerves. The two halves (leaves) are each innervated by a phrenic nerve composed of somatic motor fibers projecting from C3 to C5 cord levels. If the lung is normal and the intercostal

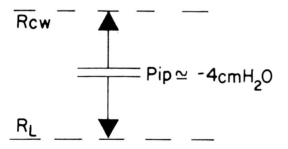

Figure 22–1. Balance of forces that determine functional residual capacity (FRC). R_{cw}, R_L are the recoil forces of the chest wall and lungs, respectively; their respective magnitudes (which are equal at FRC) are indicated by the length of the appropriate arrow. P_{ip} is the intrapleural pressure. (*From Whipp, 1982. Courtesy of Year Book Med Pub.*)

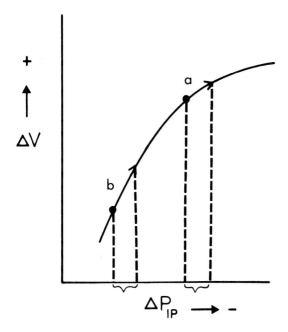

Figure 22–3. Influence of gravity on regional distribution of alveolar ventilation. Thus, apical alveoli (a) have a larger volume than basal alveoli (b) in the upright lung. However, because the apical units normally lie on a less steep portion of the compliance curve (ΔV vs ΔP_{ip}) than the basal units, they will expand from functional residual capacity (FRC = ●) to a lesser extent during normal breathing in response to a given increment in P_{ip}. Thus, the apical alveoli ventilate less than the basal alveoli. (*From Whipp, 1982. Courtesy of Year Book Med Pub.*)

muscles intact, complete denervation of the diaphragm will not seriously compromise breathing.

The intercostal muscles are arranged between the ribs. Those running down and forward are called external intercostals and have an inspiratory function; they normally are responsible for moving about 25 to 30 percent of the tidal air. Their contraction causes the ribs to move forward, upward, and outward, thus increasing the internal diameter of the thorax along the anterioposterior, vertical, and transverse axes. The movement of the rib cage forward and up is called "pump handle" motion, and the movement laterally "bucket handle" movement. The internal intercostal muscles run down and back (posterior) between the ribs and are normally inactive at rest. Their contraction pulls the ribs in a direction opposite to that resulting from external intercostal contraction, and the diameter of the thorax is altered accordingly (i.e., decreased along all axes). The intercostal muscles are innervated by the intercostal (spinal motor and sensory) nerves originating from T1 through T11 cord levels.

The mechanical events of quiet breathing are initiated by the active contraction of the diaphragm and the descent of its dome over a distance of about 2 to 3 cm from a resting position at the level of the fifth thoracic vertebra. This increases the internal diameter of the thorax mainly along the vertical axis and to a lesser degree along the transverse axis by pulling the lower ribs laterally. At the same time, the external intercostals contract with moderate force to displace mainly the upper ribs forward and up.

Quiet expiration is a passive act, initiated by relaxation of the diaphragm and external intercostals, permitting the diaphragmatic dome to ascend and the intercostals to move down and back to their resting position. In this way the thorax retracts, the lungs partially deflate, and a balance is again established between the recoil forces of the lung and thorax at the end of expiration—the resting position.

Stimulated Breathing

A far more substantial involvement of the muscles of respiration is necessary if the breathing requirement is increased (e.g., during exercise). As a result, the diaphragm descends over a greater distance (by as much as 10 cm) and the external intercostals contract with greater force than during a quiet inspiration; the contribution of the intercostals may account for some 50 percent of the tidal volume. In addition, the accessory muscles of inspiration—the scalenes and the sternomastoid—may come into play, augmenting the action of the intercostals in pulling the upper ribs forward and upward. The product of this combined muscular activity is greater thoracic expansion along all three axes, thus drawing a greater volume of air into the lungs.

The greater force required for expiration under these conditions depends on the internal intercostals, which pull the ribs down and backward, and the accessory muscles of expiration—the abdominals—which force the abdominal contents against the inferior surface of the diaphragm to push its dome to a higher resting position. This muscular activity serves to decrease the internal volume of the thoracic cavity.

Pressure Changes and the Movement of Air During the Respiratory Cycle

During quiet breathing the intrapleural pressure is negative (subatmospheric) during both inspiration and expiration. However, the degree of negativity changes during the respiratory cycle (Fig. 22–4). At the onset of inspiration the intrapleural pressure is approximately −4 cm H_2O. As the lung expands during inspiration, its tendency to recoil increases (see discussion of factors favoring lung collapse). Thus, a greater force is needed to overcome this greater recoil, and it is provided by the muscles of inspiration. As a result, the intrapleural pressure becomes more negative than at end-expiration and may reach a value of about −10 cm H_2O at the end of a quiet inspiration. As the muscles of inspiration relax and permit the lung to collapse, the intrapleural pressure becomes less negative and is restored to a value of −4 cm H_2O at the end of expiration. Thus, the intrapleural pressure is negative during a quiet respiratory cycle, becomes more negative during inspiration, and is less negative during expiration. The negative intrapleural pressure is reflected throughout the thoracic cavity, and it is thus argued that the augmented venous return characteristic of inspiration reflects the more negative intrapleural pressure in this phase of the breathing cycle.

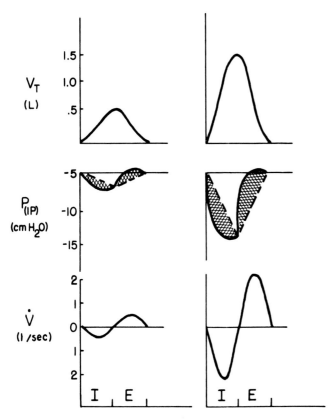

Figure 22–4. Time courses of volume (V_T), intrapleural pressure (P_{ip}), and airflow ($\dot{V}$) during inspiration (I) and expiration (E) for rest (left) and stimulated breathing (right) in a normal individual. Dashed profile on P_{ip} curve represents pressure required to generate the volume profile under static conditions (i.e., zero airflow); this is the transpulmonary pressure (P_{tp}). Shaded area on P_{ip} curve represents extra pressure needed to produce the normal airflow response and is thus equal to the alveolar pressure. (*From Whipp, 1982. Courtesy of Year Book Med Pub.*)

When inspiration is more forceful and tidal volume is increased, the intrapleural pressure becomes even more subatmospheric and may reach values of the order of −30 to −40 cm H_2O. A forceful expiration, on the other hand, can so exaggerate the reduction in intrapleural pressure with declining lung volume that it actually becomes positive or above atmospheric.

Pressure changes also occur within the alveoli during the breathing cycle (Fig. 22–4). Prior to an inspiration (i.e., at the end of a quiet expiration), when there is no movement of air into or out of the lung, the alveolar pressure is neither negative (subatmospheric) nor positive (greater than atmospheric) but is equal to atmospheric (zero), which is 760 mm Hg at sea level. At the onset of a quiet inspiration, the alveoli inflate and, as a result, the alveolar pressure becomes subatmospheric (to about −2 or −3 cm H_2O) and air is drawn down the tracheobronchial tree toward the alveoli for the exchange of oxygen and carbon dioxide. As the end of the inspiratory phase is approached, flow ceases and the alveolar pressure returns once more to zero. With a more forceful inspiration, air flow into the lungs is more rapid and thus requires a more negative alveolar pressure. Conversely, a more negative intra-alveolar pres-

sure is required to sustain flow during quiet breathing if, for some reason, the airway resistance is increased. Ordinarily, the inspiratory force required to overcome airway resistance is very small. However, there are circumstances under which the resistance to air flow increases to varying degrees. For example, Poiseuille's law predicts that a decrease in the diameter of any segment of the passageway will produce a marked increase in the resistance—to the fourth power of the radius. Increasing the length of the airway will also result in an increased resistance but to a lesser degree than decreasing the diameter. Turbulence also increases the resistance to airflow. Air normally moves down the conduits in a streamlined or laminar fashion; that is, the inner layers of air move faster than the outer ones, which molds the stream into a bullet-shaped profile. If the stream of air forms whirlpools or eddy currents or is directed at an abrupt angle to the passageways, then it is no longer laminar or streamlined and the resistance to its movement increases dramatically. Among the factors that can precipitate turbulence are multiple branchings, sharp turns, high velocities of flow, and irregular surface features on the inner walls of the airways.

As the lungs start to recoil during expiration and lung volume declines, alveolar pressure rises above atmospheric (to +2 to +3 cm H_2O, for a quiet expiration). As a result, air is forced out of the lungs and the alveolar pressure become less positive, so that by the time expiration is complete the pressure is again zero. In summary, the alveolar pressure goes from zero to negative to zero during inspiration, and from zero to positive to zero during expiration.

The intrapleural and alveolar pressure changes during breathing are altered whenever the lungs are expanded by forcing air down the airway under greater than atmospheric (positive) pressure, instead of by contracting the muscles of inspiration and "pulling" air into the alveoli. When the lungs are inflated by positive pressure, a negative intrapleural pressure is no longer required to hold them inflated by opposing their natural tendency to collapse. Rather, the lungs are now held inflated from within in the same fashion as a balloon. Naturally, the intrapleural pressure now becomes less negative during inspiration and may even assume positive values, depending upon the magnitude of the positive pressure applied at the airway opening. However, when the positive pressure is released, the lungs begin to collapse. The intrapleural pressure now becomes negative; if it reached positive values during the preceding inspiration, it first must become less positive before moving into the negative phase. On the other hand, the alveolar pressure directly reflects the degree of positive pressure applied at the airway, i.e., rising above atmospheric during inspiration, falling to equal atmospheric during expiration, and never attaining a negative value. Indeed, there is no need for a negative-pressure phase, as air is now being pushed into the lungs instead of drawn in by the pull of a negative alveolar pressure.

LUNG VOLUMES AND CAPACITIES

The various volumes and capacities of the lungs represent important functional manifestations of the mechanical properties of the lungs and chest wall. They are thus subject to alteration in conditions that are associated with abnormalities of lung recoil, chest wall recoil, and respiratory muscle function.

Conventionally four lung capacities and four lung volumes are recognized (Fig. 22–5):

- *Total lung capacity (TLC)*—the maximal volume to which the lungs and chest wall can be expanded by volitional inspiratory effort
- *Vital capacity (VC)*—the maximal volume of gas that can be exhaled by volitional effort
- *Functional residual capacity (FRC)*—the volume of gas in the lungs at the end of a normal quiet expiration
- *Inspiratory capacity (IC)*—the maximal volume of gas that can be inhaled from FRC by volitional effort
- *Tidal volume (V_T)*—the volume of gas either inhaled or exhaled during a typical respiratory cycle
- *Residual volume (RV)*—the volume of gas remaining in the lungs after a maximal volitional expiratory effort (the only volume that cannot be measured directly)
- *Inspiratory reserve volume (IRV)*—the maximal volume of gas that can be inhaled from the normal end-inspiratory position
- *Expiratory reserve volume (ERV)*—the maximal volume of gas that can be exhaled from FRC.

Certain interrelationships between the various volumes and capacities can be recognized:

$$TLC = VC + RV \qquad VC = IC + ERV$$
$$FRC = ERV + RV \qquad IC = V_T + ERV$$

It is appropriate here to consider the determinants of some of these volumes and capacities in greater detail, in view of their widespread use in the formulation of functional judgments about the mechanical properties of the respiratory system.

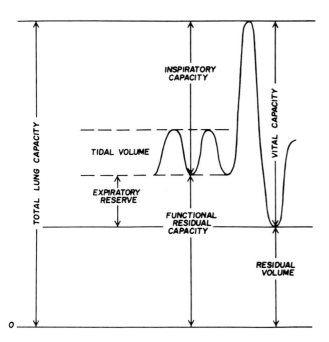

Figure 22–5. Standard lung volumes and capacities. (*From Whipp, 1982. Courtesy of Year Book Med Pub.*)

Tidal Volume

Together with the breathing frequency, V_T is an important determinant of the level of overall ventilation and, therefore, of how well arterial blood gas and acid-base homeostasis is maintained in the face of challenges, such as an increase in metabolic rate or a fall in the inspired oxygen fraction. Under basal conditions of rest or general anesthesia, for example, a normal adult would have a V_T of about 500 ml. In response to respiratory stimuli such as hypercapnia, hypoxia, and exercise, however, values of over 2 L may commonly be attained.

Functional Residual Capacity

This represents the "equilibrium volume" of the lungs and chest wall under passive conditions, at which their respective recoil forces are balanced (Fig. 22–1). During spontaneous quiet breathing, the end-expiratory lung volume is usually taken as the FRC, it being assumed that there are no forces being exerted by the respiratory muscles. A value of some 2.5 to 3.0 L would be quite reasonable for a young, healthy individual (although it should be recognized that factors such as sex, body dimensions, and age can influence FRC).

It is thus not surprising that factors affecting lung or chest wall elasticity will also affect FRC. For example, in pulmonary emphysema the degenerative changes that take place in the lung parenchyma result in a highly compliant lung having a lower-than-normal lung recoil (Fig. 22–2). As a consequence, FRC is higher than normal. In contrast, conditions characterized by a low lung compliance and a high lung recoil (pulmonary fibrosis, neonatal respiratory distress syndrome) are associated with a lower-than-normal FRC (Fig. 22–2).

During spontaneous breathing, the lungs may not necessarily return to FRC at the end of expiration, however. For example, if there is still some expiratory muscle tone at the end of expiration, the end-expiratory lung volume (EEV) may well be less than the FRC. This may explain in part why EEV is lower during muscular exercise then during the resting condition.

Total Lung Capacity

This volume is effectively dictated by the ability of the inspiratory muscles to override the recoil forces in both the lungs and the chest wall. (It is important to recognize that at these high volumes, which typically exceed the relaxation volume of the chest wall, the chest wall recoil now acts to reduce rather than increase chest wall volume.) A normal value for TLC in a young, healthy adult would be in the region of 6 L.

As discussed above for FRC, alterations in either lung or chest wall recoil are likely to influence TLC. For example, TLC is characteristically high in patients with emphysema, owing to the reduced lung recoil, but low in pulmonary fibrosis. Impaired function of the inspiratory muscles consequent, for example, to neuromuscular disorders will predispose to a lower-than-normal TLC.

Residual Volume

This volume, too, is dependent on respiratory muscle strength; in this case, that of the expiratory muscles. Thus, the expiratory muscles act in concert with the lung recoil force in attempting to reduce lung volume in the face of the opposing chest wall recoil force. A value of about 1.0 to 1.5 L can be regarded as normal for a young, healthy adult.

Predictably, RV will be lower in conditions in which lung recoil is higher than normal (pulmonary fibrosis, neonatal respiratory distress syndrome) and higher when lung recoil is reduced (emphysema). Also, expiratory muscle dysfunction will elevate RV.

Vital Capacity

In making interpretations about potential sites of respiratory-mechanical impairment, it is important to recognize that—depending on the conditions under which the VC is measured—the VC may be subject to several interpretations. Thus, it is usual for estimates of both the *forced* VC and the *slow* VC to be made; while these are effectively equal in normal individuals, the forced VC is typically less than the slow VC in conditions such as chronic obstructive pulmonary disease (COPD), in which small airway closure commonly occurs during forced exhalations.

Because the VC represents the difference between TLC and RV, the influence of altered recoil status will clearly depend on which of these two quantities is affected more. In the case of emphysema, for example, VC may not be greatly affected; this, of course, should not be taken as an indication of normal respiratory-mechanical function but rather to reflect similar degrees of impairment in both TLC and RV.

PULMONARY CIRCULATION

Structure

The lungs receive mixed venous blood from the pulmonary artery and arterial blood from the bronchial arteries. The former is principally for gas exchange, whereas the latter is entirely for the nourishment of the lung substance and is part of the systemic circulation.

The pulmonary artery originates from the right ventricle and shortly thereafter bifurcates into the two main pulmonary arteries. Each lung receives a main artery that enters at the hilum and then subdivides into a profuse network of smaller arteries, arterioles, and capillaries. Excluding capillaries, the vessels of the pulmonary circuit are rich in elastic fibers but poorly endowed with smooth muscle. Unlike the systemic circuit, the smooth muscle is evenly distributed among the vessels and not organized into distinct bands within the arteriolar walls which function as spigots for allocating blood to the capillary beds.

The pulmonary capillaries are about the diameter of an erythrocyte, with walls one cell thick and devoid of both elastic and smooth muscle fibers. As with the systemic circuit, the capillaries are the functional unit of the pulmonary system, subserving primarily the exchange of oxygen and carbon dioxide. Secondarily, these capillaries serve to nourish those lung structures distal to the terminal bronchioles, which include respiratory bronchioles, alveolar ducts, and alveoli. The approximately 300 billion pulmonary capillaries form a vascular network so profuse that it can be thought of as a vast, open lake bathing some 280 million alveoli. The capillaries of each lung empty arterialized blood into two pulmonary veins that in turn empty into the left artrium.

Dynamics

Under basal conditions, it requires about 4 seconds for blood to pass from the right to the left heart. About 1 second of this total pulmonary circulation time is spent passing through the capillaries. Under stress, the capillary circulation time can normally decrease to about 0.3 seconds without compromising gas exchange. The lungs receive the total output of the right ventricle, which is normally about 5 to 6 L/min at rest. The pulmonary blood volume is about 500 ml, with the capillaries containing some 100 ml.

The pulmonary artery blood pressure is much less than the systemic arterial pressure; the pulmonary circulation is thus often referred to as the "lesser" circulation. Some approximate pressure values, in mm Hg, are pulmonary artery 25/8 (14 mean, 20 to 30 systolic range, 7 to 12 diastolic range), arterioles/capillaries 8 to 10, pulmonary veins 6, and left atrium 5. The pressure drop or gradient from pulmonary artery to left atrium is about 9 to 10 mmHg, in contrast to the 100 mmHg fall from aorta to vena cava. This small pressure gradient across the pulmonary circuit indicates a low resistance to blood flow—an extremely important characteristic of the pulmonary circulation.

The pulmonary vascular resistance is defined as the ratio of the vascular pressure drop across the pulmonary circulation (ΔP) to the right ventricular outflow rate ($\dot{Q}_{RV}$); i.e., pulmonary vascular resistance = $\Delta P/\dot{Q}_{RV}$, where ΔP = pulmonary artery pressure − left atrial pressure. The principal factor altering resistance is vessel diameter. If the diameter is decreased, the resistance to flow will increase and vice versa.

The right ventricular output can increase from a basal 5 to 6 L/min to a maximum of about 30 L/min under stressful circumstances. Such increases in pulmonary flow will elevate the pulmonary artery pressure if the resistance in the circuit remains unchanged. However, the resistance normally decreases; this largely counters the flow increase and thus keeps the pressure within a normal range. This decrease in resistance is brought about in two ways. First, vessels that are already perfused expand in response to the increased flow, reflecting their compliant characteristics; thus, the capacitance of the pulmonary vascular bed is increased. Second, previously collapsed vessels become patent (i.e., "recruitment"). Thus, not only is the diameter of vessels increased, but also more vessels are patent; as a result, the overall cross-sectional area of the pulmonary vascular bed is greater. However, as the limits of distensibility of the pulmonary circulation are approached, further increases in right ventricular outflow can no longer continue to reduce pulmonary vascular resistance, and the pulmonary vascular pressures will start to rise, placing a strain on the right ventricle. (The right ventricle, unlike the left, is a less powerful, low-pressure pump.)

Control of Pulmonary Blood Flow

The pumping action of the right ventricle is the main factor controlling pulmonary blood flow, because, within broad limits, the lungs receive whatever the right heart ejects. The lungs are the only organ receiving the total cardiac output (aside from the normally small right-to-left shunt related to the bronchial and myocardial circulations); and despite wide fluctuations in this output, the pressure remains fairly constant because of the passive compensatory changes in resistance discussed above.

The potential also exists for active control of the pulmonary vascular resistance. The poorly developed smooth muscle within the pulmonary arteries and veins receives fibers from both divisions of the autonomic nervous system. The release of norepinephrine—a sympathetic neurotransmitter—vasoconstricts pulmonary vascular smooth muscle, whereas acetylcholine—a parasympathetic neurotransmitter—dilates. The magnitude of change in diameter resulting from the discharge of either division is, however, a clinically insignificant factor in the direct control of pulmonary blood flow. In contrast, it should be recognized that the autonomic nervous system can play an important *indirect* role in altering pulmonary blood flow by directly altering heart rate and stroke volume: sympathetic discharge serves to increase both heart rate and stroke volume, whereas parasympathetic influences can lower heart rate (though to a lesser degree, and with little effect on stroke volume).

Breathing also affects the delivery of blood to the lungs by altering venous return: during inspiration pulmonary blood flow is increased, whereas it is decreased during expiration. This reflects the more negative intrapleural pressure during inspiration, serving to draw a greater volume of blood into the thorax and thus to the heart and lungs (i.e., ΔP is increased). Conversely, during a spontaneous expiration and also during positive-pressure inspiration, venous return and pulmonary blood flow become compromised as the intrapleural pressure becomes less negative or even positive (above atmospheric). It should be pointed out that a further mechanism could also contribute: during inspiration, the lung substance surrounding the pulmonary vessels exerts an increased radial traction when the lung expands, which increases vessel diameter and thus decreases its resistance. However, this effect appears to be largely offset by an increase in the resistance of vessels situated close to the alveoli: as the alveoli expand during inspiration, these vessels become elongated and therefore narrower; the converse occurs during expiration. As a consequence, the overall pulmonary vascular resistance changes little with the phase of respiration.

Regional Distribution of Pulmonary Blood Flow

The lungs possess an intrinsic mechanism for controlling the regional distribution of the pulmonary blood flow, so that local deviations in the matching of alveolar blood flow and ventilation are minimized. Thus, blood can be diverted away from underventilated alveoli having a low alveolar

P_{O_2} (P_{AO_2}) to areas of the lung that are better ventilated and thus have a higher P_{AO_2}. In this way, perfusion is more evenly matched with ventilation, and the shunting of mixed venous blood to the left heart is reduced. The stimulus for triggering this flow shift is related to the low P_{AO_2}, which exerts a direct vasoconstrictive effect on the smooth muscle of adjacent pulmonary vessels (i.e., independently of autonomic nervous system innervation).

Owing to the effect of gravity, blood entering the lung is not evenly distributed to all of the pulmonary capillaries. In the sitting or standing posture, the perfusion to the apex of the lung is less than to the middle or basal segments because the low-pressure right ventricle cannot ordinarily (i.e., at rest) generate enough contractile force to pump blood to that height against the force of gravity. In addition, as the apical alveoli are overinflated relative to alveoli in the dependent regions of the lung, the vascular resistance of adjacent alveolar vessels is increased (see above). As a result, the pulmonary arterial pressure at the apex of the lung is relatively low, and may actually become subatmospheric during diastole; the pulmonary capillary and venous pressures will be even lower (more subatmospheric). Assuming air flow to be zero, the alveolar pressure will be atmospheric and will therefore exceed pulmonary artery pressure during diastole. This will lead to vessel collapse during diastole, and no flow will occur (Fig. 22–6). This region of the lung has been termed "zone 1." It should be emphasized that conditions which compromise pulmonary artery pressure or right ventricular outflow may lead to the generation of a zone 1 region during systole.

In the midlung region ("zone 2"), both the effects of gravity and direct vessel compression are less than in the apical region. As a result, pulmonary artery pressure now exceeds atmospheric in both systole and diastole, and is therefore greater than pulmonary alveolar pressure. How-

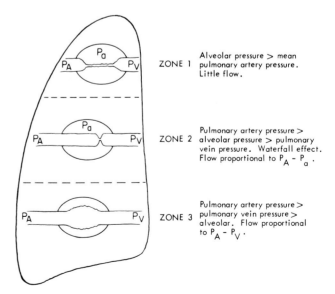

ZONE 1   Alveolar pressure > mean pulmonary artery pressure. Little flow.

ZONE 2   Pulmonary artery pressure > alveolar pressure > pulmonary vein pressure. Waterfall effect. Flow proportional to $P_A - P_a$.

ZONE 3   Pulmonary artery pressure > pulmonary vein pressure > alveolar. Flow proportional to $P_A - P_V$.

Figure 22–6. Effects of gravity on pulmonary circulation in the upright lung. Pa = pulmonary arterial pressure; Pv = pulmonary venous pressure; P_A = pulmonary alveolar pressure. (*From Whipp, 1982. Courtesy of Year Book Med Pub.*)

ever, pressure in the pulmonary capillaries and veins tends to be subatmospheric, and thus these segments will collapse (Fig. 22–6). This causes the pressure upstream of the collapsed segments to increase, as blood is still entering the pulmonary arteries, and these segments are thus forced open to allow blood flow. There is, however, a loss of energy as the blood flows through the previously collapsed segments and vascular pressures again become subatmospheric, leading to recollapse. This cycle of collapse → open → recollapse leads to "fluttering" of the vessel walls.

In the basilar lung segments, perfusion is markedly increased because the effects of gravity are minimal. Here, all the pulmonary vascular pressures (arterial, capillary, venous) are greater than alveolar pressure ("zone 3," Fig. 22–6). Thus, collapse does not occur. This regional distribution of pulmonary perfusion applies regardless of posture. That is, in varying degrees, the most superior part of the lung will conform to zone 1 (if pulmonary artery pressure becomes subatmospheric) no matter what the position, and the most inferior will be zone 3. For example, in the lateral position, the most superior areas in the uppermost lung are zone 1 (or zone 2) and the most inferior parts of the lowermost lung, zone 3. Under conditions such as exercise, in which cardiac output (and therefore right ventricular outflow) is greatly increased, zones 1 and 2 may be converted to zone 3. That is, at all levels of the lung the pulmonary vascular pressure becomes greater than atmospheric, and therefore alveolar, pressure.

OXYGEN TRANSPORT

Oxygen transport includes all the steps involved in moving oxygen from the atmosphere to the mitochondria in the various organs and tissues of the body. This is often referred to as the "oxygen cascade," reflecting the movement of oxygen along a series of partial pressure gradients. We will describe oxygen transport in three sections: transport to the alveoli, transport by the blood, and transport to the tissues.

Ventilation is the process by which oxygen exchanges between the external environment and the alveolar gas. Thus, by way of the pressure gradient between the mouth and the alveolar space, air and therefore oxygen molecules move by bulk flow through the airways (toward the alveoli in inspiration; toward the mouth in expiration). However, with the progressive branching of the airways that occurs as the alveoli are approached, the overall cross-sectional area of the respiratory tree also increases. As a result, the velocity within any single airway declines progressively (i.e., the overall airflow is "shared" between a greater number of airway units) and actually becomes zero in the vicinity of the respiratory bronchioles or alveolar ducts. Clearly, therefore, whereas the rate at which oxygen molecules are distributed *toward* the alveoli depends on the overall rate of airflow, the rate at which they are delivered *into* the alveoli depends on their ease of diffusion, which is governed primarily by the oxygen partial pressure gradient between the respiratory bronchioles and the interior of the alveoli.

It is appropriate at this point to consider the factors that dictate the partial pressure (P) or tension of a particular gas (in this case, oxygen). For example, if we were to breathe

pure oxygen at sea level, the partial pressure of oxygen (P_{O_2}) would be 760 torr (where 1 torr is the pressure required to support a column of mercury 1 mm high when the mercury is of standard density and subject to standard acceleration; this unit is synonymous with mm Hg in respiratory physiology). However, a healthy, unanesthetized individual does not usually breathe pure oxygen but rather air that is a mixture of gases. The component gas pressures are determined in accordance with Dalton's law, which states that in a gas mixture, the pressure exerted by each individual gas in a given space is independent of the pressures of the other gases in the mixture. That is to say, each gas behaves as though it were the only gas present and the total pressure of a mixture of gases is therefore the sum of the individual gas pressures. For a gas X, this can be expressed as:

$$P_X = F_X \cdot P_{TOTAL}$$

where P_X is the partial pressure of X and F_X is the fractional concentration (i.e., [X]/100), and P_{TOTAL} is the total pressure of the gas mixture. Dry atmospheric air at sea level has a total pressure of 760 torr and its major constituents are 79.03 percent nitrogen, 20.93 percent oxygen, and 0.04 percent carbon dioxide. The corresponding partial pressures of the components are $P_{N_2} = 600$ torr, $P_{O_2} = 159$ torr, and $P_{CO_2} = 0.3$ torr. As an individual inspires, the nose, mouth, and pharynx humidify the incoming gas. This addition of water vapor to the inspired gas serves to lower the partial pressures of the remaining components, in accordance with Dalton's law. At a normal body temperature of 37C, fully humidified inspired gas will have a water vapor pressure of 47 torr, regardless of the atmospheric pressure. Since the total gas pressure at sea level equals 760 torr and water vapor exerts 47 torr pressure, the difference (713 torr) is available for the sum of the partial pressures of oxygen, nitrogen, and carbon dioxide. Therefore, the P_{O_2} of moist inspired air in the trachea (P_{IO_2}) is 149 torr (i.e., 20.93/100 × 713), P_{IN_2} is 563 torr, and P_{ICO_2} is 0.3 torr.

By the time the inspired gas reaches the alveoli, the alveolar P_{O_2} (P_{AO_2}) is only about 100 torr. This decrease in P_{O_2} is due to the mixture of the inspired gas with the gas making up the functional residual capacity (FRC), which has a lower P_{O_2} because it has already given up some of its oxygen to the perfusing blood. The FRC serves as an important reservoir of oxygen which minimizes the otherwise wide swings that would occur in arterial P_{O_2} (P_{aO_2}), owing to the delivery of fresh air being confined to the inspiratory phase of the breathing cycle.

Although the greater proportion of the inspired tidal volume reaches the alveolar space and participates in the exchange of oxygen (and carbon dioxide), the final 150 ml or so of necessity remains in the conducting airways where no significant gas exchange takes place. This volume—also known as the anatomic dead space—is thus the first to be exhaled, later followed by gas from the alveolar space. As a result, the P_{O_2} of the exhaled tidal volume (termed the mixed expired P_{O_2}, $P_{\bar{E}O_2}$) is greater than P_{AO_2}, and $P_{\bar{E}CO_2}$ is less than P_{ACO_2}. Typical normal values for $P_{\bar{E}O_2}$ and $P_{\bar{E}CO_2}$ at rest are 120 and 28 torr, respectively.

A close approximation of P_{AO_2} can be determined by the alveolar air equation:

$$P_{AO_2} = P_{IO_2} - \frac{P_{ACO_2}}{R} + \left(P_{ACO_2} \cdot F_{IO_2} \cdot \frac{1-R}{R} \right)$$

in which P_{AO_2} is the alveolar partial pressure of oxygen, P_{IO_2} is the inspired partial pressure of oxygen, P_{ACO_2} is the alveolar partial pressure of carbon dioxide (usually assumed to equal arterial P_{CO_2}), F_{IO_2} is the fractional concentration of oxygen in inspired gas, and R is the respiratory exchange ratio (given by the ratio of pulmonary carbon dioxide output to oxygen uptake) which equals the respiratory quotient under steady-state conditions. The expression

$$P_{ACO_2} \cdot F_{IO_2} \cdot \frac{1-R}{R}$$

is equal to 2 torr when the P_{ACO_2} is 40 torr, F_{IO_2} is 0.2093, and R is 0.8 (i.e., a normal diet), and thus this term is often neglected in clinical determinations of P_{AO_2}. This equation permits the nurse anesthetist to calculate the P_{AO_2} for a patient breathing gas of any F_{IO_2}. With knowledge of the P_{aO_2}, it is thus possible to estimate the alveolar-arterial P_{O_2} difference, $P_{(A-a)O_2}$, which has a normal range of 5 to 10 torr on room air and approximately 10 to 60 torr with pure oxygen (i.e., F_{IO_2} 1.0).

Gas is exchanged across the alveolar capillary membrane by the process of diffusion, the driving force for which is the P_{O_2} difference between alveolar gas and blood in the pulmonary capillary. Mixed venous blood, which normally has a P_{O_2} of 40 torr at rest, is delivered to the pulmonary capillary circulation by the pulmonary artery. As the alveolar P_{O_2} is normally 100 torr, this establishes a driving force for oxygen diffusion of 60 torr at the beginning of the pulmonary capillary. Diffusion equilibrium between the blood and gas phases is normally reached well before blood leaves the capillary circulation, so that the P_{O_2} of pulmonary end-capillary blood is 100 torr. Downstream of the pulmonary capillary circulation, venous blood from the larger airways and from the myocardium normally drains into the arterialized blood (by way of the bronchial veins and thebesian veins, respectively) and thus lowers the P_{O_2}. Normally, however, such anatomic shunts are only a small fraction of the cardiac output and thus the reduction in P_{O_2} is modest: arterial P_{O_2} is normally in the region of 90 to 95 torr. With increasing age, this value is likely to be lower, however; and it is possible to predict the magnitude of this effect by means of equations derived from large groups of healthy individuals in different age ranges, e.g. (Nunn, 1977),

$$P_{aO_2} \ (torr) = 102 - 0.33 \times age \ (yr)$$

The amount of oxygen dissolved in the plasma is governed by Henry's law, which states that the amount of gas that can be dissolved in a liquid is proportional to the partial pressure of the gas to which the liquid is exposed. For example, 1 ml of plasma at 37C carries 0.00003 ml of oxygen per torr P_{O_2}. Therefore, arterial blood with a P_{O_2} of 100 torr carries 0.3 ml of oxygen per 100 ml of blood. With a normal cardiac output and a normal oxygen consumption of 250 ml/min in a resting individual, a minimum of 5 ml of O_2/100 ml of blood would have to be dissolved in the blood to meet the body's metabolic demands. Clearly, therefore, the carriage of oxygen bound chemically to hemo-

globin is needed to insure adequate rates of oxygen delivery to the tissues.

Hemoglobin, which is contained within the red blood cells, has a molecular weight of 16,700. Each molecule consists of four subunits; each subunit consists of a polypeptide chain having a complex three-dimensional structure and incorporating an iron-containing heme group to which a single oxygen molecule can combine reversibly (as long as the iron remains in the ferrous form). This process of oxygenation (not to be confused with oxidation) is governed by the affinity of the hemoglobin subunit for oxygen; this depends, in turn, on the three-dimensional structure of the particular subunit and that of the surrounding three subunits in the hemoglobin molecule.

The oxygenation (and deoxygenation) of the hemoglobin (Hb) molecule is given by the following general equation, which indicates that four steps are involved (one for each subunit):

$$Hb_4 + 4\ O_2 \rightleftharpoons Hb_4(O_2)_4$$

This can be simplified, however:

$$Hb + O_2 \rightleftharpoons HbO_2$$

The complete oxygenation of hemoglobin to oxyhemoglobin (HbO_2) requires 1.34 ml of oxygen/g of Hb (values as high as 1.39 may be cited). This corresponds to 20.1 ml O_2/100 ml blood for a normal blood hemoglobin concentration of 15g/100 ml blood, and is termed the oxygen capacity. Clearly, therefore, in conditions that are characterized by increased levels of circulating hemoglobin (e.g., polycythemia), the oxygen capacity will be greater than normal; this will provide an increased potential for tissue oxygen delivery at a given cardiac output. In contrast, the oxygen capacity is reduced when hemoglobin levels are lower than normal, as in anemia. It is possible to allow for such alterations in oxygen capacity by expressing the amount of oxygen combined with hemoglobin as an oxygen saturation (S_{O_2}). Thus, at a particular P_{O_2},

$$S_{O_2} = \frac{O_2\ bound\ to\ Hb}{O_2\ capacity} \times 100\%$$

The amount of oxygen carried by the blood both in physical solution and in combination with hemoglobin is termed the oxygen content. Owing to the combining characteristics of the hemoglobin molecule, the relationship between the oxygen content (or the oxygen saturation) and P_{O_2} of blood—the oxygen dissociation curve—is not linear but rather is S-shaped, or sigmoid (Fig. 22–7). When the hemoglobin molecule is in the deoxygenated form, it has a relatively low affinity for oxygen. Thus, as P_{O_2} is increased from zero, only a small proportion of hemoglobin subunits become oxygenated; this is reflected in the shallow slope of the oxygen dissociation curve in this low-P_{O_2} range. However, once a single combination occurs in a hemoglobin molecule, small conformational changes in the three-dimensional structure of the polypeptide chains result; the effect is to facilitate oxygen combination at the remaining three binding sites (this is termed cooperative interaction). As a result, the dissociation curve is strikingly steepened over the P_{O_2} range of 10 to 50 torr. However, as P_{O_2} increases toward the normal arterial level of 90 to 100 torr, fewer

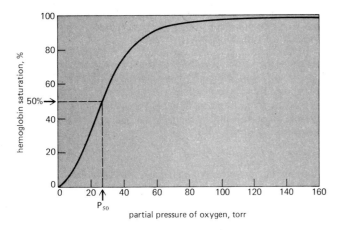

Figure 22–7. Oxygen-hemoglobin dissociation curve expressing oxygen (hemoglobin) saturation as a function of P_{O_2}. P_{50} represents the P_{O_2} at which oxygen saturation is 50%. (*From Levitsky, 1986. Courtesy of McGraw-Hill.*)

and fewer vacant sites remain for oxygen binding, and thus the oxygen dissociation curve starts to plateau.

The sigmoid shape of the oxygen dissociation curve has important functional implications for oxygen transport. A consequence of the flat, upper portion of the dissociation curve is that the amount of oxygen bound to hemoglobin is scarcely affected by moderate reductions in Pa_{O_2} that would result from conditions such as ascent to altitude or pulmonary disease. For example, blood having an arterial P_{O_2} of 95 torr and a saturation of 97 percent carries a total of 19.79 ml O_2/100 ml blood, i.e., 19.5 ml bound to hemoglobin ($20.1 \times 97/100$) and 0.29 ml in physical solution (0.003×95). This quantity is only reduced by 1.52 ml O_2/100 ml blood if the Pa_{O_2} falls to 60 torr (with $S_{O_2} = 90$ percent), i.e., 18.09 ml oxygen bound to hemoglobin and 0.18 ml dissolved, a total of 18.27 ml O_2/100 ml blood. In contrast, when arterial blood enters the capillary beds of the peripheral tissues and P_{O_2} starts to fall as a result of oxygen diffusion from the blood toward the mitochondria, a modest fall will lead to considerable unloading of oxygen from hemoglobin owing to the steep slope of the dissociation curve in this lower P_{O_2} range. Thus, while a 30 torr fall of P_{O_2} from the normal arterial point is required to unload 1.52 ml O_2/100 ml blood, the same amount of oxygen can be released from the normal resting mixed venous point ($P_{O_2} = 40$ torr and $S_{O_2} = 75$ percent) merely by a 5 torr reduction in P_{O_2}. Likewise, when mixed venous blood reaches the lung, substantial loading of oxygen from the alveolar gas into the blood can occur as the P_{O_2} of pulmonary capillary blood starts to increase.

It is important to recognize that the shape and position of the oxygen dissociation curve can be affected by a variety of factors. For example, increases in blood Pc_{O_2}, hydrogen ion concentration ($[H^+]$), and temperature—such as occur in metabolically active tissues (e.g., exercising skeletal muscle)—cause a rightward shift of the dissociation curve. As a result, less oxygen will be bound to hemoglobin at a particular P_{O_2}. This unloading action is thought to facilitate the delivery of oxygen to sites having increased metabolic oxygen requirements. Conversely, at the lungs, where

blood Pc_{O_2} and $[H^+]$ are lower as a result of carbon dioxide exchange, the oxygen dissociation curve will be shifted to the left; this should enhance the combination of oxygen with hemoglobin at a given P_{O_2}.

An index of the magnitude of such shifts in the oxygen dissociation curve is provided by the P_{50}, or the P_{O_2} at which the blood oxygen saturation is 50 percent. Under standard conditions (pH = 7.4, $Pc_{O_2} = 40$ torr, t = 37C), the P_{50} is normally about 27 torr. A rightward shift of the dissociation curve will result in an increased P_{50}, and a leftward shift in a decrease.

The actions of carbon dioxide and hydrogen ions on the oxygen dissociation curve—referred to collectively as the Bohr effect—are thought to reflect the action of hydrogen ions (in the case of carbon dioxide, these are formed by hydration) combining with basic amino acid residues on the hemoglobin polypeptide chains. This, in turn, influences the affinity of the hemoglobin subunits for oxygen.

The blood levels of 2,3-diphosphoglycerate (2,3-DPG)—an end product of red cell glycolysis—also may affect the position of the oxygen dissociation curve. An end product of red blood cell glycolysis, 2,3-DPG levels are increased during conditions of chronic hypoxemia. A raised 2,3-DPG concentration has been shown to shift the oxygen dissociation curve to the right (i.e., increasing the P_{50}); the reduced affinity of hemoglobin for oxygen is thought to improve tissue oxygen delivery in the face of hypoxemic conditions. Therefore, in a clinical context, it is crucial to recognize that blood which has been stored for some time in a blood bank has a low 2,3-DPG concentration and thus a relatively high affinity for oxygen. The transfusion of such blood could be expected to initially impair oxygen delivery to vital organs; within about 4 hours, however, the 2,3-DPG concentration of transfused blood has typically returned to normal (Valeri, 1975).

Other factors influence hemoglobin-oxygen binding through effects on the shape of the oxygen dissociation curve. Carbon monoxide (CO), for example, resembles oxygen in being able to combine reversibly at the heme groups of the hemoglobin molecule. Thus, oxygen and carbon monoxide compete for available binding sites; and as the affinity of hemoglobin for carbon monoxide is about 210 times greater than for oxygen, a substantial proportion of the binding sites will be occupied by carbon monoxide at even low levels of Pc_O (as might result from the inhalation of cigarette smoke or automobile exhaust fumes). For example, at a blood Pc_O of 1 torr and a P_{O_2} of 100 torr, hemoglobin is almost completely saturated with carbon monoxide. The influence of carbon monoxide on oxygen delivery is further exacerbated by the oxygen dissociation curve being less sigmoid, which effectively moves the curve to the left. Thus, at a given blood P_{O_2}, less of the bound oxygen (already at a lower than normal level because of the carbon monoxide-hemoglobin combination) will be released from the hemoglobin. Heavy smokers may have about 6 to 8 percent of their hemoglobin bound to carbon monoxide; this is thought to decrease the average tissue P_{O_2} by about 5 torr. This should not have serious consequences in healthy individuals, at least under resting conditions; however, it may well pose a problem with borderline oxygen supply resulting from coronary insufficiency.

Certain drugs including nitrites and sulfonamides oxidize the ferrous ions in hemoglobin to the ferric form, which renders the hemoglobin molecule unable to carry oxygen. This form of hemoglobin is called methemoglobin. Clearly, such drugs represent a potential threat to the maintenance of tissue oxygen delivery at rates compatible with metabolic demands.

Oxygen delivery to the peripheral tissues is dictated by the cardiac output and the arterial oxygen content, and thus may be compromised under conditions in which a reduction in one variable (e.g., cardiac output) is not offset by an increase in the other (oxygen content). It is evident from the preceding discusson that arterial oxygen content will be lowered in the face of a fall of arterial P_{O_2}, a diminished availability of oxygen-binding sites on hemoglobin, and a reduced affinity of hemoglobin for oxygen.

In anemia, for example, arterial oxygen content is low owing to reduced levels of circulating hemoglobin, even though Pa_{O_2} may be normal. Were an anemic individual also to be hypoxemic (i.e., low Pa_{O_2}), arterial oxygen content could fall to levels that would cause tissue P_{O_2} to encroach on the critical levels for sustained aerobic metabolism. Thus, with a Pa_{O_2} of 100 torr but a hemoglobin concentration of only 10 g/100 ml blood, a resting individual would have an arterial oxygen content of 13.35 ml/100 ml blood and—with a normal peripheral oxygen extraction of 5 ml/100 ml blood—a mixed venous oxygen content of 8.35 ml/100 ml blood, which corresponds to a mixed venous and, therefore, tissue P_{O_2} of less than 10 torr. With even mild hypoxia, tissue P_{O_2} would fall even lower (were it not for the increased cardiac output that often is seen in such conditions). This is the primary reason that the canceling of elective surgery should be seriously considered for patients whose hemoglobin concentration is less than 10 g/100 ml blood.

Under hypermetabolic conditions such as exercise, the increased oxygen requirement of the working muscles is normally met by an increase in cardiac output, rather than by an increase in arterial oxygen content. Thus, although ventilation also increases during exercise, it should be emphasized that the arterial blood is normally near full saturation, and thus any further increase in Pa_{O_2} would be of little significance.

The final step in the oxygen cascade involves diffusion of oxygen from capillary blood in the tissues to the surrounding interstitial fluid and ultimately to the mitochondria. Oxygen is consumed within the mitochondria during the oxidation of carbohydrates and fatty acids, producing the high-energy intermediary adenosine triphosphate (ATP).

CARBON DIOXIDE TRANSPORT

Carbon dioxide transport can also be viewed as a "cascade" of steps that resemble those making up the oxygen cascade but which operates in the reverse direction—from tissues to the atmosphere. During aerobic metabolism, carbohydrate and fat are oxidized to yield ATP, together with the end products carbon dioxide and water. For example, a resting individual with an oxygen consumption of 250 ml/min who is metabolizing solely carbohydrate will produce carbon dioxide also at a rate of 250 ml/min (giving a respiratory quotient [RQ] of 1.0); in contrast, the metabolism of fatty acids will result in a carbon dioxide production of about 175 ml/min (i.e., RQ $\simeq$ 0.7). Normally, however, the dietary substrate is a mixture of fat and carbohydrate (RQ $\simeq$ 0.8) which would yield a resting carbon dioxide production of $\simeq$ 200 ml/min.

Under conditions in which aerobic mechanisms cannot satisfy tissue demands for energy production (e.g., skeletal muscle during heavy exercise; the brain during cerebral hypoxemia), anaerobic (i.e., not requiring oxygen) mechanisms of ATP production may come into play; these involve the breakdown of carbohydrate to lactic acid. A significant proportion of the lactic acid so produced is buffered (or neutralized) by sodium bicarbonate in both tissue fluids and blood; this yields carbon dioxide and sodium lactate. Hence, the carbon dioxide produced by metabolism is supplemented by that resulting from the buffering of lactic acid, increasing the demands for the transport of carbon dioxide to—and its subsequent clearance from—the lungs.

Owing to tissue carbon dioxide production, the P_{CO_2} within the peripheral tissues is relatively high and carbon dioxide molecules thus diffuse down a partial pressure gradient to enter the capillary circulation. At rest, this results in a P_{CO_2} of 46 torr in the mixed venous blood returning to the lungs; this value is higher during exercise because of the increased metabolic rate in the working muscles.

The rate of carbon dioxide delivery to the lungs is dictated by the venous return and the carbon dioxide content of mixed venous blood. As is the case for oxygen, carbon dioxide is transported by blood both in physical solution and in chemical combination. The amount of dissolved carbon dioxide is governed by the P_{CO_2} in plasma and by the solubility coefficient for carbon dioxide (0.03 mmol/L/torr), as defined by Henry's law (see above). As carbon dioxide is some 20 times more soluble in plasma than oxygen, a greater proportion is thus transported in this form (i.e., $\simeq$ 5 percent); for example, at a normal Pa_{CO_2} of 40 torr, 1.2 mmol/L of carbon dioxide is carried in physical solution, compared with 1.38 mmol/L in mixed venous blood at rest (P_{CO_2} = 46 torr).

The chemical combination of carbon dioxide in blood is more complex than that of oxygen and involves three different forms: carbonic acid (H_2CO_3), bicarbonate ions (HCO_3^-), and carbamino compounds. Carbonic acid is formed from the hydration of carbon dioxide molecules:

$$CO_2 + H_2O \rightleftharpoons H_2CO_3$$

This reaction takes place slowly in plasma but is catalyzed within the red blood cells by the enzyme carbonic anhydrase. Once formed, carbonic acid dissociates readily into hydrogen ions and bicarbonate ions, and thus only a very small amount of carbon dioxide is transported as carbonic acid:

$$H_2CO_3 \rightleftharpoons H^+ + HCO_3^-$$

The full reaction sequence is given by:

$$CO_2 + H_2O \rightleftharpoons H_2CO_3 \rightleftharpoons H^+ + HCO_3^-$$

The bulk of HCO_3^- formation thus takes place in the red blood cells and proceeds according to the law of mass action with a dissociation constant (K), which equals

$$\frac{[H^+] \times [HCO_3^-]}{[H_2CO_3]}$$

As $[H_2CO_3]$ is proportional to the concentration of dissolved carbon dioxide, the dissociation constant may be redefined as:

$$K' = \frac{[H^+] \times [HCO_3^-]}{[CO_2]_{dissolved}}$$
$$= \frac{[H^+] \times [HCO_3^-]}{\alpha \times P_{CO_2}}$$

where α is the solubility coefficient for carbon dioxide. At a given P_{CO_2}, the extent to which the hydration of carbon dioxide and subsequent dissociation of carbonic acid proceeds is limited by the concentrations of H^+ and HCO_3^- ions; if the means exist to remove one or both of these reaction products, the formation of HCO_3^- can thus continue. For example, newly formed H^+ ions are buffered within the red blood cells largely by imidazole residues of the hemoglobin molecules. In addition, HCO_3^- ions diffuse across the red cell membrane to the plasma, where $[HCO_3^-]$ is lower owing to the slower rate of HCO_3^- formation.

The above equation defining the dissociation constant K' can be reformulated by taking logarithms of both sides,

$$\log K' = \log [H^+] + \log \frac{[HCO_3^-]}{\alpha \times P_{CO_2}}$$

and rearranging:

$$-\log [H^+] = -\log K' + \log \frac{[HCO_3^-]}{\alpha \times P_{CO_2}}$$

Since $-\log [H^+]$ is pH and $-\log K'$ is pK' (equal to 6.1 in plasma), then:

$$pH = pK' + \log \frac{[HCO_3^-]}{\alpha \times P_{CO_2}}$$

This important relationship between pH, P_{CO_2}, and $[HCO_3^-]$ is known as the Henderson-Hasselbalch equation and is widely used in the analysis of primary respiratory and metabolic acid-base disturbances and the secondary consequences of the compensatory mechanisms that they invoke.

To preserve electrical neutrality across the red cell membrane in the face of the efflux of HCO_3^- ions from the red blood cells (RBC), there is a corresponding influx of anions (the cell membrane being largely impermeable to cations) principally in the form of chloride (Cl) ions, according to the Gibbs-Donnan equilibrium:

$$\frac{[HCO_3^-]_{plasma}}{[HCO_3^-]_{RBC}} = \frac{[Cl^-]_{plasma}}{[Cl^-]_{RBC}}$$

This is termed the chloride shift or the Hamburger shift.

These reactions result in approximately 90 percent of the total transported carbon dioxide being in the form of HCO_3^- ions and carried mostly in the plasma (although they are formed largely within the red cells).

The remaining 5 percent of the carbon dioxide is carried as carbamino carbon dioxide in combination with amino (NH_2) groups of the hemoglobin molecules in the red cells, together with an additional small amount in association with plasma proteins. Thus:

$$R = NH_2 + CO_2 \rightleftharpoons R - NH \cdot COO^- + H^+$$

It is possible to construct a carbon dioxide dissociation curve (Fig. 22–8) that is analogous to the oxygen-hemoglobin dissociation curve (Fig. 22–7) which relates the total carbon dioxide content of blood (i.e., physically dissolved and chemically combined forms) to the P_{CO_2}. In contrast to the oxygen dissociation curve, the carbon dioxide dissociation curve is essentially linear over the physiologic range. As a result, the capacity for the blood to load and unload carbon dioxide is reasonably independent of the prevailing P_{CO_2}; i.e., there are no significant changes in the slope of the dissociation curve between, for example, the normal arterial and mixed venous points (c.f., Fig. 22–7).

As is the case for oxygen, the ability of blood to transport carbon dioxide is not merely a function of the P_{CO_2}. The oxygenation status of hemoglobin also exerts an influence: at a given P_{CO_2}, deoxygenated blood can carry more carbon dioxide than can fully oxygenated blood (Fig. 22–8). This is termed the Haldane effect. It reflects the greater H^+-buffering power of the deoxygenated hemoglobin molecule, which thus allows greater HCO_3^- formation, and also the greater availability of amino side chains on hemoglobin for carbamino carbon dioxide formation. The contributions of the various chemically combined forms of carbon dioxide to the total amount of carbon dioxide *transported* in blood at a particular level of oxygenation are thus not the same as those that relate to the total amount of carbon dioxide *exchanged* at the lungs with concomitant loading of oxygen into the blood: 30 percent of the exchanged carbon dioxide comes from carbamino carbon dioxide, 60 percent from HCO_3^- ions, and 10 percent from dissolved carbon dioxide.

As blood flowing through the pulmonary capillary bed changes its composition from mixed venous to arterialized, the oxygenation of hemoglobin encourages the unloading of carbon dioxide. Conversely, as discussed in the preceding section, the unloading of carbon dioxide (causing a lowering of blood P_{CO_2} and $[H^+]$ to their arterial values) encourages the loading of oxygen onto hemoglobin. Hence, the trans-

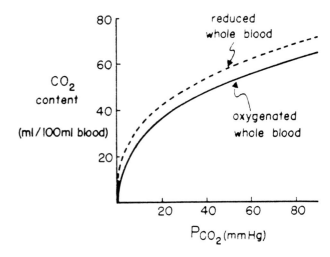

Figure 22–8. Carbon dioxide dissociation curve, expressing carbon dioxide content as a function of P_{CO_2} for oxygenated (—) and deoxygenated (- - - - -) blood. (*From Whipp, 1982. Courtesy of Year Book Med Pub.*)

port of oxygen and carbon dioxide in blood are mutually dependent.

Within the pulmonary capillary bed, the initial driving pressure for the diffusion of carbon dioxide molecules from blood to alveolar gas is provided by the difference between mixed venous and arterial P_{CO_2} (i.e., 46 and 40 torr, respectively, at rest, or 6 torr). Although this P_{CO_2} difference is an order of magnitude smaller than the corresponding P_{O_2} difference (i.e., 40 and 100, respectively, torr at rest, or 60 torr), the diffusion of carbon dioxide is as effective as that of oxygen, owing to its greater solubility in plasma. The bulk flow of gas during expiration subsequently clears carbon dioxide from the respiratory tree, thus completing the final step in the carbon dioxide cascade.

DIFFUSION

The mechanical events that occur during the process of ventilation provide the force that serves to move air into and out of the lungs by bulk flow. However, the movement of oxygen and carbon dioxide molecules within the alveoli and across the alveolar-capillary membrane relies upon diffusion. Diffusion is a passive process that does not involve the expenditure of body energy stores, requiring only a driving pressure or partial pressure difference. Thus, gas molecules will move from an area of high partial pressure to an area that has a lower partial pressure. This movement is a consequence of the gas molecules exhibiting random motion. As molecules will collide more frequently in a region of high concentration than in one of low concentration, the net effect is for molecules to move toward the region of low concentration until there is no longer a concentration difference between the two regions. Clearly, therefore, the rate of diffusion depends on the magnitude of the concentration (or partial pressure) gradient between these regions.

The density of the gas also influences its rate of diffusion. Graham's law states that, for a given partial pressure gradient, a light gas will diffuse more readily through a gaseous medium than will a dense gas, specifically in inverse proportion to the square root of the density. Thus oxygen (molecular weight [MW] 32) is relatively more diffusible than carbon dioxide (MW 44):

$$\frac{\text{rate of } O_2 \text{ diffusion}}{\text{rate of } CO_2 \text{ diffusion}} = \frac{\sqrt{MW\ CO_2}}{\sqrt{MW\ O_2}} = \frac{\sqrt{44}}{\sqrt{32}} = \frac{6.6}{5.6} = 1.18$$

Thus, oxygen diffuses some 18 percent more rapidly than carbon dioxide in alveolar gas.

Relative to the duration of the respiratory cycle, the diffusion of oxygen and carbon dioxide between the alveolar ducts and the alveolar-capillary interface is sufficiently rapid that there are negligible differences in both P_{O_2} and P_{CO_2} within the alveolar gas volume. For example, diffusion of gas in a normal alveolus (diameter approximately 100 μ) is thought to be 80 percent complete in 0.002 seconds if the diffusion distance is 0.5 mm. However, in conditions such as emphysema, where destruction of alveolar walls results in the formation of large air sacs, the distance required for diffusion of gas molecules between the alveolar duct and the gas-exchanging surface may be too great to allow diffusion equilibrium to occur in the time available.

As a result, P_{O_2} and P_{CO_2} gradients will be present within the alveolar gas, leading to inefficient exchange of oxygen and carbon dioxide and thus to arterial hypoxemia and hypercapnia.

In diffusing from alveolar gas to pulmonary capillary blood, oxygen molecules must cross a series of anatomic barriers (and likewise for carbon dioxide, which diffuses in the opposite direction). These include the layer of pulmonary surfactant lining the alveoli, the alveolar epithelium, the interstitial tissue layer that exists between the alveolar and capillary membranes, the capillary endothelial membrane, plasma in the pulmonary capillary, the red blood cell membrane and, finally, the interior of the red blood cell for ultimate binding to the hemoglobin molecule. Despite the number of structures involved, the alveolar capillary membrane is very narrow (normally, about 0.2 μ).

The rate of gas transfer across the alveolar-capillary interface depends on several factors: the diffusion coefficient of the gas, its partial pressure difference across the interface, and the physical dimensions of the interface. Thus, for a gas X, its rate of diffusion is defined as:

$$\dot{V}_X = D_X \cdot \frac{A}{\ell} \cdot \Delta P_X$$

where D_X is the diffusion coefficient of the gas, ΔP_X is the partial pressure difference across the interface, A is the surface area of the interface, and ℓ is the path length for diffusion. Factors that speed the rate of diffusion will lead to a more rapid attainment of diffusion equilibrium across the interface; conversely, factors slowing the rate of diffusion will prolong the time required for equilibrium to occur.

In a liquid medium, such as plasma, an important determinant of the diffusion coefficient (D) is the solubility (α) of the gas in the medium. Defining solubility as the number of molecules of gas that can be dissolved in 1 ml of water at 37C for a gas pressure of 1 atmosphere (or 760 torr), the solubilities for carbon dioxide and oxygen are 0.592 and 0.0244, respectively. Thus, carbon dioxide is approximately 24 times more soluble than oxygen. The other major determinant of the diffusion coefficient is the gas density. Hence, $D_X = \alpha_X / \sqrt{MW_X}$ and therefore:

$$\frac{\text{rate of } CO_2 \text{ diffusion}}{\text{rate of } O_2 \text{ diffusion}} = \frac{\alpha_{CO_2}}{\alpha_{O_2}} \times \frac{\sqrt{MW_{O_2}}}{\sqrt{MW_{CO_2}}}$$
$$= \frac{0.59}{0.024} \times \frac{5.6}{6.6}$$
$$= 20.7$$

In contrast to the alveolar gas phase, carbon dioxide thus diffuses 20 times more rapidly across the alveolar-capillary membrane than does oxygen, for a given partial pressure difference between blood and gas.

The difference between the P_{O_2} of the mixed venous blood (normally about 40 torr at rest) entering the pulmonary capillary bed from the pulmonary artery and the P_{O_2} of alveolar gas (normally 100 torr) provides the initial driving pressure for diffusion of oxygen into the blood; i.e., 60 torr, in this case. As oxygen molecules diffuse into the pulmonary capillary blood, the blood P_{O_2} rises progressively and normally reaches the alveolar value (i.e., 100 torr) within 0.25 to 0.30 seconds (Fig. 22–9). Thus, diffusion equilibrium

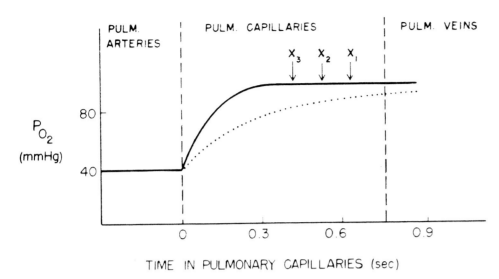

Figure 22–9. Time course of pulmonary capillary P_{O_2} in normal lung (—) and lung with a diffusion impairment (- - - - -). Effect of progressive increases in cardiac output, which reduce pulmonary capillary transit time (to X_1, X_2, and X_3) but do not normally encroach on time required for attainment of diffusion equilibrium. (*From Whipp, 1982. Courtesy of Year Book Med Pub.*)

between alveolar gas and pulmonary capillary blood is established well before the blood reaches the end of the pulmonary capillary bed (at rest, the vascular transit time is normally about 0.8 seconds). Most of the oxygen that enters the pulmonary capillary blood does so at the beginning of the capillary bed, where the difference between P_{O_2} in the gas and blood phases is greatest; this is evident in the rapid rate of blood P_{O_2} increase in the early stages of the gas exchange process (Fig. 22–9). As the capillary P_{O_2} rises and the P_{O_2} difference between gas and blood becomes narrower, the rate of oxygen diffusion slows progressively until—beyond the point of diffusion equilibrium—no more oxygen is taken up (i.e., as the alveolar and pulmonary capillary oxygen pressures are now equal, there is no longer a driving pressure for diffusion).

In the case of carbon dioxide, diffusion equilibrium between the blood and gas phases is normally also attained reasonably rapidly. At rest, the initial driving pressure for exchange, given by the difference between mixed venous P_{CO_2} and alveolar P_{CO_2}, is about 6 torr (i.e., 46 torr minus 40 torr, normally). This is an order of magnitude less than the corresponding driving pressure for oxygen. The small carbon dioxide driving pressure, however, is more than offset by the substantially greater diffusibility of carbon dioxide relative to oxygen. As a result, impairments that influence gaseous diffusion across the alveolar-capillary interface are likely to affect oxygen exchange before carbon dioxide exchange, leading in turn to arterial hypoxemia.

Diffusion equilibrium will be attained sooner in conditions that are associated with more rapid rates of oxygen or carbon dioxide diffusion across the alveolar-capillary interface. In contrast, factors that cause a slowing of oxygen or carbon dioxide diffusion will delay the attainment of diffusion equilibrium; if these effects are sufficiently marked, blood will reach the end of the pulmonary capillary bed before equilibrium can occur; i.e., pulmonary end-capillary P_{O_2} will be less than alveolar P_{O_2}, and pulmonary end-capillary P_{CO_2} will be greater than alveolar P_{CO_2}. Thus, diffusion impairment predisposes to arterial hypoxemia and arterial hypercapnia (or carbon dioxide retention).

With increased metabolic rate (e.g., with exercise, hyperthermia, or administration of hypermetabolic drugs),

the mixed venous P_{O_2} falls and the mixed venous P_{CO_2} rises because of the increased rates of tissue oxygen consumption and carbon dioxide production. This will serve to widen the oxygen and carbon dioxide driving pressures for diffusion across the alveolar-capillary membrane and, in turn, cause more rapid rates of gas exchange. Conversely, when the driving pressure is reduced, the rate of diffusion will be slowed. This can occur in hypoxemic conditions (e.g., at high altitude, with inhalation of hypoxic gas mixtures, and in pulmonary disease states) where, because of the sigmoid shape of the oxygen dissociation curve (Fig. 22–7), a given arteriovenous oxygen content difference (normally 5 vol% at rest) will be associated with a smaller corresponding arteriovenous P_{O_2} difference if the arterial point falls on the lower, steeper portion of the dissociation curve. Thus, the difference between mixed venous and alveolar oxygen pressures will also be smaller.

Alterations in both the surface area of the alveolar-capillary interface and the path length for diffusion between gas and blood phases can affect the rates of oxygen and carbon dioxide diffusion. The surface area for gas exchange can be increased under conditions in which the efficiency of regional gas exchange in the lungs is improved. This may occur on going from rest to exercise in the upright posture, as the increased cardiac output results in a more uniform perfusion of the pulmonary capillary bed (at rest in the upright posture, gravitational influences lead to a pooling of pulmonary capillary blood toward the base of the lung) and therefore a greater homogeneity of the regional alveolar ventilation-to-pulmonary blood flow ($\dot{V}_A/\dot{Q}$). This is discussed at length elsewhere in this chapter. In contrast, pathologic conditions that increase the heterogeneity of the regional $\dot{V}_A$-to-$\dot{Q}$ matching (e.g., COPD) or that lead to a reduction in the number of functioning pulmonary capillaries (e.g., pulmonary vascular occlusive disease) compromise the surface area available for diffusion of oxygen and carbon dioxide between alveolar gas and pulmonary capillary blood.

Several pathologic conditions can lead to an increased path length for diffusion of oxygen and carbon dioxide across the alveolar-capillary interface. For example, in pulmonary alveolar proteinosis, an extrusion of proteinaceous material into the alveolar space occurs, thus limiting the alveolar volume and increasing the diffusion distance across the alveolar-capillary interface. The formation of edema in the lungs has a similar consequence.

It is important to recognize that although factors such as the initial driving pressure for diffusion and the geometry of the alveolar-capillary interface may be normal, diffusion impairment can result under conditions in which the pulmonary capillary transit time is shortened. Modest progressive reductions in transit time (e.g., from X_1 to X_2 to X_3, Fig. 22–9), as might be encountered during exercise at progressively greater work rates, will not affect the P_{O_2} of pulmonary end-capillary blood as long as the transit time does not encroach on the time required for diffusion equilibrium to be attained. Should such encroachment occur, however, the blood P_{O_2} will not have sufficient time to attain the alveolar value, and arterial hypoxemia will ensue. This form of diffusion impairment may occur in response to marked increases in cardiac output (e.g., during severe exercise in highly fit athletes), or under conditions such as pulmonary vascular occlusive disease in which the pulmonary capillary bed is compromised to such a degree that blood at a given cardiac output must traverse the fewer number of competent capillaries in a shorter period of time. More importantly, diffusion impairment may frequently occur in the face of only a modest increase in cardiac output (and therefore a modest decrease of pulmonary capillary transit time) when this is accompanied by a decreased driving pressure for diffusion, a decreased surface area for exchange, or an increased path length for diffusion.

Thus, diffusion impairment is characterized by arterial hypoxemia and a widened alveolar-to-arterial P_{O_2} difference, which reflects the lack of diffusion equilibrium between alveolar gas and pulmonary end-capillary blood.

DEAD SPACE

Simply stated, dead space is that portion of the air in the respiratory tract where no gas exchange takes place. In other words, it is wasted ventilation because it does not add oxygen to the blood nor does it remove carbon dioxide. The total respiratory dead space is called the physiologic dead space, which is the sum of the anatomic dead space and the alveolar dead space.

Anatomic Dead Space

This represents the volume of air contained in the respiratory tree down to the level of the terminal bronchioles which does not exchange oxygen and carbon dioxide with mixed venous blood. The anatomic dead space [V_D(anat)] is normally about 150 ml in a healthy adult.

Various techniques have been used to measure the volume of the anatomic dead space. These include measuring the volume of displacement of a cast (e.g., latex or plastic) made from the respiratory tree of a cadaver. A second approach, often used clinically, is the use of standard predictive tables, which take account of factors such as age, sex, lung volume, and tidal volume; as a "rule of thumb," in adults the volume of the anatomic dead space in milliliters is equal to the body weight in pounds.

A more precise approach is that developed by Fowler, which requires simultaneous monitoring of airflow and the concentration of a gas such as carbon dioxide, nitrogen, or helium throughout an expiration. For example, after a single inspiration of 100 percent oxygen (i.e., a nitrogen-free gas), a characteristic profile of the exhaled [N_2] is normally generated (Fig. 22–10). In an ideal situation, [N_2] would be expected to remain at zero from the onset of expiration until such time as the volume of the anatomic dead space (which contains 100 percent oxygen in this instance) had been exhaled; thereafter, [N_2] would rise abruptly and instantaneously to the appropriate alveolar value (this reflecting the composition of gas in the alveolar volume during the previous breath, influenced by the inhalation of the oxygen and the simultaneous uptake of oxygen by the blood), at which it would remain until the start of the next inspiration. In reality, however, the transition between the dead space and alveolar phases is not instantaneous (although it is reasonably rapid) (Fig. 22–10). This is a result of some alveoli having shorter airways and therefore smaller regional dead spaces than others; alveolar gas from these alveoli will thus start to "contaminate" the dead space gas that is still being exhaled from other regions. Accurate estimation of the anatomic dead space therefore requires inclusion of the dead space contribution to this transitional phase. This is accomplished by superimposing a hypothetical transition between the dead space and alveolar phases that is instantaneous; this transition point corresponds to the exhaled volume at which the areas of regions A and B are exactly equal (Fig. 22–10). In other words, it is assumed

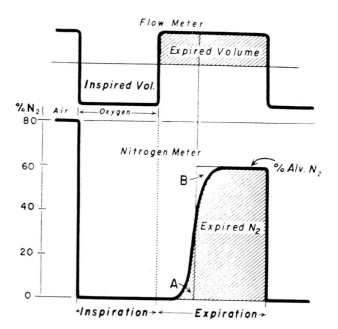

Figure 22–10. Single-breath analysis for measurement of anatomic dead space. Upper panel: idealized airflow profile, which for simplicity indicates a constant flow rate in inspiration and expiration (c.f., Fig. 22–4). Lower panel: corresponding profile of respired nitrogen (N_2) concentration, after a single breath of 100 percent oxygen. See text for further details. (*From Comroe, et al, 1962. Courtesy of Year Book Med Pub.*)

that all the exhaled nitrogen has come from the alveolar compartment, whose exchange characteristics are uniform.

An alternative approach is the carbon dioxide proportion technique pioneered by Bohr. The method assumes that the total amount of carbon dioxide exhaled (V_{CO_2}) in the tidal volume (V_T) yields a mixed expired carbon dioxide fraction ($F\bar{E}_{CO_2}$). Thus,

$$V_{CO_2} = V_T \cdot F\bar{E}_{CO_2}$$

and

$$V_{CO_2} = V_A \cdot F_{A_{CO_2}}$$

where V_A and $F_{A_{CO_2}}$ are the volume and fractional concentration of carbon dioxide for alveolar gas. Therefore,

$$V_T \cdot F\bar{E}_{CO_2} = V_A \cdot F_{A_{CO_2}}$$

Substituting for V_A ($= V_T - V_{D_{(anat)}}$) and rearranging:

$$V_{D_{(anat)}}/V_T = \frac{F_{A_{CO_2}} - F\bar{E}_{CO_2}}{F_{A_{CO_2}}}$$

Then transforming fractional concentration to partial pressure by multiplying by (barometric pressure $-$ 47):

$$V_{D_{(anat)}}/V_T = \frac{P_{A_{CO_2}} - P\bar{E}_{CO_2}}{P_{A_{CO_2}}}$$

The volume of the anatomic dead space is important in determining how effective a particular level of minute (or total) ventilation ($\dot{V}_E$) is in promoting gas exchange. Thus, the volume of inspired air that actually enters the alveolar compartment each breath is given by:

$$V_A = V_T - V_{D_{(anat)}}$$

and the corresponding alveolar ventilation by:

$$V_A \times f = (V_T \times f) - (V_{D_{(anat)}} \times f)$$

or

$$\dot{V}_A = \dot{V}_E - \dot{V}_{D_{(anat)}}$$

when f is the breathing frequency, $\dot{V}_A$ is the alveolar ventilation, and $\dot{V}_{D_{(anat)}}$ is the ventilation of the anatomic dead space.

Thus, in the face of an increase in the antomic dead space, the alveolar ventilation can be preserved (and appropriate levels of oxygen and carbon dioxide exchange therefore maintained) if $\dot{V}_E$ is caused to increase; this can be accomplished by an increase in V_T or f, or both. It is important to recognize that although an increase in the volume of the anatomic dead space can lead to hypoventilation of the alveolar compartment and hence a fall in $P_{A_{O_2}}$ and an increase in $P_{A_{CO_2}}$, this of itself will not impair the gas-exchanging characteristics of the lungs. Any fall in $P_{A_{O_2}}$, for example, is exactly reflected in the arterial P_{O_2}. As a result, arterial hypoxemia would prevail, but the alveolar-to-arterial P_{O_2} difference would not be widened.

A variety of factors can influence the volume of the anatomic dead space. For example, the anatomic dead space is larger at the end of inspiration than at the end of expiration, reflecting the greater traction exerted on the airways by the surrounding lung parenchyma at higher lung volumes. This volume-dependency of the anatomic dead space is of the order of 20ml/L of lung volume. The position of

the head can also influence the anatomic dead space: an increase of as much as 20 percent may occur with hyperextension. A change in posture from sitting to semireclining can cause the anatomic dead space to decrease by some 20 percent; a further decrease of similar magnitude accompanies the adoption of the supine posture.

Intubation leads to a reduction in the anatomic dead space because about half of the volume of the conducting airways is bypassed.

Mechanical or apparatus dead space in an anesthesia circuit can be thought of as an extension of the patient's anatomic dead space. The apparatus dead space is the volume of gas contained primarily in the face mask, endotracheal tube, and connectors up to the Y-piece. The Y-piece is considered the end point of the apparatus dead space because this is the point in an anesthesia circuit where the inhaled and exhaled gases no longer traverse the same pathway. The mechanical dead space and thence the wasted ventilation can be kept to a minimum during anesthesia by not placing extensions between the face mask or endotracheal tube and the Y-piece.

Certain drugs, such as hexamethonium, atropine, and trimetaphan, can induce an increase in the anatomic dead space. This is a consequence of their bronchodilating actions. Conversely, bronchoconstricting agents would be expected to reduce anatomic dead space.

Physiologic Dead Space

Because the physiologic dead space [$V_{D_{(phys)}}$] reflects not only the volume of the anatomic dead space but also that of the alveolar dead space, it typically receives more attention than does the anatomic dead space in the clinical setting. A modification of the Bohr equation (see above) is used to estimate the physiologic dead space; this includes the assumption that the total alveolar volume (V_A) comprises a pure dead space component [$V_{D_{(alv)}}$] and a gas-exchanging component (V_A') with uniform characteristics. Thus:

$$V_{D_{(phys)}} = V_{D_{(anat)}} + V_{D_{(alv)}}$$

and

$$V_T = V_A' + V_{D_{(phys)}}$$

As discussed earlier, the volume of carbon dioxide exhaled is given by:

$$\dot{V}_{CO_2} = V_T \cdot F\bar{E}_{CO_2}$$

and therefore

$$\dot{V}_{CO_2} = V_A' \cdot F_{A'_{CO_2}}$$

where $F_{A'_{CO_2}}$ is the fractional concentration of carbon dioxide in the alveolar gas-exchanging compartment. Thus:

$$V_T \cdot F\bar{E}_{CO_2} = V_A' \cdot F_{A'_{CO_2}}$$

Using a similar development to that presented earlier, the physiologic dead space fraction of the breath is expressed by:

$$V_{D_{(phys)}}/V_T = \frac{P_{A'_{CO_2}} - P\bar{E}_{CO_2}}{P_{A'_{CO_2}}}$$

Making the further assumption that the P_{CO_2} in arterial blood equals $P_{A'CO_2}$:

$$V_{D(phys)}/V_T = \frac{P_{aCO_2} - P_{\bar{E}CO_2}}{P_{aCO_2}}$$

In normal, healthy adults, the alveolar dead space is negligible and therefore the volumes of the physiologic and anatomic dead spaces are similar. At rest, the physiologic dead space represents about 30 percent of the tidal volume. This fraction decreases somewhat under conditions such as exercise, in which an increased cardiac output provides a more even perfusion of the lungs (i.e., reducing or even abolishing "zone 1" in the nondependent regions) and thus reducing the (already low) alveolar dead space volume. A similar effect can be accomplished by adopting the supine posture, which reduces the influence of gravity on the lungs as their vertical height is reduced from some 30 cm to about 20 cm. Hence, perfusion of the nondependent regions of the supine lung does not require such a high pulmonary artery pressure as in the upright lung.

Conversely, conditions such as hemorrhage or atropine administration accentuate the zone 1 characteristics of the lung. This is consequent to a lowering of pulmonary artery pressure, and thus leads to an increase in the volume of the alveolar dead space. In patients with COPD the alveolar dead space is also increased, owing to regions of alveolar ventilation-to-perfusion mismatch, which develop as a result of regional pulmonary tissue destruction and airway obstruction. Pulmonary embolism has a similar effect because of regional obstruction in the pulmonary capillary bed.

General anesthesia leads to an increase in the alveolar dead space; the underlying causes are unclear, however. The alveolar dead space may also be accentuated with artificial ventilation in the lateral decubitus position, in which there is a preferential distribution of ventilation to the nondependent lung (especially when the pleural membranes are opened in thoracotomy) while the pulmonary capillary perfusion is distributed primarily to the dependent lung. Thus, the dependent lung will have a low $\dot{V}_A/\dot{Q}$ ratio whereas the nondependent lung will have a high ratio.

SHUNT

By analogy with dead space, shunt may be regarded as that portion of the cardiac output that does not participate in gas exchange. Likewise, the total shunt may be viewed as the sum of the anatomic and alveolar shunts.

Not all tissues and organs contribute blood to the venous return. A few, such as the larger airways of the respiratory tree and the myocardium, drain instead into the circulation downstream of the pulmonary capillary bed (i.e., after gas exchange has taken place). This component constitutes the anatomic shunt. Normally, such contributions amount to less than 5 percent of the total cardiac output. The addition of this venous blood to the arterialized stream causes a small though significant reduction in P_{O_2} between the end of the pulmonary capillary bed and the systemic arterial circulation (typically, a few torr). The prominence of the anatomic shunt can be increased substantially in clinical conditions characterized by the presence of an intracardiac right-to-left shunt (atrial or ventricular septal defects, for example).

The alveolar shunt represents the fraction of the cardiac output that perfuses the pulmonary capillary bed but is directed to nonventilated alveoli. In the normal individual, the alveolar shunt is negligible. It can, however, assume considerable significance in pulmonary disease states where factors such as airway obstruction can lead to regional collapse (atelectasis).

The magnitude of the shunt can be estimated in a fashion analogous to that used for dead space estimation. It is assumed that the cardiac output ($\dot{Q}t$) is made up of two uniform components: a pure shunt having a mixed venous content ($C\bar{v}_{O_2}$) and a pure alveolar component having a homogeneous composition equal to that of pulmonary end-capillary blood (Cc'_{O_2}). Thus:

$$\dot{Q}t = \dot{Q}s + \dot{Q}alv$$

where $\dot{Q}s$ and $\dot{Q}alv$ represent the flow rates through the shunt and the exchanging portion of the pulmonary capillary bed, respectively. The rate at which oxygen is transported by the cardiac output into the systemic arterial circulation is given by:

$$\dot{Q}_{O_2} = \dot{Q}t \cdot C_{aO_2}$$

where C_{aO_2} is the arterial oxygen content, or

$$\dot{Q}_{O_2} = (\dot{Q}s \cdot C\bar{v}_{O_2}) + (\dot{Q}alv \cdot Cc'_{O_2})$$

where $C\bar{v}_{O_2}$ and Cc'_{O_2} are the oxygen contents in mixed venous and pulmonary end-capillary blood. Thus:

$$\dot{Q}t \cdot C_{aO_2} = (\dot{Q}s \cdot C\bar{v}_{O_2}) + (\dot{Q}alv \cdot Cc'_{O_2})$$

Rearranging this yields the shunt fraction of the cardiac output:

$$\frac{\dot{Q}s}{\dot{Q}t} = \frac{Cc'_{O_2} - C_{aO_2}}{Cc'_{O_2} - C\bar{v}_{O_2}}$$

The arterial and mixed venous oxygen contents can be measured by means of direct blood sampling. An indirect estimate of the Cc'_{O_2} is obtained by assuming that the alveolar P_{O_2} (which can be measured directly or derived from the alveolar air equation as described in the discussion of oxygen transport) equals the P_{O_2} of pulmonary end-capillary blood, and then using a standard oxygen dissociation curve to obtain the corresponding oxygen content.

When pulmonary artery catheterization is not available for the sampling of mixed venous blood, the shunt fraction may be estimated from the iso-shunt diagram of Nunn. The diagram depicts graphically the relationship between arterial P_{O_2} and F_{IO_2} for a series of different shunt fractions (Fig. 22–11). These are presented as iso-shunt bands, which are sufficiently wide to accommodate variations of P_{aCO_2} and hemoglobin concentration in the ranges 25 to 40 torr and 10 to 14 ml O_2/100 ml blood, respectively, assuming the arterial-mixed venous oxygen content difference is 5 ml O_2/100 ml blood; because the arterial-mixed venous oxygen content difference is not measured directly, it is usual to refer to the shunt as the "virtual shunt" in this context.

Hence, from knowledge of a patient's P_{aO_2} and F_{IO_2}, it is possible to (1) predict the magnitude of the shunt

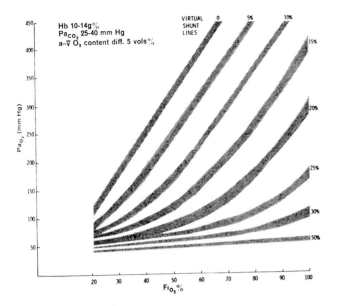

Figure 22–11. Iso-shunt chart which indicates the relationship between arterial Po₂ and inspired O₂ concentration for a range of shunt fractions (0–50%). (*From Benatar SR, Hewlett AM, Nunn JF: The Use of Iso-Shunt Lines for Control of Oxygen Therapy. Br J Anaesth 45:713, 1973.*)

and then (2) predict the level of F_{IO_2} required to achieve a particular arterial oxygen tension. These predictions rely on the assumptions that shunt is the primary gas-exchange defect and that the magnitude of the shunt is independent of Po₂. For example, a patient with a Pao₂ of 170 torr at an F_{IO_2} of 0.5 will have a predicted shunt fraction of 10 percent. This, in turn, predicts that an F_{IO_2} in the region of 0.3 is required to achieve a Pao₂ of 100 torr; it is advisable, of course, to check the accuracy of predictions in a clinical setting by drawing an arterial blood sample. It is crucial to recognize, however, that the iso-shunt technique should not be used under conditions in which the arterial-mixed venous oxygen content difference is likely to change, as would occur with alterations in either the oxygen consumption or the cardiac output.

The degree to which arterial Po₂ is reduced in the presence of a shunt will depend primarily on the size of the shunt. Also important is the location of the pulmonary end-capillary and mixed venous points on the oxygen dissociation curve. For example, assuming that the gas-exchanging portion of the lung is operating effectively, the end-capillary point will be on the upper, flat portion of the curve (e.g., Pc'_{O_2} = 100 torr, Cc'_{O_2} = 20 ml O₂/100 ml blood), whereas the mixed venous point (e.g., $P\bar{v}_{O_2}$ = 40 torr, $C\bar{v}_{O_2}$ = 15 ml O₂/100 ml blood) will lie on the lower, steep portion (Fig. 22–7). Admixture of these bloods will yield "arterialized" blood of an intermediate oxygen content; e.g., for numerical simplicity, with 50 percent of the cardiac output being shunt, the resulting Cao_2 would be the arithmetic mean of Cc'_{O_2} and $C\bar{v}_{O_2}$, or 18 ml O₂/100 ml blood. This arterial point would, of necessity, lie below the end-capillary point on the steeper portion of the dissociation curve, which would accentuate the corresponding fall of Po₂. Thus, the presence of a shunt will cause a lowering of arterial Po₂ relative to the alveolar Po₂ [and thence

a widened (A-a) Po₂ difference], even though pulmonary end-capillary Po₂ may be normal.

VENTILATION-PERFUSION DISTRIBUTION

Considerations of effective pulmonary gas exchange and therefore the provision of a normal arterial Po₂ and Pco₂ should also incorporate the regional distribution of alveolar ventilation to pulmonary capillary perfusion (i.e., $\dot{V}_A/\dot{Q}$) throughout the lungs. Thus, it is not sufficient that the *overall* levels of $\dot{V}_A$ and $\dot{Q}$ are approximately equal (i.e., yielding an overall $\dot{V}_A/\dot{Q} \simeq 1.0$); the regional rates of alveolar ventilation and perfusion should also be well matched.

The consequences of variations in $\dot{V}_A$ and $\dot{Q}$ on Pao₂ and Paco₂ can be illustrated by the following simple example, in which the lung is described as a single uniform compartment. Let us assume that at rest, $\dot{V}_A$ and $\dot{Q}$ both equal 5L/min. This yields a $\dot{V}_A/\dot{Q}$ of 1.0, and normal values for Pao₂ and Paco₂ of 100 torr and 40 torr, respectively.

Now assume that the airway is abruptly and completely obstructed, so that no fresh air enters the alveoli during the subsequent inspiration. The uptake of oxygen into blood and the release of carbon dioxide into the trapped gas of the alveolar compartment will continue by diffusion until the respective oxygen and carbon dioxide driving pressures for diffusion between the gas and blood phases are abolished; i.e., the alveolar Po₂ will fall progressively and the alveolar Pco₂ will rise to eventually attain their respective mixed venous values. Thus, Pao₂ will equal 40 torr and Paco₂ will equal 46 torr. And as $\dot{V}_A$ is now zero, $\dot{V}_A/\dot{Q}$ = 0/5 = 0. This situation corresponds to a total alveolar shunt (see previous discussion).

At the other extreme, we can assume that the pulmonary capillary bed is completely obstructed (e.g., by a pulmonary embolus). Thus, although the alveoli are ventilated normally (i.e., $\dot{V}_A$ = 5L/min), there can be no exchange of oxygen or carbon dioxide with blood. Thus, $\dot{V}_A/\dot{Q}$ = 5/0 = ∞, with the alveolar gas tensions being equal to the inspiratory gas tensions; i.e., Pao₂ = 159 torr and Paco₂ = 0. This condition represents a total alveolar dead space.

Clearly, all possible combinations of $\dot{V}_A/\dot{Q}$ between total shunt ($\dot{V}_A/\dot{Q}$ = ∅) and total dead space ($\dot{V}_A/\dot{Q}$ = ∞) could exist regionally within the lungs. For example, a condition characterized by a lower than normal $\dot{V}_A$ (i.e., hypoventilation) would yield a $\dot{V}_A/\dot{Q}$ of less than 1.0 (but greater than zero) and values for Pao₂ between 100 and 40 torr, and for Paco₂ between 40 and 46 torr. Conversely, with a greater than normal $\dot{V}_A$ (i.e., hyperventilation), $\dot{V}_A/\dot{Q}$ would be greater than 1.0 but less than infinity, Pao₂ would lie between 100 and 159 torr, and Paco₂ would lie between 40 and 0 torr.

As discussed earlier, even the lungs of a normal, healthy individual show evidence of an uneven regional distribution of both alveolar ventilation and perfusion, owing to the influence of gravity. Thus, as shown in Figure 22–12, both $\dot{V}_A$ and $\dot{Q}$ are distributed preferentially to the dependent regions of the lung (i.e., the base in the upright posture). This effect, however, is more striking for $\dot{Q}$ than for $\dot{V}_A$. Thus, while the nondependent regions have a low $\dot{V}_A$ and a low $\dot{Q}$, the $\dot{V}_A/\dot{Q}$ is higher than the average value for the whole lung. These hyperventilated areas therefore

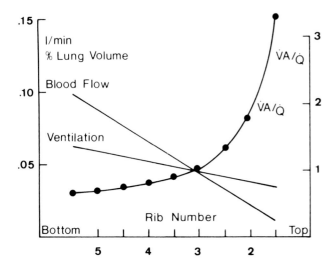

Figure 22–12. Distribution of ventilation, perfusion, and ventilation-perfusion ratios down the lung. (*From West, 1979. Courtesy of Blackwell Scientific.*)

have a P_{O_2} in alveolar gas and pulmonary end-capillary blood that is higher than normal and a corresponding P_{CO_2} that is lower than normal. Conversely, the dependent regions of the lung have higher levels of $\dot{V}_A$ and $\dot{Q}$ relative to the rest of the lung, and therefore a low $\dot{V}/\dot{Q}$. These areas are thus hypoventilated, having a lower than normal P_{O_2} and a higher than normal P_{CO_2} in both alveolar gas and pulmonary end-capillary blood.

The mean alveolar P_{O_2} and P_{CO_2} are determined by the arithmetic mean of their regional partial pressures, weighted by regional volume. (Because regional volume variations are far less prominent than the corresponding perfusion changes in the normal lung, we will assume their influence to be relatively minor in the present context.) Thus, although P_{AO_2} at the base of the lung is low and that at the apex is high (and conversely for P_{ACO_2}), admixture of alveolar gas from these different regions of the lung will normally yield typical average values of about 100 torr for P_{AO_2} and 40 torr for P_{ACO_2}.

In the average arterial gas tensions, the situation is complicated by the more marked differences in regional perfusion and, in the case of oxygen, the sigmoid character of the oxygen dissociation curve (Fig. 22–7). Thus, the composition of the arterial blood will be biased in favor of the relatively highly perfused dependent regions; i.e., with a relatively high carbon dioxide content and a low oxygen content, which, in turn, yields an arterial P_{CO_2} that is slightly higher than the average P_{ACO_2}, and an arterial P_{O_2} that is somewhat less than the average P_{AO_2}. This effect is exacerbated for oxygen where the arterialized (i.e., end-capillary) blood from the hyperventilated nondependent regions will lie on the upper, flat portion of the oxygen dissociation curve whereas that from the dependent regions will lie on the lower, steeper portion. The arterial oxygen content resulting from their admixture will thus yield a P_{O_2} that is biased toward the lower, basal value (i.e., the average arterial point, of necessity, also will lie on a steeper portion of the dissociation curve).

In cardiorespiratory disease states, the degree of re-

gional maldistribution for $\dot{V}_A$ and $\dot{Q}$ can be quite striking, leading to wide regional variations in $\dot{V}_A/\dot{Q}$. This is characteristic, for example, of COPD and pulmonary vascular occlusive disease. This situation can result in extreme degrees of arterial hypoexmia, together with a substantial widening of the alveolar-to-arterial P_{O_2} difference.

HYPOXIA

Hypoxia represents a condition in which the P_{O_2} of a particular region (e.g., inspired air, alveolar gas, arterial blood, peripheral tissues) is below the normal air-breathing value at sea level. Hypoxemia is a special case of hypoxia defined as a decrease in blood P_{O_2} below normal levels. Five categories of hypoxia are conventionally recognized: hypoxic hypoxia, anemic hypoxia, stagnant hypoxia, histotoxic hypoxia, and overutilization hypoxia. We will briefly describe each type and discuss its amenability to oxygen therapy.

Hypoxic Hypoxia

This refers to any condition that leads to a lowering of arterial P_{O_2}. If the lung has normal gas-exchange function, this may result from a deficiency of oxygen in the atmosphere or from alveolar hypoventilation.

Ascent to altitude is characterized by a reduction in the ambient P_{O_2} owing to the lower barometric pressure (even though F_{O_2} is normal). Administration of 100 percent oxygen can be used to restore alveolar and arterial P_{O_2} towards normal levels.

In the clinical setting, there are some obvious causes of a decreased F_{IO_2} related to the administration of anesthesia. For example, F_{IO_2} may be reduced consequent to the diluting effects of anesthetic gases (e.g., nitrous oxide) on the inspirate. Mechanical failures of the oxygen supply system to the anesthesia machine and disturbances in the setting of the oxygen flowmeter can also drastically reduce the F_{IO_2}. Thus, an oxygen supply failure alarm ("fail-safe") system on an anesthesia machine does not guarantee an adequate F_{IO_2} since it senses pressure only: it is not only possible to administer less than 21 percent oxygen with a "fail-safe" system, but it is also possible to deliver gases without any oxygen, provided there is oxygen pressure exerted on the diaphragm of the "fail-safe" valve.

Hypoventilation is another cause of a lowered P_{AO_2}. This can generally be corrected by oxygen inhalation. In the clinical setting, a variety of factors may lead to hypoventilation. For example, the tongue, which relaxes under anesthesia, may fall back on the posterior pharynx and partially or completely occlude airflow. This is easily corrected by hyperextension of the head or by intubation; however, it should be emphasized that intubation does not guarantee a patent airway; the endotracheal tube can become kinked, blocked with secretions, or it may enter a main-stem bronchus when the patient's position is changed. (Auscultation of the patient's chest to determine equal bilateral breath sounds is thus mandatory whenever there is a position change under anesthesia.) Foreign material like blood and vomitus may also obstruct the airway, and must therefore be removed immediately by suctioning the pharynx. Laryngospasm is another cause of hypoventilation. General central nervous system depressant drugs, such as barbiturates, narcotics, and volatile anesthetics typically exert a depressant action on overall ventilation and therefore on alveolar ventilation; under such conditions, assisted ventilation is mandatory to prevent hypercapnia and hypoxia. Likewise, assisted ventilation should be standard practice whenever a neuromuscular blocking drug is used during anesthesia. In the context of anesthesia, diffusion hypoxia is a distinct possibility during the first 5 to 10 minutes of emergence from nitrous oxide anesthesia. This is caused by the rapid outward diffusion of nitrous oxide from pulmonary capillary blood which leads to a lowering of the P_{AO_2}; it can be prevented by administering 100 percent oxygen for at least 5 minutes after nitrous oxide has been discontinued.

Diffusion impairment, right-to-left shunt, and $\dot{V}_A/\dot{Q}$ mismatch all resemble alveolar hypoventilation in causing arterial hypoxemia. In addition, however, the alveolar-to-arterial P_{O_2} difference is also widened. Thus, the magnitude of the alveolar-to-arterial oxygen difference serves as an important practical index of gas exchange function. It is important to recognize that the alveolar-to-arterial oxygen difference normally increases with age in healthy individuals; e.g., it is 5 to 6 torr in the range 20 to 30 years, approximately 10 torr for 40 to 50 years, and 15 to 20 torr in excess of 60 years.

In the case of a diffusion impairment, inhalation of oxygen can correct the hypoxemia by increasing the P_{AO_2} substantially and thus widening the initial driving pressure for diffusion from the gas phase to the blood phase. This, in turn, speeds the rate of oxygen diffusion, so that the P_{O_2} in pulmonary capillary blood rises more rapidly. Likewise, the arterial hypoxemia that results from regional mismatching of $\dot{V}_A$ and $\dot{Q}$ can also be reduced (though not abolished) by oxygen inhalation. This reflects a far more rapid rate of delivery of individual oxygen molecules to the poorly ventilated regions (i.e., with a low $\dot{V}_A/\dot{Q}$).

In contrast, however, oxygen administration cannot increase P_{aO_2} in the presence of a true shunt. Indeed, this observation provides firm evidence that a shunt is present. On occasion, the magnitude of a shunt may actually be increased in the face of sustained oxygen-breathing, thus causing further widening of the alveolar-to-arterial P_{O_2} difference. This is the consequence of absorption atelectasis, a condition in which oxygen molecules are absorbed by pulmonary capillary blood at a greater rate than they can be delivered to the alveoli from the inspirate; it is often encountered in COPD. Thus, alveolar collapse results and the magnitude of the alveolar shunt is increased.

Anemic Hypoxia

Anemic hypoxia is caused by a decrease in the levels of circulating hemoglobin available for oxygen combination. This may occur either because there is an insufficient amount of hemoglobin or there is an inability of the hemoglobin to actually transport oxygen. Anemia is the most frequent cause of this type of hypoxia and may result from hemorrhage, hemolysis, or decreased formation of red cells. Although the anemic patient may be treated by means of oxygen inhalation, it is preferable to address the causes of the anemia itself.

Various agents interfere with the reversible binding of oxygen to hemoglobin. For example, prilocaine (Citanest), a local anesthetic, may oxidize the ferrous porphyrin complex of hemoglobin to produce methemoglobin, which is not able to combine with oxygen. Other drugs causing methemoglobinemia include nitrites, chloroquine, primaquine, and diaminodiphenylsulfone. Ralston and Shnider (1978) describe the use of intravenous administration of methylene blue (e.g., 1 to 5 mg/kg) as an effective antidote for methemoglobinemia. The combination of carbon monoxide with hemoglobin to form carboxyhemoglobin also interferes with oxygen transport.

Stagnant Hypoxia

Stagnant hypoxia occurs when there is a reduced blood flow to the point at which oxygen cannot reach the sites of tissue metabolism. This type of hypoxia can be generalized (resulting from a decrease in cardiac output) or localized (as a result of partial or complete vascular occlusion within a particular tissue). Typically, the P_{aO_2} is normal, whereas the $P_{\bar{v}O_2}$ is reduced. The most appropriate form of treatment for stagnant hypoxia should relate to the primary cardiovascular impairment; oxygen administration may be of some benefit in some situations, whereas in others it is of little consequence because P_{aO_2} is normal.

Histotoxic Hypoxia

Histotoxic, or cytotoxic, hypoxia occurs when there is a failure of the cells to utilize oxygen. The classic example occurs with cyanide poisoning. Cyanide chemically combines with cytochrome oxidase in the mitochondria and therefore interferes with oxidative phosphorylation. Because the venous blood does not release oxygen to the tissues in histotoxic hypoxia, the $P_{\bar{v}O_2}$ is almost the same value as the P_{aO_2}. Oxygen therapy is ineffective in this type of hypoxia; appropriate treatment relies on rapid administration of the specific antidote.

Overutilization Hypoxia

Overutilization hypoxia occurs when tissue demands for energy production increase above normal, such that the tissues are not able to extract and use a sufficient amount of oxygen from blood. Conditions associated with an increased oxygen consumption may lead to overutilization hypoxia. Examples include hyperthyroid crisis, shivering, excessive fever, and malignant hyperpyrexia. Again, oxygen therapy can be useful and should be combined with appropriate treatment of the underlying disorder.

CONTROL OF VENTILATION

Internal homeostasis of oxygen, carbon dioxide, and hydrogen-ion levels in the face of varying metabolic demands is maintained by a matching of cellular oxygen consumption and carbon dioxide and hydrogen production to whole-body oxygen uptake and carbon dioxide and hydrogen-ion elimination. In human beings, the lungs represent the major, if not exclusive, site at which whole-body oxygen and carbon dioxide exchange occurs. The elimination of hydrogen-ions is subserved chronically by the renal system; however, acute metabolic acidosis or alkalosis can be corrected (partially, at least) by appropriate ventilatory compensation.

Accordingly, the primary function of the ventilatory control system is to preserve the oxygen, carbon dioxide, and hydrogen-ion homeostasis of arterial blood and cerebral fluids. This is effected by ventilatory chemoreflexes that emanate from the ventral medullary surface and from the carotid bodies. A second important element of ventilatory control is thought to involve selection of an appropriate tidal volume-breathing frequency combination. Ventilatory mechanoreflexes originating from the lungs and the airways are particularly important in this respect.

Spontaneous ventilation is produced by the rhythmic discharge of the motor neurons that innervate the respiratory muscles. The muscles of respiration do not have the property of inherent rhythmicity that the heart muscle does but rather are dependent on their nerve supply to bring about contraction. The periodic nature of inspiration and expiration is initiated and controlled by diffuse collections of neurons located in the medulla and pons, whose functions appear to be closely integrated. These regions receive neural and chemical inputs from sensing elements placed strategically in the body and also from higher centers such as the hypothalamus, the limbic system, and the cerebral cortex. Considerable capability normally exists for influencing breathing volitionally (or consciously), even to the extent of overriding the more fundamental control processes. This is demonstrated by activities such as breath holding while swimming underwater and by speaking. Furthermore, the maximal level of ventilation that a normal individual can generate volitionally typically exceeds the highest level observed during the severest exercise. Also, on emerging from general anesthesia, patients are often able to breathe quite forcefully in response to instruction, even though the Pa_{CO_2} may be very low (and therefore presumably restraining the activity of the central and peripheral chemoreceptors).

Brainstem Mechanisms

Considerable insight into the role of the brainstem in the control of breathing has derived from studies employing sequential brainstem transections in anesthetized animals (Fig. 22–13). If the brainstem is sectioned at the junction of the pons and the midbrain, there is no effect on breathing pattern. In contrast, transection at the junction of the pons and medulla is associated with a pattern of breathing that, although rhythmic, is less smooth in the transition between inspiration and expiration (and vice versa) and is also more rapid. All breathing movements are completely abolished with transection at the junction of the medulla and the spinal cord. On the basis of these observations, it was concluded that the medulla was responsible for the generation of respiratory rhythmicity, with the pons exerting a modulating influence. Further insight into the involvement of the pons was indicated by means of a midpontine transection which, when coupled with bilateral cervical vagotomy, caused a sustained inspiratory effort (also termed apneusis); with the vagi intact, however, the transection resulted in

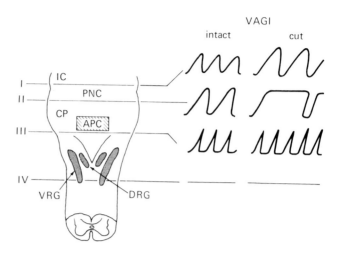

Figure 22–13. Effects of transections at various brainstem levels. APC = apneustic center; CP = cerebellar peduncle; DRG = dorsal respiratory group; IC = inferior colliculus; PNC = pneumotoxic center; VRG = ventral respiratory group. (*From Berger, Mitchell, et al. Reprinted by permission of N Engl J Med 297:140, 1977.*)

a slower rhythmic pattern of breathing characterized by a longer-than-normal inspiratory duration (i.e., apneustic breathing). Thus, the fundamental rhythmogenic mechanisms of the medulla appear to be subject to a strong inspiratory drive from the caudal pons; the periodic interruption of this drive by either rostral pontine or vagal afferent influences ensures that breathing retains its rhythmic character.

More recent techniques involving the identification and mapping of respiratory-related cells within the brainstem have provided a more precise picture of the neuronal basis for the generation and modulation of respiratory rhythm. The medulla contains both inspiratory and expiratory neurons, which are located in the reticular formation beneath the floor of the fourth ventricle. It is thought that the rhythmic discharges of these neurons produce the rhythmic pattern of breathing. These neurons are not located in discrete areas but rather are anatomically intermingled. However, two dense bilateral concentrations of respiratory neurons have now been identified in the medulla: the dorsal respiratory group (DRG) and the ventral respiratory group (VRG) (Fig. 22–14).

The DRG is located in the nucleus of the tractus solitarius. It is composed primarily of inspiratory cells, which project to the spinal cord and stimulate the contralateral phrenic neurons to initiate contraction of the diaphragm. DRG cells also project to the VRG and the pons. The DRG receives afferent projections from sources such as the glossopharyngeal and vagus nerves. It is thought that the DRG plays a primary role in respiratory motor control and respiratory phase switching and may be the site of medullary respiratory rhythmogenesis.

The VRG is located in the nucleus ambiguus and the nucleus retroambigualis. It is composed of both inspiratory and expiratory neurons, which project to phrenic, intercostal, and abdominal motoneurons. The VRG has two divisions, the cranial division and the caudal division. The cranial division, composed of neurons in the nucleus ambiguus, primarily innervates the laryngeal musculature by way

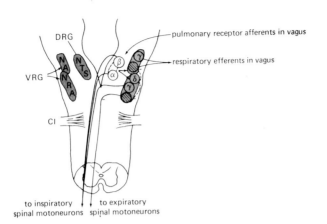

Figure 22-14. Schematic representation of medullary respiratory groups. C1 = first cervical dorsal root; DRG = dorsal respiratory group; NA = nucleus ambiguus; NRA = nucleus retroambigualis; NTS = nucleus tractus solitarius; VRG = ventral respiratory group. (*From Berger, Mitchell, et al. Reprinted by permission of N Engl J Med 297:140, 1977.*)

of the recurrent laryngeal nerves. The caudal division, composed of neurons in the nucleus retroambigualis, has various projections: to the contralateral nucleus retroambigualis and to spinal respiratory motoneurons, for example. The VRG is thought to be the final integrating site for respiratory-related activity in the brainstem.

Two pontine areas are recognized in the context of brainstem respiratory control: the apneustic center and the pneumotaxic center. The apneustic center is located in the caudal pons and is thought to be responsible for the generation of the sustained inspiratory activity that leads to apneusis. This activity of the apneustic center appears to be restrained by activity from the more rostral pneumotaxic center and from the vagus nerves. Thus, the apneustic center appears to represent an important integrating site for mechanisms involved in inspiratory termination.

The pneumotaxic center is located in the rostral pons within the nucleus parabrachialis medialis. Consistent with the pneumotaxic center's postulated role as a modulator of respiratory rhythm, electrical stimulation of its dorsal region can hasten the onset of inspiration, whereas stimulation in the ventral region hastens expiration.

Modulation of Brainstem Mechanisms

A variety of regions are able to influence the level and pattern of ventilation. As mentioned earlier, these include higher centers of the central nervous system as well as reflex inputs. Their precise contribution to ventilatory control will vary with the prevailing conditions; here, we concentrate on those mechanisms thought to be important in maintaining respiration at rest.

Central Chemoreceptors. These are located superficially on the ventral medullary surface within bilateral rostral and caudal regions. They are thought to be stimulated by increases in the P_{CO_2} or [H+] of the local extracellular fluid; it is the hydrogen ion, however, that is thought to represent

the primary stimulus to the receptor, with the carbon dioxide molecule exerting its effect via its hydration to H+ and HCO_3^-. Because carbon dioxide molecules can diffuse freely between cerebral extracellular fluids and cerebral capillary blood (by way of the blood-brain barrier), the central chemoreceptors are also responsive to increases in arterial P_{CO_2}. However, as the blood-brain barrier is relatively impermeable to hydrogen ions, the central chemoreceptors are unable to respond to metabolically induced alterations in arterial pH. It is important to point out that the central chemoreceptors are anatomically and functionally distinct from the medullary respiratory centers; the latter are located more deeply within the medullary tissue and have no chemosensory properties.

The primary reflex consequence of central chemoreceptor stimulation is hyperpnea.

Carotid Body Chemoreceptors. The carotid bodies are paired structures located at the bifurcation of the common carotid arteries. Chemoreceptors contained within the carotid bodies project to the brainstem respiratory centers by way of the carotid sinus nerve (nerve of Hering), a branch of the glossopharyngeal nerve (IXth cranial nerve). Analogous chemosensory structures, the aortic bodies, are located in the region of the aortic arch and innervated by the vagus nerve; however, their primary reflex function in humans involves cardiovascular rather than ventilatory control.

The carotid receptors are responsive to increases of arterial P_{CO_2} and [H+] and to decreases of arterial P_{O_2}. (As for the central chemoreceptors, the stimulatory action of the carbon dioxide molecule is thought to be exerted via the hydrogen ion formed in its hydration.) Furthermore, the presence of arterial hypoxemia normally potentiates the carotid chemoreceptor responsiveness, resulting in a larger increase in discharge frequency for a given increment in Pa_{CO_2} or [H+].

The reflex action of the carotid chemoreceptors is primarily to increase ventilation. In humans, the carotid bodies appear less important than the central chemoreceptors in establishing resting levels of ventilation. However, the integrity of the carotid bodies is essential if a compensatory hyperpnea is to accompany either arterial hypoxemia or arterial metabolic acidosis.

Pulmonary Mechanoreceptors. Three major categories of vagally innervated pulmonary mechanoreceptor are recognized with regard to the control of ventilation and, in particular, its pattern. These are the pulmonary stretch receptor, the irritant receptor, and the J-receptor.

Stretch Receptors. These are located in the smooth muscle of the airways and are stimulated by lung inflation. Their major reflex action is to inhibit inspiration, an effect that is known as the Hering-Breuer inflation reflex. Thus, as the lungs inflate with inspiration, these receptors are activated to terminate inspiration (they may also bring about bronchodilation, tachycardia, and vasoconstriction). There is some controversy concerning the significance of this reflex during eupnea in humans, because the strength of the reflex is weak in the tidal range. However, it may assume greater importance at the higher tidal volumes characteristic of stimulated breathing. The role of the inflation reflex may thus be to prevent overinflation of the lungs. It is believed that halothane sensitizes these receptors, thus bringing about an earlier termination of inspiration and therefore an increased breathing frequency.

Irritant Receptors. These are so called because they are stimulated by inhaled dust, smoke, cold air, histamine, and irritant gases (including diethyl ether, but not halothane). They may also be stimulated by mechanical influences, including rapid changes in lung volume. These receptors are located in the airway epithelium, particularly of the larger airways; they exhibit rapidly adapting discharge characteristics. The reflex consequences of irritant receptor stimulation range from cough, bronchoconstriction, and laryngeal constriction to hyperpnea. It has been argued that they are involved in the Hering-Breuer deflation reflex (whereby a decrease in lung volume may evoke hyperpnea) and Head's paradoxical reflex (whereby lung inflation prolongs an inspiratory effort, rather than terminating it).

J-receptors. Juxtapulmonary-capillary receptors, so called because of their location within the alveolar-capillary interstitial space, are stimulated by pulmonary congestion and pulmonary edema, likely through an increase in the interstitial fluid volume. Their reflex actions include tachypnea, hypotension, and bradycardia. The J-receptors are not thought to contribute significantly to the normal control of breathing.

Ventilatory Response to Carbon Dioxide

Carbon dioxide is a potent stimulus to ventilation. The carbon dioxide responsiveness of the ventilatory control system can be assessed by means of a carbon dioxide-inhalation procedure, in which, for example, an individual inhales a series of gas mixtures, each having a different $F_{I_{CO_2}}$, until a steady state is reached. The ensuing relationship between ventilation ($\dot{V}_E$) and arterial P_{CO_2} is linear over a substantial range of hypercapnia (though at arterial carbon dioxide pressures in excess of about 60 to 70 torr, the response may start to plateau because of a depressant effect of severe hypercapnia on neural function) (Fig. 22–15). The slope of this relationship, $\Delta\dot{V}_E/\Delta P_{a_{CO_2}}$, represents the ventilatory carbon dioxide-responsiveness. A normal value for a healthy, normoxic individual (i.e., $P_{a_{O_2}} \sim 90$ to 100 torr) is about 3 L/min/torr; this has been reported to be lower in older people.

However, the value of the carbon dioxide-responsiveness depends crucially on the background level of arterial P_{O_2}, recalling that hypoxia serves to potentiate (or increase) the carbon dioxide-responsiveness of the carotid body chemoreceptors. Thus, Figure 22–15 indicates that the slope of the ventilatory response to inhaled carbon dioxide is least during hyperoxia and greatest during hypoxia. This hypoxia-induced potentiation of ventilatory carbon dioxide-responsiveness is, therefore, generally ascribed to the carotid body chemoreceptors. Furthermore, in humans, hyperoxia (when sufficiently extreme) is thought to actually silence the carotid body chemoreceptors, so that they no

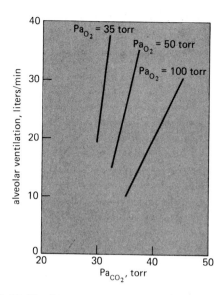

Figure 22–15. Ventilatory response to arterial P_{CO_2} at various levels of arterial P_{O_2}. (*From Levitsky, 1986. Courtesy of McGraw-Hill.*)

longer respond to the imposed carbon dioxide stimulus; the ventilatory carbon dioxide-responsiveness is then thought to represent solely that of the central chemoreceptors.

In the context of carbon dioxide-responsiveness, there are some points that should be borne in mind in relation to anesthesia. A variety of drugs and anesthetics result in hypoventilation (i.e., $P_{a_{CO_2}}$ is increased, while $P_{a_{O_2}}$ is reduced). Furthermore, the $\dot{V}_E$-$P_{a_{CO_2}}$ relationship is typically less steep and is shifted to the right: $\dot{V}_E$ does not increase as much as normal in response to a given increase in $P_{a_{CO_2}}$.

A second issue is related to the possibility that apnea may occur if a patient has a very low $P_{a_{CO_2}}$ consequent to a period of marked hyperventilation. It is thus important to ensure that prior to removing a patient from a ventilator, the level of ventilation is appropriate to maintain a reasonably normal $P_{a_{CO_2}}$; in this way, the patient's spontaneous level of ventilation should be adequate for clearance of the anesthetic agent.

Ventilatory Response to Hypoxia

Inhalation of a hypoxic gas mixture normally causes an increase in ventilation, owing to the fall of $P_{a_{O_2}}$. As was the case for carbon dioxide, it is thus possible to define the $\dot{V}_E$–$P_{a_{O_2}}$ relationship by having an individual breathe a series of gas mixtures, each with a different $F_{I_{O_2}}$, until a steady state is attained. Recognizing that the hypoxia-induced hyperpnea will also cause a fall of $P_{a_{CO_2}}$ and therefore interfere with the full expression of the hypoxic stimulus (i.e., the low $P_{a_{CO_2}}$ will reduce the extent of the potentiation between carbon dioxide and hypoxia at the carotid bodies and also reduce the degree of central chemoreceptor stimulation), it is important to maintain $P_{a_{CO_2}}$ during the hypoxic exposures by adding an appropriate amount of carbon dioxide to the inspirate.

The relationship between $\dot{V}_E$ and $P_{a_{O_2}}$ is typically hyperbolic (Fig. 22–16) and is taken to represent the hypoxic responsiveness of the carotid chemoreceptors: after surgical removal or inactivation of the carotid bodies, the ventilatory response to hypoxia is absent. Three aspects of the $\dot{V}_E$–Pa_{O_2} relationship deserve attention: (1) there is little ventilatory response to decreasing arterial P_{O_2} until a substantial level of hypoxia has been achieved; (2) the hypoxic responsiveness increases progressively as arterial P_{O_2} falls; and (3) the hypoxic responsiveness that obtains over a particular range of arterial P_{O_2} is potentiated (or increased) by arterial hypercapnia (a manifestation of the complex interaction that occurs between carbon dioxide and hypoxia at the carotid chemoreceptors). Thus, in clinical conditions where a patient's carbon dioxide-responsiveness is abnormally low (e.g., COPD), care should be taken when oxygen is administered: if the Pa_{O_2} is raised excessively, the carotid chemoreceptors will be silenced and ventilation would thus fall to very low levels (in the extreme, the patient would become apneic).

NONRESPIRATORY FUNCTIONS OF THE LUNG

Air Conditioning

The extremely vascular mucosal lining of the nose, mouth, and portions of the pharynx serves to warm and moisten the inhaled air so that, by the time it reaches the alveoli, it approximates body temperature and 100 percent relative humidity; only a minor contribution comes from the tracheobronchial tree, however. These mucosal vessels can, in turn, conserve heat and moisture by extracting the air

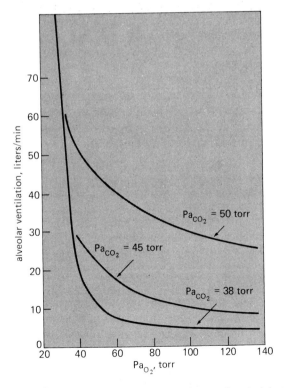

Figure 22–16. Effects on ventilation with changes in arterial oxygen pressures. (*From Levitsky, 1986. Courtesy of McGraw-Hill.*)

as it is exhaled. This process continues to function in the face of wide variations in the temperature and moisture content of the inspirate.

Filtration and Cleansing

A further important function of the upper airway is the filtering of particulate matter from the inhaled air. The first line of defense is provided by the large, stiff hairs within the vestibule just inside each side of the nose, which filter particles larger than about 10 μ in diameter.

Next, as air enters the nasal cavity proper, particulate matter (which tends to travel in a posterior direction) collides with the irregular walls of the nasal cavity (i.e., the turbinates). After colliding, these particles fall to the floor of the cavity and become entrapped in the overlying coat of mucus. This turbulent precipitation is the most effective mechanism for filtering inhaled air, as most particles between 2 and 10 μ in diameter are removed in this fashion. After being precipitated out, these particles are conveyed posteriorly toward the mouth by the systematic flow of the mucous coat, to be either swallowed or expectorated. This mucous layer is mostly water and is secreted by underlying goblet cells in quantities totaling as much as 100 ml per day.

The movement of particulate matter also involves the action of cilia, which extend out of this mucous sheet from ciliated epithelial cells. Excluding the anterior nares, oropharynx, and tracheobroncial tree distal to the terminal bronchioles, cilated epithelium lines the entire respiratory tract.

Cilia are complex, if primitive, hair-like structures that beat in a precise, methodical, wave-like fashion toward the oral cavity. They extend out of a lake of mucus that is critical to their normal functioning. They lash, whip-like, with considerable force and without any known innervation to initiate their movements. Their activity can be depressed, usually reversibly, by factors that include dyeing the overlying mucous layer, anesthesia, surgery, hypoxia, hypercapnia, and drugs (most notably, atropine, which dries the mucous blanket).

Coughing and Sneezing

Another protective function of the upper airway is the cough-sneeze reflex. Each of these reflexes is preceded by a forceful expiration against a closed glottis. After a buildup of pressure behind the glottis, it suddenly opens to permit an explosive expulsion of air, at velocities that approach supersonic.

Smell and Taste

A final nonrespiratory function of the upper airway is the sense of smell; this is also what we perceive as taste. In humans, this special sense is probably more esthetic than protective in character.

Vascular Reservoir

The lung functions as a blood reservoir in conjunction with several others throughout the body (e.g., the large systemic veins). A reservoir is a volume of blood that can be quickly mobilized into the general circulation to meet an immediate need somewhere within the closed vascular system, i.e., to maintain pressure and, it is hoped, perfusion. The potential significance of any particular reservoir is directly related to the volume of blood it contains and to the ease or promptness with which it can be mobilized when needed. A reservoir is obviously not a stagnant pond or lake of blood; rather, it is a dynamic reserve volume where there is constant flow in and out, comparable to a body of water just behind a spillway over a dam.

About one-half of the pulmonary vessels do not function in gas exchange at rest, and thus may be classified as reserve units. This represents about 300 ml that can be immediately furnished to the left ventricle to buffer the occasional transient discrepancy between venous return and cardiac output.

Blood Filtering

Whereas the upper airway filters tidal air, the pulmonary vascular system filters blood. Thus, the lung protects the systemic circulation from various potentially harmful organic and inorganic substances. The capillary is the structure that serves as the filter, and it may be sacrificed in the process. However, the loss of capillaries in this manner is easily compensated for by the tremendous number of reserve units normally available. Moreover, some capillary filters may become patent again after a time.

Substances filtered by the pulmonary capillaries include cancer cells, fibrin clots, fat cells, bone narrow, gas bubbles, crenated red blood cells, platelets, white cells, and other debris in whole blood.

Besides acting as a filter, the lung also protects itself. Phagocytes—including leukocytes and macrophages—can engulf both particulate matter and bacteria that escape the mucociliary boundary that defends the proximal airway.

Metabolic Functions

Considerable metabolic activity goes on within the lung. For example, certain types of alveolar epithelial cells synthesize a complex phospholipid called pulmonary surfactant. When this substance is extruded onto the surface film lining the alveoli, it decreases the surface tension to enhance lung compliance and lessen the inherent tendency of the lungs to collapse. This enables the lung to inflate with greater ease. Moreover, lowering the surface tension aids in keeping the alveoli dry, and so counters the tendency for pulmonary edema formation. As surfactant is synthetized late in intra-uterine life, premature infants (less than about 30 weeks' gestation) may have abnormally high alveolar surface tensions, inordinately low compliance, and therefore an inability to adequately inflate enough alveoli to sustain life; this condition is known as fetal respiratory distress syndrome.

Other substances synthesized within the lung include histamine, serotonin, bradykinins, prostaglandins, proteins, mucopolysaccharides, hydroxytryptamine, and acetylcholine. Many of these are vasoactive: it is postulated, for example, that the release of histamine in response to hypoxemia may be the factor that initiates pulmonary hyp-

oxic vasoconstriction. Finally, enzymes in the lung catalyze the conversion of angiotensin I to angiotensin II.

The significance of the lung's metabolic activity is threefold: (1) apart from considerations of oxygen and carbon dioxide exchange, analysis of arterialized blood within the pulmonary vein cannot be totally depended upon to reflect the chemistry of systemic venous blood; (2) a given drug may exert different effects, depending upon whether it is given intravenously or intra-arterially; and (3) lung disease may disturb more than oxygen and carbon dioxide exchange.

BIBLIOGRAPHY

Berger AJ, Mitchell RA, et al: Regulation of respiration. N Engl J Med 297:92–97, 138–143, 194–201, 1977.

Churchill-Davidson HC: A Practice of Anaesthesia, 5th ed. Chicago, Year Book Med Pub, 1984.

Comroe JH, Jr: Physiology of Respiration, 2nd ed. Chicago, Year Book Med Pub, 1974.

Cunningham DJC: The control system regulating breathing in man. Q Rev Biophys 6:433, 1974.

Fishman AP: Assessment of Pulmonary Function. New York, McGraw-Hill, 1980.

Gilman AG, Goodman LS, et al: The Pharmacological Basis of Therapeutics, 7th ed. New York, Macmillan, 1985.

Harris EA, Kenyon AM, et al: The normal alveolar-arterial oxygen tension gradient in man. Clin Sci Mol Med 46:89–104, 1974.

Hyatt RE, Black LF: The flow-volume curve: A current perspective. Am Rev Respir Dis 107:191, 1973.

Kronenberg RS, Drage CW: Attenuation of the ventilatory and heart rate responses to hypoxia and hypercapnia with aging in normal man. J Clin Invest 52:1812, 1973.

Levitzky MG: Pulmonary Physiology, 2nd ed. New York, McGraw-Hill, 1986.

Loeschcke HH: Central chemosensitivity and the reaction theory. J Physiol (Lond) 332:1–24, 1982.

McDonald DM: Peripheral chemoreceptors: structure-function relationships of the carotid body. In Hornbein TF (ed): Regulation of Breathing. New York, Marcel Dekker, 1981, pp. 105–319.

Macklem PT, Mead J: The physiological basis of common pulmonary function tests. Arch Environ Health 14:5, 1967.

Martin JT: Positioning in Anesthesia and Surgery. Philadelphia, Saunders, 1978.

Mitchell RA, Berger AJ: Neural regulation of respiration. Am Rev Respir Dis 111:206, 1975.

Newsom Davis J: Control of the muscles of breathing. In Widdicombe JG (ed): Respiratory Physiology, M.T.P. International Review of Science—Physiology Series. Baltimore, University Park Press, 1974, Vol. 2.

Nunn JF: Applied Respiratory Physiology, 2nd ed. London, Butterworth, 1977.

Otis AB: Quantitative relationships in steady-state gas exchange. In Fenn WO, Rahn H (eds): Handbook of Physiology. Washington, D.C., American Physiological Society, 1964.

Otis AB: The work of breathing. In Fenn WO, Rahn H (eds): Handbook of Physiology. Washington, D.C., American Physiological Society, 1964.

Paintal AS: Vagal sensory receptors and their reflex effects. Physiol Rev 53:159–227, 1973.

Rahn H, Farhi LW: Ventilation perfusion and gas exchange—the $\dot{V}_A/\dot{Q}$ concept. In Fenn WO, Rahn H (eds): Handbook of Physiology. Washington, D.C., American Physiological Society, 1964.

Ralston DM, Shnider SM: The fetal and neonatal effects of regional anesthesia in obstetrics. Anesthesiology 48:34–64, 1978.

Rehder K: Anesthesia and the respiratory system. Can Anaesth Soc J 26:451–462, 1979.

Rossier PH, Buhlmann A: The respiratory dead space. Physiol Rev. 35:860, 1955.

St. John WM: Central nervous system regulation of ventilation. In Davies DG, Barnes CD (eds): Regulation of Ventilation and Gas Exchange. New York, Academic Press, 1978.

Torrance RW: Prolegomena. In Torrance RW (ed): Arterial Chemoreceptors. Oxford, Blackwell Scientific, 1968.

Valeri CR: Blood components in the treatment of acute blood loss: use of freeze-preserved red cells, platelets, and plasma proteins. Anesth Analg 54:1–14, 1975.

West JB: Pulmonary Pathophysiology: The Essentials. Oxford, Blackwell Scientific, 1977a.

West JB: Ventilation/Blood Flow and Gas Exchange. Oxford, Blackwell Scientific, 1977b.

West JB: Respiratory Physiology: The Essentials, 2nd ed. Baltimore, Williams & Wilkins, 1979.

Whipp BJ: The respiratory system. In Ross G, (ed): Essentials of Human Physiology. Chicago, Year Book Med Pub, 1982, pp. 287–357.

Whipp BJ, Ward SA, et al: Reflex control of ventilation by peripheral arterial chemoreceptors in man. In Acker H, O'Regan RG (eds): Physiology of the Peripheral Arterial Chemoreceptors. Amsterdam, Elsevier. 1983, pp. 299–324.

Widdicombe JG: Reflex control of breathing. In Widdicombe JG (ed.): Respiratory Physiology, M.T.P. International Review of Science—Physiology Series. Baltimore, University Park Press, 1974, Vol. 2.

23

Endocrinology and Anesthesia for Endocrine Diseases

Bruce Skolnick

Most students reading this book would quickly associate the name Ernest Starling with a law describing the response of the heart to the blood filling it. However, Starling also made a very important contribution concerning what fills the blood, for he was the first person to use the term **hormone** to designate a chemical messenger that is secreted by a gland into the bloodstream and carried to a distant organ, where it influences the function of that organ. The word **hormone** is derived from a Greek term meaning "to stir up." Although too much or too little of a given hormone stirs up trouble in the body, the authors hope that the amount of information in this chapter devoted to hormones and anesthesia will be just the right amount to "stir up" the interest of the students reading it.

The study of hormones and the glands that secrete them is known as endocrinology. Endocrine glands are distinct from exocrine glands, because their chemical products pass into the bloodstream rather than into ducts, as do the secretions of the exocrine glands. However, the point should not be missed that some glands, such as the pancreas, are properly considered to be both endocrine and exocrine in function. Insulin and glucagon, the most important of the pancreatic hormones, are secreted by the islets of Langerhans into the portal venous blood. The acinar cells of the pancreas, the exocrine portion, secrete bicarbonate and digestive enzymes into the pancreatic duct.

Despite the fact that the individual endocrine glands are scattered over numerous locations, they collectively are considered to be a single system. This is because it is the rule rather than the exception that, if a given physiologic function is controlled by one endocrine gland, it is almost always also controlled by at least one other gland. An example would be endocrine regulation of blood pressure, which is directly or indirectly influenced by the pituitary, the hypothalamus, the kidney, and the thyroid. Other physiologic functions that are of importance to the anesthetist and that are controlled by multiple endocrine glands include temperature regulation, metabolism, and the blood concentrations of glucose, calcium, sodium, and potassium.

This chapter will be divided into two portions. The first will deal with certain topics common to the understanding of the endocrine system in general. The second portion will be devoted to a more thorough discussion of those endocrine glands that are the most important to the anesthetist.

CHEMICAL CLASSIFICATION OF HORMONES

Hormones can be grouped into three main categories according to their chemical composition:

1. Proteins or polypeptides
2. Amino acids or amino acid derivatives
3. Steroids

Proteins and Polypeptides

Most of the hormones in the body are composed of proteins or polypeptides. A peptide bond is a special junction formed between two amino acids, and when several amino acids are joined together by such bonds, the resulting molecule is called a polypeptide. Most biochemists restrict the use of the term *polypeptide* to chains of only a few amino acids, leaving the designation *protein* to refer to much longer chains of amino acids. However, the two terms are often used to refer to the same molecule. In this chapter, *polypeptide* refers to hormones of ten amino acids or less whereas *protein* refers to larger hormones.

About 20 different amino acids are used in the synthesis of the protein hormones in the body. Each such hormone has a unique sequence of these amino acids, and it is in part this uniqueness that allows hormones made of the same building blocks to influence different physiologic parameters. Some protein hormones share similar sequences of amino acids in a portion of their molecules, and the result is that under certain circumstances they may cause similar responses. A good example would be the pituitary hormones adrenocorticotropic hormone (ACTH) and melanocyte-stimulating hormone (MSH), both of which share an identical sequence of seven amino acids and when secreted in excess can cause pigmentation of the skin.

The same hormone in different species often has slight differences in the amino acid sequence. These differences become important when hormone deficiencies are treated by replacement therapy with the hormone from another species. A difference of only a single amino acid can lead to an immune response against the exogenous hormone, particularly if extended treatment is necessary, as in insulin replacement in diabetics. Because the chemical synthesis of a large protein is at present both costly and time-consuming, the solution to the problem of immune response lies in the tremendous advances that have been made in genetic engineering. It has now become possible to produce in the laboratory strains of microorganisms that will synthesize large protein hormones with the identical amino acid sequence found in humans. Human insulin produced by bacteria has been the first such hormone to become commercially available, but other such products are certain to follow. The easy availability of more hormones will make the treatment of endocrine disorders infinitely easier.

Chemical synthesis of a hormone with an altered amino acid sequence is sometimes used to provide an inhibitor of an endogenous hormone. The idea is that the resulting hormone resembles the natural hormone closely enough so that it can competitively bind to the receptor sites on the target organ, preventing attachment of the normal hormone. If the altered molecule has been prepared properly, it is possible for it to bind to the receptor sites without stimulating the target organ cells. Such inhibitors have been prepared for blocking angiotensin II receptors and may become available for other hormone systems in the future.

Amino Acids or Amino Acid Derivatives

Although there are only a few hormones classified as amino acids or amino acid derivatives, some are of utmost importance to the anesthetist. These hormones include thyroid hormone and the adrenal catecholamines epinephrine and norepinephrine. Because of the small size of these hormones, it has been relatively easy to prepare blockers for some of them, particularly for the catecholamines. Similarly, it has been possible to prepare physiologically active analogues of these hormones. In some cases, it has been possible to prepare analogues that have only a selected number of the normal physiologic effects of the original hormone. An example of this would be the compound phenylephrine, which stimulates α-adrenergic receptors but has little effect on β-adrenergic receptors.

Steroid Hormones

The steroid hormones are compound ring structures (Fig. 23–1) with slight modifications such as a ketone or hydroxyl group here or there. The steroid hormones include the adrenal glucocorticoids and mineralocorticoids and the sex steroids estrogen, progesterone, and testosterone. The physiologically active form of vitamin D, 1,25-dihydroxycholecalciferol, is actually a hormone and is similar in structure to the steroids. As a result of their hydrocarbon skeleton, the steroids are very lipid soluble, which makes it easy

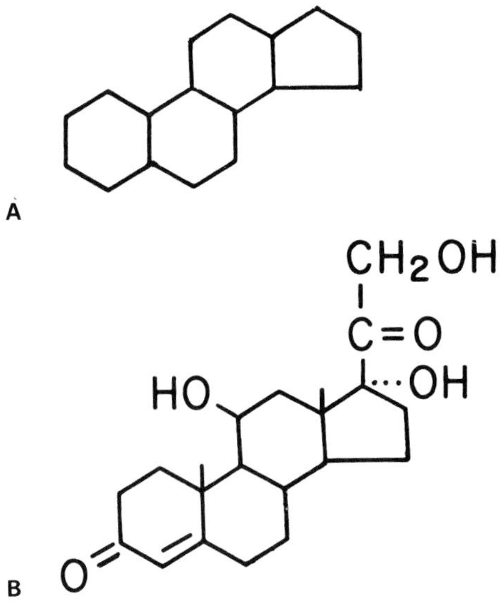

Figure 23–1. A. The carbon skeleton of the steroid hormone. **B.** The complete structure of cortisol.

for them to pass across cell membranes. The steroids are another class of compounds that have been synthesized in the laboratory. This has been particularly important for the glucocorticoids, which are so widely used in many areas of medicine. In addition, it has been possible in some instances, by producing small structural differences, to increase the potency of a steroid hormone with regard to one of its physiologic actions while at the same time either not affecting or decreasing its potency with regard to other actions. An example would be the adrenal steroids, for which *both* glucocorticoid and mineralocorticoid activity are a feature of several of the secreted compounds. It has been possible with slight alterations to accentuate one or the other of these activities. Such an increase in potency has obvious clinical advantages because it allows a more specific attack to be made in correcting hormonal deficiences.

PROTEIN BINDING OF HORMONES IN THE PLASMA

Many hormones, including all of the steroids and some of the amino acid-derived hormones, are carried in the plasma bound to carrier proteins. There are a number of advantages to such binding. Particularly in the case of a steroid hormone, the hydrophobic nature of the molecule makes it difficult for an adequate concentration of the hormone to be dissolved in the plasma. However, a steroid easily attaches to the hydrophobic portion of the binding proteins, increasing the plasma concentration of the hormone. A second advantage of protein binding relates to the fact that it is the free hormone in the plasma that stimulates the target organ and that hormones are constantly being metabolized in the target organ, in the liver, or in other organs. The amount of the free hormone is maintained by the equilibrium that exists between the protein-bound hormone and the free hormone in the plasma. As the free-hormone concentration is decreased by metabolism, it is quickly replaced by bound hormone diffusing away from the protein.

Another advantage of having hormones bound to carrier proteins in the plasma lies in the prevention of excretion of the hormones in the urine. The smaller hormones in the free form are small enough to be filtered across the glomerular capillaries in the kidneys. Large proteins, however, cannot be filtered across the capillaries. If a small hormone is bound to a large carrier protein, then it too is protected from being filtered in the glomerulus. The larger protein hormones are by themselves too big to be filtered in the glomerulus, so with regard to handling by the kidneys it is inconsequential that the large protein hormones are not bound to carrier proteins.

MEASUREMENT OF HORMONE CONCENTRATIONS

In the early days of endocrinology, the only type of assay available for measuring the concentration of a hormone in a blood or tissue sample was the bioassay. A bioassay involves observation of some type of biologic response after treatment of a living organism or excised tissue with an aliquot of the sample being examined. Examples of bioassays are the measurement of blood glucose concentration after injection into an animal of a sample containing insulin and the observation of cornification of the vaginal epithelium in rats after treatment with a sample containing estrogen. Bioassays are in most cases much less sensitive than the competitive binding and radioassays that are now available for most of the common hormones. Therefore, bioassays are now used infrequently.

The basic features of a radioassay are quite simple. First, a binding protein or antibody is prepared against a hormone. Then a radioactive preparation of the hormone is produced and a known amount is mixed with the binding protein in such a way that the degree of radioactivity of the solution is known. Finally, a sample of fluid containing an unknown concentration of the hormone is mixed with the solution containing the binding protein-radioactive hormone complex. The hormone in the unknown solution then competes for binding sites on the protein and decreases the radioactivity found on the protein in direct proportion to the concentration of the hormone in the unknown. From the decreased radioactivity, it is possible to calculate the concentration of the hormone in the unknown. Such radioassays are exquisitely sensitive and have been prepared for most of the known hormones.

HORMONE METABOLISM

Hormones are continuously being secreted (although not always at the same rate). What prevents a buildup of hormone concentration in the blood over a period of time? Such an event is avoided because of mechanisms for the metabolism or breakdown of hormones. Although each hormone is metabolized in a distinct way, a few generalizations can be made regarding this aspect of endocrine physiology. The organs that are most active in the breakdown of hormones are the liver and the kidneys. Other organs, including the target organs of some hormones, may be involved to a lesser extent.

The protein hormones are inactivated by enzymatic cleavage of the polypeptide chain. Thyroid hormone is inactivated by deiodination and deamination. It may also be converted in the liver to inactive sulfate and glucuronide conjugates (glucuronide is a slightly modified glucose molecule). Metabolism of steroids primarily takes place in the liver and generally involves a two-step process: (1) a slight alteration of the steroid molecule itself and (2) conjugation of the steroid to either sulfate or glucuronic acid. The significance of this alteration and conjugation is that the molecule is more polar and dissolves to a greater degree in the plasma without being bound to plasma protein. Consequently, the conjugates can be filtered and excreted more easily by the kidneys.

Understanding of the metabolism of catecholamines is particularly important for the anesthetist. However, because this topic is discussed in detail in most pharmacology texts, only a basic discussion will appear here. The catecholamines are inactivated by two different enzymes, monamine oxidase (MAO) and catechol-O-methytransferase (COMT). MAO catalyzes the oxidation of the catecholamines and is found in high levels in the liver, kidneys, and the ends of neurons that use catecholamines as neurotransmitters. COMT attaches a methyl group to a catecholamine and is found primarily in the liver and kidneys. The oxidized and methylated catecholamines may then be further oxidized or conjugated to sulfate or glucuronic acid. These metabolites are excreted by the kidneys.

An understanding of hormone metabolism is important in the diagnosis of endocrine disease, particularly with regard to the steroids and catecholamines. As a consequence of the metabolism of these hormones, a certain normal pattern of the metabolites appears in the urine. By observing changes in this pattern, the locus of a disease may be pinpointed.

The epinephrine secreted by the adrenal medulla increases the contractility of cardiac muscle, yet it has no such effect on skeletal muscle. Angiotensin II is a hormone that stimulates the secretion of aldosterone from the adrenal cortex, whereas the same angiotensin II is a potent stimulating agent for the contraction of vascular smooth muscle. How can a given hormone such as epinephrine have a certain effect on one tissue and have no effect on other tissues? How can a hormone such as angiotensin II have one effect on a given tissue and an entirely different effect elsewhere? The answer to these questions lies in the specificity of hormone action brought about by the presence or absence of specific receptors in the target organs. If no receptors for a hormone are present in an organ, any action by the hormone is impossible. The situation is analogous to a key needed to unlock a door. If a key fits into the keyhole and it is the right key, the door may be unlocked. If there is no keyhole, the key is useless in unlocking the door. Epinephrine excites the heart because there are receptors for the hormone on the cardiac muscle cells. Epinephrine has no effect on skeletal muscle because no receptors are present in that tissue. The situation of a single hormone having different effects on different target organs would be like the same key fitting into similar locks on doors opening into different rooms. Thus, angiotensin II can have one effect on the adrenal cortex and an entirely different effect on vascular smooth muscle.

MECHANISMS OF HORMONE ACTION

Once a hormone has interacted with a receptor, how does it influence the function of the cell? The topic addressed here is known as the mechanism of hormone action. Although other mechanisms probably exist, the two most common mechanisms of action of hormones are referred to as the second-messenger hypothesis and the mobile receptor hypothesis.

The Second-Messenger Hypothesis

Most of the protein hormones and the amino acid or amino acid-derived hormones work by the second-messenger hypothesis (Fig. 23–2). Most of these hormones are either too large or too polar to pass through the cell membrane. The result is that the only way such hormones can affect a cell is if they bind to a receptor molecule on the surface of the cell membrane. Activation of the receptor increases the activity of an enzyme known as adenyl cyclase, which converts adenosine triphosphate (ATP) into cyclic adenosine monophosphate (cAMP). In most cases, cAMP then changes the activity of enzymes within the cell, thereby altering cellular metabolism. The hormone can therefore be considered a "first messenger," bringing a signal from a distant endocrine gland, and the cAMP is the "second messenger," relaying the signal within the cell. The cAMP that is formed remains as an influence on cellular metabolism unless it is broken down by an enzyme known as phosphodiesterase. Phosphodiesterase activity is physiologically altered by hormones and can also be affected by certain drugs, such as the methylxanthines (caffeine falls into this category).

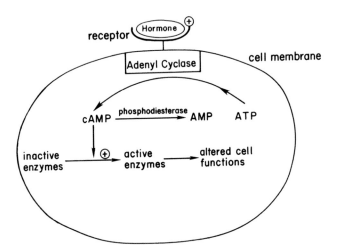

Figure 23–2. The second-messenger hypothesis: The hormone binds to the receptor on the cell membrane, activating adenyl cyclase, which in turn alters cellular functions. Adenyl cyclase converts ATP to cAMP, which activates cellular enzymes. cAMP is destroyed by the enzyme phosphodiesterase.

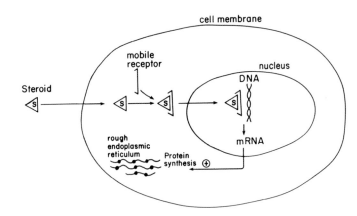

Figure 23–3. The mobile receptor hypothesis: The steroid hormone passes across the cell membrane and binds to the "mobile receptor." This hormone-receptor complex then passes into the nucleus, stimulating mRNA synthesis. The mRNA goes back out to the cytoplasm and calls for synthesis of specific proteins.

The Mobile Receptor Hypothesis

Because the steroid hormones are quite lipid soluble, they readily pass across the cell membrane, alleviating the need for a receptor located on the outer surface of the membrane (Fig. 23–3). Instead, a steroid hormone binds to a receptor protein in the cytoplasm, and the hormone-receptor complex then moves into the nucleus. The movement of the complex is the basis of the name *mobile* receptor hypothesis. Once in the nucleus, the steroid binds to DNA, stimulating the synthesis of a particular messenger RNA (mRNA) molecule (or set of molecules). The mRNA passes back out into the cytoplasm, where it becomes associated with rough endoplasmic reticulum and calls for the synthesis of a particular protein or group of proteins. The synthesized proteins may be structural proteins or enzymes, but whatever the particular proteins synthesized in a given cell under steroid stimulation, the change in cell structure or metabolism is specifically dependent on which proteins are synthesized. All of the steroid hormones are believed to act via the mobile receptor hypothesis.

CONTROL OF ENDOCRINE SECRETION

What are the factors that control the secretion of hormones? In the case of most hormones, secretion is prominently (in some instances exclusively) influenced by other hormones. All of the anterior pituitary hormones are controlled by releasing hormones or release-inhibiting hormones, which are secreted by cells in the hypothalamus into the hypothalamohypophyseal portal vessel. The releasing hormones then pass down to the pituitary gland to stimulate or inhibit the secretion of the appropriate hormones. Of the six anterior pituitary hormones—growth hormone (GH), ACTH, thyroid-stimulating hormone (TSH), follicle-stimulating hormone (FSH), luteinizing hormone (LH), and prolactin—all but prolactin in turn are important regulators of the secretion of hormones from their target organs. Secretion of the releasing hormones and the anterior pituitary hormones is controlled in a feedback fashion (usually negatively) by the hormones of the pituitary target organs. Further examples of control of hormonal secretion by other hormones include stimulation of aldosterone secretion from the adrenal cortex by angiotensin II and regulation of secretion of insulin and glucagon by gastrointestinal hormones. The adrenal medullary catecholamines affect secretion of a number of other hormones and may be either excitatory or inhibitory, depending on the target organ and whether α- or β-adrenergic receptors are stimulated.

Another major method of control of hormonal secretion is by intermediary metabolites in the blood. Perhaps the best-known example is the stimulation of insulin secretion from the pancreas in response to a rising blood glucose concentration. Glucose inhibits the secretion of glucagon from the pancreas and growth hormone from the anterior pituitary. Amino acids stimulate the secretion of insulin, glucagon, and GH. Free fatty acids inhibit the secretion of glucagon and GH. Ketone bodies stimulate the secretion of insulin and inhibit secretion of glucagon. It is likely that secretion of other hormones is also affected by intermediary metabolites such as glucose, amino acids, and fatty acids.

The concentrations of inorganic ions in the blood are key factors controlling a number of hormones. High potassium (within the physiologic range) and low sodium (probably not within the physiologic range) stimulate secretion of aldosterone by the adrenal cortex. The total osmostic pressure of the plasma is monitored by osmoreceptors in the hypothalamus, and when this pressure is elevated, secretion of antidiuretic hormone (ADH) increases. Renin secretion by the juxtaglomerular apparatus is inversely proportional to the rate of transport of Na^+ or Cl^- out of the distal convoluted tubule. The secretion of parathyroid hormone and calcitonin, two hormones responsible for calcium metabolism, is regulated by Ca^{2+}. Parathyroid hormone secretion is inversely proportional to plasma Ca^{2+} concentration, whereas the secretion of calcitonin is proportional to plasma Ca^{2+}. 1,25-Dihydroxycholecalciferol (commonly referred to as vitamin D), which is secreted by the kidneys and is involved in control of plasma Ca^{2+} and PO_4^{3-} concentrations, is secreted in response to low PO_4^{3-} concentrations. Finally, acid in the lumen of the duodenum increases the secretion of the hormone secretin, which among other actions stimulates the secretion of bicarbonate by the pancreas to neutralize the acid in the duodenum.

Direct neural control of hormone secretion is of importance with regard to regulation of some hormones. The adrenal medulla secretes epinephrine and norepinephrine in response to neural activity in the preganglionic sympathetic axons reaching the gland. The adrenal medulla can therefore be considered a part of the sympathetic nervous system, functioning as a mass of postganglionic sympathetic neurons that release epinephrine and norepinephrine into the bloodstream as hormones to act on target organs rather than as neurotransmitters to act on postsynaptic cells. Other hormones that have secretion regulated by the nervous system include renin, the hypothalamic releasing hormones, and the posterior pituitary hormones oxytocin and vasopressin.

EFFECTS OF A HORMONE: PHYSIOLOGIC VERSUS PHARMACOLOGIC

When discussing the effects of a hormone, it becomes very important to distinguish whether the concentration being considered is at a level within the normal range found in the body, which would be a physiologic concentration, or at a level far in excess of what might be found, which would be a pharmacologic concentration. The reason it is important to know whether physiologic or pharmacologic concentrations are present is that the effects of a hormone may not be the same at the different concentrations. Several of the hormones frequently dealt with by anesthetists have different effects at physiologic and pharmacologic concentrations. At physiologic concentrations, ADH has as its major effect the stimulation of water reabsorption in excess of solute in the collecting ducts of the kidney. The result is that a smaller volume of more concentrated urine is produced. Another action that has been attributed to ADH is constriction of blood vessels, and for this reason ADH has also been called vasopressin. Constriction of blood vessels is an effect of ADH at pharmacologic concentrations, and it is questionable whether such an effect ever occurs at concentrations within the physiologic range. However, vasoconstriction as a result of exogenous ADH must be kept in mind and may be a contraindication to use if a patient has coronary artery or other vascular disease.

Another group of hormones of which physiologic and pharmacologic effects are frequently confused are the glucocorticoids. Glucocorticoids are among the most prescribed drugs, but they are given most often because of their effects at pharmacologic doses. At physiologic concentrations, the glucocorticoids have such effects as increased glycogenesis and gluconeogenesis in the liver, a permissive action for many of the effects of glucagon and the catecholamines, inhibition of ACTH secretion by the pituitary, maintenance of the ability to excrete a water load by the kidneys, alterations of lymphatic organs and of blood cells, and provision of a resistance to stress. Although treatment with glucocorticoids is often necessary for maintenance of these functions, glucocorticoids are also frequently given at higher, pharmacologic doses to inhibit an inflammatory response.

STRESS AND HORMONES

We are all familiar with the word *stress* and the unpleasant connotations that it conjures up. Physiologists sometimes describe stress as those stimuli that increase the secretion of ACTH. Although the ability to secrete ACTH and the glucocorticoids that are secreted in response to the ACTH is essential for life, we have very little understanding of exactly why these hormones are necessary for the response to stress. Many other hormones are secreted in response to stress, including ADH, GH, glucagon, and the adrenal catecholamines. Again, the benefit of increasing the plasma concentrations of these hormones is not fully understood. Perhaps the changes in the endocrine environment confer on the individual some metabolic advantage that is beneficial in combating the effects of stress.

TYPES OF ENDOCRINE DISEASE

Endocrine disease is quite simply manifested in two forms: excess or deficiency. However, the underlying pathologic condition may stem from several sources. Tumors are a common cause of hormonal excess, and symptoms may be directly or indirectly an indication of the site of the tumor. For example, an excess of glucocorticoids may be due directly to an adrenal tumor or indirectly to an ACTH-secreting pituitary tumor. If a particular endocrine gland secretes more than one hormone, a tumor of that gland may secrete excess amounts of one or any combination of the hormones normally secreted, depending on the particular cell type involved.

Some endocrine disorders are autoimmune diseases. In Graves' disease of the thyroid gland, antibodies are produced against the TSH receptors on the follicular epithelial cells in the thyroid, resulting in stimulation of the cells and the ensuing hyperthyroidism. Autoimmune diseases are known to exist for other endocrine glands, and they may result in either hormonal excess or deficiency, depending on the exact component against which the antibodies are formed. It has been suggested that diabetes mellitus (the juvenile form) may be an autoimmune disease.

Congenital enzyme deficiencies are the basis of another important category of endocrine pathology. An example is congenital adrenal hyperplasia. Androgens may be secreted by the same cells of the adrenal cortex that secrete the glucocorticoids, and the androgens are in fact intermediates in the pathway for glucocorticoid synthesis. The major regulator of both androgen and glucocorticoid secretion by the adrenal cortex is ACTH from the pituitary. When the glucocorticoid concentration of the blood reaches a certain level, there is a negative feedback effect on the hypothalamus–pituitary axis, shutting down the secretion of ACTH. However, the adrenal adrogens do not inhibit ACTH secretion, even when present in high concentrations. If there is an enzymatic deficiency in the adrenal cortex in the synthetic pathway between the androgens and the glucocorticoids, secretion of glucocorticoids will be low and ACTH secretion will rise. The increased ACTH will stimulate the adrenal cortex, but because glucocorticoids cannot be formed, the androgens will be secreted in excess but a deficiency in the glucocorticoids will remain. There are a number of such enzyme deficiency diseases in the adrenal cortex, and the patient's symptoms depend on which enzyme in the synthetic pathway is inadequate.

Another form of endocrine disease is a result of target organ insensitivity to a hormone. In nephrogenic diabetes insipidus, ADH is present but does not increase the uptake of water from the collecting ducts since these structures do not respond to ADH as they should. As a result, a large volume of dilute urine is formed. In maturity-onset diabetes, the B cells that secrete insulin from the pancreas may have normal morphology and insulin content and may secrete the hormone, but the number of receptors for insulin on the cell membranes of target organ tissues may be decreased. This paucity of receptors may account for the inability to handle a glucose load.

Dietary problems can also contribute to endocrine disease. Perhaps the best known of such diseases is hypothyroidism due to insufficient dietary iodine. The dietary iodine is needed for the synthesis of thyroid hormone, and if it is lacking, the thyroid gland cannot produce enough hormone for normal thyroid function to occur. The gland may hypertrophy in an attempt to bring hormone synthesis back to normal levels. Simply supplementing the diet with iodine alleviates this type of hypothyroidism.

HORMONES AS NEUROTRANSMITTERS

The student should be aware that several hormones are also found as neurotransmitters. By definition, to be a hormone a compound must be released by a cell and then pass into the bloodstream to act on a target organ some distance away. To be a neurotransmitter, a compound must be released by a neuron and diffuse across a synaptic gap to act on a postsynaptic cell, usually another neuron, a muscle cell, or a glandular cell. The terms *hormone* and *neurotransmitter* are functional terms and do not place a limit on the chemical nature of the compound involved. The most widely known example of a hormone playing double duty as a neurotransmitter is norepinephrine, which is secreted as a hormone by the adrenal medulla and is found as the neurotransmitter of most postganglionic sympathetic neurons and in several locations in the central nervous system. Epinephrine and to a much lesser extent dopamine are also secreted by the adrenal medulla and are found as well as neurotransmitters in the brain. Dopamine also serves as a hormone released by the hypothalamus into the hypothalamohypophyseal portal vessel to inhibit secretion of the hormone prolactin from the pituitary. Somatostatin is a polypeptide that acts as a hormone in two locations. It is found in the islets of Langerhans in the pancreas, where it may be involved in the control of insulin and glucagon secretion; and it is secreted by the hypothalamus, from which it passes to the pituitary to inhibit the secretion of GH. Somatostatin is also found as a neurotransmitter in the pain pathway in the spinal cord and elsewhere in the brain. Finally, a great deal of attention has in recent years been given to a family of compounds known collectively as opioid peptides. These compounds, which include the enkephalins, are known to be secreted as hormones by the pituitary gland, and they are found in neuronal endings in many parts of the brain and spinal cord, where they may act as neurotransmitters. Although the enkephalins are known to have an analgesic effect when injected into certain parts of the brain and are found in high concentrations in pain pathways in the spinal cord and brain, the significance of these compounds is not yet fully understood. It is certainly possible that the enkephalins may be found to play an important role in controlling pain, so anesthetists may expect to hear much more about these compounds in future years.

THE THYROID GLAND

The thyroid gland consists of two elongated lobes (right and left) joined close to their inferior poles by an isthmus (Fig. 23–4A). Occasionally, a pyramidal lobe is seen extending upward from the isthmus toward the thyroglossal duct and foramen cecum of the tongue. Wrapped around the junction between the larynx and the trachea, the thyroid has an important anatomic relationship with the recurrent laryngeal nerves, the major nerves controlling laryngeal function. The recurrent laryngeal nerves are located on either side, between the thyroid and the trachea. This anatomic relationship is important to keep in mind when the thyroid is manipulated during surgery, since physical

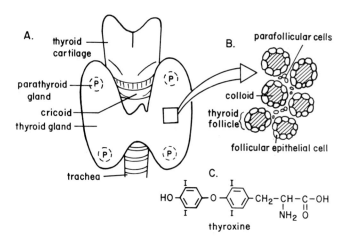

C.

$$HO-\overset{I}{\underset{I}{\bigcirc}}-O-\overset{I}{\underset{I}{\bigcirc}}-CH_2-CH-\overset{O}{\overset{\shortparallel}{C}}-OH$$
$$\underset{NH_2}{}$$

thyroxine

Figure 23–4. A. Gross anatomy of the thyroid gland. **B.** Histology of the thyroid gland. **C.** Thyroxine.

trauma to the recurrent laryngeal nerves may result in laryngeal dysfunction.

Histologically the thyroid gland is composed of fluid-filled spheres called follicles, each of which is covered by a single layer of follicular epithelial cells (Fig. 23–4B). The fluid of the follicles, which is known as thyroid colloid, contains "extracellularly" stored thyroid hormone. This extracellular storage of thyroid hormone is in great enough quantities that handling of a hyperactive gland during surgery may cause enough release of the hormone to cause the systemic hyperthyroid state described as a thyroid storm (discussed below).

Thyroid hormone can be classified chemically as an amino acid that has been iodinated (Fig. 23–4C). Four or three atoms of iodine may be added to the molecule, resulting in tetraiodothyronine (T_4) or triiodothyronine (T_3), respectively. Eighty percent of the hormone secreted is in the tetraiodinated form, and this is the molecule commonly known as thyroxine. It should be noted, however, that T_3 may be the physiologically active form of the hormone and that T_4 is converted to T_3 peripherally before any effect is seen.

An important aspect of thyroid physiology is that the gland avidly concentrates iodide from the plasma for synthesis into thyroid hormone. Secretion of thyroid hormone is in part regulated by the availability of iodide from the diet. If a dietary deficiency of iodide exists, the thyroid gland will enlarge in an attempt to accumulate more iodide in order to produce an adequate amount of hormone. Such an enlargement constitutes an iodine-deficient goiter. The term *goiter* implies only that the thyroid is enlarged and denotes nothing regarding the thyroid state of an individual. In the presence of a goiter, an individual can be hypothyroid, euthyroid, or hyperthyroid with respect to the normal physiologic state.

The main regulator of thyroid gland function is TSH from the anterior pituitary (Fig. 23–5). TSH stimulates both the synthesis and secretion of thyroid hormone. The radioimmunoassay currently available for measuring the TSH levels in the blood is very accurate, and a knowledge of the concentration of TSH acting on the thyroid gland is important in being able to make an informed diagnosis regarding thyroid function. Thyrotropin-releasing hormone (TRH) is secreted by the hypothalamus into the hypothalamohypophyseal portal vessel and stimulates the secretion of TSH. Both TRH and TSH are controlled in a negative feedback fashion by thyroid hormone in the blood.

It should be noted that most of the thyroid hormone in the blood is bound to a carrier protein, thyroid-binding globulin (TBG), which is produced in the liver. However, it is the unbound thyroid hormone that is responsible for the physiologic effects and for the feedback control over TRH and TSH secretion. For unknown reasons, when the concentration of estrogen in the blood increases, such as in women who are taking contraceptives or who are pregnant, the liver responds by producing more TBG. More thyroid hormone then becomes associated with the carrier protein, and the concentration of free thyroid hormone drops. This drop results in release of the negative feedback on the pituitary and hypothalamus, resulting in increased TSH secretion. The rise in TSH stimulates secretion of thyroid hormone until the point that the free thyroid hormone concentration in the blood has risen enough so that a new feedback effect can be exerted on the pituitary–hypothalamus system. What has happened is that the total amount of thyroid hormone in the blood has increased. However, it is only the protein-bound fraction that has actually risen. The free thyroid hormone concentration is restored to its previous level. It is therefore important when measuring thyroid hormone clinically to distinguish between total thyroid hormone and free thyroid hormone. Again, it is the free thyroid hormone in the blood that is physiologically active and exerts the negative feedback effects on the pituitary–hypothalamus system.

Although the thyroid hormone is not a steroid, it acts

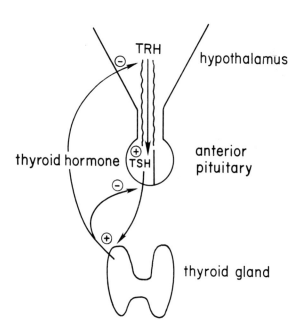

Figure 23–5. Regulation of thyroid hormone secretion.

by entering the cell and binding to receptors associated with the DNA in the nucleus. New mRNA is synthesized, calling for the synthesis of protein in the cytoplasm. It is the specific enzymatic action of the thyroid-induced proteins that is responsible for the effects of the hormone. A well-known action of thyroid hormone is the stimulatory effect it has on the metabolic rate. This effect may in part be due to an increase in the activity of Na^+–K^+ ATPase. The energy released when the ATP is hydrolyzed may be responsible for the increased generation of heat caused by thyroid hormone. Thyroid hormone is also involved in regulation of carbohydrate and lipid metabolism and is important in normal growth and development.

Hypothyroidism

Most of the symptoms of hypothyroidism can be traced directly to the effects of the decreased metabolic state on the particular organ involved. The overall metabolic rate is often decreased. Neurologic symptoms of hypothyroidism may include slowing of mental function, slowing of stretch reflexes, loss of motivation, depression, poor memory, and somnolence. The accumulation of osmotically active proteins and mucopolysaccharides in the skin and elsewhere results in the condition known as myxedema, a nonpitting edema that is particularly evident externally as puffiness around the eyes and on the dorsa of the hands and feet. The skin may be dry, cold, and pale, although hypercarotenemia may cause yellowing. Internally the myxedema may cause thickening of the mucous membranes of the larynx and pharynx, as well as enlargement of the tongue. These features lead to a husky voice, which when added to slow motor control of the laryngeal muscles make the slow speech of a myxedema patient very characteristic. Gastrointestinal function is often slowed, resulting in constipation. Gastric emptying may be delayed, and segments of intestine may be impacted with stool. Significant changes may also be seen in cardiovascular function. Cardiac output and contracility may be decreased, possibly because of the myxedematous infiltration that occurs. The heart sounds may be muffled, and low voltage and repolarization abnormalities may be seen in the electrocardiogram (ECG). The response of the heart to circulatory stress may be insufficient, and stress may put further strain on the already diseased organ. Total blood volume may be decreased, making hypothyroid patients vulnerable to hypovolemic shock.

Younger patients may be hypotensive, but older patients may exhibit diastolic hypertension. Cardiovascular reflexes may be defective, including decreased heart rate and blood pressure responses in the Valsalva maneuver and baroreceptor dysfunction. Respiratory abnormalities may include depressed hypercapnic and hypoxic ventilatory drives, decreased maximum breathing capacity, and decreased diffusion capacity for carbon monoxide. Pleural effusions are also common. There are many more symptoms of hypothyroidism, and it should be stressed that those symptoms described above are for overt hypothyroidism. In less severe cases, the symptoms may not be quite as dramatic. The most advanced state of hypothyroidism is myxedema coma, which can develop as a result of undiagnosed or neglected hypothyroidism. A patient with myxedema coma exhibits hypoventilation, respiratory acidosis, hypothermia, hypoglycemia, low serum sodium and high serum lactate levels, cachexia, inappropriate ADH secretion, and progressive stupor ending in a comatose state (Werner, 1978).

Early detection and treatment of hypothyroidism in infants or children who are hypothyroid is critical in order to avoid permanent brain damage caused by abnormal development. In adults, early hypothyroidism is often misdiagnosed as a psychiatric problem. Treatment of hypothyroidism basically involves replacement of the thyroid hormone.

Anesthesia for Hypothyroid Patients. Whenever possible, treatment with thyroid hormone at a daily dose of 100 to 200 mg should be begun before bringing a patient with mild hypothyroidism to surgery. The more severe the hypothyroid state, the greater the danger of increased sensitivity to a number of drugs. Patients who are overtly hypothyroid may metabolize drugs at a slower rate, so a given dose may act longer. Because of the potential for the development of hypothyroid coma after general anesthesia, elective surgery should be postponed until severely hypothyroid patients have been made euthyroid. Thyroid hormone replacement in hypothyroid patients who have ischemic heart disease carries the risk of exacerbating angina or even precipitating myocardial infarction, perhaps by increasing the metabolic demands of the heart. In such patients, incomplete thyroid hormone replacement may have to be accepted (Murkin, 1982).

The increased incidence of adrenocortical insufficiency in hypothyroid patients is the basis for steroid replacement with hydrocortisone in preparation of such a patient for surgery.

Prudent anesthetic management of hypothyroid patients requires close attention to the underlying pathologic condition. Because of the decreased rate of drug metabolism and an already depressed central nervous system, preoperative sedation should not be given. When feasible, regional nerve blocks are preferable over general anesthesia. Due to the delayed gastric emptying that may be present in a hypothyroid patient, endotracheal intubation should be performed with cuffed tubes, and in severe cases awake intubation may be preferable (Abbott, 1967). Because of the hypovolemic state of hypothyroid patients, central venous pressure should be monitored during any major surgery. Possible decreases in blood volume should be considered when deciding on an induction agent. A controlled induction, with smaller incremental doses, is preferable to large bolus injections. The agent of choice for anesthesia is nitrous oxide and oxygen under controlled ventilation (Pender et al, 1981). Hypocapnia should be avoided. Because of the danger of prolonged recovery from anesthesia or even hypothyroid coma, narcotics including fentanyl and morphine are contraindicated. As for muscle relaxants, succinylcholine has been found to have a normal duration of action in hypothyroid patients (Kim and Hackman, 1977). Because of the underlying defects in metabolism, hypothyroid patients may be particularly prone to develop hypothermia. Since hypothermia increases mortality in hypothyroid patients, body temperature should be monitored throughout anesthesia and postoperatively. Warming blankets, peritoneal lavage, increased operating room temperature, and warmed intravenous solutions can all be used to maintain body temperature. Care must be taken to avoid hypovolemic shock, which may result from peripheral vasodilation when using warming blankets.

After surgery, respiration must be closely watched in hypothyroid patients, since respiratory failure may develop as a result of hypothermia or because of the use of narcotics.

Hyperthyroidism

Hyperthyroidism is generally expressed as a hypermetabolic state of both individual organs and the body as a whole. The basal metabolic rate (BMR) is often increased, and a slight increase in body temperature may be seen, perhaps because of the increased BMR. Many hyperthyroid patients show heat intolerance. If the caloric intake is not increased to keep pace with the increased BMR, metabolism of endogenous protein and fat will occur, and weight loss results. Another consequence of the increased metabolic rate is the possibility of vitamin deficiencies because the need for vitamins exceeds the intake. The chronic depletion of liver glycogen in hyperthyroid patients leads to abnormal susceptibility to liver failure. Because the liver is a site of thyroid hormone metabolism, hepatic failure due to hyperthyroidism may actually worsen the hyperthyroid state. A change may occur in the bowel habits (including diarrhea), and increased thirst and urination may also be seen. Nervous system changes in hyperthyroidism may include nervousness, irritability, restlessness, emotional instability, depression, and difficulty in sleeping. Reflexes may be brisk, and a fine tremor of the extended hands or a coarse tremor and jerking of the trunk may be seen. Movements may be rapid and jerky, and muscle weakness is sometimes present. The skin temperature is usually elevated, and the skin is often soft and moist as a result of excess sweating. Reticuloendothelial involvement may be seen as a relative lymphocytosis, neutropenia, a palpable spleen, and hyperplasia of lymphatic tissue. One form of hyperthyroidism, Graves' disease, is thought by some to be an autoimmune condition and is sometimes associated with other autoimmune disorders. Mild anemia is also a common finding in hyperthyroidism.

Ocular involvement in hyperthyroidism is often apparent in the form of exophthalmos as a result of swelling of the orbital contents. The underlying cause of exophthalmos is not clearly understood. It seems unlikely that thyroid hormone itself is directly responsible for exophthalmos, since this manifestation of hyperthyroidism sometimes becomes worse after the thyroid gland is removed. It has been suggested that a breakdown product of TSH from the pituitary may be the compound directly responsible. In addition to the protrusion of the eyes that is most characteristic of exophthalmos, pain, injection of the conjunctivae, tearing, sensation of a foreign body in the eye, diplopia, loss of visual acuity, and discordant extraocular muscles may also be part of the ocular symptoms of a hyperthyroid patient.

An understanding of the cardiovascular consequences of hyperthyroidism is of utmost importance for the anesthetist. The increased metabolic state of the tissues of the body requires an increased supply of oxygen and hence an increased blood flow. This is one factor increasing the demands made on the heart. A second factor is that vasodilation occurs in the skin because of the increased body temperature, approximating an arteriovenous fistula. Thus, cardiac output in hyperthyroidism must increase even in the resting state in order to keep pace with the increased metabolic demands of the tissues and the increased blood flow to the skin. The cardiac output may not increase sufficiently, leading to a condition known as high-output failure. Excess thyroid hormone has direct effects on the heart, including tachycardia and a tendency to create dysrhythmias. There is likely an interaction between the effects of thyroid hormone on the heart and those of the catecholamines, and it has been well documented that β-adrenergic blockers are of tremendous value in reducing the cardiac problems in hyperthyroidism.

Anesthetic Management of Hyperthyroid Patients. The most important consideration in the anesthetic management of a hyperthyroid patient is, whenever possible, to bring the patient back to the euthyroid state before surgery is begun. There is great risk involved in anesthetizing a hyperthyroid individual, and it is only in emergencies that surgery should be performed under such conditions. The drugs that are used to bring about the euthyroid state function in three basic ways:

1. To suppress uptake of iodine by the thyroid gland and decrease synthesis of thyroid hormone
2. To decrease secretion of thyroid hormone by the gland
3. To interfere with the peripheral action of the hormone on the tissues of the body.

The thionamides are the most frequently used antithyroid agents. Carbimazole (given at an initial dose of 30 mg/day) is generally preferred over propylthiouracil (initial dose 300 mg/day). Both of these compounds prevent the incorporation of iodine into thyroid hormone and inhibit later stages in thyroid hormone synthesis. Potassium perchlorate, which blocks uptake of iodine by the gland, has been used when problems develop with other drugs. However, the perchlorate treatment may lead to anemia, and it is not the drug of choice. The main problem encountered in suppression of thyroid hormone synthesis with the thionamides is that it may take up to 8 weeks for the euthyroid state to be reached. In addition, these antithyroid drugs may cause an increase in the size of a goiter. Thus, it may be preferable to stop treatment with these antithyroid drugs 2 weeks before the surgery and switch the patient to iodide tablets (60 mg/day). The iodide prevents secretion of thyroid hormone by the gland and, as an added benefit, also decreases the size and vascularity of the gland. Radioiodine may also be used to decrease the size of the thyroid. A subtotal thyroidectomy may be performed as an alternative to the drug treatments described above. If there is insufficient time available to bring the patient to a euthyroid state, the β-adrenergic blocking drug propranolol should be used to decrease the risks inherent in performing surgery on a hyperthyroid individual. The propranolol will help to control tachycardia and dysrhythmias, and its use should be continued into the postoperative period.

Because anxiety is a prominent characteristic of hyperthyroid patients, premedication is very useful, and in the absence of airway obstruction any premedication can be used. If the patient has been brought to the euthyroid state, the anesthetic agent may be chosen on general medical grounds. Particularly if a patient still shows signs of hyperthyroidism, there may be an increase in the requirement for the anesthetic agent. Such a situation may be due to the faster metabolic clearance of the anesthetic by the hypermetabolic tissues. If exophthalmos is present, special care should be taken to keep the patient's eyes from becoming too dry during surgery. This may be done by applying protective drops or by maintaining the eyelids in the closed position.

Thyroid Storm. The most severe manifestation of hyperthyroidism is the condition referred to as thyroid storm or thyrotoxic crisis. This relatively rare condition arises as a result of excess thyroid hormone acting on the tissues and is characterized by the presence of the previously described signs of hyperthyroidism pushed to the extreme. The body temperature may rise to 41C (106F). Profuse sweating may occur, leading to severe dehydration. Cardiovascular problems include sinus tachycardia, tachyarrhythmias, and large increases in systolic and pulse pressure. Particularly in patients with preexisting heart disease, signs of congestive heart failure may appear. Other signs of thyrotoxicosis include nausea, vomiting, tremor, restlessness, and delirium. A comatose state with hypotension develops as the condition worsens. The thyroid storm frequently occurs in a patient who is hyperthyroid but has not been diagnosed as such. The episode of thyroid storm can be brought on by stress such as surgery or infection.

If not treated vigorously, a thyroid storm is frequently fatal. The proper treatment must consist of combating the symptoms of the excess thyroid hormone already present, as well as attempting to prevent further release of hormone. Administration of propranolol may be useful in alleviating some of the cardiovascular problems.

A vigorous attempt should be made to lower the body temperature, and fluid balance and respiratory parameters should be closely watched. Thionamides and iodide should be given to prevent further production of thyroid hormone. A patient who developed a thyroid storm during surgery should be watched carefully during the postoperative period.

CALCIUM METABOLISM AND THE PARATHYROID GLAND

Ionized calcium is essential for the normal function of many physiologic processes, including muscle contraction, nerve function, secretory activity by endocrine and exocrine glands, and blood clotting. It is important that the total plasma Ca^{2+} level (ionized plus protein-bound) be maintained in the normal range of 9 to 10.5 mg/100 ml. If the Ca^{2+} concentration falls, muscle cell membranes become hyperexcitable and there is an increased tendency for tetany to develop. Latent tetany may be seen at a plasma Ca^{2+} of less than 8 mg/100 ml. Should plasma Ca^{2+} fall to less than 7 mg/100 ml, tonic contractions may occur. Tetany of the laryngeal muscles, known as laryngospasm, is particularly likely to occur when plasma Ca^{2+} falls. The asphyxia that results from laryngospasm underscores the need to maintain plasma Ca^{2+}. Acute hypercalcemia can also develop into an emergency situation, with symptoms that may include nausea, vomiting, polyuria, and coma. Moderate but chronic elevation of plasma Ca^{2+} may lead to kidney failure and kidney stones.

The regulation of the plasma Ca^{2+} concentration on a day-to-day basis is coordinated primarily by two hormones, parathyroid hormone and 1,25-dihydroxycholecalciferol. A third hormone, calcitonin, may be involved to a lesser extent. Other hormones that may play a role in calcium metabolism in special situations include GH, glucocorticoids, estrogen, and thyroxine. The discussion that follows is primarily concerned with the effects of parathyroid hormone, 1,25-dihydroxycholecalciferol, and calcitonin on plasma Ca^{2+}. The major actions of these hormones are summarized in Table 23–1.

Parathyroid Hormone

Parathyroid hormone (PTH) is a polypeptide secreted by the chief cells of the parathyroid glands. The main action of PTH is to increase plasma Ca^{2+} by the mobilization of Ca^{2+} from bone stores and by increasing the reabsorption of filtered Ca^{2+} by the kidney tubules. PTH also increases the formation of 1,25-dihydroxycholecalciferol by the kidneys, and the actions of this hormone (discussed below) increase the plasma Ca^{2+}. PTH also decreases plasma phosphate by increasing the excretion of phosphate in the urine.

Secretion of PTH is regulated in a negative feedback fashion by Ca^{2+}. When the plasma Ca^{2+} drops, secretion of PTH by the parathyroid glands is increased, and this PTH then restores the plasma Ca^{2+} to normal. As the plasma

TABLE 23–1. SUMMARY OF ENDOCRINE REGULATION OF Ca^{2+} METABOLISM

Hormone	Bone	Kidney	Intestines
Parathyroid hormone (PTH)	↑ Mobilization of Ca^{2+}	↑ Reabsorption of Ca^{2+} ↑ Formation of 1,25-dihydroxycholecalciferol ↑ Excretion of PO_4^{3-}	
1,25-Dihydroxycholecalciferol	↑ Mobilization of Ca^{2+} ↑ Mobilization of PO_4^{3-}		↑ Transport of Ca^{2+} into blood
Calcitonin	↓ Mobilization of Ca^{2+}		

Ca^{2+} rises, the secretion of PTH is decreased, thereby limiting the level reached by plasma Ca^{2+}. Magnesium ions also exert an effect on PTH secretion, with low plasma Mg^{2+} inhibiting it.

One of the consequences of hypoparathyroidism is hypocalcemic tetany, which is due to hyperexcitability of muscle cell membranes. The condition is demonstrated by contraction of the facial muscles after a tap on the facial nerve in front of the ear. This response is known as Chvostek's sign. Additional evidence of hypocalcemic tetany is Trousseau's sign, which consists of extension of the fingers and flexion of the wrist and thumb (carpopedal spasm). It may be necessary to occlude the blood supply to the limb for 3 minutes in order to demonstrate Trousseau's sign. The greatest danger of hypocalcemic tetany is the occurrence of laryngospasm, which can lead to asphyxia.

Hypoparathyroidism occurs frequently after thyroidectomy because the parathyroid glands were unintentionally removed. Hypoparathyroidism also occurs after the parathyroids have been removed to treat *hyper*parathyroidism. Treatment of acute hypocalcemia after parathyroidectomy is by IV injection of 10 ml of 10 percent calcium gluconate over a 5- to 10-minute period. If the plasma magnesium concentration is low, it may also be necessary to give magnesium to eliminate tetany. Chronic hypocalcemia is treated by a combination of oral calcium salts and vitamin D.

The most common cause of hyperparathyroidism is primary hyperparathyroidism due to increased secretion of the chief cells in the parathyroid gland. Hypercalcemia is generally produced in response to primary hyperparathyroidism. Ectopic hyperparathyroidism, such as seen in carcinoma of the breast, lung, and pancreas, is also accompanied by hypercalcemia. Hyperparathyroidism secondary to chronically low plasma Ca^{2+}, as seen in chronic renal failure or intestinal malabsorption, is not accompanied by hypercalcemia. The untoward effects of hyperparathyroidism are due to the hypercalcemia that is produced. These effects may include renal failure and calculi, hypertension, ECG abnormalities (prolonged P-R interval and shortened Q-T interval), vomiting, peptic ulcer, pancreatitis, muscle weakness, bone pain and demineralization, gout, lethargy, and coma. The treatment of acute hypercalcemia due to hyperparathyroidism includes hydration and the administration of a diuretic and electrolytes. However, at present, parathyroidectomy is the only feasible permanent treatment for hyperparathyroidism. Before parathyroidectomy is performed to relieve hypercalcemia, causes other than hyperparathyroidism must be ruled out. Other potential causes of hypercalcemia include malignancies, vitamin D intoxication, and adrenal insufficiency.

1,25-Dihydroxycholecalciferol

1,25-Dihydroxycholecalciferol is a sterol-derived compound properly considered to be a hormone secreted by the kidneys. It is formed in the kidneys by hydroxylation of 25-hydroxycholecalciferol, a compound that is produced in the liver from cholecalciferol. Cholecalciferol, also known as vitamin D_3, is ingested in the diet and is formed in the skin by the influence of sunlight on 7-dehydrocholesterol. This sequence of reactions is summarized in Figure 23–6. Note that 25-hydroxycholecalciferol is actually converted

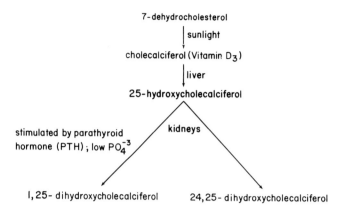

Figure 23–6. Formation of 1,25-dihydroxycholecalciferol.

into two different dihydroxy compounds, 1,25 and 24,25. The 1,25 compound is the physiologically active form that influences calcium and phosphorous metabolism. The 24,25 form is an inactive metabolite. The amount of the 1,25 compound produced is increased under the direct influence of PTH and low plasma PO_4^{3-}.

1,25-Dihydroxycholecalciferol acts primarily on intestine and bone, and its overall effect is to increase the plasma Ca^{2+} and PO_4^{3-}. The action on the intestine is to increase the transport of Ca^{2+} from the lumen into the blood. The action of 1,25-dihydroxycholecalciferol on bone is to increase the mobilization of Ca^{2+} and PO_4^{3-} from the bone stores. As will be recalled from the previous discussion, PTH also has a direct effect on bone to mobilize Ca^{2+}. Thus, both 1,25-dihydroxycholecalciferol and PTH increase plasma Ca^{2+}.

What is commonly known as a dietary deficiency of vitamin D is actually a deficiency of one of the precursors of 1,25-dihydroxycholecalciferol. However, the pathologic condition that develops is expressed as a decreased secretion of 1,25-dihydroxycolecalciferol by the kidneys. Such a deficiency may also be caused by a lack of exposure to sunlight and is made worse by a diet low in calcium. Whatever the cause of decreased secretion of 1,25-hydroxycholecalciferol, the result is a softening of the bones. The condition is known as rickets in children and osteomalacia in adults. It should be noted that there are many other causes of rickets and osteomalacia besides a dietary deficiency, for example, renal disease and vitamin D resistance. In children, a lack of 1,25-dihydroxycholecalciferol decreases absorption of Ca^{2+} from the intestine, which in turn leads to poor mineralization of bone. In adults, because the amount of Ca^{2+} brought in from the intestine is insufficient to maintain plasma Ca^{2+}, existing bone is demineralized. In both rickets and osteomalacia, plasma Ca^{2+} is maintained by mobilization of bone Ca^{2+} under the influence of PTH. However, the anesthetist should be aware that a patient with rickets or osteomalacia is prone to develop hypocalcemic tetany. In addition, problems in airway management may be encountered as a result of bone abnormalities consequent to demineralization.

Calcitonin

Calcitonin is a protein hormone secreted by the parafollicular cells of the thyroid gland, the cells surrounding the follicular epithelial cells that secrete thyroid hormone (see Fig. 23–4B). Calcitonin is secreted in response to high plasma Ca^{2+}. The action of calcitonin is to decrease mobilization of Ca^{2+} from existing bone. Although it would make a complete picture to say that the physiologic role of calcitonin is to oppose the ability of PTH and 1,25-dihydroxycholecalciferol to raise plasma Ca^{2+}, the evidence for such a role does not exist. A calcitonin deficiency condition has yet to be identified, and patients with an excess of calcitonin secretion do not have problems in calcium metabolism. Thus, the true role (if one exists) of calcitonin in calcium metabolism is not known at present.

Parathyroidectomy

Parathyroidectomy is the only long-term treatment presently available for primary hyperparathyroidism. Normally, four parathyroid glands are present, but about 10 percent of the population are believed to have fewer or more than four. The parathyroid glands are small, commonly described individually as being the size of a split pea. Each gland measures only about 1 mm by 3 mm by 5 mm and weighs about 35 mg. In most cases, the four parathyroids are located one each behind the two upper and two lower poles of the thyroid gland (see Fig. 23–4A). The parathyroids may lie on or within the substance of the thyroid gland. However, parathyroid tissue may be located elsewhere, including as low as the superior mediastinum. The anesthetist should be prepared to cope with a pneumothorax during a parathyroidectomy, particularly if mediastinal exploration is performed. A parathyroidectomy may be a prolonged surgical procedure for any of the following four reasons:

1. The small size of the glands
2. The difficulty in distinguishing the parathyroid glands from surrounding tissue in a surgical field
3. The variation in location of the glands
4. The need to identify and examine all four parathyroid glands to determine possible involvement in hyperparathyroidism

Anesthesia for Parathyroidectomy. Preoperative care of a patient scheduled for parathyroidectomy should include careful management of fluid and electrolyte balance. Prior to surgery the vocal cords should be examined. There is no particular agent of choice for the anesthetic. However, because of the common occurrence of renal problems in hyperparathyroidism, agents such as enflurane, which may have adverse effects on the kidneys, may be contraindicated. Despite the presence of hypercalcemia in hyperparathyroid patients, the use of muscle relaxants generally has not been reported as causing any particular problems. Because of its effects on calcium in the heart, digitalis, if it is necessary, should be used with caution.

Endotracheal intubation should be carefully established so that the traction of the neck tissues may be performed without compromising the airway. Because physical trauma to the recurrent laryngeal nerves is possible during surgery, the vocal cords should be carefully examined at the end of a parathyroidectomy. The hyperparathyroid patient may have osteoporosis, so special care should be taken when the patient is positioned. The head-up position, although

it increases the possibility of air embolism, may be preferable to maintain a surgical field free of blood.

The major postoperative problem after parathyroidectomy is hypoparathyroidism, manifested by hypocalcemia. Such hypocalcemia is initially demonstrated by the neuromuscular hyperexcitability encountered in Chvostek's and Trousseau's signs and paresthesias located circumorally or in the extremities. The hypocalcemia is usually noticed 24 to 28 hours postoperatively. Treatment must be initiated to avoid frank tetany and laryngospasm. Treatment consists of administration of calcium gluconate, which may be necessary for several days until parathyroid tissue left after the surgery resumes function. If hypoparathyroidism persists, treatment is maintained with calcium salts and vitamin D therapy.

THE PANCREAS AND DIABETES

The pancreas is a flattened, elongated organ extending from the concavity of the duodenum on the right to the hilum of the spleen on the left. The pancreas is both an exocrine gland and an endocrine gland. Approximately 98 to 99 percent of the weight of the pancreas is composed of the acinar cells, which serve an exocrine function by secreting enzymes and bicarbonate into the pancreatic duct. These secretions then pass into the duodenum, where they play an important role in digestive processes. The 1 to 2 percent of the pancreatic cells with an endocrine function exist as clusters of cells known as the islets of Langerhans. The most important hormones secreted by these cells are insulin (from the B cells), glucagon (from the A cells), and somatostatin (from the D cells). As will be discussed in detail below, insulin and glucagon are intimately involved in control of intermediary metabolism. Somatostatin has been proposed to have a regulatory role in the secretion of insulin and glucagon.

It has been estimated that almost 5 percent of the U.S. population has diabetes, a disease characterized by a real or relative lack of insulin. As will be discussed later in this section of the chapter, the pathology behind the diabetes is not always the same. Because the disease is so common and because it complicates the administration of anesthesia, an understanding of the actions of insulin and the consequences of an insulin deficiency is of utmost importance for the anesthetist. Knowledge of certain basic aspects of intermediary metabolism is necessary for understanding the pathology involved in diabetes. Therefore, the following three topics will be discussed to give the student the ability to administer anesthesia in an informed fashion to diabetic patients:

1. The major events of intermediary metabolism and the effects of insulin and other hormones on these events
2. Diabetes and control of blood glucose
3. Anesthesia for diabetic patients

Metabolism and Its Control by Hormones

In a discussion of the subject of metabolism, three groups of substrates must be considered: carbohydrates, lipids (fats), and proteins. A knowledge of carbohydrate metabolism and lipid metabolism is important for understanding the development of hyperglycemia and ketoacidosis, respectively. Because knowledge of these conditions is important in proper anesthetic management of diabetic patients, carbohydrate and lipid metabolism is discussed in some detail below. A few relevant points regarding amino acid and protein metabolism will also be interspersed in this discussion.

The entry of substrates into the cell is the initial event in all metabolic pathways. Carbohydrates are generally transported into the cell as monosaccharides (i.e., glucose), fats as free fatty acids, and protein as single amino acids. Insulin stimulates the transport into the cell of all three substrate types in many organs. An absolute or relative lack of insulin and the resulting decrease in glucose transport into the cells constitute the main event producing hyperglycemia in diabetes. It should be noted that other hormones, particularly GH and the glucocorticoids, inhibit glucose transport into the cells, and an excess of these hormones may cause hyperglycemia. Once inside the cell, a substrate may be stored for later use, metabolized for energy, or converted into another type of substrate.

Carbohydrate Metabolism. In many tissues, particularly liver and muscle, glucose can be stored in a polymerized form as glycogen (Fig. 23–7). Glycogen synthesis is stimulated by insulin. Breakdown of a glycogen back to glucose is stimulated by other hormones, notably glucagon, epinephrine, and norepinephrine. The lack of insulin in diabetes decreases glycogen synthesis and allows glycogen breakdown to occur unopposed. Most of the glucose produced

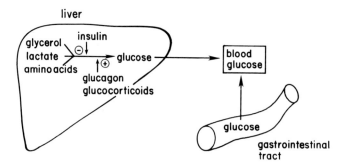

Figure 23–8. Gluconeogenesis and sources of blood glucose.

in this fashion in the liver diffuses out of the cells and adds to the hyperglycemia already present because of decreased transport of glucose into the cells.

Glucose can be metabolized by two pathways, the hexose monophosphate shunt and glycolysis. The hexose monophosphate shunt produces ribose for nucleic acid synthesis and coenzymes for lipid metabolism. However, this pathway is relatively unimportant in the present discussion and will not receive further attention.

Glycolysis is the pathway by which glucose is converted to pyruvate (aerobically) or lactate (anaerobically). The pyruvate is converted to acetyl-CoA and runs through the tricarboxylic acid (TCA) cycle for production of the reduced form of nicotinamide-adenine dinucleotide (NADH). Oxidation of NADH in the electron transport chain then yields ATP. An alternative use for the acetyl-CoA produced from glucose is the synthesis of fatty acids, which are in turn synthesized into triglycerides (see Fig. 23–7). This pathway, which is particularly important in liver and adipose tissue, is stimulated by insulin. Thus, insulin can be considered a hormone of storage, promoting synthesis of both glycogen and triglycerides from glucose. Insulin also promotes protein synthesis from amino acids in muscle and other tissues.

Most of the glucose in the blood comes directly from food that has been digested in the gastrointestinal tract. However, an additional source of glucose in the blood is that which is produced by the liver via gluconeogenesis (Fig. 23–8). Gluconeogenesis is the synthesis of "new glucose" from glycerol, lactate, and amino acids. This additional output of glucose becomes important in starvation, particularly since the brain relies on glucose as its primary energy source. Gluconeogenesis also increases in uncontrolled diabetes, and the glucose released into the blood adds to the hyperglycemia caused by the lack of glucose transport into the cells. Gluconeogenesis is inhibited by insulin and stimulated by glucagon and the glucocorticoids.

Lipid Metabolism. The triglycerides are carried in the blood as part of a lipoprotein complex. They are split into their component glycerol and fatty acids by the enzyme lipoprotein lipase. This enzyme is found in the endothelial cells of the capillaries and is particularly active in adipose tissue (Fig. 23–9). The activity of the enzyme is increased by insulin.

Depending on the tissue and the nutritional state of the individual, once inside the cell fatty acids are either resynthesized into triglycerides for intracellular storage or are metabolized for energy (see Fig. 23–9). The enzymatic

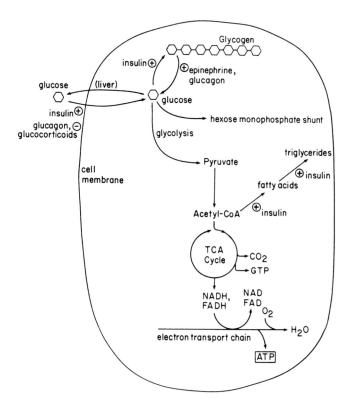

Figure 23–7. Summary of carbohydrate metabolism.

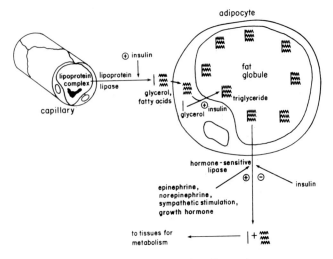

Figure 23–9. Metabolism in adipose tissue.

pathways leading to the synthesis of triglycerides for storage are particularly important in adipose tissue and liver and are activated by insulin. Triglyceride synthesis is increased in the nourished state if insulin is present and is decreased in starvation and in uncontrolled diabetes.

Those tissues such as adipose and liver, which store triglycerides, also have the capability of breaking down the triglycerides into the component fatty acids and glycerol. This process is known as lipolysis. The enzyme responsible for lipolysis, hormone-sensitive lipase, is stimulated by epinephrine, norepinephrine, and GH. In adipose tissue, the enzyme is also stimulated by increased sympathetic activity, which may be the main mechanism for lipolysis under physiologic conditions. Lipolysis via hormone-sensitive lipase is *blocked* by insulin (see Fig. 23–9). This fact is demonstrated by the release of fatty acids that can occur when there is a lack of insulin, such as in diabetes. As will be discussed below, it is the body's failure to properly metabolize large numbers of fatty acids that leads to ketoacidosis in diabetes.

In summary, the amount of lipids held in storage is controlled by two opposing enzyme systems, lipoprotein lipase and hormone-sensitive lipase. (The student should not be confused by the poor choice used in naming hormone-sensitive lipase—both enzymes are "sensitive" to hormones, but in different ways.) Lipoprotein lipase facilitates storage of triglycerides by providing the cells with a source of free fatty acids, and hormone-sensitive lipase breaks down the triglycerides, releasing the glycerol and the fatty acids into the blood. Lipoprotein lipase activity is increased by insulin. Hormone-sensitive lipase activity is increased by the catecholamines, glucagon, and GH and is decreased by insulin. It can therefore be seen that by promoting storage and preventing breakdown, insulin plays a key role in regulating the fat stores of the body.

Fat is an important component in the typical American diet, providing about 35 percent of the daily caloric requirement. Fatty acids are metabolized two carbons at a time to acetyl-CoA, which is then run through the TCA cycle. In certain situations, such as in uncontrolled diabetes, there is an excess of fatty acids and the ability of the cells to burn all of the acetyl-CoA is overcome. Particularly in the liver, the acetyl-CoA is converted into ketone bodies. Small

amounts of ketone bodies can be metabolized by the tissues, but when the supply exceeds this capability the ketone concentration in the blood increases. Two of the three "ketone" bodies, β-hydroxybutyric acid and acetoacetic acid, contain a carboxylic acid group (Fig. 23–10). If the H^+ released from these compounds is not adequately buffered, ketoacidosis results. Ketoacidosis is a severe complication of diabetes, and its treatment in relationship to anesthesia will be discussed below.

Diabetes Mellitus and Control of Blood Glucose

The disease known as diabetes mellitus has classically been subdivided into two separate forms, juvenile onset and maturity onset. Although the average age of onset of the juvenile form is 12 years and most maturity-onset cases appear after the age of 35, there is some crossover of occurrence between the two forms. It is therefore better to categorize the types of diabetes as either insulin dependent (most juvenile-onset diabetics are of this type) or insulin independent (most maturity-onset diabetics are of this type).

Insulin-dependent diabetes is characterized by pathologic changes in the B cells of the pancreatic islets that decrease the amount of insulin secreted. Insulin-dependent diabetics are more prone to develop ketoacidosis when the disease goes out of control. There are suggestions (Walker and Cudwoith, 1980; Palmers and Asplin, 1983) that at least some cases of insulin-dependent diabetes may be characterized as an autoimmune response resulting in the destruction of the B cells. Control of insulin-dependent diabetes is simplified by a regulated diet. However, the key distinguishing feature of insulin-*dependent* diabetes is that exogenous insulin is required for controlling the disease.

Insulin-independent diabetics are commonly obese. Their plasma insulin concentration may be normal or even elevated. These individuals show a decreased sensitivity to insulin that may be related to a reduced number of insulin receptors on cell membranes, particularly in adipocytes. Insulin-independent diabetics are prone to hyperglycemia but do not usually proceed into ketoacidosis, possibly because the amount of insulin present is sufficient to prevent lipolysis. Many insulin-independent diabetics can bring

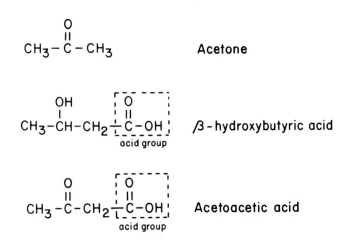

Figure 23–10. The ketone bodies.

their disease under control by losing weight and continuing dietary regulation. However, many insulin-independent diabetics must also take an oral hypoglycemic agent such as a sulfonylurea. The sulfonylureas, which include tolbutamide, stimulate insulin secretion (remember that in insulin-independent diabetics the pancreas may still have the ability to secrete normal amounts of insulin). Less commonly used are phenethylbiguanides which increase the utilization of glucose by the tissues. Although many insulin-independent diabetics rely on the oral hypoglycemic agents, these drugs have fallen into disfavor. The sulfonylureas can have adverse cardiovascular effects, and the biguanides cause lactic acidosis.

The goal in the control of diabetes is to keep the blood glucose concentration within normal limits as much as possible, since both hyperglycemia and hypoglycemia have adverse effects on the patient. Except in an absolute emergency, surgery should not be performed on a patient in hyperglycemia (with or without ketoacidosis) or hypoglycemia. Administration of anesthesia itself is greatly complicated by these conditions and should not be attempted until the patient's metabolism has been brought under control. The discussion below will describe the sequelae and treatment of hyperglycemia (with and without ketoacidosis) and hypoglycemia in the awake patient. The special problems encountered in controlling blood glucose in the perioperative period will be considered in a following section.

Hyperglycemia. Hyperglycemia may occur in any situation in which there is a relative or actual deficiency of insulin in the blood. The prime cause of the hyperglycemia is the failure of glucose to be transported into the cells. However, further increases in blood glucose occur because of the increased breakdown of glycogen and gluconeogenesis, which can occur in the liver when not enough insulin is available.

As the blood glucose concentration increases, the amount of glucose filtered in the glomeruli of the kidneys also increases, and eventually the ability of the tubules to reabsorb the glucose will be exceeded. The result is an osmotic diuresis and glycosuria (diabetes mellitus is from the Greek words *diabetes*, "a siphon," and *mali*, "honey"). However, more than just glucose is lost in the urine. As the urine flow increases, electrolytes, including sodium and potassium, are also excreted in increasing amounts. An additional consequence of the diuresis is hypovolemia, and when the plasma volume becomes very low renal function is further impaired. The patient attempts to replace the lost water by increasing the intake of water (polydipsia).

Hyperglycemia can become so severe that the extreme hyperosmolality that results may draw water out of the neurons in the brain, inducing neurologic abnormalities. Initial signs include altered mentation, areflexia, and hallucinations. The neurologic signs may proceed to seizures and ultimately coma, a condition known as hyperglycemic, hyperosmolar, nonketotic coma (HHNKC). HHNKC is more likely to occur in older insulin-independent diabetics and is rare in insulin-dependent patients. An infection or dehydration often precedes the development of HHNKC, and HHNKC frequently occurs in nondiabetic patients, particularly the elderly.

Treatment of hyperglycemia requires insulin to move glucose into the cells. Because K$^+$ may have been lost in the diuresis and because insulin directly stimulates movement of K$^+$ into the cells, it is advisable to give K$^+$ when treating hyperglycemia with insulin. If K$^+$ is not given, hypokalemia may be an unwanted result of the insulin treatment. If full-blown HHNKC has developed and hypotension has occurred, it will also be necessary to replace the lost fluids, preferably with 0.45-percent saline. The blood glucose concentration in HHNKC is often greater than 600 mg/ml, and serum osmolality may exceed 330 mOsm/L. Small doses (10 to 20 U/hr) of intravenous regular insulin will initially be effective toward lowering the blood glucose to 300 mg/100 ml, and 300 to 400 units may be required in the first 24 hours in the average patient (Moorthy, 1983). To avoid cerebral edema and other problems, the osmolality should be brought down slowly to below 320 mOsm/L in approximately 4 to 6 hours (Maw, 1975; Miller and Walts, 1980).

Hyperglycemia as a result of anxiety and the stress of surgery itself is difficult to avoid. Surgery increases the secretion of GH, ACTH, the glucocorticoids, epinephrine, norepinephrine, and glucagon. These hormones collectively act to increase blood glucose by antagonizing the utilization of glucose normally stimulated by insulin, by increasing gluconeogenesis, or by increasing glycogen breakdown in the liver. Sympathetic nervous system stimulation during surgery also increases glycogen breakdown. The degree of increase of blood glucose due to these endocrine and neural factors is proportional to the length and severity of the surgery.

Development of Ketoacidosis. Ketoacidosis in diabetics is almost always preceded and accompanied by hyperglycemia. Although there is an overabundance of glucose extracellularly in hyperglycemia, there is a paucity of it inside the cells. More commonly in insulin-dependent diabetics than in insulin-independent diabetics, other metabolic events begin to take place as the blood glucose rises. Perhaps as a means of supplying an alternate source of substrate for energy produced through metabolism, lipolysis is increased in adipose tissue. The large number of fatty acids released into the blood cannot be completely metabolized by the other tissues, and an excess of ketone bodies is generated in the liver and released into the blood. Ketoacidosis will ensue if the lipolysis and ketone body generation continue. The lipolysis that occurs is a direct consequence of the absence of insulin, and insulin replacement returns fat metabolism to normal. It is not fully understood why insulin-independent diabetics are less prone to develop ketoacidosis than insulin-dependent diabetics. It may be that the amount of insulin present in the insulin-independent individual is sufficient to prevent lipolysis (even though it may not be sufficient to prevent hyperglycemia).

Of the three types of ketone bodies produced, one, acetone, is very volatile and may be detected on the breath of a patient in ketoacidosis. The other two ketone bodies, β-hydroxybutyric acid and acetoacetic acid, contain carboxylic acid groups and must be buffered to prevent the blood pH from dropping (see Fig. 23–10). As the ketones increase in concentration, the ability to buffer the acids is exceeded and the plasma pH may drop to 7.2 or below. This may produce the deep and rapid pattern of respiratory movements known as Kussmaul's breathing. Below a plasma pH of 7.1, ventilation decreases.

The way in which the kidneys handle the ketoacidosis adds to the seriousness of the situation. The excess of ketone bodies is filtered in the glomeruli of the kidneys. Initially, the ketone bodies are excreted in the urine accompanied by either H^+ or NH_4^+. However, as more ketones are filtered, Na^+ and K^+ are also used as accompanying cations and are lost in the urine in increasing amounts. Despite the loss of K^+ in the urine, hyperkalemia may be present. The hyperkalemia is due to a movement of K^+ from inside to outside the cells as a result of insufficient insulin. The ketonuria contributes to the osmotic diuresis caused by the hyperglycemia that may be present and thus increases the degree of dehydration, hypovolemia, and hypotension.

A patient in ketoacidosis will present with thirst, polyuria, glycosuria, ketonuria, dehydration, hypovolemia, and hypotension. The patient may experience nausea and vomiting, and bowel sounds may be sparse or even absent. There may be severe abdominal pain that may mimic an acute abdomen as encountered in appendicitis. However, when the abdominal pain is caused purely by ketoacidosis, it will disappear completely with appropriate treatment of the ketoacidosis (Campbell et al, 1975). Muscle tone is decreased and reflexes are depressed. Central nervous system signs may include headache, drowsiness, stupor, and coma.

Treatment of Ketoacidosis. Treatment of ketoacidosis includes a three-pronged attack: (I) insulin replacement, (II) fluid replacement, and (III) potassium replacement.

I. The need for treatment with insulin in a patient in ketoacidosis is paramount, since only insulin can bring the underlying metabolic abnormality under control. Insulin will have the following effects in returning the patient to a physiologic state:
   A. Insulin will bring blood glucose down to normal levels by
      1. stimulating glucose transport into the cells,
      2. increasing glucose metabolism by the cells,
      3. decreasing gluconeogenesis in the liver, and
      4. increasing glycogen synthesis and decreasing glycogen breakdown in the liver.
   B. Insulin will lower the plasma concentration of ketone bodies by
      1. increasing uptake of ketones by the cells
      2. decreasing ketogenesis in the liver
      3. decreasing lipolysis in adipose tissue
      4. increasing lipid synthesis in adipose tissue and liver.
   C. Insulin will move K^+ into the cells, alleviating the hyperkalemia that may have been present (this is also the reason why K^+ must be given to prevent *hypo*kalemia).

      The preferred route of administration of insulin to treat ketoacidosis is a continuous intravenous infusion of short-acting insulin at a rate of 5 to 6 U/hr. Administration via a syringe pump is much preferable to a drip, since insulin adheres to plastic tubing and the amount of tubing is minimized by using a syringe pump. Alternative plans for administration of insulin in ketoacidosis combine intravenous infusion

with intramuscular injections (Hayes, 1982). The effectiveness of the insulin should be monitored by hourly analysis using reagent strips to measure the blood glucose (Dextrostix) and ketone bodies (Ketostix). The dose of insulin given can be adjusted according to the results of these tests. The results obtained from the reagent strips should be compared periodically with determinations made from blood sent to the clinical laboratory. Monitoring hyperglycemia and ketoacidosis by measurement of urine glucose and ketones is unwise, because catheterization is necessary in order to obtain freshly formed urine for accurate determinations. Diabetics are particularly prone to urinary tract infections, especially after catheterization. In addition, the hypoglycemia that may occur as a result of excess insulin administration cannot be detected by urine glucose measurements.

II. Fluid replacement is best achieved using isotonic saline. Rapid replacement of fluids should be avoided (Maw, 1975; Miller and Walts, 1980). A recommended rate of replacement is to give the first liter in 30 minutes, the second liter in 1 hour, a third liter in the next 2 hours, and 500 ml every 4 hours (Ahern and Walker, 1980).

III. As indicated above, potassium must be given when treating ketoacidosis because of the amount lost in the urine and to avoid the hypokalemia that would result from movement of the ion into the cells. A recommended rate of administration of potassium is 13 mmol in the first liter of intravenous fluid. This should be doubled if the plasma potassium falls below 4 mmol/L, and it should be stopped if the level rises to above 6 mmol/L (Ahern and Walker, 1980). Monitoring the ECG will be useful in following the course of the potassium treatment.

   Since treatment with insulin and fluids will usually correct the acidosis, administration of bicarbonate is generally unnecessary. Bicarbonate may even be detrimental since it may cause alkalosis some time into the recovery from the acidosis. However, if the blood pH is less than 7.0, 50 mmol of bicarbonate may be given with potassium (Hayes, 1982).

Hypoglycemia. Hypoglycemia among diabetics occurs most often in insulin-dependent patients and in insulin-independent patients taking long-acting oral hypoglycemic agents (the sulfonylureas). The basic cause of hypoglycemia in either case is an excess of insulin relative to the needs of the individual. The result is an increased movement of glucose into the cells and a decrease in the concentration of glucose in the blood. In the case of insulin-dependent diabetics, hypoglycemia may be a result of too strong an insulin injection, an unusual alteration in dietary habit, or participation in unanticipated exercise. Among insulin-independent diabetics, hypoglycemia is most likely to occur as a result of altered food intake or an incorrect dosage of the oral hypoglycemic agent. These factors are particularly prevalent in elderly patients who are chronically malnourished, have existing arteriosclerosis, have underlying renal or hepatic disease, or are taking drugs (such as alcohol and propranolol) that by themselves may cause hypoglycemia. Patients with arteriosclerosis are prone to hypoglycemic episodes since they may already have marginal cerebral blood flow. Renal and hepatic disease contribute to hypoglycemia because the kidneys and the liver are very important in the degradation of insulin. If these organs are diseased, the insulin that is in the blood will be effective longer and thus the possibility for hypoglycemia is increased. In addition, the liver stores a large amount of glycogen. If the amount of glycogen stored is decreased (as it often is in hepatic disease), the ability of the liver to break down glycogen into glucose and release it into the blood is decreased. Thus, one of the key homeostatic mechanisms for maintaining the blood glucose concentration and preventing hypoglycemia will have been lost.

The student should be aware that there are many other causes of hypoglycemia other than those that have been discussed here. Additional potential causes include abnormal gastric function, the presence of an insulin-secreting tumor, and hypofunction of endocrine organs (deficiencies of glucocorticoids, glucagon, and catecholamines). A more detailed discussion of hypoglycemia and its causes may be found in a textbook of clinical endocrinology.

Recognition of Hypoglycemia. The symptoms of hypoglycemia generally first appear when the blood glucose concentration falls to less than 45 mg/100 ml. However, the blood glucose level at which a given patient shows signs of hypoglycemia is variable and is influenced by factors such as the rate at which the blood glucose falls and the actual level and duration of hypoglycemia.

The clinical signs of hypoglycemia are initially neurologic. The brain is heavily dependent on glucose as an energy source, so that any deprivation will affect neural function. The initial signs may include tremor, sweating, nervousness, weakness, hunger, palpitations, tachycardia, diaphoresis, blurred vision, diplopia, mental confusion, violent behavior, and inappropriate affect. If the hypoglycemic episode continues, coma may ensue. Death may result from failure of the cardiorespiratory control centers in the brain stem.

Treatment of Hypoglycemia. If the individual is conscious and cooperative, hypoglycemia can be treated by simply having the person swallow some glucose (which may be given in the form of juice or a couple of sugar cubes)—10 to 20 g of glucose should be sufficient. In a patient who is unable to swallow, 25 g of glucose should be given intravenously. In a violent patient, 1 mg of glucagon may be injected subcutaneously for initial treatment, followed by oral or intravenous glucose.

If the hypoglycemia was not too long in duration, in most cases a return to normoglycemia will reverse the patient's signs and symptoms. The recovery may be immediate, as in mild cases of hypoglycemia, or it may take a period of days if the hypoglycemia was severe. Particularly in patients taking long-acting oral hypoglycemic agents, care must be taken that there is not an immediate recurrence of hypoglycemia. Because prolonged hypoglycemia may cause neuronal death and thus permanent brain damage, it is extremely important to initiate treatment of hypoglyce-

mia as soon as the condition is recognized. If a patient remains unconscious even after treatment for hypoglycemia, it may be that cerebral edema has developed. In such a case, mannitol may be given intravenously to reduce the edema.

Except when the urgency of the situation demands it, patients who are hypoglycemic should not be anesthetized for surgery until the blood glucose has been normalized. There are two reasons why hypoglycemia should be corrected before administering anesthesia. The first and most important reason is that prolonged hypoglycemia can cause permanent brain damage. The second reason is that most of the neurologic and behavioral symptoms that are present in the awake individual are not present in an anesthetized patient. This makes the diagnosis of hypoglycemia much more difficult and therefore increases the risk of brain damage if a hypoglycemic episode occurs intraoperatively.

If a patient is in need of emergency surgery, hypoglycemia can be treated by an IV bolus of up to 50 ml of 50 percent dextrose, followed by establishment of an IV line of 10 percent dextrose. Although reversal of symptoms should occur quickly, a second bolus injection may be needed. Because the hypoglycemia was most likely caused by an excess of insulin or of an oral hypoglycemic agent, the patient should be monitored closely in case the hypoglycemia recurs. Because of the inherent difficulty of recognizing hypoglycemia under anesthesia, the optimal intraoperative blood glucose concentration range is 150 to 250 mg/ml. This is slightly higher than the normal blood glucose of 100 mg/ml, but it decreases the possibility of a hypoglycemic episode. Should the blood glucose fall below 150 mg/100 ml intraoperatively, more glucose can be given (or if insulin is being administered, the amount of insulin given can be decreased). If the blood glucose exceeds 250 mg/100 ml, the delivery of glucose to the patient should be decreased or the administration of insulin increased or both.

Control of Blood Glucose Perioperatively. The key to proper metabolic management of a diabetic patient undergoing surgery is frequent measurement of blood glucose, with insulin and glucose being given to the patient as needed to maintain the blood glucose within the desired range. Blood glucose measurement should be made before surgery, hourly during surgery, and hourly postoperatively until oral feeding has been resumed. The importance of monitoring the patient carefully postoperatively cannot be overemphasized. Any prolonged abnormal blood glucose level following surgery will make intraoperative vigilance totally meaningless.

Glucose oxidase (Dextrostix®) is suitable for glucose measurement, although care must be taken that the determinations are accurate. This may be done by periodically comparing the glucose oxidase values with those derived from blood samples sent to the clinical laboratory. The amount of insulin or glucose that must be administered to maintain blood glucose can then be based in confidence on the glucose oxidase measurements. Should hyperglycemia occur, testing for ketone bodies with ketone oxidase (Ketostix®) should also be performed. Periodically in the past, the recommendation has been made that insulin and glucose administration during surgery be based on a sliding scale dependent on urinary glucose. However, the urinary glucose concentration value is at best a late reflection of blood glucose and therefore is an unreliable basis on which to manage a patient.

The two most important factors to be considered in determining the best means of management of the blood glucose in a diabetic patient undergoing surgery are (1) the patient's history with regard to means of blood glucose control and (2) the duration and nature of the surgery. A variety of regimens for managing diabetics during anesthesia have been postulated. A few possible guidelines for blood glucose management are offered below.

Insulin-Independent Diabetics. A patient whose diabetes is successfully controlled by diet alone needs no special metabolic management for minor surgery (Hayes, 1982). A patient whose diabetes is treated by long-acting oral hypoglycemic agents should be switched to short-acting agents a few days before minor surgery. No hypoglycemic agent should be given the morning of the operation, and treatment should be resumed when the patient is able to eat. If it should become necessary to give a carbohydrate-containing infusion during the surgery, then insulin should also be given to prevent hyperglycemia from developing.

An insulin-independent diabetic patient scheduled for a major surgical procedure should be switched from oral hypoglycemic agents to regular insulin several days before surgery. Such a patient should then be treated in the same manner as an insulin-dependent patient undergoing major surgery (discussed below).

Insulin-Dependent Diabetics. In managing an insulin-dependent diabetic patient during surgery, it is important for the anesthetist to have as much control over the blood glucose as possible. This is particularly true with respect to the ability to respond quickly to changes in blood glucose. It is important to be as certain as possible about the length of action of any administered insulin. No intermediate- or long-acting insulin should be given before or during surgery, since the duration of a hypoglycemic episode that occurs perioperatively may be prolonged.

It is important that the route by which insulin is administered be the most reliable with respect to time of action. Because of the many factors that may influence cutaneous blood flow during and after surgery (i.e., stress, temperature regulatory mechanisms, and anesthetics and other drugs), it is inadvisable to administer insulin subcutaneously. For example, a sudden increase in cutaneous blood flow may cause an increased release of insulin from a subcutaneous insulin depot, resulting in a hypoglycemic episode. Therefore, the best route by which to give insulin is intravenously. This may be done through a regular intravenous line or via a syringe pump. There has been some concern about the fact that some insulin adheres to the administration tubing. Obviously, the shorter the tubing used the less adhesion will occur. A delivery of up to 90 percent of the available insulin has been demonstrated when a constant infusion pump with a plastic syringe is used (Taitelman et al, 1977).

It is preferable to use separate intravenous delivery systems for insulin and for glucose so that adjustments of the two to maintain blood glucose can be made independently. Unless it is necessary to combat severe hyperglyce-

mia, it is best not to use large bolus injections of insulin. Such injections result in uncertainty in blood glucose management by increasing the likelihood of hypoglycemia in the short run. In addition, because the half-life of insulin in the circulation is only 5 minutes, there may be a need for further injections when the insulin from the first injection is no longer effective.

The actual amounts of glucose and insulin that should be given will vary from patient to patient. Miller and Walts (1980) have suggested a glucose infusion of 2 ml/kg/hr of 5 percent dextrose (which is approximately 100 mg/kg/hr) piggyback into a non–dextrose-containing fluid. These authors recommend not giving insulin preoperatively and, if blood glucose exceeds 250 mg/dl, administering single injections of IV insulin, 1 to 2 U/hr. If blood glucose drops below 150 mg/dl, more glucose can be given.

Another recommended plan (Hayes, 1982) in treating insulin-dependent diabetics perioperatively is to begin glucose and insulin administration at the time of the first missed meal at the following rates: 5 percent dextrose infusion delivering 1 L/8 hr and an infusion (syringe pump recommended) of short-acting insulin at the rate of 1 to 3 U/hr.

Another recommendation (Taitelman et al, 1977) (based on a study of insulin-dependent patients undergoing orthopedic procedures) is to give 5 percent dextrose at the rate of 500 ml during the first hour after induction and at the rate of 125 ml/hr during the following 4 hours. In this study, insulin was administered either preoperatively as two-thirds of the regular dose of neutral protamine Hagedorn (NPH) insulin subcutaneously or via an infusion pump at the rate of either 1 U/hr or 2 U/hr (1 U/hr if the patient normally received 20 U/day or less and 2 U/hr if the normal dose was greater than 20 U/day). For those patients receiving 2 U/hr, diabetic control was better (on average) than for those receiving the subcutaneous shot. In those patients receiving 1 U/hr, diabetic control was equivalent to that of patients receiving the subcutaneous treatment.

Although recommendations regarding perioperative management of diabetics have been made and some specific examples of treatment have been cited, it is important to remember that the insulin and glucose needs of every patient will be unique. These needs will be a function of the normal means of metabolic control and will be influenced by the nature of the surgery. Trouble can best be avoided by close attention to the metabolism of the patients as monitored by frequent determinations of blood glucose and appropriate adjustments in the amounts of insulin and glucose given.

Anesthesia for Diabetic Patients. The most important consideration in the handling of a diabetic patient in the perioperative period is the maintenance of the metabolic state. If the blood glucose is maintained within normal limits and ketoacidosis is avoided, anesthesia may in most cases be handled as it would be for a nondiabetic patient. Some general anesthetics themselves have hyperglycemic effects, but the degree is relatively minor compared with the hyperglycemia caused by the surgical intervention. Thus, if a general anesthetic is needed, the choice of which one to use can be made on general medical grounds. Spinal and local anesthesia have very little effect on blood glucose. Therefore, with regard to consideration of the metabolic management of a diabetic patient in surgery, spinal or local anesthesia may be preferable to general anesthesia when possible. Muscle relaxants and premedications generally have little effect on blood glucose. It should be noted that a major part of the physiologic response to combat hypoglycemia involves a sympathetically mediated breakdown of glycogen in the liver. Any diabetic who is taking β-blockers such as propranolol may show a deficient response to a declining blood glucose and be more inclined to develop hypoglycemia when an excess of insulin has been given perioperatively.

THE ADRENAL GLANDS

The adrenal glands are composed of two embryologically and functionally distinct glands, the adrenal cortex and the adrenal medulla. The adrenal cortex is derived from mesoderm and secretes three types of steroid hormones— mineralocorticoids, glucocorticoids, and androgens. The adrenal medulla is derived from ectoderm and is functionally an important part of the sympathetic nervous system, secreting the catecholamines norepinephrine and epinephrine. The adrenal cortex is wrapped around the medulla like a shell.

The adrenal glands sit one atop each kidney. The right adrenal has a close relationship with the inferior vena cava, the right crus of the diaphragm, and the liver. The left gland is close to the tail of the pancreas, the peritoneum, the stomach, and the left crus of the diaphragm. The adrenals have a very rich blood supply, receiving branches from the phrenic and renal arteries and from branches directly off of the aorta. The venous return is to the inferior vena cava on the right and the renal vein on the left. A unique aspect of the venous drainage of the adrenal cortex is that the blood drains through sinusoids into the adrenal medulla before passing into the adrenal vein. This fact is functionally important because the glucocorticoids secreted by the adrenal cortex are necessary for the synthesis of epinephrine from norepinephrine by the adrenal medulla.

Although they are anatomically related, the adrenal cortex and adrenal medulla are quite distinct in the physiologic parameters that each affects in the body. This section of the chapter will deal with the adrenal cortex.

The Adrenal Cortex

The adrenal cortex consists of three histologically distinct layers, which from the outer surface inward consist of the zona glomerulosa, the zona fasciculata, and the zona reticularis. The zona glomerulosa secretes primarily mineralocorticoids, whereas the inner two zones secrete both glucocorticoids and androgens. Although many other hormones are secreted in lesser amounts, the major hormones secreted by the adrenal cortex are aldosterone, cortisol, corticosterone, and dehydroepiandrosterone. Aldosterone is a mineralocorticoid, cortisol and corticosterone are glucocorticoids, and dehydroepiandrosterone is an androgen. Small amounts of estrogen may also be secreted by the adrenal cortex.

Aldosterone. The major action of aldosterone is on the kidney, where it increases the reabsorption of Na^+ in exchange for K^+ and H^+ in the distal convoluted tubules

and collecting ducts. Water is reabsorbed with the sodium, thereby expanding the extracellular fluid volume. The amount of K^+ and H^+ in the urine increases under the influence of aldosterone. It should be noted that aldosterone has no effect on Na^+ reabsorption in the proximal convoluted tubule or loop of Henle of the nephron.

Aldosterone also affects the ionic composition of saliva, gastric secretions, and sweat, although these actions are minor compared with the actions on the kidneys.

Secretion of Aldosterone. There are four factors that regulate the secretion of aldosterone: ACTH, the plasma concentrations of Na^+ and K^+, and the renin–angiotensin system. The role of ACTH in regulation of aldosterone secretion is of some importance, but it is not the major factor. Low plasma Na^+ concentrations increase the secretion of aldosterone, although it is doubtful that the low level of Na^+ needed for the secretion is reached under physiologic conditions. Increased plasma K^+, within levels reached on a normal diet, increases aldosterone secretion in the renin–angiotensin system.

Renin is a protein hormone secreted by the juxtaglomerular cells of the kidney. These cells are located in the afferent arterioles, in close association with the distal convoluted tubules. Renin is secreted in response to the following factors:

1. Decreased pressure in the afferent arteriole such as might occur in hypotension, hemorrhage, dehydration, or renal artery stenosis
2. Decreased passage of Na^+ and Cl^- in the distal tubules
3. Stimulation of the sympathetic nerves to the kidneys
4. Prostaglandins.

Renin acts on a globulin secreted by the liver to produce angiotensin I (Fig. 23–11). Angiotensin I is a decapeptide and is shortened to angiotensin II by converting enzyme, which is high in activity in the lungs. Angiotensin II is the physiologic end point of the renin–angiotensin system, acting to increase the secretion of aldosterone from the adrenal cortex (angiotensin II also causes constriction of arterioles, increasing blood pressure). The aldosterone that is secreted then acts on the kidney to increase sodium re-

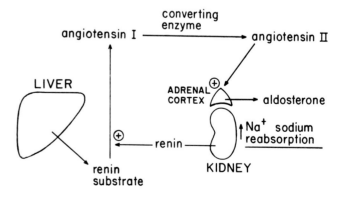

Figure 23–11. Control of aldosterone secretion by the renin–angiotensin system: Renin increases production of angiotensin I from renin substrate, which is converted to angiotensin II. Angiotensin II increases aldosterone secretion from the adrenal cortex.

sorption, restoring the blood pressure or state of hydration to normal and shutting off the original stimulus for renin secretion.

Excess Aldosterone Secretion. An excess of aldosterone (or other adrenal cortex hormones with mineralocorticoid activity) leads to an elevation of diastolic blood pressure because of the extracellular fluid volume expansion that occurs. Because of the exchange of K^+ for Na^+ when the resorption of Na^+ increases in the kidney, the excretion of K^+ increases and hypokalemia develops. A metabolic alkalosis develops, both because of increased H^+ excretion by the kidney (in exchange for Na^+ reabsorption) and because of movement of H^+ into the cells to replace K^+ that has been lost. In addition to diastolic hypertension, hypokalemia, and alkalosis, other signs and symptoms of hyperaldosteronism may include muscle weakness, fatigue, tetany (due to the lowering of plasma Ca^{2+} by the alkalosis) paralytic ileus, and headache. The hypokalemia may cause impaired renal function leading to polyuria and polydipsia. The hypokalemia may also contribute to the appearance of cardiac arrhythmias, including flattened T waves, prominent U waves, prolongation of the QT intervals, and depression of ST segments (Maddi and Gabel, 1980). The hypokalemia also results in altered insulin secretion in many patients, and glucose tolerance may be impaired.

For unknown reasons, an excess of aldosterone is in most cases self-limiting in its effect on Na^+ reabsorption, an occurrence known as the escape phenomenon. The significance of the escape phenomenon is that many patients with hyperaldosteronism will develop hypertension, but fewer than 10 percent of the patients develop edema (Weinberger et al, 1979).

Hyperaldosteronism may be primary, due usually to adrenal hyperplasia or adenoma, or secondary, due to activation of the renin–angiotensin system. Primary hyperaldosteronism is known as Conn's syndrome. Primary and secondary hyperaldosteronism can be distinguished from each other in part by considering the plasma levels of aldosterone, renin, and angiotensin. In primary hyperaldosteronism, the plasma level of aldosterone is high but the levels of renin and angiotensin are not. In secondary hyperaldosteronism, the plasma levels of all three of these hormones are elevated. In either primary or secondary hyperaldosteronism, measurement of the excretion of metabolites of aldosterone in the urine may be more useful than determination of the plasma concentration of the hormone itself.

Treatment of Hyperaldosteronism. Treatment of primary hyperaldosteronism may be managed medically with spironolactone, an aldosterone antagonist that inhibits the Na^+–K^+ exchange mechanism in the kidney. It may also be necessary to administer potassium supplements to correct the hypokalemia. Medical treatment of secondary hyperaldosteronism can be achieved with a drug such as indomethacin, which inhibits the synthesis of prostaglandins and thus decreases the secretion of renin by the kidney. An alternative medical treatment for secondary hyperaldosteronism involves administration of potassium and triamterene (which inhibits the secretion of K^+ by the kidneys). Spironolactone may be given, and propranolol has been used to block the secretion of renin (Block and Montgomery, 1982).

The value of surgery for treatment of hyperaldosteronism depends on the specific pathology involved. Surgical removal is called for in the presence of an adenoma or carcinoma secreting aldosterone. After removal of an adenoma, blood pressure is significantly reduced in most patients (Biglieri et al, 1970; Hunt et al, 1975) and the electrolyte abnormalities are reversed in virtually all patients (Ferris et al, 1978). In patients with idiopathic hyperaldosteronism or hyperplasia, the results of surgery are poor. If bilateral adrenalectomy is being considered, it should be recognized that the problems involved in total replacement of all the adrenal hormones may be worse than medical management of the isolated aldosterone excess (Shipton and Hugo, 1982).

Anesthesia for Primary Hyperaldosteronism. The key preoperative consideration in preparing a patient with primary hyperaldosteronism for surgery is correction of any existing hypokalemia and hypertension. The acid–base status of the condition should also be carefully considered. The choice of the anesthetic may be made on general medical grounds. Because of the proximity of the adrenal glands to the pleural cavity, respiratory management should include tracheal intubation and controlled respiration. Right atrial pressure or pulmonary artery pressure should be monitored by an appropriately placed catheter to assess intravascular fluid volume.

After surgery for hyperaldosteronism, it may be necessary for the patient to receive a mineralocorticoid such as fludrocortisone. If extensive manipulation of the adrenals was necessary during surgery or if a considerable amount of adrenal tissue was removed, a glucocorticoid may also be necessary postoperatively.

Additional considerations regarding adrenal surgery may be found later in the section of this chapter on anesthesia for patients with Cushing's syndrome.

The Glucocorticoids. The two major glucocorticoids secreted by the adrenal cortex are cortisol and corticosterone. The amount of cortisol secreted is about seven times greater than the amount of corticosterone secreted. Because the effects of cortisol and corticosterone are fairly similar, in this section of the chapter the more general term *glucocorticoid* will be used to describe the actions of both hormones. The term *glucocorticoid* is an appropriate name, since these hormones are involved in the control of intermediary metabolism. However, as will be discussed in the following paragraphs, the glucocorticoids also affect many other functions.

Effects on Intermediary Metabolism. The glucocorticoids have a number of important effects on the metabolism of carbohydrates, fat, and protein. The overall action the glucocorticoids have on carbohydrate metabolism is to increase the blood glucose concentration, acting in opposition to insulin. The glucocorticoids decrease utilization of glucose by many peripheral tissues. In the liver, glucocorticoids increase the formation of glucose from amino acids and glycerol by the process known as gluconeogenesis. Although the glucocorticoids increase the amount of glycogen stored in the liver, the extent of the decreased utilization of glucose in other tissues and the gluconeogenesis in the liver is such that the blood glucose concentration rises. Patients with an excess of glucocorticoids may show altered glucose tolerance curves and may even be classified as diabetic because of the glucocorticoids.

The glucocorticoids increase the breakdown of proteins in a number of tissues. Many of the amino acids released are converted to glucose in the liver (gluconeogenesis). An excess breakdown of protein may be deleterious, causing wasting and weakness in skeletal muscle, osteoporosis in bone, creatinuria, and a negative nitrogen balance.

Glucocorticoids promote deposition of fat, but in excess a characteristic redistribution known as truncal obesity occurs. In this condition, the fat depots in the abdomen, trunk, shoulders, and cheeks are enlarged but those in the extremities are smaller.

Effects on Water and Electrolyte Metabolism. The glucocorticoids have important actions on the kidney, facilitating the excretion of a water load. The glucocorticoids increase glomerular filtration and decrease reabsorption of water by the renal tubules, both actions that increase the volume of urine formed. A patient who has adrenal cortical insufficiency will be unable to excrete a water load in the same amount of time as a normal person and may develop water intoxication. The glucocorticoids also exert a weak mineralocorticoid activity on the kidney, increasing the reabsorption of sodium and increasing potassium excretion.

Permissive Actions and the Cardiovascular System. In order to comprehend the effects of the glucocorticoids on the cardiovascular system, a phenomenon known as the "permissive" actions of the glucocorticoids must be understood. There are a group of physiologic functions not directly controlled by the glucocorticoids but which in the presence of other stimulatory factors (such as other hormones) are "permitted" to occur by the glucocorticoids. The permissive actions of the glucocorticoids include many of the functions stimulated by the catecholamines, some gastrointestinal functions, and nervous system activity.

Perhaps the most important permissive actions of the glucocorticoids are those involved in cardiovascular function. The glucocorticoids maintain vascular reactivity to the catecholamines and are thereby important in blood pressure regulation.

Effects on Hematologic and Lymphatic Tissue. Glucocorticoids decrease the number of circulating basophils, eosinophils, and lymphocytes but increase the number of erythrocytes, platelets, and neutrophils.

Pharmacologic Effects of the Glucocorticoids. Many of the more familiar effects of the glucocorticoids on the inflammatory response and the immune system occur only at pharmacologic doses of the hormones. The glucocorticoids decrease the amount of histamine released by mast cells in the response to antigen–antibody complexes. Since histamine is responsible for many of the unpleasant manifestations of allergic reactions, this action of the glucocorticoids is very important.

The glucocorticoids are believed to stabilize lysosomal membranes. Lysosomes are cellular organelles that basically are membrane-lined bags of very powerful proteolytic enzymes. Release of these enzymes may cause damage in the tissues, so by stabilizing lysosomal membranes the glucocorticoids help prevent such damage.

The glucocorticoids decrease the activity of fibroblasts and so may be of use in the prevention of keloid formation and adhesions after surgery.

A note of caution is necessary in the consideration of the use of glucocorticoids in any situation in which a bacterial infection may be present. Although the glucocorticoids may in some cases relieve many of the symptoms of such infections, including fever, toxin effects, and the effects of released histamine, the hormones do not have bactericidal actions. Thus, inappropriate use of glucocorticoids in the presence of a bacterial infection may relieve the symptoms but will allow the infection to spread.

Regulation of Secretion of the Glucocorticoids. Secretion of the glucocorticoids is under the control of ACTH, which is secreted by the anterior pituitary (Fig. 23–12). Under the influence of ACTH, the adrenal cortex (the zona fasciculata and the zona reticularis) secretes increasing amounts of glucocorticoids. In the absence of ACTH, the secretion of glucocorticoids is decreased. In a situation in which ACTH is absent for a prolonged period of time, the adrenal cortex atrophies and fails to secrete an adequate amount of glucocorticoids when ACTH is again present. After a period of absence of ACTH stimulation, it may take some time for the adrenal cortex to readapt to appropriate responsiveness to ACTH.

Secretion of ACTH is increased by corticotropin-releasing hormone (CRH). CRH is produced in the hypothalamus and secreted into the hypothalamohypophyseal portal vessel, down which it passes to the anterior pituitary, where it increases ACTH secretion (see Fig. 23–12). Secretion of CRH is increased in a number of stressful situations by neural inputs that act on the hypothalamus.

The glucocorticoids exert feedback to directly inhibit the secretion of both CRH from the hypothalamus and ACTH from the pituitary (the decrease of CRH secretion further decreases the secretion of ACTH). This situation

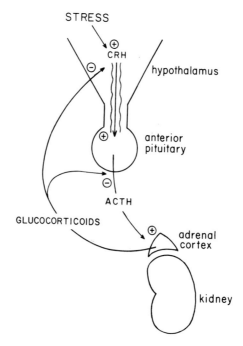

Figure 23–12. Regulation of glucocorticoid secretion.

is a classic negative-feedback cycle. It should be clear that a problem in the secretion of glucocorticoids may be primary, as in the case of adrenal disease, or secondary, due to a problem in the hypothalamus or pituitary. For example, hyposecretion of glucocorticoids in the presence of normal or high levels of ACTH is a sign of adrenal disease. On the other hand, hyposecretion of glucocorticoids accompanied by low levels of ACTH is an indication of pituitary or hypothalamic disease.

Circadian Rhythm of Glucocorticoid Secretion. The secretion in stressful situations of CRH, then ACTH, and finally the glucocorticoids is superimposed on a basal level of secretion. A characteristic of this basal level of secretion is the circadian rhythm that exists. The peak secretion of glucocorticoids with respect to the circadian rhythm occurs in the early morning hours. In determining the status of adrenal function, it is important to take the circadian rhythm into account.

Excess Secretion of Glucocorticoids: Cushing's Syndrome. An excess secretion of glucocorticoids from the adrenal cortex causes a characteristic condition known as Cushing's syndrome. Many of the clinical findings in Cushing's syndrome can be described as an exaggeration of the normal actions of the hormones.

The protein catabolism encountered in Cushing's syndrome leads to skeletal muscle weakness and wasting, osteoporosis, purpura, and ecchymoses. Wound healing is very poor. Because of the decreased peripheral utilization of glucose and increased gluconeogenesis in the liver, glucose tolerance may be abnormal in about 20 percent of cases and characteristic of diabetes in 10 percent of cases. Alterations in fat metabolism lead to truncal obesity, with a characteristic moon face appearance, pendulous abdomen, and fat hump on the back (sometimes described as a buffalo hump).

Arterial hypertension is present in most patients with Cushing's syndrome, and heart failure and other circulatory problems may result. The glucocorticoids may cause hypertension because of effects on blood vessels or because of mineralocorticoid effects that may be exerted. Sodium is retained, and hypokalemia may also be present.

Other abnormalities encountered in Cushing's syndrome include hirsutism, menstrual abnormalities, acceleration of EEG rhythms, mental disturbances, and an increased incidence of infections.

TREATMENT OF CUSHING'S SYNDROME. Treatment of Cushing's syndrome depends on the type of pathology involved. If the cause is excess ACTH secretion by the pituitary, radiation therapy or partial transsphenoidal hypophysectomy would be the appropriate treatment. If the pathology is in the adrenal gland, removal of the involved gland (or glands) is the only long-term treatment that has been successful. Medical suppression of hypersecreting adrenals with agents such as DDD or aminoglutethimide has not been very successful.

ANESTHESIA FOR PATIENTS WITH CUSHING'S SYNDROME. Careful attention must be paid to preoperative treatment of a number of the medical problems that may exist in a patient with excess secretion of glucocorticoids. The underlying abnormalities in intermediary metabolism may necessitate treatment with insulin and glucose in the perioperative period. Existing hypertension may be treated with diuretics. The patient may be hypokalemic as a consequence of some mineralocorticoid action of the excess adrenal hormones, so potassium supplementation should be given preoperatively. The acid–base state of the patient should be evaluated and corrected, if necessary. Osteoporosis is a common occurrence in patients with Cushing's syndrome, and evidence of this condition should be sought preoperatively from radiographs. Awareness of the possibility of existing osteoporosis underscores the care that should be taken in positioning a patient with Cushing's syndrome to avoid fractures.

Preoperative medications and the anesthetic agent may be chosen on general medical grounds. Because muscle weakness and hypokalemia are characteristic of Cushing's syndrome, the dose of a muscle relaxant used should initially be low (Tasch, 1983). The status of the neuromuscular block should be monitored periodically with a nerve stimulator.

Mechanical ventilation is recommended during adrenal surgery for two major reasons. First, the combination of muscle weakness and truncal obesity in Cushing's syndrome may make spontaneous respiration difficult during surgery. The second reason is related to the position of the adrenal glands in front of the posterior diaphragmatic recess of the pleura. The possibility of pneumothorax is increased, and mechanical ventilation will be necessary to deal with the situation intraoperatively. It is advisable to examine a chest x-ray in the recovery room to be sure that a pneumothorax has not occurred.

Even if some adrenal tissue is left intact after adrenal surgery (as it would be in partial or unilateral adrenalectomy), it will be necessary to begin treating the patient with glucocorticoids intraoperatively. The reason for this is that the remaining adrenal cortical tissue becomes hypoactive in the presence of the hyperactive tissue secretions during the long period preceding diagnosis of the disease. For the same reason, treatment with glucocorticoids will immediately be necessary postoperatively. It may also be necessary to administer a mineralocorticoid postoperatively.

Adrenal Androgens. Steroid hormones classified as androgens are secreted by the adrenal cortex in both males and females. The adrenal androgen secreted in the largest amount is dehydroepiandrosterone, although this hormone has less than 20 percent of the activity of the gonadal androgen testosterone. The function of the adrenal androgens is not clearly understood. Androgens are generally referred to as the "male" sex hormones. However, this categorization may be inappropriate in the case of the adrenal androgens, since the amount of hormones secreted in females is normally as high as two-thirds of what it is in males. Thus, it seems unlikely that the adrenal androgens are serving an exclusively male function. It is possible that the adrenal androgens have a predominately metabolic function in both sexes, promoting actions such as protein synthesis and growth. The adrenal androgens may also be involved in sexual maturation at puberty.

When the adrenal androgens are secreted in excess, problems arise and the androgenic nature of the hormones becomes most apparent. Excess adrenal androgens result in the condition known as the adrenogenital syndrome. In females, this condition is characterized by an increasingly masculine appearance, including clitoral enlargement, the development of a masculine distribution of body hair, and baldness. Excess adrenal androgens in adult males cause accentuation of male secondary characteristics and in prepuberal males cause precocious development of these characteristics.

The adrenogenital syndrome may be a result of an adrenal tumor or an enzyme deficiency in the pathway for synthesis of the adrenal hormones. An understanding of how the condition develops in the presence of an enzyme deficiency is based on a knowledge of the synthetic pathway for adrenal hormone synthesis and of the control of adrenal cortex secretion by ACTH from the pituitary. As discussed earlier in this section of the chapter, secretion of glucocorticoids from the adrenal cortex is stimulated by ACTH, and the glucocorticoids in turn exert feedback to inhibit the secretion of ACTH. If glucocorticoids are not secreted by the adrenals, ACTH secretion remains elevated. If an enzyme deficiency exists in the synthetic pathway for the glucocorticoids, the continuous stimulation by ACTH that results from a lack of feedback inhibition causes a buildup of the intermediates in the synthetic pathway for the glucocorticoids. In the normal state, some of these intermediates are synthesized into androgens. If there is a buildup of the intermediates, as would occur in the presence of an enzyme deficiency, there is an increased production of the adrenal androgens and the adrenogenital syndrome may result (Fig. 23–13). Treatment of such an enzyme deficiency is by the administration of cortisol. Since cortisol inhibits the secretion of ACTH, the buildup of synthetic intermediates in the adrenal cortex declines and the secretion of androgens also drops.

The adrenogenital syndrome may be accompanied by either an excess or deficiency of mineralocorticoid secretion, and if a deficiency exists, it may be necessary to treat the patient with a mineralocorticoid as well as cortisol.

Adrenal Cortical Hypofunction. Adrenal cortical hypofunction, a condition known as Addison's disease, may potentially involve any or all of the hormones normally secreted. The situation demands attention when there is a deficiency in glucocorticoids or mineralocorticoids or both. Adrenal hypofunction may be a result of any of the following conditions:

1. Primary adrenal disease due to such factors as enzyme deficiencies, physical trauma, infection, or adrenalectomy.
2. Secondary involvement due to hypothalamic or pituitary hypofunction. If CRH is secreted in insufficient quantities from the hypothalamus or if ACTH secretion from the pituitary is lacking, glucocorticoids will not be secreted from the adrenal cortex. Atrophy of the zona fasciculata and zona reticularis (the areas secreting the glucocorticoids and androgens) will occur, and the adrenal becomes insensitive to stimulation by ACTH at a later time.
3. Suppression of the adrenal cortex secondary to prolonged treatment with exogenous glucocorticoids used for anti-inflammatory or anti-immune system

actions. Exogenous glucocorticoids inhibit secretion of CRH and ACTH, and, as described above, when ACTH is low for a prolonged period the adrenal cortex will be insensitive to stimulation by ACTH when administration of exogenous glucocorticoids is discontinued. Even while exogenous glucocorticoids are being given, suppression of the adrenal gland will result in an inadequate secretory response in stressful situations.

SIGNS AND SYMPTOMS OF ADRENAL HYPOFUNCTION. A major concern in patients with adrenal hypofunction is hypotension. Although a deficiency of aldosterone may cause hypotension due to loss of fluids and electrolytes in the kidneys, a lack of glucocorticoids plays an important but poorly understood role in the ability to maintain blood pressure. Faintness and dizziness are consequences of the hypotension. If aldosterone is deficient, hyponatremia and hyperkalemia are likely to occur and metabolic acidosis may develop.

Weight loss, anorexia, weakness, and anemia are common complaints in adrenal hypofunction. Depression and fatigue are accompanying mental symptoms. The glucocorticoid deficiency will result in a tendency to develop hypoglycemia because of decreased gluconeogenesis in the liver and anti-insulin activity in other tissues. If there is a deficient secretion of adrenal androgens, loss of body hair may be seen.

If the adrenal hypofunction is primary in nature, an increase in ACTH secretion will occur because of a release from the negative feedback normally mediated by the glucocorticoids. ACTH has a certain degree of MSH activity, and abnormal, spotty pigmentation results.

ANESTHESIA FOR PATIENTS WITH ADRENAL HYPOFUNCTION. Provided that adrenal hormone replacement is adequate to compensate for the surgical stress, there are no special instructions regarding anesthetic management of a patient with adrenal hypofunction. However, hormone replace-

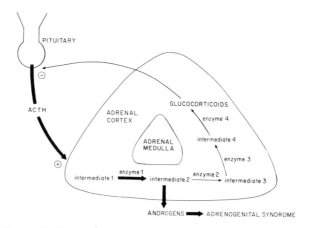

Figure 23–13. The adrenogenital syndrome. A deficiency in enzymes 2, 3, or 4 leads to a buildup of synthesis intermediates and decreased production of glucocorticoids. The lack of glucocorticoids removes the inhibition of secretion of ACTH from the pituitary. The increased secretion of ACTH stimulates the adrenal cortex, and the ensuing increased secretion of androgens causes the adrenogenital syndrome.

ment is of immense concern because of the potentially fatal consequences of inadequate coverage.

The normal adrenal gland responds to the stress of surgery by an increased secretion of glucocorticoids. The exact ways by which the glucocorticoids benefit the patient are unknown, but it is known that hypotension, cardiovascular collapse, and ultimately death may ensue if glucocorticoids are not present. That is why if there is any doubt about whether or not to give glucocorticoids to a patient who may have adrenal hypofunction, it is better to err on the side of too much than too little.

Because treatment with glucocorticoids for anti-inflammatory or immunosuppressive purposes depresses the pituitary–adrenal system, glucocorticoids should be given preoperatively to a patient who has been on steroid therapy. However, agreement on what degree of previous treatment calls for supplementation in the perioperative period is not universal. One opinion is that supplemental corticosteroids should be given to any patient who has been treated for more than 1 month in the past 6 to 12 months (White and Kumagai, 1979). Another opinion is that supplementation should be given to patients who have been treated with steroids within the previous 2 months (Millar, 1980). Still another opinion is that supplementation should be given to surgical patients who have received adrenal steroid treatment for a period of 4 days or longer during the preceding 6 months (Vandam and Moore, 1960). In patients already on a glucocorticoid regimen at the time of surgery, the hormone replacement should be continued. A recent study has indicated that an increase in the dose of corticosteroids at the time of surgery in patients already on a low-dose regimen seems unnecessary and is undesirable because of possible side effects (Symreng et al, 1981).

REFERENCES

Abbott TR: Anaesthesia in untreated myxoedema: Report of two cases. Br J Anaesth 39:510, 1967.

Ahern RS, Walker BA: Diabetes in relation to anaesthesia. In Gray TC, Nunn JF, Utting JE (eds): General Anaesthesia, 4th ed. Longdon, Butterworth Pub., 1980, pp. 797–806.

Block GW, Montgomery AD: Adrenal disease. In Vickers MD (ed): Medicine for Anaesthetists, 2nd ed. Oxford, Blackwell Scientific Publications, 1982, pp. 451–496.

Biglieri EG, Schambelan M, Slaton PE, et al: The intercurrent hypertension of primary aldosteronism. Circ Res 27:195, 1970.

Campbell JW, Duncan LJP, Innes JA, et al: Abdominal pain in diabetic metabolic decompensation. Clinical significance. JAMA 233:166, 1975.

Ferris JB, Beeves DG, Brown JJ, et al: Low-renin (primary) hyperaldosteronism: Differential diagnosis and distinction of the subgroups within the syndrome. Ann Heart J 95:641, 1978.

Hayes TM: The endocrine pancreas. In Vickers MD (ed): Medicine for Anaesthetists, 2nd ed. Oxford, Blackwell Scientific Publications, 1982, pp. 497–514.

Hunt TK, Schambelan M. Biglieri EG: Selection of patients and operative approach in primary aldosteronism. Ann Surg 182:353, 1975.

Kim JM, Hackman L: Anesthesia for untreated hypothyroidism: Report of three cases. Anesth Analg 56:299, 1977.

Maddi R, Gabel RA: Anesthetic consideration for adrenalectomy. In Brown BB (ed): Anesthesia and the Patient with Endocrine Disease. Philadelphia, Davis, 1980, pp. 1–9.

Maw DSJ: Emergency mangement of diabetes mellitus. Anaesthesia 30:520, 1975.

Millar RA: Pituitary and adrenal glands in relation to anaesthesia. In Gray TC, Nunn JF, Utting JE: General Anaesthesia, 4th ed. London, Butterworth Pub., 1980, pp. 807–824.

Miller J, Walts LF: Perioperative management of diabetes mellitus. In Brown BB (ed): Anesthesia and the Patient with Endocrine Disease. Philadelphia, Davis, 1980, pp. 91–103.

Moorthy SS: Metabolism and nutrition. In Stoelting RK, Dierdorf SF (eds): Anesthesia and Co-Existing Disease. New York, Churchill-Livingstone, 1983, pp. 485–521.

Murkin JM: Anesthesia and hypothyroidism: A review of thyroxine physiology, pharmacology, and anesthetic implications. Anesth Analg 61:371, 1982.

Palmers JP, Asplin CM: Insulin antibodies in insulin-dependent diabetics before insulin treatment. Science 222:1337, 1983.

Pender JW, Fox M, Basso LV: Diseases of the endocrine system. In Katz J, Benumof J, Kadis LB (eds): Anesthesia and Uncommon Diseases. Philadelphia, Saunders, 1981, pp. 155–220.

Shipton EA, Hugo JM: Primary aldosteronism and its importance to the anaesthetist. S Afr Med J 62:60, 1982.

Symreng T, Karlberg BE, Kagedal B, et al: Physiological cortisol substitution of long-term steroid-treated patients undergoing major surgery. Br J Anaesth 53:949, 1981.

Taitelman V, Reece EA, Bessman AN: Insulin in the management of the diabetic surgical patient, continuous intravenous infusion vs. subcutaneous administration. JAMA 237:658, 1977.

Tasch MD: Endocrine diseases. In Stoelting RK, Dierdorf SF (eds): Anesthesia and Co-Existing Disease. New York, Churchill-Livingstone, 1983, pp. 437–483.

Vandam LD, Moore FD: Adrenocortical mechanisms related to anesthesia. Anesthesiology 21:531, 1960.

Walker A, Cudwoith, AG: Type I (insulin dependent) diabetes multiplex families: Mode of genetic transmission. Diabetes 29:1036, 1980.

Weinberg MH, Clarence EG, Hollifield JW, et al: Primary aldosteronism: Diagnosis, localisation, and treatment. Ann Intern Med 90:386, 1979.

Werner SC: Myxedema coma. In Werner SC, Ingar SH (eds): The Thyroid: A Fundamental and Clinical Text. New York, Harper & Row, 1978, pp. 970–973.

White VA, Kumagai LF: Preoperative and meabolic considerations. Med Clinic North Am 63:1321, 1979.

BIBLIOGRAPHY

Brown BR (ed): Anesthesia and the Patient with Endocrine Disease. Philadelphia, Davis, 1980.

Ezrin C, Gadden JO, Volpe R (eds): Systematic Endocrinology, 2nd ed. New York, Harper & Row, Pub., 1979.

Friesen SR, Bolinger RE (ed): Surgical Endocrinology, Clinical Syndromes. Philadelphia, Lippincott, 1978.

Ganong WF: Review of Medical Physiology, 11th ed. Los Altos, Lange, 1983.

Gray TC, Nunn JF, Utting JE (eds): General Anaesthesia, 4th ed. London, Butterworth Pub., 1980.

Katz J, Kadis LB, Benumof, J (eds): Anesthesia and Uncommon Diseases: Pathophysiologic and Clinical Correlations, 2nd ed. Philadelphia, Saunders, 1981.

Oyama T: Anesthetic Management of Endocrine Disease. New York, Springer-Verlag, 1973.

Stoelting RK, Dierdorf SF (eds): Anesthesia and Co-Existing Disease. New York, Churchill-Livingstone, 1983.

Traynor C, Hall GM: Endocrine and metabolic changes during surgery: Anaesthetic implications. Br J Anaesth 53:153, 1981.

Vickers MD (ed): Medicine for Anaesthetists, 2nd ed. Oxford, Blackwell Scientific Publications, 1982.

Williams RH (ed): Textbook of Endocrinology, 6th ed. Philadelphia, Saunders, 1981.

Yao FF, Artusio JF (eds): Anesthesiology, Problem-oriented Patient Management. Philadelphia, Lippincott, 1983.

Part V
PARENTERAL THERAPY

24

Coagulation and Blood Component Therapy

Lorraine M. Jordan

Blood component therapy plays an important role in anesthesia practice. The principles of transfusion therapy indicate that the patient should be given blood products when needed. The patient is assessed and the blood products are selected based on the status and needs of the patient. The purpose of blood component therapy is to meet the needs of the patient with the least amount of risk.

Selection of the blood component is not always easy. Since there are approximately 20 different blood products currently available to fulfill the needs of the patient, it is vital that anesthetists are aware of the indications, contraindications, and potential side effects of the blood component chosen. Blood products are generally used to meet three needs: (1) increased oxygen transport; (2) expansion of blood volume; and (3) control of bleeding.

HEMOSTASIS

When the integrity of a blood vessel is broken, the injured area of the vessel attracts platelets which have formed from megakaryocyte cells in the bone marrow to the injured site and activates plasma coagulation proteins (Fig. 24–1). This leads to the initial clot formation which is referred to as primary hemostasis. Secondary hemostasis is when an insoluble fibrin clot is formed.

During primary hemostasis many steps lead up to the clot formation. When the vessel is damaged, the smooth muscle wall contracts, which alters the surface of the endothelium and facilitates the adhesive quality of the damaged membrane, and prothrombin activator is formed in response to the ruptured vessel. When the vessel is injured, collagen is exposed and offers a surface at which the platelets can adhere. As these platelets adhere to the collagen, platelet granules are formed and adenosine diphosphate is released (ADP). The ADP and other chemical agents cause the surface of the platelets to adhere to each other forming a plug of platelets. Platelets adhere to the site and a cascade

of events occurs to form a clot (Fig. 24–2). The platelets adhere to the subendothelial collagen layer of the vessel and the platelet plug is formed. Figure 24–3 illustrates the process of platelet activation beginning with platelet adhesion through the fibrin formation.

Secondary hemostasis occurs when the insoluble fibrin clot is formed. The formation of this clot occurs when the coagulation proteins are activated to form a fibrin network.

The general sequence of events in blood coagulation begins with prothrombin activator forming in response to rupture of the vessel. After the prothrombin activator is released, it acts as a catalyst to convert prothrombin to thrombin. Extrinsic or intrinsic prothrombin activator and calcium convert the prothrombin to thrombin. Thrombin then converts fibrinogen into fibrin threads to form the clot under the influence of calcium and fibrin stabilizing factors.

The extrinsic pathway for initiating clotting begins with the formation of prothrombin activator. The extrinsic pathway is illustrated in Figure 24–4. The intrinsic pathway begins with trauma to the vessel initiating a cascade of events leading to activation of factor Xa. The intrinsic coagulation pathway is illustrated in Figure 24–5. The major difference in the pathways is that the extrinsic pathway responds very rapidly within 15 seconds after the vessel is damaged while the intrinsic pathway is much slower and responds in 2 to 6 minutes.

There are several drugs which inhibit platelet function and ultimately hemostasis. Drugs inhibit hemostasis at different phases of the process. Some of these drugs are listed in Table 24–1. Chronic ingestion of any of these drugs may pose a problem during the operative course for the patient. Bleeding may be difficult to control in the intraoperative and postoperative period due to the effect of these drugs inhibiting hemostasis.

There are laboratory tests which can assess a patient's degree of hemostasis. The tests are highlighted in Table 24–2. The tests listed in this table are divided into categories based on secondary hemostasis and fibrinolysis. These tests

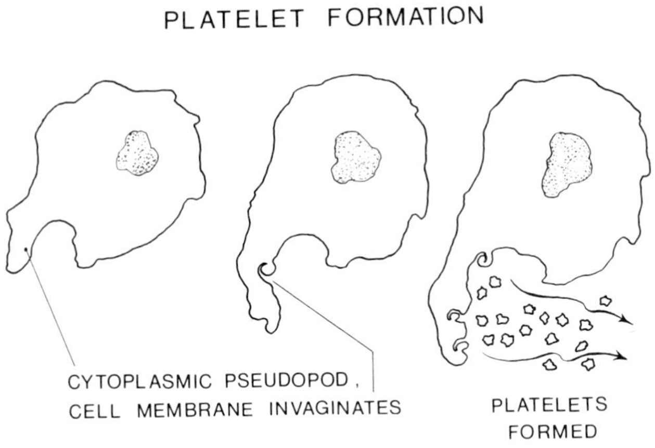

PLATELET FORMATION

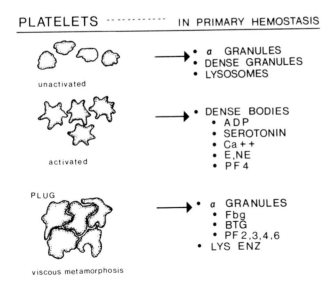

CYTOPLASMIC PSEUDOPOD,
CELL MEMBRANE INVAGINATES

PLATELETS
FORMED

Figure 24-1. Platelet production.

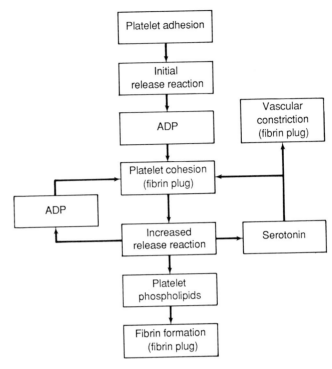

Figure 24-3. Steps in platelet activation. (*From Henry RL. In Murano G, Bick RL (eds): Basic Concepts of Hemostasis and Thrombosis. Boca Raton, CRC Press, 1980.*)

can be conducted to assess the bleeding tendency of the patient. These tests should be ordered based on the physical status and condition of the patient. This baseline data will help to identify potential problems that may occur in the operating room, allowing for better evaluation and treatment of bleeding problems which may develop during the operative course.

COMPATIBILITY TESTING

The extent of compatibility testing is based upon the urgency of the situation. Complete testing should be the goal of the transfusion service to establish compatibility and avoid an antigen–antibody reaction. Establishing the patient's blood type is essential to avoid devastating agglutination and hemolysis of the donated blood. An incompatibility

PLATELETS --------- IN PRIMARY HEMOSTASIS

- *a* GRANULES
- DENSE GRANULES
- LYSOSOMES

unactivated

- DENSE BODIES
  - ADP
  - SEROTONIN
  - Ca + +
  - E,NE
  - PF 4

activated

PLUG

- *a* GRANULES
  - Fbg
  - BTG
  - PF 2,3,4,6
- LYS ENZ

viscous metamorphosis

Figure 24-2. Platelets in primary hemostasis.

reaction occurs when antibodies are activated and the complement causes hemolysis of the red blood cells. The two major antigen systems that are most often tested are the blood group (ABO) system and the Rh or D antigen. Other blood group antigens do exist and can cause reactions, however, these reactions are usually less devastating than an ABO or Rh mismatch.

The patient's blood group (ABO) is determined by the antigen on the surface of the red blood cell. Antibodies also exist in the serum of the different blood types. Therefore, typing a patient's blood based on the ABO blood group includes typing the surface of the red blood cell as well as the serum of the different blood types.

One example of blood typing is a person who has type O blood who has neither A or B antigens on the surface of the cell and has anti-A and anti-B serum antibodies. This means that type O blood can be given to an individual with Type A, B, AB, and O. Individuals with type O blood are known as "universal donors." Just the opposite is true of individuals who have type AB blood and are known as "universal recipients." Type AB blood recipients are able to receive blood from all of the blood groups without having a hemolytic reaction. The typing of a blood group is illustrated in Table 24–3.

The other form of testing is RH (D) testing. The majority of individuals are Rh (D)-positive. A person is classified as Rh (D)-positive when the Rh-antigen on the surface is either C, D, or E. When the Rh-antigen on the surface of the red blood cell is either c, d, or e, the individual is Rh(D)-negative.

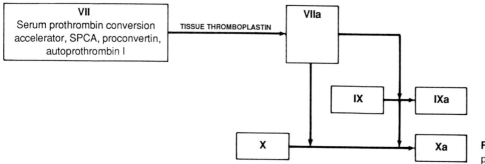

Figure 24–4. Extrinsic coagulation pathway.

In emergency situations, in which the sustenance of life depends upon immediate blood therapy, most experts recommend uncrossmatched group O packed red blood cells for initial resuscitation fluid therapy. This finding was confirmed in a study by Schwab et al (1986) in which 99 patients had clinical signs of class III or class IV hemorrhage and were treated with uncrossmatched group O packed cells. Schwab concluded that using uncrossmatched group O packed cells was a safe form of blood component therapy in the immediate resuscitative period.

CROSSMATCHING AND SCREENING

Crossmatching is performed to determine the potential for blood transfusion reaction. The patient's serum and donor's red blood cells are mixed together to detect the potential of a hemolytic transfusion reaction. Crossmatching, which usually takes an hour's laboratory time, helps to ensure optimal safety of the transfused blood. This technique is being used less and less in routine practice because of limited blood supplies and the amount of time the laboratory needs to spend on testing. Crossmatching is done for patients who are likely to receive a transfusion.

Screening is mixing together the patient's serum and panel (commercially supplied) red blood cells to detect potential hemolytic transfusion reactions. A patient's blood is typed and screened for both ABO and Rh compatibility to ascertain that the most commonly found antibodies are not present. Type and screen without a complete crossmatch does not ensure complete compatibility of the blood to less frequently found antigens. Oberman et al studied 13,950 patients and found that only 8 had "clinically significant" antibodies following complete crossmatch that were not detected during the antibody screening. Screening of blood is used when the patient may need a blood transfusion during the operative course. Blood will be available for transfusion if necessary, but it is not held in reserve for the patient.

Negative antibody screening occurs when there are no irregular antibodies present to the more common red blood cell antigens. This indicates that there is little or no difficulty in crossmatching of compatible blood. However, if the positive antibody screen occurs, then the irregular antibody indicates the probable absence of red blood cell antigen and the possibility of difficulty in obtaining compatible blood. Additional blood screening is indicated if a positive antibody screen occurs.

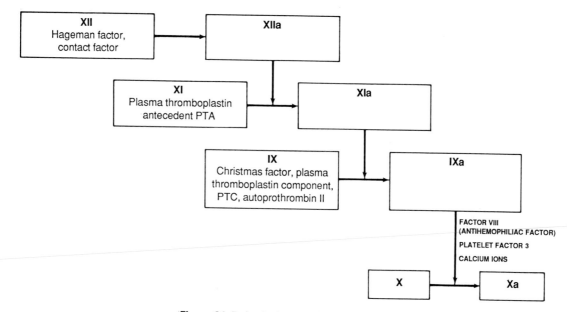

Figure 24–5. Intrinsic coagulation pathway.

TABLE 24–1. DRUGS INHIBITING HEMOSTASIS

Primary hemostasis (platelet function)
- Aspirin
- Penicillins
- Nonsteroidal anti-inflammatory agents
- Antihistamines

Secondary hemostasis
- Heparin
- Oral anticoagulants

Fibrinolysis
- Epsilon aminocaproic acid

BLOOD COMPONENTS

The utilization of blood component therapy must be based on many factors. Military casualties studies have shown that a patient can lose up to 30 to 40 percent of blood volume without requiring red blood cell replacement. However, this statement is based on the fact that blood volume is replaced by other means such as with plasma substitutes and electrolytes.

Blood component therapy is becoming more and more popular in the clinical arena. The advantages of component therapy include decreased cost and the capability to administer only the component necessary to meet the needs of the patient. Whole blood can be separated into many components. The flow diagram in Figure 24–6 illustrates the many components that can be derived from a unit of whole blood. The blood components that will be discussed in this chapter are outlined in Table 24–4. This table will be used as a guide to discuss blood component therapy.

PRODUCTS USED FOR RED BLOOD CELL CONTENT

Blood products differ in the forms and indications for usage. The major differences in blood products are highlighted in Table 24–5. These blood products are compared with each other in this table to offer an overview and compliment the information which will be presented.

TABLE 24–2. LABORATORY EVALUATION OF SECONDARY HEMOSTASIS AND FIBRINOLYSIS

Secondary hemostasis
- Factor activities and assays
- Prothrombin time (PT)
- Activated partial thromboplastin time (aPTT)
- Thrombin time (TT)
- Fibrinogen

Fibrinolysis
- Thrombo-Wellco test
- Protamine sulfate test

TABLE 24–3. ABO BLOOD GROUP ANTIGENS AND ANTIBODIES

Blood Type	Red Blood Cell Surface Antigen	Serum Antibodies
A	A	Anti-B
B	B	Anti-A
AB	A and B	No ABO antibodies
O	No ABO surface Antigen	Anti-A and anti-B

WHOLE BLOOD

With the development of component therapy, there has been a tremendous decline in the use of whole blood, because whole blood contains leukocytes, platelets, and plasma antigens which may result in a febrile or allergic transfusion reaction. However, in certain situations the use of whole blood as form of treatment is indicated. Whole blood is used for treating massive hemorrhages and for exchange transfusions of an infant, child, or adult.

Whole blood differs from that of the patient in that there is anticoagulant–preservative solution in the bag. The anticoagulant–preservative solution most often used today is citrate-phosphate-dextrose with adenine (CPD–A1), which chelates ionized calcium and prevents activation of the coagulation system prolonging the life of the red blood cells.

A unit of whole blood contains 513 ± 45 ml of blood of which 63 ml of CPD-A1 has been added. The hematocrit of the unit is about 40 percent. The shelf life of a unit of blood with CPD–A1 stored at 4C is 35 days. At this time 70 percent of the red blood cells present are recoverable in the circulation and survive normally. During this storage time there is a progressive loss of components and an accumulation of hydrogen and potassium ions in the plasma.

RED BLOOD CELLS

Packed Red Blood Cells

Most red blood cells have hematocrits between 70 and 80 percent. Packed red blood cells (PRBC) differ from whole blood in that the red blood cells are separated from the plasma. The high hematocrit has a high viscosity and therefore, problems with flow can develop during administration of the product. Clinicians often add 0.9 percent of isotonic saline to the red blood cells to markedly decrease the viscosity of the blood and increase the flow. The utilization of a Y-shaped blood administration set will facilitate the addition of the saline to the blood.

Each unit of packed red blood cells contains from 190 to 390 ml of which 155 to 270 ml are erythrocytes. Each unit of packed red blood cells is anticipated to raise the hemoglobin 1 gm/dl, and the hematocrit 3 percent in a 70-kg adult. The shelf life of packed red blood cells is 35 days if collected into CPD–A1 and stored at 4C.

Packed red blood cells are effective in treating anemias when the oxygen-carrying capacity has dropped because

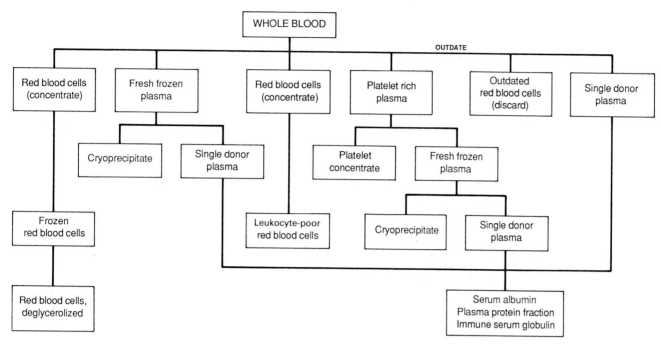

Figure 24–6. A flow diagram of the separation of whole blood into components. Single donor plasma can be manufactured into blood derivatives, such as albumin, plasma protein fraction and immune serum globulin. Fresh frozen plasma can be processed by pharmaceutical firms into coagulation factor concentrates. (*Reproduced with permission from Kennedy MS: Essentials of immunohematology and blood therapy. In Zuspan FP, Quilligan EJ, (eds): A Practical Manual of Obstetrical Care, St. Louis, CV Mosby Co, 1981.*)

of the low hemoglobin levels and when time does not permit a more conventional treatment of anemia such as iron replacement or hematopoiesis.

Leukocyte-Poor Red Blood Cells

Leukocyte-poor red blood cells are red blood cells in which the leukocytes have been removed. Leukocyte-poor red blood cells are indicated in those individuals who have severe febrile reactions when transfused with red blood cells or whole blood. There are different techniques to remove leukocytes from the red blood cells. The most common method is by inverted centrifugation, which removes over

TABLE 24–4. COMMON BLOOD COMPONENTS

- Whole blood
- Erythrocyte (RBC) preparations
  Packed RBC (plasma removed)
  Leukocyte-poor RBC (plasma and white cells removed)
  Washed RBC (plasma and other elements removed)
  Deglycerolized RBC
  Frozen RBC (plasma removed)
- Plasma
  Stored plasma
  Fresh frozen plasma
- Platelet
- Leukocyte concentration
- Cryoprecipitate
- Albumin
- Factor concentrates

70% of all leukocytes and platelets. This method of preparation has a volume of 180–250 ml, with a shelf life of 35 days in CPD–A1, when stored at 4C.

Washed Red Blood Cells

Washed red blood cells are indicated for patients who have febrile transfusion reactions to leuykocyte-poor red blood cells or any serious allergic reaction to blood. Washed red blood cells are prepared by washing one or more liters of isotonic saline through the red blood cells. About 93 percent of the leukocytes are removed. The shelf life of washed red blood cells is 24 hours after preparation with storage at 4C.

Deglycerolized Red Blood Cells

Deglycerolized red blood cells are used to store rare donor units of blood, autologous blood, and units of blood for special purposes. This process of preparing the red blood cells allows for storage of the blood in the frozen state for 3 years or more. The red blood cells are preserved and stored by adding a cryoprotective agent. The disadvantage of the process is that the units are depleted of all plasma, platelets, granulocytes, and almost all lymphocytes. Because of the preparation and purity of the blood, this product is used primarily for intrauterine transfusions and severely immunosuppressed patients.

After the blood has been thawed and washed the glycerolized red blood cells have a shelf life of only 24 hours.

TABLE 24–5. DIFFERENCES IN COMPOSITION OF MAJOR BLOOD PRODUCTS

	Normal Whole Blood	Citrated Whole Blood	Citrated PRBCs[a]	Frozen PRBCs	Fresh Frozen Plasma
pH	7.4	6.6–6.9	6.6–6.9	6.6–7.2	6.6–6.9
PCO_2	35–45	180–210	180–210	0–10	180–210
Base deficit (mEq/L)	0	9–15	9–15	?	9–15
K^+ (mEq/L)	3.5–5.0	18–26	18–26	1–2	4–8
Citrate	None	—	—	None	—
Factors V, VIII	Normal	20–50% Normal	20–50% Normal	None	85–100% Normal
Fibrinogen	Normal	Normal	Normal	None	Normal
Platelets	240,000 400,000	None	None	None	None
2,3-DPG	Normal	3% Normal	3% Normal	Nearly normal	—
Hematocrit	35–45	35–45	60–70	50–95	—
Temperature	37C	4–6C	4–6C	4–6C	Cold

[a] Citrated whole blood and citrate packed red blood cells (PRBCs) have the same chemical composition, but citrated PRBCs have considerably less plasma volume.
(*Modified from Miller RD: A.S.A. Refresher Courses 1:101, 1973.*)

The units should be stored at 4C. Each unit has a volume of 180 to 250 ml with a hematocrit of 50 to 70 percent.

Frozen Red Blood Cells

Frozen red blood cells (FRBC) are a pure red cell preparation containing no citrate, white cells, platelets, or plasma. FRBCs are used for patients who have a history of febrile transfusion reactions and for those who have rare blood types. The risk of transmitting hepatitis with FRBC is less due to the processing of the blood. The major disadvantage of FRBCs is the high cost of the product. Between 20 and 30 percent of the red blood cells are lost during preparation and in the first 24 hours posttransfusion. Once the frozen cells are reconstituted the shelf life of unit is 24 hours.

To help highlight some of the clinical indication and approximate content and shelf life of the products, refer to Table 24–6.

PLATELET, LEUKOCYTE, AND PLASMA COMPONENTS

Plasma

Stored Plasma. Stored plasma is obtained from whole blood during the first 72 hours of storage. Stored plasma is to be kept a 4C for 35 days in the liquid state or it can be kept in the frozen state (−30C) for 12 months. Stored plasma is used to replace volume and protein for patients. It has also been used to prime extracorporeal pumps, for plasma exchange, and for burned patients.

Fresh Frozen Plasma. Fresh frozen plasma (FFP) is prepared from fresh whole blood within 6 hours of collection. After preparation, the unit is stored at −18C or below to preserve the labile plasma coagulation factors. FFP contains adequate factor V and VIII levels to treat coagulation deficiencies. Each bag of FFP contains 400 mg of fibrinogen and 200 units of factor V and factor VIII. FFP is given based on ABO compatibility but no Rh compatibility.

FFP has been used for volume replacement, treating coagulopathies, treating disseminating intravascular coagulation (DIC), replacing coagulation factors in patients with liver disease, and treating thrombocytopenia purpura. However, the primary indication for the use of FFP is labile coagulation factors. The use of FFP is recommended (2–3 U for every 10–15 U of whole blood) in the treatment of massive transfusion therapy.

As prepared the volume of FFP is 200 to 275 ml per bag of which 40 to 45 ml represent citrate anticoagulant. There is only a single donor hepatitis risk. FFP must be thawed before administration. After FFP is thawed, the plasma should be stored at 4C and given within 24 hours after thawing. The shelf life for FFP is 1 year.

Platelet Concentrations

Platelets are obtained from two sources: random-donor and single-donor platelet concentrations. Single-donor platelet concentrations are produced by apheresis. Random donor platelet concentrates are prepared by centrifuging whole blood from platelet-rich plasma. Single-donor platelet concentrates contain 3 to 8×10^{11} platelets while random-donor platelet concentrates contain 5.5 to 8×10^{10} platelets.

Single-donor platelet concentrations may be necessary for patients who have developed antibodies that cause destruction of transfused platelets. HLA-compatible platelet concentrations are prepared by harvesting platelets from single-donor platelet concentrations by automated apheresis.

Platelets are necessary to maintain normal bleeding

TABLE 24–6. PRODUCTS USED FOR RED BLOOD CELL CONTENT*

Blood Component	Clinical Indications	Approximate Composition[a]			Shelf Life
		RBC	Plasma	WBC	
Whole blood	Exchange transfusion or massive transfusion	155–270 ml	180–305 ml	25×10^8	35 days[b]
Red blood cells	Chronic anemia, surgical blood loss or hemorrhage	155–170 ml	40–115 ml	25×10^8	35 days[b]
Leukocyte-poor red blood cells	Repeated febrile transfusion reactions and anemia, surgical blood loss or hemorrhage	125–215 ml	30–90 ml	5×10^8	35 days[b]
Saline-washed red blood cells	Febrile transfusion reactions or IgA deficiency with antibody and anemia, surgical blood loss, or hemorrhage	140–240 ml	Nil	1×10^8	24 hours
Deglycerolized red blood cells	Autologous transfusion, rare donor blood, IgA deficiency with antibody, transplant candidates, or febrile transfusion reactions	140–240 ml	Nil	0.5×10^8	24 hours

RBC = erythrocytes; WBC = leukocytes.
[a] Calculated.
[b] CPD–A1, for CPD the shelf life is 21 days.
(From Kennedy MS: Essentials of immunohematology and blood therapy. In Zuspan PF, Quilligan EJ (eds): A Practical Manual of Obstetrical Care. St. Louis, CV Mosby, 1981.)

times. A platelet count above 100,000/mm³ is usually adequate to cause hemostasis. Most clinicians believe that a level of 50,000 to 75,000 platelets/mm³ is an acceptable lower level for surgery. When a platelet count of 10,000/mm³ is reached there is a high likelihood of spontaneous bleeding that may be life threatening to the patient. A unit of random-donor platelet concentrate usually increases the platelet count by 5,000 to 10,000/μl. However, a unit of single-donor concentrate raises the platelet count 50,000 to 100,000/μl.

It is not uncommon during surgery that the platelet count may drop due to the increased utilization of the plug formation and dilution of blood components. However, this is usually not a problem because the body has adequate bone marrow reserve to respond to a mild reduction of platelets. Platelets are often supplemented when treating massive hemorrhage. Replacement of platelets (approximately 5 U) for each 10 to 15 units of stored red blood cells or whole blood administered is recommended. Platelets are indicated for patients who have severe aplastic anemia, who have thrombocytopenia (due to leukemia or massive blood transfusions), or who are undergoing a cardiopulmonary bypass. The amount of increase in platelet count from infused platelets is influenced by factors such as infection, platelet alloantibodies, splenomegaly, and fever.

Random-donor platelet concentration can be stored for 72 hours at room temperature and 48 hours at 4 degrees centigrade. However, single-donor platelet concentrates should only be stored for 24 hours because the apheresis procedure is considered "open" and after 24 hours the incidence of contamination of the unit is increased. Plasma should be given through a standard 170-μm blood filter set.

Leukocyte Concentrates

Some chemotherapeutic agents suppress the bone marrow production. Therefore, these patients on chemotherapy may develop neutropenia. Insufficient granulocytes make it difficult for the body to protect itself from infections and leukocyte therapy may help these patients. Leukapheresis removes leukocytes, granulocytes, erythrocytes, platelets, and lymphocytes from the donor. The administration of leukocyte concentrations has not been proven to be as effective as once thought. Leukocyte antibodies are stimulated by the transfusion. The administration of leukocyte concentrates is usually limited to cases of bone marrow transplants, cases of gram-negative septicemia or infection that is not responsive to antibiotics, and cases of granulocyte counts of less than 500/μl.

The volume of the product varies according to the apheresis techniques used. Since the process of apheresis is an "open" technique, the product should be discarded after 24 hours.

CRYOPRECIPITATE

Cryoprecipitate is a major source of fibrinogen and is used in the treatment of hemophilia (factor VIII deficiency), hypofibrinogenemia, von Willebrand's disease, and rare cases of factor XIII deficiency. Cryoprecipitate contains factor I (fibrinogen), factor VIII, and factor XIII. A single unit of cryoprecipitate contains approximately 100 clotting units of factor VIII and 250 mg of fibrinogen. The unit contains 10 to 15 ml of cryoprecipitate to which diluent volume is added, resulting in a total volume of 25 to 35 ml. Cryoprecipitate is kept frozen at $-18C$ to preserve factor VIII activity for 1 year. Transfusion of cryoprecipitate should occur within 6 hours after thawing or 4 hours after pooling. Cryoprecipitate is ABO-type specific whenever possible. Cryoprecipitate is the only product which contains concentrated fibrinogen and because of a single donor decreases the risk of carrying hepatitis.

Table 24–7 highlights the clinical indications and blood components discussed in this section.

ALBUMIN

Albumin is used to help expand circulating blood volume when oxygen-carrying capacity is adequate. Albumin has a molecular weight of 65,000 and maintains capillary osmotic pressure. Not only does the albumin help to maintain capillary osmotic pressure but it also service as a carrier protein for various drugs, hormones, enzymes, and metabolites. The body produces 50 grams of albumin daily.

There are three types of albumin solutions: 5 percent albumin, 25 percent albumin, and plasma protein fraction (PPF). The risk of hepatitis does not exist with the administration of albumin, because during the preparation process the albumin is heated to 60C for 10 hours thereby destroying the hepatitis virus. The patient does not have to have a blood typing done prior to receiving albumin. The broad use of albumin has decreased because of the expense of this product. The trend seems to be to use crystalloids rather than albumin to expand volume.

FACTOR CONCENTRATIONS

Factor VIII

Factor VIII has a half-life of 4 to 8 hours. The product does not have to be ABO typed for administration of the concentrate. The factor VIII is highly concentrated and can be stored at refrigerator temperatures. The two major disadvantages of using the product is that a high risk of hepatitis may be implicated with the product due to the fact that it is derived from a pooled sample and there have been reported abnormal liver functions following its administration. Factor VIII is used to treat patients with hemophilia A and with von Willebrand's disease. Both diseases are alterations in factor VIII.

Factor IX

Factor IX contains not only factor IX but also factors II and VII, and factor X is an assayed product for factor IX. This product is used most frequently for hemophilia B (factor IX deficiency), Christmas disease, rare congenital factor deficiencies of factors II, VII, and X, and for reversal of the effects of coumadin anticoagulation therapy in life threatening hemorrhage. The major disadvantage of factor IX administration is that there is a high risk of hepatitis transmission with the blood product.

The selection and successful treatment of blood derangements is based on use of appropriate blood components. In Table 24–8, coagulation factor deficiencies are listed and the component treatment is indicated.

SYNTHETIC COLLOIDS

Synthetic colloid agents for blood volume expansion are dextran, gelatin, hydroxyethyl starch, polyvinylpyrrolidone, and stroma-free hemogolobin. These isotonic electrolyte solutions are able to act as plasma proteins to provide osmotic pressure. Colloid preparations are used in clinical situations to treat acute hypovolemic shock.

Dextran and hydroxyethyl starch are nonprotein colloid volume expanders. A disadvantage to these agents is that ABO blood grouping can be interfered with by the roleaux

TABLE 24–7. PLATELET, LEUKOCYTE, AND PLASMA COMPONENTS

Blood Component	Clinical Indications	Approximate Composition		Shelf Life and Storage Temperature
		Plasma	Platelets	
Random donor platelet	Thrombocytopenia with hemorrhage, severe thrombocytopenia or functional platelet disorders with hemorrhage	30 ml (4C) 50 ml (20–24C)	$> 5.5 \times 10^{10}$	48 hours at 4C 72 hours at 20–24C
Single donor platelet concentrate by apheresis	Refractory to random donor platelet concentrate and severe thrombocytopenia or hemorrhage with thrombocytopenia or functional disorder	300–500 ml	$3–8 \times 10^{11}$	24 hours at 20–24C
Leukocyte concentrate by apheresis	Severe neutropenia, fever, and infection unresponsive to antibiotics	300–700 ml	$3–8 \times 10^{11}$ (Granulocytes $= 1 \times 10^{10}$)	24 hours at 4C or 20–24C
Fresh frozen plasma	Multiple coagulation deficiencies	200–275 ml	Nil	1 year at $-18C$ 24 hours at 4C
Single donor plasma	Plasma expansion	200–275 ml	Nil	5 years at $-18C$ 24 hours at 4C
Cryoprecipitate	Factor VIII deficiency, factor XIII deficiency, von Willebrand's disease or hypofibrinogenemia	10–15 ml	Nil	1 year at $-18C$ 6 hours at 20–24C

(*From Kennedy MS: Essentials of immunohematology and blood therapy. In Zuspan PF, Quilligan EJ (eds): A Practical Manual of Obstetrical Care. St. Louis, CV Mosby, 1981.*)

TABLE 24–8. BLOOD PRODUCTS FOR TREATMENT OF COAGULATION FACTOR DEFICIENCIES

Fibrinogen deficiency	Cryoprecipitate Stored plasma
Factor V deficiency	Fresh frozen plasma
Factor VII deficiency	Factor IX complex (II, VII, IX, X) Stored plasma
Factor VIII deficiency	Factor VIII concentrate (AHF) Cryoprecipitate Fresh frozen plasma
von Willebrand's disease	Cryoprecipitate Fresh frozen plasma
Factor IX deficiency	Factor IX complex (II, VII, IX, X) Stored plasma
Factor XIII deficiency	Stored plasma

(From Blajchman MA, Sheppard FA, Perrault RA: Clinical use of blood, blood components and blood products. Can Med Assoc J 121:33, 1979.)

formation with dextran and the agglomeration of the red cells with starch. Dextran is used to treat normovolemic hemodilution occurring in major surgical procedures. Gelatin has also been used to treat polycythemia and thrombocytanemia.

Some of the disadvantages of these products are that all of the preparations can produce some incompatibility reactions. The symptoms may vary from histimine release to anaphylaxis. Ennis and Lorenz (1985) have reported a high incidence of adverse reactions to colloid therapy while others, such as Ring and Messmer (1977), have reported relatively low adverse reactions to colloid therapy. Belcher and Lennox (1984) reported that there were no untoward effects attributable to hydroxyethyl starch administration in 27 patients undergoing cardiac surgery. The study concluded that hydroxyethyl starch is a safe, cheap, and effective plasma substitute for volume replacement. Some of the potential side effects of colloid synthetic solutions are highlighted in Table 24–9.

ISSUES IN TRANSFUSION THERAPY

Citrate Intoxication and Hyperkalemia

Stored bank blood has three different anticoagulant preservatives: acid–citrate–dextrose (ACD), citrate–phosphate–dextrose (CPD), and citrate–phosphate–dextrose with adenine (CPD–A1). The preservative most frequently used is CPD–A1. The purpose of the preservative is to anticoagulate the blood, maintain red cell viability, and maintain normal hemoglobin function. The anticoagulate chelates the ionized calcium and inhibits the coagulation cascade. The addition of dextrose to phosphate citrate and citric acid prolongs red cell viability by generating adenosine triphosphate (ATP).

Stored blood has excess acidity due to the citric acid and lactic acid generated during ATP utilization. Massive transfusions (replacing the patient's blood volume one or more times) may lead to metabolic acidosis. Most of the time this metabolic acidosis is not treated. Treating metabolic acidosis may further decrease the oxygen delivery to the tissues, result in increased sodium loads, and impair calcium mobilization.

During massive transfusion, hyperkalemia may de-

velop. Plasma potassium levels are increased in stored blood. Miller (1974) states that serum potassium levels may be as high as 19 to 30 mEq/L in blood stored after 21 days. However, the clinically diagnostic signs of hyperkalemia (peak T waves) are the indicator to determine if calcium should be given.

Calcium

When administering large amounts of citrated blood there is a decrease in ionized calcium levels. Calcium is mobilized rather rapidly from the bones to supply the body with adequate calcium to continue physiologic functioning. Howland, Schweizer, and Carlon have indicated that routine empiric supplementation of calcium is not necessary during massive transfusion. However, Allen recommends the routine administration of 1 gram of calcium gluconate for every 2 to 3 units of blood. The utilization of calcium should be determined by laboratory values to support the administration of the drug. Miller (1986) states that rarely is calcium administration necessary with transfusion therapy.

Since citrate intoxication is caused by citrate binding calcium, the characteristics of citrate intoxication are signs of hypocalcemia. The signs of hypocalcium are hypotension, narrow pulse pressure, and elevated left ventricular, end-diastolic, and central venous pressures.

Hypothermia

The potential of rendering a patient hypothermic during massive transfusion therapy is one of great concern. Cold blood can cause cardiac arrhythmias as well as contribute to hypothermia. Hypothermia increases oxygen and energy requirements. The metabolism of anesthetic agents and narcotics is impaired by the cold. Hypothermia impairs the metabolism of citrate and of lactate, which could lead to hypocalcemia and metabolic acidosis. The cold temperature also promotes the release of potassium from the intracellular space. Therefore, the use of a blood warmer is recommended to maintain normothermia of the patient. The patient's exposure during the surgical procedure, especially during abdominal cases, helps to contribute to a decreased

TABLE 24–9. SYNTHETIC COLLOIDS AVAILABLE FOR BLOOD VOLUME EXPANSION SIDE EFFECTS

Synthetic Colloid	Potential Side Effects
Dextran	Erythrocyte rouleaux Hemostatic abnormalities
Gelatin	Erythrocyte rouleaux
Hydroxyethyl starch	Erythrocyte rouleaux Hemostatic disorders Prolonged retention Hyperamylasaemia
Polyvinylpyrrolidone	Erythrocyte rouleaux Prolonged retention in the reticuloendothelial system
Stroma-free hemoglobin	Renal damage Hypercoagulability from residual membrane lipids

(From Blajchman MA, Sheppard FA, Perrault RA: Clinical use of blood, blood components and blood products. Can Med Assoc J 121:33, 1979.)

temperature. The importance of maintaining temperature becomes even more relevant when administering large amounts of blood to patients with a great deal of body exposure during surgery. The problem of hypothermia during massive transfusions can be compounded by further insensible heat loss from exposure during a large abdominal case.

One of the problems associated with administration of blood via a blood warmer is the impedance of flow rates when rapid infusion is necessary. There are many different blood warmers available on the market. The blood warmer that offers the least amount of impedance of flow, therefore, is the best choice for rapid administration of blood.

HEMOLYTIC TRANSFUSION REACTIONS

Hemolytic transfusion reactions are difficult to assess under general anesthesia. The patient is asleep and unable to communicate the experiencing of any of the signs and symptoms of a hemolytic transfusion reaction. The clinical signs that a patient exhibits during a transfusion reaction may vary. Signs and symptoms that may develop during a reaction are fever, chills, flushing, dyspnea, pain in the back or chest, hypotension, shock, oliguria, anuria, DIC, and hemoglobin present in the urine and plasma (Table 24–10). During anesthesia, the symptoms that may be recognizable are hemoglobinuria, hemolysis, and hypotension. The treatment of hemolytic transfusion reactions focuses on maintaining adequate renal function.

Miller (1986) states that a minimal urinary output of 75 ml/hr is desired to maintain adequate renal function. This goal is minatained by administering fluids and diuretics to help facilitate renal function. The exact mechanism of decreased renal function is not certain. However, it is hypothesized that a form of acid hematin precipitates in the distal tubules actually blocking the tubules thereby impairing renal function.

The recommended procedure in treating a hemolytic transfusion reaction is described in Table 24–11. The treatment is to stop the infusion of the blood, maintain an adequate urinary output, alkalinize the urine, assay urinary and plasma hemoglobin, determine coagulation levels, return unused blood to the blood bank, send a sample of the patient's blood to be tested for antibodies, and avoid hypotension. Hypotension will decrease renal perfusion which may cause a decrease in renal function, potentially leading to renal failure. Therefore, adequate hydration and optimal renal function during a hemolytic transfusion reaction are absolutes.

TABLE 24–10. HEMOLYTIC TRANSFUSION REACTION: SIGNS AND SYMPTOMS

- Fever, chills, flushing
- Dyspnea
- Pain: chest and/or back
- Hypotension, shock
- Oliguria, anuria
- DIC
- Hemoglobin in plasma and urine

(From Harrigan C, Cantrell, ME: Unit VI: Anesthesia for emergency surgery; hemostasis and blood replacement therapy. In Current Concepts in Inhalation Anesthesia. Philadelphia, Ted Thomas, 1986.)

TABLE 24–11. STEPS FOR THE TREATMENT OF HEMOLYTIC TRANSFUSION REACTION

1. *Stop the transfusion.*
2. Maintain the urine output at a minimum of 75 to 100 ml/hr by the following methods:
   a. Generously administer fluids intravenously and possibly mannitol, 12.5 to 50 g, given over a 5- to 15-minute period.
   b. If intravenously administered fluids and mannitol are ineffective, then administer furosemide, 20 to 40 mg, intravenously.
3. Alkalinize the urine; since bicarbonate is preferentially excreted in the urine, only 40 to 70 mEq/70 kg of sodium bicarbonate is usually required to raise the urine pH to 8, whereupon repeat urine pH determinations indicate the need for additional bicarbonate.
4. Assay urine and plasma hemoglobin concentrations.
5. Determine platelet count, partial thromboplastin time, and serum fibrinogen level.
6. Return unused blood to blood bank for recrossmatch.
7. Send patient blood sample to blood bank for antibody screen and direct antiglobulin test.
8. Prevent hypotension to ensure adequate renal blood flow.

(From Miller RD, et al: Anesthesia Vol 2. New York, Churchill Livingstone, 1986, pp. 1329–1369.)

INFECTIOUS DISEASES

Non-A Non-B Hepatitis

Viral hepatitis is the most frequently occurring disease that is transmitted by blood transfusions. However, the risk of acquiring hepatitis is rather low. There are many viruses that can be passed through blood transfusions. Some of the viruses that are common are: non-A non-B (NANB) hepatitis viruses, hepatitis B virus, cytomegalovirus and human immunodeficiency virus (HIV). Table 24–12 has these four types of viruses listed and describes the clinically significant features of the viruses.

The majority of transfusion recipients who become infected with viral hepatitis have NANB hepatitis. The frequency of occurrence of NANB hepatitis is between 4.5 and 18 percent of those receiving transfusions. Clinically, patients who have NANB hepatitis may become icteric, fatigued, and anorexic. However, the majority of patients remain asymptomatic. Clinical evaluation of posttransfusion hepatitis is defined as a transient twofold elevation of serum alanine aminotransferase (ALT) in at least two consecutive tests (5 days apart) performed from 2 to 26 weeks after transfusion. ALT levels may be elevated with or without jaundice and for reasons other than hepatitis. Therefore, the patient must have studies done to rule out other disease processes such as congestive heart failure or alcoholism.

Hepatitis B is caused by a DNA virus. The majority of patients who develop hepatitis B are asymptomatic (85–95%). Five to ten percent of the patients who have hepatitis B surface antigen (HBsAg) which forms on the outer core of the virus develop chronic hepatitis or become carriers.

Delta hepatitis is recognized as a cause of fulminant hepatitis with hepatitis B. Screening for HBsAg helps to decrease the risk of transmitting delta hepatitis.

TABLE 24–12. FEATURES OF DIFFERENT TYPES OF POSTTRANSFUSION HEPATITIS[a]

Feature	B	NANB	Delta	CMV
Proportion	6–15%	75–90%	Unknown	2–17%
Donor screening tests	HBsAg	ALT (SGPT), anti-HBcAg	HBsAg	Anti-CMV
Carrier rate	5–10%	2–6%	1%	6–12%
Patients at risk	Any	Any	Hepatitis B carriers, persons with hemophilia, intravenous drug abusers	Immunosuppressed, low-birth-weight premature infants
Average incubation period, wk (range)	13 (2–26)	7 (2–26)	Unknown	5 (3–6)
Clinical outcome	85–95% asymptomatic, 5–10% chronic hepatitis, 1–3% fatal	60% asymptomatic, 25–50% chronic hepatitis	Fulminant hepatitis	Usually asymptomatic, rarely fatal

[a] ALT, alanine aminotransferase; CMV, cytomegalovirus; HBcAg, hepatitis B core antigen; HBsAg, hepatitis B surface antigen; NANB, non-A non-B.
(*From Coffin CM: Current issues in transfusion therapy. 1. Risks of infection. Postgrad Med 80(8):219–224, 1986.*)

Cytomegalovirus (CMV) infections are spread by infected leukocytes in donor blood. The largest population at risk for contracting CMV are the immunosuppressed patients and premature, low birth weight babies.

To help prevent the transmission of hepatitis, careful screening for HBsAg of the donated blood and use of volunteer donors reduces risk factors associated with viral hepatitis. Aach, Szmuness, and Mosley (1981) have suggested that all blood donors should be screened for ALT to reduce the risk of transmission of NANB hepatitis. The incidence of hepatitis is related to the number of transfusions an individual receives. Therefore, unnecessary transfusions should be avoided to help decrease the transmission of viral hepatitis.

Acquired Immunodeficiency Syndrome

Acquired immunodeficiency syndrome (AIDS) is a disease caused by a virus or group of viruses known as a human lymphocytotropic virus, type III (HTLV-III). AIDS can be transmitted by blood transfusions. The clinical symptoms range from no symptoms to a severe immunodeficiency that could lead to death. The time from transfusion to diagnosis of AIDS may be as soon as 4 months after transfusion to as long as 84 months after transfusion. The AIDS virus can be transferred by whole blood, red blood cells, platelets, plasma, and cryoprecipitate. The incidence of AIDS transmitted by blood transfusion is 2 percent of all who have contracted the disease. To prevent the spread of AIDS, there is blood screening for donors with antibodies to HIV and an effort is made to persuade donors identified as being high risk not to donate blood. However, the number of false–negative tests are not known and the reliability of the test is not absolute.

PARASITIC INFECTIONS

The parasitic infection most frequently transmitted by blood transfusions in the United States is malaria. The two most common organisms in transfusion-associated malaria are *Plasmodium malariae* and *Plasmodium falciparum*. Patients most at risk for acquiring malaria are those who receive many transfusions, those who undergo immunosuppressive therapy, and those who have had a splenectomy.

PULMONARY DYSFUNCTION

The incidence of pulmonary dysfunction following massive transfusions is high. Many factors may be associated with the pulmonary dysfunction following transfusions. Unfiltered debris found in transfused blood may cause pulmonary vascular obstruction which could lead to adult respiratory distress syndrome. A study was conducted by research teams in Vietnam who found that in 1 unit of blood filtered with a 170-μm filter there were up to 4 g wet weight particles per unit of stored blood. The other factors that are considered to cause adult respiratory distress include chest and abdominal compliance injury, circulatory overload, hypoxemia resulting from hypovolemic shock, sepsis, and extensive use of colloids rather than crystalloid for rapid volume replacement.

Hypoxemia

Hypoxemia has been associated with massive transfusions due to embolization. Particulate debris has been found in the pulmonary capillaries after massive transfusion. However, studies by Colline et al (1968) have indicated hypoxemia may be associated with the type of injury rather than the amount of blood transfused. These two variables are difficult to delineate in the studies.

Red cells that are transfused can improve the oxygen-carrying capacity. However, the blood that is stored in CPD-A1 causes an increase in the 2,3-diphosphoglycerate levels. The addition of 2,3-diphosphoglycerate to blood causes a shift in the oxygen dissociation curve to the right. The shift to the right indicates a decrease in the hemoglobin–oxygen affinity and oxygen is more readily released to the tissue (Fig. 24–7).

Sepsis

The reticuloendothelial system is depressed following trauma, major surgery, burns and after hemorrhage. The depression of the reticuloendothelial system may be related

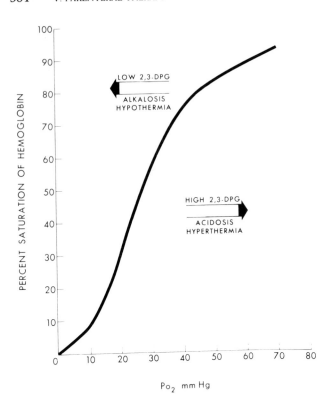

Figure 24–7. Factors that shift the oxygen dissociation curve. (*From Miller RD: The oxygen dissociation curve and multiple transfusions of ACD blood. Management of patients for radical cancer surgery. In Howland WS, Schweizer O (eds): Clinical Anesthesia, Vol 9. Philadelphia, FA Davis, 1972, pp. 43–52.*)

TABLE 24–13. CHANGES THAT OCCUR DURING BLOOD STORAGE

- Decreased pH
- Decreased 2,3-diphosphoglycerate
- Decreased platelets, leukocytes
- Decreased factors V and VIII
- Decreased plasma sodium and bicarbonate

- Increased plasma potassium
- Increased plasma ammonia
- Increased plastic particles
- Increased histamine and serotonin

- RBC shape

(*Modified from Miller RD: A.S.A. Refresher Courses 1:101, 1973.*)

to several factors such as blockage of the reticuloendothelial system due to debris and endogenous adrenocortical hormone secreted as a result of shock.

Not only is the reticuloendothelial system depressed but studies by Snyder et al (1981) found that fibronectin levels are also decreased under these stressful situations. Fibronectin has been identified as playing a major role in opsonization of tissue debris, soluble fibrin, and gram-positive bacteria. Mosher and Furcht (1981) stated that fibronectin plays a major role in the lung fluid balance during bacterial sepsis. This is demonstrated by an increased pulmonary vascular permeability.

Coagulopathies

Abnormal bleeding times are often attributed to massive transfusions. Many of the problems, such as deficiencies in platelets and labile coagulation factors, are associated with the dilutional effect of transfusion therapy. Episodes of intravascular coagulation and fibrinolysis have occurred following massive transfusions. Stored blood has many missing vital components, such as platelets and ionized calcium, and has low levels of factors V and VIII (Table 24–13). Therefore, during massive transfusion, the utilization of blood component therapy to meet the needs of the patient should be continually assessed.

Platelets in whole blood no longer function after 48 hours when stored at 4C. Platelet function is further inhib-

ited by depressed ionized calcium and alterations in pH and temperature. Because of this, massive transfusions may led to dilutional thrombocytopenia. Dilutional thrombocytopenia is one of the most common causes of hemorrhagic diathesis in patients who receive massive transfusions. When the platelet count is less than 100,000 cells/mm^3 the tendency for developing bleeding problems is likely. When bleeding problems develop after several transfusions, assessment of a platelet count may be necessary to determine the appropriate intervention.

Disseminated intravascular coagulation (DIC) has been reported after massive transfusions. DIC is an abnormal activation of the coagulation system. The treatment of DIC is with heparin in an attempt to counteract the hypercoagulability of the blood. DIC is believed to cause a release of tissue thromboplastin due to acidotic tissue. This results in consumption of coagulation factors.

CONCLUSION

The administration of blood components carries risks. Therefore, when administering blood and blood components the advantages of therapy must outweigh the risks. Myhre (1980) studied the number of fatalities reported to the Food and Drug Administration due to transfused blood and blood products. Of those fatalities, 61 percent were due to clerical errors. The second most common problem that developed due to blood transfusions was posttransfusion hepatitis. About 33 percent of the total fatalities from blood transfusions resulted from hepatitis. The majority of fatalities due to blood transfusions can be prevented by careful screening and judicious administration of blood components.

REFERENCES

Aach RD, Szmuness W, Mosley JW, et al: Serum alanine aminotransferase of donors in relation to the risk of non-A, non-B hepatitis in recipients: The transfusion-transmitted viruses study. N Engl J Med 304(17):989–994, 1981.

Attar S, Boyd D, Layne F, et al: Alterations in coagulation and fibrinolytic mechanisms in acute trauma. J Trauma 9:939, 1969.

Belcher P, Lennox SC: Avoidance of blood transfusion in coronary artery surgery: A trial of hydroxyethyl starch. Ann Thorac Surg 37(5):365–370, 1984.

Bick RL: Disseminated intravascular coagulation and related syndromes: etiology, pathophysiology, diagnosis, and management. Am J Hematol 5:265–282, 1978.

Blajchman MA, Sheppard FA, Perrault RA: Clinical use of blood, blood components and blood products. Can Med Assoc J 121:33, 1979.

Blajchman MA, Herst R, Perrault RA: Blood component therapy in anaesthetic practice. Can Anaesth Soc J 30(4):382–389, 1983.

Blood, Blood Components and Derivatives in Transfusion Therapy. Washington, DC, American Association of Blood Banks, 1980.

Blumberg BS: Polymorphisms of the serum proteins and the development of iso-precipitins in transfused patients. Bull NY Acad Med 40:377, 1964.

Blumberg N, Laczin J, McMican A, et al: A critical survey of fresh-frozen plasma use. Transfusion 26(6):511–513, 1986.

Blume KG, Beutler E, Bross KJ, et al: Bone-marrow ablation and allogeneic marrow transplantation in acute leukemia. N Engl J Med 302:1041–1046, 1980.

Breckenridge RL, Solberg LA, Pineda AA, et al: Treatment of thrombotic thrombocytopenic purpura with plasma exchange, antiplatelet agents, corticosteroid, and plasma infusion: Mayo Clinic experience. J Clin Apheresis 1:6–13, 1982.

Bunker JP, Bendixen HH, Murphy BS: Hemodynamic effects of intravenously administered sodium citrate. N Engl J Med 266:372–377, 1962.

Coffin CM: Current issues in transfusion therapy. 1. Risks of infection. Postgrad Med 80(8):219–224, 1986.

Collins JA: The causes of progressive pulmonary insufficiency in surgical patients. J Surg Res 12:685, 1969.

Collins JA: Problems associated with the massive transfusion of stored blood. Surgery 75(2): 274–292, 1974.

Collins JA, Gordon WC, Hudson, TL, et al: Inapparent hypoxemia in casualties with wounded limbs: Pulmonary fat embolism? Ann Surg 167:511, 1968.

Connell RS, Swank RL: Pulmonary microembolism after blood transfusions: An election microscopic study. Ann Surg 177:40, 1973.

Derrick JB: AIDS and the use of blood components and derivatives: The Canadian perspective. Can Med Assoc 131(1):20–22, 1984.

Ellison, N: Blood component therapy in the operating room. Current Rev Nurse Anesth 2:Lesson 15, 1980.

Ennis M, Lorenz W: Hypersensitivity reactions induced by anaesthetics and plasma substitutes. In Dean, Luster, Munson, Amos (eds): Immunotoxicology and Immunopharmacology. New York, Raven Press, 1985, p. 457.

Feinstein DI: Diagnosis and management of disseminated intravascular coagulation: the role of heparin therapy. Blood 60:284–287, 1982.

Gazzard BG, Henderson JM, Williams R: The use of fresh frozen plasma or a concentrate of factor IX as replacement therapy before liver biopsy. Gut 16:621–625, 1975.

Goldfinger D: Febrile transfusion reaction: What blood component should be given next? Vox Sang (6):400–401, 1983.

Guyton A: Textbook of Medical Physiology, 6th ed, Philadelphia, W. B. Saunders, 1981.

Harrigan C, Cantrell, ME: Unit VI: Anesthesia for emergency surgery; hemostasis and blood replacement therapy. In Current Concepts in Inhalation Anesthesia. Philadelphia, Ted Thomas, 1986.

Hehne HJ, Nyman D, Burri H, Wolf G: Management of bleeding disorders in traumatic hemorrhagic shock states with deep frozen fresh plasma. Eur J Intensive Care Med 2:157–161, 1976.

Hester JP, McCredie KB, Freireich EJ. Platelet replacement therapy: A clinical assessment. In Greenwalt TJ, Jamieson GA (eds): The Blood Platelet in Transfusion Therapy. New York, Alan R Liss, 281–294, 1978.

Holley PW, Polesky HF, Saeed SM: Components. In Taswell HF, Saeed SM (eds): Principles and Practice of Quality Control in the Blood Bank. Washington, DC, American Association of Blood Banks, 1980, pp. 63–97.

Howland WS, Schweizer O, Carlon GC, et al: The cardiovascular effects of low levels of ionized calcium during massive transfusion. Surg Gynecol Obstet 145:581, 1977.

Kahn RA: Diseases transmitted by blood transfusion. Hum Pathol 14(3):241–247, 1983.

Kennedy MS: Essentials of immunohematology and blood therapy. In Zuspan PF, Quilligan EJ (eds): A Practical Manual of Obstetrical Care. St. Louis, CV Mosby, 1981.

Kennedy MS, Adkins S, Wansky J: Blood Components, Safe Transfusion, a Technical Workshop. Washington DC, American Association of Blood Banks, 1981.

Lowe KC: Blood transfusion or blood substitution? Vox Sang 51(4):257–263, 1986.

Lucas CE, Ledgerwood AM: Clinical significance of altered coagulation tests after massive transfusion for trauma. Am Surg 47:125–130, 1981.

Mallory TH, Kennedy MS: The use of banked autologous blood in total hip replacement surgery. Clin Orthop 117:254–257, 1976.

Mannucci PM, Franchi F, Dioguardi N: Correction of abnormal coagulation in chronic liver disease by combined use of fresh-frozen plasma and prothrombin complex concentrates. Lancet 2:542–545, 1976.

Mannucci PM, Federici AB, Sirchia G: Hemostasis testing during massive blood replacement: A study of 172 cases. Vox Sang 42:113–123, 1982.

McCullough J, Crosby WH: Contempo '80: Hematology. JAMA 243:2188–2190, 1980.

Mendelson JA: The selection of plasma volume expanders for mass casualty planning. J Trauma 14:987, 1974.

Messmer K: Acute preoperative hemodilution: An alternative to transfusion as donor blood. In Lewis (ed): Dextran—30 Years. Uppsala, Almqvist & Wiksell, 1977, p. 93.

Miller RD: Medical intelligence complications of massive blood transfusions. Anesthesiology 39(1), 82–92, 1973.

Miller RD, et al: Anesthesia Vol 2 New York, Churchill Livingstone, 1986, pp. 1329–1369.

Moore SB: Management of transfusion in the massively bleeding patient. Hum Pathol 14(3):267–270, 1983.

Moseley RV, Doty DB: Death associated with multiple pulmonary emboli soon after battle injury. Ann Surg 171:336, 1970.

Moseley RV, Doty DB: Changes in the filtration characteristics of stored blood. Ann Surg 171:329, 1970.

Mosher DF, Furcht LT: Fibronectin: Review of its structure and possible functions. J Invest Dermatol 77:175, 1981.

Myers TJ, Wakem CJ, Ball Ed, Tremont SJ: Thrombotic thrombocytopenic purpura: Combined treatment with plasmapheresis and antiplatelet agents. Ann Int Med 92:149–155, 1980.

Myhre BA: Fatalities from blood transfusion. JAMA 24:1333–1335, 1980.

Nilsson L, Hedner U, Nilsson IM, Robertson B: Shelf-life of bank blood and stored plasma with special reference to coagulation factors. Transfusion 23(5):377–381, 1983.

Oberman HA, Barnes BA, Friedman BA: The risk of abbreviating the major cross match in urgent or massive transfusion. Transfusion 18:137, 1978.

Perkins HA: Transfusion-associated AIDS. Am J Hematol 19(3):307–313, 1985.

Peterman TA, Jaffe HW, Feorino PM, et al: Transfusion-associated acquired immunodeficiency syndrome in the United States. JAMA 254(20):2913–2917, 1985.

Pisciotto P, Rosen D, Silver H, et al: Treatment of thrombotic thrombocytopenic purpura: Evaluation of plasma exchange and review of the literature. Vox Sang 45:185–196, 1983.

Richter W, Messmer K, Hedin H, Ring J: Adverse reactions to plasma substitutes: incidence and pathomechanisms. In Watkins, W (ed): Adverse Response to Intravenous Drugs. London, Academic Press, 1978, p. 49.

Ring J, Messmer K: Incidence and severity of anaphylactoid reactions to colloid volume substitutes. Lancet *i*: 466–469, 1977.

Rosario MD, Rumsey EW Jr, Arakaki G, et al: Blood microaggregates and ultrafilters. J Trauma 18:498, 1978.

Saba TM, Blumenstock FA, Scoville WA, et al: Cryoprecipitate reversal of opsonic alpha$_2$-surface-binding glycoprotein deficiency in septic surgical and trauma patients. Science 201:622, 1978.

Saba TM, Jaffe E: Plasma fibronectin (opsonic glycoprotein): Its synthesis by vascular endothelial cells and role in cardiopulmonary integrity after trauma as related to reticuloendothelial function. Am J Med 68:577, 1980.

Schwab CW, Civil I, Shayne JP: Saline-expanded group O uncrossmatched packed red blood cells as an initial resuscitation fluid in severe shock. Ann Emerg Med 15(11):1282–1287, 1986.

Sherman LA: Alterations in hemostasis during massive transfusion. In Nusbacher J (ed): Massive Transfusion. Washington, DC, American Association of Blood Banks, 1978, p. 53.

Silbert JA, Bove JR, Dubin S, Bush WS. Patterns of frozen plasma use. Conn Med 45:507–511, 1981.

Snyder EL (ed): Blood Transfusion Therapy: A Physician's Handbook. Arlington, American Association of Blood Banks, 1983, pp. 59–64.

Snyder AJ, Gottschall JL, Menitove JE: Why is fresh-frozen plasma transfused? Transfusion 26(1):107–112, 1986.

Snyder EL, Mosher DF, Hezzey A, et al: Effect of blood transfusion on in vivo levels of plasma fibronectin. J Lab Clin Med 98:336, 1981.

Sohmer PR, Dawson RB: Transfusion therapy in trauma. A review of the principles and techniques used in the M11.MS program. Am Surg 45:109, 1979.

Spector I, Corn M, Ticktin HE: Effect of plasma transfusions on the prothrombin time and clotting factor in liver disease. N Engl J Med 275:1032–1037, 1966.

Standards for Blood Banks and Transfusion Services, 10th ed. Washington, DC, American Association of Blood Banks, 1981.

Tawes RL Jr, Scribner RG, Duval TB, et al: The cell-saver and autologous transfusion: An underutilized resource in vascular surgery. Am J Surg 152(1):105–109, 1986.

Thompson HW, Lasky LC, Polesky HF: Evaluation of a volumetric intravenous fluid infusion pump for transfusion of blood components containing red cells. Transfusion 26(3):290–292, 1986.

Umlas J: Coagulation and component therapy in trauma and surgery. In Nusbacher J, Berkman EM (eds): Hemotherapy in Trauma and Surgery. Washington, DC, American Association of Blood Banks, 1979, p. 31.

Widmann FK (ed): AABB Technical Manual, 9th ed. Arlington, VA, Am Assoc of Blood Banks, 1985.

Wiklund L, Thorien L: Intraoperative blood component and fluid therapy. Acta Anaesthesiol Scand Suppl 82:1–8, 1985.

Wilson RF, Mammen E, Walt AJ: Eight years of experience with massive blood transfusions. J Trauma 11:275–285, 1971.

Zuckerman A: A review. Current status of the immunology of blood and tissue protozoa. II. Plasmodium. Exp Parasitol 42:374, 1974.

25

Fluid and Electrolyte Therapy

Lorraine M. Jordan

*T*he management of fluids and electrolytes is an essential part *of the anesthetic care of the surgical patient. The surgical procedure can impose great stress on the fluid and electrolyte status of the patient. This chapter will outline fluid derangements and their treatment.*

ANATOMY OF BODY FLUIDS

The isotope tracer techniques are perhaps the most accurate means of measuring the different fluid compartments of the body. There is a wide range of normal values based on the person's age, weight, body size, and sex. The compartments remain relatively constant throughout life, once adulthood is reached, as long as the patient remains in a normal steady state. This state is referred to as *dynamic equilibrium*. Dynamic equilibrium attempts to maintain the composition of fluids in balance regardless of the intake and output of fluids.

TOTAL BODY WATER

Total body water (TBW) is the water in the intracellular and extracellular compartments. Water accounts for between 50 and 70 percent of total body weight. Using deuterium oxide (D_2O) or tritiated water for measurement of TBW, the average value for young adult males is 60 percent of body weight, and for young adult females 50 percent. The average volume of the total body water is 42 L. The amount of total body fluid in adults is based on the percentage of body fat. Fat contains little water, and lean body mass has more body fluid. Obese persons have as much as 25 to 30 percent less TBW than do lean persons of the same height and average weight.

Age has a significant effect on TBW. Moore and Ball have shown that TBW as a percentage of total body weight decreases steadily with age. As age increases, TBW decreases to as low as 52 percent for males and 47 percent for females. Just the opposite is true for infants. In premature infants, TBW is approximately 90 percent of the total body weight. The full-term infant has approximately 70 to 80 percent TBW compared with total body weight. As an infant becomes older, there is a gradual reduction of TBW. The 1-year-old has a TBW of approximately 65 percent. The TBW remains relatively constant throughout childhood and puberty. TBW ranges from 500 to 600 ml/kg for an average adult (Table 25–1).

The TBW is divided into two compartments:

- Intracellular fluid (ICF)
- Extracellular fluid (ECF)

Intracellular Fluid

ICF is the water within the body's different cells. The ICF makes up 30 to 40 percent of the body weight. The largest amount of ICF is in the skeletal muscle mass. ICF contains large amounts of potassium, magnesium, and phosphate ions and small amounts of sodium and chloride. The principal cations of ICF are potassium and magnesium, and the principal anions are proteins and phosphates.

Extracellular Fluid

ECF is the body water outside the cells. The ECF helps to maintain the internal environment of the body. It provides nutrients and removes waste from the cells. The ECF comprises 20 percent of the body weight and 25 percent of TBW. ECF is further categorized into two major types—the intravascular volume (plasma), which totals 5 percent of body weight, and the interstitial volume (fluid between the cells), which totals 15 percent of body weight (Fig. 25–1).

Approximately 80 percent of the ECF is interstitial fluid. Interstitial fluid includes lymph and the extracellular portion of dense connective tissue and the transcellular compartment. Transcellular water includes fluid such as cerebrospinal fluid, intraocular fluid, joint fluid, salivary fluid, and mucous secretions of the respiratory and gastrointestinal tract. This nonfunctional component represents approximately 10 percent of the interstitial fluid volume and should not be confused with "third-space fluid" found in burns

TABLE 25–1. APPROXIMATE VALUES OF TOTAL BODY FLUID AS A PERCENTAGE OF BODY WEIGHT IN RELATION TO AGE AND SEX

Age	Total Body Fluid (% body weight)
Full-term newborn	70–80
1 year	64
Puberty to 39 years	Men: 60
	Women: 52
40 to 60 years	Men: 55
	Women: 47
More than 60 years	Men: 52
	Women: 46

(*From Metheny N: Quick Reference to Fluid Balance. Philadelphia, Lippencott, 1984.*)

and soft tissue injury. The interstitial fluid also possesses a functional equilibrating component in which dissolved substances move through spaces.

The plasma is approximately 20 percent of the ECF and is the fluid portion of the blood. The plasma interchanges continuously with the interstitial fluid through pores exchanging oxygen and other metabolic substances as the plasma passes through the capillaries. Colloid osmotic pressure minimizes the loss of plasma from the circulatory system through the capillary pores.

ELECTROLYTES

Continuous interactions occur between the various body fluid compartments. To aid in understanding some of these

changes, an explanation of the terminology follows.

Electrolytes are electrically charged particles within the body fluids. These charged particles are ions. The term *ion* describes chemical reactivity. The ions possess negative (anions) and positive (cations) charges. ICF and ECF have different concentrations of ions. The chemical reactivity of ions in each compartment is expressed as mEq/L (Fig. 25–2).

Molecules of substances found in fluid compartments are expressed in mg/100 ml or in g/1000 ml of fluid. The number of particles per unit volume is expressed in moles as mol or millimoles as mmol.

One millimole is 1/1000 of a mole. A mole is the molecular weight of a substance expressed in grams. One mole of $CaCl_2$ is 110 g of $CaCl_2$. To determine the number of grams in $CaCl_2$, the sum of the atomic weight of Ca and Cl is determined. The atomic weight of Ca is 40 and Cl is 35. The sum of the atomic weights is known as molecular weight. An example follows for $CaCl_2$:

$$\text{Atomic weight of Ca} = 40$$
$$\text{Atomic weight of Cl} = 35$$
$$\text{Atomic weight} + \text{atomic weight} = \text{molecular weight}$$
$$40 + 35(2) = 110$$
$$110 \text{ g} = 1 \text{ mol of } CaCl_2$$

If 1 mol of a substance is mixed with 1 L of water, the solution would be expressed as 1 mol/L.

Osmolarity

Osmolarity is an expression of total solute concentration of body fluids. The solute concentration exerts a pressure that is attributed to the number of osmotically active particles in solution. The osmole (Osm) is a unit of measure used to quantify osmolarity. The osmotic pressure of body fluid is often expressed in a smaller unit, the milliosmole (mOsm). An example is sodium chloride. Sodium chloride (NaCl) dissociates into Na^+ and Cl^-, which constitute 2 mOsm.

SOLIDS
40% by weight

FLUID
60% by weight (42 liters)

Total body fluid volume in liters equals 60% of the body weight in kilograms (60% X 70 = 42 liters)

Cellular fluid
40% of body wt, 28 liters

Cellular fluid volume
(0.40 X 70 = 28 liters)

ECF
20% of body wt, 14 liters

Extracellular fluid volume (0.20 X 70 = 14 liters)

ISF, 15%, 10.5 liters

Interstitial fluid volume
(0.15 X 70 = 10.5 liters)

Plasma, 5%, 3.5 liters

Plasma fluid volume
(0.05 X 70 = 3.5 liters)

Figure 25–1. Fluid compartments and the amount of fluid in a 70-kg (154-lb) young adult male. (*From Metheny N: Quick Reference to Fluid Balance. Philadelphia, Lippencott, 1984.*)

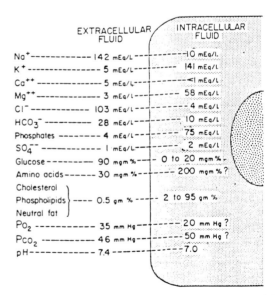

Figure 25–2. Chemical compositions of extracellular and intracellular fluids. (*From Guyton A: Textbook of Medical Physiology, 5th ed. Philadelphia, Saunders, 1976.*)

Calcium (Ca^{2+}) and magnesium (Mg^{2+}) are divalent ions. Divalent ions carry two charges in the molecule. Therefore, 1 mmol of a divalent cation equals 2 mEq. If an element is monovalent, such as sodium (Na^+), 1 mmol of a monovalent ion is equivalent to 1 mEq.

There remains an ionic difference between the two compartments of ICF and ECF. The ICF and ECF are separated by a semipermeable membrane. The osmotic pressure exerted is dependent on the number of osmotically active particles. The number of substances that fail to pass through the semipermeable membrane contribute to the effective osmotic pressure. Sodium is the principal cation of ECF and is the major contributor of osmotic pressure, whereas the dissolved proteins in the plasma are responsible for the osmotic pressure between the plasma and the interstitial fluid compartment.

The osmotic pressure of the ECF and ICF is essentially equal. The number of osmotically active particles in the ECF and ICF is 290 to 310 mOsm. The semipermeable membrane between ECF and ICF is freely permeable to water and allows the two compartments to maintain essential osmotic equilibrium. The osmotic pressure of compartments can become altered. A change in osmotic pressure of ECF and ICF compartments will lead to changes in fluid volume. For example, a loss of sodium from the ECF would cause an efflux of H_2O from the ECF to the ICF.

Osmosis is the net movement of water across a semipermeable membrane, from higher concentration to lower concentration. The greatest exchange of fluid occurs within the ECF compartment.

BODY FLUID CHANGES

Disorders in fluid balance can be categorized as disturbances in:

- Volume
- Concentration
- Composition

Volume Changes

Volume changes that occur are either a volume deficit or a volume excess.

Volume Deficit. ECF volume deficit is frequently referred to as fluid deficit, hypovolemia, and dehydration. An ECF volume deficit is due to a loss of water and electrolytes, a greater loss of fluid than intake of fluid. The body loses fluid from the kidneys, skin, lungs, and gastrointestinal tract. The adult typically excretes 1 to 2 L of urine per day. The skin loses water through perspiration, which varies widely with the temperature of the environment. Insensible loss of water through the skin occurs by evaporation. The loss of fluid via the lungs occurs at a rate of 300 to 400 ml every day. This loss can increase greatly with an increased respiratory rate and tidal volume. The body loses 100 to 200 ml of fluid daily through the gastrointestinal tract. Therefore, the average adult requires at least 2000 ml of water per day as maintenance.

ECF volume deficit may be caused by vomiting, diarrhea, loss of nasogastric secretions, and fistula drainage. During surgery, the patient loses a great deal of ECF via evaporation, blood loss, and third spacing due to surgical trauma. Other causes of ECF loss include burns, peritonitis, intestinal obstruction, and sequestration of fluid from soft tissue injury.

Two systems primarily affected by volume changes are the cardiovascular and nervous systems. The cardiovascular system displays such signs as a postural decrease in systolic blood pressure in excess of 10 mm Hg, increased heart rate, flat neck veins in supine position, and a decreased central venous pressure. Other signs and symptoms noted when there is an ECF deficit are oliguria (less than 20 to 40 ml/hr), nausea, vomiting, weight loss, a depressed anterior fontanel in infants, an increase in specific gravity of the urine, longitudinal wrinkles in the tongue, dry skin, weakness, and apathy.

A severe loss of ECF may lead to shock or cardiovascular collapse, as well as permanent renal damage. The decrease in ECF may lead to hypotension and inadequate perfusion of the kidneys. Inadequate perfusion of the kidneys may cause the nephrons and tubules to deteriorate and to become permanently damaged.

Volume Excess. Excess of ECF volume is often caused by fluid excess, which develops when fluid input exceeds output. The kidneys are unable to rid the body of excess water and electrolytes. Volume excess often develops from overloading the body by oral or parental administration of excessive quantities of fluid or as a result of renal failure. Excess ECF indicates an increase in both plasma and interstitial fluid volume.

Some signs generally encountered with volume excess include circulatory overload manifested by pulmonary hypertension, dyspnea, cyanosis, coughing, frothy sputum, elevated pulmonary artery wedge pressure, ascites, effusions into third spaces, peripheral edema, bounding pulse, distended neck veins, moist rales, and increases in central venous pressure and blood pressure. Volume excess in the elderly often presents as congestive heart failure. Patients more susceptible to volume overload are those with chronic heart failure, chronic renal failure, excessive adrenocortical hormones, and excessive administration of IV fluids, especially isotonic solutions.

The treatment for volume excess includes fluid restriction, administration of diuretics, restriction of sodium intake, administration of oxygen, high Fowler's position, and decreasing the work load of the heart by the administration of vasodilators and positive-pressure ventilation. Positive-pressure ventilation increases the intraalveolar pressure, forcing the fluid out of the alveoli.

Changes in Serum Concentration

Sodium. Sodium (Na^+) is the most abundant cation of the ECF, and is the most important ion exerting osmotic pressure on the cellular membrane. Concentrations of sodium in the ECF range from 135 to 145 mEq/L. Sodium is a primary determinant of ECF and water distribution.

Sodium is regulated in part by the kidneys. It helps

to maintain normal composition of ECF, as well as chemical-electrical equilibrium. Sodium also mediates action potentials within the nerves and muscles. The regulation of sodium in the body is controlled by the secretion of antidiuretic hormone (ADH) and aldosterone.

ADH is secreted by the hypothalamic posterior pituitary. The secretion of ADH causes an increase in water reabsorption by the kidneys, decreasing urinary output and increasing urinary concentration. The reabsorption of water in the kidneys occurs at the collecting tubules.

The production and release of ADH are influenced by receptors in the hypothalamus known as osmoreceptors. The osmoreceptors are sensitive to osmotic pressure of the plasma. ADH assists in regulation of osmotic pressure.

Aldosterone is a hormone secreted by the adrenal cortex. It is a mineralocorticoid that exerts effects on the kidneys, stimulating reabsorption of sodium and excretion of potassium ions.

Hyponatremia. Hyponatremia is low sodium concentration in the ECF. Hyponatremia may be due to excessive loss of sodium via vomiting, diarrhea, diuretics, and loss through body cavities such as peritonitis, draining ascites, and burns. Sodium deficit may also result in excessive intake of water. The resulting water intoxication dilutes the serum sodium. Examples of serum sodium dilution include excess water intake, depressed renal blood flow, repeated water enemas, congestive heart failure with water retention, and parental administration of electrolyte-free solutions. The hyponatremic state lends itself to an osmotic shift out of the ECF compartment and into the ICF compartment. This shift of fluid causes fluid depletion in the ECF compartment and leads to hypovolemia. A severe shift of fluid causes cerebral edema, leading to the development of neurologic symptoms.

The clinical signs associated with hyponatremia due to sodium loss are weakness, confusion, nausea, vomiting, neurologic signs, postural hypotension, and lethargy. Some serious neurologic symptoms that may develop are loss of reflexes, the Babinski's sign, and seizures. These signs develop when the serum sodium drops below 115 mEq/L.

The treatment of sodium deficiency is aimed at restoration of sodium in the ECF compartment. Treatment may entail oral sodium intake and intravenous fluid replacement of sodium with 3 percent or 5 percent sodium chloride. The treatment may require free-water fluid restriction in an effort to increase the sodium in the ECF compartment.

The disease state frequently associated with hyponatremia is Addison's disease, which results from degeneration of the adrenal cortex and leads to aldosterone deficiency. The decrease of aldosterone secretion is followed by the loss of sodium. Addison's disease may lead to hypovolemia and cerebral edema if left untreated. The treatment of Addison's disease includes corticosteroid supplements and controlled salt intake. If Addison's disease remains untreated, death will result.

Another syndrome in which there is an inappropriate secretion of ADH is associated with the dilution of sodium and with water gain. The inappropriate secretion of ADH is often associated with certain tumors frequently found in the bronchus of the lung or in the basal regions of the brain. The effects of ADH are a decrease in sodium concentration in the ECF and a slight increase in ECF volume. The inappropriate secretion of ADH leads to very concentrated urinary output and a loss of sodium. Treatment includes correcting the serum sodium levels and alleviating water retention. Restriction of fluid alone may not provide adequate relief, and a diuretic may be a necessary adjunct. The use of 3 or 5 percent intravenous NaCl is suggested for treatment of decreased sodium levels.

The administration of oxytocin may also lead to water intoxication. The hormone oxytocin has an intrinsic antidiuretic effect, leading to an increase in water reabsorption. Therefore, a patient in labor and on a continuous drip of oxytocin needs to be continually assessed for signs of water intoxication. The symptoms of water intoxication must be carefully assessed and must not be mistaken for signs of eclampsia. The best diagnostic aid is a serum sodium determination.

Hypernatremia. Hypernatremia is an increased sodium concentration in the ECF. Some causes of hypernatremia include decreased water intake, excessive loss of body fluids particularly via the bronchial tree, increased aldosterone, and excessive administration of sodium-containing fluids. Often the excessive retention of sodium occurs in the chronically ill patient in whom water is also retained. The retention of sodium by the kidneys is an effort by the body to restore the plasma volume. However, the attempt to restore adequate plasma volume by the renin-angiotensin-aldosterone mechanism results in retention in the interstitial space. Accumulation in the interstitial space leads to edema, ascites, and pleural effusion.

Hypernatremia can be caused by overzealous administration of sodium bicarbonate during resuscitative efforts. Another cause of hypernatremia that the anesthetist may encounter is a hypertonic saline abortion. The hypertonic saline may accidentally enter into the maternal circulation via direct access or by amniotic fluid absorption, possibly elevating the serum sodium.

Signs of hypernatremia include furrowed tongue, restlessness, lethargy, increased deep tendon reflexes, sticky mucous membranes, flushed skin, and thirst.

The treatment of hypernatremia is to limit sodium intake and administer diuretics and water.

Potassium. Most potassium within the body is found in the intracellular compartment, where it is the major cation. Potassium plays a vital role in the transmission of nerve impulses and the contraction of muscle. Potassium moves freely between the intracellular and extracellular compartments. The sodium–potassium pump controls the movement of potassium between the cells and the ECF. The normal value of serum potassium is 3.5 to 5.5 mEq/L.

The normal dietary intake of potassium is 50 to 100 mg daily. However, 80 percent of the potassium is excreted via the renal system and the other 20 percent is lost through the bowel and sweat glands. The normal range of potassium secreted through the kidneys is 40 to 80 mEq/24 hr. The kidneys excrete a large amount of potassium daily and do not conserve potassium; therefore, a daily intake of potassium is vital for body functions.

The regulation of potassium is influenced by dietary intake. A high dietary intake of potassium is reflected in an increase in the excretion of potassium. Renal failure inhibits the secretion of potassium and allows the serum levels of potassium to reach potentially fatal levels. A low potassium level may result from diarrhea, surgical stress, or acidosis. Another means of controlling potassium is by the regulation of aldosterone. The release of aldosterone facilitates potassium secretion and sodium reabsorption. Increased potassium intake stimulates the renin-angioten-sin-aldosterone mechanism, and the kidney increases tubular potassium secretion. If the extracellular potassium concentration is low, a decrease in aldosterone production results, conserving potassium at the tubular level. Both excesses and deficits alter the resting membrane potential of the cell.

Hypokalemia. Hypokalemia is defined as low serum levels of potassium. Many of the causes of hypokalemia are iatrogenic. Hypokalemia is frequently evidenced in patients on diuretic therapy. Because hypertension is becoming relatively common and one of the modalities of treatment is the use of diuretics, the frequency of hypokalemia in the surgical patient has increased. Other factors leading to hypokalemia are starvation, diarrhea, loss of body fluids particularly gastric secretions, crushing injuries, primary aldosteronism, reduced renal absorption, and stressful situations (fever, sweating, thyroid storm). Prolonged administration of some antibiotics such as sodium carbenicillin and sodium penicillin may also lead to hypokalemia. Hypokalemia also occurs in patients undergoing surgery. In the first 2 postoperative days, the patient may lose 100 mmol of potassium and continues to lose 25 mmol/day in the immediate postoperative period.

Hypokalemia is frequently associated with metabolic alkalosis. Respiratory and metabolic alkalosis results in an increased renal excretion of potassium. Hydrogen and potassium compete for exchange with sodium in the renal tubule. Therefore, potassium is excreted in exchange for sodium. Hypokalemia results in alkalosis from an increase in hydrogen ion excretion, compensating with a lower potassium concentration. Movement of hydrogen ions into the cell results in a potassium loss responsible for alkalosis. Chloride depletion often accompanies hypokalemia.

Signs and symptoms of hypokalemia result from an alteration of the body systems. The neuromuscular dysfunctions that are due to hypokalemia are anorexia, weakness, loss of muscle tone, and loss of muscle reflexes. The cardiovascular system displays signs of a weak pulse, arrhythmias, decreased intensity of heart sounds, and a decrease in blood pressure when hypokalemia is evident. The electrocardiogram (ECG) will display a low to flattened T wave, depressed ST segment, and predominant U wave (Fig. 25–3). Cardiac arrest may eventually follow. The gastrointestinal tract decreases peristalic movement, and abdominal distension may result. A pseudodiabetic glycosuria may result because of an inability to move glucose across the cell membrane.

Hypokalemia is treated by replacing the potassium and correcting the reason for its loss. If mild hypokalemia is

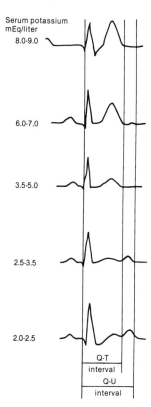

Figure 25–3. Effect of serum potassium levels on ECG. Hyperkalemia initially causes the T wave to increase in magnitude. With increasing serum potassium levels, the ST segment becomes depressed, the U wave disappears, and the QRS duration and P-R interval increase. With serum potassium levels greater than 10 mEq/L, ventricular fibrillation often ensues. Hypokalemia broadens and lowers the magnitude of the T wave, increases the magnitude of the U wave, and causes the T and U waves to fuse. It should be noted that, with respect to the heart rate, the Q-T interval and Q-U interval do not increase. With severe hypokalemia, ST segment depression is observed. (*With permission from Wilson RF [ed]: Principles and Techniques of Critical Care. Philadelphia, F.A. Davis Co., 1976, p. 29.*)

evident, replacement of potassium may be given by dietary or oral supplements.

Decreased serum potassium levels may threaten the patient's life, and potassium may be given at a rate of 40 mEq/hour in intravenous fluid. ECG monitoring should be continuous when administering intravenous potassium. In crisis situations, rapid administration of potassium is potentially dangerous. However, close and constant monitoring is essential. During rapid potassium replacement, a rapid rise in potassium can predispose the patient to hyperkalemia. In cases of large potassium deficit, replacement and restoration of normal serum values may take days to weeks.

Hyperkalemia. Hyperkalemia is an excess of potassium in the ECF volume. A common cause of hyperkalemia is renal failure and an inability of the kidneys to excrete potassium. Life-threatening situations such as crushing injuries, burns, and myocardial damage allow a sudden release of potassium into the ECF. The sudden release of potassium into the

ECF compartment can lead to diastolic cardiac arrythmias, a flaccid myocardium, and cardiac arrest. Other factors associated with hyperkalemia include transfusion of aged blood, adrenocortical insufficiency (Addison's disease), and too rapid or excessive administration of potassium.

Hyperkalemic signs are associated with nerve and muscle function. The muscular system demonstrates signs of weakness and flaccid paralysis. The myocardium becomes flaccid in states of hyperkalemia, and arrhythmias and cardiac arrest develop. The conduction system throughout the myocardium is affected, and the ECG demonstrates high, tented T waves. P waves disappear, the QRS complex widens, and bradycardia develops (see Fig. 25–3). Heart block may occur during a severe state of hyperkalemia. The gastrointestinal tract of a patient in a hyperkalemic state demonstrates signs of hyperactivity: nausea, vomiting, intestinal colic, and diarrhea.

The treatment of hyperkalemia entails reduction of serum potassium levels. Restriction of potassium administration and intake is one corrective measure. The use of a cation-exchange resin helps to prevent hyperkalemia in certain patients. The treatment of severe hyperkalemia may include the intravenous administration of calcium gluconate, sodium bicarbonate, or regular insulin and hypertonic dextrose. The administration of 5 to 20 ml of 10 percent calcium gluconate or chloride temporarily reverses the chronotropic effects on the myocardium. Continuous ECG will display the altered conduction through the Purkinje's fibers, and, should bradycardia develop, the infusion should cease. Sodium bicarbonate raises the pH and drives the potassium into the cell. Administration of sodium bicarbonate should be used carefully in reversing hyperkalemia because of the potential for sodium excess; furthermore, the effects of the drug last a few hours. Intravenous administration of regular insulin, a hypertonic dextrose, stimulates the synthesis of glycogen, resulting in the uptake of potassium. Insulin drives the potassium into the cell but should be limited to 1 unit/5 g of glucose to prevent a rebound of hypoglycemia. For the chronically hyperkalemic patient, other means of potassium excretion are needed. Treatment of these patients may include cation-exchange resins, peritoneal dialysis, and hemodialysis.

Calcium. Calcium is the most abundant cation in the body. It is found in the protoplasm and is present in large proportions in the bone and teeth. Calcium is involved with cellular permeability, neuromuscular activity, and normal blood clotting mechanisms. The normal daily intake of calcium is 1 to 3 g. The body cannot store calcium, and daily consumption of calcium is therefore necessary to sustain adequate calcium levels in the body. Intake of 1 g of calcium is considered adequate for the average adult, but children and pregnant women require larger amounts (1.5 to 2g/day). The normal serum level is 8.6 to 10.5 mg/100 ml. About 50 percent of serum calcium exists in the ionized form, which is responsible for neuromuscular function. Calcium has a reciprocal relationship with phosphorus. Parathyroid hormone and calcitonin facilitate the transfer of calcium from bone to plasma and therefore raise the plasma level of calcium. The normal urinary calcium content is 100 to 250 mg/24 hr.

Calcium disturbances are generally not encountered in the postoperative patient, in whom routine calcium supplementation is seldom indicated. Surgical hypoparathyroidism, acute pancreatitis, excessive administration of citrated blood, and maternal diabetes all are circumstances that may require a calcium supplement.

Hypocalcemia. Hypocalcemia is a low serum level of calcium. Common causes of hypocalcemia include hypoparathyroidism, removal of the parathyroid glands, acute pancreatitis, vitamin D deficiency, and chronic administration of cimetidine.

The symptoms of hypocalcemia include tingling and numbness of the fingers, toes, and the circumoral region; cramps in the extremities; hyperactivity of deep tendon reflexes; Trousseau's sign; Chvostek's sign; and mental confusion leading to convulsions. The ECG manifests a prolonged QT interval and ST segment (Fig. 25–4).

The sign of hypocalcemia that particularly concerns anesthetists is the spasm of laryngeal muscles leading to airway obstruction. Hypocalcemia can result from accidental damage to the parathyroid glands, potentially occurring in patients undergoing a thyroidectomy or a radical neck dissection.

Treatment is aimed at restoration of calcium to normal values. Acute management of hypocalcemia includes intravenous administration of calcium gluconate or calcium chloride. The administration of calcium on a routine basis after massive blood transfusions is controversial. Monitoring calcium levels during massive transfusions is a guide for calcium replacement. The ECG and observation of the QT interval are rough guidelines in assessing serum calcium levels.

Mild calcium deficit may be treated with oral supplements and vitamin D. Vitamin D enhances the absorption of calcium by the gastrointestinal tract.

Hypercalcemia. Hypercalcemia may result from hyperparathyroidism, malignant neoplastic disease, overuse of calcium-containing antacids, and prolonged immobilization.

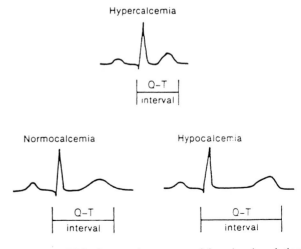

Figure 25–4. ECG changes by serum calcium level variations. (*With permission from Wilson RF [ed]: Principles and Techniques of Critical Care, Philadelphia, F.A. Davis Co., 1976, p. 26.*)

Clinical signs of hypercalcemia are vague. Symptoms of hypercalcemia that may be encountered are fatigue, anorexia, nausea, vomiting, urinary calcium stones, somnambulism, stupor, polydipsia, polyuria, and thirst. The two major causes of hypercalcemia are hyperparathyroidism and cancer with bony metastasis. The ECG displays a shortened ST segment and QT interval.

Acute hypercalcemia may be treated with 0.45 percent NaCl or 0.9 percent NaCl to dilute the serum calcium and aid in urinary excretion. Other measures of treatment used to lower serum calcium include chelating agents, steroids, and hemodialysis.

Magnesium. Magnesium is necessary as a catalyst for intracellular enzymatic reactions. The majority of magnesium is in the intracellular compartment. The extracellular magnesium concentration ranges from 1.5 to 2.5 mEq/L. An increase in extracellular concentrations of magnesium depresses the nervous and skeletal muscular systems. Magnesium imbalance is not a frequent cation imbalance. The normal dietary intake of magnesium is approximately 20 mEq daily. A large amount of magnesium is lost in the urine. The regulation of magnesium is not well understood.

Hypomagnesemia. Magnesium deficiency has been associated with chronic alcohol abuse, gastrointestinal irritability, diuretics, primary aldosteronism, acute pancreatitis, diabetic acidosis, hyperthroidism, and the use of certain drugs such as gentamicin and cisplatin. Magnesium depletion is characterized by neuromuscular and central nervous system hyperactivity. Coarse tremors, muscle cramps, hyperactive reflexes, tachycardia, paresthesias of the feet and legs, and arrhythmias all are clinical signs of magnesium deficiency. Hypomagnesemia on the ECG demonstrates a prolonged PR interval, wide QRS complex, ST depression, and broadened and flattened (inverted) T waves.

Hypomagnesemia is treated by restoring the magnesium levels. Oral administration of magnesium salts can be given for mild depletion. Severe depletion may be treated with intravenous magnesium sulfate or magnesium chloride. A dose of 2 mEq/kg of body weight in 24 hours is given for severe depletion, providing the renal function is within normal limits. Vital signs should be carefully monitored when administering magnesium supplement. In the event of a rapid rise in plasma magnesium levels, calcium gluconate and calcium chloride should be available to counteract the adverse effects.

Hypermagnesemia. Renal failure is one of the major causes of hypermagnesemia. Other conditions associated with hypermagnesemia are Addison's disease, untreated ketoacidosis, and hypothyroidism. Clinical signs of hypermagnesemia include lethargy, loss of deep tendon reflexes, flushing, hypotension, depressed respirations, bradycardia, and ECG changes. The ECG displays an increased PR interval, widened QRS complex, and prolonged QT interval.

In severe hypermagnesemia, treatment is the administration of calcium gluconate or calcium chloride to antagonize the action of magnesium. Correcting acidosis and limiting magnesium intake will aid in lowering the serum level. If conventional means of correcting magnesium are not successful, hemodialysis may be used.

Normal Exchange of Fluid/Electrolytes

The body attempts to maintain a homeostatic environment. The internal and external environments of the body fluids attempt to maintain stable conditions, in which the responses of compensatory mechanisms may be activated. The regulatory system assists in keeping the fluctuations of body fluids and electrolytes at a minimum. The internal environment is maintained by the kidneys, brain, lungs, skin, and gastrointestinal tract. Surgical stress may alter the internal environment.

Water Exchange. The body exchanges the fluid and electrolyte requirements on a daily basis. The average needs of a 60- to 80-kg man are outlined in Table 25–2.

Daily water losses include 250 ml in the stool, 800 to 1500 ml as urine, and approximately 600 to 900 ml as insensible loss. Insensible water losses occur from the lungs by the humidification of inspired air and through the skin

TABLE 25–2. WATER-EXCHANGE (60- TO 80-kg MAN)

H₂O Gain—Routes	Average Daily Volume (ml)	Minimal (ml)	Maximal (ml)
Sensible			
Oral fluids	800–1500	0	1500/hr
Solid foods	500–700	0	1500
Insensible			
Water of oxidation	250	125	800
Water of solution	0	0	500
H₂O Loss—Routes			
Sensible			
Urine	800–1500	300	1400/hr (diabetes insipidus)
Intestinal	0–250	0	2500/hr
Sweat	0	0	4000/hr
Insensible			
Lungs and skin	600–900	600–900	1500

(From Sabiston DC: Textbook of Surgery: The Biological Basis of Modern Surgical Practice, 11th ed. Philadelphia, Saunders, 1977.)

by evaporation. The insensible water loss that occurs is approximately 500 ml/m² of body surface. However, this insensible loss can become greatly increased under conditions of hypermetabolism, hyperventilation, and fever. This loss through the breathing circuit during anesthesia is a major concern that must be considered particularly during long cases.

The minimal urinary output for a patient who has been totally restricted of fluids is 500 to 800 ml of urine. This is the minimal amount of urinary excretion necessary to rid the body of products of catabolism.

There are two variables that help in the regulation of body fluids. The sensation of thirst is the body's sensory drive for fluid replacement. A person experiences thirst by a feeling of deprivation of fluid intake demonstrated by dry mucous membranes and decreased salivary secretions. The second variable associated with thirst is the secretion of ADH. A change in the tonicity of ECF inhibits the release of ADH, and water reabsorption by the renal tubules occurs. The sensation of thirst may be induced by pharmacologic means such as the administration of atropine and can also be stimulated by withholding fluids or by hemorrhage. Many factors influence the thirst mechanism.

FLUID AND ELECTROLYTE THERAPY

Parenteral Solution

The selection of parenteral solution should be based on the needs of the individual patient. The type and amount of parenteral solution should be carefully reviewed and estimated according to the physical status and weight of the patient. Some important factors to be considered when reviewing fluid requirements are the renal function of the patient, the cardiovascular status of the patient, daily maintenance requirements based on weight or body surface area, and the present fluid status of patient prior to fluid therapy. Maintenance fluids provide replacement of normal fluid loss, such as loss via the lungs, urine, and skin. Maintenance fluids are isotonic. The purpose of replacement fluids is

to correct a loss of isotonic fluid from the body. The loss of isotonic fluid may include ascites and interstitial edema. Table 25–3 can be used as a guide to the most appropriate fluid therapy for maintenance or replacement therapy.

Rate of Fluid Administration

The rate of fluid administration varies considerably, depending on the type of fluid loss, the severity of the fluid loss, and the cardiac and renal status of the patient. Replacement of severe fluid loss can be treated with isotonic solution at a rate of 2000 ml/hr or as indicated by the vital signs.

Patients who are ill and have compromised body functions will not tolerate rapid fluid loss and replacement as well as patients who are in good physical condition. Therefore, patients who have cardiovascular and renal disease will not tolerate shifts in fluid as well as healthy patients. Fluid administration must be monitored with special care in infants and in the elderly.

Preoperative Fluid Therapy

The majority of surgical patients have been fasting 8 to 10 hours prior to surgery. Therefore, patients coming to surgery are depleted of solutes and water as a result of normal body function. In general, adult patients have intravenous fluids started prior to induction of anesthesia to replace these losses and to provide access to the circulatory system.

An adequate assessment of preoperative fluid and electrolyte balance and subsequent correction are necessary for successful surgical intervention. Observation and an accurate history of the patient's fluid intake are a means of appraising a patient's fluid status. If the patient's fluid status indicates abnormalities in fluid balance, these should be corrected before entering the surgical suite. Abnormalities of fluid balance can easily be categorized into three classes: volume, concentration, and composition. Guidelines for administering fluids on the day of surgery are illustrated in Table 25–4.

TABLE 25–3. COMMERCIALLY AVAILABLE FLUIDS FOR PARENTERAL USE

Symbol	Type	Dextrose (mg/ml)	Sodium (mEq/L)	Other Cations (mEq/L)	Chloride (mEq/L)	Other Anions (mEq/L)
D5W	Maintenance	50	—	—	—	—
D4MLR	Maintenance	40	26	K, 0.8; Ca, 0.5	22	Lactate, 5.5
D5NaCl 0.45	Maintenance	50	77	—	77	—
LR	Replacement	—	130	K, 4; Ca, 3	109	Lactate, 28
D5LR	Replacement	50	130	K, 4; Ca, 3	109	Lactate, 28
0.9% NaCl	Replacement	—	154	—	154	—
D5NaCl	Replacement	50	154	—	154	—
Normosol-R	Replacement	—	140	K, 5; Mg, 3	90	Acetate Gluconate, 50
Plasmalyte	Replacement	—	140	K, 5; Mg, 3	98	Acetate, 27 Gluconate, 23
5% NaCl	Special purpose	—	855	—	855	—

Abbreviations used: D5W = 5% dextrose in water USP; D4MLR = 4% dextrose in modified lactated Ringer's solution; D5NaCl 0.45 = 5% dextrose in half-strength saline USP; LR = lactated Ringer's solution (also known as Hartman's solution); D5LR = 5% dextrose in lactated Ringer's solution; 0.9% NaCl = 0.9% sodium chloride solution USP (frequently called isotonic saline, "normal saline," or simply "saline" and abbreviated NS); D5NaCl = 5% dextrose in 0.9% sodium chloride solution USP; 5% NaCl = 5% sodium chloride solution (also called hypertonic saline). (*From Miller RD: Anesthesia, 2nd ed. New York, Churchill Livingstone, 1986.*)

TABLE 25–4. GUIDELINES FOR ROUTINE FLUIDS ON THE DAY OF SURGERY

Step 1
  Start intravenous, replace insensible loss with maintenance-type solutions, 2 ml/kg/hr, for interval since last oral intake.
Step 2
  Change to replacement-type solutions for intraoperative insensible losses. Administer LR, Normosol-R, or in some cases NaCl, 2mg/kg/hr.
Step 3
  Estimate surgical trauma and add appropriate volume of replacement-type solution to that given in Step 2:
  Minimal trauma, add 4 ml/kg/hr.
  Moderate trauma, add 6 ml/kg/hr.
  Extreme trauma, add 8 ml/kg/hr.
Step 4
  Give appropriate colloid solution for each volume of blood lost over 20 percent of the patient's estimated blood volume.
Step 5
  Monitor vital signs and urine output. Adjust fluids to keep urine output at 1 ml/kg/hr.

(From Miller RD: Anesthesia, 2nd ed. New York, Churchill Livingstone, 1986.)

Volume Changes. Disturbances in the ECF compartment are the most common fluid disturbances in the preoperative patient. Withholding fluids prior to surgery causes depletion of ECF because of continuous sensible and insensible losses. This deficit may be strictly volume related, and there may be no derangement of concentration or composition. The diagnosis of severe volume depletion in the ECF compartment is demonstrated clinically by tachycardia and hypotension.

In third-space loss, fluid is sequestered into a nonfunctional space from the extracellular compartment. Third-space loss may occur in patients who have ascites, burns, massive crush injuries, and gastrointestinal inflammation and swelling. A sequestration of fluid into the third space may require replacement treatment to combat the potential for hypotension and tachycardia. The nonfunctional loss of fluids may also occur in patients who have considerable swelling and tissue trauma due to surgical manipulation. Third space sequestration also occurs in patients who have bowel obstructions and injury to the peritoneum.

Estimating fluid deficit is difficult and can best be accomplished by evaluating clinical signs. A mild deficit represents approximately 4 percent of the body weight, a moderate deficit is 6 to 8 percent, and a severe loss is a loss of 10 percent of the body weight. When a patient has an extracellular volume deficit of 6 to 8 percent, orthostatic hypotension can generally be observed. Signs of ECF loss are manifested by tachycardia, dry mucous membranes, hypotension, furrowed tongue, apathy, oliguria, collapsed veins, poor skin turgor, cool and dry skin, and subnormal temperature.

Restoration of ECF balance is the target of treatment and is directed at achieving stable vital signs and adequate urinary output. Urinary output should be 30 to 50 ml/hr or 1/2 to 1 ml/kg/hr as a general guideline. The use of a balanced salt solution such as lactated Ringer's is a good choice to replace the pure ECF loss without causing derangements in concentration or composition.

Concentration Changes. The two primary factors involved in concentration changes are the serum sodium concentration and the serum osmolality. The initial and major concern is the replacement of fluid volume, and the concentration abnormality can be corrected at a slower rate.

Serum sodium evaluation is one of the best indicators of concentration in the ECF. A volume deficit is often associated with increased serum sodium. The increased sodium is due to a decrease in extracellular electrolyte-free water and an increase in dissolved substances in the plasma. Elevated serum sodium levels can be corrected with hypotonic solutions.

Hyponatremia may be present in increased, decreased, or normal ECF volume. Therefore, the treatment varies according to the condition in which hyponatremia exists.

In the hyponatremic patient with a normal ECF volume, the suggested action is observation and detection of the cause of the underlying sodium loss. This type of condition may develop from failure of the kidneys to conserve sodium. The neonate is a sodium loser because the kidneys have an inability to conserve sodium. Inappropriate secretion of ADH and early stages of renal disease may also result in sodium loss with normal ECF volume.

Hypervolemia hyponatremia is caused by excess water retention. Anesthesia staff are particularly concerned with hypervolemia hyponatremia caused by transurethral resections and the administration of oxytocin (Pitocin) with D_5W during labor. The D_5W acts as an antidiuretic, and water is not excreted but absorbed. Treatment of hypervolemia hyponatremia is with administration of hypertonic salt. The hypertonic salt solution will cause volume expansion in the extracellular space.

Hypovolemia hyponatremia often occurs when there is fluid loss through the gastrointestinal tract. This condition may be corrected with the administration of hypotonic fluids such as lactated Ringer's and 0.9 percent normal saline.

Composition. Composition abnormalities are an imbalance of electrolytes and blood gases. The electrolyte disturbance most frequently encountered in the preoperative patient is hypokalemia, which can easily be corrected with the administration of potassium chloride. If the rapid addition of potassium is considered, continuous ECG monitoring should be performed. Acid–base balance is also subject to compositional disturbance and should be considered preoperatively, intraoperatively, and postoperatively.

Intraoperative Fluid Management

Preoperative patients require appropriate replacement of fluid and electrolytes to circumvent a hypotensive episode during the induction of anesthesia. The preoperative fluid loss can be as great as 1.5 to 2.0 ml/kg/hr for an adult. (For children this loss is even greater.) The ECF loss should be replaced with hypotonic solution before the induction of anesthesia if there are not further derangements of fluid disturbances. The fluids most often considered are saline, lactated Ringer's, and dextrose and water. These fluids offer water and electrolytes in the solution.

The loss of fluids during anesthesia must be assessed. Unhumidified gases, high flows, evaporation, surgical

TABLE 25–5. TYPICAL REQUIREMENTS FOR MAINTENANCE FLUIDS

Age	Amount (ml/kg/hr)
Adult	1.5–2
Child	2–4
Infant	4–6
Neonate	3

(From Miller, RD: Anesthesia, 2nd ed. New York, Churchill Livingstone, 1986.)

trauma, and fever all contribute to the loss of fluids in the surgical patient. Several suggested methods of determining maintenance fluids are listed in Tables 25–5 and 25–6.

Because infants have a greater surface area, they also have a greater amount of insensible water and less circulating blood volume. Preoperative and intraoperative fluid maintenance for the pediatric population is a challenge.

Replacement of Blood Loss. A great deal of controversy surrounds the issue of when to initiate the replacement of blood. Under normal circumstances, the average adult can tolerate very well a blood loss of 500 ml or 10 percent of the estimated blood volume. However, a loss of 15 percent of the blood volume should be considered the point of careful consideration for replacement. A guide that can be used to determine the need for a blood transfusion is based on the hematocrit as a means of determining the allowable blood loss.

An example for calculating allowable blood loss follows:

An average adult male weighs 70 kg and has a hematocrit of 40 percent, and an estimated blood volume of 70 ml/kg. What is the allowable blood loss for this patient?

$$\text{Estimated blood volume (EBV)} = 70 \times 70$$
$$\text{EBV} = 4900$$

TABLE 25–6. INTRAOPERATIVE FLUID REQUIREMENTS

1. Basic formula
   a. Deficit: baseline hourly fluid requirement

4 ml/kg/hr	1–10 kg
2 mg/kg/hr	11–20 kg
1 ml/kg/hr	21–up

   multiplied by the number of hours NPO
   b. Maintenance: crystalloid solution such as Ringer's lactate at a rate of 5 to 15 ml/kg/hr
   c. Losses
      Ringers's lactate can be used if hematocrit remains above 30% at 3 ml/1 ml of blood
2. Overall formula (rough estimates)

10 ml/kg	1st hour
7 ml/kg	2nd hour
5 ml/kg	3rd hour
3 ml/kg	4th hour

   for fluid replacement
3. Surface area formula

Surface area (m²)	0.1	0.2	0.3	0.4	0.5	0.6	0.7	0.8	0.9	0
Weight (lb)	3	6	12	18	24	30	36	42	50	60

   Minimum rate, 60 ml/m²/hr
   Maximum hourly rate, 20 ml/kg/hr

Calculated estimated red cell mass (ERCM) = EBV times patient's preoperative Hct
$$\text{ERCM} = 4900 \times 0.40$$
$$\text{ERCM} = 1960$$
Estimated red cell mass desired (ERCM d) = EBV times acceptable low Hct (30 percent)
$$\text{ERCM d} = 4900 \times 0.30$$
$$\text{ERCM d} = 1470$$
Allowable red cell loss (ARCL) = ERMC − ERMC d
$$\text{ARCL} = 1960 - 1470$$
$$\text{ARCL} = 490$$
Allowable blood loss (ABL) = 2 times ARCL
$$\text{ABL} = 2 \text{ times } 490$$
$$\text{ABL} = 980$$

Therefore, the allowable blood loss for this patient is 980 ml of blood, which conceivably will lower the patient's hematocrit to 30 percent.

When estimating blood loss, it is important to realize that the operative blood loss seen on the field may not be the total amount of blood that is lost. Some authorities suggest that above the estimated loss observed on the field an additional amount of 15 to 40 percent should be added.

Crystalloids are often used to replace the blood loss due to surgery. When replacing blood loss with crystalloids, the ratio of fluid replacement to loss is 3 ml crystalloids to 1 ml blood loss. Another alternative to replacement of blood loss is the use of Plasmanate-type solutions. Plasmanate is a good volume expander, but the major disadvantage of this fluid is its inability to carry oxygen.

As surgical procedures have become more complicated, the use of blood products has increased. However, particularly because of concerns about transmitting acquired immunodeficiency syndrome (AIDS) and hepatitis, there is a trend not to use blood transfusions unless necessary. Approximately 14 percent of all surgical patients receive blood transfusions, and 50 percent of all blood transfused in the hospital is given in the operating room suite.

The loss of blood during a surgical procedure is not the only fluid loss. Loss through evaporation and ECF volume depletion must be considered in the replacement of fluid in the operative course. It bears repeating that loss of ECF into the third space due to surgical trauma and manipulations also must be considered in the replacement of fluids.

Immediate Postoperative Period

The recovery room evaluation should include the preoperative fluid status, the amount of fluid lost and given during surgery, and clinical assessment of vital signs and urinary output. It is clinically desirable to establish normal pulse and blood pressure. Additional insidious fluid loss in the recovery room can result from bleeding at the surgical site, internal bleeding, evaporation, and loss through external draining devices. Signs of ECF deficit resulting from fluid loss are primarily manifested by circulatory instability.

The replacement of fluids in the postoperative period often requires the administration of hypotonic solutions and, if necessary, isotonic salt solution combined with packed red cells to replace surgical losses. Continuous monitoring of the patient in the postoperative period includes assessing blood pressure, heart rate, urinary output, level of consciousness, pupil size, airway patency, respiratory patterns, body temperature, and skin color. Sharp observation and skilled response to the patient in the recovery room contribute to successful postoperative management.

Replacement Therapy.   The different types of blood and therapy with blood products are discussed in Chapter 24.

Indications for Replacement Therapy. The values obtained in the operating room when assessing blood loss are rough estimates. Therefore, vital signs, hematocrit, and all other available data are assessed to determine fluid balance. A patient who has been NPO for a long period of time may have an ECF deficit and often is hemoconcentrated. Such a patient may have a very high but misleading hematocrit. Hypotension occurring in a hypovolemic patient may be erroneously related to a deep stage of anesthesia. A significant fall in blood pressure may not occur until 40 percent of the patient's blood volume is lost. Therefore, the use of blood pressure as the only indicator of volume status may be a late sign. Tachycardia, another symptom of hypovolemia, may be due to stimulation on intubation, surgical stimulation, or the use of pharmacologic agents and therefore may not be solely a particularly reliable sign of blood and fluid loss.

SUMMARY

The proper management of fluid and electrolyte disturbances is very challenging for the anesthetist. A thorough understanding of fluid management is critical to achieving successful overall patient well-being.

BIBLIOGRAPHY

Goudsouzian N, Karamanaian A: Physiology for the Anesthesiologist, 2nd ed. E. Norwalk, Appleton-Century-Crofts, 1984.

Guyton A: Textbook of Medical Physiology, 5th ed. Philadelphia, Saunders, 1976.

Jenkins MT, Gliesecke AH, Johnson ER: The postoperative patient and his fluid requirements. Br J Anaesth 47:143–150, 1975.

Metheny N: Quick Reference to Fluid Balance. Philadelphia, Lippincott, 1984.

Metheny N, Snively WD: Nurses' Handbook of Fluid Balance, 4th ed. Philadelphia, Lippincott, 1983.

Miller RD: Anesthesia, 2nd ed. New York, Churchill Livingstone, 1986.

Moore FD, Ball MR: The Metabolic Response to Surgery. American Literature Series 132. Springfield, Ill., Chas. C Thomas, 1952.

Reed GM, Sheppard VF: Regulation of Fluid and Electrolyte Balance, 2nd ed. Philadelphia, Saunders, 1977.

Sabiston DC: Textbook of Surgery: The Biological Basis of Modern Surgical Practice, 11th ed. Philadelphia, Saunders, 1977.

Still JA, Modell JH: Acute water intoxication during transuretheral resection of the prostate using glycine solution for irrigation. Anesthesiology 38:98–99, 1973.

Vander AJ, Sherman JH, Luciano DS: Human Physiology—The Mechanisms of Body Function. New York, McGraw-Hill, 1970.

Part VI
ANESTHESIA AND THE SUBSPECIALTIES

26

Pediatric Anesthesia

Stanley L. Loftness

ANATOMIC AND PHYSIOLOGIC DIFFERENCES BETWEEN CHILDREN AND ADULTS

The anesthetist's approach to the pediatric patient requires knowledge of the conditions that are unique to children and awareness of the pediatric patient's lack of physiologic reserve. Although physiologic considerations in the newborn and infant are totally different from those of the adult, after the age of 6 months, pediatric physiology is remarkably similar to that of adults. Normally pediatric patients maintain their physiologic parameters and laboratory values within the "normal" range. However, when pediatric patients are subjected to stress, the ability to compensate may be impaired by their decreased reserve. Thus, in order to avoid unnecessary problems during anesthesia, it is important to know the physiologic limits and reserves of various systems. With this knowledge, it is then possible to select various techniques and equipment that will help to minimize these physiologic fluctuations.

Respiratory

The differences between the adult and pediatric respiratory systems are often the most appreciated but also the least understood. The anesthetist soon realizes that the pediatric airway is much more difficult to manage that of the adult. As a result of small nares, a large tongue, a small mandible, a small oral cavity, and short mandibular to hyoid distances, the pediatric patient's airway obstructs very easily (Fig. 26–1). This is usually the result of relaxation of the tongue muscles, allowing the tongue to fall against the posterior pharynx. This implies that the best way to relieve this obstruction is to move the tongue anteriorly. This is most reliably accomplished by displacing the mandible and the attached tongue forward, by lifting the angle of the mandible, and keeping the mouth open slightly. Another common error in the management of the pediatric airway is application of pressure in the submandibular soft tissue, displacing the tongue upward against the soft palate, obliterating the nasal as well as the oral airway. The anesthetist should make sure that the fingers are placed on the bone of the mandible and not on the soft tissues.

THE PEDIATRIC AIRWAY

Even using mandibular displacement, it is extremely problematic to intubate infants younger than 6 months. In this age-group, routine prophylactic intubation is often indicated.

In the adult, the narrowest part of the airway is the vocal cord opening. Since this is triangular in shape, an endotracheal tube with a cuff placed in the midtrachea may be necessary to provide an adequate airway seal. In children younger than 10 years, however, the narrowest part of the airway is the cricoid ring, with a soft tissue funnel, the conus elasticus, extending from the vocal cords to the cricoid area. This funnel will mold to an appropriately sized round endotracheal tube, providing an adequate seal without the need for a cuff.

The rapidity with which hypoxia develops in infants and children is often frightening. A study of the lung volumes of children and adults (Table 26–1) demonstrates that each is roughly proportional to weight. Infants and children are different in their reduced alveolar number, lower closing volumes, higher oxygen consumption, and increased carbon dioxide production in relation to weight. The result of these differences is a higher minute ventilation and the more rapid development of hypoxia when gas exchange is inadequate. Pulse oximetry, a continuous monitor of oxygen saturation, is becoming routine in infants and children. This monitor allows for the rapid appreciation of hypoxia. Although the peak inspiratory pressures required to provide for adequate positive-pressure ventilation in children are usually the same (15 to 20 cm H_2O) as required in adults, meticulous attention must be paid to maintenance of airway patency and frequency of respiration. Enriching the ambient oxygen concentration will help provide a larger physiologic reserve.

The control of respiration is also altered in children. Periodic breathing and a blunted hypoxic ventilatory response are quite common in the first 6 months of life. Sudden infant death syndrome (SIDS) is also most prevalent in this age-group and is probably related to an immature respiratory control mechanism. The use of anesthetic agents, both inhalational and intravenous, exacerbates these

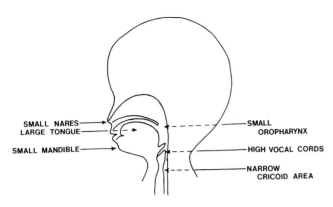

SMALL NARES
LARGE TONGUE

SMALL MANDIBLE

SMALL
OROPHARYNX

HIGH VOCAL CORDS

NARROW
CRICOID AREA

Figure 26–1. The pediatric airway.

respiratory control problems and makes apnea and hypoventilation common. Assisted or controlled ventilation is often required to avoid these problems. There is some evidence that children less than 47 weeks total conceptual age may be more prone to apnea or hypoventilation in the postoperative period, and they therefore should be monitored overnight.

Cardiovascular

In utero, the fetal cardiovascular system is designed to bypass the pulmonary circulation. After birth, the pulmonary vascular bed rapidly opens and the shunts that detoured blood around it close. Although these shunts are usually completely closed within the first 24 hours of life, they may persist well into childhood as a patent ductus arteriosus or patent foramen ovale. In addition, congenital defects in the atrial and ventricular septum may occur. Although these shunts usually permit blood to pass from the systemic circulation to the pulmonary circulation, in situations such as pulmonary outflow obstruction or high pulmonary vascular resistance, they may shunt desaturated blood into the systemic circulation or allow even small venous air emboli to reach the coronary circulation or the brain. This so-called paradoxical air embolus can occlude small vessels and may result in cardiac arrest or cerebral vascular insufficiency. Careful attention must be paid to removing small air bubbles in fluid administration systems to avoid this potential problem.

In a child, the cardiac output as related to weight is often two times that of an adult. This adaptation serves

to meet the increased metabolic demands of children. Cardiac output is the product of heart rate and stroke volume. Since stroke volume cannot be altered appreciably in children, cardiac output is dependent on heart rate. Therefore, any factor that results in bradycardia should be avoided or quickly corrected. Two of the most often encountered situations are vagal stimulation during intubation and hypoxia. The first can be avoided by ensuring adequate depth of anesthesia prior to manipulation of the airway or by the prior administration of atropine. The second requires careful maintenance of adequate minute ventilation and ambient oxygen concentration.

Children have a larger blood volume per kilogram of body weight than adults, but the absolute quantity of blood is much smaller (Table 26–2). Unfortunately, the rate of blood loss during procedures does not differ with size. Therefore, meticulous hemostasis and careful quantitation of blood loss are essential in avoiding hypovolemia. Tachycardia is often the earliest sign of hypovolemia in children because of their rate-limited cardiac output. Anesthetic agents may obtund this normal physiologic response.

Thermoregulation

Temperature control is one of the more prevalent problems in pediatric anesthesia. Anesthesia has a poikilothermic effect on any patient, and this is exaggerated in infants because of an increased ratio of body surface area to weight and poor cutaneous vasomotor control. Surface heat loss by means of radiation, conduction, and convection is enhanced. In addition, newborns and infants are unable to shiver adequately to generate heat, even when awake. Therefore, body temperature drops rapidly in the usual cool environment of the operating room. Since even moderate degrees of hypothermia (32 to 35C) have profound depressant effects on respiratory drive and prolong recovery from anesthesia, careful temperature regulation is essential. Core body temperature needs to be monitored in all pediatric patients, and environmental heat loss should be minimized. Effective means for altering body temperature should be readily available. These should include the ability to increase room temperature up to 85 to 90F, circulating warm-water blankets, and heating lights.

Renal

The kidneys mature to their adult physiologic status within the first 6 weeks of life. Prior to this time, the kidneys lack the ability to maximally concentrate or dilute the urine. This makes the neonate extremely susceptible to both dehydration and fluid overload. Maintenance fluid requirements are higher in children than in adults when computed by weight (Table 26–3). Calculation should be made of both the preoperative deficit and intraoperative requirement, and these should be meticulously replaced.

Adult fluid administration systems can easily result in the injudicious administration of too large a quantity of fluid. The use of pediatric calibrated drip chambers can help avoid this problem.

TABLE 26–1. LUNG VOLUMES[a]

	Adult	Child	Neonate
V_A (ml/kg/min)	60	80	100–150
Frequency (min)	10	20	40
TLC (ml/kg)	80	70	60
FRC (ml/kg)	34	32	30
RV (ml/kg)	17	19	20
Vt (ml/kg)	7	7	6

[a] TLC = total lung capacity; FRC = functional residual capacity; RV = residual volume.

TABLE 26–2. CARDIOVASCULAR DATA

	Heart Rate	BP (mm Hg)	Blood Volume ml/kg	Hemoglobin g/100 ml
Newborn (0–6 weeks)	120	60/40	80	16–18
Infant (6 weeks–6 months)	110	90/60	75	10–11
Child (6 months–6 years)	100	100/70	70	12–14
Adult	80	120/70	60–65	12–14

Metabolic

The major metabolic consideration in infants is to provide sufficient glucose substrate to prevent hypoglycemia. The normal glucose metabolic rate is approximately 4 mg/kg/min. Infusion of a 5 percent glucose-containing solution (D5) at maintenance rates will provide sufficient substrate to meet normal metabolic demands. Stressed infants may require substantially greater amounts of glucose, which may be met by an increased infusion rate or by increasing the concentration of glucose in the solution. In the normal infant, infusion of boluses of 5 percent glucose solutions at rates substantially greater than maintenance can result in hyperglycemia, which must be considered and guarded against.

Pharmacologic

Children have a larger extracellular fluid space and total body water content than do adults. This results in a larger volume of distribution for many drugs. Balancing this is the increased sensitivity of children to many drugs. The net result is that the drug dose for children is usually proportional to that of adults, when calculated on the basis of weight. Two particularly problematic classes of drugs are the central nervous system (CNS) depressants and the neuromuscular blocking agents. CNS depressants can often have an exaggerated or prolonged effect on the level of consciousness and on the respiratory center. Titration of these drugs to effect rather than the use of arbitrary formulas will help avoid undesired consequences. Neuromuscular blocking agents, particularly the nondepolarizing drugs, can have unpredictable responses both in degree and duration of effect. These unpredictable responses can present as a "resistance" or "sensitivity" to the drug. This is especially true in the neonate. Titration of the drugs to desired

effect is essential when prolonged blockade is important. It is essential to assure the return of full muscle strength prior to extubation. Lack of adequate attention to this can easily result in postoperative hypoventilation and hypoxia.

PRELIMINARY CONSIDERATIONS IN INFANTS AND CHILDREN

To provide a safe anesthetic for the pediatric patient, it is essential to conduct a thorough preoperative evaluation. This should include a comprehensive history from the parents and a physical examination of the child. Special attention should be paid to the areas discussed in the paragraphs that follow.

Preoperative Evaluation

Given that the airway in children is often the most troublesome system under anesthesia, special attention should be paid to its evaluation. A history of croup, snoring, or difficulty breathing during colds can provide some evidence of potential problems. On physical examination, look for a small receding chin, unusually large tongue, or short neck. In addition, it is important to try to elicit a history of recent colds. The congestion and secretions associated with an intercurrent respiratory infection can make airway management extremely difficult. There is also an increased likelihood of airway reactivity predisposing to laryngospasm or bronchospasm. Generally, parental observation should be trusted over a brief physical examination. Elective surgery should be postponed if history or physical examination discloses significant findings.

The child's hydration status should also be evaluated (Table 26–4). NPO time, last voiding, and physical appearance should all be considered.

It is important to rehydrate children adequately prior to induction of anesthesia. Failure to accomplish this can result in life-threatening hypotension. In older children such as those with appendicitis, a urine specific gravity should

TABLE 26–3. MAINTENANCE OPERATING ROOM FLUID REQUIREMENTS[a]

	Fluid requirement/24 hr	Type of Fluid
Premature (first day)	70 ml/kg	D5-D10 + 1/4 NS
Full term infant	150 ml/kg	D5-D10 + 1/4 NS
	100 ml/kg	D5 + 1/2 NS
Child over 10 kg	1000 ml + 50/kg over 10 kg	D5 + LR
Adult over 20 kg	1500 ml + 20/kg over 20 kg	NS or LR

[a] NS = normal saline.

TABLE 26–4. DEHYDRATION CRITERIA

Physical Sign	% Dehydration
Dry mouth and mucous membranes, infrequent voiding	5
Sunken eyes or fontanelle, lethargy, poor capillary filling	10
Tenting of the skin, anuria, hypotension	15

be 1.020 or less prior to surgery. In infants, a urine specific gravity of 1.010 or greater generally indicates dehydration.

Cardiovascular status should be evaluated, including pulse, blood pressure, auscultation of the heart, and examination of capillary refill. If there is any question of an undiagnosed heart murmur or congenital heart lesion, appropriate consultation should be requested.

Preoperative Preparation

In the preparation of the pediatric patient, perhaps the most important preoperative consideration is psychologic. From a child's point of view, only dying animals are "put to sleep." Children undergoing anesthesia are said to "take naps." This sums up nicely the difference in approach necessary for the pediatric patient. Children less than 5 years of age, because of incompletely developed reasoning ability and defense mechanisms, are the most prone to psychologic trauma. Areas of concern are (1) fear of pain, (2) separation from parents, security objects, and a familiar environment, (3) fear of mutilation, and (4) the loss of control over themselves.

Anesthetists must be forthright and honest in their discussions with children. The language and terminology must be in words that are appropriate for the child's age, and the anesthetist must prepare the child for all the events and procedures that he or she will undergo. Surprises like shots only exacerbate the feeling of loss of control. A child's favorite toy or object can provide reassurance during these difficult events (Fig. 26–2).

Once the psychologic aspects have been addressed, attention can focus on other aspects of preparation. NPO status is vitally important to the safe conduct of anesthesia. As long a time as possible should ideally be allowed to assure complete stomach emptying. The small pediatric patient, however, is at risk for developing hypoglycemia and dehydration. Table 26–5 lists NPO guidelines for routine surgery.

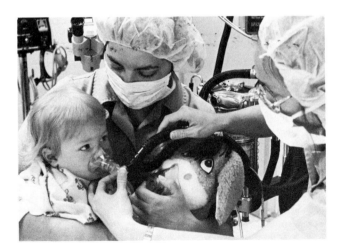

Figure 26–2. A child undergoing induction. Notice that the child's security object is with her, that she is in a sitting position, and that eye contact is maintained between the child and the anesthetist.

TABLE 26–5. NPO GUIDELINES

	Solids (hr)	Clear Liquids (hr)
Newborns (0–6 weeks)	12	4
Infants (6 weeks–6 months)	12	4
Children over 6 months	8	4

Premedication should then be considered. With proper psychologic preparation and a gentle and caring operating room staff, most children can be safely anesthetized without premedication. This has the advantage of a faster emergence and shorter recovery room stay. Particularly anxious children should be given the benefit of sedation. This can be in the form of (1) PO diazepam (0.1 to 0.25 mg/kg suspension), (2) PO chloral hydrate (20 to 60 mg/kg), or (3) IM barbiturates (pentobarbital, 2 to 4 mg/kg) and/or narcotics (morphine, 0.05 to 0.15 mg/kg). All have been used successfully, and the choice usually depends on the anesthetist's experience and preference.

In children younger than 6 months, hypotension and bradycardia are not uncommon during induction with potent inhalational agents. This can be prevented, to some degree, by premedication with atropine (0.02 mg/kg) IM 20 minutes prior to induction.

Pediatric Anesthesia Delivery Systems

Three different types of anesthesia circuits are in frequent use in pediatrics. They are (1) the Jackson–Rees modification of the Ayre's T-piece, (2) the Bain circuit, and (3) the pediatric circle (Fig. 26–3). The first two have the advantage of low weight, almost no resistance to breathing, and minimal dead space. They both, however, require high gas flows to avoid rebreathing (approximately two and one-half times minute ventilation). Humidification of gases may be necessary, particularly during extended anesthesia. This is to avoid the possible deleterious effects of dry gases on the tracheobronchial epithelium and the thermal energy cost required for local humidification. The pediatric circle offers a slightly higher resistance to breathing and usually requires the use of controlled ventilation in very small infants. The lower gas flow that the pediatric circle allows can offer a significant savings in total anesthetic use. When flows of less than 3 L/minute are used, additional humidification is probably unnecessary.

Temperature Regulation

The most effective means of maintenance of body temperature in children is manipulation of the environmental temperature. When the operating room temperature exceeds 30C (85F), very little heat loss occurs. Although this is extremely uncomfortable for the surgeons and operating room personnel, it is usually necessary in premature and newborn infants. Operating under an overhead radiant warmer can also be effective. For larger infants and children, the use of a warming mattress under the child is often sufficient to maintain body temperature and to allow the operating room suite to be at a more comfortable temperature. When the child's body temperature is falling, warming the intra-

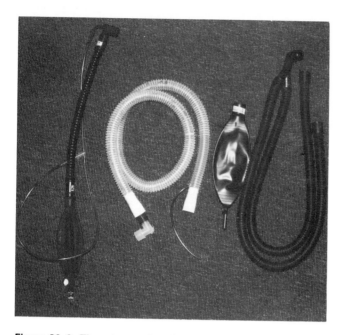

Figure 26–3. Three types of pediatric anesthesia circuits. From left to right: Jackson–Rees modification of the Ayre's T-piece, Bain circuit, and the pediatric circle with 1-L bag.

TABLE 26–6. ENDOTRACHEAL TUBE SIZE (mm)

Premature infants	2.5
Newborn infants	3.0
Infants less than 6 months	3.5
Infants 6 months to 1 year	4.0
Children older than 1 year	(16 + age)/4

type of mask is extremely useful in smaller children and in infants.

Endotracheal tubes should preferably be clear, implantation-tested plastic, and uncuffed in children younger than 10 years. Appropriate endotracheal tube size can be determined from Table 26–6.

Intravenous equipment should include the following (Fig. 26–5):

- Small intravenous catheters
- Pediatric administration sets with 60 drops per ml
- Pediatric calibrated fluid chambers
- Injection sites close to the catheter site

Available monitoring equipment should include the following (Fig. 26–6):

- Electrocardiogram for observation of heart rate and rhythm
- Precordial or esophageal stethoscope
- Rectal or nasopharyngeal temperature probe
- Blood pressure cuff with Doppler or oscillotonometer
- Pressure manometer in the anesthetic circuit
- Oxygen analyzer in the anesthetic circuit
- Transcutaneous P_{O_2}, arterial, and central venous pressure monitoring as indicated
- Pulse oximetry and end-tidal CO_2 monitor are excellent adjuncts when possible. Pulse oximetry provides the anesthetist with moment to moment changes in oxygen saturation of the blood. This knowledge can be life saving in the conduct of pediatric anesthesia.

venous fluids, using a heated humidifier in the anesthetic circuit, employing radiant warming lights, as well as raising the environmental temperature can be beneficial.

Equipment

An assortment of different types and sizes of laryngoscope blades are necessary to assure easy intubation of the entire spectrum of pediatric patients (Figure 26–4). Straight blades generally are the most successful in small infants and children.

A collection of appropriate size masks must be available prior to induction of anesthesia. The Rendell–Baker–Soucek

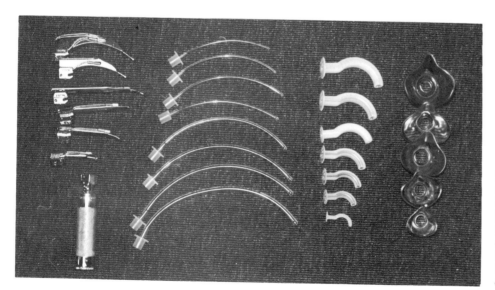

Figure 26–4. Pediatric airway equipment. From left to right: laryngoscope blades—#0, 1, 2 Miller, #1½ Wis–Hipple, #2, 3 Macintosh; uncuffed endotracheal tubes—2.5 to 6.0 mm by half sizes; oral airways—40 to 100 mm; Rendell–Baker–Soucek masks, #00, 0, 1, 2, 3.

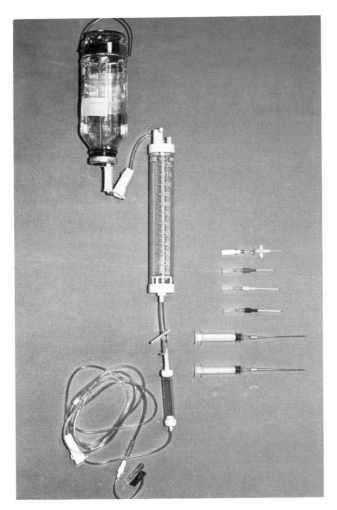

Figure 26–5. Intravenous administration equipment; 250-ml bottle of D5 LR (5% dextrose in lactated Ringer's solution); volumetric administration set; pediatric microdrip administration set; T-connector; size 24, 22, 20, 18, 16, 14 gauge catheters.

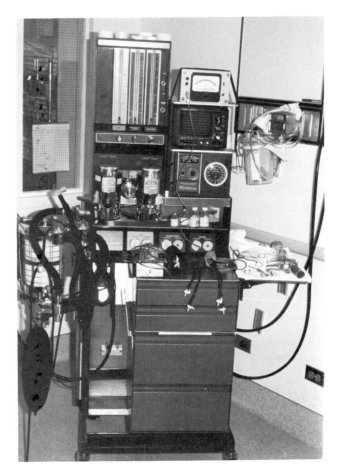

Figure 26–6. Monitoring equipment. From top to bottom: temperature monitor, electrocardiogram, O₂ analyzer. On top of anesthesia machine: Doppler and assorted BP cuffs, precordial stethoscope. In circle system: manometer.

The appropriate width of the blood pressure cuff is two-thirds the distance from elbow to shoulder.

ANESTHETIC MANAGEMENT IN INFANTS AND CHILDREN

Induction

Placement of noninvasive monitors such as the electrocardiogram, blood pressure cuff, and precordial stethoscope is a first priority when the child enters the operating room. Induction of anesthesia in children requires great gentleness. This is because of both their high level of apprehension and their extremely sensitive airways. Children younger than 7 years tend to find a mask induction less anxiety provoking than the needle stick required for an intravenous or intramuscular technique. Hypnotic techniques and candy- or fruit-scented masks can facilitate the child's acceptance of inhalational induction. Children older than 7 years can comprehend the limited discomfort involved in the placement of an intravenous catheter and may find it prefer-

able to a mask induction. Alternately, methohexital can be given per rectum (PR) (20 to 30 mg/kg) or ketamine (4 to 8 mg/kg) given IM. All these techniques are safe in routine elective surgery, and each can have its place.

Intravenous Lines

Starting intravenous lines in children is a skill perfected through practice. Although veins can usually be found over the hands and feet, it is useful to remember that scalp veins and the external jugular vein are usually prominent even in obese children. Intravenous catheters range in size from 24 to 12 gauge and must be selected on the basis of vein size. Metal scalp vein needles usually are not adequately secure for anesthetic use. Intravenous lines should generally be used in all but the very briefest surgery (less than 10 to 20 minutes).

Endotracheal Intubation

Endotracheal intubation should be performed whenever maintenance of an airway is difficult, impractical, or will not allow for adequate ventilation. Some general guidelines are listed in Table 26–7.

TABLE 26–7. INTUBATION CRITERIA

TABLE 26–7. INTUBATION CRITERIA

- Children less than 6 months of age
- Surgical field avoidance
- Controlled ventilation
- Full stomach/aspiration risk situations
- Cases with major blood loss
- Procedures longer than 2 hours

Tracheal intubation can be accomplished through the use of inhalation anesthesia sometimes facilitated by the use of neuromuscular relaxants. A check should be made to assure that gas leaks around the endotracheal tube at 20 cm H_2O or less. Stylets are not usually necessary but can be helpful when the cephalad placed vocal cords are difficult to visualize. The endotracheal tube should be placed midway between the vocal cords and the carina. In children, an approximation of the tracheal length can be derived by converting the internal diameter (ID) of the endotracheal tube in millimeters to centimeters (e.g., 3.5 mm ID tube = 3.5 cm cord to carina distance). One manner of facilitating the correct placement of the endotracheal tube is by using tubes with measured marks proximal to the distal end. Placement of the mark at the level of the vocal cords will generally assure a proper position in the trachea.

Maintenance

Maintenance of anesthesia can be accomplished with inhalation, intravenous, or combined techniques. Inhalation techniques are very popular among pediatric anesthetists. This is both a function of ease of use and the somewhat unpredictable sensitivity of children to the respiratory depressant effects of narcotics. Halothane is the most widely used inhalation anesthetic agent, probably because of its superior acceptance by patients for mask induction. Isoflurane, which has acquired increasing acceptance as a maintenance inhalation agent because of its decreased myocardial sensitization, may be inappropriate as an induction agent because it frequently causes laryngospasm. Nitrous oxide, as a result of its rapid uptake and distribution and analgesic properties, is complementary when used in combination with potent inhalation anesthetics. Its concentration should never exceed 66 percent in order to maintain a margin of safety in the oxygen concentration.

Intravenous narcotics are used in much the same manner as they are in adults, although doses tend to be somewhat less because of the respiratory sensitivity. Shorter-acting agents such as fentanyl are becoming more popular because of their ease of titration and pharmacologic reversibility.

Muscle relaxants are used in titrated doses based on a mg/kg body weight basis (Table 26–8). Pancuronium is the most commonly used agent because tachycardia is usually beneficial in children, although not in adults.

Great care must be used in establishing complete reversal prior to extubation, because even minor residual blockade can easily lead to airway obstruction in children. Typical reversal doses might be neostigmine (0.07 mg/kg) or edrophonium (0.75 mg/kg) and atropine (0.02 mg/kg).

Ketamine has a much more prominent role in children than in adults, the incidence of postoperative delirium is less, and the maintenance of airway-protective effects and ventilatory drive may be very beneficial. Preoperative antisialogogue agents should be administered to avoid the secretory stimulation effects of ketamine and ensure airway patency.

Blood Loss and Fluid Replacement

Fluid and blood losses must be rigorously monitored and replaced. Hypovolemia occurs much more rapidly because of the small total intravascular volume in children. Tachycardia, especially with hypotension, should generally be assumed to be a sign of hypovolemia until proved otherwise. The measurement of blood loss in children requires meticulous attention to the operative field, weighing of sponges, and the use of suction cannisters with graduations appropriate for small amounts. Loss of red cell mass should be replaced with either whole blood or packed cells, and all blood products should be warmed prior to administration. Hypocalcemia secondary to citrate absorption occurs occasionally when replacement exceeds one blood volume, and administration of calcium chloride (20 mEq/kg) should be considered if hypotension persists despite adequate volume replacement.

In addition to administering maintenance fluid requirements intraoperatively, preoperative fluid deficit may be replaced by infusion rates double or triple those of maintenance. During intraabdominal or intrathoracic cases, up

TABLE 26–8. MUSCLE RELAXANTS

Drug	Intubation Dose (mg/kg)	Surgical Relaxation Dose (mg/kg)	Side Effects
d-Tubocurarine	0.6, IV	0.2–0.6, IV	Hypotension, bronchospasm
Gallamine	3–4, IV	1–3, IV	Tachycardia
Pancuronium	0.1–0.15, IV	0.04–0.07, IV	Tachycardia
Metocurine	0.3, IV	0.1–0.3, IV	
Atracurium	0.5, IV	0.2–0.4, IV	
Vecuronium	0.1, IV	0.02–0.05, IV	
Succinylcholine	1–3, IV or IM		Bradycardia with repeat bolus IV

TABLE 26–9. EXTUBATION CRITERIA

- Good respiratory effort
- Good cough and gag
- Good muscle strength
- Eye opening

to 10 ml/kg/hour of additional fluid should be administered to replace insensible and third-space losses.

Emergence

In general, the emergence times for children are similar to those in adults and are dependent on duration and depth of anesthesia. Special attention must be paid to assure the return of adequate pharyngeal muscular tone prior to extubation. In order to be reasonably sure of a successful extubation, the criteria listed in Table 26–9 should be met.

Adequacy of muscle strength is often best assessed by the ability of the child to flex the legs onto the abdomen. Extubation should be performed at the end of a full inspiration and under positive pressure to ensure that pharyngeal secretions are not aspirated.

Immediately after extubation, it is usually necessary to help hold the airway open during the first few breaths. Once a sustained pattern of respiration has been observed, children will usually be able to maintain the airway on their own.

RECOVERY ROOM CARE OF INFANTS AND CHILDREN

Recovery room care is vitally important in anesthesia for infants and children. On admission to the recovery room, the patient's anesthetic management and current status must be reviewed with the staff. Vital signs should be taken and recorded on the anesthetic record. Assessment must be made of the airway, adequacy of ventilation and oxygenation, CNS status, and airway protective reflexes. Postoperative airway obstruction and hypoventilation occur with some frequency. Signs of airway obstruction are listed in Table 26–10.

Assessment then needs to be made of the cardiovascular system. This should include pulse, blood pressure, capillary filling, and urine output. Pediatric patients are prone to the rapid development of hypovolemia. This can be due to continued blood loss, inadequate fluid replacement intraoperatively, and third spacing in the postoperative period. Recovery room personnel must be alert to the various signs of hypovolemia.

The level of observation necessary to recover the pediatric patient usually requires a larger number of personnel, and frequently longer recovery room stays.

Children often need to be restrained in the recovery period. This is both to assure that they do not remove their intravenous cannula or dressings and to prevent them from falling out of the bed.

Prior to discharge from the recovery room, the child should have a postanesthesia recovery room score of 8 for overnight stay and 10 for discharge home (Table 26–11).

SPECIAL CONSIDERATIONS IN THE NEONATE

Anesthesia for neonatal surgery is difficult and is fraught with complications in the best of circumstances. When possible, it should only be carried out in pediatric centers. When anesthetizing the neonate, some additional areas of concern include those discussed in the paragraphs that follow.

The neonate during the first hours and days of life may not have completed the switch from intrauterine to extrauterine circulation. Residual shunting may persist through the foramen ovale or patent ductus arteriosus. This may at times result in the addition of desaturated venous blood to the arterial circulation. The existence of hypoxia or acidosis can perpetuate these shunting problems. Halogenated agents should be used in small amounts (less than 1 percent) and with extreme caution. Peripheral vasodilatation and myocardial depression are such common occurrences with the use of these agents that many pediatric anesthetists prefer to use small doses of narcotics as their only anesthetic agent. Muscle relaxants may also help in providing a good surgical field without the need for high concentrations of potent inhalational agents.

Neonatal respiratory control is normally a precarious situation; as a general rule, no reliance should be placed on spontaneous ventilation under anesthesia. All neonates should be intubated for surgery, and ventilation controlled by the anesthetist. Respiratory rate should be maintained in the range of 50 to 60 breaths per minute and inspiratory pressure limited to 20 cm H_2O or less if possible. The neonatal lungs are extremely fragile, and excessive pressure can

TABLE 26–10. SIGNS OF AIRWAY OBSTRUCTION

- Cyanosis
- Grunting
- Retractions
- Nasal flaring
- Tachycardia

TABLE 26–11. POSTANESTHESIA RECOVERY SCORE

Moves purposefully	2
Moves involuntarily	1
Not moving	0
Regular respirations—coughs, cries	2
Distressed or periodic respirations	1
Requires ventilation	0
Pink	2
Pale, dusky, blotchy, other	1
Cyanotic	0
BP ± 20% preop level	2
BP ± 20–30% preop level	1
BP ± 50% preop level	0
Awake	2
Responding	1
Not responding	0

easily result in a pneumothorax. Postoperatively, the safest approach is to continue controlled ventilation in the intensive care unit until complete recovery from all aspects of the anesthetic can be documented.

Neonatal oxygenation must also be closely monitored. Both hypoxia and hyperoxemia can pose a problem. As a result of the neonate's small pulmonary reserve for oxygen, hypoxia occurs rapidly whenever ventilation is compromised. Even surgical manipulation in the abdomen can cause significant hypoventilation and consequent hypoxia. Neonates of less than 47 weeks' total conceptual age may have immature retinas. Even brief periods during which the Pa_{O_2} exceeds 100 mm Hg have been associated with the development of retrolental fibroplasia. This can result in interference with the retinal maturation process. As a result of both these problems, neonates should be maintained on their preoperative Fi_{O_2} at the beginning of surgery. The use of a trancutaneous Pa_{O_2} monitor, pulse oximetry, or blood gas sampling should dictate changes in intraoperative oxygen administration.

The management of fluids in the neonate must be extremely cautious. Attention must be paid to the potential for the development of hypoglycemia. This is accomplished first by the administration of the same dextrose concentration as the child is receiving preoperatively and, second, by the use of glucose monitoring intraoperatively. Fluids should be given by continuous infusion pumps or by syringed aliquots.

Rigorous temperature control is critical in the neonate. Operating room temperature must be elevated to the 30C range, warming blankets must be used, and fluids often must be heated prior to administration. Only through the use of all these adjunctive techniques can precipitous temperature drops be avoided. Consideration of temperature must extend to the transport of the child to and from the operating room. Warm blankets and heated mattresses can help prevent temperature losses of 2 to 3 degrees during these periods.

SUMMARY

The conduct of anesthesia in the pediatric population can be as safe as that in the adult. Safe anesthesia, however, requires increased vigilance during all points of contact between the anesthetist and the child.

BIBLIOGRAPHY

Loftness SL, Lockhart CH: Pitfalls in the use of anesthetic agents in children. Int Anesthesiol Clin 23:201–226, 1985.

Gregory GA: Pediatric Anesthesia. New York, Churchill-Livingstone, 1983.

Jones AE, Pelton DA: An index of syndromes and their anesthetic implications. Can Anaesth Soc J 23:207–226, 1976.

Steward DJ: Manual of Pediatric Anesthesia, 2nd ed. New York, Churchill-Livingstone, 1985.

27

Obstetric Anesthesia and Analgesia

Norman H. Blass and Jonathan H. Skerman

Obstetric anesthesia and analgesia have recently become sub-jects of renewed interest to personnel in the field of obstet-rics. Nurse anesthetists have had to perform obstetric analgesia for many years, since the majority of anesthesiologists have gener-ally shunned the delivery suite. However, with the knowledge that good obstetric anesthesia is often a necessity for providing optimal obstetric care to assure a healthy mother and baby, there has evolved this important aspect of anesthetic education.

The chapter is divided into seven categories.

- *Physiologic changes during pregnancy*
- *Maternal and fetal pharmacology*
- *Anesthesia for vaginal delivery*
- *Anesthesia for cesarean section*
- *Anesthesia for abnormal obstetrics*
- *Maternal complications of obstetric anesthesia*
- *Evaluation and resuscitation of the newborn*

PHYSIOLOGIC CHANGES DURING PREGNANCY

Pregnancy produces profound physiologic changes in all major organ systems.

The cardiovascular system shows alteration as early as the fifth to eighth week of gestation. Cardiac output starts to increase in early pregnancy and reaches its zenith at approximately 30 to 34 weeks of gestation, then declines toward term. There has been some dispute about the rate of decline in maternal cardiac output as term approaches. It is now known that many factors modify cardiac output. Some of these factors are the age of the patient, the maternal position (especially near term), the pain of uterine contrac-tions, bearing down efforts or Valsalva maneuvers, the type of delivery, and the type of anesthesia/analgesia.

The cardiovascular system imposes significant de-mands on the pregnant mother, but these demands are usually well tolerated during gestation. However, the partu-rient with heart disease or reduced cardiac reserve may not be able to meet the increased requirement during preg-nancy or labor.

During pregnancy, the red blood cell volume and total blood volume and the total plasma volume all increase. Since the increase in the total blood volume is greater than the red cell volume, physiologic anemia ensues. The total blood volume is usually 40 percent above the nonpregnant state but is ordinarily well tolerated by the gravida.

There is a slight fall in both the systolic and diastolic pressure during the midtrimester of pregnancy, but a return to the nonpregnant or early trimester level usually occurs in the last trimester. The white blood cell count also in-creases during pregnancy. The reason for this is not obvious, but the increase may be estrogen induced. When attempting to evaluate leukocytosis as an indicator of infection, the shift to the left of the white blood cell count is more impor-tant than the actual rise in the blood count itself.

There is a question about whether pregnancy produces a hypercoagulable state in the parturient. It is known that there is a change in the coagulation mechanism, with an increase in fibrinogen, prothrombin, Factors VII, VIII, IX, and X, and augmentation of the fibrolytic inhibitors. There is decreased concentration of Factors XI and XIII, however a triggering mechanism is needed to begin the coagulation mechanism.

Respiratory System

The enlarging uterus produces a mechanical change in the configuration of the abdomen and a concomitant rise in the diaphragm of approximately 4 cm. There is an increase in the transverse and anterior-posterior diameter of the thoracic cage plus an outward and upward movement of the rib cage. This produces alterations in the lung volume during pregnancy. These alterations in lung volume usually occur at approximately 4 to 5 months of gestation, so that at term the expiratory reserve volume, the residual volume, and the functional residual capacity are reduced 20 to 25 percent from the nonpregnant state. However, the respira-tory capacity increases so that there is compensation. Min-ute alveolar ventilation is increased. This is produced by a mild increase in the respiratory rate and a greater increase in the depth of the ventilatory tidal volume. There is hyperventilation producing a mild respiratory alkalosis.

A decrease in the functional residual capacity at term is a constant finding. This decrease is exaggerated by the supine or Trendelenburg's position, which is usually assumed by the patient on the delivery or operating table. The accentuation does not occur in the sitting position.

The decrease in the functional residual capacity and the increased alveolar ventilation facilitate washout of anesthetic gases, producing rapid induction of general anesthesia, especially with the more volatile inhalation agents. The reduced functional residual capacity and the low Pa_{CO_2} in the pregnant patient can lead to a rather precipitous decline in Pa_{O_2} during periods of apnea. Preoxygenation prior to the induction of general anesthesia and before intubation is thus essential to minimize the risk of hypoxemia.

Maternal Pa_{O_2} is increased because of the increased alveolar ventilation. Nevertheless, airway closure occurs at normal tidal volume range in many parturients approaching term. This is particularly prevalent in the supine position and may lead to ventilation-perfusion abnormalities and reduced Pa_{O_2}.

Hyperventilation and mechanical positive-pressure ventilation may reduce uterine blood flow and fetal oxygenation. Similarly, the distraught hyperventilation of uncontrolled labor patients may be detrimental to the fetus, and it is not unusual to see maternal carbon dioxide levels as low as 20 to 25 mm Hg and pH levels as high as 7.65.

Central Nervous System

The dosage of local anesthetics used in conduction anesthesia during pregnancy should be less than that during the nonpregnant state. Epidural veins are swollen, leading to a diminution in the size of the epidural and subarachnoid spaces. This is the cause of the reduced size of the epidural and subarachnoid spaces and the amount of the local anesthetic required.

There is an increase in cerebrospinal fluid pressure, and this is probably the reason for the high dermatome level of spread of local anesthetics during pregnancy.

There is a reduction in minimal alveolar concentration (MAC) during pregnancy. The cause is not known, but it may be related to the sedative effects of progesterone.

Gastrointestinal Tract

As the pregnancy progresses, the enlarging uterus pushes the intestines and the stomach cephalad. This contributes to the increase in the risk of regurgitation and pulmonary aspiration. There is a rise in intragastric pressure, particularly when the patient is in the lithotomy or modified lithotomy position; and there is a decrease in the gastroesophageal sphincter tone. The motility of the stomach is reduced, and there is an increase in gastric contents as well as a lowered gastric pH. During labor, anxiety and pain also tend to reduce the motility of the stomach, delaying emptying time even further and increasing gastric acidity and volume.

The administration of an antacid to women in labor has been shown to increase the gastric pH, although pulmonary aspiration of particulate matter is still possible. Clear antacids such as 0.3 M sodium bicitrate have become the accepted standard. Measures recommended to minimize the risk of maternal aspiration are as follows:

1. Avoid general anesthesia if possible.
2. Administer prophylactic antacid.
3. Rapid-sequence induction of anesthesia when indicated, using intubation with cricoid pressure and a cuffed endotracheal tube.
4. Administration of intravenous atropine or glycopyrrolate not only as an anticholinergic agent but to increase the tone of the gastroesophagaeal junction.
5. Avoid positive-pressure ventilation prior to intubation and inflation of the endotracheal tube cuff.

Although results of many liver function tests are altered during pregnancy, the appropriate dose of drugs such as succinylcholine is safe to use.

Renal, Endocrine, and Metabolic Changes

Progesterone contributes to the dilatation of the smooth muscle of the kidney, pelvis, and ureters starting as early as the third month of gestation. As the pregnant uterus enlarges, the growing uterus encroaches on the ureters, producing a mechanical cause of the kidney dilatation.

There is a gradual increase in renal blood flow and glomerular filtration, leading to a lowering of blood urea nitrogen (BUN) and creatinine. A patient whose creatinine and BUN are in the normal range for nonpregnant females may be abnormal when pregnant. The anesthetist must be aware of this prior to the administration of potentially nephrotoxic drugs.

Since tubular reabsorption of increased amounts of glucose filtered by the glomerulus is relatively fixed, glycosuria during pregnancy is not uncommon.

Pregnancy induces increased activity of the endocrine system. The pituitary gland enlarges during pregnancy, producing more adrenotropic and thyrotropic hormones along with prolactin.

The elevated basal metabolic rate during pregnancy has been attributed to pregnancy per se, but studies have shown that this apparent hypermetabolic state is produced by the needs of the fetus for increased oxygen.

There is an increase in thyroxin-binding globulin produced by the excess amount of estrogen in the pregnant state, and there is an increase in the size of the thyroid gland over the nonpregnant state. During pregnancy, results of thyroid function tests must be interpreted carefully.

The adrenal gland produces more aldosterone, and the parathyroid glands show enlargement. The pancreas is stimulated to increase insulin production, but this is in response to the diabetogenic action of pregnancy.

Maternal metabolism and oxygen consumption increase steadily throughout gestation, and metabolism of protein, fat, and carbohydrate is altered.

MATERNAL AND FETAL PHARMACOLOGY

Most drugs administered to a pregnant woman readily cross the placenta, although a few of large molecular size do not.

Although it is true that more consideration is given to drugs administered to the mother during labor and delivery, a number of studies have shown that there is a tendency for pregnant women to take medications throughout pregnancy. The number of drugs taken by any patient during pregnancy averages from 5 to 10, 80 percent of these without a physician's knowledge or supervision.

The drugs most frequently used during labor and delivery are analgesics, sedatives, tranquilizers, and local and general anesthetics. It is axiomatic that almost all medication can be found in the fetus within minutes of administration to the mother.

For years it was believed that the placenta was a barrier to the passage of drugs from mother to baby. However, it is known that nonionized, fat-soluble, low-molecular-weight drugs are transferred rapidly.

Most muscle relaxants in the usual dosage pass poorly from the mother to fetus, but in doses of high magnitude they readily cross the placenta. Anesthetic gases, narcotics, and barbiturates pass readily. Nitrous oxide will approach 80 percent of the maternal level in about 10 minutes. Pregnancy-induced hypertension (toxemia) and other maternal diseases may interfere with this so-called placental barrier and may allow even a more rapid and complete transfer.

Fetal brain concentration of medication can be reduced by giving an intravenous dose at the time of a uterine contraction so that there will be less drug going to the fetus because of the placental vasoconstriction. Fetal liver metabolism and the dilution of drugs in the fetal circulation prior to their reaching the fetal brain also contribute to a lessening of the anesthetic effect.

Whether any drug that is given to the mother has an adverse effect on the fetus or the mother can only be determined by direct observation. Ideally, maternally administered analgesics should provide maternal pain relief without any adverse effects on the newborn. We have not achieved this goal, but research efforts of this nature are ongoing. It behooves us, however, to use the minimum amount of anesthetic agents and other drugs to produce any desired effect.

ANESTHESIA FOR VAGINAL DELIVERY

Most women have a great deal of discomfort during labor and delivery. The pain of the first stage of labor is the pain resulting from dilatation and effacement of the cervix as well as uterine ischemia because of uterine contractions. In the second stage of labor, there is the addition of pain resulting from the stretching of the vagina and perineum. The degree of discomfort that a parturient may have cannot be accurately predicted.

Ideally, analgesia for labor and delivery should alleviate the pain of labor for the mother and not interfere with the mechanics or progress of labor. There should be no undue risk to the mother or to the fetus. Early bonding between the mother and baby should be possible, and adequate working conditions for the obstetrician should not be ignored.

Obstetric analgesia may be provided by using techniques such as acupuncture, hypnosis, and natural childbirth, all of which may play a satisfactory role but do not

belong in the confines of this chapter. There are many satisfactory books on these subjects.

Analgesia for labor and delivery can be provided by systemic medications such as narcotics, sedatives, tranquilizers, and inhalation analgesia; local anesthetics and regional anesthesia are also used. It is important to remember that all systemic medications used for analgesia or to relieve anxiety rapidly cross the placenta.

Tranquilizers, hypnotics, and amnestics may all be given to the mother to alleviate anxiety, but they assist little in the relief of pain. Use of these drugs with concomitant narcotics may cause the patient to become disoriented and uncontrollable during painful contractions. These drugs mostly are additive in their depressant effects on both the mother and newborn.

Systemic narcotics are frequently used to lessen the pain of the first stage of labor. Equal analgesic doses of narcotics cause equal maternal and neonatal depression. The primary difference in the narcotics used is the duration of their action in the mother. Thus longer-acting narcotics such as meperidine are indicated early in labor, whereas fentanyl and alphaprodine are more appropriate toward the end of labor.

Naloxone is a specific narcotic antagonist with no narcotic action of its own. It is effective in both the mother and newborn. Rarely should it be given to the mother before delivery unless another form of analgesia is begun, because it will rapidly antagonize any narcotic analgesia at a time when it is most needed. The neonatal dose of naloxone is 0.5 mg to 0.10 mg intramuscular (IM) or intravenous (IV). Its duration of action is only about 1 hour, and renarcotization may follow its use. The use of naloxone, however, in patients who are chronic narcotic users or in their newborn children may produce rapid symptoms of narcotic withdrawal. Recent evidence has shown that naloxone may cause problems in patients with cardiovascular disease and probably should be used most cautiously in cardiac compromised parturients. Doses of meperidine as low as 50 mg have been associated with decreased Apgar scores at birth and depressed neurobehavioral function. Depression in the newborn may be minimal if delivery occurs within the first hour following intramuscular injection. However, drugs given by the intravenous route may still be associated with newborn depression when delivery rapidly follows drug administration.

Intermittent Inhalation Analgesia

Intermittent inhalation analgesia involves administration of subanesthetic concentrations of inhalation agents to the mother. Inhalation drugs such as methoxyflurane may be self-administered throughout labor and delivery. It is used during contractions in a concentration of 0.2 to 0.6 percent in air by means of a hand-held device such as the Duke or Cyprane inhaler. Nitrous oxide (30 to 40 percent in oxygen with or without a small added concentration of methoxyflurane) can give satisfactory analgesia for delivery. The use of enflurane in concentrations of 0.5 to 0.8 percent with oxygen has also been effective as an analgesic agent for delivery. However, one must be cautious in administering enflurane because of the ease of rapid deepening to general anesthesia. When inhalation analgesia is combined with a pudendal block or local infiltration of the perineum, adequate analgesia for episiotomy and forceps delivery can be obtained.

The administration of nitrous oxide with contractions may not be satisfactory, because the peak effect of concentration is not reached until 50 seconds after inhalation has begun. Better relief of pain is obtained with continuous administration of 50 percent nitrous oxide and oxygen in the delivery room before the delivery and continued through the expulsion of the placenta and postpartum examination of the vagina and cervix.

Inhalation analgesia causes little neonatal depression even when used for long periods of time. Uterine activity is not depressed, and when inhalation agents are properly administered, the mother remains awake. She maintains the urge to push and can protect her own airways, which minimizes the threat of pulmonary aspiration of stomach contents. However, the depths of analgesia can be rapidly altered and anesthesia may ensue. It is therefore essential that inhalation analgesia be constantly supervised. The mother should be able to answer questions and remain cooperative.

Low-dose ketamine in the range of 0.25 mg/kg to 0.3 mg/kg of maternal body weight provides effective analgesia for vaginal delivery with little or no neonatal depression. There is a minimal amount of hallucinatory response and very little increase in salivation. Ketamine produces profound analgesia and amnesia and as such does take away the mother's ability to relate to her newborn and thus does decrease bonding. As far as the fetus is concerned, there is no hypotonia and apparently no thermoregulatory inhibition, nor is there any decrease in the baby's Apgar score. This particular type of analgesia is most satisfactory in those patients who do not want to view the birth of the baby because they are giving the baby up for adoption or because there is fetal demise and they do not want to be aware of the delivery. In a normal vaginal delivery, low-dose ketamine probably does not contribute much because of the amnesia it produces and today may even be contraindicated by this fact alone.

General anesthesia is rarely required for normal vaginal delivery. It abolishes the bearing down reflex, and it is associated with neonatal depression correlating with the depth of the anesthetic and the elapsed time until delivery. General analgesia, when administered, removes from the mother the awareness of her newborn and definitely increases the risk of pulmonary aspiration. The parturient is particularly prone to aspiration because her stomach usually is not empty even if she has not eaten for a long period, and the enlarged uterus plus the lithotomy position causes a marked rise in intragastric pressure.

When general anesthesia is necessary, it is mandatory to intubate the trachea with a cuffed endotracheal tube. It may be placed either as an awake intubation or immediately after rapid-sequence induction with correct cricoid pressure (Sellick's maneuver) applied from the time of induction to the time of intubation. General anesthesia for the parturient without intubation is totally unacceptable anesthetic practice.

General anesthesia is indicated when acute fetal dis-tress occurs and prompt vaginal delivery is impossible. It may be used in a patient who becomes uncontrollable during delivery or when regional anesthesia is contraindicated or refused and operative obstetrics is required. It is often indicated when depression of uterine activity is required. Such uterine relaxation may be necessary to abolish a tetanic uterine contraction or to allow internal uterine manipulation, as in the extraction of a second twin. For uterine relaxation, halothane and probably enflurane and isoflurane may be used because they cause rapid relaxation of the uterus, but accompanying this relaxation of the uterus there is always the danger of hemorrhage. After the baby has been delivered, the halothane, enflurane, or isoflurane should be discontinued. If it is necessary to maintain general anesthesia, a nitrous oxide–oxygen/narcotic technique will be satisfactory.

Regional Anesthesia

Conduction anesthesia is suitable for vaginal delivery, and there are distinct advantages associated with the use of regional anesthesia for both mother and fetus. Maternal airway reflexes usually remain intact provided severe hypotension or reactions to local anesthetics are avoided. The mother remains awake and can react to her newborn early in the postpartum period. There is a decrease in the need for narcotics or sedatives, and regional anesthesia usually eliminates the need for general anesthesia and its potentially depressant effect on the neonate. When properly administered, regional anesthesia is associated with minimal or no neonatal depression.

There is some evidence that nontoxic doses of some local anesthetics, particularly mepivacaine, when used in a continuous lumbar epidural block, may be associated with a prolonged half-life in the neonate. Chloroprocaine and bupivacaine do not seem to cause this problem.

Repeated doses of an amide type of local anesthetic are associated with increased blood levels of the drug in the mother and fetus, probably associated with their prolonged elimination and extended half-life and high protein-binding capabilities. This is not a problem with the ester type of local anesthetics such as procaine and chloroprocaine because of their short half-life and rapid metabolism in the bloodstream.

Chloroprocaine has been implicated in creating neurotoxic reactions when injected into the subarachnoid space. Recent research has shown that the chloroprocaine itself is probably not the causative factor, but rather that the high concentration of the preservative sodium bisulfite was the noxious agent.

Bupivacaine in high concentrations (0.5 and 0.75 percent) injected intravascularly as large boluses has been blamed for a large number of cardiovascular arrests in parturients who were unable to be resuscitated. Action by the Food and Drug Administration subsequently led to the banning of the use of 0.75 percent bupivacaine in all obstetric suites.

These controversies further emphasize the need for vigilance when administering epidural blocks, through either the needle or a catheter. Negative aspiration of blood or spinal fluid should always be used with an appropriate test dose volume of suitable local anesthetic. This test, in and of itself, is not always conclusive of appropriate needle/catheter placement. Fractionated, intermittent doses of the agent of choice are absolutely essential, along with continuous observation and communication with the patient.

When regional anesthesia is used, maternal monitoring is required in both the labor room and the delivery room. A reliable, large-bore intravenous line must be in place. It is mandatory that the airway be kept patent, and someone must always be available to treat any untoward reaction, whether it is due to a high level of anesthetic block, hypotension, or intravascular or accidental intrathecal injection.

Paracervical block is produced by infiltration submucosally of a local anesthetic into the fornix of the vagina lateral to the cervix. It provides relatively rapid relief of pain and is associated with minimal maternal side effects; but it gives no perineal relief, even though the block does not interfere with the second stage of labor.

Unfortunately, paracervical block may cause fetal bradycardia and can lead to fetal acidosis and sometimes even fetal demise. These effects are thought to be secondary to rapid placental passage of the drug, decreased uterine blood flow caused by absorption in the uterine arteries, as well as the direct uterine vasoconstrictive effect created by the local anesthetic. These effects are minimized by the use of small amounts of less toxic anesthetics and by injecting carefully into the parametrium.

Paracervical block is best avoided when the fetus is at risk and when the use of continuous fetal electronic heart monitoring is indicated. Studies have shown that after paracervical blocks, parturients had decreased baseline variability in fetal heart rate and some also had variable decelerations.

Bilateral lumbar sympathetic blocks at the L2 level eliminate uterine pain alone. Because the block is rather difficult to perform and is somewhat painful during its administration, it is rarely used in obstetrics today.

Pudendal nerve block will alleviate most of the vaginal and perineal pain associated with delivery. It provides no uterine pain relief and will not provide analgesia for uterine manipulation. Pudendal block does, however, provide adequate analgesia for an episiotomy repair. Supplemented with inhalation analgesia, it may provide sufficient analgesia for low forceps delivery or low forceps rotation. Since purdendal block does not produce complete pelvic analgesia, the bearing down reflex usually is not abolished.

If local anesthetic toxicity is avoided, the block has a minimal depressant effect on the mother and newborn and is not associated with maternal hypotension. It is a safe and effective block and is usually administered in the delivery room shortly before delivery by the obstetrician.

Subarachnoid block is one of the more versatile types of regional anesthesia available for use in obstetrics. Various names are given to this anesthetic technique, such as saddle block, subarachnoid block, or spinal anesthesia, but all are essentially the same technique. A saddle block, giving alleviation of pain from S1 to S5, is no longer deemed a satisfactory method for delivery since a true spinal anesthetic with a T10 sensory level block alleviates all pain of labor and delivery and will allow uterine manipulation. Use of 40 to 50 mg of lidocaine (5 percent in dextrose 7.5 percent) will give a satisfactory block for most operative vaginal procedures. For a longer duration of block, tetracaine (1 percent in dextrose 10 percent) in the range of 4 mg will give a satisfactory dermatome level and a block lasting approximately 2 to 2½ hours.

The major drawbacks of subarachnoid analgesia include a large degree of maternal hypotension (particularly if adequate rapid prehydration of intravenous fluids is not infused prior to initiation), "total spinal," abolishment of the urge to bear down, possible prolongation of the second stage of labor, and postdural puncture headache. Severe and sudden hypotension leading to maternal cardiovascular collapse is a leading cause of maternal mortality. Prophylaxis includes left uterine displacement along with preblock hydration of an intravenous balanced salt solution. Treatment consists of the above plus the use of a primary acting central vasopressor like ephedrine (10 to 20 mg) intravenously and a high Fi_{O_2}.

Vasoconstrictors such as methoxamine and phenylephrine will correct hypotension but will cause a further decrease in uterine blood flow and compromise the fetus since they are α-adrenergic agents.

Total spinal block may lead to apnea and probably loss of consciousness and cardiovascular collapse. It may be prevented by limiting the dose of local anesthetic to between two-thirds or even one-half of that used in a non-pregnant woman and not injecting the medication during a contraction. Treatment consists of correction of the hypotension and the protection of the upper airway with an endotracheal tube and ventilation (i.e., intermittent positive-pressure ventilation with 100 percent oxygen).

Even though subarachnoid analgesia abolishes the bearing down reflex, the mother can be coached to push, and forceps delivery is easily performed.

Postdural puncture headache occurs very commonly in the parturient, probably because of the increased pressure of cerebrospinal fluid and the venous engorgement discussed earlier. Prophylaxis includes the use of a small-gauge spinal needle (25, 26, or 27 gauge), adequate postpartum hydration, and use of a tight abdominal binder when a parturient assumes the upright position. Treatment consists of all of the above plus bed rest in the supine position (the prone position is even more efficacious), hydration, and appropriate analgesics. If severe headache persists, an epidural blood patch may be indicated. Maintaining the supine position after postdural puncture does not prevent headaches.

Lumbar epidural analgesia is becoming more popular than ever for vaginal delivery. The use of a continuous catheter technique, specifically localized for segmental anesthesia and with a T10 to T12 sensory block, is efficacious. This allows a mother to have a relatively pain-free labor and still maintain her motor ability. She can easily push for the vaginal delivery. When the baby is to be delivered, anesthesia of the vagina and perineum can be achieved. This allows all necessary obstetric maneuvers.

Segmental lumbar epidural anesthesia has mostly replaced caudal anesthesia. The perineal analgesia that caudal provides is out of logical sequence and requires more local anesthetic, is less reliable, and technically may be more difficult to perform.

Lumbar epidural anesthesia can be extended cephalad and caudad to provide satisfactory levels for cesarean section. If the dose is not accidentally placed in the subarachnoid space, postspinal cephalalgia is avoided. Continuous epidural analgesia frequently eliminates the necessity for depressant drugs that are used during labor and delivery. The mother is awake, mostly pain free and cooperative.

Many obstetric anesthesiologists are today using continuous-infusion pumps to maintain continuous local anesthetic infusions of lower-concentration solutions of the customarily used local anesthetics. The technique is very effective, even at the extremely low concentrations used in maintaining adequate analgesia for the pain of labor and contractions. A "top-up" dose prior to delivery provides superb anesthesia for either a forceps delivery or episiotomy repair.

The important added advantages are that the low-dose concentrations seem to cause no change in the labor pattern or curve. There is no prolongation of labor, and even if, as often occurs with a primigravida, there should be acute pain in the early stages of an extended labor, the possibility of accumulation leading to toxic levels is minimized.

The facilitated ease of maintenance does not mean that the patient needs any less observation or monitoring, but safety is certainly enhanced. Furthermore, low-dose continuous infusion eliminates the magnitude of changes that occur as analgesia wanes.

A most exciting recent development has been the use of epidural opiods in labor, usually in conjunction with extremely low-concentration local anesthetic solutions. Many different research protocols (both animal and human) are being tried with varying dosages of morphine, fentanyl, or sufentanil to investigate the quality of analgesia, effects on the progress of labor, and effects on the fetus. The most recent results from Europe, along with our own investigations, seem to indicate that fentanyl, although ineffective alone for labor, is extremely beneficial when mixed with local anesthetics producing no apparent untoward side effects.

Postoperative pain relief after surgery has similarly been shown to be extraordinarily effective with epidural administration of narcotics without need for parenteral medications, although vigilance is essential and close monitoring of these patients is mandatory because of the variable side effects that may occur in a small percentage of patients.

Hypotension after epidural anesthesia is usually slower in onset than after a subarachnoid block; however, its severity can be just as marked. Prevention and treatment are the same as in subarachnoid injection of local anesthetic, and hypotension may be avoided by giving a test dose of 3 to 4 ml of local anesthetic, waiting 2 to 3 minutes, and then checking the dermatome level before giving the remainder of the local anesthetic in fractionated or incremental doses. Epidural anesthesia requires five to ten times the amount of local anesthetic to produce the same level of anesthesia as spinal anesthesia. Unrecognized subarachnoid injection usually results in a very high or total block.

Epidural analgesia of the perineum does decrease the urge to bear down and may result in an increased tendency for forceps delivery. There may also be an increase in the incidence of persistent posterior presentations.

A disadvantage of lumbar epidural anesthesia as compared with subarachnoid anesthesia is that a larger dose of anesthetic agent is required. The blood levels of local anesthetic in the mother and fetus rise with each subsequent injection, particularly when using an amide type of local anesthetic. When large amounts of local anesthetic are required, the use of a rapidly metabolized anesthetic such as 2-chloroprocaine might be indicated.

The parturient in labor deserves as good if not better anesthetic care than a patient for surgery, particularly because the anticipated life expectancy of both mother and fetus totals more than 120 years. Failure to provide this care during labor, delivery, and the postpartum period can lead to tragedy such as the death of a young mother or the birth of a stillborn or brain-damaged child.

ANESTHESIA FOR CESAREAN SECTION

The type of anesthesia for cesarean section should be determined by the reason for the surgery, any underlying medical problems, and the presence of complicating anatomic abnormalities.

There are guidelines on which to base the choice of regional or general anesthesia. If the patient has had an uneventful labor and the fetus has shown no signs of depression of heart rate patterns, then the choice between epidural, spinal, or general anesthesia is essentially a decision agreed on by the patient, obstetrician, and anesthetist. (An example of this type of situation would be a young mother with cephalopelvic disproportion, after a trial of labor without progress.)

If the fetus has shown signs of hypoxia and has had changes in fetal heart rate patterns, late decelerations, prolonged tachycardia, or loss of beat-to-beat variability, then general anesthesia is preferable to either spinal or epidural anesthesia. General anesthesia maintains uterine perfusion more uniformly than regional, with less chance of hypotension. In the face of an emergency procedure and a possibly mildly dehydrated acidotic mother with a hypoxic fetus, maternal hypotension is probably an unjustified risk to the fetus.

Anesthesia for cesarean section for a prolapsed cord or for the patient with potential hemorrhage such as in placenta previa, is again preferably general anesthesia. One of the most important factors in this choice is the longer time required for a regional anesthetic to be performed and to take effect. This is often noxious to the fetus. The second consideration is the sympathetic blockade produced by regional anesthesia in the face of possible hemorrhage.

In the extremely obese patient (weight greater than 250 lb or 100 kg), general anesthesia is preferable because of the decrease in vital capacity and other respiratory parameters associated with the supine position and the decrease in functional residual capacity associated with the supine position, pregnancy, and obesity. This judgment will be tempered somewhat by the obstetrician doing the operative procedure and the time required to empty the uterus.

Prior to giving a general anesthetic to an extremely obese patient, the anesthetist must be certain that he or she will be able to intubate the patient without undue difficulty. If this cannot be accomplished, an awake intubation definitely should be considered.

Conduction Anesthesia for Cesarean Section (Spinal or Epidural)

It is important to preload the patient with between 1500 and 2000 ml of intravenous fluids (non–glucose-containing crystalloid) prior to initiating the block, but this does not pertain if the patient is cardiac compromised. The block should be instituted with the patient either in the right lateral decubitus position or sitting position. After the block is given and the patient has been placed supine, the operating table should be tilted approximately 10 degrees to the left and a wedge should be placed under the patient's right hip. The blood pressure should be checked every 30 seconds until stable and thereafter at a minimum of every 5 minutes. A dull safety pin should be used to determine the dermatomal level of anesthesia. If the systolic blood pressure begins to fall from its preanesthetic level, it is advisable that the uterus be displaced further to the left and an intravenous fluid bolus of crystalloids be given. Ephedrine in increments of 10 to 12 mg should be given intravenously. No longer does one wait until the systolic blood pressure drops below 100 mm Hg (or 20 percent less than the preanesthetic block level) before instituting ephedrine as a vasopressor. If the patient is toxemic and is running a diastolic blood pressure in the range of 100 to 120 mm Hg, the limit of the drop in blood pressure should not be below 90 to 100 mm Hg (diastolic).

It is important to realize that the dose of local anesthetic necessary to achieve a T4–T5 level is approximately two-thirds to one-half the dose normally used in a nonpregnant patient. The compression of the subarachnoid space by engorged epidural veins, the pressure of the uterus on the pelvic veins, and the hypertrophy of the vertebral veins all lead to diminution of the epidural space. This produces the alteration in dosages of local anesthetic solutions required for cesarean section.

Epidural anesthesia is being used more often for cesarean section, particularly after being administered for pain relief during labor and then extended for cesarean section. The dosage required is again usually two-thirds that for the normal nonpregnant woman, and the blood pressure must be taken every 5 minutes for the first 15 to 20 minutes after injection. The dermatomal level that should be achieved is T4–T5.

General Anesthesia for Cesarean Section

General anesthesia for cesarean section requires the same preliminary maneuvers as for conduction anesthesia. A large-bore intravenous line should be adequately secured, and the patient, after being placed on the operating table, should be oxygenated for 4 to 5 minutes because of the increased oxygen demands of pregnancy, along with the increased risk of hypoxia. While the patient is lying on the operating table, the table should be tilted 10 degrees to the left and a wedge placed under her right hip.

There is considerable controversy about precurarization 3 minutes prior to the administration of succinylcholine used to facilitate intubation in the rapid-sequence induction. One school of thought claims the use of a nondepolarizing muscle relaxant prior to succinylcholine will help prevent an increase in intragastric pressure and the fasciculations produced by succinylcholine. The other school of thought is that a parturient rarely complains of muscle soreness from excessive fasciculations and that the increased time delay to the onset of action of the succinylcholine is too heavy a price to pay in an already compromised situation. We recommend that precurarization *not* be used.

After the patient is completely prepared and draped, thiopental sodium (Pentothal) in the amount of 3 to 4 mg/kg is given as a bolus intravenously (up to a maximum of 250 mg), and this is followed by succinylcholine in the range of 80 to 100 mg. With the sodium pentothal, cricoid pressure should be instituted. The reservoir bag should not be squeezed. The face mask should be kept on the patient's face.

Once the endotracheal tube is passed into the trachea and the cuff has been inflated slightly beyond the vocal cords, then the operation can begin. To maintain muscle relaxation throughout the procedure, a succinylcholine drip or a nondepolarizing muscle relaxant may be used.

It is accepted practice today for the halogenated inhalational agents such as halothane (0.5 percent), isoflurane (0.75 percent), or enflurane (1.0 percent) to be used prior to abdominal delivery of a fetus to provide supplemental anesthesia and to help in prevention of the mother's recall if skin incision to delivery time should be extended. At these concentrations, uterine bleeding is not magnified. After clamping and cutting of the cord, the halogenated agents most often should be discontinued and a narcotic agent such as fentanyl and an amnestic such as diazepam are then used to deepen the anesthesia.

If general anesthesia has to be used in an emergency situation when the mother or fetus may already be severely compromised, it is the authors' opinion that after the rapid-sequence induction already described, 100 percent oxygen only with the addition of one of the above agents in low concentrations may contribute toward a better outcome (as long as delivery is rapid). The high Fio_2 delivered without nitrous oxide would seem to cause less depression to either mother or fetus, with the extremely low concentration of the halogenated agent preventing maternal recall.

Endotracheal intubation is mandatory when general anesthesia is chosen for cesarean section. However, it must be anticipated that the anesthetist may be unable to intubate the trachea. It is therefore necessary to have a plan to fall back on to protect the patient from developing hypoxia. Cricoid pressure must be maintained. The patient should be turned head down with her face toward the side, and an airway should be inserted. Oxygenation should be established by face mask while maintaining the cricoid pressure. The patient should be ventilated with 100 percent oxygen, the nitrous oxide turned off, and the anesthetic allowed to wear off. Local or regional anesthesia should be carried out as a safer alternative, or an awake oral intubation should be considered. If the operation is an emergency and there is no time to consider another form of anesthetic technique, the patient should be ventilated using nitrous oxide–oxygen and anesthesia maintained with an agent such as enflurane

(Ethrane) or isoflurane to establish surgical anesthesia with spontaneous ventilation, after the succinylcholine has worn off. If a nondepolarizing muscle relaxant has been used, then ventilation has to be continued by the anesthetist. The operation should be allowed to proceed via the face mask, but cricoid pressure must be maintained.

ANESTHESIA FOR ABNORMAL OBSTETRICS

Abnormal obstetrics may be defined as situations in which conditions unfavorable to the mother or the fetus already exist or are predicted and anticipated. Women with pregnancy-induced hypertension (toxemia), antepartum or postpartum hemorrhage, preterm labor, or abnormal presentation all fall within this category. There are a myriad of medical conditions that may influence the management of the pregnant patient. Such conditions include diabetes mellitus, congenital and acquired heart disease, preexisting renal disease, and chronic hypertension.

Pregnancy-Induced Hypertension (Preeclampsia, Eclampsia)

It is important for the anesthetist to understand the physiologic factors that alter the condition of the toxemic patient: renal and hepatic involvement, hypovolemia, anemia, and electrolyte imbalance. Classically, the patient presents with hypertension, peripheral edema, and albuminuria. Pathophysiologically, there is generalized arterial spasm and general vasoconstriction, with swelling of the renal glomeruli and epithelial cells leading to reduction of the capillary lumen and a subsequent decrease in glomerular filtration rate and renal blood flow. There is vascular hyperactivity, with an increased pressor response to angiotensin, probably from the shift of sodium into the arterial wall. In approximately 7 to 8 percent of the patients, there is a decrease in platelets, fibrinogen, and prothrombin, leading to a potential disseminated intravascular coagulopathy.

The central nervous system becomes edematous, irritable, and sensitive to all depressant drugs. The blood–placenta barrier may be rendered even more ineffective because of a decrease in the uterine blood flow. Hypovolemia is a common occurrence despite the presence of peripheral edema. It is noteworthy that blood pressure may be very sensitive to autonomic blockade from epidural anesthesia. There also is frequent uterine irritability, which may lead to a marked response to small doses of oxytocin (Pitocin).

Treatment, prior to the termination of pregnancy, is bed rest, with the patient on her side, a low-salt diet, and some sedation. If the patient requires an antihypertensive drug, a direct vasodilator such as hydralazine usually is effective. Magnesium sulfate is given for control of central nervous system irritability, and the dosage is determined by serum magnesium levels and tendon reflexes.

If vaginal delivery is planned, the patient should labor on her side, and if the diagnosis is severe pregnancy-induced hypertension, central venous pressure monitoring would be indicated, since the hypovolemia that is present can be quite marked. Coagulation studies should be performed, and the patient should receive magnesium sulfate as indicated. Crystalloid solutions are quite useful in com-

bating the severe vasoconstriction that exists. Serial hematocrits may be useful in determining if treatment is improving the patient's condition.

Recent work has verified that there are often gross fluid shifts in these parturients with pregnancy-induced hypertension. Effective and judicious use of volume expanders such as albumin or human plasma protein function (Plasmanate), along with continuous monitoring of central venous pressures, is essential and assists in shifting extravascular fluids back to the intravascular compartment, raising the central venous pressure to nearly normal levels without compromising the already altered blood pressures.

Epidural anesthesia, well administered, without epinephrine, provides satisfactory analgesia for labor if the above criteria are met. It will help to eliminate the stressful, painful contractions and can be used to correct the blood pressure elevation. It is necessary that the central venous pressure be at a level of approximately 5 to 8 cm H_2O and that the coagulation profile and platelet count be normal prior to initiating the block. A pudendal block may also be a suitable adjunct for vaginal delivery.

For cesarean section, epidural anesthesia is excellent if there are no blood volume problems, bleeding, or convulsions. Spinal anesthesia is never the anesthetic technique of choice and is contraindicated because of the probability of a rather severe drop in blood pressure that would be detrimental to the fetus. General anesthesia is preferred to spinal anesthesia. If general anesthesia is used, endotracheal intubation and preoxygenation are again mandatory.

If a parturient with severe pregnancy-induced hypertension requires emergent delivery via general anesthesia, protection against increasing the already hypertensive state with laryngoscopy and intubation procedures will often necessitate an infusion of a potent antihypertensive agent such as nitroglycerin for protection, despite the fact that hydralazine and magnesium sulfate may have already been given. Nitroprusside is probably contraindicated in these parturients because the degradation products following placental transfer can cause cyanide toxicity for the neonate.

During laryngoscopy, the blood pressure will increase but will usually not exceed prenitroglycerin levels. By preventing marked exacerbations of hypertension, intracranial hemorrhage and pulmonary edema may be avoided. If circumstances allow, it would probably be better if such severely affected parturients be managed and treated at a tertiary care facility or a high-risk obstetric center where every resource is immediately available.

Acute Intrapartum Hemorrhage

Hemorrhage is the most common cause of obstetric shock, but the blood pressure may not decrease nor the pulse rate increase until a liter or more of blood has been lost. Placenta previa and abruptio placenta are the most common causes of external hemorrhage.

Placenta previa, which may be total, partial or marginal, occurs in approximately 0.4 percent of pregnancies and has a greater incidence in the multipara. It is painless and is frequently accompanied by malpresentations and prematurity.

The diagnosis of placenta previa is determined by the

patient's history of painless vaginal bleeding, the use of ultrasonography, and the "double setup." This consists of a pelvic examination performed in the operating room while prepared for a stat cesarean section, since the vaginal examination may cause uncontrollable bleeding. General anesthesia and cross-matched blood should be immediately available prior to this procedure.

Abruptio placenta, which is often associated with toxemia, may present with mild to moderate bleeding or with a stormy onset, severe pain, and continuous heavy bleeding. There is significant risk of fetal death and maternal shock. Extensive infarction of the placenta with the release of thromboplastin and activation of the clotting mechanism can lead to a defect in clotting, hypofibrinogenemia, and disseminated intravascular coagulopathy.

The anesthetic management of patients with hemorrhage reflects the effects and manifestations of hypovolemia and loss of oxygen-carrying capacity. This usually precludes the use of spinal or epidural anesthesia. For vaginal delivery of a patient with partial placenta previa or partial abruptio placenta, pudendal block, nitrous oxide, and oxygen with the use of low-dose ketamine can be recommended. High FiO_2 should be used. When cesarean section is indicated, general anesthesia with endotracheal intubation is the anesthetic of choice. Ketamine and oxygen are an excellent general anesthetic combination. If there is a need to increase uterine tone, as in abruption, one should consider lower doses of thiopental sodium as an induction agent since ketamine is known to increase uterine tone.

Medical Conditions Associated with Obstetrics

Diabetes Mellitus. The current thoughts about the management of the insulin-dependent pregnant patient include strict control of maternal hyperglycemia and the maintenance of the maternal blood glucose concentration between 80 mg/100 ml and 120 mg/100 ml.

Problems encountered in the diabetic patient during pregnancy include an increased tendency to ketoacidosis in the last half of pregnancy, alterations in insulin dosage, and the fact that pregnancy itself is diabetogenic. There is an increased risk of preeclampsia and hydramnios.

As far as the fetus is concerned, macrosomia and death in utero are relatively common if the diabetic parturient is not carefully supervised throughout her pregnancy. Placental pathology with premature aging of the placenta is not uncommon and may lead to hypoxia in utero.

Anesthetic care includes intelligent fluid therapy during labor and delivery. If cesarean section is indicated, an insulin technique that is time tested consists of half the usual A.M. dose of insulin and an intravenous infusion of 5 percent dextrose just prior to the delivery. However, hypoglycemia has been a problem in the baby because of the release of insulin produced by stimulation of the infant's pancreas. A newer insulin technique that seems to be an improvement is the microinsulin technique used by endocrinologists. This maintains strict maternal blood glucose control and has just about eliminated hypoglycemia in the neonate.

It is now advocated by neonatologists and understood by anesthesia personnel that the mother not receive a bolus of dextrose prior to receiving an epidural anesthetic for cesarean section. It is again important to avoid aortocaval compression by careful positioning of the parturient. If cesarean section is necessary, it has been shown that both epidural and general anesthesia are satisfactory. Spinal anesthesia may increase the acidosis that is encountered in the fetus.

It is noteworthy that once the baby is delivered, the mother may become adiabetic for several days.

Heart Disease. The incidence of heart disease in pregnant women is relatively small but is a major nonobstetric cause of death. Patients who have left-to-right shunts usually tolerate labor and delivery without any major problems, unless a drop in blood pressure causes a reversal in the shunt. Patients with a right-to-left shunt have a higher incidence of fetal wastage. Myocardial infarction is rare in pregnant women but does occur and can lead to fatalities.

In rheumatic heart disease, the valvular lesions can cause decreased cardiac response to the demands of pregnancy and labor. Mitral stenosis is the most common lesion associated with rheumatic heart disease, and it produces increased pulmonary blood volume and decreased cardiac output throughout pregnancy. It is important to minimize increases in the central blood volume and avoid marked increases in pulmonary artery pressure.

When a patient with rheumatic heart disease enters the hospital in labor, her clinical status, as represented by either the New York Heart Association classification or the American Heart Association should be ascertained. If the patient is in category 1 or 2 (almost no limitation of activity and no evidence of congestive heart failure), then she should be treated with caution; but the usual standards of care are sufficient. On the other hand, patients who have marked symptoms probably should be monitored with an arterial line and a pulmonary artery catheter.

Anesthesia for vaginal delivery in a patient with rheumatic heart disease would be best carried out with segmental epidural anesthesia to lessen the stress of labor and to relieve the anxiety of labor with its effects on the heart. Ephedrine should be avoided and, if possible, so should excess fluids. If general anesthesia is necessary, drugs that produce tachycardia such as pancuronium, meperidine, and ketamine should be avoided.

The pregnant patient with congenital heart disease presents the problem of reversal of a left-to-right shunt. The systolic pressure must be maintained, and the stress and the strain of delivery should not be allowed to create further impositions on the heart. Continuous segmental lumbar epidural anesthesia and spinal anesthesia for delivery are both therefore useful.

Pulmonary Disease. In patients with pulmonary disease such as bronchial asthma, the anesthetic management that should be used is regional anesthesia. Reactive airways are liable to bronchospasm under rapid-sequence induction of general anesthesia with endotracheal intubation.

For patients with nonasthmatic chronic obstructive pulmonary disease, regional anesthesia is satisfactory. If there is reduced total lung volume and reduced vital capacity, then general anesthesia may be more effective and safer for cesarean section.

MATERNAL COMPLICATIONS OF OBSTETRIC ANESTHESIA

It would be impossible to list all the potential complications that may follow obstetric anesthesia. This discussion is limited to acute complications that may develop intrapartum or postpartum and that the anesthetist may be called on to recognize or treat immediately.

Hypotension

Hypotension as a consequence of obstetric anesthesia usually is a sequela of conduction anesthesia techniques (i.e., spinal or epidural anesthesia). The development of hypotension may be defined as blood pressures falling 20 percent below the initial baseline blood pressures or systolic pressure decreases below 100 mm Hg.

Prevention is preferable to treatment. The patient in labor should not be allowed to labor on her back because of the consequences of aortocaval compression, which can lead to supine hypotensive syndrome. A mild to moderate drop in blood pressure can usually be corrected by placing the patient in a slight head-down lateral position and giving a rapid infusion of fluids, preferably crystalloid. Oxygen tends to reduce nausea and vomiting associated with the hypotension and may aid in transplacental oxygenation of the fetus. Ephedrine given in small incremental doses of 10 to 12 mg at the initial onset of the hypotension usually eliminates the syndrome rather rapidly and helps prevent hypoxia of the fetus.

Approximately 1 out of 10 or 12 pregnant women in the last trimester of pregnancy, when placed in the supine position, sustains these significant reductions in blood pressure. There is definite obstruction of the vena cava and the aorta by the gravid uterus when the patient lies supine. The majority of parturients compensate for this by shunting blood from the lower extremities through the azygos veins and the paravertebral circulation into the superior vena cava and then into the right atrium. There is an accompanying increase in sympathetic tone and peripheral vascular resistance. However, approximately 30 percent of women who have conduction anesthesia (spinal or epidural) have significant hypotension, since the sympathetic blockade produced by the conduction anesthetic tends to eliminate the compensatory mechanisms of the body. Treatment consists of placing the patient on her left side, placing a wedge under her right hip, giving an infusion of fluids, and administering oxygen. If she is to be transported to the delivery or operating room, she should always be placed in the lateral position, not on her back.

Postdural Puncture Headache

Although not considered dangerous, the postdural puncture headache (often called a postspinal headache) is one of the most annoying and bothersome complications of anesthesia. Postdural puncture headache occurs twice as frequently in the postpartum patient as in a nonpregnant woman of equivalent age. Apparently, the incidence of headache is related to the size of the needle. The 26- or 27-gauge needle has helped to reduce the incidence and severity of these headaches. It is stated that the cause of the headaches is the loss of cerebrospinal fluid via the puncture site and a subsequent drop in cerebrospinal pressure. The headache is generally located in the frontal or occipital areas and is relieved when the patient lies flat. It is aggravated in an upright position.

Conservative therapy in the manner described may very often eliminate the problem. An abdominal binder should be placed over the site of puncture because it may help to increase the tone and peripheral vascular resistance. A rapid infusion of 250 ml/hour infused for a period of 8 hours with a Foley catheter in place, with the patient being kept supine or flat (denied bathroom privileges), very often relieves the problem. Appropriate analgesics should be used, and if severe headache persists, an epidural blood patch will usually provide immediate relief.

If there is an accidental dural puncture during lumbar epidural anesthesia, place the epidural catheter either one lumbar space above or below the area of the dural puncture. This should be followed by a small bolus of normal saline (3 ml to 4 ml), which is placed into the epidural space through the needle at the site of puncture prior to withdrawal of the needle. Keep the catheter in place after the delivery. Use a continuous infusion of sterile saline at a rate of 8 to 10 ml/hour for approximately 24 hours. This is an attempt to reduce the incidence of postpartum headache from about 75 to 10 percent.

Pulmonary Aspiration

Anesthesia complications are a leading cause of maternal mortality. Approximately 30 to 40 percent of the patients who die from anesthesia during labor or delivery die from pulmonary aspiration. Several predisposing factors make pulmonary aspiration a great risk in the parturient.

1. General anesthesia may be required with great urgency—for example, in the event of a prolapsed cord or fetal distress or if acute hemorrhage should be present.
2. The patient may have had a meal just prior to admission or even after the onset of labor. Pregnant patients have delayed gastric emptying time, with retention of food and solids, particularly after the onset of labor. Sedation, anxiety, and pain also delay gastric emptying.
3. Hiatus hernia has been demonstrated radiographically to exist in 20 percent of all women in the last trimester of pregnancy.
4. Increased intraabdominal pressure produced by the pregnant uterus is aggravated by the lithotomy position; the fasciculations from succinylcholine may also predispose to regurgitation and vomiting.

Pathophysiologically, particulate matter may cause difficulty, and acid aspiration, particularly if the pH is below 2.5, causes a chemical burn. If the pH is less than 1.2, actual necrosis occurs. There may be a high mortality even if the pH is less than 1.75.

When the aspiration syndrome occurs, there is intense bronchospasm and an increase in lower airway resistance. There is a rapid fall in arterial blood pressure and an initial rise in pulmonary artery blood pressure followed by a return to normal. This is then followed by a fall in the pulmonary artery pressure. Acute pulmonary edema ensues, with a large loss of plasma into the lungs. The resultant decrease in plasma volume allows a consequent hemoconcentration to occur. There is a progressive fall in the Pao_2, pH, and a moderate rise in the $Paco_2$. Right-sided aspiration is favored by the bronchial configuration. If the patient is in Trendelenburg's position, the apical segment of the upper lobe and the apical segment of the lower lobe are more frequently involved. Infection is an infrequent but serious complication, but most patients are afebrile and the chest usually clears in 7 to 10 days, if the patient survives.

When the patient aspirates solid material, there is massive collapse of the lung independent of the pH, with airway obstruction and atelectasis. There is no free fluid in the pleural or pericardial cavities, but there is a rise in the $Paco_2$ despite less exudation or fluid loss.

The clinical picture of aspiration may occur during induction, maintenance of anesthesia, or recovery from anesthesia. Trivial amounts of acid will cause severe illness. The syndrome itself may occur immediately after the aspiration or may be delayed several hours. The patient becomes restless, dyspneic, tachypneic, and cyanotic; her blood pressure falls rapidly, and she progresses into shock. Generalized bronchospasm, rales, and rhonchi with sanguineous secretions of bloody frothy sputum from the frank pulmonary edema are noted. Chest x-rays show mottled densities, as in pulmonary edema or bronchopneumonia.

The clinical picture of a patient who has aspirated solid particles depends on the size of these particles. Acute bronchospasm and often massive atelectasis of a lobe or entire lung may occur. Cyanosis, tachycardia, dyspnea, and mediastinal shift can develop.

Treatment. Prevention is preferable to actual treatment. Although it is not guaranteed that local or regional anesthesia will circumvent pulmonary aspiration, it does lower the incidence. It is important to ensure that patients do not eat during labor. The use of a nasogastric tube or the induction of vomiting for patients in labor is very controversial.

Antacids definitely cause a rise in the pH of gastric contents and help alleviate the potential for acid aspiration. Antacids do not eliminate pulmonary aspiration. It has been suggested that there is a danger of aspirating particulate-matter antacids and producing particulate-matter aspiration. Nevertheless, it is wise to give antacids to patients in labor and prior to cesarean sections to raise the pH. Whether to use a particulate-matter antacid or a clear antacid is debatable, but an antacid should be used. Even with the use of a clear antacid, if general anesthesia is to be used, it is essential that the patient be intubated with a cuffed endotracheal tube, and cricoid pressure be applied and maintained from the moment induction is begun.

Awake intubation should not be ignored or neglected in the case of a patient with a difficult airway.

Recent research studies using H_2-blockers such as cimetidine and ranitidine in conjunction with a new gastric emptying drug, metoclopramide, have been producing interesting but controversial results. Metoclopramide, for example, is ineffective if narcotics were previously administered. The intravenous administration of H_2-blockers may be contraindicated, since they can produce biliary dysfunction. The oral route and intramuscular route (the night before and the morning of), if elective cesarean section is to be performed, appears to be beneficial in all respects. It should be emphasized that these are useful adjuncts to our armamentarium and that they should not be considered a substitute for prevention and vigilance.

The management of the actual aspiration, if it should occur, consists of clearing the airway immediately with the head down in a lateral position, the right side being preferred. The pH of the vomitus should be tested, the patient should be oxygenated, and the airway secured with endotracheal intubation prior to suction. If solid material is aspirated, immediate bronchoscopy may be required. Artificial ventilation with 100 percent oxygen, positive end-expiratory pressure, and chest therapy may be necessary. If there is hypovolemia, cardiovascular support based on central venous pressure, arterial blood gases, and the wetness of the lungs should all be taken into account. The use of steroids is controversial, but there is no evidence that steroids help the patient. Antibiotics probably should not be used unless infection supervenes.

Total or High Spinal Anesthesia

High spinal or total spinal anesthesia can occur after an accidental injection of an epidural dose into the subarachnoid space or a miscalculation in the injection of local anesthetic into the subarachnoid space. Epidural anesthesia predisposes to a massive total spinal, since the dose of local anesthetics used in epidural anesthesia is 5 to 10 times that of spinal anesthesia.

Patients with a high spinal characteristically suffer from difficulty in breathing, tingling in the fingers of the hand, difficulty in coughing, nausea, and possible vomiting. If the dermatome level reaches T1–T2 or even T3, bradycardia may ensue.

Total spinal anesthesia leads to vascular hypotension, cessation of respiration, and unconsciousness.

Treatment of a massive subarachnoid injection consists of administering fluids to support the circulation, immediate intubation with an endotracheal tube, and ventilation with 100 percent oxygen. Blood pressure, circulation, and respiration should be maintained until the effects of the block are terminated. A vasopressor may be necessary.

Intravenous Injection of Local Anesthetics

A toxic level of local anesthesia may follow from an accidental injection of a local anesthetic into a vein or may be the end result of an accumulation of local anesthetic after prolonged administration. An anesthetist usually encounters the former. This occurs when local anesthetic has been injected into a vein instead of into the epidural space. It may occur via the epidural needle or the epidural catheter. The engorged nature of the veins and the fact that there are numerous veins in the epidural space predispose to this situation. There are no valves in the veins of the epidural space, and the local anesthetic therefore easily reaches the brain and the heart, producing the symptoms of toxicity. Patients may complain of sleepiness, ringing in the ears (tinnitus), circumoral numbness, or a funny taste in the mouth. Grand mal seizures may rapidly follow. There may be bradycardia and cardiovascular collapse. The drop in blood pressure is due to both the lowering of cardiac output and to peripheral vasodilatation.

Prevention is preferable to treatment and consists of making sure the epidural catheter is placed in the midline, not in the lateral portion of the epidural space. Careful aspiration of the catheter before injection of any local anesthetic and the use of a test dose help to prevent problems and do decrease their incidence, although they do not guarantee safety. Treatment consists of turning the mother to a lateral position, giving 100 percent oxygen, and immediate intubation if indicated. Utilization of a barbiturate such as thiopental (50 mg) or intravenous diazepam aids in terminating convulsions. Succinylcholine will control the outward manifestations of the convulsions, but an electroencephalogram still reveals convulsive activity and this is not the treatment of choice. Maintenance of circulation and cardiovascular stability by vasopressors or fluids may be necessary. With a convulsion, there is a tremendous increase in oxygen demand and oxygen is mandatory.

EVALUATION AND RESUSCITATION OF THE NEWBORN

A newborn's first breath usually occurs 20 to 30 seconds after the appearance of its nose. The stimulus for initiation of this first breath is unknown, but within 90 seconds rhythmic respirations usually occur under the control of the medullary centers.

It is best if someone other than the obstetrician is available to resuscitate a compromised infant. The baby should have its mouth and nose cleared of secretions, since 80 percent of infants are obligatory nasal breathers. The baby should be kept dry to reduce heat loss and then placed in an infrared warming device. The Apgar score, a means of determining five variables consisting of the heart rate, respiratory effort, muscle tone, reflex irritability, and color should be evaluated and scored 0 to 2, at 1- and 5-minute intervals. If the 1-minute Apgar score is between 5 and 7, the baby should be stimulated and kept dry and should have oxygen blown over its face. If the Apgar score is 3 to 4, the baby should be stimulated, kept dry, and ventilated with oxygen by bag and mask. If the Apgar score is 0 to 2, the baby's trachea should be intubated, the lungs ventilated with oxygen, and cardiac resuscitation initiated.

Acute neonatal asphyxia may manifest first with an accelerated heart rate and then an abrupt decrease. Proper resuscitation can bring a rise in heart rate followed in several minutes by spontaneous breathing.

An infant heart rate of less than 100 is an indication for active, vigorous resuscitation.

When ventilating a baby, the adequacy of ventilation is determined by equal expansion of its chest, an increase in the heart rate to normal, improvement of color, and equal bilateral strong breath sounds in the axilla. The ventilatory pressure should be maintained at between 25 to 30 cm H_2O, but if the lungs remain stiff, higher pressures may be necessary.

If meconium is present, an endotracheal tube should be used as a suction catheter. Laryngoscopy should be performed to see if there is meconium present at or below the vocal cords, and if so, the baby should be suctioned. If there is no meconium present, then just visualization alone is sufficient.

Cardiac massage should be performed if the heart rate is less than 60/minute. This is done by compressing the sternum two-thirds the distance to the vertebral column at a rate of 80 to 100 times a minute with the thumbs placed at the junction of the middle third of the body. Observe pupil size rather than palpate for pulses.

If pH determination shows evidence of metabolic acidosis, administer 2 to 3 ml of sodium bicarbonate into the umbilical vein and continue the ventilation. If the pH is below 7.10 despite ventilation, try to correct one-fourth of the metabolic component with the initial sodium bicarbonate.

It is important to maintain volume, since 60 percent of asphyxiates in utero are volume depleted and the correction of acidosis may reveal unrecognized hypovolemia. To detect hypovolemia, check arterial pressure, capillary filling, the color of the baby, and the pulse. Treatment consists of giving blood, 10 ml/kg; albumin, 25 percent, 1 g/kg; crystalloid solution, 10 ml/kg; or plasma, 10 ml/kg. Evaluate the blood pressure regularly.

Recognizing those infants who need special observation or therapy and placing them in intensive care nurseries will definitely reduce perinatal mortality, particularly among premature infants.

BIBLIOGRAPHY

Abboud TK, Sarkis F, Blikian A, et al: Lack of adverse neurobehavioral effects of lidocaine. Anesthesiology 57:A404, 1982.

Abboud TK, Shnider SM, Dailey PA, et al: Intrathecal administration of hyperbaric morphine for the relief of pain in labour. Br J Anaesth 56:1351–1360, 1984.

Albright GA: Cardiac arrest following regional anesthesia with etidocaine or bupivacaine (editorial). Anesthesiology 51:285–287, 1979.

Blass NH: Regional anesthesia in the morbidly obese parturient. Reg Anaesth 4(1):20–22, 1979.

Blass NH: Anesthesia for the morbidly obese. In Katz J, Benumof J, Kadis LB (eds): Anesthesia and Uncommon Diseases: Pathophysiology and Clinical Correlations, 2nd ed. Philadelphia, Saunders, 1981, pp. 450–462.

Bonica JJ: Maternal physiological and psychological changes. Clin Obstet Gynecol 2(3):469–495, 1975.

Brazelton TB, Parker WB, Zuckerman B: Importance of behavioral assessment of the neonate. Curr Probl Pediatr 7(2):71, 1976.

Cohen SE: Why is the pregnant patient different? Semin Anesth 1(2):73–82, 1982.

Cohen SE: Why is the pregnant patient different? Refresher Courses Anesth 11:45–58, 1983.

Cohen SE, Jasson J, Talafre L, et al: Does metoclopramide decrease the volume of gastric contents in patients undergoing cesarean section? Anesthesiology 61:604–607, 1984.

Cohen SE, Wyner J: Endocrine disease. In James FM (ed): Obstetric Anesthesia—The Complicated Patient. Philadelphia, Davis, 1982, pp. 139–170.

Conklin KA, Murad SHN: Pharmacology of drugs in obstetric anesthesia. Semin Anesth 1(2):83–100, 1982.

Craig DB, Toole MA: Airway closure in pregnancy. Can Anaesth Soc J 22:665–672, 1975.

Crandell JT, Kotelko DM: Cardiotoxicity of local anesthetics during late pregnancy. Anesth Analg 64:204, 1985.

Datta S, Alper MH: Anesthesia for cesarean section. Anesthesiology 53:142, 1980.

Datta S, Brown WU Jr: Acid base status in diabetic mothers and their infants following general or spinal anesthesia for caesarean section. Anesthesiology 47:272, 1977.

Datta S, Corke BC, Alper MH, et al: Epidural anesthesia for cesarean section: A comparison of bupivacaine, chloroprocaine and etidocaine. Anesthesiology 52:48–51, 1980.

Datta S, Kitzmiller JL: Anesthetic and obstetric management of diabetic and pregnant women. Clin Perinatol 9(1):154–166, 1982.

Dick-Reed G: Childbirth Without Fear. New York, Harper & Row, 1959.

Eckstein KL, Marx GF: Aortocaval compression and uterine displacement. Anesthesiology 40:92–96, 1974.

Gibbs CP: Anesthesia for the high risk parturient. IARS Review Course Lectures 58(7):49–61, 1984.

Gibbs CP, Banner TC: Effectiveness of Bicitra as a preoperative antacid. Anesthesiology 61:97, 1984.

Gibbs CP, Gabbe SG: Diabetes. In James FM (ed): Obstetric Anesthesia—The Complicated Patient. Philadelphia, Davis, 1982, pp. 171–184.

Gissen AJ, Datta S, Lambert D: The chloroprocaine controversy. Is chloroprocaine neurotoxic? Reg Anesth 9(4):135–145, 1984.

Gutsche BB: Maternal physiologic alterations during pregnancy. In Shnider SM, Levinson G (eds): Anesthesia for Obstetrics. Baltimore, Williams & Wilkins, 1979, pp. 3–11.

Hodgkinson R, Glassenberg R, Joyce TH, et al: Comparison of cimetidine (Tagamet) and antacid for safety and effectiveness in reducing gastric acidity before elective cesarean section. Anesthesiology 59:86–90, 1983.

Holmes F: The supine hypotensive syndrome: Its importance to the anesthetist. Anaesthesia 15:298, 1960.

Howard BK, Goodson JH, Mengert WF: Supine hypotensive syndrome of late pregnancy. Obstet Gynecol 1:371, 1953.

Hughes SC, Rosen MA, Shnider SM, et al: Maternal and neonatal effects of epidural morphine for labor and delivery. Anesth Analg 63:319–324, 1984.

James FM III, Crawford JS, Hopkinson R, et al: A comparison of general anesthesia and lumbar epidural analgesia for elective caesarean section. Anesth Analg 56:228, 1977.

James FM III, Greiss FCJ, Kemp RD: An evaluation of vasopressor therapy for maternal hypotension during spinal anesthesia. Anesthesiology 33:25, 1970.

Joyce TH III: Cardiac disease. In James FM (ed): Obstetric Anesthesia—The Complicated Patient. Philadelphia, Davis, 1982, pp. 87–101.

Joyce TH, Debnath KS, Baker EA: Preeclampsia: Relationship of CVP and epidural analgesia. Anesthesiology 51:S297, 1979.

Kitzmiller JL, Cloherty JP, Younger D, et al: Diabetic pregnancy and perinatal morbidity. Am J Obstet Gynecol 131:560, 1978.

Kotelko DM, Dailey PA, et al: Epidural morphine analgesia after cesarean delivery. Obstet Gynecol 63:409–413, 1984.

LeBoyer F: Birth Without Violence. London, Wildwood House, 1975.

Metcalfe J, Ueland K: Maternal cardiovascular adjustments to pregnancy. Prog Cardiovasc Dis 16:363–374, 1974.

Moore DC, Spierdijk J, Van Kleef JD, et al: Chloroprocaine neurotoxicity: Four additional cases. Anesth Analg 61:155, 1982.

Ostheimer GW: Newborn resuscitation. Semin Anesth 1(2):168–176, 1982.

Ostheimer GW, Morrison JA, Lavoie C, et al: The effect of cimetidine on mother, newborn and neonatal neurobehavior. Anesthesiology 57:A405, 1982.

Philip BK: Complications of regional anesthesia for obstetrics. Reg Anaesth 8(1):17–30, 1983.

Ramanathan S, Masih A, Rock I, et al: Maternal and fetal effects of prophylactic hydration with crystalloids or colloids before epidural anesthesia. Anesth Analg 62:673–678, 1983.

Rawal N, Wattwil M: Respiratory depression after epidural morphine—an experimental and clinical study. Anesth Analg 63:8–14, 1984.

Redick LF: Epidural analgesia. Clin Perinatol 9(1):63–76, 1982.

Reisner LS, Hochman BN, Plumer MH: Persistent neurologic deficit and adhesive arachnoiditis following intrathecal 2 chloroprocaine. Anesth Analg 59:452, 1980.

Roberts RB, Shirley MD: Reducing the risk of acid aspiration during cesarean section. Anesth Analg 53:859, 1974.

Scanlon JW, Brown WV, Weiss JB, et al: Neurobehavioral responses of newborn infants after maternal epidural anesthesia. Anesthesiology 40:121–238, 1974.

Schaer HM: History of pain relief in obstetrics. In Marx GF, Bassel GM (eds): Obstetric Analgesia and Anesthesia. Amsterdam, Elsevier North Holland, 1980, pp. 12–16.

Sellick BA: Cricoid pressure to control regurgitation of stomach contents during induction of anesthesia. Lancet 2:404, 1961.

Shnider SM: Vasopressors in obstetrics. Reg Anaesth 8(1):74–80, 1983.

Skaredoff MN, Ostheimer GW: Physiologic changes during pregnancy: Effects of major regional anesthesia. Reg Anaesth 6(1):28–40, 1981.

Skerman JH, Gupta A, Jacobs MA, et al: Continuous infusion of epidural fentanyl for postoperative pain relief following cesarean section. In Abstracts of Scientific Papers, Society for Obstetric Anesthesia and Perinatology, Washington, DC, 1985, p. 95.

Skerman JH, Thompson BA, Goldstein MT, et al: Combined continuous epidural fentanyl and bupivacaine in labor: A randomised study. Anesthesiology 63:A450, 1985.

Ueland K, Metcalfe J: Circulatory changes in pregnancy. Clin Obstet Gynecol 18:41–50, 1975.

Wright JP: Anesthetic considerations in preeclampsia–eclampsia. Anesth Analg 63:590–601, 1983.

28

Cardioperipheral and Thoracic Anesthesia

Cathy A. Mastropietro

CORONARY ARTERY SURGERY

Introduction

When symptoms occur from inadequate oxygen delivery to the myocardium, the result is said to be ischemic coronary heart disease. In a vast majority of patients, the cause is an atherosclerotic narrowing of the coronary arteries; in the remainder, the cause is embolism, inflammatory changes, or vasospasm.

Extensive coronary artery narrowing can exist without symptoms. The asymptomatic individuals are classified as the coronary atherosclerotic, whereas those who present with symptoms are classified as the coronary artery diseased (Vanden Belt and Ronan, 1979).

The incidence of coronary artery disease (CAD) is vastly increasing. It has been estimated that 600,000 individuals develop CAD annually. It has been the major cause of deaths between the ages of 45 and 54 and the most common cause of death in males between the ages of 35 and 44. The increase in incidence, sudden onset of symptoms, and tragic nature of the disease has caused warranted concern by both the medical profession and the lay public.

There are several risk factors associated with the development of coronary atherosclerosis. These include (1) genetic susceptibility, (2) obesity and carbohydrate tolerance, (3) hemodynamic and local arterial factors, and (4) stress (Table 28–1).

Atherosclerosis refers to a thickening and hardening of medium- or large-sized arteries. It is an unevenly distributed progressive process that mostly affects the population of the more industrialized areas, such as North America, Europe, and the Soviet Union.

The disease process rarely involves small arteries and should not be confused with the term arteriosclerosis, which rarely has notable clinical effects. The feature that sets atherosclerosis apart from other forms of arteriosclerosis is the lipid component, which in the advanced plaque is often represented by a central necrotic core that is rich in cholesterol esters and is often accompanied by visible cholesterol crystals (Braunwald, 1980). This part of the lesion, which on gross examination is usually soft and grumous, is responsible for the name of the disease process, derived from the Greek stem "athera," meaning gruel or porridge (Braunwald, 1980).

Atherosclerotic plaques more frequently involve the abdominal aorta, especially around the ostia of its major branches. Renal arteries are usually spared from plaque except at their ostia; coronary arteries show the most intense involvement within the first six centimeters.

Plaques are composed of plaque cells, arterial smooth muscle cells, and lipid. There are several theories proposed to explain the pathogenesis of plaques. The most accepted one is the insudation theory, which suggests that there is increased passage and accumulation of plasma constituents from the arterial lumen into the intima, promoting a type of low-grade inflammatory edema. Elevated serum lipoproteins assist in carrying cholesterol, in the form of low-density lipoprotein, into the arterial system; chronically elevated levels are always associated with progressive atherosclerosis. Endothelial injury often plays a major part in accelerating atherosclerosis because it results in encrustation of platelets and monocytes, which in turn exposes the intimal and medial arterial smooth muscle cell to the peptides that stimulate cell proliferation (Braunwald, 1980).

Clinically, the formation of plaque produces symptoms resulting from stenosis caused by its space-occupying tendencies or because of its embolic properties. Ulceration in the area of the plaque leads to thrombus formation, and if the occurrence takes place in the coronary system, occlusion or infarction results. In larger vessels, such as the aorta, occlusion is not the problem. Weakening of the aortic wall occurs, resulting in aneurysm formation and embolization to distal arteries.

Educating the public on how to reduce risk factors has resulted in some decline in statistics; however, the incidence and mortality rates remain high. Prevention, early detection, and medical or surgical intervention is essential to longevity.

TABLE 28–1. RISK FACTORS ASSOCIATED WITH THE DEVELOPMENT OF CORONARY ATHEROSCLEROSIS

1. Genetic susceptibility: inherited traits
2. Obesity, carbohydrate tolerance: hypercholesterolemia, hypertriglyceridemia, diabetes mellitus
3. Hemodynamic and local arterial factors: hypertension, cigarette smoking
4. Stress: psychological and personality factors ("Type A" personality)

It is not within the realm of this chapter to discuss the medical approach to CAD. Surgical intervention and the anesthetic principles of management will be the focal point.

Functional Anatomy of Coronary Circulation

The coronary arteries arise from the sinuses of Valsalva just above the aortic arch. The left coronary artery (a. coronaria sinistra) arises in the left posterior aortic sinus (of Valsalva) and after a short course under the left atrium, bifurcates into the anterior descending branch (LAD) and

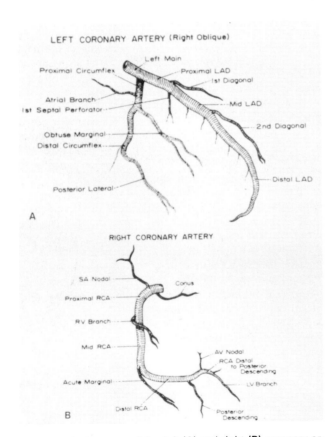

Figure 28–1. Anatomy of the left **(A)** and right **(B)** coronary arteries showing the nomenclature recommended by the American Heart Association. AV = atrioventricular, LAD = left anterior descending, LV = left ventricular, RCA = right coronary artery, RV = right ventricular, SA = sinoatrial. (*From King SB III, Douglas JS: Coronary arteriography and left ventriculography. In The Heart, 4th ed, 1978. Courtesy of McGraw-Hill.*)

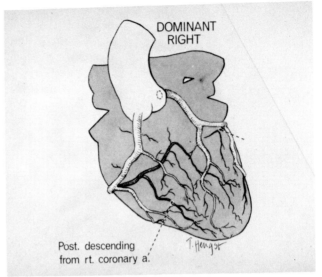

Figure 28–2. Right coronary artery dominance. (*From Cooley DA, Norman JC: Techniques in Cardiac Surgery, 1975. Courtesy of Texas Medical Press.*)

the circumflex (Gray, 1973). The LAD is a continuation of the left main coronary artery and courses down the anterior interventricular sulcus, around the apex of the heart, into the posterior interventricular sulcus, supplying perforating branches to the anterior right and left ventricular walls. A large diagonal branch to the anterior left ventricle is frequently found as a branch of the LAD. The circumflex runs posteriorly into the atrioventricular groove, with its marginal branch supplying the left lateral ventricular wall and most of the left atrium (Fig. 28–1).

The right coronary artery (a. coronaria dextra) arises in the right atrioventricular groove. The first branch turns toward the base of the pulmonary artery. (The sinoatrial node artery arises from the proximal right coronary artery in 55 percent of all hearts, in the remainder from the circum-

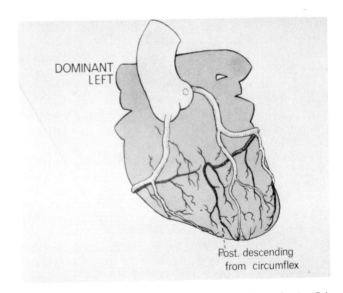

Figure 28–3. Left coronary artery dominance. (*From Cooley DA, Norman JC: Techniques in Cardiac Surgery, 1975. Courtesy of Texas Medical Press.*)

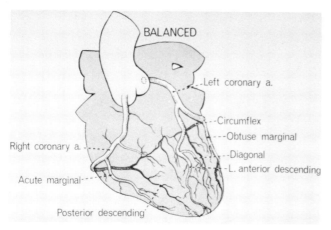

Figure 28–4. Balanced coronary artery dominance. *(From Cooley DA, Norman JC: Techniques in Cardiac Surgery, 1975. Courtesy of Texas Medical Press.)*

TABLE 28–2. ANATOMIC BLOOD SUPPLY TO CARDIAC CHAMBERS

Artery	Area Supplied
Left anterior descending	Anterior right and left ventricular wall
Diagonal	Anterior left ventrical wall
Circumflex	Lateral left ventricular wall, most of left atrium
Right coronary artery	Right atrium, right ventricular wall

Pathophysiology

When atherosclerosis becomes symptomatic, the degree is usually extensive, because a 75 percent stenosis is required before flow is decreased. Lesions may be found in one or several vessels.

Generally, the LAD and circumflex arteries are affected in their proximal areas, whereas the right coronary artery lesion can be proximal or distal. Whether a lesion is proximal or distal in the LAD is important because of its anatomic structures. THe LAD gives rise to its major branches as it descends. Conversely, the main right coronary artery branches are in its periphery and proximal or distal lesions are less compromising. (Figure 28–5 illustrates a coronary arteriogram with triple vessel disease.)

The LAD is most commonly affected, followed by the right, left circumflex, and left main coronary artery (Vanden Belt and Ronan, 1979). The subendocardial region of the left ventricle is more prone to ischemic damage because of ventricular contraction and compression of subendocardial vessels. The coronary vessels are initially epicardial, perforate the myocardium, and then become subendocardial arterioles. Perfusion to subendocardial areas depends on diastolic time. If left ventricular end-diastolic pressure (LVEDP) (pulmonary capillary wedge pressure) is greatly increased or diastolic pressure decreased, the gradient declines and subendocardial ischemia occurs. Tachyarrhythmias will shorten diastolic time and decrease subendocardial perfusion. Figure 28–6 illustrates zones of predilection of atherosclerotic lesions.

flex.) It follows the sulcus, first to the right margin of the heart, then left on the diaphragmatic surfaces, ending in two or three branches that supply the right atrium and ventricle. In 90 percent of hearts, the right coronary artery crosses the crux, supplies a branch to the atrioventricular junction and continues on in the posterior atrioventricular sulcus as the posterior descending artery (Gray, 1973; Vanden Belt and Ronan, 1979). In the remaining 10 percent, the circumflex branch of the left coronary crosses the crux, supplies the atrioventricular junction and gives rise to the posterior descending artery (see Fig. 28–1) (Gray, 1973).

Coronary artery dominance is determined by which artery crosses the crux. When the right crosses, the coronary circulation is referred to as right dominant, and when the circumflex crosses, the circulation is referred to as the left dominant (Fig. 28–2, 28–3, 28–4). Even though this terminology exists, it should be remembered that it is the left coronary artery that supplies the major mass of the myocardium in most individuals (85 percent).

Venous drainage occurs via the great cardiac veins, the thebesian, and the anterior cardiac veins. Table 28–2 provides a summary of anatomic blood supply to cardiac chambers.

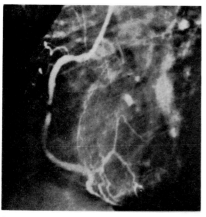

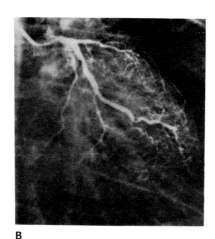

Figure 28–5. A. Right coronary arteriogram; there is a significant stenosis of the midportion of the right coronary artery. **B.** Left coronary arteriogram; there is profound disease of the anterior descending coronary artery followed by a stenosis; the circumflex origin is also stenosed.

A   B

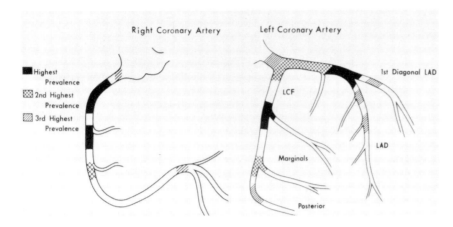

Figure 28–6. Zones of predilection of the atherosclerotic lesion in the left and right coronary arteries. LAD = left anterior descending artery. LCF = left circumflex artery. (*From Vanden Belt RJ, Ronan JA, et al: Cardiology: A Clinical Approach, 1979. Courtesy of Yearbook Med. Pub.*)

Physiologic Principles

In the normal heart there exists a delicate balance between myocardial oxygen supply and demand. The oxygen demands of the heart may vary constantly, and normally the heart can accommodate these changes. The arterial-venous oxygen difference across the myocardial capillary bed is normally wide; therefore, the heart must rely on increased flow rather than more oxygen extraction when demand increases (Berne and Levy, 1977). The heart with obstructive lesions cannot increase flow and thus slight alterations in cardiovascular dynamics will shift the myocardial demand: supply ratio. The result is myocardial ischemia.

As illustrated in Figure 28–7, oxygen supply is dependent on coronary blood flow, oxygen delivery, and heart rate.

Coronary Blood Flow. Coronary blood flow, and thus myocardial perfusion, is the result of the aortic pressure that is generated by the heart itself. Changes in aortic pres-

sure directly evoke changes in coronary blood flow. The resting coronary blood flow is 225 ml/min or 4 to 5 percent of the total cardiac output.

In addition to providing the bulk pressure that drives blood through the coronary vessels, the heart influences its blood supply by the squeezing effect of the contracting myocardium on the vessels that course through it (extravascular compression) (Berne and Levy, 1977). This force is so great during ventricular systole that blood flow in the left coronary artery is briefly reversed. Maximal left coronary inflow occurs in early diastole when the ventricles are relaxed (LVEDP) and extravascular compression is absent.

Flow in the right coronary artery follows a similar pattern, but because of lower pressure developed during systole by a thinner right ventricle, reversal of flow does not occur in early systole and systolic blood flow constitutes a greater proportion of total right coronary flow (Berne and Levy, 1977).

Changes in cardiac metabolic activity also play a role in coronary blood flow. Increased metabolic activity of the heart results in a decrease in coronary resistance and vice versa, probably through the local action of the metabolic by-product adenosine. Abrupt changes in perfusion pressure will produce abrupt changes in coronary blood flow (Figure 28–8) (Berne and Levy, 1977).

Oxygen Delivery. Oxygen delivery is determined by the oxygen saturation and the hematocrit. Oxygen content of the arterial blood depends on normal amounts of hemoglobin with normal (2,3 DPG), pH, and Pa_{CO_2} levels. Decreased Pa_{CO_2}, decreased 2,3 DPG, and alkalemia will shift the oxygen dissociation curve to the left, thus allowing hemoglobin to hold on to its oxygen. Increased Pa_{CO_2}, increased 2,3 DPG, and acidemia cause shifts to the right and hemoglobin to readily give up its oxygen.

Heart Rate. Tachycardia and bradycardia influence oxygen supply by affecting coronary blood flow. A change in heart rate is accomplished chiefly by shortening or lengthening diastole. With tachycardia, the proportion of time spent in systole (restricted inflow) increases. However, this mechanical reduction in mean coronary flow is overridden by the coronary artery dilation associated with increased metabolic activity of the more rapidly beating heart. With

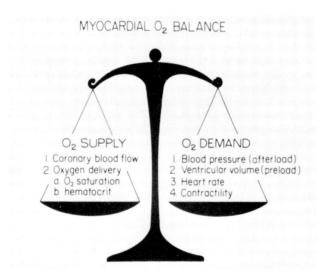

Figure 28–7. The myocardial oxygen balance is demonstrated. The two sides of the balance are the oxygen supply and the oxygen demand; the factors that affect them are shown. (*From Kaplan JA: Cardiac Anesthesia, 1979. By permission of Grune & Stratton and the author.*)

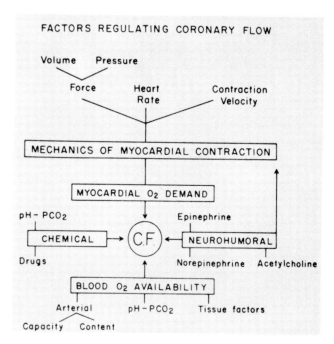

Figure 28–8. Factors affecting coronary flow (CF) through neuro-metabolic pathways. The factors are arranged in four groups: chemical, blood oxygen availability, neurohumoral, and myocardial oxygen demand. These are further broken down into subcategories. Note in particular the factors that affect myocardial mechanics. Note also that neurohumoral agents (the catecholamines in particular) exert effects on the coronary circulation both directly in the arteriole and indirectly through induced changes in mechanical modalities of contraction. (*From Hurst JW, Logue B: The Heart, 5th ed., 1966. Courtesy of McGraw-Hill.*)

bradycardia the opposite is true: restriction of coronary inflow is less (more time in diastole), but so are the metabolic oxygen requirements of the myocardium (Vanden Belt and Ronan, 1979). According to the adenosine hypothesis, a reduction in myocardial oxygen tension produced by low coronary blood flow, hypoxemia, or increased metabolic activity of the heart leads to a breakdown of adenine nucleotides to adenosine, which diffuses out of the cardiac cells and induces dilation of the coronary resistance vessels (Berne and Levy, 1977). This dilation increases coronary blood flow. Normally, only small amounts of adenosine are released and dilating effects are minimal.

Thus, factors that will increase oxygen supply are (1) increased aortic diastolic pressure, (2) decreased LVEDP, (3) decreased arterial resistance, and (4) increased PaO$_2$.

Myocardial Oxygen Demand. Referring to Figure 28–7, one can see that the primary influences on myocardial oxygen demand are (1) ventricular wall tension (influenced by ventricular systolic pressure—afterload—and ventricular volume or end-diastolic volume—preload), (2) heart rate, and (3) contractility. *Alterations* in these variables elevate myocardial oxygen demand to a level that cannot be supplied by obstructed coronary arteries.

Preload is defined as the degree of end-diastolic myocardial fiber length. Variations in preload affect myocardial

function, forming the basis for the Frank-Starling curve (Vanden Belt and Ronan, 1979). As the length of the fiber increases, so does the degree of contraction because of alterations in the troponin-tropomyosin complex. This property of myocardium is referred to as heterometric autoregulation, i.e., the ventricle can normally eject whatever volume is presented to it (Fig. 28–9) (Vanden Belt and Ronan, 1979).

Afterload (the pressure the heart works against) refers to the tension or stress in the ventricular wall during systole. One major determinant of afterload is the aortic pressure of impedance encountered by the ventricle during ejection. (Vander Belt and Ronan, 1979). If a failing ventricle compensates by failing to take advantage of the Frank-Starling curve, it has to work against the same aortic and intraventricular pressure, but with the increased radius, wall tension is increased, with augmentation of myocardial oxygen requirements (Vanden Belt and Ronan, 1979).

Increases in myocardial *contractility* alter myocardial oxygen demand by increasing peak tension and increasing the rate of rise to tension.

Alterations in *heart rate* obviously influence myocardial demand, i.e., slow rhythms decrease demands, whereas rapid rhythms will increase demand in proportion to the increase in rate.

The anesthesia team plays a vital role in the management of patients with CAD. An understanding of the principles of care is essential to be able to provide an atmosphere that promotes the least possible physiologic or psychological stress to the patient. This is accomplished by maintaining a balance in the patient's supply:demand ratio.

Preoperative Workup

Preoperative Interview. In 1967, the first aortocoronary bypass surgery was performed by Favalora. At present, there are approximately 700,000 revascularization procedures performed annually (Kaplan 1979).

With the number of surgeries progressively on the rise, it is obvious that the anesthesia team plays a vital role in

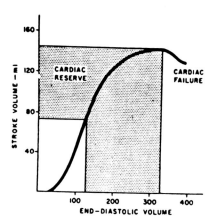

Figure 28–9. The ventricular function curve. As the end-diastolic volume increases, so does the force of ventricular contraction. Thus the stroke volume becomes greater up to a critical point, after which stroke volume decreases (cardiac failure). (*Courtesy of Datascope Corporation.*)

the total care of the patient. The preoperative interview, imperative for all surgical procedures, has a tremendous impact on the cardiac patient. Experiencing preoperative anxiety can be detrimental to these patients if allowed to persist. Catecholamine release, with a concomitant hypertension and tachycardia, increases myocardial oxygen demand.

A detailed, unhurried explanation of the preoperative, intraoperative, and postoperative events is of paramount importance because the fear of anesthesia is just as great as the fear of the actual surgery. It is not uncommon for anginal attacks, with increased blood pressure and heart rate, to occur immediately during the preinduction period. The incidence of such attacks can be reduced by informing the patient and family of upcoming events. Table 28–3 lists minimal preoperative studies used in evaluating the cardiac patient.

The preoperative evaluation begins by taking a thorough history, because it is imperative to determine the pathologic condition of cardiac and other organ systems. The specific inquiries and laboratory examinations should

TABLE 28–3. MINIMAL PREOPERATIVE STUDIES USED IN EVALUATING THE CARDIAC PATIENT

Function	Factors to Consider
Angina	Type
	Severity
	Medication
	Dosage
ECG	Presence of arrythmias
	Myocardial ischemia
	Cardiac catheterization report
Left ventricular	Ejection fraction
	Left ventricular end-diastolic pressure
	Cardiac output
	Cardiac index
Peripheral vascular	Carotid stenosis
	Aortoiliac disease
	Renal vascular disease
Respiratory	Pulmonary function studies
	Arterial blood gas analysis
	Chest x-ray
Renal/hepatic	Blood, urea, nitrogen
	Serum creatinine
	Prothrombin time
	Partial thromboplastin time
	Platelet and bleeding times
Fluid compartment volume	State of hydration
	Electrolyte values
	Pulmonary artery pressure
	Pulmonary wedge pressure
	Pulmonary mean pressure
Chronic medications	Type
	Dosage
	Side effects
General appearance	Dyspneic
	Exercise tolerance
	Retinopathy
	Xanthoma

be designed to determine the kind of functional impairment that the patient suffers with regard to his heart and peripheral vascular system, oxygen-carrying capacity, pulmonary exchange, renal and hepatic function, and body compartment volumes.

First and foremost, the severity of the cardiac dysfunction must be determined. Ventricular dysfunction is a cardiac disorder that reduces cardiac output, stroke volume, and arterial pressure to an extent that they are insufficient for metabolic needs (Lappas and Powel, 1977). Not only does this determination give some indication of the degree of ventricular function, but it also gives clues to any coexisting disease.

Angina. Angina pectoris is regarded as stable when it has not changed in frequency, duration, or time of appearance of precipitating factors during the preceding 60 days. Stable angina may be (1) mild (of brief duration, not markedly interfering with the patient's life-style) or (2) disabling (occurring at less than the usual daily activity level but not at rest) (Kaplan, 1979).

Unstable angina describes a whole group of syndromes varying from the above definition (Kaplan, 1979). The patients experience chest pain; however, serum enzyme evidence is lacking.

Variant angina is a term used to describe pain that occurs at rest, not with strenuous exercise.

The examiner must determine the type of angina that presents, if it is relieved by medication, such as nitroglycerin, and the dosage needed for relief. Shortness of breath, exercise limitations, arrythmias, or signs of pulmonary hypertension should be looked for. Xantheloma or retinopathy are common. An S_4 murmur is often present in anginal patients.

Electrocardiogram. Electrocardiogram findings may not be conclusive. Nonspecific R-ST segment or T-wave abnormalities are common. Typically during myocardial ischemia a horizontal or down-sloping depression of the R-ST segment is present.

Left Ventricular Function. The degree of left ventricular function should also be determined. The ejection fraction (end-diastolic volume minus end-systolic volume divided by end-diastolic volume) is a useful measure of ventricular function and is currently the most reliable. A normally contracting ventricle will eject 67 percent of end-diastolic volume with each beat. Ejection fractions of 0.40 to 0.55 are common in patients with previous infarction who are asymptomatic. When the values range between 0.25 and 0.40, symptoms occur with exercise, and if less than 0.25, symptoms occur at rest (Kaplan, 1979).

Another useful method of assessing ventricular function is wall motion, which is determined by echocardiography or cardiac catheterization. The ventricular wall is classified as hypokinetic (decreased motion), akinetic (absent motion), or dyskinetic (paradoxical motion).

Resting LVEDP is another indicator of ventricular function. The normal value is 12 mm Hg, and levels above 18 usually indicate poor ventricular function.

The cardiac output and index provide some knowledge

of ventricular function. The cardiac output is the best indicator of overall cardiac performance. Abnormally low values indicate cardiac decompensation.

Patients scheduled for revascularization procedures can be divided into two groups: (1) those with good left ventricular function evidenced by normal cardiac output, LVEDP less than 12 mm Hg, and an ejection fraction of greater than 0.55, and (2) those with poor ventricular function evidenced by decreased cardiac output, LVEDP greater than 19 mm Hg, ejection fraction less than 0.40, and symptoms of congestive heart failure. These patients have had previously detected infarctions.

Peripheral Symptoms. One should automatically assume that peripheral vascular disease accompanies coronary atherosclerosis. Carotid stenosis is common. The management of combined carotid stenosis and coronary bypass remains controversial. However, the carotid status of these patients must be evaluated and managed accordingly.

The presence of aortoiliac disease should be determined before bypass in the event that use of the intraaortic balloon is necessary.

Respiratory Status. The most common respiratory insult is chronic obstructive lung disease, and symptoms are compounded by large doses of crystalloid therapy and hemodilution, hypothermia, and cardiopulmonary bypass itself. Pulmonary function studies and arterial blood gas analysis should be performed preoperatively to provide a baseline for reference. The oxygen content of arterial blood is dependent on the amount of hemoglobin, the amount of 2,3 DPG, and a normal acid-base status. Any abnormalities in these areas should be corrected before elective surgery commences.

Renal and Hepatic Function. Renal vascular disease presents problems with urinary output from ischemic kidneys. Also, vast fluctuations in blood pressure can be expected with renal artery lesions.

Renal function can be determined by blood urea nitrogen and serum creatinine levels. Abnormally high levels may indicate renal impairment and should be further evaluated.

Coagulation studies are mandatory preoperative assessment screening studies. The prothrombin (PT), partial thromboplastin time (PTT), platelet count, and bleeding time should be evaluated. The importance of these values being normal is obvious for the patient undergoing cardiopulmonary bypass, because of the large doses of anticoagulants administered.

Fluid Compartment Volume. Special attention should be paid to the patient's hydration. Patients with congestive heart failure have peripheral pooling of water and pulmonary congestion. They are usually taking diuretics, which may provoke electrolyte imbalance. In addition, diuretics exacerbate the decline in plasma volume common in CAD and hypertension (Kaplan, 1979). Patients may require volume expansion prior to induction.

Infection. Provided the patient can wait, any preexisting infection should be treated. The reticuloendothelial system functions poorly in post-cardiopulmonary-bypass patients, and they are prone to infections. Preoperative prophylactic use of antibiotics is essential.

Chronic Medications. The cardiac patient is usually taking several medications to provide him or her with some comfort. These may include beta blockers to reduce myocardial contractility, heart rate, and systemic hypertension; nitroglycerin for anginal relief; calcium channel blockers for arrythmias; diuretics; vasodilators; cardiac glycosides; and sedatives.

The general rule of thumb is to maintain blood levels of these medications preoperatively, so as not to interfere with the supply:demand ratio.

Anesthetic Management

Preoperative Medication. The goal of preoperative medication is to provide enough sedation to obtund heightened anxiety levels for the patient arriving in the operating room suite. The anxiety experienced by these patients is often unexpressed and frequently denied, accentuating angina or the possibility of myocardial infarction. The heightened sympathetic response associated with stress must be obliterated. Choice of medication is an individual preference. If the patient's drug therapy already includes a sedative, the prescriber might want to continue this regimen to maintain constant blood concentrations.

It should be kept in mind that belladonna administration must be minimal, so that the cardioaccelerator effect of these drugs is avoided.

Preinduction. The ideal anesthetic induction provides comfort to the patient, stability of circulatory dynamics, and absence of excitement. Regardless of the technique selected, it is imperative that these patients be in surgical planes of anesthesia prior to stimulation to prevent tachyarrythmias and hypertension. The anesthetist must remember that patients with low cardiac outputs will have a decreased circulation time and thus a delayed onset of action of intravenous agents. On the other hand, in the presence of low cardiac output, inhalation agents will rapidly come into equilibrium with alveolar gas, and onset of anesthesia will be more rapid.

The ultimate goal in managing a patient with myocardial ischemia is prevention of an intraoperative infarction.

Monitoring. Changes in oxygen supply-demand balance by alterations in circulatory dynamics can be determined by using the appropriate monitoring devices. Effective monitoring sounds the alarm when something goes awry, provides some clue to the reason, and may help determine the appropriate treatment.

Minimal monitoring for the patient undergoing coronary revascularization should include electrocardiogram, esophageal temperature, direct arterial pressure, central venous pressure, serum electrolytes and pH, and urinary output. In addition, cardiac output, pulmonary artery pressure,

TABLE 28-4. NORMAL VALUES FOR MEASURED AND CALCULATED HEMODYNAMIC PARAMETERS

Parameter	Value	
Central venous pressure	10–15 mm Hg	
S$\bar{\text{v}}$o$_2$	75%	
Cardiac output	4–8 L/min	
Systemic vascular resistance	800–1600 units (dynes)	
Pulmonary vascular resistance	75–200 units (dynes)	
Rate pressure product	<12,000	
Triple index	<150,000	
Stroke volume	60–100 ml/beat	
Cardiac index	2.5–4.0 L/min/m^2	
Left ventricular stroke work index	45–75 g/m^2/beat	
Right atrial pressure	0–7 mm Hg	
Right ventricular pressure	Systolic	15–25 mm Hg
	Diastolic	0–8 mm Hg
Pulmonary artery pressure	Systolic	15–25 mm Hg
	Diastolic	8–15 mm Hg
	Mean	10–20 mm Hg
Pulmonary capillary wedge pressure	6–12 mm Hg	
Left ventricular end-diastolic pressure	8–12 mm Hg	
Left atrial pressure	5–10 mm Hg	

wedge pressures, and venous oxygen saturation (S$\bar{\text{v}}$o$_2$) are being used with increasing frequency as monitoring aids to determine hemodynamic alterations (Table 28–4).

Electrocardiogram. The electrocardiogram (ECG) readily alerts the anesthetist to changes in rate, rhythm, or segment. It can also provide some information about myocardial ischemia. A five-lead system should be attached to the patient; it will reflect leads I, II, III, aV$_R$, aV$_F$, aV$_L$, and V$_5$. Arrythmias are best determined in lead II, whereas ischemia is more readily detected in V$_5$. Lead II parallels the P-wave vector, thus differentiating ventricular from supraventricular arrythmias. The presence or absence of the P wave is especially important in the assessment of the hemodynamic effect of the atrial kick (Naples, 1981).

Lead V$_5$ monitors the myocardium in areas most susceptible to ischemic change. Typically, the ECG change noted in ischemia is a down-sloping depression of the R-ST segment of 1 mm and 0.08 seconds duration. The electrophysiology of the ST segment changes in myocardial ischemia has not been completely clarified, but an altered ion transport across the myocardial cell membrane apparently is the underlying cause of the change in current, responsible for the ST segment shift induced by ischemia (Braunwald, 1980).

Arterial cannulation is essential to denote beat-to-beat changes in arterial pressure. Arterial access also allows ease of acquiring blood samples for frequent blood gas analysis.

Central Venous Pressure. Central venous pressure values represent right heart filling pressure. Radiographic examination should be used to assess proper placement. A sudden increase in venous pressure may indicate obstruction of cannula drainage and requires immediate correction. The central venous pressure does not directly indicate left heart filling pressure, and it may not be reliable in patients with left ventricular dysfunction, but can be used as a rough estimate of this measure.

Oximetric or Swan-Ganz Catheter. The newest invasive monitoring modality in use today is the oximetric catheter. This catheter, which is placed in the pulmonary artery, determines the oxygen saturation of mixed venous blood, or S$\bar{\text{v}}$o$_2$. S$\bar{\text{v}}$o$_2$ is a valuable measure of oxygen transport and should be used in conjunction with cardiac output, hemoglobin concentration, and Pao$_2$ to adequately assess tissue oxygenation.

Normal S$\bar{\text{v}}$o$_2$ is dependent on arterial oxygen saturation, hemoglobin concentration, cardiac output, and tissue oxygen demands.

The normal range of S$\bar{\text{v}}$o$_2$ is 65 to 80 percent. Decreases (40 to 60 percent) may be indicative of abnormal hemodynamics with reduced cardiac output, hypotension, elevated systemic vascular resistance, arrythmias, abnormal oxygen demand—as with shivering or pyrexia—or abnormal oxygen supply—caused by anemia or obstruction—or reduced pulmonary venous oxygen saturation (Jamison et al, 1982).

Marked increases (85 to 95 percent) may indicate elevated cardiac output but frequently represent catheter wedging (Jamison et al, 1982).

Measurements of S$\bar{\text{v}}$o$_2$ are valuable in early detection of hemodynamic disturbances and predicting the adequacy of the body's cardiac output in meeting oxygen demands, thus avoiding irreversible stages of metabolic acidosis.

The oximetric catheter can also serve as a pulmonary artery catheter. The pulmonary artery (Swan-Ganz) catheter monitors pressures on the right side of the heart. It is a flow-directed catheter that is placed in the pulmonary artery.

At the onset of systole, right ventricular pressure begins to rise, closing the tricuspid valve. As ventricular pressure rises above pulmonary artery diastole pressure, the pulmonic valve will open. With pulmonic valve opening, blood leaves the ventricle and pressure in the pulmonary artery becomes greater than systolic. As the amount of blood ejected from the ventricle decreases, pulmonary artery pressure decreases and the pulmonic valve closes. Ventricular relaxation (diastole) begins and pressure in the ventricle becomes lower than the pulmonary artery pressure and atrial pressure. The tricuspid valve opens. As diastole progresses, the atrium continues to contract, forcing the remaining blood into the ventricle. The ventricle contraction begins again and the cycle is repeated.

The Swan-Ganz catheter measures pulmonary artery pressure, systolic, diastolic, and mean pressures, pulmonary capillary wedge pressure (PCWP), cardiac output, and central venous pressure.

The systolic pressure is measured during ventricular contraction and represents the highest pressure in a chamber during this time period. The balloon is deflated during this measurement. Pulmonary artery systolic pressure is normally 15 to 25 mm Hg.

The diastolic pressure records the lowest pressure dur-

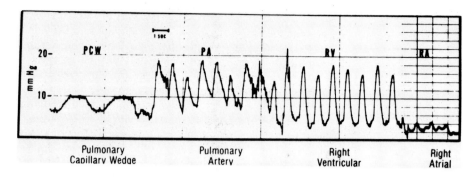

Figure 28–10. Wave patterns that can be determined by Swan-Ganz catheter. (*Courtesy of Datascope Corporation.*)

Pulmonary Capillary Wedge   Pulmonary Artery   Right Ventricular   Right Atrial

ing ventricular relaxation. Normal value is 8 to 15 mm Hg.

The mean pulmonary artery pressure is 10 to 20 mm Hg. The PCWP reflects pressure when a distal branch of the pulmonary artery is occluded by the balloon; this measurement is of great clinical significance. It is used to determine the presence of pulmonary congestion or fluid shifts from pulmonary capillaries into interstitial tissue and alveoli. The PCWP closely reflects left atrial pressure and can serve as an indicator of left ventricular filling pressure. Normal value is 6 to 12 mm Hg. Various wave forms can be seen in Figure 28–10.

The Swan-Ganz catheter can also be used to measure cardiac output. The most commonly used method is by means of a thermodilution technique, which uses temperature changes in the pulmonary artery as an indicator of circulatory volume. Cardiac output is determined by stroke volume and heart rate, and measurement of cardiac output allows for calculation of several other important hemodynamic parameters. These include systemic vascular resistance (SVR), peripheral vascular resistance (PVR), stroke volume (SV), and cardiac index (CI) (Table 28–5).

Central hemodynamics are best assessed by measuring CI, mean right atrial pressure, and PCWP. These values will vary with different disease processes (Table 28–6). Prompt recognition and proper identification of variation from normal values is critical to begin appropriate management.

Primary indications for use of an oximetric or Swan-Ganz catheter are ventricular dysfunction, recent myocardial infarction, altered chamber pressures, or whenever there is an anticipated alteration in preload or afterload (Naples, 1981). In patients with CAD, two distinct situations exist in which LVEDP (PCWP) can be evaluated: (1) myocardial ischemia causing left ventricular dysfunction, resulting in elevated LVEDP; (2) elevated LVEDP causing increased

myocardial oxygen consumption (MVO_2) and decreased oxygen supply resulting in subendocardial ischemia (Naples, 1981).

It should be remembered that patients with abnormal cardiac anatomy should not have pulmonary artery lines inserted. These patients include those with ventricular or atrial septal defects. Complications can occur after the use of pulmonary arterial catheters. These include balloon rupture, endocarditis, pulmonary artery perforation, thrombosis, and intracardiac knotting. Complications can be minimized by a sound background knowledge in the use of these catheters.

The myocardial oxygen demand should also be monitored closely. Since Rohde demonstrated, in 1912, that MVO_2 varies directly with the heart rate times peak developed pressure, extensive investigation into the relative effects of pressure, SV, and heart rate on oxygen consumption has been carried out (Kaplan, 1979). Rohde theorized that the rate pressure product (systolic blood pressure times heart rate) correlates with MVO_2. A value greater than 12,000 increases oxygen demand. Control of heart rate lessens the chance of myocardial ischemia.

Triple index (systolic pressure times heart rate times PCWP), and the tension time index (heart rate times area under the systolic portion of the aortic pressure curve) have also been used to determine oxygen demand, but the rate pressure product (RPP) seems to be more reliable.

Induction of Anesthesia. Choice of anesthesia for coronary revascularization should be made on the basis of the patient's left ventricular function, i.e., good versus poor cardiac performance. If normal ventricular function is present with CAD, the incidence of reflex response to stimulation, i.e., hypertension or tachycardia, is increased. Controlled myocardial depression is necessary to prevent

TABLE 28–5. FORMULAS FOR CALCULATING VARIOUS HEMODYNAMIC PARAMETERS

Parameter	Normal Value	Formulas
Central venous pressure (CVP)	5–12 cmH₂O	mm Hg = CVP 1.36
Mean arterial pressure (MAP)	70–90 mm Hg	Diastolic + ⅓ pulse pressure
Cardiac index (CI)	3.4	Cardiac output/body surface area[a]
Stroke volume (SV)	60–100 ml/beat	Cardiac output/heart rate × 1000
Peripheral vascular resistance (PVR)	200	Mean pulmonary artery pressure (MPAP) − Left atrial pressure (LAP) (or Pulmonary capillary wedge pressure [PCWP])/Cardiac output × 80
Systemic vascular resistance (SVR)	1150	MAP − CVP (mm Hg)/Cardiac output × 80

[a] Body surface area is determined by use of the Dubois nomogram.

TABLE 28–6. PATHOPHYSIOLOGIC EFFECTS ON CARDIAC INDEX, RIGHT ATRIAL PRESSURE, AND PULMONARY CAPILLARY WEDGE PRESSURE (PCWP)

	Cardiac Index	Right Atrial Pressure	PCWP
Normal	2.3–3.5	1–5 mm Hg	6–12 mm Hg
Hypovolemia	↓	↓	↓
Pump or heart failure	↓	↑	↑
Tamponade	↓	↑	↑

sympathetic nervous system activity and subsequent increases in myocardial oxygen requirements. If left ventricular function is depressed, the induction technique must prevent a further depression in hemodynamic status.

Selection of the induction agent varies according to vital sign lability and user preference. Commonly used non-narcotic drugs are thiopental, diazepam, lorazepam, and the newest induction agent, etomidate. Thiopental sodium, an ultra-short-acting barbiturate, possesses myocardial depressant properties and vasodilating effects. Therefore, hypotension may ensue, and doses large enough to prevent contact stimulation may not be achievable. For this reason, thiopental is frequently used in conjunction with sedatives or narcotics. Dosage is 4 mg/kg.

Etomidate is a nonnarcotic, nonbarbiturate, short-acting induction agent. The hypnotic effect begins in 1 minute with a three-to-five-minute duration. Induction dose varies from 0.2 to 0.5 mg/kg, with the average dose being 0.3 mg. Etomidate is a unique hypnotic agent in that it provides excellent cardiorespiratory stability. There is little cardiovascular depression and the effect on MV_{O_2} is minimal. Another advantage to its use is that there is no histamine release.

Diazepam, a benzodiazepine derivative, is an antianxiety agent that acts on the limbic system, thalamus, and hypothalamus to produce calming effects. It possesses transient cardiovascular depressor effects and no peripheral autonomic blocking action, thus providing somnolence with minimal hemodynamic changes. Usual adult dosage ranges from 0.2 to 0.5 mg/kg. Peak action occurs in seven to ten minutes after administration.

Diazepam also produces anterograde amnesic effects by affecting the storage period of memory—the stage during which information is encoded and entered into memory. It is postulated that diazepam causes a decrease in hippocampal activity. The hippocampus is responsible for repetitive firing necessary for memory storage.

Lorazepam is also a benzodiazepine with antianxiety and sedative effects. Injections of doses of 2 to 4 mg intravenously provide somnolence, relief of preoperative anxiety, and lack of recall of events related to the day of surgery.

Should the patient be unable to tolerate any degree of myocardial depression, a narcotic can be used. Fentanyl in high dose (50 to 100 μg/kg) is commonly used. The advantage to this technique is that there are minimal effects on myocardial performance. The pharmacokinetics of fentanyl will be discussed later.

As mentioned previously, the goal of induction is to provide the patient some degree of relaxation, progressing to a surgical plane of anesthesia that will, upon noxious stimulation, propagate minimal hemodynamic change.

Muscle relaxation must be adequate before endoscopy. Table 28–7 compares muscle relaxant properties. Because of the length of cardiac surgery, long- or intermediate-acting muscle relaxants seem to be the drugs of choice. This is not to say that a short-acting relaxant, such as succinylcholine, can't be used for induction, followed by a nondepolarizing agent for maintenance. However, if succinylcholine is used, the dosage should be large enough to prevent the need for additional drug, because the risk of arrythmias is increased with consecutive doses.

Pancuronium bromide is very popular as a muscle relaxant for these procedures. The degree of muscle relaxation is profound and effects are of long duration. Pancuronium-induced tachycardia and hypertension must be avoided. The cardiovascular effects of pancuronium are thought to be due to inhibition of vagal tone and a direct or indirect beta-adrenergic effect. This does not seem to be as great a problem with narcotic inductions as with other techniques, with the exception of sufentanil, which does not appear to protect the heart against adverse tachyarrythmias. The narcotic-induced bradycardia appears to override the tachyarrythmic effects of pancuronium. If pancuronium is used to provide skeletal muscle relaxation for intubation, doses of 0.06 to 0.1 mg/kg are recommended. The onset and duration of action is dose-dependant. Doses suitable for endotracheal intubation have an onset in 30 seconds and peak at 3 minutes. The maintenance dose is 0.1 mg/kg.

Metocurine is an intermediate-acting muscle relaxant that structurally resembles d-tubocurarine. Its effects are at the myoneural junction, but it does not produce autonomic ganglionic blockade as tubocurarine does. Histamine release occurs less frequently. Intubation doses appear adequate at 0.2 to 0.4 mg/kg, followed by 0.5 to 1 mg for maintenance. Onset of action occurs in 1 to 4 minutes and lasts 35 to 60 minutes. The main excretory pathway for metubine is via the kidneys; thus caution must be exercised with those patients who have coexisting renal disease.

Atracurium besylate is an intermediate-acting, nondepolarizing skeletal muscle relaxant. The duration of blockade is approximately one-third to one-half that of pancuronium, metubine, or tubocurarine in equipotent doses. An intubation dose of 0.4 to 0.5 mg/kg produces relaxation of 35 to 45 minutes duration. There are no adverse clinical effects on the heart; however, some histamine may be released with larger doses, so caution should be used in patients where an exaggerated response may be anticipated. Neuromuscular blockade is enhanced with the use of inhalation anesthetic agents as with other nondepolarizing relaxants. Maintenance doses of 0.08 to 0.10 mg/kg are recommended for prolonged surgical procedures. It should be remembered that because the rate of degradation of tracurium is dependent on temperature (Hoffman elimination) and pH, significant reductions in body temperature will affect the half-life. Flynn et al, found that a reduction in temperature of 37C to 23C increased the half-life at least two-fold (Flynn, 1983).

The depth of anesthesia and degree of muscle relaxation

TABLE 28–7. COMPARISON OF MUSCLE RELAXANTS

	Effect on Pulse Rate	Effect on Blood Pressure	Histamine Release	Broncho-constriction	Sympathetic Ganglion Blockade	Metabolism and Elimination	Usual Mode of Administration	Type of Neuromuscular Blocking Drug	Time to Maximum Effect	Duration of Action (to 90% Return of Twitch Known)	Reversal with Edrophonium, Pyridostigmine, or Neostigmine	Recommended Dose
Vecuronium bromide	No clinically significant change	No clinically significant change	None reported	None reported	None	Minimal reliance on kidney; bile main route of excretion	Intravenous	Nondepolarizing neuromuscular blocking agent	3–5 min	45–65 min	Yes	0.04–0.1 mg/kg
Pancuronium bromide	Slight rise or no change	None or slight rise on surgical stimulation	Minimal	Some reported cases	None	Metabolites and unchanged pancuronium mainly excreted in the urine and to a lesser extent in the bile	Intravenous	Nondepolarizing neuromuscular blocking agent	3–5 min	45+ min	Yes	0.04–0.1 mg/kg
Gallamine	Tachycardia, which may last after end of relaxation	None or slight rise	Minimal	None	None	100% unchanged in kidney	Intraveous	Nondepolarizing neuromuscular blocking agent	2.5–3 min	45+ min	Yes	1 mg/kg
d-Tubocurarine (d-TC)	None	Moderate incidence of hypotension	Considerable	Occasionally seen	Present and contributes to hypotension	Redistributed, taken up by liver; 33% in urine	Intravenous	Nondepolarizing neuromuscular blocking agent	3–5 min	60+ min	Yes	0.3–0.6 mg/kg
Succinylcholine chloride	Bradycardia in some patients; cardiac arrhythmias and asystole	Variable effects may cause hypertension	Minimal	Some reported cases	None	Broken down rapidly by pseudocholinesterase; liver may also play a role	Intravenous intramuscular	Depolarizer	1.25–1.5 min	5–8 min	No–not under usual circumstances	0.75–1.5 mg/kg
Atracurium	Minimal change	Minimal change	30% incidence at dose of 0.5 mg/kg; 50% incidence at 0.6 mg/kg; 20% decrease in blood pressure and 8% increase in pulse rate	Some reported cases	None	Hofmann elimination and ester hydrolysis	Intravenous	Nondepolarizing neuromuscular blocking agent	3–5 min	60–70 min	Yes	0.3–0.5 mg/kg

Courtesy of Organon Pharmaceuticals.

can be tested by urinary catheter insertion. If no change in hemodynamics occurs with insertion, the patient is ready for intubation. The patient is preoxygenated during the entire preparatory period of a bolus of lidocaine 1 to 1.5 mg/kg is injected prior to endoscopy. The use of laryngeal tracheal anesthesia spray is optional.

The competent anesthetist will have adjunctive drugs on hand such as nitroglycerine, nitroprusside, or propranolol to counteract any hypertension or tachycardia associated with endotracheal intubation.

Maintenance of Anesthesia. When significant myocardial depression is a desired response, as in the case of patients who have normal ventricular function, the inhalation anesthetics are the drugs of choice. All inhalation anesthetics in significant concentrations depress myocardial function. Potent inhalation anesthetics will suppress reflex response to noxious stimulation, provide muscle relaxation, and allow for early extubation.

Inhalation Agents. Eger (1983) suggests that enflurane and halothane produce a dose-related depression of contractility, whereas isoflurane and nitrous oxide do not. When selecting an inhalation agent, or any agent, for that matter, the reader should remember that the young surgical patient usually responds to stress by increasing heart rate, whereas the elderly one usually responds by elevating arterial pressure.

HALOTHANE. Halothane is a haloalkane that produces significant myocardial depression. In a study performed by Hilfiker et al, halothane-nitrous oxide anesthesia was associated with a significant decline in oxygen consumption of the left ventricle, together with a corresponding decrease in coronary blood flow, both of which decreased the hemodynamic load on the myocardium and decreased contractility (Hilfiker et al, 1983). Even though coronary perfusion was decreased, myocardial lactate (index of myocardial ischemia) was not measurable. Halothane seems to prevent disturbances in myocardial oxygen balance mainly by attenuating or preventing tachycardia, hypertension, and sympathetic hyperactivity caused by noxious stimuli during anesthesia and surgery (Hilfiker et al, 1983). It has been suggested that data concerning the effects of halothane on the ischemic myocardium are inconsistent, and controversy exists as to whether anesthesia with myocardial depressants is beneficial for the ischemic heart (Merin, 1980).

ENFLURANE. Enflurane is a haloether that dilates both resistance vessels and coronary vessels and in this sense is more potent than halothane. Enflurane will decrease mean arterial pressure and reflexly increase heart rate to maintain cardiac output. Left ventricular filling pressure decreases because of a reduction in afterload. Enflurane also reduces coronary perfusion pressure. There is a critically low perfusion pressure at which coronary autoregulation is lost. In patients with normal coronary arteries, this occurs at a mean aortic pressure of approximately 60 mm Hg. In patients with coronary atherosclerosis, autoregulation may be lost at a higher perfusion pressure because of the pressure fall over a stenosis (Reiz, 1983). Delaney et al compared the myocardial

function of halothane and enflurane and concluded that both agents decrease arterial pressure, but by different mechanisms. Halothane decreases cardiac output and SVR whereas enflurane decreases only SVR. (Delaney et al, 1980). Halothane increases both PCWP and central venous pressure (CVP), but enflurane does not, suggesting greater myocardial depression with halothane. Halothane decreases the contractile state, heart rate, and afterload and so presumably decreases MV_{O_2}, while slightly increasing preload; on the other hand, enflurane reduces afterload only (Delaney et al, 1980).

ISOFLURANE. Isoflurane also is a haloether. Ethers generally increase stability of cardiac rhythm. It has been reported that cardiac output is sustained with isoflurane by an increase in heart rate, which compensates for a reduction in SV. This increase in heart rate is probably due to beta-adrenergic stimulation. Cardiac responses that occur with isoflurane represent an imbalance between autonomic sympathetic and parasympathetic influences on the heart (Balasoraswathi et al, 1982). Isoflurane causes depression of both preganglionic sympathetic and vagal nerve activity, with a greater effect on the vagus (Balasoraswathi et al, 1982). There is a marked decrease in PVR, with only a slight decline in mean arterial pressure. The sympathoadrenal responses associated with isoflurane are elevated plasma epinephrine levels in conjunction with increased heart rate and decreased plasma norepinephrine levels, with decreased SVR. The efficiency of the heart (the rate of MV_{O_2} to external work) appears to be greater with enflurane and halothane than with isoflurane (Eger, 1983). Because halothane decreases arterial pressure by reducing cardiac output without a decrease in PCWP, and isoflurane reduces arterial pressure by decreasing SVR, some authors feel that isoflurane is superior to halothane in controlling intraoperative hypertension.

NITROUS OXIDE. Nitrous oxide (N_2O) can be used as a supplement to both inhalant and narcotic anesthetics. Generally, the depressant effects of nitrous oxide are mild. However, in the patient with poor cardiac performance, the degree of myocardial depression and hypotension can be severe. The use of nitrous oxide also carries the risk of expanding air spaces. If cardiac chambers or saphenous grafts are not devoid of air, these spaces can expand with the use of nitrous oxide. Nitrous oxide potentiates truncal rigidity induced by narcotic analgesics and limits the inspired oxygen concentration to the extent of its own concentration in the inspired gas mixture (Miller, 1981).

Inhalation anesthetics do have disadvantages, the most severe of which is postoperative shivering, with a concurrent increase in oxygen demand, caused by heat loss from vasodilation. In addition, they provide very little analgesia in the postanesthesia period. A summary of the hemodynamic effects of inhalation agents can be seen in Table 28–8.

Intravenous Agents. The patient with poor ventricular function is unable to tolerate minimal myocardial depression. Anesthetic techniques based on the opiates as primary agents produce minimal cardiac depression and thus remain

TABLE 28–8. HEMODYNAMIC EFFECTS OF INHALATION AGENTS (NOTE MAC DIFFERENCES)

	Preload	Afterload	Contractility	CO	O₂ Consumption	MAP	HR	SVR	PCWP	CVP
Halothane (1.25 MAC)	↓	↓	↓	↓	↓	↓	↓	↓	↓	↑
Enflurane (1 MAC)	—	↓	↓	+ ↓	↓	↓	↑ −	↓	—	↑
Isoflurane (2 MAC)	—	↓	↓	↓	↓	↓	↑	↓	—	—
Nitrous oxide (50%)	↑ −	↑	↓	↓	↓	—	− ↓	↑	↑	− ↑

CO = Cardiac output; CVP = Central venous pressure; HR = Heart rate; MAC = Minimal alveolar concentration; MAP = Mean arterial pressure; PCWP = Pulmonary capillary wedge pressure; SVR = Systemic vascular resistance.

popular for those patients with reduced myocardial function. The first narcotic to be used for these procedures was morphine sulfate. One major disadvantage to its use is histamine release, which produces some change in hemodynamic status. Morphine, although still in use, has given way in popularity to fentanyl, which is ten times more potent and produces less histamine release.

FENTANYL. Fentanyl was introduced in 1968 as the first synthetic morphinomimetic. At equianalgesic doses, side effects are minimal because fewer fentanyl molecules are available to reach sites other than intended opiate receptors. Protection against stress, more rapid recovery, and a shorter duration of respiratory depression are the major advantages of fentanyl. Fentanyl is highly lipophilic, rapidly penetrating cell membranes. Peak brain levels occur in minutes. With intravenous administration, the initial concentration of fentanyl in plasma is directly proportional to dose. The highest concentration is produced immediately but declines rapidly because of tissue uptake and biotransformation. Even though the plasma concentrations fall rapidly after a single injection, tissue concentration remains high. Because the tissues already contain some fentanyl, they will take up a smaller proportion of subsequent doses during the distribution phase. Hence, plasma levels will decline less during the distribution phase, and they will remain above the threshold concentration for progressively longer times after each dose because of their slow decline during the elimination phase. Therefore, repeated intravenous bolus doses of the same size should produce progressively more intense and prolonged effects (Hug, 1981).

When attenuation of the response to surgical stress is desired, doses of 50 to 100 μg/kg (0.05 to 0.1 mg/kg or 1 to 2 ml/kg) intravenous drip is administered with oxygen and a muscle relaxant until surgical planes are reached. The advantage of this technique is protection of the myocardium from excess oxygen demand. Some authors do report an increase in arterial pressure and SVR during stimulation, thus increasing the potential of myocardial ischemia. In doses of such magnitude, truncal rigidity can occur, and it is best to anticipate this side effect. Pretreatment with a nondepolarizing relaxant helps to curtail this effect. There have been several reports documenting such large doses. It may be necessary to supplement with nitrous oxide or an inhalant at this time, not only to decrease the stress response, but also to obliterate intraoperative awareness.

Fentanyl will decrease cardiac output and mean arterial pressure. There is no change in SVR. Fentanyl does not control hormonal releases while on pump. Elevated cortisol, antidiuretic hormone, and catechol levels have been reported.

SUFENTANIL. Sufentanil citrate, a new synthetic opioid analgesic, is five to ten times as potent as fentanyl but has the same duration of action and a much greater margin of safety. Sufentanil has an immediate onset of action, with limited accumulation. There is rapid elimination from tissue storage, which allows for a more rapid recovery compared with fentanyl. Sufentanil decreases cortisol and antidiuretic hormone levels but produces the same effect on catechol as fentanyl. Dosage for coronary artery bypass procedures is 20 to 25 μg/kg. Recovery is from 3 to 6 hours.

de Lange et al compared the effects of fentanyl to sufentanil for coronary artery surgery. Their study concluded that sufentanil had properties similar to fentanyl but, in addition, appeared more effective in preventing intraoperative hypertension and tachycardia, reducing MVo₂, and producing less postoperative depression, indicating that sufentanil provides greater protection against the stress response (de Lange et al, 1981). Sufentanil will increase the incidence of chest rigidity and this effect is proportional to speed of administration. The reoccurrence of narcotics in the circulation during the recovery period has been reported. Causes of reoccurrence include elevated central nervous system activity or elevated plasma concentrations from intestinal reabsorption or shift from muscle to circulation.

ALFENTANIL. Afentanil is a new, short-acting narcotic that is structurally related to fentanyl but with only one-third its potency and duration. The use of alfentanil during coronary artery surgery has been studied. Episodes of intraoperative hypertension, primarily during sternotomy or sternal spread were common, probably due to the extremely short duration of action of alfentanil, suggesting that a continuous drip and/or supplementation with other agents may be necessary to eliminate this hazard. Figure 28–11 compares the chemical structure of fentanyl, sufentanil, and alfentanil. Lofentanil is also an analgesic analog of fentanyl. It is 50 times more potent and has a long duration of action. It possesses strong respiratory depressant properties and for this reason is desirable when prolonged respiratory support

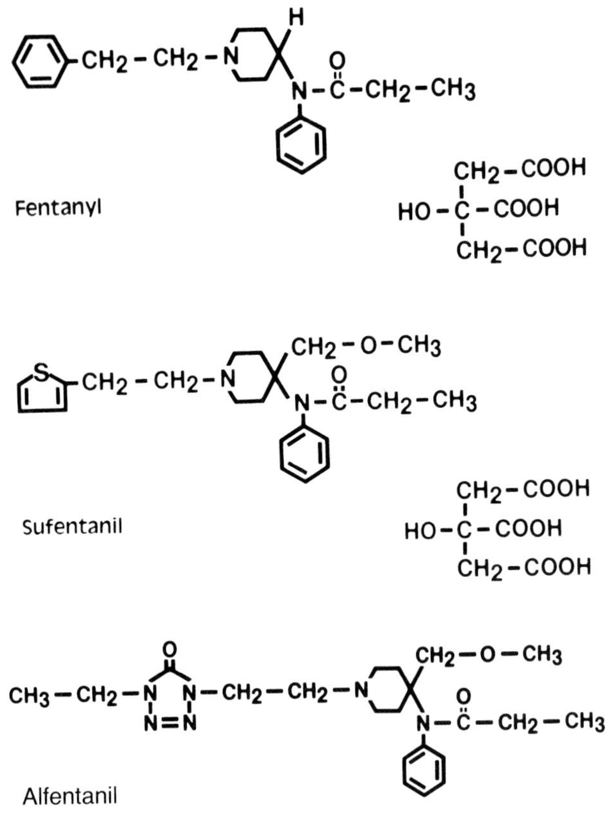

Figure 28–11. A comparison of the chemical structures of fentanyl, sufentanil, and alfentanil.

is indicated. Use in coronary artery surgery has not been thoroughly studied.

The role of chronic propranolol therapy on cardiovascular dynamics and narcotic requirements has been studied. The findings suggest that patients on preoperative beta blocking agents require less narcotic and supplements than those who are not. Also, these patients appeared to exhibit a lower incidence of hypertension and tachycardia than those not receiving beta-blocking drugs (Stanley, 1982).

Surgical Intervention

The impact of coronary artery bypass surgery on the survival of patients with CAD has been a subject of debate since its inception. The setting in which bypass grafting is performed certainly influences the statistical analysis of this debate. Successful intraoperative management—reflected in low rates of mortality, perioperative infarction, and other postoperative complications—and short hospital convalescence will depend not only on surgical skill and judgment, but also on the availability of competent anesthesia personnel, efficient extracorporeal support, the best possible myocardial preservation techniques, and a minimal period of myocardial ischemia consistent with optimal revascularization (Orkin and Cooperman, 1983).

The consensus is that in those patients with angina pectoris and a 50 percent narrowing of the left main coronary artery, bypass surgery results in better survival than medical treatment. In patients with chronic angina pectoris who

undergo bypass surgery, 60 to 70 percent will obtain complete anginal relief and 80 to 90 percent will note symptomatic improvement in the early postoperative period (Smith et al, 1983).

Larrieu published statistics on the current status of coronary bypass surgery (Larrieu, 1981). His results show that patients with left main coronary artery stenosis who had surgical intervention had survival rates of 86 to 88 percent at three years postoperatively, those with triple vessel disease had quite similar statistics, and those with double vessel ranged from 69 to 96 percent.

There exist no supportive data reflecting increased survival rates in patients surgically treated for single vessel disease, unless severe left main lesions are present. Medical treatment allowed for a 90 percent survival rate.

Extracorporeal Circulation and Cardiopulmonary Bypass

The ultimate objective of extracorporeal circulation in open heart surgery is to provide essentially normal organ perfusion while the surgeon has optimal conditions for cardiac procedures of indefinite duration (Pierce, 1969). The concept of extracorporeal circulation is more than 150 years old, but it was not until 1951 that it was used with open heart surgery.

Extracorporeal circulation involves the diversion of venous blood through an external device that returns the blood to the arterial side of the circulation. In its most advanced form, the device consists of a pump to provide the motive force, an oxygenator to add oxygen and remove carbon dioxide, a heat exchanger to promote hypothermia or normothermia, filters to trap bubbles and debris, and pressure transducers to monitor its function (Orkin et al, 1983). Basically, extracorporeal bypass reroutes all the blood returning to the right atrium away from the heart and lungs.

For total cardiopulmonary bypass, i.e., when the lungs are completely bypassed, the entire systemic venous return to the heart must be collected and delivered to an oxygenator via gravity drainage. After heparinization, a 32 and 36 French cannula or two 51 French single cannulas, depending on surgeon preference, are used to cannulate both the superior and inferior venae cavae. Cannulation of the superior vena cava is performed using the right atrial appendage as access. The apex of the appendage is excised and the cannula introduced into the right atrium and directed into the superior vena cava approximately 2 to 3 cm. A similar procedure is used for the inferior vena cava. Once both cannulas are secured, they are connected to a ½-inch Y connector and then to a ½-inch venous tubing leading to the oxygenator. These cannulas are clamped during insertion of the aortic cannula.

Cannulation of the ascending aorta (antegrade flow) is the most common technique for patients undergoing total cardiopulmonary bypass. However, if previous surgery was performed, or if there are anatomic problems with the aorta, the femoral artery can then be cannulated (retrograde flow). If this method is used, perfusion to that extremity is minimal and complications secondary to decreased perfusion and retrograde flow can occur. The most common problem with femoral artery cannulation is dissection of the artery. When cannulating the ascending aorta for cardiopulmonary bypass, a vascular clamp first is applied longitudinally to the ascending aorta and an aortotomy is performed; the cannula is then inserted and secured. Air is evacuated from the cannula and from the arterial line leading to the pump. The clamps on the venous lines are released and blood flows by gravity to the oxygenator, which is a minimum of 30 cm below the level of the heart. After equilibrium between drainage and inflow is achieved, snares are applied to occlude blood flow to the lungs, and total bypass begins. The use of a sump suction to further empty the heart is optional. The time bypass began, mean pressure, CVP, temperature, arterial and venous gases, and activated clotting times should be recorded.

Equipment. The pump component of the extracorporeal circuit should provide the equivalent of a basal cardiac output. Early on, these were designed to provide a pulsatile flow imitating physiologic flow through the circulatory system. However, the size of the cannulas and connectors altered this flow and as a result, the pulsing was ineffective. Consequently, pulsatile flow, although considered essential for long-term isolated organ perfusion, has not been thought to be essential for routine cardiopulmonary bypass (Dunn and Kirsch, 1974). To date, the use of a continuous-flow nonpulsatile pump is common. The roller head pumps are driven in a circular motion, milking the blood-filled pump tubing. This tubing is securely attached so that there is no net movement of the tubing. It is this compression of the tubing that drives the blood forward. These rollers may also be used to aspirate blood from the surgical field. Three to four pumps are necessary: one for arterial inflow, one to vent or empty the heart, and one to two to maintain a dry surgical field. Venous blood is drained by gravity. Figure 28–12 illustrates the pump roller head system and the entire cardiopulmonary bypass circuit.

The integrity of the red cell is usually well maintained with the roller pump because of the low-pressure nonturbulent flow. Red cell damage can be attributed to the negative

pressure provided by the pump suction. Thus, the amount of hemolysis will depend on the amount and duration of suction used. Tissue lysosomes and blood left in the pericardial cavity for prolonged periods also contribute to cell damage (Kaplan, 1979).

The oxygenator not only supplies oxygen, as the name implies, but also eliminates carbon dioxide. Two main types of oxygenators are in existence today. The first is the bubble oxygenator, which provides a gas interface; the other is the membrane oxygenator, which lacks a gas interface. It should be mentioned that the membrane is somewhat more sophisticated and more physiologic because it causes less damage to red blood cells. Its main disadvantage is that it is not economical.

In the bubble oxygenator, ventilating gases, oxygen and carbon dioxide, are passed through multiple perforations in a diffusing plate, giving rise to bubbles that exit into the venous blood at the bottom of what is usually a columnar reservoir (Hammond and Barley, 1974). This produces turbulence, which drives the blood into a "debubbling section." The perforations in the diffusing plate and the bubble size are controlled so that bubbles are just the right size for appropriate gas transfer.

Oxygenation in the bubbler is not membrane limited as in the normal lung or membrane oxygenator but depends upon the gas-blood surface contact area, the thickness of the film, the mean red cell transit time, and the partial pressure of oxygen used (Dorsen et al, 1971). The gas-blood interface surface contact area is usually in the range of 15 m^2 (Bartlett et al, 1959). Large bubbles are used to provide a more efficient, thicker film. The red cells' mean transit time is usually of 1 to 2 seconds (normally 0.1 to 0.75 seconds). Thus, the flow of gas should equal the flow of blood to allow for carbon dioxide elimination and oxygen uptake.

The bubble oxygenator, by means of gravity, conducts venous blood to the bottom of the reservoir where a stream of bubbles passes over it. The bubbles produce turbulence and froth, which increases the gas-bubble contact, leading to increased gas exchange. An exhalation port at the debub-

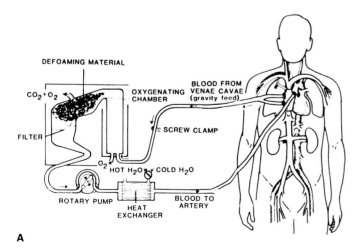

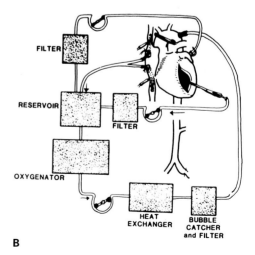

Figure 28–12 A. Blood is drained from the venae cavae by gravity. As it enters the oxygenator, a mixture of CO_2 and O_2 is implemented. The process of defoaming, debubbling, heating, or cooling then occurs. Propulsion is obtained by a rotary pump, and the blood is returned antegrade via the aorta. **B.** Blood loss is kept to a minimum by returning all blood to a filtered cardiotomy reservoir via a pericardial suction vent to assist in further drainage of the heart.

bling site allows for exhaust gases to escape—especially inhalation anesthetics. When gas exchange is complete, the blood descends into the heat exchange and finally into the arterial system.

Oxygenators are ventilated with 100 percent oxygen, but controversy exists over the detrimental effects of such high oxygen tensions, suggesting that physiologic oxygen tensions are less traumatic with regard to enzyme systems and the degree of hemolysis.

In the membrane oxygenators, instead of the blood-gas interface, blood passes between layers of membrane with the gas phase on the other side. The membrane oxygenator is popular because of its increased efficiency. There are two types, hollow fiber and the micro porous (thin Teflon or polypropylene sheets). Gas exchange through a membrane device is limited by characteristics of the membrane and the degree of mixing of blood on either side (Bartlett et al, 1971). The silicone membranes have carbon dioxide:oxygen transfer capacities of 5:1 to 6:1 rather than lower ratios and thus more closely resemble the lung (Kaplan, 1979). There is less risk of disruption of red blood cell integrity; however, once again this is influenced by the rigorous nature of the sump suction and by pericardial suctioning.

Volatile anesthetic agents can be added to the oxygenators by incorporating a flow- and temperature-compensated vaporizer into the gas line. It should be kept in mind that hemodilution, hyperthermia, and low flows all alter the expected response, and concentrations must be adjusted accordingly.

The tubing used in the circuit should have the following characteristics. It should be clear, chemically inert, pliable, and accommodate small priming volumes. In addition, it should be thrombus-resistant. In essence, the tubes must withstand prolonged assault by the roller pump and also provide optimal physiologic conditions, such as minimal overhydration from priming solutions and safety from thrombi formation.

The filter, placed on the arterial side, is designed to trap the smallest of particles. This may include red blood cells, platelets, and leukocytes, fat, silicone, air, and any other debris. The introduction of filters has contributed to the reduction of organ dysfunction.

The heat exchanger is a system where blood and water (housed in a stainless steel or aluminum container) flow in opposite directions. The cooling and warming is provided by a hot and cold water system that will change the temperature of the blood as it passes over it. The pump flow rates vary somewhat from team to team, with an average rate of about 2,400 ml/m^2/min. This is roughly 50 to 70 ml/kg/min. Although the tissue oxygen need may be considered the most basic requirement, it is calculated in terms of blood flow. Basal cardiac output is approximately 3,000 ml/m^2 of body surface/min. This provides for a full oxygen uptake at an average arteriovenous oxygen difference of about 4.4 volumes percent (Pierce, 1969). If blood flow is low, blood flow redistribution with resultant ischemia to some organs may occur. This increase in oxygen extraction interferes with normal oxygen consumption, and metabolic acidosis can occur. Therefore, the adequacy of extracorporeal flow should be determined by monitoring blood gases and acid-base balance.

Priming. Solutions used to prime the heart-lung machine vary with the institution. Some use a dextrose-and-water solution, others a balanced electrolyte solution with a plasma expander, such as dextran (or, more recently, hetastarch), and an osmotic diuretic like mannitol. Hetastarch is an artificial colloid derived from amylopectin with colloidal properties similar to albumin.

An all-blood priming solution is used by a few institutions. The total amount of solution ranges between 1,500 to 2,400 ml and should be as close to extracellular fluid composition as possible so as not to increase the patient's metabolic requirement. It is believed that the priming solutions that provide hemodilution are most physiologic.

The trend today is to add blood only if the patient is severely anemic, having the circuit maintain only a 30 to 40 percent blood volume of the patient. The hematocrit levels should not be below 20 to 25 percent because lower values result in severe hypotension caused by changes in blood viscosity. A reduction in oxygen-carrying capacity accompanies hematocrit reduction; however, this is compensated for by the use of hypothermia during bypass.

Hemodilution does not proceed without some ill effects. Oncotic pressure changes, caused by alterations in serum protein, can expand the extracellular fluid compartment. This is in accordance with Starling's hypothesis that fluid balance (absence of flow in either direction) is achieved when osmotic and hydrostatic forces at the compartment membrane are equal. If these are not equal, fluid moves in the direction of the superior force. Changes in electrolyte values can occur. Low serum potassium levels are a common occurrence, partly because of inappropriate aldosterone response, partly because of the use of diuretics, and partly because of hyperventilation. Serum potassium levels should be monitored frequently during cardiopulmonary bypass. A reduction in calcium, magnesium, phosphate, and zinc can accompany hemodilution.

Changes in calcium levels may be significant in altering mean arterial pressure, and calcium administration may be necessary to overcome hypotension, particularly at the outset of perfusion.

Anticoagulation. Heparin should always be administered through a well-functioning central line. Heparin works by producing a thrombin-antithrombin complex, which in the presence of the cofactor will deactivate thrombin. Heparin is protein-bound and thus is readily distributed in the plasma volume. Its effects vary from individual to individual both in onset and in half-life. Factors that affect the pharmacologic action of heparin are age, body temperature, and lean body mass.

The method of calculation of heparin dosage is still a matter of controversy. Some institutions use a fixed-dose technique, i.e., 3 to 4 mg/kg or 90 mg/m^2, while others use a dose-response method based on the activated clotting time (ACT). Calculation by dose-response method appears to be more accurate and is used by the majority of institutions today. This method allows for individualized heparin and protamine dosage calculations. A baseline ACT is drawn prior to heparin administration and immediately after administration and every 15 to 30 minutes thereafter. The procedure for constructing and using the dose-response curve is illustrated in Figure 28–13. As depicted, the heparin

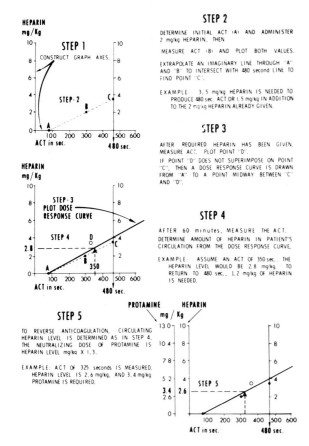

Figure 28–13. Dose-response curve for heparin and protamine dosage calculations. ACT = activated clotting time. (*From Bull B, Hyse WM, et al: J Thorac Cardiovasc Surg 69:686, 1975.*)

essary. Protamine injection should be slow to avoid a hypotensive episode. This decline in arterial pressure may be associated with the release of vasoactive drugs, such as histamine and serotonin. Severe anaphylactic reactions have been documented with protamine administration.

On Bypass. Once the circuit has been primed, the patient appropriately heparinized, and surgical access attained, bypass commences. The anesthetist immediately notes and records ACT levels, mean arterial pressure, heart rate, urinary output, and CVP. The depth of anesthesia, degree of muscle relaxation, and pupil size should also be evaluated.

The perfusionist and anesthetist must work very closely to maintain desired hemodynamics. If drug administration is necessary, it is done via the pump. Drugs would most likely be additional heparin, anesthetic, vasopressor, or a vasodilator. Mean arterial pressure is usually maintained between 60 to 80 torr. Increases or decreases can be altered by changes in flow or altering total peripheral resistance, since mean pressure equals cardiac output times total peripheral resistance.

Pump flow is maintained at 2 to 2.5 L/min/m^2 of body surface area (BSA) but can be varied according to blood gases or temperature. The CVP should be very low or at zero when on bypass. The CVP catheter should be placed in the superior vena cava above the venous return line so that obstructed venous return from the head can be determined (Pierce, 1969), because persistent elevated venous pressure can lead to cerebral edema. PCWP, pulmonary artery and left atrial pressure also should be at zero. Elevations suggest left ventricle distention. If the pulmonary artery pressure rises above 15 mm Hg while on bypass, there is cause for concern. Appropriate measures must be taken to decompress distended ventricles.

The urinary output while on bypass should be maintained above 1 ml/kg/hr. Careful observation should be made for hemolysis of red blood cells. If this is noted, the urinary output should be maintained at a higher level with diuretics or by alkalinization with tromethamine (THAM) or bicarbonate. However, with the new hybrid oxygenators in use today, hemolysis is seldom seen.

Several blood studies are performed routinely during cardiopulmonary bypass, usually at 15-minute intervals. These include arterial blood gases, hematocrit, venous oxygen, electrolytes, blood sugar in diabetics, and ACT. The hematocrit is maintained between 20 and 30 percent. Arterial gases should be at normal range while on bypass. Venous Po$_2$, obtained from the oxygenator, ranges from 40 to 45 torr. Causes of abnormal values were discussed above. Electrolyte values can change abruptly because of hemodilution and the use of cardioplegic solutions that are hyperkalemic. Any alterations in electrolytes should be remedied.

Revascularization of coronary arteries requires a quiet, dry operative field. Many methods can be used to stop heart motion. A normal contracting myocardium can be slowed or fibrillated by core and topical cooling. If spontaneous fibrillation does not occur, this can be achieved by electric current, but is best avoided because of increased oxygen consumption and possible muscle destruction.

The most commonly used method of obtaining circulatory arrest to the heart is by aortic cross-clamping. This

dose in mg/kg is on the vertical axis and the ACT in seconds on the horizontal axis. Three graphs are plotted—the pre-heparin ACT, the ACT immediately postheparin, and the ACT prior to protamine administration. By plotting the curves, dosages can be determined, eliminating excessive anticoagulation or heparin reversal (Bull et al, 1975). The ACT drawn every 15 to 30 minutes should have a value above 480. If not, additional heparin should be given. It should be remembered that the ACT is temperature- and heparin-dependent, so during the hypothermic period and with hemodilution the ACT may increase unreliably. Tinker (1983) recommends against using the ACT as a criterion for heparin administration during hypothermia. However, if the bypass procedure does not exceed two or three hours, additional heparin should not be necessary. The rapid infusion of crystalloid with resultant hemodilution can significantly lengthen ACT. The effect is usually transient, lasting only the first 30 minutes of bypass (Bull et al, 1975).

The dosage for heparin reversal with protamine sulfate is also determined by the ACT. Because of its hypotensive tendency, protamine should be given slowly, over a 30-minute period, and not before stability of vital signs is ensured. The current practice of protamine administration is to administer smaller doses over a longer period of time. It is suggested that this dose should be less than the first heparin dose. Successive doses may be administered if nec-

procedure produces a static heart with no flow through its arteries. The disadvantage of aortic cross-clamping is anoxia to the myocardium. The time frame for anoxia can be reduced under hypothermic conditions produced by core and surface cooling. Oschner and Mills (1978) state seven minutes of core cooling, achieved by progressively lowering the perfusate temperature in increments of one, two, and three minutes and concomitant surface cooling with a cold isotonic solution at 7C probably allows more than 40 minutes of myocardial protection.

Hypothermia. Adequate myocardial preservation remains the key determinant of successful cardiac procedures. Although myocardial ischemia can occur at any time intraoperatively, the most common cause is inadequate preservation during cardiopulmonary bypass. One of the key elements in maintaining myocardial protection is maintaining myocardial temperature below 15C during ischemic arrest. This is accomplished by systemic hypothermia plus the direct application of cold cardioplegia.

The heart is relatively more active metabolically at any given temperature level than other major organs, including the brain. The working myocardial cell maintains a tight coupling between energy production and energy utilization; thus adenosine triphosphate (ATP) is produced relative to need, while oxygen and substrate are consumed in the precise amounts needed to resynthesize ATP. In the normal myocardial cell, the three main reactions utilizing ATP are: (1) myosin ATPase involvement in the development of wall tension, (2) calcium and magnesium ATPase involvement in the sequestration of calcium that enters the cell with each beat and as the calcium that is liberated from the sarcoplasmic reticulum in the activation of contractile protein, and (3) sodium plus potassium ATPase involvement in sodium efflux (Engeilman and Levitsky, 1981).

Approximately 50 to 60 moles of ATP are produced per minute per gram of heart during these three reactions; the value increases ten-fold during moderate cardiac effort (Engeilman and Levitsky, 1981). It is estimated that 60 percent of the ATP utilization is markedly decreased. A reduced flux of adenosine diphosphate (ADP) in the mitochondria is associated with reduced flux of citric acid cycle intermediates, high citrate levels (which inhibit glycolysis), high levels of nicotinamide adenine dinucleotide (NADH) (as electron transport is slowed), and acetyl-CoA levels are elevated, resulting in a limiting effect on fatty acid beta oxidation.

During cardioplegia, glucose utilization and pyruvate dehydrogenase activity are decreased, so metabolite formation is inhibited.

By provision of systemic hypothermia, oxygen consumption and thus metabolic requirements are decreased. It has been estimated that oxygen consumption is decreased by 25 percent at 25C. Profound hypothermia is provided by perfusing cold blood, followed by the infusion of a cold cardioplegic solution and then topical cooling. Perfusion cooling is performed rapidly, dropping the temperature to 22 or 25C. Once the heart fibrillates, the aorta is cross-clamped and cardioplegic infusion into the aortic root is begun at 4C and a volume of 10 ml/kg. In addition, the heart is bathed in a cold solution at 4C.

Although these methods are very successful in reducing myocardial consumption, they are not without side effects. Hypothermia causes several physiologic manifestations. There is a reduction in cerebral blood flow that is directly proportional to the decrease in temperature—6.7 percent for each degree Celsius (Orkin and Cooperman, 1983). Nerve impulse conduction and neuromuscular transmission is reduced, thus affecting the dosages of muscle relaxant. (Nondepolarizing drug dosage should be decreased.) The oxyhemoglobin curve shifts to the left; thus the partial pressure of oxygen in tissues must fall before hemoglobin gives up oxygen. Systemic blood pressure decreases. Renal blood flow is decreased, with a concomitant decrease in urinary output. Splanchnic flow is impaired, resulting in decreased drug metabolism. Clotting factors are impaired, and hypothermia enhances the stability of blood and serum lipids, thus reducing the risk of hematologic disruption after bypass.

Chemical cardioplegia protects the myocardium against inadequate cooling. The cardioplegic solution must be at 2 to 4C to be effective. The composition of chemical cardioplegic solutions varies somewhat, but most often the agent responsible for cardioplegia is potassium chloride in concentrations of 12 to 30 mEq/L. Table 28–9 lists several examples of various solutions in use.

The use of cardioplegic solutions is based on the following principles:

1. Rapid asystole to prevent breakdown of high-energy phosphate groups;
2. hypothermia to lower energy demands without inducing cold injury;
3. membrane stabilization to prevent breakdown of sodium potassium, and calcium membrane pumps;

TABLE 28–9. VARIOUS CARDIOPLEGIC SOLUTIONS IN USE

Solutions		Components		Quantities	
Sodium	120.0 mEq	Lactated Ringer's	1000 cc	Lactated Ringer's	1000 cc
Potassium chloride	16.0 mEq	Potassium chloride	20 mEq	Potassium chloride	25.0 mEq
Magnesium	32.0 mEq	Procainamide	1 g	Sodium chloride	152.0 mEq
Calcium	2.4 mEq	Dextrose 50%	30 cc	Magnesium sulfate	20.0 mEq
Chloride	160.0 mEq	Regular insulin	20 U	Calcium chloride	4.5 mEq
Sodium bicarbonate	10.0 mEq			Dextrose	2.0 g
				Sodium bicarbonate	25.0 mEq

4. hyperosmolarity to prevent intracellular edema; and
5. acid buffering to counteract intracellular acidosis from anerobic metabolism (Engeilman and Levitsky, 1981).

Rapid asystole is produced by potassium chloride. Potassium causes asystole during diastole by depolarizing the cell membrane. The amount of potassium required to produce asystole appears to be directly proportional to the myocardial temperature (Engeilman and Levitsky, 1981).

Hyperosmolarity (provided by glucose or mannitol) in the range of 350 to 400 mOsm appears to combat myocardial swelling associated with the sodium ion shifts secondary to ischemia during aortic cross-clamping (Engeilman and Levitsky, 1981).

Buffers such as tromethamine (THAM), bicarbonate, and histadine are necessary to overcome the effects of inhibited glycolysis, thus allowing some ATP formation, and to prevent decreased enzymatic activity caused by variant pH ranges.

Once myocardial temperature reaches 10 to 12C, asystole occurs within seconds. Myocardial temperature and ECG activity must be monitored so as to recognize increases in metabolic demands caused by an upward shift in temperature. These values are checked every 15 to 20 minutes and reinfusing of cardioplegic solution begun if necessary, usually at the completion of each distal anastomosis. Clinical studies indicate that despite the infusion of large volumes of hyperkalemic cardioplegic solution, serum potassium levels rarely exceed 5.5 mEq/L because increased urinary excretion of potassium rapidly compensates for the exogenous administration (Engeilman and Levitsky, 1981).

Some problems that may occur during chemical cardioplegia administration include: a solution that is not cold enough, insufficient delivery to the myocardium because of valvular disease or coronary artery stenosis, and heat gain from environmental influences. Some studies have also demonstrated nonhomogenous cooling, incomplete protection, and delayed reperfusion when significant coronary stenosis is present. It is wise to use a myocardial temperature probe to monitor temperature to be certain that the solution is achieving proper cooling.

There are some proponents of cold-blood cardioplegia who urge that this technique provides oxygenation and substrate delivery during aortic cross-clamping. Blood cardioplegia should be administered at 20C; otherwise red cell sludging and possible activation of cold agglutins can occur. (Patients should have a cold agglutin test preoperatively if blood cardioplegia is used.) Studies have determined that the myocardial preservation is equivalent to that provided by crystalloid solutions; however, patients with abnormal left ventricular function (ejection fraction below 40 percent) or prolonged aortic cross-clamp seem to have more favorable results with cold blood than crystalloid. It must be emphasized that the temperature must be 20C because lower temperatures interfere with oxygen delivery (Katz et al, 1981).

Revascularization. The approach to revascularization depends on coronary artery distribution, i.e., whether or not there is left dominance, right dominance, or a balanced

system. With right coronary dominance, circulation is provided to both right and left ventricles posteriorly and to the interventricular septum via a descending artery. With left dominance, the posterior left ventricle and interventricular septum are supplied by the circumflex. The right coronary is short. With a balanced system, one descending branch from each coronary provides the circulation. There is no limit to the number of bypass grafts that can be performed, but the most frequent is the triple bypass, i.e., to the right coronary, to the LAD, and to the obtuse marginal branch of the circumflex. This should supply enough blood flow to the left ventricle and interventricular septum.

The greater saphenous vein is preferred for supplying graft material and is prepared as the sternum is being opened. Once the site of anastomosis is determined and the graft cut to size, the distal end is sewn, followed then by the proximal end of each graft. Air should be evacuated from the grafts as the clamp on the aorta is released.

Once revascularization has been completed, the patient is rewarmed. Approximately five minutes before aortic clamp removal, the perfusion temperature is raised to 30C. After the clamp is removed, the temperature is raised to 38C and the room is warmed. Bypass continues until the esophageal temperature is 37C.

Removal of the aortic clamp allows oxygen, blood, and substrate to fill the myocardium. During aortocoronary bypass, myocardial ATP levels may be very high, but once the heart starts its own beat, the ATP levels fall rapidly, probably because of energy requirements for contraction.

There has been some evidence that mitochondrial distortion may occur after reperfusion to ischemic hearts.

Possible causes of this injury include: loss of magnesium and increase in mitochondrial calcium uptake, decrease in ATP levels critical to enzymatic performance, accumulation of long-chain fatty acid acyl-CoA esters, and loss of critical enzymes from the postischemic cell (Engeilman and Levitsky, 1981).

Usually, once the patient's temperature reaches 37C, the heart will resume its normal beat. If not, the patient is defibrillated. Pump flow is gradually reduced, while careful watch is made of arterial pressure, ECG, and heart size. The adequacy of volume replacement is usually determined by each of these parameters, plus left atrial pressure, central venous blood gases, acid-base status, and serum potassium levels. Because of the large volumes of cardioplegic solution, it may be necessary to give sodium bicarbonate or calcium chloride through the pump to resume myocardial function.

Withdrawal from cardiopulmonary bypass should be slow (approximately 15 to 20 minutes) and stability of vital signs sustained before cannulas are removed. Reinstitution of anesthetic agents and muscle relaxants may be necessary at this time. Depressant agents should be avoided as should nitrous oxide because of air embolism potentials.

As cardiovascular dynamics are restored, reversal of anticoagulation is instituted. The protamine dosage is calculated according to the dose-response curve described earlier. At this time, the sump tubing should be removed so as not to suction protamine into the remaining pump volume.

Postvascularization. Low output states may be present after revascularization procedures. Symptoms include low arterial pressure and cardiac output. Initial treatment should be a fluid challenge to determine if hypovolemia is the underlying cause. If cardiac output does not increase with adequate preload, one must assume that left ventricular failure is present, provided normal pH, $PaCO_2$ and cardiac rhythm exist.

The pharmacologic treatment of ventricular failure is two-fold: (1) reduce the workload of the heart, and (2) increase myocardial contractility (Naples, 1981).

There are relatively standard regimens of drug administration for the patient who does not wean from bypass easily. As previously noted, there are four major determinants of myocardial performance: preload, afterload, heart rate, and contractility or the inotropic state. Preload and inotropic properties determine myocardial contractile performance, whereas afterload and heart rate are mechanical factors that affect myocardial performance (Smith and Kampine, 1980).

Circulatory supportive measures should be directed at alterations in ventricular preload, ventricular afterload, or ventricular contractility.

When discussing preload, there are several terms that can be used interchangeably. Preload refers to the venous side of the circulatory system. It is synonomous with left ventricular volume. Other terms that correlate with preload are left ventricular end-diastolic pressure (LVEDP) and diastolic filling pressure.

When calculating preload, one is essentially measuring left atrial pressure or capillary wedge pressure. Normal value is 14 to 16 mm Hg. Preload is therefore determined by Swan-Ganz catheter or left atrial pressure.

Afterload, on the other hand, reflects the arterial side of the circulatory system and is synonomous with resistance—how much effort the ventricle must work against to obtain a functional cardiac output. Afterload, or systemic vascular resistance (SVR), is also calculated by means of Swan-Ganz catheter. In determining SVR, it must be remembered that the CVP is measured in cmH_2O, whereas all other values are in mm Hg. (To convert cmH_2O to mm Hg, multiply the CVP by 10 and then divide by 13.)

Referring to Starling's law, a maximally dilated ventricle will eject the entire volume that it holds, so whether the volume be 10 ml or 200 ml, it will be totally ejected, provided the heart can do so. The cardiac output, or left ventricular ejection volume, is altered by (1) a failing ventricle that lacks enough force to pump, (2) by aortic resistance that the ventricle must overcome (SVR), or by (3) volume depletion.

It is essential to know the underlying pathophysiology behind a decreased cardiac output before treatment is instituted so as not to complicate the problem.

A failing left ventricle, i.e., one with poor contractile properties, is best treated with an inotropic agent such as epinephrine, dobutamine, or isoproterenol. The inotrope should be selected on the basis of its pulmonary effects. Norepinephrine will dramatically increase pulmonary artery pressure and pulmonary vascular resistance, whereas isoproterenol or dobutamine reduce pulmonary artery pressure and pulmonary vascular resistance (Table 28–10) (Katz et al, 1981).

Aortic resistance, or afterload, is best decreased by the use of a vasodilator such as nitroglycerin (NTG) that will decrease SVR and concomitantly increase stroke volume (SV). Alterations of aortic pressure will affect cardiac function because of the resistance it places on the left ventricle during emptying. These aortic pressure changes will result in changes in strength and duration of the left ventricular ejection and SV.

If the cardiac output is low because of volume depletion (decreased preload), then volume expanders are used judiciously. If preload is increased, treatment with a vasodilator and/or a diuretic is also recommended.

Vasodilating Drugs. Vasodilators are able to improve cardiac performance because of their ability to dilate peripheral arteries and veins. Five factors that determine the hemodynamic and clinical response to vasodilator drugs have been identified: (1) the direct vascular effects of the drug; (2) the activation of endogenous neurohumoral mechanisms by peripheral vasodilation; (3) the response of the left ventricle to a decrease in venous return and peripheral resistance; (4) the regional distribution of the improved peripheral blood flow; and (5) the physiologic response during exercise (Packer and Legemtel, 1982).

At present, vasodilating drugs can be divided into two categories: (1) direct-acting agents, such as hydralazine, nitroprusside, nitrates; and (2) receptor-dependent agents, such as prazosin, captopril (Phillips, 1979). The mechanism of action of direct-acting agents is unclear in that they are mediated by vascular production of potent vasodilating prostaglandins, such as prostacyclin. Receptor-dependent vasodilators have specific, definite sites of action, i.e., either postsynaptic alpha-sympathetic blockade or inhibition of angiotensin-converting enzyme.

For the purposes of this chapter, discussion will center on the myocardial responses to this type of drug therapy. In patients with dilated left ventricles and markedly elevated left ventricular filling pressures, venodilation can reduce filling pressures without reducing SV, as long as pressures remain on the flat portion of the Frank-Starling curve; excessive decreases in venous return can, however, compromise critical levels of filling pressure and decrease output. Similarly, arterial vasodilation can reduce systolic impedance and wall stress and thereby permit more effective shortening during systole. There is a limit to the degree of increased systolic ejection, and once it reaches its limit, arterial pressures will decrease without an improvement in cardiac performance (Packer and Legemtel, 1982).

It is imperative to maintain critical levels of preload and avoid vasodilator therapy in patients with normal left ventricular filling pressures to avoid significant decreases in SV. The effect of vasodilator therapy on ventricular afterload is not so clear-cut. The pharmacologic significance of afterload reduction varies with the degree of wall stress. If there is a marked increase in wall stress, reduction in afterload will shorten systole, with a resultant improvement in hemodynamic status. In contrast, depressed left ventricular function associated with low wall stress is most likely due to severe myosystolic dysfunction, which is not afterload-dependent; in these instances, efforts to reduce wall stress are futile and may be dangerous (Packer and Legemtel, 1982).

TABLE 28–10. PULMONARY VASCULAR PHARMACOPEIA

Drug	PAP	PCWP	Pulmonary Blood Flow	SAP	HR	PVR
Alpha- and beta-agonists						
1. Norepinephrine 0.10–0.20 μg/kg/min	↑	↑ to ↑↑	—**	↑↑	↓	NC* to ↑
2. Methoxamine 5–10 mg	↑	↑	—	↑↑	↓↓	—
3. Phenylephrine 50–100 μg	↑↑	—	↓	↑↑	↓↓	↑↑
4. Epinephrine 0.05–0.20 μg/kg/min	↑	NC or ↓	↑	↑↑	↑	↑
5. Dopamine 2–10 μg/kg/min	NC	NC or ↓	↑	NC or ↑	↑	NC
6. Dobutamine 5–15 μg/kg/min	—	↓	↑↑	NC or ↑	↑	↓
7. Isoproterenol 0.015–0.15 μg/kg/min	SL ↓	↓	↑↑	↓	↑↑	↓
Beta-antagonist Propranolol 0.5–2 mg	—	NC to ↑	NC to ↓	NC to ↓	↓	NC to ↑
Alpha-antagonist Phentolamine 1–3 μg/kg/min	↓	↓	↑	↓	↑	↓
Smooth muscle dilators						
1. Aminophylline 500 mg	↓	↓	—	—	↑	↓
2. Sodium nitroprusside 0.5–3 μg/kg/min	↓	↓	↑↑	NC to ↓	↑	↓
3. Nitroglycerin 0.5–5 μg/kg/min	↓↓	↓↓	NC to ↑	↓	↑	↓

HR = heart rate; NC = no change; PAP = pulmonary artery pressure; PCWP = pulmonary capillary wedge pressure; PVR = peripheral vascular resistance; SAP = systolic arterial pressure; SL = slight.
From Katz J, Benumof J, et al: Anesthesia and Uncommon Disease, 2nd ed., 1981. Courtesy of Saunders.

It is obvious that vasodilator therapy is successful only after careful scrutiny of the patient's pathophysiologic condition. Treatment must be individualized and centered on each patient's specific cardiac performance. Kaplan's inotrope-vasodilator combinations are listed in Table 28–11.

Sodium Nitroprusside. Sodium nitroprusside is a potent hypotensive agent, which causes an immediate vascular dilation in both peripheral resistance and capacitance vessels. This decrease in total peripheral resistance and increase in venous pooling result in a significant drop in blood pres-

TABLE 28–11. INOTROPE-VASODILATOR COMBINATIONS (PHARMACOLOGIC BALLOON PUMP)

1. Epinephrine-nitroglycerin
2. Epinephrine-nitroprusside
3. Dopamine-nitroglycerin
4. Dobutamine-nitroprusside
5. Norepinephrine-phentolamine
6. Epinephrine-nitroprusside-nitroglycerin

From Kaplan JA: Cardiac Anesthesia, 1979. By permission of Grune & Stratton and the author.

sure. The sharp vasodilating effect of nitroprusside appears to derive from its relationship to the nitro group, which is a smooth-muscle relaxant (Phillips, 1979). It acts directly upon vascular musculature and is independent of the autonomic, central, and peripheral nervous systems (Phillips, 1979). There is a suggested increase in cardiac and stroke index, probably caused by decreased afterload. Hypotensive effects are usually followed by reflex tachycardia. There is a slight decline in cardiac output and no impairment of contractility or increase in oxygen consumption.

The hypotensive effects of nitroprusside are caused by peripheral vasodilation as a result of a direct action on the blood vessels. This effect is augmented by ganglionic blocking agents, volatile anesthetics, and by other circulatory depressants. Nitroprusside reduces collateral flow to ischemic areas by dilating small-resistance vessels and decreasing coronary perfusion pressures, resulting in a coronary steal. The blood to the underperfused zone, which is already maximally dilated because of ischemia, is shunted to adjacent nonischemic zones, which are vasodilated by nitroprusside (Kaplan, 1983).

Nitroprusside is available in 50 mg ampules and is mixed in 250 or 500 cc of D_5W. Rate of administration will vary according to the patient's response. Dosage usually ranges from 0.5 to 10 μg/kg/minute. Usually at 3 μg/kg blood pressure can be lowered by 30 to 40 percent.

Aside from profound hypotension, the other serious side effect of nitroprusside administration is cyanide poisoning. Symptoms include metabolic acidosis, dyspnea, nausea, vomiting, dizziness, loss of consciousness, and coma. Treatment for this adverse reaction involves the administration of nitrites, which will bind with the cyanide to release cytochrome oxidase, which forms cyanmethemoglobin, a nontoxic substance. The cyanide then disassociates.

The solution should be freshly mixed and adequately protected from light during administration. Infusion should always be via infusion pump with a microdrip regulator.

Nitroglycerin. NTG is a potent systemic vasodilator whose primary effect is relaxation of vascular smooth muscle both on the arterial and venous side. When postcapillary vessels are relaxed, peripheral pooling of blood decreases venous return to the heart, reducing LVEDP (preload). Arteriolar relaxation reduces SVR and arterial pressure (afterload). The results are decreased oxygen consumption, decreased CVP, decreased PCWP, decreased PVR, and decreased SVR.

Perioperative hypertension is a common phenomenon that is associated with coronary artery bypass as well as other types of vascular operations, particularly with carotid endarterectomies, or aortic aneurysm resections. Hypertension is usually defined as blood pressure that exceeds 20 percent of the patient's normal range during hospitalization.

Control of intraoperative hypertension must be a major concern in patients who have myocardial dysfunction. Kaplan and Jones have found this is best accomplished with nitroglycerin. Their studies conclude that the use of NTG has several advantages over the use of nitroprusside, and is the drug of choice in 90 percent of their bypass procedures (Kaplan and Jones, 1979).

NTG has a rapid onset of action (approximately 2 minutes). It will provide relief from most hypertensive episodes and at the same time will treat myocardial ischemia. Nitroprusside, on the other hand, does not reduce myocardial ischemia and may contribute to an intracoronary steal syndrome. ST depression may worsen with nitroprusside. Nitroprusside is very useful in controlling hypertensive episodes that are not alleviated by NTG.

NTG is commonly employed preoperatively for the relief of angina and also to reduce myocardial oxygen demand. This medical treatment should be continued intraoperatively. If the patient is not receiving NTG intravenously, a preparation should be put on the skin (Nitrodur patch). Continuation of vasodilator therapy postoperatively is necessary if hypertension persists.

The use of nitroglycerin allows for predictable reductions in blood pressure with less chance of overshoot hypotension.* Use of an NTG specific infusion set overcomes any difficulty with titration and eliminates the need for protection from light.

NTG has direct coronary effects, not by significant increases in coronary blood flow but by redistribution of flow to the subendocardial area and increase in collateral flow. NTG also diminishes coronary artery spasm. All of these effects lead to an increase in the myocardial oxygen supply, which, combined with the decreased MVo$_2$ induced by NTG, markedly improves the myocardial oxygen balance and provides clinical improvement. NTG has been shown to improve left ventricular wall motion, leading to increases in SV and ejection fractions (Kaplan, 1983).

NTG has many clinical uses in addition to those described above. In addition to reducing oxygen consumption and hemodynamic responses, it also is useful in the control of unstable angina, especially if administered intravenously. NTG is also useful in acute myocardial infarction. Research has indicated that it reduces infarct size and the incidence of heart failure and arrythmias.

Kaplan (1983) suggests that use of NTG during cardiopulmonary bypass is less effective in reducing blood pressure in hypertensive patients than in normotensive patients and that additional doses may be required to lower mean pressure.

NTG is especially useful in patients with increased PCWP and hypotension; however, if the NTG brings about an excessive decline in systemic pressure, then one can use simultaneous supplemental doses of phenylephrine (Moore, 1983).

The use of intravenous NTG is advantageous to the anesthetist because of ease of titration and ability to control hemodynamic parameters. NTG is used routinely during coronary artery bypass. In Tables 28–12 and 28–13, Kaplan lists the intraoperative and postbypass indications for use of NTG. The most frequent use is for acute hypertension. During valvular surgery, NTG is useful in the treatment of pulmonary hypertension or to reduce systemic afterload (Kaplan, 1983).

The first commercial preparation of an intravenous preparation is Tridil. Tridil contains 10 ml of NTG. It must be diluted in either D$_5$W or normal saline. Dilution is 50 mg (10 ml) of NTG in 250 or 500 ml, which yields a concentration of 100 to 200 μg/ml. Initial dosage should be 5 μg/min with increases every three to five minutes until some response is seen.

Another intravenous preparation is available, which contains 0.8 mg of NTG per ml. When 10 ml is diluted in 250 cc of D$_5$W or 0.9 percent sodium chloride, the dosage is 30 μg/ml.

Propranolol. Propranolol is a beta-adrenergic blocker, which competes for occupation of the tubular receptor site to decrease heart rate and cardiac output, prolongs systole, and decreases arterial pressure slightly. Peripheral resis-

TABLE 28–12. INTRAOPERATIVE INDICATIONS FOR INTRAVENOUS NITROGLYCERIN

1. Hypertension > 20% above control values
2. Pulmonary capillary wedge pressure > 18–20 mm Hg
3. AC and V waves > 20 mm Hg
4. ST changes > 1 mm
5. Acute right ventricular or left ventricular dysfunction
6. Coronary artery spasm

Normal venous tracing has 3 positive waves: A, C, and V. A = right atrial contraction; C = right atrial relaxation; V = right atrial filling.
From Kaplan JA: Cardiac Anesthesia, 1979. By permission of Grune & Stratton and the author.

TABLE 28–13. INDICATIONS FOR INTRAVENOUS NITROGLYCERIN AT TERMINATION OF CARDIOPULMONARY BYPASS

1. Elevated pulmonary capillary wedge pressure
2. Elevated pulmonary vascular resistance
3. Infusion of oxygenator reservoir volume
4. Transfusion of blood products
5. Incomplete revascularization
6. Ischemia (ST-segment changes in leads II or V_5)
7. Intraoperative myocardial infarction
8. Coronary artery spasm (ST elevation, arrhythmias)

From Kaplan JA: Cardiac Anesthesia, 1979. By permission of Grune & Stratton and the author.

tance is increased compensatorily and a transient vasodilation may occur. The cardiac response to beta blockade frequently is reflected by changes in sodium excretion, whereby there is an increased total body sodium and extracellular fluid volume (Goodman and Gilman, 1985). In hypertension, beta blockers reduce blood pressure by two mechanisms: (1) reduced cardiac output and (2) reduced plasma renin activity (Kaplan, 1983).

The antiarrythmic effects of propranolol are based on its ability to decrease the rate of phase 4 depolarization in sinus node cells and, to a lesser degree, in nonspecialized atrial tissue (Kaplan, 1983). It increases sinus cycle length and atrioventricular (A-V) nodal conduction time, resulting in prolonged atrial and A-V refractory periods.

The effect of beta blockade on the heart is more marked under conditions of increased demand and sympathetic tone. Total coronary blood flow and MV_{O_2} are decreased. An internal shunting after beta-adrenergic blockade allows blood flow to ischemic areas of the heart to be altered less than to other regions (Goodman and Gilman, 1985).

In addition to cardiac responses, propranolol also produces bronchoconstriction and increased vascular tone. This vasoconstriction directly reduces blood flow to involved organs such as skin, somatic muscle, abdominal viscera, kidneys, and myocardium (Kaplan, 1983).

Propranolol is available in 1-ml ampules, which contain 1.0 mg for intravenous use. Usually, the intravenous dose is 0.5 mg increments up to 3 mg over several minutes.

Common side effects of propranolol include heart failure, A-V dissociation if used in conjunction with digitalis, and increased airway resistance; thus it is definitely contraindicated in the asthmatic or any patient with obstructive pulmonary disease.

Termination of Cardiopulmonary Bypass. If termination of cardiopulmonary bypass remains impossible after the administration of various drug combinations, insertion of an intra-aortic balloon pump (IABP) may be necessary to provide circulatory support with minimal increase in afterload.

The use of the IABP had its inception in 1969 to treat patients with left ventricular failure. Technical advances and catheter simplification have expanded its use to patients

suffering from myocardial ischemia. The two primary effects of IABP therapy are increased coronary perfusion and decreased afterload. Reduction of afterload is achieved during counterpulsation by deflating the IABP prior to ventricular ejection.

The IABP is used frequently after open heart surgery to enhance ventricular function, after acute myocardial infarction, and in cardiogenic shock secondary to myocardial infarction.

The intra-aortic balloon is usually inserted via the femoral artery and positioned with the tip of the balloon just below the subclavian artery and its base just above the renal arteries. The balloon, once properly positioned, is then connected to a gas-driven pump, which inflates and deflates the balloon at different phases of systole and diastole (Fig. 28–14).

When appropriately set, i.e., when the timing of inflation and deflation are correct, the balloon serves to augment myocardial oxygenation and reduce cardiac workload. Thus, coronary perfusion is increased and afterload decreased. To understand the theory behind the use of the intra-aortic balloon therapy, the cardiac cycle must be understood. Figure 28–15 demonstrates normal cardiac cycle. During atrial systole (1) the A-V valves are open and the atria contracted. Isovolumetric contraction (2) is characterized by closure of all four valves. During this phase, the pressure increases to exceed aortic and pulmonary end-

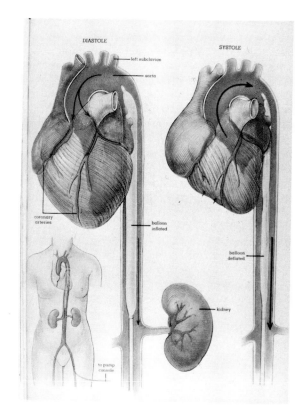

Figure 28–14. The balloon should inflate at the beginning of diastole–aortic valve closure. The balloon should deflate just prior to systole to allow the left ventricle to eject blood without interference. (*From Purcell J, Pippin L, et al: Am J Nurs 83(5):779.* © *1983, American Journal of Nursing Company.*)

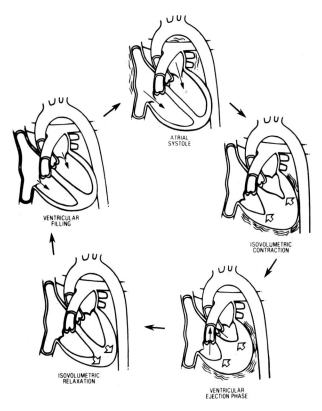

Figure 28–15. The cardiac cycle. (*Courtesy of the Datascope Corporation.*)

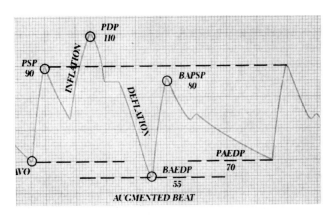

Figure 28–17. The tracing illustrates changes in arterial pressure associated with properly timed balloon inflation and deflation. AUO = aortic valve opening; BAPSP = balloon-assisted peak systolic pressure; BAEP = balloon-assisted end-diastolic pressure; PAEDP = patient's aortic end-diastolic pressure; PDP = peak diastolic pressure; PSP = peak systolic pressure.

diastolic pressure. The greatest oxygen consumption occurs here. During the ventricular ejection phase (3), the semilunar valves open and the atria fill. Isovolumetric relaxation (4) then occurs with closure of the semilunar valves, decreased ventricular pressure and increased coronary perfusion, and ventricular filling (5), the phase of diastole, is characterized by ventricular relaxation.

The most common method of activating the pump is to trigger the machine according to the R wave on an ECG. The pump will inflate the balloon in the middle of diastole, or T wave, and deflate just prior to the QRS complex, or

systole. Figure 28–16 shows an ECG with inflation and deflation patterns. Because systole and diastole cannot be observed from an ECG, an arterial wave form must be used. Balloon inflation (diastolic augmentation) should occur at the beginning of diastole, which occurs on the dicrotic notch when arterial pressure is being measured at the aortic root. Diastolic augmentation should exceed or at least equal the patient's systolic pressure.

Deflation should occur during the time of isovolumetric contraction, i.e., the beginning of systole, prior to opening of the aortic valve. During isovolumetric contraction, the left ventricle must overcome aortic root end-diastolic pressure before it can eject its volume. Because deflation occurs just prior to systole, blood fills the area vacated by the deflated balloon, decreasing aortic root end-diastolic pressure. The ventricle needn't work as hard to empty, and peak ventricular systolic pressure is reduced (Fig. 28–17, 28–18).

The use of IABP therapy is not without complications. Limb ischemia occurs in 4 to 8 percent of the patients. Excessive bleeding may occur at the insertion site. Thrombo-

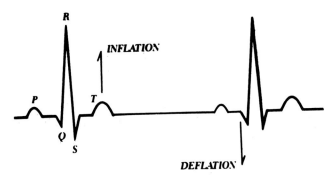

Figure 28–16. Electrocardiogram demonstrating optimal inflation and deflation timing. ECG lead should be one that maximizes R waves and minimizes other wave forms. (*From Purcell J, Pippin L, et al. Am J Nurs 83(5):778. © 1983. American Journal of Nursing Company.*)

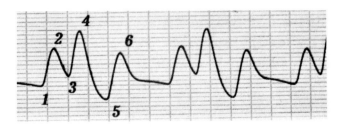

Figure 28–18. **1.** Aortic valve opening (unassisted end-diastolic pressure); **2.** peak systolic pressure (unassisted); **3.** dicrotic notch (balloon inflation); **4.** maximum pressure generated by balloon; **5.** end-diastolic pressure associated with balloon deflation (assisted end-diastolic pressure); **6.** peak systolic pressure assisted by balloon (assisted systolic pressure). (*From Purcell J, Pippin L, et al: IAPB therapy. Am J Nurs 83(5):779. © 1983, American Journal of Nursing Company.*)

cytopenia with a rapid decrease in platelets is another side effect, and migration of the catheter is common.

VALVULAR SURGERY

Anatomy of the Cardiac Valves

The interior of the right ventricle has several openings. These include the right atrioventricular orifice, the right atrioventricular valve, and the anterior, posterior, and septal cusps (Vanden Belt and Ronan, 1979). The right A-V orifice, which is an oval aperture about 4 cm in diameter, is surrounded by a fibrous ring, and protected by the tricuspid valve. The right A-V, or tricuspid, valve surrounds the orifice with a thin sheet that projects into the ventricle in three leaflets, or cusps: the anterior, posterior, and medial, or septal. The leaflets are fibrous in nature and triangular in shape. The bases attach to the fibrous ring and the apices project into the ventricular cavity. The cusps are held in place by the chordae tendineae and papillary muscles.

The chordae tendineae are strong fibrous cords that are attached to the apices of the valve cusps and are anchored to the muscular wall. There are 60 or more in number. The chordae originate in each of the papillary muscles, the posteromedial papillary muscle having six primary chordae and the antecolateral papillary muscle having about four primary chordae. The chordae subdivide into secondary and tertiary components that attach to the mitral leaflets and prevent them from prolapsing into the left atrium. If the anatomy of the chordae changes for any reason, be it in length or by rupture, the leaflets fail to approximate and regurgitation results.

The papillary muscles are round projections, two in number, the anterior and posterior papillary muscles. They are named according to the commissures that they are related to.

The interior of the left ventricle also has several openings—the left A-V orifice, the left A-V valve, and the anterior and posterior cusps. The left A-V orifice (mitral orifice) is smaller than the right and encircled by a dense fibrous ring. The bicuspid, or mitral, valve surrounds the opening. It extends down into the left ventricle in two leaflets, the anterior and the posterior. The chordae tendineae are stronger and fewer in the left ventricle than in the right, and the left has two papillary muscles, whereas the right has three. Mitral valve closure is accomplished when the anterior leaflet swings posteriorly to abut against the free edge of the posterior leaflet (Vanden Belt and Ronan, 1979). It is crucial to the competence of the mitral valve than the papillary muscles shorten during ventricular systole as ventricular size is reduced (Vanden Belt and Ronan, 1979).

The aortic valve is composed of three semilunar cusps. Between each cusp and the aortic wall, there are related sinuses, the sinuses of Valsalva, from which the coronary arteries arise. The anatomic structure of the mitral valve differs from the aortic and pulmonic (Fig. 28–19) allowing for pressure and velocity accommodations, which are higher in the pulmonic valve. These semilunar valves are responsible for preventing backflow from the aorta and pulmonary artery into the ventricles during diastole.

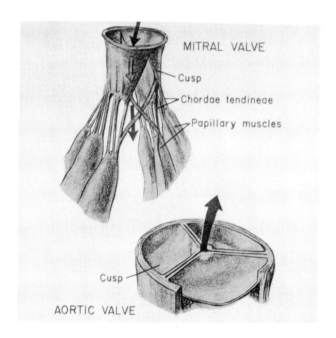

Figure 28–19. Anatomic differences between mitral and aortic valves. (*From Guyton A: Textbook of Medical Physiology, 3rd ed., 1981. Courtesy of Saunders.*)

The Cardiac Cycle. The cardiac cycle designates that period of time between the beginning of one heart contraction and the end of the next. It is initiated by impulses that begin in the sinoatrial node and travel through the entire conduction system to the ventricles. There is a delay before the passage of impulse from atria to ventricles, allowing the atria to contract earlier than the ventricles, thus augmenting ventricular contraction with an increased volume of blood.

The cardiac cycle consists of a period of relaxation (diastole) followed by a period of contraction (systole) (see Fig. 28–16).

Atrial Systole. Under normal conditions, blood flows continually from the great veins into the atria, and approximately 70 percent of this flows directly to the atria without the assistance of atrial contractions. The remaining 30 percent is pumped by atrial contraction. The heart can operate effectively without this 30 percent increase during rest but with exercise, ventricular efficiency depends on this increased volume from the atria, and the atrial contractions act as a prime for the ventricles.

Atrial systole is responsible for increases in atrial, ventricular, and venous pressures, as well as an increase in ventricular volume. Because there are no valves between the right atrium and venae cavae or the left atrium and pulmonary veins, atrial contraction can force blood in both directions (Berne and Levy, 1977).

Ventricular Systole

ISOVOLUMETRIC CONTRACTION. Immediately after ventricular contraction begins, the ventricular pressure rises abruptly, causing the A-V valves to close. An additional 0.02 to 0.03

second is required for the ventricle to build sufficient pressure to push the semilunar valves open against the pressure in the aorta and pulmonary artery. During this time, the ventricles are not emptying but are trying to generate a pressure that exceeds aortic and pulmonary end-diastolic pressure. Thus, muscle tension increases, but actual muscle fiber shortening does not occur (Guyton, 1982). It should be noted that the greatest amount of oxygen consumption occurs here.

VENTRICULAR EJECTION PHASE. When left ventricular pressure rises slightly above 80 mm Hg and the right ventricle pressure rises to slightly above 8 mm Hg, the pressure generated by the ventricles will open the semilunar valves and blood will eject from the ventricles immediately (Guyton, 1982). Ejection is divided into two phases: the shorter phase (rapid ejection) and a longer phase (reduced ejection). During the rapid phase, there is a sharp rise in ventricular and aortic pressures, an abrupt decrease in ventricular volume, and a greater aortic blood flow. The rapid phase occurs during the first one-third of the ejection. During the second two-thirds of the ejection phase, the reverse is true (Berne and Levy, 1977).

During the last portion of ventricular systole, there is no blood flow from the ventricle into the arterial circulation, even though ventricular contraction is still occurring. Both arterial and ventricular pressures fall. This time interval is called the protodiastolic phase.

It is during the ventricular ejection phase that the atria fill.

Ventricular Diastole

ISOVOLUMETRIC RELAXATION. The period between the closure of the semilunar valves and the opening of the A-V valves is termed isovolumetric relaxation and is characterized by a precipitous fall in ventricular pressure without a change in ventricular volume (Berne and Levy, 1977). An increased arterial pressure occurs, pushing blood back toward the ventricles, closing the semilunar valves. The ventricular muscle continues to relax and the ventricular pressure falls below diastolic level. The A-V valves open and a new cycle begins.

RAPID FILLING PHASE. This phase occurs immediately on opening of the A-V valves. Just as soon as systole ends and the ventricular pressure falls, the high pressures in the atria push the A-V valves open and allow blood to flow rapidly into the ventricles (Berne and Levy, 1977). The major portion of ventricular filling occurs here. As the blood flows from the atria to the ventricles, there is a decrease in atrial and ventricular pressures and a sharp increase in ventricular volume.

Figure 28–20 illustrates the events of the cardiac cycle as described by Guyton. Note how he relates the electrocardiogram to the cardiac cycle. The P wave occurs just prior to a rise in atrial pressure and represents atrial depolarization. Atrial contraction occurs. The QRS wave appears next, representing ventricular depolarization and ventricular contraction. The T wave begins slightly before the end of the ventricular contraction and represents repolarization of the ventricle.

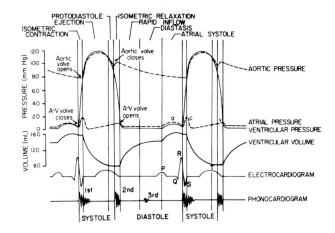

Figure 28–20. Events of the cardiac cycle. (*From Guyton A: Human physiology and mechanism of disease, 1982. Courtesy of Saunders.*)

Guyton also illustrates pressure changes that occur within the atria as the cardiac cycle proceeds. These are represented by the *a*, *c*, and *v* atrial pressure waves. Each wave denotes elevations in atrial pressure. The *a* wave is caused by atrial contraction and signifies a 4 to 6 mm Hg rise in right atrial pressure and a 7 to 8 mm Hg rise in the left (Guyton, 1982). The *c* wave occurs when the ventricles contract and is caused by (1) bulging of the A-V valves toward the atria because of increasing pressure in the ventricles and (2) pulling of the atrial muscle by contracting ventricles (Guyton, 1982). The *v* wave occurs toward the end of ventricular contraction and is the result of atrial volume buildup while the A-V valves are closed.

During diastole, the volume in each ventricle rises to 120 to 130 ml. This volume is known as the end-diastolic volume. During systole, this volume decreases to approximately 70 ml (stroke volume, SV). There remain 50 to 60 ml in each ventricle. This is the end-systolic volume. By augmentation of both of these values, SV and thus cardiac output can be increased.

Valvular Heart Diseases

Valvular heart disease, in its earliest stages, is identified by a murmur. Most murmurs are caused by obstruction or regurgitation in a cardiac valve. In general, most valvular heart disease occurs in the adult population (Vanden Belt and Ronan, 1979).

Aortic Regurgitation. Approximately three-fourths of all patients with pure aortic regurgitation are males. The disease is primarily caused by rheumatic fever, which causes shortened valve cusps, resulting in improper closure during diastole. In contrast to mitral regurgitation, in which a fraction of the left ventricular SV is delivered into the low-pressure left atrium, in aortic regurgitation the entire left ventricular SV must be ejected into a high-pressure zone, the aorta (Isselbacher et al, 1980). Although the low aortic diastolic pressure facilitates ventricular emptying during early systole, an increase of the left ventricular end-diastolic volume constitutes the major hemodynamic compensation of aortic regurgitation, and the total SV is augmented primarily through the operation of the Frank-Starling mechanism (Isselbacher et al, 1980).

Aortic insufficiency results in ventricular hypertrophy and dilation (Fig. 28–21). Hemodynamically, particularly as left ventricular function diminishes, the ejection fraction and SV decrease. There is a decreased aortic diastolic pressure and shortened isovolumetric contraction. Cardiac output is reduced slightly. There are elevated pulmonary wedge, arterial, and left atrial pressures. Coronary perfusion is decreased and myocardial ischemia ensues.

Symptoms. The interval between the first episode of acute rheumatic fever and the development of hemodynamically significant aortic regurgitation averages approximately 7 years, and this period is followed by an asymptomatic interval of approximately 10 to 20 years, during which the severity of the regurgitation usually increases (Isselbacher et al, 1980). Symptoms include palpitations, sinus tachycardia, or premature ventricular beats. Dyspnea, orthopnea, and diaphoresis are common, along with symptoms of left ventricular failure (Table 28–14). Angina, unaffected by NTG, is common to advanced stages as is systemic fluid retention.

Surgical intervention must be instituted at the appropriate time. It should be considered in patients with symptomatic free aortic regurgitation who do not respond to medical treatment.

Aortic Stenosis. Aortic stenosis occurs in about one-fourth of all patients with chronic valvular heart disease. It is most frequently found in adult males. The normal aortic valve has three cusps that are thin and movable. Disease processes affect the valve structure by causing a thickened or calcified area, which causes commissural fusion.

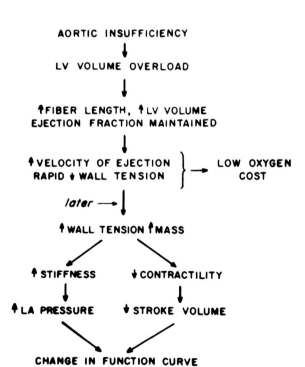

Figure 28–21. Pathophysiology of aortic insufficiency. LA = left atrium; LV = left ventricle. (*From Lowenstein E, Thomas SJ. Int Anesthesiol Clin 17:67, 1979. Courtesy of Little, Brown.*)

The primary insult with aortic stenosis lies in obstruction to the left ventricular outflow, resulting in a pressure gradient between the left ventricle and aorta during systolic ejection. The causes may be congenital, rheumatic fever that affects the aortic valve, or calcification of the aortic cusps. Besides aortic valvular stenosis, three other lesions may be responsible for obstruction to left ventricular outflow: (1) idiopathic hypertrophic subaortic stenosis, characterized by marked left ventricular enlargement, (2) discrete congenital subvalvular stenosis, caused by a fibrous ridge below the aortic valve, or (3) supravalvular aortic stenosis, which is a congenital anomaly produced by narrowing of the ascending aorta (Orkin and Cooperman, 1983).

Aortic stenosis overloads the left ventricle but does not cause dilation—that is, if there is low ventricular compliance (Orkin and Cooperman, 1983). There are two major consequences of decreased ventricular compliance: (1) higher filling pressures are needed for optimal cardiac performance, leading to pulmonary congestion if too high, and (2) normal sinus rhythm helps maintain adequate ventricular filling because the atrial kick may account for up to 40 percent of ventricular filling (Orkin and Cooperman, 1983).

Hemodynamic values such as cardiac output or SV are normal in severe stenosis at rest. As the disease progresses, cardiac output and SV decrease and elevations of the mean left atrial, pulmonary wedge, and pulmonary artery pressures are seen.

Symptoms. Murmurs usually precede onset of symptoms by several years. Aortic stenosis is rarely of hemodynamic or clinical importance until the orifice has narrowed to one-third of normal (Kaplan and Jones, 1979). In contrast to mitral stenosis, severe aortic stenosis may be present for years before clinical symptoms. When symptoms do occur, they include dyspnea, syncope, and angina. Dyspnea occurs from elevation of LVEDP, syncope from hypotension secondary to vasodilation from fixed cardiac output, and angina from myocardial oxygen supply-demand imbalance. Terminal symptoms include orthopnea, pulmonary edema, right ventricular failure, systemic venous hypertension, hepatomegaly, atrial fibrillation, and tricuspid regurgitation (Kaplan and Jones, 1979).

Aortic and mitral stenosis can exist simultaneously. If so, the symptoms of mitral stenosis prevail. Surgical intervention should be undertaken prior to the development of left ventricular failure, but not before the patient is symptomatic.

Mitral Regurgitation. The mitral valve has several anatomic structures that are responsible for closure of the valve during ventricular systole. These include (1) the anterior and posterior mitral leaflets, (2) the chordae tendineae, (3) the papillary muscles, (4) the left ventricular myocardium, and (5) the mitral annulus. Mitral regurgitation may be due to a defect in any one of these; specific disease states tend to center on certain components.

Mitral regurgitation caused by involvement of the valve leaflets occurs most commonly in rheumatic heart disease and is seen more frequently in males than females (Braunwald, 1980). It is a consequence of shortening, rigidity, deformity, and retraction of one or both cusps of the mitral

TABLE 28–14. DIFFERENCES BETWEEN ACUTE AND CHRONIC AORTIC REGURGITATION

Clinical Features

	Acute	*Chronic*
Congestive heart failure	Early and sudden	Late and insidious
Arterial pulse		
Rate per minute	Increased	Normal
Rate of rise	Normal	Increased
Systolic pressure	Normal to decreased	Increased
Diastolic pressure	Normal to decreased	Decreased
Pulse pressure	Near normal	Increased
Contour of peak	Single	Bisferiens
Pulsus alternans	Common	Uncommon
Left ventricular (LV) impulse	Near normal to moderately displaced, not hyperdynamic	Displaced hyperdynamic
Auscultation		
S_1	Soft to absent	Normal
Aortic component of S_2	Soft	Normal or decreased
Pulmonic component of S_2	Normal or increased	Normal
S_2	Common	Uncommon
S_4	Consistently absent	Usually absent
Aortic systolic murmur	Grade 3 or less	Grade 3 or more
Aortic regurgitant murmur	Short, medium-pitched	Long, high-pitched
Austin Flint	Mid-diastolic	Presystolic, mid-diastolic, or both
Peripheral arterial auscultatory signs	Absent	Present
Electrocardiogram	Normal LV voltage with minor repolarization abnormalities	Increased LV voltage with major repolarization abnormalities
Chest roentgenogram		
Left ventricle	Normal to moderately increased	Markedly increased
Aortic root and arch	Usually normal	Prominent
Pulmonary venous vascularity	Increased	Normal

Hemodynamic Features

	Acute	*Chronic* *(Without Left Ventricular Failure)*
Left ventricular (LV) compliance	Normal	Normal or increased
Regurgitant volume	Increased	Increased
LV end-diastolic pressure	Markedly increased	Normal or increased
LV ejection velocity (dP/dt)	Not significantly increased	Markedly increased
Aortic systolic pressure	Not increased	Increased
Aortic diastolic pressure	Normal to decreased	Markedly decreased
Systemic arterial pulse pressure	Slightly to moderately increased	Markedly increased
Ejection fraction	Normal or decreased	Normal
Effective stroke volume	Decreased	Normal
Effective cardiac output	Decreased	Usually normal
Heart rate	Increased	Normal
Peripheral vascular resistance	Usually increased	Normal

Echocardiographic Features

	Acute	*Chronic*
Mitral valve		
Closure point	Premature	Normal
Opening point	Delayed	Normal
E-F slope	Decreased	Normal
Fluttering	Usually present	Usually present
Left ventricle		
Internal dimension (end diastole)	Normal	Increased
Septal and free wall thickness	Normal	Normal
Septal and free wall motion	Normal	Increased
Left ventricular mass	Normal	Increased

From Morganroth J: Ann Intern Med 87:224, 228, 230, 1977.

valve as well as shortening and fusion or rupture of the chordae tendineae (Braunwald, 1980). If the leaflets are strictured by excessive tissue, the valves will prolapse into the left atrium.

Papillary muscle fibrosis, if present, will cause inadequate shortening of the papillary muscle during systole, with prolapse of the leaflets into the atrium. Regurgitation ensues. The papillary muscles receive their blood supply from the coronary vessels, so any insult to coronary perfusion can cause ischemia to the papillary muscles, with concurrent dysfunction. If severe enough, papillary muscle necrosis can occur and result in mitral regurgitation. Papillary muscle ischemia can also be caused by anemia, shock, coronary arteritis, or left ventricular aneurysm.

The chordae tendineae may be abnormal at birth or may rupture because of rheumatic fever, trauma, endocarditis, or left ventricular regurgitation. If this abnormality exists, acute regurgitation ensues.

Calcification of the mitral annulus results in a dilation of this opening and severe dilation of the left ventricle. Normally during systole, the annulus constricts and plays a very important role in valve closure. When it is calcified, mitral regurgitation occurs. This condition presents with most severe myocardial dysfunction, and these patients may not improve after valve replacement because of the increase in left ventricular afterload, which occurs with dilation of the regurgitation leak (Braunwald, 1980).

Left ventricular function can be determined by evaluating the end-systolic volume. Braunwald et al found that patients with normal end-systolic volume retained normal ventricular function postoperatively, whereas marked enlargement of the end-systolic volume usually correlated well with postoperative mortality (Braunwald, 1980).

The combined left atrial and pulmonary venous bed compliance is an important determinant of the hemodynamic and clinical picture in mitral regurgitation (Braunwald, 1980). Three major subgroups have been identified: (1) normal or reduced compliance, in which there is little enlargement of the left atrium but marked elevation of the mean left atrial pressure, with prominent systems of pulmonary congestion; (2) moderately increased compliance, which is the most common and consists of patients with variable atrial enlargement and significant elevation of left atrial pressure; and (3) markedly increased compliance, within the adult population frequently secondary to high ventricular pressure.

Pathophysiology. In patients with mitral regurgitation, the resistance to left ventricular emptying is reduced. As a result, the left ventricle decompresses itself rapidly into the left atrium early during ejection, and with a marked reduction in left ventricular size there is a rapid decline in left ventricular tension (Kaplan and Jones, 1979). Therefore, a greater proportion of the contractile activity of the left ventricle is expanded in shortening, and the cardiac output may be maintained for long periods of time.

The initial compensation to mitral regurgitation consists of more complete systolic emptying of the left ventricle; however, a progressive increase in left ventricular end-diastolic volume occurs as the severity of the regurgitation increases and the left ventricular function deteriorates (Kaplan

and Jones, 1979). Significant mitral regurgitation tends to be progressive, because enlargement of the left atrium places tension on the posterior mitral leaflet, pulling it away from the mitral orifice. Dilation of the left ventricle increases the regurgitation, which further enlarges the left atrium and ventricle, resulting in a vicious cycle (Kaplan and Jones, 1979).

Mitral regurgitation produces volume overload of the left ventricle. The volume of mitral regurgitance flow depends on the size of the regurgitant orifice as well as the pressure gradient between the left ventricle and the left atrium. Left ventricular systolic pressure and thus left ventricular-left atrial gradient are dependent on SVR and forward SV. Thus, increases in both preload and afterload and depression of contractility increase left ventricular size and enlarge the regurgitant orifice. If regurgitation is caused by something other than a rigid valve, the volume of flow is influenced by left ventricular dimensions, which in turn affect orifice size (Braunwald, 1980).

Ejection fractions must be closely examined in these patients. Values may be at normal levels and yet myocardial function may be impaired. If ejection fractions are reduced, severe myocardial dysfunction may be present. An ejection fraction under 40 percent in patients with mitral regurgitation represents massive enlargement of the left atrium and normal or slightly elevated left atrial pressure (Braunwald, 1980).

Symptoms. The symptoms that present depend on the pressure in the left atrium and the cardiac output. The left atrial pressure determines the pulmonary venous pressure and the severity of the dyspnea (Vanden Belt and Ronan, 1979). Symptoms include fatigue, dyspnea, orthopnea and nocturnal dyspnea, weight loss, exhaustion, and cachexia. Right-sided failure and associated symptoms can be seen with patients who have pulmonary vascular disease and regurgitation. Figure 28–22 summarizes the hemodynamic and physiologic changes that occur with mitral regurgitation.

Mitral Stenosis. The incidence of mitral stenosis after rheumatic fever is high; it is estimated that roughly 40 percent of all patients with a past history will develop mitral stenosis. Mitral stenosis is more prevalent in women.

Pathophysiology. Valve leaflets become thickened and fibrous or impeded by calcified deposits, the chordae tendineae shorten, the cusps become rigid, and the apex of the valve narrows. Rheumatic fever results in four types of fusion of the apparatus, leading to stenosis: (1) commisural—occurring in 30 percent, (2) cuspal—15 percent, (3) chordal—10 percent, and (4) combined—45 percent.[11] The stenotic mitral valve is usually funnel-shaped, and the orifice is frequently shaped like a fish mouth or buttonhole, with calcium deposits in the valve leaflets sometimes extending to involve the valve ring, which may become quite thick.

The basic problem in tight mitral stenosis is getting blood out of the blocked left atrium into the left ventricle during diastole. The price of moving blood rapidly is inevitably an increase in left atrial pressure, which must be shared

THE SYNDROME OF MITRAL REGURGITATION

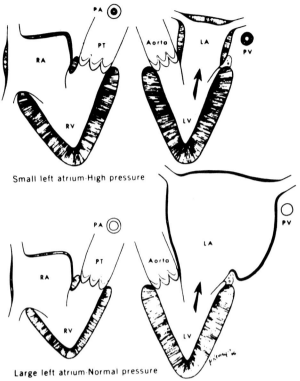

Small left atrium-High pressure

Large left atrium-Normal pressure

Figure 28–22. The extremes of the syndrome of mitral regurgitation. **Top:** Mitral regurgitation into small, hypertrophied left atrium results in pulmonary vascular changes and right ventricle hypertrophy. **Bottom:** Mitral regurgitation into large, thin-walled left atrium results in little or no change in pulmonary vessels or right ventricle. LA = left atrium; LV = left ventricle; PA = pulmonary artery; PT = pulmonary trunk; PV = pulmonary vein; RA = right atrium; RV = right ventricle. (*From Roberts WC, Perloff JK: Ann Intern Med 77:939, 1972.*)

by the pulmonary venous reservoir. Two events contribute to the left atrial pressure and hence to the important task of squeezing blood through the stenotic valve into the left ventricle: (1) Atrial systole is an active effort but is quite brief. It does not greatly shrink the atrium. Its major role may be during exercise and tachycardia. (2) More important is the leftover force of right ventricular contraction, dampened more or less by transmission through the pulmonary vascular bed (Hurst and Logue, 1970). For this to be of any benefit in stenosis, the pressure in the pulmonary bed must be very high, limiting left atrial pressure and consequently blood flow.

Normally, the orifice of the mitral valve is 4 to 6 cm². With mild stenosis, this is reduced to 2 cm². Under these circumstances, blood will flow from left atrium to left ventricle only by abnormally high pressure gradients. In patients with severe stenosis (opening reduced to 1 cm²) an even higher gradient is required to maintain a normal cardiac output. Pulmonary capillary and venous pressures are elevated and dyspnea results. Any episodes of tachycardia will augment the pressure gradient and result in an increased left atrial pressure. Thus, it is obvious that tachyarrythmias must be avoided in these patients.

The severity of mitral obstruction influences the elevation of left atrial pressure, which, in turn, determines the extent of the pulmonary congestive symptoms of dyspnea and orthopnea.

The following hemodynamic changes are associated with mitral stenosis: left ventricular diastolic pressure is normal with pure stenosis and elevated if regurgitation is present. Ejection fraction is usually normal or somewhat reduced in moderate stenosis and subnormal even at rest in the severely stenosed patient.

The clinical and hemodynamic pictures of mitral stenosis are dictated largely by the level of the pulmonary artery pressure. Pulmonary hypertension results from (1) the passive backward transmission of the elevated left atrial pressure, (2) arteriolar destruction, which is presumably triggered by left atrial and pulmonary venous hypertension, and (3) organic obliterative changes in the pulmonary vascular bed (Isselbacher et al, 1980).

Symptoms. The most common symptoms associated with mitral stenosis are dyspnea and episodes of pulmonary edema caused by chronic pulmonary congestion. Orthopnea and paroxysmal nocturnal dyspnea also occur, especially in the recumbent position, caused by rapid redistribution of blood from the periphery to the lungs. Pulmonary edema develops if there is a sudden increase in flow through the mitral orifice. Arrythmias in the form of atrial abnormalities are common when moderate stenosis is present. These include premature atrial beats, flutter, fibrillation, and paroxysmal atrial tachycardia. Hemoptysis occurs in those patients with increased left atrial pressures.

Symptoms of a more serious nature include (1) thrombi, particularly as a result of atrial fibrillation, with emboli to brain, kidneys, and spleen, (2) pulmonary emboli, particularly in those patients with increased pulmonary vascular resistance, (3) bacterial endocarditis, and (4) pulmonary infections.

Unless there is a specific contraindication, operative treatment is indicated in the symptomatic patient with pure mitral stenosis whose effective orifice is less than 1.5 cm². Mitral commissurotomy has been an excellent operation in patients without significant mitral regurgitation and without severe valvular calcification. Before commissurotomy is begun, the atrial cavity should be examined closely for thrombi. It is common practice to tie off the atrial appendage from the left atrium to avoid embolization from chronic atrial fibrillation. Emboli frequently occur when there are sudden changes from atrial fibrillation to sinus rhythm and the atria begin to contract. Valvular replacement with a prosthetic valve may be done in those cases in which commissurotomy may not be helpful, particularly in those patients with coexisting mitral regurgitation or heavy valvular regurgitation (Goodman and Gilman, 1985).

Mitral Valve Prolapse. Mitral valve prolapse has become one of the most common valvular abnormalities, affecting roughly 6 to 17 percent of the population, with the highest incidence occurring in females. This increase in occurrence is probably due more to advanced diagnostic tools than to an actual increase in prevalence. Several names have been given to this syndrome. These include midsystolic click-murmur syndrome, Barlow's syndrome, floppy valve syndrome, and redundant cusp syndrome. There are several disease entities that can predispose to mitral valve prolapse. These include rheumatic endocarditis, congestive cardiomyopathy, myocarditis trauma, lupus erythematosus, Wolff-Parkinson-White syndrome, and coronary artery disease. This list is not inclusive.

General symptoms include systolic clicks and a late systolic murmur. Clinically, these patients are asymptomatic. However, if the prolapse is severe enough, palpitations, chest discomfort, or any symptoms indicative of mitral regurgitation may present. Palpitations are often caused by arrythmias, which may be secondary to autonomic dysfunction. The arrythmias may be atrial or ventricular in nature. They may be premature beats or ventricular tachyarrythmias or bradyarrythmias. The exact cause of the arrythmias is not definite, but some theorize that they may be due to stretch of the leaflets. By far the most common arrythmia is paroxysmal supraventricular tachycardia. This is probably related to the existence of atrioventricular bypass tracts.

The pathophysiology of mitral valve prolapse is similar to that of mitral regurgitation; thus, similar hemodynamic changes will be seen. The mitral valve leaflets are myxomatous, weakening the valves' ventricular surface and thus allowing the valve to protrude toward the atrium. In most cases there is no apparent cause and consequently the prolapse is idiopathic (Vanden Belt and Ronan, 1979).

If progressive mitral regurgitation occurs and becomes severe enough, valve replacement is necessary. Surgical correction of mitral valve prolapse without mitral regurgitation but with cardiac arrythmias has also been reported to be of benefit (Braunwald, 1980).

Prosthetic Cardiac Valves

The first insertion of a valve in the mitral position was performed by Albert Starr in 1960 (Arfan, 1983). Since that time, several valves have been designed to improve hemodynamics. Currently there are four functional categories of prosthetic heart valves: (1) caged ball, (2) caged disk, (3) tilting disk, and (4) tissue valves (Fig. 28–23). Selection of the type of valve is influenced by several factors. These include age, sex, heart size, hemodynamics, or contraindications to anticoagulation therapy. For selecting a valve, several broad guidelines are suggested (Guyton, 1982).

Tissue valves are suitable for:
1. Patients with absolute contraindications to anticoagulation therapy, such as those with bleeding tendencies, athletes, patients who will not reliably take anticoagulants, women of childbearing age.
2. Patients with short life expectancies.

Mechanical valves are suitable for:
1. Patients with a long life expectancy.
2. Patients with no contraindications to coagulation therapy.
3. Patients with small left ventricles or aortic root.
4. Children.
5. Patients with chronic renal disease or altered calcium metabolism.

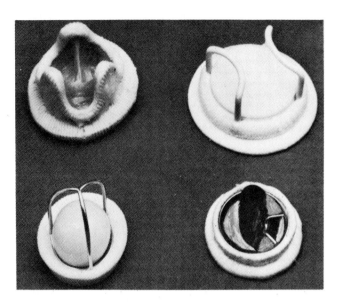

Figure 28–23. Four prosthetic heart valves. From upper left clockwise: (1) Porcine xenograft (pig aortic valve fixed in glutaraldehyde attached to sewing ring) used for aortic, mitral, or tricuspid valve replacement. (2) Caged-disk (Beall) valve used for mitral valve replacement. The lower cloth ring is designed for suturing in the atrioventricular annulus. (3) Tilting disk semicentral flow valve (Björk-Shiley) used for mitral or aortic valve replacement. The disk is shown in the full open position. Sutures are placed in the lower cloth ring. (4) Caged-ball valve with Silastic poppet (Starr-Edwards Model 1260) used for aortic valve replacement. With some modification, this valve is used in the mitral position as well. The porcine, Beall and Starr-Edwards valves are shown in the closed position. (*From Vanden Belt RJ, Ronan JA, et al: Cardiology: A Clinical Approach, 1979. Courtesy of Year Book Med Pub.*)

Indication for Placement. The proper selection of patients about to undergo valvular surgery must be made with the patient's natural history in mind. Clearly, those patients who have aortic stenosis and suddenly develop symptoms should be operated on immediately to avoid rapid deterioration and high mortality. Braunwald suggests that a drop in the mortality rate of patients with aortic stenosis from 50 to 5 percent or less has been achieved with timely aortic valve replacement (Braunwald, 1980). Patients with aortic regurgitation may have severe left ventricular dysfunction and yet be devoid of symptoms, so it is imperative that these patients be evaluated frequently to determine the best time for replacement. Generally speaking, cardiac catheterization is indicated in patients with LVEDP exceeding 5 mm Hg or more on two successive echocardiograms and replacement is recommended at this time because the majority of patients usually develop symptoms in two to three years (Henry et al, 1980).

In patients with mitral regurgitation, the presence of symptoms is a strong indication that replacement may be necessary. The degree of ventricular dysfunction may be misleading in these patients. If the ejection fractions are evaluated, a moderate reduction may indicate significant dysfunction. The full extent of the dysfunction may be apparent only postoperatively when the afterload imposed on the left ventricle increases as mitral competence is restored. Mortality rates higher than average should be expected for patients with advanced left ventricular dysfunction, as well as for those undergoing mitral valve replacement on emergency basis, such as patients with ruptured chordae tendineae (caused by bacterial endocarditis, mitral valve prolapse, trauma), postinfarction rupture of a papillary muscle, or intractable infective endocarditis (Arfan, 1983).

Mitral stenosis, on the other hand, is not as rapidly progressive as regurgitation and can be treated medically for long periods of time. If possible, commissurotomy should take preference to replacement if surgery is required. Replacement is required if the valvular opening is significantly reduced.

Complications. The complications of valve replacement are generally the same regardless of the type of valve used.

Thromboembolism. The threat of thromboemboli formation with mechanical valves is ever present; however, the incidence is rare with the tissue valve. Long-term anticoagulation therapy is required for all patients with mechanical valves, whether aortic or mitral, and should not be interrupted for elective surgical procedures of any nature. Tissue valves are generally nonthrombogenic and usually do not require anticoagulation therapy. If, however, the patient has an increased susceptibility to thromboembolism, such as atrial fibrillation, large left atrium, clots detected intraoperatively, or low cardiac output states, anticoagulation therapy should be instituted, especially if mitral replacement is being considered (Arfan, 1983).

Endocarditis. The average incidence of prosthetic valve endocarditis is 1 to 4 percent and is not significantly different in mechanical or tissue valves (Arfan, 1983). Between 36 and 53 percent of these cases are documented within two months of surgical implantation and are described as early prosthetic valve endocarditis (McClung et al, 1983). The organisms most commonly involved are *Staphylococcus aureus* or *S. epidermidis. Streptococcus* and gram-negative organisms are less commonly noted. The infection usually involves the suture line and is highly virulent, with reported mortality rates as high as 87 percent, regardless of the mode of therapy employed (Ferrans et al, 1979). Those patients who develop late endocarditis, especially with a streptococcus infection, fare better, with the mortality significantly decreased.

Tissue valve endocarditis has a higher success rate for treatment, which is believed to result from the location of the infection. Mechanical valve endocarditis usually involves the subvalvular cardiac tissue, whereas tissue valve infection is frequently limited to the cusps of the prosthesis (Ferrans et al, 1979).

Hemolysis. Formed blood element destruction is a complication of all mechanical cardiac valves and occasionally leads to the development of anemia. The incidence is related to turbulence of blood flow across the prosthesis. Laboratory evidence of hemolysis is noted more frequently in patients with aortic than with mitral stenosis, especially if a paravalvular leak is present (Ferrans et al, 1979).

Flow Obstruction. The incidence of flow obstruction is greatest in the caged disk valve design and least with the tissue valve. Roberts has demonstrated significant intimal proliferation in the aortic root of patients with the caged disk design and fibrous tissue deposition in the coronary ostia (McClung et al, 1983).

Regurgitation. The volume of backflow varies with the particular valve design. Backflow associated with prosthetic heart valves falls into two categories, (1) closure backflow (which is required to close the valve), and (2) leakage backflow (which occurs after the valve is closed) (Dellsperger et al, 1983). Regurgitation is dependent on heart rate and cardiac output. During tachycardia, closure backflow dominates, whereas, during bradycardia, leakage backflow dominates. Regurgitation varies inversely with cardiac output (Dellsperger et al, 1983). Tachycardia and decreased cardiac output puts backflow increase the energy expended tremendously, and a valve designed to reduce energy requirements by low closure backflow is desirable. The bradycardic patient requires a valve with little or no leakage backflow because the total backflow may be as high as 75 percent with leakage.

Preanesthetic Evaluation. The patient with valvular heart disease should be scrutinized closely for the degree of cardiac impairment. Symptoms such as chest pain, arrythmias, and syncope indicate difficulties with oxygen balance; dyspnea, edema, and orthopnea point to a failing myocardium.

Careful screening of laboratory results will also provide information about the depth of disease. Information about normal blood pressure, respiratory patterns, and presence of arrythmias should be noted.

Inotropic agents, diuretics, beta blockers, and vasodilators are employed in the medical management of these patients. Specific drugs and dosages should be noted in case intraoperative continuation is necessary.

Unlike the heavy sedation that is required for the patient with CAD, light premedication is preferred in this group of patients. Because of the limited cardiac reserve, these patients are very susceptible to cardiac- and respiratory-depressant drugs. Atropine must be eliminated because of its ability to increase heart rate. Selection of an anesthetic agent, once again, depends on the degree of cardiac impairment. The patients with valvular heart disease present a problem to the anesthetist because the degree of decompensation may be difficult to determine or the degree of compensation may be easily interrupted by hemodynamic change. Myocardial depression should be avoided, as well as increases in heart rate. Potent inhalation agents that depress the myocardium and provide junctional rhythms or muscle relaxants that increase heart rate obviously should not be included in the anesthetic regimen.

Anesthetizing patients with valvular heart disease requires maintenance of myocardial function, hemodynamic stability, and optimum working conditions for the surgeon

For these goals to be accomplished effectively, the nature of lesion, the stress imposed on the circulatory system, and the compensatory mechanisms must be understood.

When considering anesthesia for these cases, the anesthetist should be concerned with control of heart rate, regulation of intravascular volume, and regulation of stress imposed on the circulatory system.

Cardiac output is determined by two factors, (1) heart rate, and (2) SV, and control of output is essential. Because heart rate is one of the major determinants of MVO_2, maintenance of a normal heart rate is important because there is a decrease in myocardial oxygen delivery. Tachycardia will decrease the total time for diastole, thus decreasing the time for ventricular filling. A reduction in cardiac output follows. Selection of an anesthetic technique that will not interfere with heart rate is imperative. This is of particular concern when a muscle relaxant is being selected. Propranolol or digitalis may be necessary for optimal control of heart rate.

Usually, with a stenotic valve, SV is limited. Bradycardia will drastically reduce cardiac output because of this limited SV. SV is influenced by three factors: preload, afterload, and contractility. Because volume cannot be measured clinically, a measure of ventricular filling pressure is used. Measurement of CVP correlates well with right ventricular filling pressure and measurement of PCWP correlates well with left ventricular filling pressures. The anesthetist must remember that the relationship with volume and pressure will vary with different disease states. In aortic stenosis, the compliance is decreased, but with chronic volume overload such as with mitral or aortic regurgitation, compliance is markedly increased (Miller, 1986). In a highly compliant ventricle, large changes in volume may not be reflected accurately by changes in ventricular filling pressure, and small shifts in volume may be accompanied by large changes in ventricular filling pressures in stiff ventricles (Hug, 1981).

Mitral Stenosis. Anesthetic considerations are as follows: (1) Control of heart rate is of paramount importance. Drug therapy may be necessary to keep the rate within normal limits. (2) Ventricular filling pressures must be maintained. However, it must be remembered that both PCWP and left atrial pressure are greater than LVEDP in the presence of mitral stenosis because of the pressure gradient across the mitral valve (Kaplan, 1979; Hug, 1981). (3) If pulmonary hypertension exists, the deleterious effects of anesthetics on the pulmonary circulation must be considered. Pulmonary vasoconstriction induced by anesthetic agents causes right ventricular strain or failure and must be avoided. The use of nitrous oxide should be avoided in patients where there is suspected or determined pulmonary hypertension because of nitrous oxide's tendency to increase pulmonary artery pressure. The use of vasodilators may be considered. (4) Changes in position, especially to the Trendelenburg, are poorly tolerated because of increased blood flow to the lungs, which can result in impaired oxygenation or pulmonary edema. (5) Ventricular contractility is usually not of clinical significance (Kaplan, 1983). Table 28–15 lists the steps in the surgical procedure for replacement of a mitral valve.

TABLE 28–15. SURGICAL PROCEDURE FOR CORRECTION OF MITRAL VALVE PATHOLOGY

1. Median sternotomy.
2. Left atriotomy performed.
3. Valve excised with chordac tendineae and apices of papillary muscle.
4. Prosthesis is sutured for tying into atriotomy.
5. Valve lowered into annulus.
6. Valve holder removed, sutures tied.
7. Cannulas removed and pericardium closed.

From Cooley DA, Norman JC: Techniques in Cardiac Surgery, 1975. Courtesy of Texas Medical Press.

Mitral Regurgitation. The patient who develops acute mitral regurgitation is at considerable risk from sudden, significant changes in hemodynamic status. Of prime importance is the degree of pulmonary involvement secondary to increased left atrial pressure. If these changes exist, the same principles of pulmonary protection apply as do for mitral stenosis.

Compensating increases in sympathetic nervous system activity exist with right heart failure. Tachycardia and increased SVR exacerbate the regurgitant flow (Kaplan, 1983). Chronic mitral regurgitation has little effect on the pulmonary vasculature, and heart failure develops only late in the disease process.

The anesthetist should strive for (1) maintenance of normal heart rate, (2) afterload reduction with vasodilators to increase cardiac output and reduce SVR (3) reduction of heart size with inotropic agents if necessary, and (4) avoidance of cardiac-depressant drugs.

Aortic Stenosis (Pressure Overload on Left Ventricle). Patients who exhibit symptoms of aortic stenosis are usually considered high risks. Normal heart rate helps maintain ventricular filling and normal cardiac output. Adequate ventricular filling becomes increasingly dependent on sufficient intravascular volume and maintenance of normal sinus rhythm, which may account for up to 40 percent of ventricular filling via the atrial booster pump effect (Balasoraswathi et al, 1982).

These patients may be on diuretic therapy and thus suffer from reduced intravascular volume. Adequate hydration is essential to avoid hypotensive episodes. Also, they are especially at risk from peripheral vasodilation, which can produce sudden and profound hypotension, thus impairing both cerebral and coronary perfusion (Kaplan, 1979; Balasoraswathi et al, 1982).

Any hemodynamic change that will cause myocardial ischemia, such as tachyarrythmias or hypotension, must be avoided. Bradycardia must also be avoided, once again, because it limits SV.

Aortic Regurgitation (Volume Overload on Left Ventricle). Patients with mild-to-moderate aortic insufficiency should have a slightly elevated heart rate to reduce ventricular distention (by decreasing LVEDP) and to reduce oxygen consumption (Balasoraswathi et al, 1982). Bradycardia should be avoided because it predisposes to ventricular distention and subsequent pulmonary congestion (Balaso-raswathi et al, 1982). Blood pressures are very labile and unresponsive to vasoactive agents. Vasodilator therapy can be used if it is done judiciously and, in fact, is desirable to decrease ventricular afterload, increasing forward cardiac output and decreasing regurgitant volume.

Caution should be exercised to avoid vasoconstriction and increased SVR, which will reduce effective cardiac output. Table 28–16 lists the steps in the surgical procedure for replacement of the aortic valve.

Ventricular Septal Defect. Ventricular septal defects occur in the adult as a complication to myocardial infarction. The incidence is 1 to 2 percent (Gilboney, 1983). Ventricular septal defect is a communication that allows blood to be shunted from the left to the right ventricle. Its size determines the physiologic alterations that occur. Ventricular septal defects (VSD) are categorized as either restricted or nonrestricted. A restricted VSD is one in which the amount of blood that is shunted is regulated by the size of the defect; in the nonrestricted it is not (Gilboney, 1983). The magnitude and direction of the shunt across a VSD depends upon the size of the defect and the pressure gradient across it during the various phases of the cardiac cycle (Gilboney, 1983). When the defect is small, it offers considerable resistance to flow, and slight variations in the size of the defect are accompanied by large variations in the rate of flow (or shunting) (Braunwald, 1980). When the defect is large, it offers little resistance to flow, and small pressure differences between left and right ventricle result in shunting (Braunwald, 1980).

When left-to-right shunting exists, pulmonary blood flow is increased above normal and systemic blood flow. Both left and right ventricle are overworked, resulting in hypertrophy. As a result of elevated left atrial pressures and pulmonary venous pressures, pulmonary resistance increases and pulmonary hypertension results. The severity of increased resistance can be defined by the absolute level of the pulmonary vascular resistance (which is mean pulmonary arterial pressure minus mean left atrial pressure, divided by cardiac index [CI]) or simply of total pulmonary resistance (mean pulmonary arterial pressure divided by CI). If the pulmonary resistance is severely elevated, the flow across the septal defect is usually bidirectional and of about equal magnitude in the two directions, or may

TABLE 28–16. SURGICAL PROCEDURE FOR CORRECTION OF AORTIC VALVE PATHOLOGY

1. Median sternotomy.
2. Transverse aortotomy incision above right coronary artery.
3. Traction sutures placed at the three commissural points.
4. Interrupted sutures are placed, marking three groups of sutures for each cusp.
5. Valve holder removed after valve is seated.
6. Sutures tied.
7. Aortotomy repair.

From Cooley DA, Norman JC: Techniques in Cardiac Surgery, 1975. Courtesy of Texas Medical Press.

TABLE 28–17. SURGICAL PROCEDURE FOR CORRECTION OF VENTRICULAR SEPTAL DEFECT

1. Median sternotomy.
2. Area of infarction excised along with necrotic septal tissue creating interventricular communication.
3. Dacron patch is used to repair the septum and is placed on the left ventricular side of the septum.
4. Felt pledgets are sutured to margins of the ventricular incisions.
5. Ventriculorrhaphy closed.

From Cooley DA, Norman JC: Techniques in Cardiac Surgery, 1975. Courtesy of Texas Medical Press.

be right to left, depending on the exact relation between pulmonary and SVR (Braunwald, 1980).

Because the occurrence of VSD in the adult is rapid, it is usually seen in conjunction with cardiogenic shock.

It is best to manage these patients medically until the hemodynamic parameters are stable; then surgical intervention is desirable. The surgical procedure is described in Table 28–17. The anesthetic management consists of maintenance of these normal hemodynamic parameters with anesthetic agents and techniques that will not decrease ventricular function or increase the workload of the myocardium.

Multivalvular Disease. Multivalvular involvement is common, particularly in patients with rheumatic heart disease, and a variety of clinical and hemodynamic syndromes can be produced by different combinations of valvular abnormalities (Braunwald, 1980).

MITRAL STENOSIS AND AORTIC REGURGITATION. Approximately 10 percent of patients with mitral stenosis have severe aortic regurgitation (Braunwald, 1980). Recognition of the dual problem may be missed because of the presence of aortic regurgitation symptoms may mask those of stenosis.

MITRAL STENOSIS AND AORTIC STENOSIS. If these two disease entities coexist, the mitral stenosis and its sequelae usually mask the presence of aortic stenosis. It is vital to recognize the presence of hemodynamically significant aortic valvular disease preoperatively in patients about to undergo surgical correction of mitral stenosis, because isolated mitral commissurotomy may be hazardous in such patients; this operation can impose a sudden hemodynamic load on the left ventricle that may lead to acute pulmonary edema (Braunwald, 1980).

AORTIC STENOSIS AND MITRAL REGURGITATION. The presence of aortic stenosis and mitral regurgitation produces complications that are life-threatening. Obstruction to left ventricular outflow, on the one hand, augments the volume of mitral regurgitant flow, while the presence of mitral regurgitation, on the other, diminishes the ventricular preload necessary for maintenance of left ventricular SV in aortic stenosis (Braunwald, 1980). Significant reductions in cardiac output and symptoms of venous hypertension ensue.

AORTIC REGURGITATION AND MITRAL REGURGITATION. This combination is frequent, and the symptoms of aortic regurgitation usually manifest. When both leaks are severe, blood may reflux from the aorta all the way through both chambers of the left heart into the pulmonary veins (Braunwald, 1980).

DOUBLE VALVE REPLACEMENT. The incidence of operative mortality is high for surgical replacement of two valves in comparison to that for the replacement of one.

Idiopathic Hypertrophic Subaortic Stenosis. Idiopathic hypertrophic subaortic stenosis (IHSS) is a muscular obstruction to left ventricular outflow resulting in assymetric hypertrophy of the interventricular septum. During systole, the hypertrophied outflow tract muscle often narrows sufficiently to obstruct left ventricular ejection (Paulson, 1971). The etiology behind IHSS has not been fully determined. The incidence is higher in men than women. There is no ventricular filling, wall stiffness increases, and an increase in MV_{O_2} occurs. The obstruction usually becomes severe enough to cause left ventricular failure. Symptoms include dyspnea, angina, fatigue, and syncope.

Approximately two-thirds of the patients respond to propranolol therapy and require no surgical intervention. Propranolol reduces oxygen consumption and prevents increase in outflow obstruction that occurs with physical activity.

If beta blockade is not successful in relieving symptoms, surgical intervention is necessary. The goal is relief of obstruction, and this may be accomplished by reducing the hypertrophied myocardium or by mitral valve replacement. The myocardium is reduced by septectomy. The surgical procedure is described in Table 28–18.

With left septectomy, care must be taken not to damage the anterior leaflet of the mitral valve and to avoid injury to major construction bundles in the ventricular system (Cooley and Norman, 1976). Left bundle branch block is a common complication to this procedure.

The procedure for mitral valve replacement of IHSS is the same as for replacement required by other pathologic conditions. With replacement, conduction defects are not manifested.

Tricuspid Regurgitation. Tricuspid regurgitation is commonly associated with rheumatic heart disease; therefore it may accompany other valvular diseases. The venous pressure is frequently elevated. Atrial fibrillation is present because of mitral stenosis. These patients have a murmur over the lower left sternal border. Because of cardiac cirrhosis, splenomegaly, jaundice, and a dragging pain in the right upper quadrant may develop. The most common problem is right ventricular failure and pulmonary hypertension.

Replacement of severely leaking tricuspid valves is determined by the patient's hemodynamic status. Often, once the left-sided lesion is repaired, symptoms may be alleviated. This may not be determined until the time of surgery.

Sometimes when it is impossible for a postoperative patient to get along without the pump oxygenator, an acute increase in tricuspid regurgitation may be the cause. There is difference of opinion about how often the minimally diseased but severely leaking tricuspid valve needs to be replaced, but there is no doubt that such replacements may sometimes be lifesaving (Hurst and Logue, 1970).

Pericarditis. Pericarditis is an inflammation of the visceral or parietal pericardium or both. Some of the causes of pericarditis include acute rheumatic fever, infection, acute myocardial infarction, trauma, metastatic tumor, uremia, and tuberculosis.

The pathologic development of pericarditis is as follows. The pericardium is a double-layered sac that surrounds the heart. The inner layer (the visceral pericardium) lines the surface of the heart itself. The outer layer (parietal pericardium) is continuous with the great vessels of the heart. These two layers are separated by a potential space that contains approximately 5 ml of fluid.

When the pericardium is subject to infection or trauma, an inflammatory response occurs, with exudate formation and effusion. If the involvement is extensive, enough fluid may accumulate in the pericardial space to restrict ventricular filling. Slow fluid accumulation usually does not present a problem because the pericardium is able to accommodate to the stretch. Rapid fluid accumulation, on the other hand, can produce tamponade, which will restrict blood flow to the ventricle and cause a decrease in cardiac output. Other symptoms may include elevated venous pressure and decreased arterial pressure.

As the pericardium heals, it becomes thickened and scarred, resulting in a decrease in ventricular filling. Pericardial friction rub, venous distention, peripheral edema, and hepatomegaly ensue with this "constrictive" pericarditis.

Electrocardiographic changes include ST segment elevation similar to that associated with myocardial infarction. Atrial arrythmias, such as premature atrial contraction or atrial fibrillation are common, especially with acute pericarditis. Pericardial effusion is noted on chest x-ray.

Constrictive pericarditis is best treated surgically. If the ventricular involvement is minimal, a pericardectomy can be performed. The operative procedure can usually be done satisfactorily without the use of cardiopulmonary bypass. However, pump standby is recommended.

TABLE 28–18. SURGICAL PROCEDURE FOR CORRECTION OF IDIOPATHIC HYPERTROPHIC SUBAORTIC STENOSIS

Left Septectomy

1. Ascending aorta is excised and leaflets are retracted to visualize the muscular ridge.
2. Septum is excised with care to not damage the anterior leaflet of the mitral valve.
3. If right bundle-branch block exists, only a wedge of tissue should be removed.

Right Septectomy

1. Septum is exposed via right ventriculotomy.
2. Aortotomy is performed and left index inserted into aortic valve to prevent perforation of the septum.
3. Anterior septum is excised with care so as not to injure the pulmonary valve.

From Cooley DA, Norman JC: Techniques in Cardiac Surgery, 1975. Courtesy of Texas Medical Press.

SURGERY FOR CONDUCTION SYSTEM DEFECTS

The conduction system (Fig. 28–24) in its broadest sense comprises the entire heart; in its narrowest sense includes the sinoatrial (S-A) node and its approaches, the atrial preferential pathways, the approaches to the atrioventricular (A-V) node, the A-V bundle (bundle of His), the bundle branches, and the peripheral Purkinje nets (Chung, 1978).

The S-A node is a crescent-shaped muscle that rests between the superior vena cava and the right atrial appendage. It is located directly beneath the pericardium and contains specialized cells, P cells, which are responsible for its pacing activity.

The approaches to the S-A node consist of ordinary atrial cells, which connect to Bachmann's bundle and the atrial preferential pathways. There are three pathways: (1) the anterior pathway, which begins at Bachmann's bundle and proceeds to the superior aspect of the A-V node, (2) the middle pathway, which begins at the middle and inferior parts of the S-A node and proceeds to the superior aspect of the A-V node, and (3) the inferior pathway, which proceeds from the posterior aspect of the S-A node to the inferior portion of the A-V node.

It must be emphasized that alternate routes are available from the S-A to the A-V node without use of the preferential pathways.

Approaches to the A-V node (transitional zone) consist of a region of myocardium superior and distal to the mouth of the coronary sinus, whose fibers enter the distal portion of the A-V node (Gilboney, 1983).

The A-V node is situated by the coronary sinus and the tricuspid valve, just beneath the endocardium. The fibers are elastic in character and distally arrange themselves to form the A-V bundle. The A-V node is divided into three regions: (1) the A-N region at the crest of the A-V node, (2) the N region, which is the middle portion, and (3) the terminal portion in the N-H or bundle of His region. Tissue sample studies of the N region show this area to be incapable of automaticity, whereas the A-N and N-H

regions are capable of spontaneous depolarization but at a slower rate than the S-A node. Because of these specialized regions, these rhythms are called junctional; there is no anatomic basis for the terms upper, middle, and lower nodal rhythms (Jones, 1980).

Fibers from the A-V node then form the bundle of His, situated between the aortic valve, which divides immediately into a left and right bundle branch, which further subdivide into the Purkinje network.

The right and left bundle branches conduct to all of the right and left ventricles respectively. The left ventricle is the first to be depolarized because the left bundle branch divides sooner than the right, thus permitting a wave of depolarization to reach the left ventricle sooner than the right (Jones, 1980).

The electrical voltage causing depolarization and repolarization of the cardiac cell is dependent on the concentration of the sodium and potassium that surround the cell membrane. Sodium is the predominant extracellular ion. Potassium is primarily an intracellular ion. The cell membrane is more permeable to potassium; differences across the cell membrane create a gradient for electrical energy.

When the cell is at rest, it is polarized. Upon receipt of an impulse, the permeability of the cardiac cell membrane changes, and sodium influx occurs. This phase, termed depolarization, continues until membrane potential has been reached and muscle contraction occurs. As a result, sodium efflux follows. In an attempt to maintain homeostasis, the cell resumes its normal order, i.e., sodium outside and potassium inside, and the cell is once again polarized.

It is during the phase of depolarization that the cell is vulnerable to stimuli; however, during early repolarization, no stimulus, regardless of its strength, will propagate an impulse. This interval is termed the absolute refractory period. As repolarization continues, a strong or perpetual stimulus can initiate an impulse. This phase is termed the relative refractory phase. And toward the end of the relative refractory phase, in the supernormal phase, the smallest impulse can propagate a response.

Depolarization and repolarization states produce changes in the electrical current within the cell membrane. The changes are called action potentials and are the result of sudden changes in sodium and potassium permeability. At rest, the potential is normally −90 mV. When sufficient sodium ions have rushed into the cell carrying positive charges (reverse potential), the negative resting potential becomes obsolete. This loss of negativity (depolarization) initiates potassium efflux, removing positively charged ions from inside the cell, creating a normal negative resting potential (repolarization).

During the reverse potential, the fiber becomes positive to a +45 mV, during depolarization negative to −60 mV, and back to −90 mV during repolarization.

The electrical voltage of the cardiac cells is transmitted to the body surfaces and magnified by electrocardiography. The ECG represents a cardiac cycle. The first positive deflection is the P wave, which represents atrial depolarization, followed by a flat line, which signifies delay of impulse through the A-V node. The next is a negative deflection, the Q wave, followed by a positive R, then a negative S wave. This entire QRS complex signifies ventricular depo-

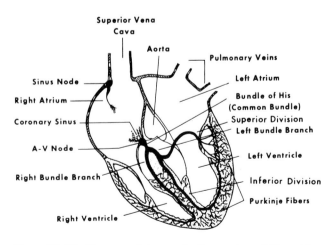

Figure 28–24. Diagram of the conduction system. A-V = atrioventricular. (*From Chung EK: Artificial Cardiac Pacing: A Practical Approach, 1978. Courtesy of Williams & Wilkins and the author.*)

Superior Vena
Cava

Aorta

Pulmonary Veins

Left Atrium

Sinus Node

Right Atrium

Bundle of His
(Common Bundle)
Superior Division
Left Bundle Branch

Coronary Sinus

A-V Node

Left Ventricle

Right Bundle Branch

Inferior Division

Purkinje Fibers

Right Ventricle

larization. The last deflection is positive, the T wave, and is preceded by a flat line, the ST segment. Both the T wave and ST segment also indicate ventricular depolarization. Figure 28–25 represents normal intervals in seconds for each of these electrical events. If prolongation occurs, it indicates a delay in the atrial or ventricular conduction system, depending on which interval is affected. ST segment and T-wave deflections are either elevated or depressed when ischemia or myocardial damage is present.

Conduction Disturbances

Abnormalities of electrical conduction can occur for many reasons. The conduction can be affected either directly or indirectly by disease processes, by drug effect, electrolyte imbalance, or as a complication of open heart surgery.

The S-A node is perfused by the right coronary artery in 60 percent of the population and by the left circumflex in 40 percent, so any disturbance in perfusion to these areas will compromise blood flow to the S-A node, causing atrial dysrhythmias.

Because of its location, the S-A node is vulnerable to the inflammatory process that is associated with pericarditis. Lupus may cause inflammatory changes that affect the S-A node.

Pharmacologically induced vagal stimulation can be responsible for bradyarrhythmias. The S-A node can also be damaged during cannulation procedures for aortocoronary bypass.

If the right coronary artery is occluded, disturbances will be seen in the A-V node, bundle of His, and bundle branches. As mentioned previously, the right coronary artery supplies the A-V node in 90 percent of hearts, whereas the remaining 10 percent is supplied by the left circumflex.

The sequence of events (sinus bradycardia, nausea and vomiting, and A-V block) frequently seen with inferior myocardial infarction can be linked to ischemia or edema of the A-V node when the right coronary artery is occluded (Jones, 1980). The block is usually transient and may be

treated pharmacologically, but if residual block occurs, artificial pacing may be necessary.

Valvular disease, primarily in the form of calcification, may intrude on normal conduction tissue and cause dysrhythmias. The location of the A-V node and the distal conduction system relative to the tricuspid valve, aortic valve, and mitral annulus make it vulnerable to disease processes in these structures (Jones, 1980). Tumors, sarcoidosis, myocarditis, and syphilis have all been known to affect normal conductivity.

Primary heart block is a degenerative disease process that is fibrotic or sclerotic in nature and is usually seen in patients over 60 years of age (Jones, 1980). Heart block is frequently induced after open heart surgery, especially after ventricular septal defect repair or aortic and tricuspid replacement because of edema or damage to the A-V node. Pacing may be required to alleviate symptoms.

Conduction defects caused by drug toxicity or electrolyte imbalance can usually be treated by withdrawing the drug or correcting the imbalance.

There are two types of conduction disorders that may require pacemaker insertion: (1) those caused by delayed impulse formation and (2) those caused by a conduction delay.

Conduction Disorders Caused by Delayed Impulse Formation

1. Sinus bradycardia occurs when the rate of the S-A node falls below 60 beats/min. It is caused by vagal stimulation, acute myocardial infarction, or degenerative disease of the S-A node. It is frequently found in athletes. Pharmacologic intervention is reserved for those people who present with symptoms. Therapy includes atropine or isoproterenol. Occasionally, a pacemaker may be required, especially if symptoms of low cardiac output persist.
2. S-A block is a disease state in which the S-A node is firing but the impulse to the atrium is blocked. It is caused by drug intoxication, infarction, ischemia, or vagal stimulation.
3. Sinus arrest occurs when the S-A node stops firing because of ischemia, infarct, diseased S-A node, vagal stimulation, or drug intoxication. Symptoms of decreased cardiac output occur and, if persistent, require a pacemaker.
4. Sick sinus syndrome: Sinus arrest, S-A block, persistent sinus bradycardia, rapid supraventricular tachycardia, and hypersensitive carotid sinus syndrome are usually classified under the term sick sinus syndrome (Jones, 1980). Not all of these arrythmias may occur. The sequence of events in this syndrome consists of a sudden onset of a supraventricular tachycardia, upon termination of which the sinus node does not return as the pacemaker for 4 to 5 seconds (Jones, 1980). Symptomatic tachyarrythmias may require pacemaker insertion.

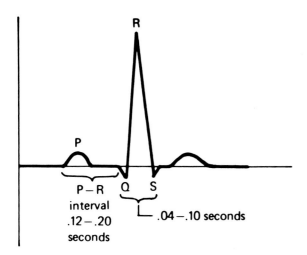

Figure 28–25. A normal electrographic complex identifying normal time intervals for the PR and QRS intervals. (*From Jones P: Cardiac Pacing, 1980. Courtesy of Appleton-Century-Crofts.*)

Conduction Delays. Blocks can occur in any of the specialized conduction tissue to interfere with A-V conduction. The degree of block varies and may be not only the result of anatomic disruption but may also be due to drug intoxication, ischemia, or metabolic processes. Heart block is probably the most common reason for pacemaker insertion.

A-V block may be either partial or complete. Incomplete, or partial, block includes first, second, and advanced block. A-V block may be transient or permanent and may vary in degree of block in the same individual. Chung classifies A-V block in Table 28–19.

First Degree A-V Block. First degree A-V block is present when the PR interval is prolonged beyond 0.20 seconds. In contrast to second and third degree block, each P wave is followed by a QRS complex at a constant PR interval (Vanden Belt and Ronan, 1979). With first degree block, A-V conduction is delayed either at the A-V junction or at the His bundle. The cause is a prolongation of the relative refractory period in the A-V junction. First degree block is the most common conduction abnormality and appears in healthy as well as diseased hearts. It is especially common in the elderly, who suffer degenerative processes of the conductive system. These patients are generally asymptomatic and require no treatment.

Second Degree A-V Block. Second degree A-V block conducts some but not all of the P waves, resulting in atrial impulses that fail to reach the ventricles, leaving absent QRS complexes. It occurs when the refractory periods of the A-V junctional tissue, both absolute and relative, are abnormally prolonged, but do not occupy the entire cardiac cycle (Chung, 1978). There are two types of second degree block:

TYPE I (WENCKEBACH OR MOBITZ I BLOCK). This block is caused by a diseased A-V node, drug effect, ischemia, vagal stimulation, or by myocardial infarction. It is characterized by a progressive lengthening of the PR interval until conduction of a QRS complex is obstructed. As a result, there are more P waves than QRS complexes. The occurrence of a blocked P wave preceded by a progressive lengthening of the PR interval is termed the Wenckebach phenomenon (Chung, 1978). Pacemaker therapy is required if there are symptoms of decreased peripheral perfusion or emergence of ventricular arrythmias caused by a slow rate.

TYPE II (MOBITZ II). Type II block does not present with a PR prolongation before a beat is dropped. There is no Wenckebach phenomenon. Its occurrence is far less frequent than

TABLE 28–19. CLASSIFICATION OF ATRIOVENTRICULAR BLOCKS

1 First degree
2. Second degree
(a) Wenckebach (Mobitz type I)
(b) Mobitz type II
(c) 2:1
3. High degree (advanced)
4. Complete (third degree)

From Chung EK: Artificial Cardiac Pacing: A Practical Approach, 1978. Courtesy of Williams & Wilkins and the author.

Mobitz I and symptoms are far more pronounced. It is associated with a high incidence of congestive failure or Adams-Stokes syndrome.

A 2:1 ratio is common. That is, one out of every two atrial impulses is blocked.

Advanced (High Degree Block). Advanced block presents as a P wave that occurs in more than a 2:1 A-V ratio; frequently seen are 4:1 or 6:1 ratios rather than odd-number ratios. In advanced A-V block, A-V junctional escape beats (and less commonly, ventricular escape beats) frequently appear as a physiologic mechanism, leading to incomplete A-V dissociation (Chung, 1978).

This is the most advanced incomplete A-V block. A-V junctional escape beats commonly control the ventricles. The atria are controlled by tachyarrythmias, such as atrial fibrillation or atrial flutter. Advanced block often results from Wenckebach or Mobitz Type II blocks.

Third Degree Block (Complete Block). Complete heart block exists when atrial impulses are not conducted to the ventricles and a pacemaker distal to the block controls the ventricles. In complete block, there is blockage at the A-V junction, the A-V bundle, or bilateral bundle branches. Independent atrial and ventricular activity occurs. The atrial rate is usually faster, with the ventricular rate usually only 20 to 40 beats per minute.

In complete A-V block, the prolonged refractory period occupies the entire cardiac cycle so that no relative refractory phase can occur.

The most common cause of complete A-V block is coronary artery disease. Other causes are acute inferior myocardial infarction, aortic stenosis, syphilis, or damage to the conduction system during cardiac surgery.

Bundle Branch Block. The His bundle gives rise to two bundle branches, the right and the left. The left bundle branch divides almost immediately into an anterior and posterior division. Therefore, the intraventricular conduction system has three pathways (fascicles): the right bundle branch, the left anterior, and the left posterior divisions. Blocks may occur in any of all of the fascicles (Fig. 28–26).

In bundle branch block, the impulse will be conducted via an intact bundle branch so that the ventricle with a blocked bundle branch will be activated later than the ventricle with the intact bundle branch (Chung, 1975). Therefore, instead of normal simultaneous activation of both ventricles, bundle branch block provides asynchronous activation of the two ventricles.

Bundle branch blocks are commonly associated with ventricular hypertrophy or with acute anterior myocardial infarction.

RIGHT BUNDLE BRANCH BLOCK (RBBB). If the right branch is blocked, the right ventricle receives its impulses late. The QRS is prolonged beyond 0.11 seconds and shows a R-S-R configuration.

LEFT BUNDLE BRANCH. If both branches of the conduction system to the left ventricle are blocked, a slow impulse spread across the ventricle is necessary for its activation. The QRS

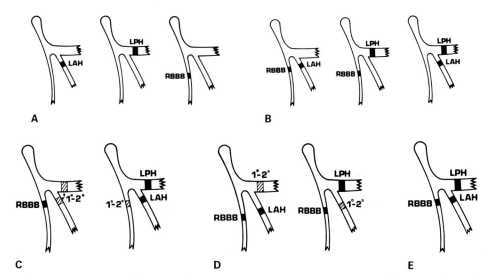

Figure 28–26. Diagrams illustrating the three forms of monofascicular block **(A)**, the three forms of bifascicular block **(B)**, incomplete trifascicular block (incomplete bilateral bundle branch block) **(C and D)**, and complete trifascicular block **(E)**. LAH = Left anterior hemiblock; LPH = left posterior hemiblock; RBBB = right bundle branch block. (*From Mangiola S, Ritota M: Cardiac Arrythmias: Practical ECG Interpretation, 1974. Courtesy of Lippincott.*)

is longer than 0.11 seconds, but there are no R waves. An abnormal sequence of depolarization from left to right septum occurs, with consequent interruption of repolarization. Thus, ST segment and T-wave abnormalities exist.

LEFT ANTERIOR HEMIBLOCK. Left anterior hemiblock (LAH) results in depolarization that travels inferiorly first and toward the right, thus inscribing a small Q in lead I and an R in lead III (Jones, 1980). The terminal forces will then spread superiorly and to the left, causing left axis deviation, an R wave in lead I, and a terminal S wave in lead III.[53] Left posterior hemiblock (LPH) produces the exact opposite phenomenon. Whereas LAH is more common than LPH, the incidence of development of advanced heart block in RBBB and LPH is 85 percent (Jones, 1980).

Treatment of Conduction Disturbances

Conduction disorders that cannot be controlled by medication may need pacemaker generation for relief of symptoms. There are several pacing generators available.

Types of Pacemaker Generations

Asynchronous. This generator is responsible only for the formation of electrical impulses and is used safely in patients who have no intrinsic ventricular activity. If used in those patients with ventricular activity, it may compete with the patient's own conduction system. If such competition occurs during the supranormal period of repolarization, ventricular tachycardia can result.

Synchronous. This generator contains two circuits, one that forms impulses, the other that acts as a sensor. When activated by an R wave, the sensing circuit either triggers

or inhibits the pacing circuit. These are classified as triggered or inhibited pacemakers. The inhibited is the most frequently used pacemaker because it eliminates competition and is energy sparing.

Sequential. This type of pacing facilitates a normal sequence between atrial and ventricular contraction, promoting the normal atrial kick.

Programmable. This is the newest type of pacemaker. As the name implies, it is programmable as well as operable on a fixed-function basis. Rate, output, and R wave sensitivity are the most common programmed areas. An advantage to the use of this type of generator is that it can overcome the interference caused by the electrocautery.

A three- and five-letter code system has been devised to simplify the naming of pacemaker generators. The letters used in this code are listed in Tables 28–20 and 28–21.

1. AOO and VOO are asynchronous generators that pace the atrium or ventricle respectively.
2. VVI is a synchrous generator that paces and senses in the ventricle. As implied, this generator is inhibited if a sinus or escape beat occurs.
3. DVI is used for A-V sequential pacing in which both the atria and ventricles are paced.

Mechanics of Pacing. Pacemakers provide the rhythm that the heart is incapable of producing. They may be either temporary (Table 28–22) or permanent (Table 28–23). Cardiac pacing consists of an external or internal power source and a lead to carry the current to the heart muscle. Batteries provide the power source. The pacing lead is a coiled wire spring that is encased in silicone to insulate it from body fluids.

TABLE 28–20. THREE-LETTER PACEMAKER CODES

Letter 1	Chamber paced
A	Atrium
V	Ventricle
D	Dual (both A and V)
Letter 2	Chamber sensed
A	Atrium
V	Ventricle
D	Dual (both A and V)
O	Asynchronous, or does not apply
Letter 3	Response to sensed signal
I	Inhibition
T	Triggering
O	Asynchronous, or does not apply

From Zaidan JR: Anesthesiology 60:321–323, 1984. Reproduced with permission.

Pacemakers are unipolar or bipolar. A unipolar lead has only one electrode, at its tip, that contacts the heart. This is the positive pole. The power source is the negative pole. If the pacemaker is temporary, a ground lead, sutured to the skin, is connected to the power source along with the pacing lead.

In the bipolar pacemaker, there are two electrodes at its tip, providing a built-in ground. There is more contact with the endocardium and the pacemaker requires lower current to pace.

The precise criteria for the use of temporary or permanent cardiac pacemakers vary slightly from institution to institution and from physician to physician. When selecting the proper mode of cardiac stimulation, the physician must have a proper awareness of the anatomy of the conduction system and the purpose of cardiac stimulation (Chung, 1978).

Ventricular Pacing

TEMPORARY VENTRICULAR PACING. Temporary ventricular pacing is indicated in short-term conduction defects until symptoms are abolished. It may be used in acute myocardial

TABLE 28–21. FIVE-LETTER PACEMAKER CODE

Letter 1	See Table 28–20
Letter 2	See Table 28–20
Letter 3	Responses to sensed signal
T	Triggered
I	Inhibited
O	Asynchronous
D	Dual (triggering and inhibition)
R	Reverse functions (activation of the generator by rapid heart rates rather than slow heart rates)
Letter 4	Programming
O	No programming
P	Programming only for output and/or rate
M	Multiprogrammable
Letter 5	Tachyarrhythmia functions

From Zaidan JR: Anesthesiology 60:321–323, 1984. Reproduced with permission.

TABLE 28–22. INDICATIONS FOR TEMPORARY PACING

1. Symptomatic second degree, high degree, and complete A-V block
2. Symptomatic bradyarrhythmias due to any mechanism as a result of acute myocardial infarction
3. Acute bifascicular or trifascicular block due to acute myocardial infarction
4. Sick sinus syndrome and brady-tachyarrhythmia syndrome
5. Symptomatic digitalis-induced bradyarrhythmias
6. Drug-resistant tachyarrhythmias
7. Carotid sinus syncope
8. Ventricular standstill
8. Before or during implantation of a permanent pacemaker
10. Therapeutic trial for intractable congestive heart failure, cardiogenic shock, and cerebral or renal insufficiency
11. Prophylactic pacing during and immediately after major cardiac surgery

A-V = antrioventricular.
From Chung EK: Artificial Cardiac Pacing: A Practical Approach, 1978. Courtesy of Williams & Wilkins and the author.

infarction when the patient exhibits conduction absences or conduction delays, to suppress tachyarrythmias, and after open heart surgery.

Transvenous pacing electrodes can be inserted into the subclavian, jugular, or basilic veins through the superior vena cava into the right atrium and through the tricuspid valve into the right ventricle. Once proper positioning has been verified, the electrode is connected to its power source and pulses will be generated.

Once the electrode is in place, a stimulation threshold must be determined. Threshold is defined as the minimum amount of electrical current necessary to produce a consistent cardiac depolarization when the inherent heart rate

TABLE 28–23. INDICATION FOR PERMANENT PACING

1. Sick sinus syndrome and brady-tachyarrhythmia syndrome
2. Mobitz type II A-V block
3. Complete or advanced A-V block
   - Due to trifascicular block
   - Congenital in origin
   - Surgically induced (irreversible)
   - Lasting more than 2–3 weeks in acute myocardial infarction
   - All other chronic and symptomatic A-V blocks
4. Symptomatic bilateral bundle branch blocks
5. Bifascicular block or incomplete trifascicular block with intermittent complete A-V block as a result of acute myocardial infarction
6. Carotid sinus syncope
7. Recurrent ventricular standstill
8. Recurrent drug-resistant tachyarrhythmias benefited by temporary pacing
9. Intractable congestive heart failure and cerebral or renal insufficiency benefitted by temporary pacing

A-V = atrioventricular.
From Chung EK: Artificial Cardiac Pacing: A Practical Approach, 1978. Courtesy of Williams & Wilkins and the author.

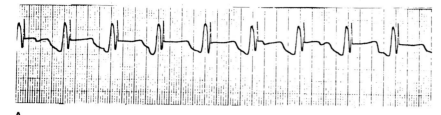

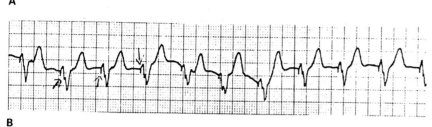

Figure 28–27. Ventricular pacing **(A)** with a unipolar catheter and 100 percent capture and **(B)** with a bipolar electrode. Note that pacer artifact in the bipolar tracing (indicated by arrows) is much more difficult to see than with a unipolar electrode. (*From Jones P: Cardiac Pacing, 1980. Courtesy of Appleton-Century-Crofts.*)

falls below a predetermined rate (Jones, 1980). If a ventricular response to stimulation is not observed on the ECG, then the current is of too low a magnitude.

Rate is predetermined according to the patient's need. If the rate falls below this predetermined figure, the demand mode will kick in and begin to pace. Figure 28–27 demonstrates unipolar and bipolar ventricular pacing patterns.

PERMANENT VENTRICULAR PACING. Permanent ventricular pacing is indicated for patients who suffer from congestive heart failure with associated dysrhythmias, postmyocardial infarction whereby the conduction system is permanently damaged, sinus arrest or sinus bradycardia with symptoms, Stokes-Adams syndrome, and fascicular block.

Atrial Pacing. Atrial pacing is designed for those patients with pure atrial arrythmias or with ventricular tachyarrythmias (Fig. 28–28). It is also of benefit to those patients with heart disease, in that it provides the atrial kick, thus increasing cardiac output. The atrial kick is lost with ventricular pacing because the atrial and ventricular contractions may not be sequential.

A major problem associated with atrial pacing is electrode instability. Because of the anatomic structure of the atrium (lack of trabeculae) the electrode cannot be secured and has a tendency to float, causing inconsistent pacing. This, plus inability to achieve a consistent atrial "demand" function and the unpredictable appearance of A-V conduc-

tion defects, has limited the use of pure atrial pacing (Chung, 1978). Consequently, an A-V sequential pacemaker was developed.

The A-V sequential pacemaker can be used both on a temporary and permanent basis. The sequential pacemaker consists of two stimulators, which are recycled by the sensing of the ventricular R wave but fire at a preset escape interval (Chung, 1978). The ventricular bipolar electrode subserves the dual function of sensing and stimulating, whereas the atrial bipolar electrode subserves stimulation only. By separately programming the two stimulators, the pacemaker is made to remain dormant while the electric R–R interval is shorter than the two escape intervals; it functions as an atrial pacer when the R–R interval is greater than the atrial escape interval, as an A-V sequential pacer when a block renders the A-V conduction period longer than the pacer's sequential interval, or as a ventricular pacer when the atrial electrode is not functioning, avoiding the danger of asystole from loss of control of the atrial electrode (Fig. 28–29) (Chung, 1978).

Permanent pacemakers may be inserted either transvenously or transthoracicly. The most serious complication of pacemaker insertion or implantation is ventricular fibrillation, especially in the asynchronous type of generator because of the R-on-T phenomenon.

Malfunction of the pacer may be due to broken or displaced electrodes or loss of generator power. Malfunctioning pacers may cause acceleration of pacing, deceleration of pacing, irregular pacing, or failure to sense and

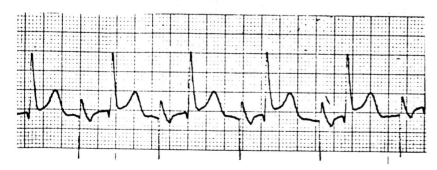

Figure 28–28. Atrial pacer firing 100 percent with 100 percent capture. (*From Jones P: Cardiac Pacing, 1980. Courtesy of Appleton-Century-Crofts.*)

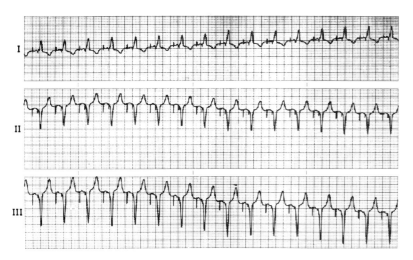

Figure 28–29. Bifocal demand pacemaker (sequential atrioventricular) rhythm. Note that there are two sets of artificial pacemaker spikes, one of which precedes the P waves, the other of which precedes the QRS complexes. (*From Chung EK: Artificial Cardiac Pacing: A Practical Approach, 1978. Courtesy of Williams & Wilkins and the author.*)

pace. The newer pacemaker generators are lithium-powered and should survive for a five-year period.

Both transvenous and transthoracic pacemakers can be inserted under local anesthesia with standby. The anesthetist must also keep in mind that there are several factors that will modify pacer function:

1. Sympathomimetic amines may increase myocardial irritability.
2. Quinidine or procainamide toxicity may cause failure of cardiac capture.
3. Hyperkalemia, advancement of heart disease, or fibrosis around the electrode may cause failure of cardiac capture.

The primary considerations for the anesthetist are patient comfort and control of dysrhythmia during insertion. Mild sedation with intravenous diazepam can be helpful in reducing anxiety. Once insertion is complete, proper functioning of the pacer should be determined. Capture is determined by the ECG tracing.

SURGERY FOR EXTRACRANIAL CEREBROVASCULAR DISEASE

It has been estimated that 500,000 victims are afflicted with strokes every year. Slightly less than half of these individuals die from this affliction, while one-fifth remain alive but disabled. The initial mortality of an ischemic stroke ranges from between 20 and 30 percent (Moore, 1983) and survivors remain at an inordinately high risk of subsequent stroke, estimated between 4.8 and 20 percent each year. Mortality in these patients is usually due to subsequent stroke or myocardial infarction.

Pathology

The causes of cerebrovascular disease of extracranial origin are usually classified as either flow-restrictive lesions or lesions with embolic potential. The most common lesion found in patients with cerebrovascular insufficiency is an athersclerotic plaque located at the carotid bifurcation, which produces symptoms by reducing blood flow to the hemisphere supplied or, more commonly, by releasing embolic material in the form of clot, platelet aggregate, or cholesterol crystals (Moore, 1983).

The carotid bifurcation appears to be prone to plaque formation because of the hemodynamic changes associated with flow through this area. The exact mechanism is not known; however, evidence derived from studies leans toward low flow velocity.

Once the intima of the vessel is injured from such alterations, platelets begin to accumulate along with lipoproteins in an effort to repair the injury. However, if the accumulation is of sufficient magnitude, plaque formation may occur and cause further injury.

Platelets play an important role in development of plaque. They may adhere to one another, to the diseased vessel, or both, leading to thrombus formation that may narrow the vessel lumen or dislodge, resulting in distal embolization.[38] Other events such as release from platelets of vasoactive substances that cause vasospasm will have an effect on lumen diameter.

When intima is injured, collagen is released and reacts with the platelets, which can initiate smooth muscle growth and intimal thickening. Platelets and collagen reactions also lead to the release of prostaglandins, specifically thromboxane A_2, a powerful vasoconstrictor, whose release aggravates plaque formation. Hemorrhage into a plaque is common and often associated with symptoms as flow restriction increases.

Clinical Symptoms. The clinical symptoms that develop in cerebrovascular occlusive disease are due to ischemia in a hemisphere or region of the brain. These symptoms can be classified into three stages: (1) transient ischemic attacks, characterized by transient episodes of sudden neurologic deficit, self-reversing in minutes to 24 hours, with no residual effects, although the risk of cerebral infarction is high if left untreated; (2) progressive stroke, characterized by a gradual increase in symptoms; and (3) complete stroke, whereby progression of symptoms has ceased but residual effects are present.

Motor symptoms include weakness or paralysis of one

or both limbs opposite the affected side. Sensory symptoms include numbness or paresthesia of the opposite limbs and side of the face.

Motor aphasia, transient loss or blurring of vision in the ipsilateral eye, confusion, or amnesia can occur with transient ischemia.

Cerebral Blood Flow

Anatomy. Blood supply to the brain is derived from arteries that originate at the aortic arch. The left common carotid arises from the aorta whereas the right arises from the innominate. The common carotid artery divides into the internal and external carotid arteries. The cerebral arteries arise from the internal carotid artery and the vertebral artery, which form the circle of Willis at the base of the brain. This anastomosis is formed anteriorly by the anterior cerebral arteries, connected by the anterior communicating, and posteriorly by two posterior cerebral arteries connected by the internal carotid on one side and the posterior communicating on the other. The posterior cerebral arteries are branches of the basilar arteries (Fig. 28–30).

The three trunks that supply each cerebral hemisphere arise from the circle of Willis. From its anterior part, the two cerebrals arise, from the anterolateral parts, the middle cerebrals arise, and from the posterior part, the posterior

cerebrals arise. Each of these main arteries branch into numerous vessels, which supply the entire brain.

The normal blood flow through the brain averages 50 to 55 ml/100 g of brain/min. This is roughly 750 ml/min or 15 percent of the cardiac output.

Physiology. Cerebral blood flow (CBF) is unique in that it has the ability to autoregulate. Autoregulation refers to the intrinsic capacity of the cerebral circulation to alter its resistance to maintain constant CBF over a range of cerebral perfusion pressure changes from 50 to 150 torr (Miller, 1986). Autoregulation may be abolished by hypercapnia, hypoxia, trauma, seizures, chronic hypertension, and deep anesthesia. For this reason, arterial pressure should not be permitted to fall below normal. Once autoregulation is lost, CBF becomes dependent upon perfusion pressure and blood volume. Any agent that is capable of producing vasodilation can modify autoregulation or cause the compensatory mechanism to be lost altogether. If such is the case, CBF becomes entirely blood-pressure-dependent. This reduction in the upper limits of autoregulation associated with anesthetic agents could potentiate a rapid elevation in intracranial pressure during episodes of extreme arterial hypertension (Miller, 1986).

CBF usually remains constant unless chemical interference takes place. CBF correlates well with the metabolic processes in the brain, and the concentrations of carbon dioxide, hydrogen ion, and oxygen have significant effects on CBF. Increases in CBF are caused by increases in P_{CO_2} and hydrogen ion and decreases in P_{O_2}.

Any substance that will increase brain acidity will increase CBF. When carbon dioxide combines with water to form carbonic acid, hydrogen ion dissociates, causing cerebral vasodilation and consequent increased CBF. The degree of vasodilation is proportional to the hydrogen ion concentration.

Increased hydrogen ion concentration greatly depresses neuronal activity; conversely, diminished hydrogen ion concentration increases neuronal activity (Engeilman and Levitsky, 1981). The compensatory vasodilation caused by rises in hydrogen ion concentration serves to flush acid and carbon dioxide away from the brain in an effort to maintain normal neuronal activity.

Hypoxia will cause a compensatory vasodilation in an effort to increase blood flow to the sensitive brain tissue. The brain uses approximately 3.5 ml of oxygen per 100 g of brain/min. If P_{O_2} levels fall below 30 mm Hg, CBF increases as a protective response.

In summary, the major factors that influence CBF are cerebral perfusion pressure (CPP = blood pressure minus intracranial pressure) and arterial blood gas tensions. It is most influenced by carbon dioxide arterial tension. CBF changes about 2 ml/100 g/min for each 1 torr change in $P_{a_{CO_2}}$; this response is attenuated below a $P_{a_{CO_2}}$ of 25 mm Hg and above a $P_{a_{CO_2}}$ of 100 torr (Table 28–24) (Miller, 1986).

Oxygen, on the other hand, has its greatest effect when $P_{a_{O_2}}$ levels are below 50 torr or above 300 torr, with maximum CBF at the lower limits of $P_{a_{O_2}}$.

CBF is markedly affected in patients with occlusive cerebrovascular disease. Areas of both high and low CBF

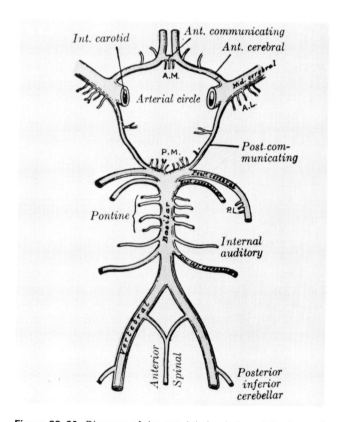

Figure 28–30. Diagram of the arterial circulation at the base of the brain. AL = anterolateral; AM = anteromedian; PL = posterolateral; PM = posteromedial ganglionic branches. (*From Gray H: Anatomy of The Human Body, 29th ed., Goss CM (ed.), 1973. Courtesy of Lea & Febiger, Philadelphia.*)

TABLE 28–24. CHEMICAL INFLUENCES ON CEREBRAL BLOOD FLOW

Chemical Influence	CBF
Hydrogen ion concentration	↑
Pao$_2$	↓
Paco$_2$	↑

have been observed to coexist with a loss of normal vasomotor responses (Miller, 1986). These take roughly four to six weeks to stabilize (Paulson, 1971). According to Miller, about one month after an occlusive vascular accident, anesthesia and surgery can be undertaken with about the same risk of inducing another stroke as existed immediately before the last episode (Miller, 1986).

Perfusion Phenomena. There are three types of perfusion phenomena associated with brain circulation:

Luxury Perfusion. This is a localized overabundant CBF associated with lactic acid production and hydrogen ion accumulation. In this situation, cerebral venous blood is hyperoxygenated, and variable losses in CBF autoregulation and carbon dioxide sensitivity occur (Miller, 1986).

Intracranial Steal Syndrome. The syndrome is a phenomenon whereby damaged areas of the brain may not react to arterial carbon dioxide changes. These damaged areas receive circulation according to perfusion pressure. Hypercarbia will thus cause vasodilation in normal cerebral vessels and divert blood from diseased to healthy areas (Wylie and Churchill-Davidson, 1972).

Robin Hood Syndrome. The syndrome occurs when normal vasculature is constricted and shunts blood to ischemic areas, increasing brain function.

Diagnosis

Carotid artery studies are either invasive or noninvasive. Noninvasive studies include the Doppler imaging technique.

Doppler Imaging. Doppler imaging uses a Doppler probe to determine stenotic lesions of the internal carotid artery. A two-dimensional image is created by moving the probe back and forth across the carotid. An image is created that normally should be smooth and without disruption. Ultrasound imaging is not possible if the vessel is severely calcified. If stenosis is present, the contour of the image is affected, and if occlusion is present, there will be absence of image from the occluded branch. Calcification of the vessels provides no image at all.

Computerized Tomography. Computerized tomography (CT) is extremely useful in determining whether symptoms are arising from pathologic causes other than extracranial cerebrovascular disease. It is routinely used as a workup in these patients before angiography. One advantage of having a CT scan available is identification of cerebral infarction and documentation of size and location.

Positive findings with these noninvasive studies warrant angiographic visualization to determine the exact location of the lesion, surgical accessibility, and whether a satisfactory distal vascular bed is present. Angiography should not be performed on a routine basis but if surgical correction is being considered or in patients who have focal neurologic symptoms and negative vascular laboratory findings.

Preoperative Evaluation

Preoperative evaluation of patients undergoing extracranial occlusive surgery is the same for any other major procedure. When thinking of atherosclerosis, one should not consider disease in various organs as separate entities, but all part of the same process, which proceeds at different rates in different parts of the arterial tree (Sabawala et al, 1970). Associated with atherosclerosis are such conditions as hypertension, diabetes mellitus, and coronary disease. Also, the majority of these patients are in their sixth and seventh decade of life and suffer the normal consequence of aging.

Administration of preoperative medication should be kept to a minimum because of the possibility of producing hypotensive episodes. Heavy sedation also masks the neurologic symptoms.

Anesthetic Considerations

With continued experience, the nurse anesthetists will find that anesthesia for this procedure is one of the most, if not the most, challenging to administer. Control of blood pressure and ensurance of cerebral protection are variables that provide a continuous challenge, and the consequence of inadequate cerebral protection is devastating.

Carotid endarterectomy may be performed under general anesthesia or local anesthesia utilizing monitored anesthesia care. However, these patients are controlled maximally under general anesthesia because the anesthetist can augment CBF and reduce cerebral metabolic demands with the selected technique. When selecting an agent, the anesthetist should look for an agent that will not produce wide fluctuations in blood pressure but that will maintain autoregulation and provide for a rapid emergence so as to be able to assess neurologic status.

The most critical time of the procedure is during induction and during the time of carotid clamping. More often than not, because of interference with baroreceptors, these patients have blood pressures that are extremely labile, and control is the anesthetist's greatest challenge. This lability in blood pressure appears to be more pronounced in those individuals who are having their second procedure.

Minimal monitoring includes ECG, esophageal stethoscope, radial artery catheter, and in many institutions, electroencephalography (EEG).

Regardless of the agent selected, the anesthetic induction must be free from sympathetic depression or stimulation. A slow approach, with care to maintain blood pressure within normal limits, is mandatory. As suggested earlier, patients with cerebrovascular insufficiency usually suffer from other vascular problems, including CAD, and must be managed accordingly. The use of a nitroglycerin patch on all major vascular procedures has proved beneficial.

Influence of Anesthetics on Cerebral Blood Flow.

When a patient is subject to anesthesia, several physiologic responses occur. Among these are changes in cerebral flow, cerebral metabolic rate, and EEG. Careful consideration of the individual effects of specific anesthetic agents is necessary to provide the patient with optimal physiologic support.

Halothane. Halothane is known to be the most potent cerebral vasodilator of all the anesthetic agents. It will progressively increase CBF until cerebral perfusion pressure falls below the autoregulatory levels. When mean arterial pressure is maintained at about 80 torr, equipotent levels of halothane, enflurane, and isoflurane elicit CBF increases of 190, 37, and 18 percent respectively (Murphy et al, 1974). All of the inhalation anesthetic agents increase CBF, and the only intravenous agent that augments flow is ketamine. With regard to cerebral metabolic rate (CMR), all inhalation agents except nitrous oxide reduce CMR, and all intravenous agents with the exception of ketamine reduce CMR (Table 28–25).

Enflurane. Enflurane and isoflurane have effects on CMR and CBF similar to halothane but are dose-dependant. Thus, with higher concentrations, CBF is increased, but not to the extent as with halothane. The epileptogenic effects of enflurane offset its advantage over halothane in amount of CBF increase. Because seizure activity can elevate the brain metabolism by as much as 400 percent, the use of enflurane, especially in high doses and with hypocapnia, should be limited in patients with seizure disorders or intracranial disease associated with reduced CBF (Miller, 1986).

Barbiturates. A dose-dependent reduction in CBF and CMR, approximately paralleling CNS depression, occurs with barbiturates (Pierce et al, 1962). If large doses of barbiturates are used, these values are reduced by approximately 50 percent, suggesting the major effect of nontoxic doses of depressant anesthetics is a reduction in the component of cerebral metabolism that is linked to brain function, with only minimal effects on metabolism related to cellular homeostasis (Miller, 1986). Thiopental has potent cerebrovasoconstrictor effects and, therefore, is of benefit when reduction in CBF is indicated.

TABLE 28–25. ANESTHETIC INFLUENCE ON CEREBRAL BLOOD FLOW (CBF) AND CEREBRAL METABOLIC RATE (CMR)

Agent	CBF	CMR
Halothane	↑	↓
Enflurane	↑	↓
Isoflurane	↑	↓
Nitrous oxide	↑	↑
Thiopentone	↓	↓
Fentanyl	↓	↓
Morphine sulfate	↓	↓
Ketamine	↑	↑

Ketamine. All intravenous agents are vasoconstrictors, the degree being dose-related, with the exception of ketamine. Ketamine is unique because of its cerebroexcitatory ability. Associated with this activation is a 50 percent increase in CBF and a less than 20 percent increase in overall $CMRO_2$ (Dewson et al, 1971). It is a potent cerebrovasodilator, thus increasing intracranial pressure.

Muscle relaxants are not known to alter cerebral blood flow.

Induction

Whatever the agent or technique selected for induction, the process must be carried out with minimal alterations in the patient's hemodynamic status. Maintaining a blood pressure that is normotensive or slightly above is recommended. Once anesthetic levels have been achieved, the anesthetist should strive to maintain CBF. The means by which this is accomplished depends on whether a shunt is used during the procedure. Intraoperative blood pressure control, especially during the period of arterial clamping, is essential. If necessary, agents such as nitroprusside or vasopressors should be used judiciously to maintain an optimal blood pressure range.

Two primary options are available to monitor cerebral perfusion during trial clamping of the carotid artery and before deciding to use an internal shunt; these are measurement of internal carotid artery back pressure and intraoperative use of EEG (Moore, 1983). Currently, most procedures are either selectively or routinely shunted.

Whichever the case, satisfactory maintenance of blood pressure during carotid artery clamping is of paramount importance. There is controversy as to the desirable levels of arterial pressure. Some authors feel that increased pressure is readily transmitted through the dilated arterioles in the area of cerebral ischemia, increasing capillary pressure and could cause protein leakage and cerebral edema (Miller, 1986). In addition, the deleterious effects of hypertension on the patient with myocardial ischemia cannot be overemphasized.

Previously, there existed some debate as to the benefit of hypercapnia or hypocapnia during arterial clamping. Currently, the accepted technique is to maintain a $Paco_2$ at slightly lower than normal (35 torr).

Regardless of the precautions taken to maintain adequate CBF, there is no technique that is totally safe. Some surgeons routinely use a shunt in order to maximize cerebral blood flow during clamping, but its use is not without deleterious effects, because of the possibility of embolism or intimal damage.

There are some techniques that can be used to judge the degree of cerebral perfusion. These include measurement of stump pressure and EEG. Stump pressures have been used to evaluate circulation to the side of the brain that is occluded. Stump pressures are obtained by placing a needle into the carotid artery and measuring the mean pressure. Most authors will agree that stump pressure changes correlate well with EEG changes; however, EEG changes are highly respected as the best indicator of alterations in CBF. Unfortunately, the complexity and cost of the EEG limits its use.

Surgical Procedure

The first surgical procedure to correct extracranial occlusive disease was performed by DeBakey and colleagues in 1953. A carotid artery stenosis is demonstrated in Figure 28–31 and surgical anatomy in Figure 28–32.

With the patient in the supine position, the head is turned away from the operative side and the head flexed to reduce venous pressure and thus minimize bleeding. Incision is made along the anterior border of the sternocleidomastoid muscle. The jugular vein is seen through the carotid sheath and mobilized until the common facial vein is observed. This vein serves as a landmark for the carotid bifurcation. Care must be taken to protect the vagus and recurrent laryngeal nerves.

The common carotid is then mobilized to provide sufficient length of exposure of the lesion. As exposure nears the bifurcation, local infiltration to the carotid body with lidocaine may be necessary to prevent reflex bradycardia. Once the artery has been sufficiently exposed, the patient is heparinized.

Back pressure readings are then obtained to determine whether a shunt is necessary. Back pressures are determined by placing a 22-gauge needle into the common carotid, clamping the common carotid proximal to the needle, and clamping the external carotid, thus permitting internal carotid artery pressure readings. Readings are accomplished

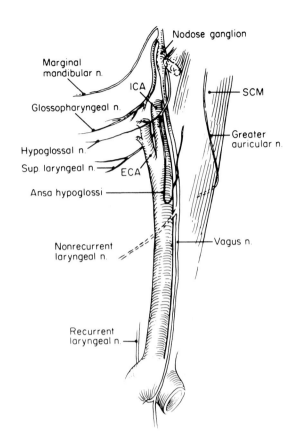

Figure 28–32. Surgical anatomy and relationship of structures encountered during exposure of the carotid bifurcation. ECA = external carotid artery; ICA = internal carotid artery; n = nerve; SCM = sternocleidomastoid. (*From Moore WS (ed.): Vascular Surgery: A Comprehensive Review, 1983. By permission of Grune & Stratton and the author.*)

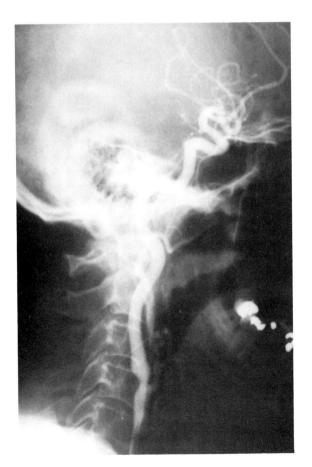

Figure 28–31. Carotid arteriogram demonstrating severe carotid stenosis.

by means of tubing connected to a pressure transducer. If the pressure readings are less than 25 mm Hg, the surgeon should consider the use of a shunt.

With the common, external, and internal arteries clamped, an arteriotomy is made, and plaque removal beings. Once all plaque and debris has been removed, the arteriotomy is closed primarily or with a patch if the lumen has been compromised. Flow is reestablished to the external carotid first, and then to the internal. Heparin is reversed with protamine and the wound closed.

Complications

The most common problem after carotid endarterectomy is hypo- or hypertension. The incidence of hypertension is high, especially among those patients who are not well controlled preoperatively. Strong evidence suggests that interference with the baroreceptor mechanism is responsible for blood pressure fluctuations. Hypertension is critical in these patients and should be treated promptly with vasodilators such as sodium nitroglycerin. Diastolic pressures should be maintained below 100 mm Hg.

Hypotension is usually the result of inadequate hydration before surgery. This is especially true if arteriography has been performed in the previous 24 hours. The use of vasoconstrictor drugs may be necessary if blood pressure is not returned to normal after administration of fluids. Caution should be exercised with the use of vasoconstrictors in the presence of hypovolemia.

The most frequent cause of neurologic deficit, either intra- or postoperatively, is emboli. Intraoperative emboli are caused by artery mobilization, shunt insertion, or after arteriotomy closure. Emboli that occur postoperatively are likely to be due to fibrin and platelet aggregates formed in the endarterectomized segment (Moore, 1983).

Another complication of carotid surgery is airway obstruction caused by edema, hematoma formation, or damage to the recurrent laryngeal nerves. Extubation should not be performed until respiratory status has been carefully assessed; reintubation may be extremely difficult because of deviation of the trachea from edema or hematoma and may necessitate emergency tracheotomy.

SURGERY FOR ARCH VESSEL OCCLUSIVE DISEASE

Arch vessel reconstruction is indicated in patients with extremity ischemia or hemispheric or vertebrobasilar symptoms. With subclavian artery occlusive disease, a bypass graft from the carotid to the subclavian artery is made. A subclavian steal syndrome is illustrated in Figure 28–33.

Primary anesthetic considerations are the same as for carotid surgery. The pulse will be diminished or absent on the affected arm and monitoring devices should be placed on the unaffected side.

SURGERY ON THE ABDOMINAL AORTA AND ITS BRANCHES

Anatomy

The abdominal aorta (aorta abdominalis) begins at the aortic hiatus of the diaphragm, ventral to the caudal border of the body of the last thoracic vertebra, and descending ventral to the vertebral column, ends on the body of the fourth lumbar vertebra, a little left of midline, by dividing into the two common iliac arteries (Gray, 1973).

The branches of the abdominal aorta may be divided into three sets: visceral, parietal, and terminal (Fig. 28–34) (Gray, 1983).

1. Visceral:
   A. Celiac
   B. Superior mesenteric
   C. Inferior mesenteric
   D. Middle suprarenals
   E. Renals
   F. Testicular
   G. Ovarian
2. Parietal:
   H. Inferior phrenics
   I. Lumbars
   J. Middle sacral
3. Terminal:
   K. Common iliacs

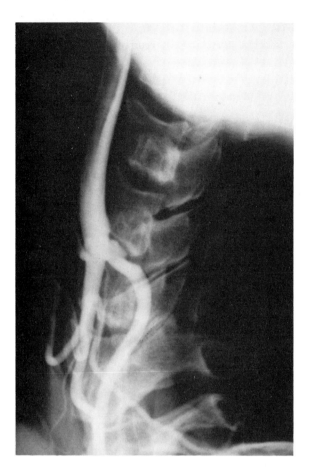

Figure 28–33. Subclavian steal syndrome. The subclavian is obstructed before the vertebral artery branch. Blood travels up the internal carotid through the vertebral artery to provide circulation to the arm.

Abdominal Aortic Aneurysm

True aneurysms or atherosclerotic occlusive disease can occur along the aorta or in any of its branches. A true aneurysm is one whose walls, although dilated and deformed, contain elements of the original vessel wall. The process usually affects middle-aged or elderly people and is thought to be due to congenital defects, degenerative changes, dissection aortitis, or trauma (Moore, 1983).

Aneurysms confined to the infrarenal abdominal aorta are the most common aortic aneurysm and true aneurysms of this area are almost entirely due to atherosclerosis (Szelagyi et al, 1972). The natural course of this disease has been well established as one that progresses to rupture and death in about half of the patients within a year of diagnosis and in 91 percent at unpredictable times within five years (Szelagyi et al, 1972). Surgical intervention, when electively performed, provides for mortality ranges of 3 to 5 percent (Crawford et al, 1981).

Early detection and surgical intervention are the keys to successful treatment. These patients generally present with abdominal or back pain and a pulsating abdominal mass. Diagnosis is confirmed by aortogram (Fig. 28–35). Once diagnosis has been established, replacement graft should be considered. Generally speaking, replacement is

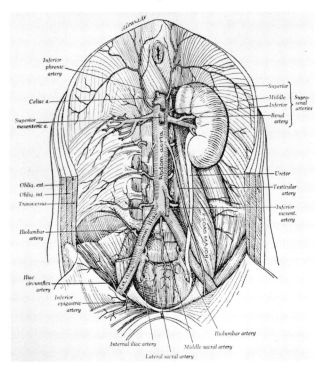

Figure 28–34. The abdominal aorta and its principal branches. (*From Gray H: Anatomy of The Human Body, 29th ed., Goss CM (ed.), 1973. Courtesy of Lea & Febiger.*)

indicated when the aneurysm is twice the size of the distal or proximal uninvolved aorta (Crawford et al, 1981). Abdominal aneurysms frequently rupture and are a source of emboli, leading to lower extremity ischemia (Fig. 28–36). In 60 percent of cases, the aneurysms are located 2 to 5 cm below the origin of the renal arteries and extend down to, but do not include, the aortic bifurcation (Moore, 1983). In 40 percent of patients, the common iliac arteries are involved either by aneurysmal disease or by associated atherosclerotic occlusive disease (Moore, 1983). Approximately 15 percent of patients undergoing aneurysm resection have associated narrowing of iliac vessels.

Aortoiliac Occlusive Disease

Atherosclerotic occlusive disease is a common cause of ischemic symptoms in the lower extremities. Initially, symptoms include intermittent claudication of muscles of the thigh, hips, buttocks, and calf and progress to impotence and diminished pulses. The risk factors for these patients are the same for other atherosclerotic processes, i.e., smoking, diabetes, hypertension, and elevated serum cholesterol levels.

The initial lesions of aortoiliac occlusive disease appear to begin at the terminal aorta and the proximal portion of the common iliac arteries or at the bifurcation of the common iliacs and progress slowly. The ultimate anatomic result

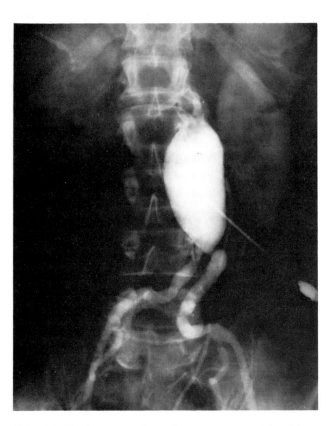

Figure 28–35. Aortogram illustrating an aneurysm of the abdominal aorta.

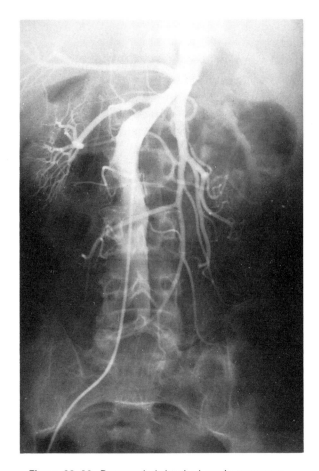

Figure 28–36. Ruptured abdominal aortic aneurysm.

of progressive aortoiliac atherosclerosis is occlusion of the distal abdominal aorta, with progression of a thrombus up to the level of the renal arteries (Fig. 28–37) (Moore, 1983).

The indications for surgery are disabling claudication and ischemia at rest, manifested by rest pain in the foot, ischemic ulceration, or pregangrenous skin changes (Moore, 1983).

Preoperative Assessment. The anesthetic evaluation includes adequate assessment of other systems. Generally speaking, these patients should be managed as though occlusive disease exists in all arterial systems. Because these patients are older, impairment of renal, cardiac, and respiratory systems is common and the possibility of complication is high.

As many as 30 percent of all American adults and approximately 50 percent of patients with vascular disease have hypertension of unknown etiology (DeBakey et al, 1965). Most of these patients present with extremely labile blood pressures preoperatively, demonstrating the need for adequate antihypertensive regimens. Chronic hypertension presents several problems to the anesthetist in major procedures such as this. Patients with uncontrolled hypertension, when anesthetized, suffer a greater reduction in systemic vascular resistance and a marked fall in mean

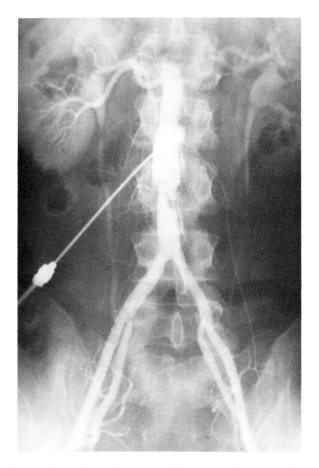

Figure 28–37. Abdominal aorta with severe atherosclerotic occlusive disease.

arterial blood pressure and are subject to a higher incidence of arrhythmias and ischemia (Miller, 1986).

Patients with diastolic hypertension usually have a reduced plasma volume, leading to lability of blood pressure under anesthesia. The importance of using a Swan-Ganz catheter to determine the status of intravascular volume cannot be overemphasized for these patients.

In addition to antihypertensive agents, diuretics are common therapy for the patient with elevated arterial pressure. Electrolyte imbalance may accompany their use. Except in the case of an emergency procedure, electrolyte imbalances, intravascular volume depletion, and hypertension should be corrected preoperatively. Controversy still exists as to whether to continue antihypertensive medication preoperatively, but it appears that withholding the medication has become more the exception than the rule.

The most common cause of death after elective vascular surgery of the aorta or its major branches is myocardial infarction (Miller, 1986), and 33 to 49 percent of the deaths are secondary to an infarction that occurs perioperatively (Morris and DeBakey, 1968). Careful preoperative assessment of myocardial status is indicated.

Renal status is another area of importance in the preoperative evaluation. Careful analysis of renal laboratory studies should be made to determine if a prerenal condition exists. Several causal factors are associated with postoperative renal failure in these patients: (1) arterial dye studies, (2) mechanical occlusion of renal vessels during surgery, (3) renal trauma, and (4) dehydration. If laboratory values are borderline, special precautions to protect the kidneys should be taken, such as adequate hydration and diuresis.

Anesthetic Considerations. The anesthetic agent is selected by the administrator and should be one that he or she is most comfortable with.

Each of the agents available, whether inhalation or narcotic, has advantages and disadvantages. Use of inhalation agents risks myocardial depression in higher concentrations, whereas use of intravenous agents risks hypertension and tachycardia. Both inhalation and intravenous agents offer the advantage of allowing for administration of high oxygen concentrations.

Some authors advocate low concentrations of inhalation agents with the use of a vasodilator to overcome hypertensive episodes. Others suggest intravenous agents with supplemental doses of inhalant or vasodilators to combat hypertension. Continuous epidural or spinal anesthesia is used in some centers, the advantage being absence of vasospasm secondary to sympathetic blockade and prolonged postoperative analgesia with minimal respiratory depression (Miller, 1986).

Cardiovascular compromise is the major cause of complications and death in patients undergoing surgery of the abdominal aorta. For this reason, the need for extensive monitoring of hemodynamic status cannot be overemphasized. Minimal monitoring should include ECG, esophageal probe (for temperature and heart sounds), direct arterial pressure, CVP, arterial blood gas samples, pulmonary artery and wedge pressures. Each of the above parameters will provide information about sudden changes in physiologic status.

The pulmonary artery catheter has been a major break-through for monitoring under anesthesia. Besides providing pulmonary artery and right arterial pressures, this instrument has made possible monitoring of left ventricular filling pressure (via pulmonary artery wedge pressure) and, thus, left ventricular function as well as cardiac output determinations on a moment-to-moment basis (Miller, 1986). Furthermore, measurements of pulmonary artery or mixed venous oxygen tension are an extremely sensitive index of the adequacy of cardiac output for total body metabolic needs (Stanley and Isern, 1979).

Upon insertion of each of these instruments, baseline values should be obtained and used as guidelines for therapy throughout the case.

The primary concern of the anesthetist throughout the surgical procedure should be adequate hydration. As mentioned previously, such factors as chronic hypertension, arteriography, age, and poor nutrition predispose these patients to inadequate intravascular volumes. The pulmonary artery catheter provides information about the hydration of the patient. The need for volume replacement can be assessed before surgical insult. It is essential to maintain "patient normal" volume replacement or slightly above because of the hemodynamic changes associated with aortic occlusion and release. Furthermore, blood loss during these operations can be significant and poorly tolerated by the patient with marginal myocardial function. Expansion of intravascular volume can be accomplished by use of balanced salt solutions or by the plasma volume expanders. Once the anesthetist feels confident about the patient's hydration, blood loss can be replaced on a volume to volume basis.

The most critical part of the surgical procedure is the time during aortic occlusion and release. Aortic occlusion produces a variety of changes in the cardiovascular status of the patient. The degree of change is dependent on several variables. These include intravascular volume status, myocardial function, degree of collateral circulation around the occlusion, the anesthetic agent, and metabolic status of the patient. Infrarenal occlusion above and below an abdominal aneurysm will generally produce a change in arterial pressure because the vascular bed proximal to the occlusion still constitutes 70 percent of the total circulatory bed, including circulation to all major organs (Sabawala et al, 1970). Backflow of blood from the severed distal aortic segment usually appears, indicating the presence of collateral circulation. Ischemia of the lower extremities can therefore be expected only with prolonged occlusion and with lumbar artery involvement (Sabawala et al, 1970).

Upon occlusion of the aorta, a transient rise in blood pressure and pulse rate should be expected. In an effort to reduce myocardial afterload during clamping, to permit fluid volume loading of the patient, and to avoid declamping hypotension, the use of nitroglycerin is advocated before and during aortic cross-clamping.

Because aortic cross-clamping can produce hemodynamic changes consistent with ischemia, the V_5 lead should be used, it being most sensitive to ischemic changes.

Aortic occlusion results in absence of circulation to the lower extremities and distal organs, producing metabolic acidosis that becomes evident when the clamps are re-moved. Analysis should be performed at regular intervals to evaluate the metabolic state of the patient. Metabolic acidosis is due to accumulation of nonvolatile acids. Arterial sampling in uncompensated acidosis should show the following: (1) decreased pH, (2) decreased plasma bicarbonate, (3) normal or increased carbon dioxide, (4) base deficit, and (5) decreased standard bicarbonate.

If left untreated, several processes will evolve: the myocardium becomes depressed, reducing cardiac output, peripheral vasoconstriction may occur, the oxyhemoglobin curve is shifted to the right, the respiratory center is stimulated, hyperkalemia occurs, and response to sympathetic stimulation, whether direct or indirect, decreases. Acidosis interferes with normal enzymatic activity and can produce changes at the cellular levels.

Thus, acidosis, if present, must be corrected to provide normal hemodynamic and cellular function. Corrective treatment should be aggressive and immediate, using sodium bicarbonate. The dosage of bicarbonate can be calculated as follows:

$$\text{Dose (mEq)} = \frac{\text{Base excess} \times \text{body weight in kg}}{3}$$

One half of the calculated dose should be given slowly and samples drawn to determine correction. The administration of bicarbonate to correct a metabolic acidosis presents a carbon dioxide load for the lungs to excrete, and efficient buffering of a metabolic acidosis depends on adequate pulmonary ventilation (Wylie and Churchill-Davidson, 1972).

Aortic occlusion is associated with a reduction in renal blood flow. The exact mechanism by which renal cortical blood flow is reduced has not been well defined. Several theories exist regarding its etiology. Flow may be impaired by arterial pressure changes, direct trauma, embolization of plaque, or because of a renin-angiotensin response. The administration of an osmotic diuretic should help overcome the renin-angiotensin response.

Even with judicious care, transient oliguria or renal failure may occur and can be a major cause of death after successful surgery (Sabawala et al, 1970). Oliguria may be the result of preoperative dehydration, effects of anesthetics, and related pharmacopeia and hypovolemia, all of which play a role in increasing secretion of antidiuretic hormone.

The kidney may be protected by administration of large volumes of fluid just before clamping and by administration of a diuretic such as mannitol 12.5 to 25 g, or furosemide 10 to 20 mg prior to clamping.

Mannitol is completely excreted by the kidney, together with a volume of obligatory water of about 5 ml/g mannitol (Sabawala et al, 1970). Because it requires water for excretion, mannitol should not produce diuresis in dehydrated patients, nor should it dehydrate patients in whom sufficient volumes of obligatory water are available or supplied by infusion (Barry and Berman, 1961). The erythrocyte is most sensitive to changes in osmotic pressure, and it is suggested that one-half of obligatory water comes from this source (Brewster, 1984). The fall in hematocrit, without change in hemoglobin or red blood cell count leads to a reduction in viscosity, decrease in renal vascular resistance, and an increase in renal blood flow (Sabawala et al, 1970).

Excessive blood loss can create serious problems for the anesthetist, particularly when rapid transfusion is necessary. The risk of throwing these elderly patients into frank congestive failure is ever present. Generally speaking, blood should be replaced volume for volume. The Haemonetics Cell Saver currently in use has provided intraoperative autotransfusion during sudden excessive blood loss. Intraoperative autotransfusion has obvious advantages: immediate availability, normothermia, and none of the hazards inherent to use of homologous bank blood (Duncan et al, 1974). Autotransfused blood contains only washed, packed red cells suspended in saline solutions and is essentially devoid of other blood components. Coagulation factors must be replenished and heparin-neutralized when large volumes of salvaged red blood cells are transfused. Autotransfusion is not without complication. Air embolism and hemolysis with associated renal dysfunction and microembolism have been reported (Duncan et al, 1974).

Excessive administration of stored whole blood always risks reaction and decreased coagulation function. After administration of four to five units of whole blood, fresh-frozen plasma should be administered to enhance coagulation function. The administration of calcium with massive transfusion remains a controversial issue.

There are at least three indications for administration of large volumes of intravenous fluid in vascular surgery: (1) elimination of discrepancies between the volumes of circulating blood and blood in the vascular bed caused by large blood loss or release of an occluding clamp, (2) dilution of radiopaque dyes, and (3) prevention of postoperative oliguria.

Some advocate the use of crystalloid solutions whereas others advocate the use of hypertonic sodium solutions. Proponents of hypertonic sodium solutions feel that sodium, being largely confined to the extracellular compartment, in hypertonic solution will expand extracellular fluid space by extracting water from cells (Earley et al, 1972). Several authors have postulated that, in addition to its role in the restoration of the functional extracellular fluid space, sodium itself has a beneficial effect upon oxidative phosphorylation in the shock state.

Once reconstruction of the aorta has been performed, circulation to the lower extremities can be reestablished. When the aortic occlusion clamp is released, a vasoactive substance may be liberated and a hypotension phenomenon may occur. "Declamping shock" has been attributed to many factors including the duration of occlusion, the amount of acid metabolites generated during occlusion, abruptness of declamping, sympathetic tone of the venous system, lack of sufficient collateral blood flow during cross-clamp, anesthetic agents and depth of anesthesia, presence of associated cardiorespiratory problems, actual blood loss before and during cross-clamp, and inadequacy of left ventricular filling pressure before cross-clamp (Lunn et al, 1979).

The most common cause of hypotension after release of the clamp appears to be an inadequate circulating volume. This can be avoided by increasing left ventricular filling pressure. One approach is to infuse lactated Ringer's solution in a volume significant enough to increase PCWP 3 to 4 torr above preanesthetic values during cross-clamping (Lunn et al, 1979).

As previously mentioned, the majority of the total blood volume is proximal to the occlusion, and excessive blood loss can occur without being reflected by hemodynamic change. Hypovolemia is also due to evisceration of bowel necessary for aortic exposure; the small bowel dilates and significant fluid loss occurs (Sabawala et al, 1970). Thus, when aortic occlusion is discontinued, a smaller blood volume is available to fill the vascular bed. Overhydration will contract this vascular bed, eliminating decreases in cardiac output and venous return. Even after satisfactory replacement of the vascular volume as determined by pulmonary artery pressure, hypotensive episodes frequently occur in the postoperative period because of third space shift. It may take several hours for stabilization of fluid compartments.

Ruptured Abdominal Aneurysm

Because of the highly lethal nature of a ruptured aneurysm, the key to resuscitation is speed. These patients present in frank circulatory collapse and rapid cessation of blood loss is imperative. This is only accomplished by aortic clamping and it is not until clamping occurs that beneficial results from resuscitative measures can be seen.

Induction of anesthesia is on an emergency basis, with care taken to avoid cough, strain, or fasciculation. Once relaxation has been established, it should be noted that additional bleeding may occur from removal of the tamponade caused by a rigid abdominal wall.

Rapid replacement of fluids and blood to expand the vascular bed is essential to prevent death in these patients. Although hypotension or circulatory collapse exists, contraction of the vascular bed with vasoconstrictors should be avoided so as to provide for maximum volume replacement.

Blood loss usually proceeds at a rate faster than availability or replacement can occur. Volume expanders and crystalloid solutions are recommended until adequate blood replacement can occur. Rapid massive blood administration is not without consequence and all principles governing massive transfusions should be followed.

Even though all resuscitative measures may be taken, the rate of mortality is high for this group of surgical patients. These patients succumb to massive blood loss, myocardial failure or infarction, irreversible hypotension, or renal failure.

Renal Artery Revascularization

The renal arteries leave the aorta at L-2. Occlusion or stenosis of the renal arteries results in hypertension and renal failure (Fig. 28–38). Renovascular hypertension is thought to account for 5 to 10 percent of the hypertensive population. The presence of renovascular hypertension should be suspected when severe hypertension, uncontrolled by drug therapy, exists. This form of hypertension usually affects the young adult who lacks family history of hypertension.

The most common cause of renal vascular hypertension is atherosclerotic narrowing of the renal artery. Reduced pulse pressure distal to a stenotic lesion in the main or segmental artery activates the renin-angiotensin system,

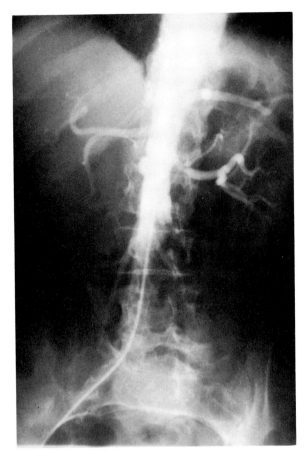

Figure 28-38. Renal artery stenosis.

resulting in increased renin production by the ischemic kidney (Brewster, 1984). The macula densa and juxtaglomerular apparatus are the two intrarenal sites that exert a control on blood pressure. The macula densa is the intrarenal sensor of sodium concentration and thereby exerts a control in renin production in the juxtaglomerular apparatus (Brewster, 1984). The juxtaglomerular cells are sensors on intra-arteriolar perfusion pressure. Reduced perfusion pres-

sure causes an increased release of renin by these cells (Moore, 1983) and the renin angiotensin system is activated (Fig. 28-39).

Theory suggests that there are three mechanisms whereby renin release is regulated:

1. Intrarenal arteriolar baroreceptor mechanism: causes renin secretion to increase when the intra-arteriolar pressure at the juxtaglomerular cell decreases.
2. Macula densa process: renin secretion is inversely proportional to the rate of sodium transport across this area of the distal tubule.
3. Sympathetic nervous system: increases renin secretion by increasing circulatory catecholamines and by renal sympathetic nerves.

Diagnosis is made, not only by a demonstrable lesion but also by selective renal vein renin productions. A renal vein: renin ratio of 1:1.5 is considered positive (Brewster, 1984). Surgical correction of these lesions provides good results in the cure or correction of hypertension. Preferred methods of surgical revascularization include aortorenal bypass, splenorenal bypass, hepatorenal bypass, or renal endarterectomy.

Anesthetic Considerations. Anesthetic considerations for these procedures are the same as for any major abdominal vascular surgery, with special attention to preservation of renal tissue.

Antihypertensive therapy must be continued to the time of surgery. Alpha-methyldopa appears to be the drug of choice, producing little effect on hemodynamics when combined with anesthesia. It reduces both central and peripheral norepinephrine levels and is known to interact with anesthetic agents dose-relatedly, lowering minimal alveolar concentration (MAC) of anesthetics required for analgesia (Brewster, 1984).

Because the aortic occlusion clamp is placed above the renal arteries, special precautions need to be taken for kidney preservation. Local hypothermia may be applied. Mannitol or furosemide are given to promote diuresis and to overcome the renin-angiotensin response. In addition, some centers use a renal perfusion fluid consisting of chilled Ring-

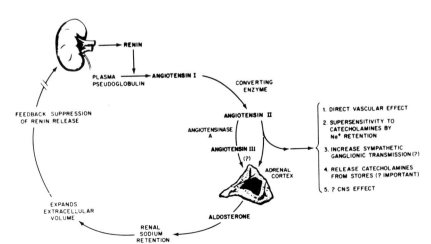

Figure 28-39. Summary of renin-angiotensin-aldosterone pharmacology. (*From Brenner BM, Rector FC: The Kidney, 1976, Vol. 2. Courtesy of Saunders.*)

er's lactate (3C), mannitol, heparin, and methylpredniso-lone during this period of renal ischemia (Brewster, 1984).

Manipulation of the stenosed artery may cause a renin-angiotensin response, and drugs should be available to overcome this reaction.

Although most inhalation agents are to some extent biotransformed and the products of metabolism often elimi-nated by the kidney, these drugs do not rely on renal excre-tion for reversal of their therapeutic effects; thus all inhal-ants, with the exception of methoxyflurane and enflurane, can be used in mild or moderate renal failure (Katz et al, 1981).

The action of narcotics is intensified with renal disease. With regard to muscle relaxation, the only absolute contrain-dications are gallamine and decamethonium, which are ex-creted almost entirely by the kidney.

Patients suffering from renal disease and on antihyper-tensive therapy are generally hypovolemic and caution must be taken not to cause a reduction in arterial pressure. The best therapy for hypotensive episodes is volume expansion, because all vasopressors will result in some degree of renal compromise.

Ultra-short-acting barbiturates produce few side effects in the patient with renal compromise. Belladonna alkaloids such as atropine and hyoscyamine are excreted unchanged by the kidneys and should be avoided or dosage modified. Scopolamine is almost entirely metabolized and is the drug of choice if a belladonna is indicated.

Aortoduodenal Fistula

Aortoduodenal fistula is characterized by gastrointestinal bleeding, which can be exsanguinating. Rupture usually occurs on the left side into the retroperitoneal space, but it can occur on the right into the retroperitoneal space, the duodenum, vena cava, or iliac vein (Moore, 1983). Treat-ment consists of control of bleeding by graft replacement and repair of the duodenum.

These patients are septic with all of the sequelae that accompany this shock-like state. Blood loss is usually exces-sive and requires massive transfusions. Swan-Ganz cathe-ters are beneficial in determining hemodynamic status.

Hepatodecompression

Portal hypertension is the result of obstruction to splanchnic blood flow. Diagnosis is usually made on a basis of a past history of cirrhosis accompanied by esophageal variceal bleeding. About 30 percent of patients with varices will bleed. Approximately 70 percent who have bled from varices die within one year and 60 percent rebleed massively in one year (Katz et al, 1981). The pathogenesis of esophageal varices relates to the development of collateral vessels be-tween the high-pressure splanchnic circulation and the low-pressure systemic circulation (Moore, 1983). A number of collateral pathways develop in an attempt to decompress the portal system, but regardless of their number and size, they are rarely able to bring about complete portal decom-pression (Moore, 1983).

Signs and Symptoms. Ascites is very common in portal hypertension and is due to redistribution of fluid between plasma and extracellular fluid and also to excessive renal reabsorption of salt and water (Moore, 1983). Abnormal laboratory findings include elevated lactic dehydrogenase, serum glutamic-oxaloacetic transaminase, serum glutamic-pyruvic transaminase, globulin, bilirubin, and prothrombin time. Hypoalbuminuria exists. Hypersplenism, if present, is accompanied by decreases in white cell count and plate-lets. Anemia is common.

Treatment. To date, surgical intervention is not the treat-ment of choice in the management of these patients, but if selected, the following procedures may be used: Portal caval shunt is indicated only when esophageal hemorrhage is present. This procedure anastomoses the portal vein to the inferior vena cava, shunting blood away from the portal system.

Mesocaval shunt directs blood from the superior mes-enteric vein to the inferior vena cava. Because it is easier technically, this shunt is indicated in emergency manage-ment of variceal bleeding.

Distal splenorenal, or the Warren, shunt was developed in an effort to avoid total diversion of portal blood flow, preventing further hepatocellular damage. The splenic vein is anastomosed to the left renal vein.

Anesthetic Management. Although ideally bleeding is controlled before surgery, emergency surgery to control bleeding may be necessary. Tamponade with a Blakemore tube is usually necessary; once inserted the tube remains in place until after induction. These tubes are usually an-chored into position in such a way that they obstruct the anesthetist during intubation. Even with the tube inserted, these patients must be managed as full stomach. Awake intubation is encouraged.

Blood loss is extreme and, if possible, only fresh blood should be given to provide the clotting factors needed. Hypertonic salt solutions should be avoided because these patients conserve sodium. Large volumes of crystalloid and plasma expanders should be on hand. Generally, because of poor nutritional habits, these patients are anemic, which predisposes them to thrombocytopenia or granulocytope-nia. Vitamin K, potassium, glucose, and protein usually need to be replenished.

Anesthetic agents that will not further compromise the liver should be employed. The anesthetist is thus limited to the use of nonmetabolized inhalation agents or to intrave-nous agents. Muscle relaxants that are not metabolized via the liver should be used.

Because these patients are prone to bleeding, induction should be as atraumatic as possible to avoid oral and pharyn-geal bleeding. Bony prominences should be padded to pre-vent ecchymosis from pressure areas.

THORACOABDOMINAL AORTIC ANEURYSM

Aneurysms of this type are more frequent than previously considered; it has become apparent that many patients with aneurysms of the thorax have abdominal extension of the disease or have separate lesions located in the abdomen (Fig. 28–40) (Crawford and Cohen, 1982).

Aneurysms that involve segments of both the descending thoracic and abdominal aorta in continuity, i.e., true thoracoabdominal aortic aneurysms, are considered with abdominal aortic aneurysms that involve the upper segment from which visceral vessels arise, because they pose similar problems in treatment (Moore, 1983). Visceral artery reconstruction may be necessary because over 20 percent of patients have occlusive disease in these arteries.

The causes of aneurysms of this nature are chronic dissection, arteriosclerosis, and medial degenerative disease, with the latter two being the most common (Moore, 1983).

They occur more commonly in the middle-aged and elderly, with high incidences of associated coronary artery, pulmonary, and renal disease. Treatment is graft replacement.

Preoperative Management.
The preoperative and anesthetic regimen described is that used by the Baylor College of Medicine.

Hydration is very important in these patients, and in an effort to minimize renal dysfunction, 5 percent dextrose with Ringer's lactate solution with 25 g mannitol/1000 ml is given at 150 ml per hour for 12 hours before and after

aortography (Moore, 1983). Blood urea nitrogen and creatinine levels should be within normal limits. All patients are placed on digitalis. Electrolytes, serum blood gases, and arterial pressures should be within normal limits.

Anesthetic Management.
Monitoring consists of Swan-Ganz catheter, right atrial catheter, and two radial artery lines to evaluate cardiac hemodynamics, blood gases, electrolytes, acid-base balance, and plasma colloidal osmotic pressure (Crawford and Saleh, 1980). Four peripheral lines are used. A double-lumen tube is used to aid in operative exposure and to avoid pulmonary or cardiac injury.

The patient is placed on the right side at a 60- to 80-degree angle. The abdominal component of the thoracoabdominal incision is midline and is curved across the costal arch into intercostal space, appropriately located according to the extent of the descending thoracic aorta involvement (Moore, 1983).

CVP, PCWP, and cardiac output are kept within normal limits. Mannitol 25 g is given postinduction. Blood replacement is by component technique, using packed red cells, fresh-frozen plasma, platelets, and albumin. A unit of albumin and two units of fresh-frozen plasma are given at the onset of surgery. A unit of fresh-frozen plasma is given after the third transfusion and then alternated with two units of red cells. Fresh platelets, 10 to 16 units, are given

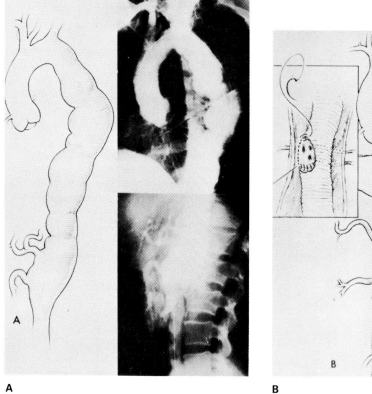

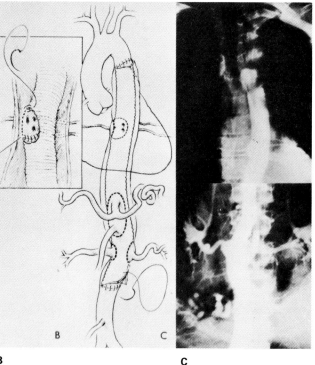

A   B   C

Figure 28–40. Illustration of treatment of fusiform degenerative thoracoabdominal aortic aneurysm by graft. **A.** Aortogram made before operation showing nature and extent of aneurysm. **B.** Technique of graft replacement. **C.** Aortogram made after operation showing graft in place. (*From Crawford ES, Saleh SA: Operative Techniques in Vascular Surgery, 1980. By permission of Grune & Stratton and the authors.*)

rapidly when flow is restored through the graft (Crawford and Saleh, 1980).

Sodium nitroprusside is used to maintain normal cardiac hemodynamics during aortic clamping.

After visceral vessel anastomosis, the head of the operating room table is lowered, the graft is filled with blood to expel air, and then the aorta is reclamped (Crawford and Cohen, 1982).

Restoration of circulation is slow, and once achieved, the table is elevated to its original position.

Extra-anatomic Arterial Reconstruction

Although conventional aortic reconstruction for occlusive disease is in most instances performed with low mortality, extra-anatomic vascular reconstruction may be necessary for life or limb salvage when conventional approaches cannot be used.

These procedures are considered for the severely debilitated, the septic, or the patient with an infected vascular prosthesis. Patients with occlusions of the distal aorta or proximal iliacs may then be treated with femoral to femoral, axillofemoral, or iliofemoral reconstruction. With proper patient and donor vessel selection, operative mortality rates are low; nevertheless patency rates descend after a five-year period.

The protocol for anesthetic management of these pa-tients depends on the physiologic status of the patient and his or her general overall presentation. The surgical procedure itself is less taxing because the aorta is not occluded and the special considerations for aortic occlusion are not necessary.

Blood loss may be significant, particularly if there is anatomic difficulty in exposure. The general condition of these patients may necessitate the need for Swan-Ganz monitoring, which allows for ease of administration of large volumes of fluid or blood without fear of subjecting the patient to congestive heart failure.

Femoral-Popliteal-Tibial Occlusive Disease

Arteriosclerosis may involve the common femoral artery and its branches, the above-the-knee or below-the-knee popliteal artery, any of the infrapopliteal arteries, including their terminal branches, or any combination of these arteries (Moore, 1983).

Primary considerations for the anesthetist are selection of an anesthetic agent. Surgical procedures of this nature become longer in duration the further distal the reconstruction becomes. The goal of the anesthetist is to provide optimal anesthesia with the lowest concentrations possible. Fluid replacement should be carefully monitored, taking into account the insensible loss during such long cases. Blood loss usually is not excessive, unless unforeseen developments occur (Fig. 28–41).

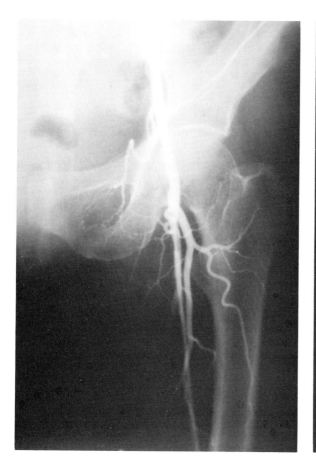
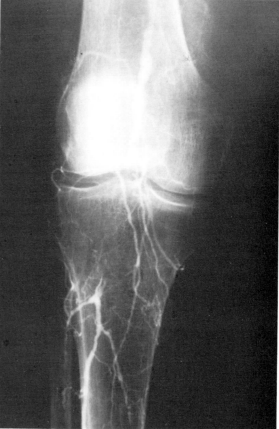

Figure 28–41. Femoral-popliteal occlusive disease.

SURGERY FOR LUNG DISEASES

Anatomy

Respiratory Anatomy. The terms respiration and ventilation are often used interchangeably, but a difference does exist between the two. Ventilation is the mechanical movement of air in and out of the lung, whereas respiration is an actual exchange of oxygen and carbon dioxide in the lung and at the cellular level. This process of respiration is carried out by means of the respiratory apparatus.

Functional Anatomy

The Upper Airway. The upper airway consists of the nose, oropharynx, larynx, and trachea. The nose is lined with a vascular membrane, which contains cilia to humidify and filter air. The pharynx is divided into three areas, the nasopharynx, oropharynx, and laryngopharynx. The nasopharynx, which lies above the soft palate, maintains separation of the nasal and oral cavity during swallowing. The oropharynx extends from the soft palate to the epiglottis and protects the opening to the larynx during swallowing. The laryngopharynx extends from the upper border of the epiglottis to the lower border of the cricoid cartilage, where it becomes the esophagus. The larynx extends from the epiglottis to the level of C-6, where it connects with the trachea. Its primary purpose is to prevent the entry of food into the respiratory system. This is accomplished primarily by the epiglottis and also by apposition of the vocal cords. The area between the vocal cords is the most common site of upper airway obstruction because it is the narrowest portion of the upper respiratory tract.

The trachea is 10 to 12 cm long and extends from the cricoid cartilage (C-6) to the carina (T-5) where it bifurcates into the right and left main-stem bronchi. It is 16 mm in diameter and is composed of 16 to 20 tracheal cartilages, which form U-shaped rings encompassing two-thirds of the anterior portion of the trachea (Gray, 1973). The trachea has a capacity of 30 ml constituting 20 percent of anatomic dead space (Goudsouzian and Karamanian, 1984).

Lower Airway. The lower respiratory system is that portion below the trachea, i.e., the lungs and their components.

The different levels of the lower respiratory tract can be described as generations (1 to 23) beginning with the trachea and ending with alveolar sacs (Fig. 28–42).

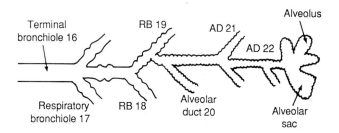

Figure 28–42. The terminal air passages. (The numbers indicate generations.) (*From Goudsouzian NG, Karamanian A: Physiology for the Anesthetist, 1977. Courtesy of Appleton-Century-Crofts and the authors.*)

TABLE 28–26. BRONCHOPULMONARY SEGMENTS

	Right Lung	Left Lung
Upper lobe	Apical	Apical-posterior
	Anterior	Anterior
	Posterior	
Middle lobe	Lateral	Superior
	Medial	Inferior
Lower lobe	Superior	Superior
	Medial basal	Anteromedial basal
	Anterior basal	Lateral basal
	Lateral basal	Posterior basal
	Posterior basal	

From Wilson RF: Principles and Techniques of Critical Care. Upjohn Company, 1975. Reproduced with permission.

THE BRONCHI (GENERATIONS 2 TO 11). The right bronchus is wider and shorter than the left and thus more readily accepts foreign bodies and endotracheal tubes. The right bronchus gives rise to three smaller bronchi, one to each of the lung's lobes. The superior lobe bronchus arises above the pulmonary artery, whereas the middle and inferior lobe bronchi branch off below the pulmonary artery. Each secondary bronchus divides into two to five segmental, or tertiary, bronchi.

The left bronchus is smaller in diameter and much longer than the right. It passes under the aortic arch, crosses over to the esophagus, thoracic duct, and descending aorta (Gray, 1973). It gives rise to two smaller bronchi for the superior and inferior lobes. These secondary bronchi then also divide into segmental, or tertiary, bronchi (Table 28–26). The right lung accounts for 55 percent of the total ventilation and the left for 44 percent (Wilson, 1976).

As the bronchi leave the hilum, they become progressively smaller (distal bronchioles) until the terminal bronchioles, the smallest airways without alveoli, are reached. The portion of the airway from the trachea to the terminal bronchioles is called the conducting airway. Its function is to conduct gas to the area of exchange. There is no gas exchange in this section of the airway and so anatomic dead space exists. The volume of dead space is 150 ml.

THE BRONCHIOLES. The bronchioles (generations 12 to 16) characteristically lack cartilages, and it is readily assumed that they are easily compressed. However, this compression is prevented because the bronchioles are embedded in the lung parenchyma, and the elastic recoil of the alveolar septa keeps them open. Therefore, the caliber of the bronchioles is directly related to lung volumes, and they are not influenced by intrathoracic pressures as are the larger bronchi. Until the 16th generation of air passages, the bronchi are supplied by the systemic vascular tree via the bronchial circulation; beyond this, nourishment is derived via the pulmonary circulation (Goudsouzian and Karamanian, 1984). The respiratory bronchioles (generations 17 to 19) are transitional zones between the bronchioles and alveolar ducts. They contain few alveoli.

THE ACINUS. The acinus (the basic pulmonary unit) contains the structures involved in gas exchange and is supplied by the first order respiratory bronchiole (Fig. 28–43). It begins immediately following the terminal bronchiole and has three succeeding orders of bronchioles, each containing more alveoli. The last, or third order, bronchiole is followed by the alveolar duct (generations 20 to 22), which is completely lined with alveoli, and then the alveolar sacs (generation 23). The distance from the terminal bronchiole to the alveolar sac is about 5 mm. This region is called the respiratory zone and constitutes most of the lung volume, approximately 2500 ml (West, 1974).

Microscopic Anatomy. The distal bronchioles contain bands of elastin, which are important in elastic recoil of the lung. They also contain organelles holding surfactant.

The alveoli in a normal lung number 200 to 600 million. The epithelial lining of the alveoli contains two types of cells. Type I cells are attached to the basement membrane and play a passive role in the diffusion of alveolar gases. Type II alveolar cells contain the phospholipid surfactant, which functions to reduce alveolar surface tension and to prevent atelectasis. The alveolar wall, situated between two contiguous alveoli, is made up of two layers of alveolar epithelium, each on a separate basement membrane enclosing the capillary vascular network. These capillaries are embedded between the elastic and collagen fibers and between the smooth muscles and nerves. Therefore, a gas molecule passing from inside the alveolus to the blood has to cross the following layers: (1) a single layer of alveolar epithelial cells with its basement membrane, (2) a space containing elastic and collagen connective tissue, and (3) the basement membranes and endothelial cells of the capillaries (Goudsouzian and Karamanian, 1984).

The Pulmonary Circulation and Physiology

The pulmonary circulation is unique in that it has a double arterial supply from the pulmonary arteries and the bronchial arteries. The circulation begins at the right and left

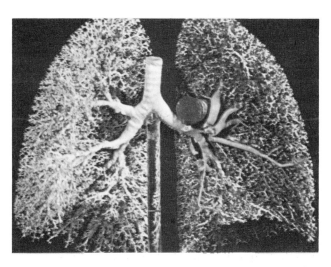

Figure 28–44. The pulmonary circulation. (*From Shields TW: General Thoracic Surgery, 1972. Courtesy of Lea & Febiger, Philadelphia.*)

pulmonary arteries, which transfer mixed venous blood from the right side of the heart to the pulmonary capillaries for gas exchange. The arteries, veins, and bronchi initially run close together, but toward the periphery of the lung, the veins move away to pass between the lobules, whereas the arteries and bronchi travel down the centers of the lobules to the terminal bronchioles (West, 1974). At this point they branch into capillaries that form a dense network in the walls of the alveoli (Fig. 28–44). The capillaries are just wide enough to accommodate a red blood cell and form a continuous sheet of blood in the alveolar wall (West, 1974).

The pulmonary artery receives the entire right heart output. However, the resistance in this system is low. Each red cell spends approximately one second in the capillary network crossing two to three alveoli. The anatomy for gas exchange is so efficient that this short second allows for complete equilibrium between oxygen and carbon dioxide, between alveolar gas and capillary blood (West, 1974). In addition to the circulation provided by the pulmonary arteries, the bronchial arteries carry arterial blood from the conducting airways to the terminal bronchioles. The right lung has one bronchial artery whereas the left usually has two.

The oxygenated blood is carried from the pulmonary capillary bed by small pulmonary veins, which emerge as four large veins to drain into the left atrium. The azygos and hemiazygos veins may absorb some of the venous drainage from the bronchi. The flow through the bronchial circulation is a mere fraction of that through the pulmonary circulation and the lung can function fairly well without it, as is seen with lung transplantation (Wilson, 1976).

Pressures in the pulmonary circulation are very low. The mean pressure in the main pulmonary artery is only about 15 mm Hg; the systolic and diastolic pressures are about 25 and 8 mm Hg, respectively, implying a pulsatile flow (West, 1974). The systemic pressures, on the other hand, are much higher (mean aortic pressure is 100 mm Hg) to direct the flow of blood to various organs. The pulmonary circuit is not concerned with the distribution of blood

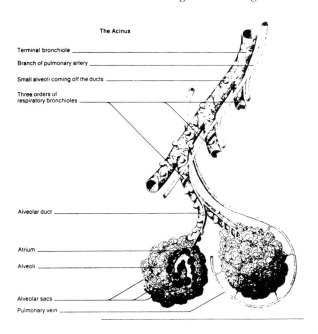

The Acinus

Terminal bronchiole

Branch of pulmonary artery

Small alveoli coming off the ducts

Three orders of
respiratory bronchioles

Alveolar duct

Atrium

Alveoli

Alveolar sacs

Pulmonary vein

Figure 28–43. Illustration of the acinus (basic pulmonary unit). (*From Wilson R: Principles of Critical Care. The Upjohn Company, 1975. Reproduced with permission.*)

from one area to another and requires pressures sufficient only to provide adequate gas exchange. In other words, even though the lung accepts the entire cardiac output, the work of the right heart is minimized because the only blood that it directs is that supplying the lung itself.

Unique to the pulmonary circulation is the fact that the capillaries are surrounded by gas and easily collapse or expand, depending on the pressures in and around them. The pressures within the capillaries are very close to alveolar pressures but can succumb to rises in alveolar pressures and collapse (Kaplan, 1983). The pressure difference between the inside and outside of the vessels is called the transmural pressure (West, 1974).

The pressure around the pulmonary arteries and veins is less than alveolar pressure so they are capable of increasing their diameter as the lung expands. The capillaries and blood vessels differ markedly in terms of their ability to change caliber and have therefore been labeled alveolar and extraalveolar vessels. Alveolar vessels include capillaries, arterioles, and venules; their calibers depend on the alveolar pressure and the pressures within them. Extraalveolar vessels, arteries and veins, run through the lung parenchyma; their caliber is dependent on lung volumes (West, 1974).

The amount of vascular resistance that occurs in the pulmonary circulation is one-tenth that of the systemic system and measures 1.7 mm Hg/L/min or approximately 100 dynes. Vascular resistance is defined as (input pressure − output pressure)/blood flow. The pulmonary vascular resistance is low, once again, because of the small area to which blood is distributed compared with the systemic circulation. Even though this resistance is small, it has the capability of becoming smaller as the pressure within the pulmonary circulation rises. According to West, this fall in pulmonary resistance is produced by two mechanisms: (1) recruitment and (2) distention. Increasing pressure within the pulmonary vessels begins the flow of blood through capillaries that are closed or have no blood flow. With increased blood flow, the overall resistance is decreased. This is recruitment. In addition, as the pressure rises, the caliber of the vessels increases, lowering resistance. This is distention (West, 1974). Large lung volumes lower vascular resistance whereas low lung volumes reduce caliber and increase vascular resistance. Distensibility is influenced strongly by the presence of smooth muscle in the vascular walls, and anything that will influence contraction of smooth muscle will increase pulmonary resistance. Drugs such as serotonin, histamine, and norepinephrine vasoconstrict when lung volumes are low. Relaxation of bronchial smooth muscle is seen with acetylcholine and isoproterenol (Miller, 1986; Kaplan, 1983).

Distribution of Blood and Ventilation. The distribution of blood flow in the lung is unequal. This distribution varies with position and is highly influenced by gravity. West divides perfusion to the lungs into three zones (West, 1977) (Fig. 28–45). Zone 1 encompasses the apex of lung where no flow exists, zone 2, the middle portion of lung with increased flow, and zone 3 the base of the lung, which has maximum flow.

Distribution of ventilation is also dependent on gravity.

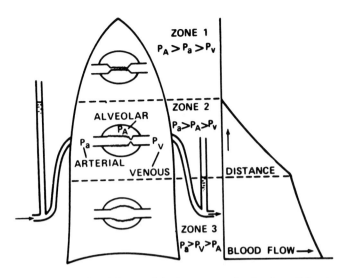

Figure 28–45. Model to explain the uneven distribution of blood flow in the lung based on the pressures affecting the capillaries. (*From West JB, Dollery CT, et al: J Appl Physiol 19:713, 1964.*)

Whereas the blood flow per unit volume decreases rapidly up the lung, the change in ventilation is not nearly so marked (West, 1977). Change of posture from the erect to the supine position abolishes this uneven distribution.

The areas of the lung being ventilated need not necessarily be perfused and vice versa. This inequality of ventilation to perfusion can be expressed as $V_A:Q$, the ventilation:perfusion ratio. The normal value is 0.85 derived from 5.1 L/min total ventilation and 6 L/min total blood flow. This ratio describes the degree of overperfusion or underventilation and determines the gas exchange in any lung unit.[76]

Hypoxic Pulmonary Vasoconstriction. Hypoxic pulmonary vasoconstriction (HPV) is a local compensatory mechanism peculiar to the lungs whereby contraction of the smooth muscle of the arterioles occurs in the presence of a decline in P_{O_2} of alveolar gas. This contraction or vasoconstriction diverts blood flow from the hypoxic area of the lung to areas with normal P_{O_2} levels. HPV is due either to a direct action of alveolar hypoxia on the pulmonary vasculature or due to an alveolar hypoxia-induced release of vasoactive substances (Bohr, 1977). This diversion of blood flow enhances gas exchange by bypassing unoxygenated regions and adjusting regional ventilation:perfusion ratios. Hypoxic ventilation or atelectasis of one lung or one lobe generally causes a 30 to 40 or 50 to 60 percent diversion of blood from the hypoxic to the nonhypoxic lung (Zarslow et al, 1981). This is vital in minimizing the transpulmonary shunt during disease of one lung, one-lung anesthesia, and inadvertent intubation of a main-stem bronchus (Kaplan, 1983; Grant et al, 1980). HPV is inhibited by several factors. Certain inhalation agents, such as nitrous oxide, halothane, methoxyflurane, enflurane, and isoflurane, inhibit HPV (Benumoff and Wahrenbock, 1975). All systemic vasodilator drugs probably inhibit HPV (Benumoff, 1979). Large hypoxic compartments (Benumoff, 1981) and decreases in P_{ACO_2} and P_{aCO_2} below 30 mm Hg inhibit HPV (Benumoff, 1976). Infections, hypothermia, and clinical conditions that increase pulmonary vascular pressure such as mitral stenosis, volume overload, vasopressors and ligation of pulmonary vessels will all inhibit HPV (Finlayson, 1980; Zarslow et al, 1981; Benumoff, 1981).

Preoperative Evaluation

Of all thoracotomies, 40 to 60 percent are associated with respiratory complications and overall mortality can run as high as 15 percent (Kaplan, 1983). The risk factors associated with thoracic surgery are age, obesity, and underlying heart and lung disease. The severity of lung disease must be determined to provide some clue as to the likelihood of development of complications. The assessment of respiratory function should begin with a thorough medical history and physical examination. A tobacco history is one of the most important predictors of postoperative pulmonary difficulty (Finlayson, 1980). This can be determined by calculating the number of pack/years, that is, the number of packs smoked per day multiplied by the number of years smoked (Ayres, 1975). Any increase in pack/year will obviously increase the risk for chronic lung disease as well as malignancy.

Chronic Obstructive Lung Disease. Chronic lung disease can be determined by the presence of chronic productive cough, dyspnea, wheezing, or asthmatic attacks.

Chronic respiratory insufficiency results in an inability to maintain adequate Pa_{O_2} and Pa_{CO_2} levels at normal activity and may either be nonrespiratory or respiratory in origin. Nonrespiratory causes include: (1) central nervous system disorders caused by drugs, infection, or trauma, (2) peripheral nervous system diseases such as polio or Guillain-Barré syndrome, (3) myopathies, which include myasthenia gravis or multiple sclerosis, or (4) chest wall abnormalities from obesity, surgery, or scoliosis (Wilson, 1976). Respiratory causes include: (1) upper airway obstruction, (2) chronic bronchitis, (3) parenchymal diseases, such as emphysema, (4) vascular problems such as congestive heart failure or pulmonary embolism, and (5) chronic pleural inflammation (Wilson, 1976).

Of these, emphysema and chronic bronchitis are the most common causes of chronic respiratory insufficiency.

Emphysema. Emphysema is an irreversible condition characterized by abnormal enlargement of air spaces distal to the terminal bronchioles; it is also associated with destructive changes of the interalveolar septal walls. Destruction of the connective tissue responsible for much of the elastic recoil of the lung results in large alveolar sacs with little elastic recoil (Shapiro and Harrison, 1975). A resultant increase in residual volume with small-airway changes leads to increased airway resistance (Shapiro and Harrison, 1975). The many types of emphysema are classified according to the area of the acinus involved. Centrilobular emphysema involves the respiratory bronchioles in the proximal portions of the acinus and is usually found only in smokers. Other classifications include paraseptal, panlobular, or irregular emphysema.

Asthma. Asthma is usually a reversible respiratory condition characterized by an acute episodic respiration from bronchial smooth muscle constriction, mucosal edema, and accumulation of bronchial secretions (Wilson, 1976). The pathophysiology is a result of a lack of adenylcyclase from the cell membrane, leading to a reduction in the formation of 3'5' cyclic adenosine monophosphate from adenosine triphosphate. A beta blockade occurs, with resultant hyperirritability of the bronchial tree (Wilson, 1976).

Chronic Bronchitis. This disease process is characterized by a chronic increase in mucous secretions of the tracheobronchial tree. Edema and ciliary dysfunction also occur. The underlying pathology is associated with smoke and air pollution, infection, or allergies.

The physiologic effects of chronic obstructive pulmonary disease (COPD) are many. They include: metabolic alkalosis; pulmonary hypertension; polycythemia; and hepatic congestion. Chest X-ray reveals fibrotic changes, increased anterior-posterior diameter, and increased vascular markings. ECG may show right axis deviation and right ventricular hypertrophy. The effects on ventilation are due to a gaseous alveolar distention and are as follows: increased functional residual capacity (FRC) and decreased expiratory reserve volume (ERV), inspiratory reserve volume (IRV), and vital capacity (VC). Alveolar dead space is increased, resulting in an increased carbon dioxide retention and a decreased Pa_{O_2} (Shapiro et al, 1975; Wilson, 1976). (Carbon dioxide levels above 70 mm Hg inactivate the respiratory center's response to Pa_{CO_2}, and respiration becomes hypoxic-dependent.)

The metabolic effects associated with COPD are the result of hypercarbia and hypoxia. Metabolic alkalosis is most frequently seen. The increased carbon dioxide retention increases chloride excretion and bicarbonate reabsorption by the kidneys. The circulatory changes include pulmonary hypertension and right heart failure or cor pulmonale. Pulmonary hypertension develops because of an increasing constriction of the pulmonary arterioles and a reduction in pulmonary capillary bed size (Wilson, 1976; Zarslow et al, 1981). The physical signs of right ventricular failure and pulmonary hypertension include right ventricular heave, palpable pulmonary artery pulsation, accentuated pulmonary component of the second heart sound, peripheral edema, hepatomegaly, jugular vein distention, and hepatojugular reflex (Miller, 1986). Wide fluctuations in stroke volume and blood pressure may occur during the respiratory cycle as a result of forced expirations (Wilson, 1976).

Polycythemia develops from chronic hypoxia. If the hematocrit reaches levels above 55 percent, the tendency to develop thrombosis within the pulmonary arterial tree increases. Leukocytosis may indicate active infection. Congestive heart failure may cause elevations of blood urea nitrogen and serum creatinine and accompanying hepatic congestion may cause abnormal liver function tests (Miller, 1986).

The ECG not only detects rhythm disturbances but also can reflect COPD by demonstrating clockwise rotation, right axis deviation, or right ventricular hypertrophy. The anterior-posterior diameter of the chest is usually increased on x-ray, and fibrotic changes or increased vascular markings are common. Tracheal deviation or obstruction can be detected by chest x-ray, providing information about potential difficulty with intubation. Potential ventilatory problems can exist with pleural effusions, pulmonary edema, or lung consolidation. Spread of infection must be a concern if an abscess or bullous cyst exists. The chest x-ray may not be diagnostic in that it may be normal in the severely obstructed patient. As many as 10 percent of patients with chronic diffuse infiltrative lung disease may have normal chest roentgenograms (Epler et al, 1978).

The cardiac status of the patient must also be evaluated (see discussion earlier in this chapter). Chronic medications should be reviewed, continued, or withheld if necessary.

Preoperative Preparation

The primary purpose of the preoperative evaluation and preparation of the patient is to avoid or at least lessen the incidence of postoperative complications; there exists a strong correlation between preoperative respiratory dysfunction and postoperative complications.

The degree of pulmonary disease can be ascertained by the use of pulmonary function studies. Routine spirometry, particularly forced expiratory volume (FRC_1) and lung volumes with residual volume/total lung capacity (RV/TLC) are fairly sensitive indicators of the likelihood of perioperative difficulty and can identify prospectively up to 80 percent of the potential complications (Ferrans et al, 1979). Patients with an FEV_1 below 2 liters or RV/TLC greater than 40 percent should stop smoking and receive bronchodilator therapy for at least 48 to 72 hours and then be retested (Kaplan, 1983).

Patients with preexisting infections should be treated with antibiotic or antimicrobial therapy and elective surgery delayed until the infection no longer exists.

Overt respiratory failure associated with body water imbalance should be corrected by the use of diuretic therapy. Conversely, dehydration, which results in interstitial or intracellular water loss, needs to be corrected by enteral or parenteral fluid therapy because dehydration may compromise the efficiency of the mucociliary host defense system.

Patients with esophageal tumors may demonstrate abnormalities in serum potassium, calcium, and chloride values as a result of excessive vomiting. Needless to say, elective surgical procedures should be postponed until these levels are within normal limits, which may take anywhere from 12 to 48 hours.

Obesity, especially morbid obesity, is a problem that cannot be corrected easily or rapidly preoperatively. Rapid, sudden weight loss may be detrimental to respiratory function by reducing forced vital capacity. Normally, the obese patient suffers from chronic hypoxemia resulting from a lowered FRC (Stalnecker et al, 1980). Anesthesia will further decrease the FRC by as much as 10 to 25 percent (Marshall and Wyche, 1972).

Smoking should be stopped before surgery and the earlier the better to resolve small-airway abnormalities. A significantly noticeable improvement in small-airway function, sputum production, and mucociliary transport is usually evident after 6 to 14 weeks of smoking cessation (Buist

et al, 1976). Cessation for as short a time as 48 hours has been shown to decrease carboxyhemoglobin levels (Davis et al, 1979).

Bronchodilator Therapy. The tracheobronchial tree is supplied by both sympathetic and parasympathetic nerves. If the sympathetic nerves are stimulated, bronchial relaxation occurs whereas the opposite effect, bronchoconstriction, is evidenced with parasympathetic stimulation. The sympathetic nervous system is believed to accomplish bronchodilation by releasing epinephrine at the receptor site, stimulating beta-2 receptors and causing relaxation of bronchial muscle (Fig. 28–46). On the other hand, alpha-receptors mediate vasoconstriction and may be involved in bronchoconstriction (Fig. 28–47). Pharmacologic manipulation of bronchial smooth muscle tone involves specific intervention at various points of the complex neurohumoral mechanism controlling muscle tone (Nadel, 1977).

The smooth muscle cells of the tracheobronchial tree contain an intracellular messenger enzyme called adenosine monophosphate (cAMP). Increased levels of this enzyme catalyze a series of chemical events that result in relaxation of muscle fibers. Bronchodilating drugs cause an increase in cAMP levels, either by increased production or decreased breakdown (Nadel, 1977). In general, catecholamines increase the production of cAMP and other bronchodilators decrease the breakdown of cAMP (Miller, 1986). Table 28–27 classifies bronchodilating agents.

It is essential that appropriate bronchodilator therapy be instituted several days preoperatively to maximize pulmonary function.

Premedication. The use of anticholinergics remains a controversial issue in the preoperative protocol for patients

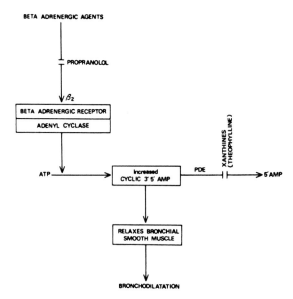

Figure 28–46. Beta-adrenergic pathways through which cAMP is increased in the bronchial smooth muscle cell, leading to bronchodilation. AMP = adenosine monophosphate; ATP = adenosine 5' = triphosphate; PDE = phosphodiesterase. (*From Webb-Johnson DC, et al: Reprinted by permission of N Engl J Med 297:476–482, 1977.*)

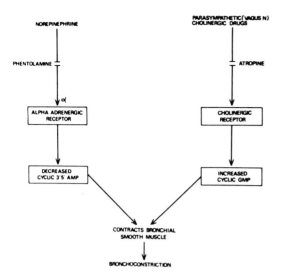

Figure 28–47. Alpha-adrenergic and cholinergic pathways through which cAMP is decreased, or cGMP is increased, in bronchial smooth muscle cell, thus causing bronchoconstriction. cAMP = cyclic adenosine monophosphate; cGMP = cyclic guanine monophosphate. (*From Webb-Johnson DC, et al: Reprinted by permission of N Engl J Med 297:476–482, 1977.*)

TABLE 28–27. CLASSIFICATION OF BRONCHODILATORS

I. Bronchoactive autonomic drugs
  A. Sympathomimetics
    1. Catecholamines
      a. Epinephrine
      b. Isoproterenol
      c. Isoetharine
      d. Ephedrine (indirect acting)
    2. Resorcinols [not metabolized by catechol-O-methyl transferase (COMT); B_2 specificity]
      a. Terbutaline
      b. Metaproterenol
    3. Saligenin
      a. Salbutamol (B_2 specificity)
    4. Others
      a. Protokylol (Ventaire)
      b. Ethylnorepinephrine (Bronkephine)
      c. Methoxyphenamine (Orthoxine)
  B. Parasympatholytic
    1. Anticholinergic
      a. Atropine
      b. Ipratroprium (SCH-1000)
II. Methylxanthines
  A. Phosphodiesterase inhibitors
    1. Theophylline ethylenediamine (aminophylline)
III. Antimediator drugs
  A. Glucocorticoids
    1. Hydrocortisone
    2. Methylprednisolone
    3. Beclomethasone
    4. Triamcinolone
    5. Betamethasone
  B. Antihistamines
  C. Bischromes
    1. Cromolyn
IV. Prostaglandins

From Kaplan JA: Thoracic Anesthesia, 1983. Courtesy of Churchill Livingstone.

undergoing thoracic procedures. Some studies reveal complications such as laryngospasm and coughing associated with excessive secretions. Conversely, other investigators feel that the drying effects of anticholinergics increase complications by decreasing the transportability of bronchial mucus because of increased viscosity (Kaplan, 1983). Generally speaking, the amount of secretion is thought to increase in those who are obese and in those who smoke.

Atropine dilates air passages, the larger ones more than the smaller, and reduces airway resistance. It improves airway conductance in COPD and in allergic states because there is an element of intrinsic bronchoconstriction in these situations that is mediated by the parasympathetic nervous system (Butler et al, 1960).

Glycopyrrolate produces the same drying effects with less incidence of cardiac dysrhythmia. It is twice as potent as atropine and provides little central nervous system stimulation. Opiates in large doses can increase the incidence of postoperative respiratory depression and therefore they are eliminated from the protocol for thoracic surgery. Benzodiazepines are useful premedicants. They produce mild depression of the respiratory system while providing relief of anxiety. Cardiovascular effects are minimal and the amnesia effect is certainly advantageous.

Anesthesia

Each of the inhalation anesthetics exerts its own specific effects on the respiratory system, which raises concerns for the patient undergoing thoracic surgery. The major parameters of an agent's influence on the respiratory centers are: tidal volume (V_T), respiratory rate, minute volume, and effective alveolar ventilation (Stoetling and Eger, 1969).

Inhalation Anesthetics

Nitrous Oxide. Nitrous oxide exerts little effect on the respiratory center in analgesic doses. The V_T, respiratory rate, and minute volume are unaffected. Effective alveolar ventilation is decreased.

Because of its weak anesthetic properties, nitrous oxide must be supplemented with other anesthetic agents so that awareness is avoided.

Nitrous oxide is rapidly taken up by the alveoli, and oxygen given with it will be concentrated (concentration effects) as the nitrous oxide enters the blood, leaving relatively more oxygen in the alveoli and raising the Pa_{O_2}, thereby improving oxygenation (Sheffer et al, 1972).

Upon emergence the reverse is true. Nitrous oxide will rapidly dilute the oxygen left in the alveoli and if they are not properly oxygenated, diffusion hypoxia may be produced (Yacoub et al, 1976). Nitrous oxide depresses the respiratory response to hypoxia, however, and so may add to the diffusion hypoxia syndrome (Eckenoff and Helrich, 1958; Kaplan, 1983). On the other hand, the response to hypercapnia is not depressed by nitrous oxide, and respiration may be increased (Wallace and Sadove, 1962).

Nitrous oxide appears to produce little or no effect on bronchial musculature but does depress mucociliary flow in the trachea, which may increase airway resistance because of the accumulation of secretions (Kaplan, 1983).

The untoward effect of nitrous oxide that causes the most concern is its ability to trap in gas enclosed spaces. Nitrous oxide is thus contraindicated in any process in which it could potentiate an increased volume such as pulmonary blebs, cyst, pneumothorax, and even hemothorax. Mediastinal shift results if the volume expansion is significant. After a pneumonectomy, the hemithorax contains free air. The possibility of mediastinal shifts exists if a chest tube is not used.

Halothane. Halothane rapidly obtunds laryngeal and pharyngeal reflexes. Secretory activity of the glands lining the respiratory tract is depressed, as well as ciliary activity. Bronchial relaxation occurs, resulting in a reduction in airflow resistance and an increase in conductance, which is an advantage in those patients subject to bronchospasm, such as asthmatics. Halothane decreases V_T dose-relatedly. Minute volume and effective alveolar ventilation are also decreased. Respiratory rate is increased, possibly because of sensitization of the stretch receptors in the lungs (Stoelting and Eger, 1969).

A depression of the ventilatory response to hypoxemia occurs at concentrations as low as 0.1 MAC and, when it occurs in those patients who are hypoxic-drive dependent, is a cause for concern postoperatively (Gelb and Knell, 1978). At concentrations of 1.0 to 1.5 percent, the apneic threshold rises, and as anesthetic depth increases, the Pa_{CO_2} rises, causing release of catecholamines (Hickey et al, 1971; Kaplan, 1983).

It is believed that halothane depresses HPV resulting in a venous admixture (Weinreich et al, 1980). This may be of clinical significance during one-lung anesthesia because if HPV is depressed in the nondependent lung, shunting of blood is probable (Kaplan, 1983). The degree of shunting is thought to be significant. Even though this HPV does occur, Kaplan suggests that the use of halothane is acceptable in one-lung anesthesia provided a fraction of inspired oxygen (FI_{O_2}) of 1.0 is used (Kaplan, 1983).

Enflurane. Enflurane is a profound respiratory depressant, which may produce respiratory acidosis with increasing doses. There is a reduction in V_T and alveolar ventilation. Respiratory rate increases and mucociliary flow is depressed. Enflurane is thought to relax constricted airways and thus conductance, although cases of bronchospasm have been reported.

The ventilatory response to hypoxia is also greatly depressed by enflurane, more so than with halothane (Knell et al, 1975). The effects on HPV are similar to those of halothane—it inhibits HPV in anesthetic ranges.

Isoflurane. Isoflurane is also a profound respiratory depressant. V_T, minute volume, alveolar ventilation, and respiratory rate are decreased. Mucociliary activity is also depressed.

A depression of the ventilatory response to Pa_{CO_2} increases or Pa_{O_2} decreases is apparent with isoflurane as with other inhalation agents. Depression is evident at 0.1 MAC. Lung compliance and FRC are thought to decrease slightly and pulmonary resistance increases. HPV is significantly decreased by isoflurane in animal studies (Kaplan,

1983). Addition of nitrous oxide to isoflurane decreases the degree of respiratory depression.

Intravenous Anesthetics. Fentanyl and related compounds produce potent respiratory depressant effects. Both V_T and respiratory rate are decreased. This decline in respiratory rate is opposite to the effect observed with inhalation agents, where a compensatory increase in rate occurs. There is no apparent effect on HPV. In addition to the depressant effects produced by narcotics, lung compliance is decreased and truncal rigidity may occur. The occurrence and degree of truncal rigidity are accentuated by rapidity of injection.

Droperidol produces minimal effects on the respiratory center.

Ketamine. Ketamine produces minimal respiratory effects. It has bronchodilating properties, which are thought to be due to beta-adrenergic stimulation secondary to increased catecholamine levels. Ketamine is thought to increase both pulmonary artery pressure and pulmonary vascular resistance and may be contraindicated in pulmonary hypertension (Gooding et al, 1977; Kaplan, 1983).

One-Lung Anesthesia

Physiology. In one-lung ventilation, the nondependent lung (up lung) is nonventilated; thus blood flow to this lung becomes shunt flow in addition to whatever shunt flow might exist in the dependent lung (down lung) (Kaplan, 1983). The term shunt refers to blood that finds its way into the arterial system without going through ventilated areas of lung (West, 1974). Thus, one-lung ventilation creates an obligatory right-to-left transpulmonary shunt through the nondependent lung, which is not present during two-lung ventilation (Kaplan, 1983). Pa_{O_2} measurements in one-lung ventilation are lower than during two-lung ventilation, but carbon dioxide levels do not appear to be affected. A single overventilated lung can eliminate enough carbon dioxide but cannot take up enough oxygen to compensate for the nonventilated lung. In addition, there is a great disparity between the venous-to-arterial oxygen and carbon dioxide tension differences and a shunt will cause a larger change in Pa_{O_2} than in Pa_{CO_2} (Kaplan, 1983).

The absolute indications for one-lung-ventilation anesthesia include the need for prevention of contamination of the other lung by infected material or blood, when the distribution of ventilation between the lungs must be controlled, as with lung cysts or bronchopleural fistula, or for one-sided bronchopulmonary lavage.

The relative indications for the use of one-lung anesthesia are to facilitate surgical exposure in thoracic aneurysm repair, pneumonectomy, and upper lobectomy (the most difficult lobe to remove). However, this technique is advantageous in procedures such as segmental resections, removal of other lobes, or esophageal surgery (Lappas et al, 1977; Kaplan, 1983).

Although the benefits of one-lung anesthesia in terms of isolation of a diseased lung or for optimization of surgical exposure are obvious and often mandatory, a large alveolar-to-arterial oxygen pressure difference [$P(A - a)_{O_2}$] is a necessary consequence of this intervention. (Torda et al, 1974). The greatest reason for this difference is that the transpulmonary shunt continues because there is perfusion to nonventilated lungs. The venous blood of the nonventilated lung mixes with oxygen from the ventilated lung, lowering the arterial oxygen tension. This degree of hypoxemia varies with the amount of perfusion to the nonventilated lung (Torda et al, 1974; Kerr et al, 1974).

Several factors will influence the degree of perfusion to the deflated lung. These include the condition of the dependent lung, the degree of HPV, the degree of manual insult, such as compression or retraction of the atelectatic lung, and the method used to ventilate the dependent lung. If the dependent lung is diseased with COPD, alterations in both ventilation and perfusion may occur, depending on the degree of insult. Perfusion to the deflated lung is also influenced by the degree of HPV. HPV will minimize the amount of transpulmonary shunting by diverting blood flow. The dependent lung may become diseased intraoperatively from long periods in the lateral decubitus position, leading to fluid accumulation or atelectasis secondary to extended periods of low FRC and low V_T and to hydrostatic effects.

The method by which the dependent lung is ventilated will influence the degree of perfusion to the deflated lung. The influence of positive end-expiratory pressure (PEEP) and F_{IO_2} will affect HPV and the degree of atelectasis. By maintaining a positive pressure during expiration, the FRC will be increased. This effect is desired to prevent atelectasis but may not be welcomed when its effects on blood flow are considered. If FRC is low and then increased to a normal value, pulmonary vascular resistance should decrease, with a resultant increase in blood flow. But if a normal FRC is increased, pulmonary vascular resistance is increased and a considerable amount of blood will be shunted through the ventilated lung.

Other factors, such as a diminished cardiac output and an inadequately functioning endotracheal tube, can also lead to hypoxemia.

The minute volume plays a major role in controlling the carbon dioxide level during one-lung anesthesia whereas several factors control oxygenation. These include the efficiency of the ventilated lung, the amount of residual gas in the nonventilated lung, the cardiac output, and also the inspired oxygen tension.

The degree of efficiency of the ventilated lung is vital to maintenance of adequate oxygenation. Large V_T (10 ml/kg) with 100 percent oxygen during anesthesia usually improve ventilation. However, in some instances, oxygenation with 100 percent will not provide adequate ventilation because of the cumulative effects of shunting in the ventilated lung and increase in blood flow through the nonventilated lung. The amount of residual gas left in the unventilated lung is usually absorbed in five to ten minutes, provided blood flow is present (Nunn, 1969). Thus, there is little effect on the shunt fraction after the first ten minutes. Low cardiac outputs and low F_{IO_2} will, for obvious reasons, influence the degree of oxygenation.

The patient undergoing a thoracic procedure suffers many consequences from the nature of the surgery itself. Among these are the insult from a general anesthetic, which

is complicated by a lateral decubitis position, an open pleural space, and one-lung ventilation.

Collapse of an operated lung provides easier exposure to intrathoracic structures, limiting the damage to lung tissue from excessive traction (Peltola, 1983). Atelectasis in one lung is usually tolerated well in the majority of patients because of pulmonary vascular adaptation, but the risk of hypoxia is always present.

The major alterations in ventilation and perfusion that cause arterial oxygen desaturation and increased intrapulmonary shunting during one-lung ventilation are largely influenced by position and position changes (Peltola, 1983).

Awake Supine Closed Chest. When the awake patient assumes the supine position, the FRC is reduced as a result of the pressure of the abdominal contents against the diaphragm. When this position is changed to the lateral decubitus position, the FRC is reduced more in the lower lung than the upper lung because the dome of the lower diaphragm is pushed higher into the chest than the upper and is more sharply curved. As a result, the lower diaphragm is able to contract more efficiently during spontaneous respiration and thus the lower lung is always better ventilated than the upper lung (Fig. 28–48). Gravitational pull provides better perfusion to the lower lung. The preferential ventilation to the lower lung then is matched by its increased perfusion so that ventilation:perfusion ratios of the two lungs are not greatly altered when the awake patient assumes the lateral position (Miller, 1981).

When the patient is turned from supine to lateral, the cardiac output may drop because of a diminished venous return secondary to pooling in the dependent lung.

Anesthetized Closed Chest. When the anesthetized patient is positioned in the lateral decubitus position, the dependent lung receives more perfusion than the nonde-

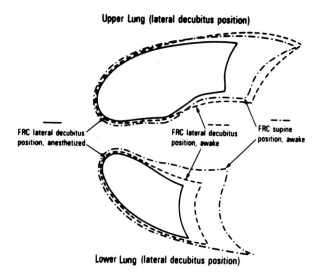

Figure 28–48. Schematic of the lungs at functional residual capacity (FRC) during supine position, awake; lateral decubitus position, awake; and lateral decubitus position, anesthetized. Note the greater loss in FRC in the lower lung in the lateral decubitus position when awake and anesthetized. (*From Miller RD: Anesthesia, 2nd ed, 1986. Courtesy of Churchill Livingstone.*)

pendent lung because of gravitational influences. Significant changes in ventilation also occur. In this position, the upper lung in the spontaneously ventilated anesthetized patient receives most of the V_T. This major change is due to (1) a decrease in FRC bilaterally and loss of lung volume, (2) interference with the contracting diaphragm by muscle relaxants, (3) the mediastinum impeding lower lung expansion, (4) the weight of the abdominal contents pushing against the diaphragm, which is largest in the dependent lung, and (5) methods to improve operative access, such as supporting rolls, which may jeopardize lower lung expansion (Kaplan, 1983).

The nondependent lung is well ventilated and poorly perfused, and the dependent lung is well profused but poorly ventilated, indicating ventilation:perfusion mismatch. Ventilation to the dependent lung can be improved by adding PEEP to both lungs (Rheder et al, 1973). Consideration should be given to the fact that PEEP may also increase the shunt fraction.

Anesthetized Open Chest. Opening of the pleural cavity causes the lung to collapse and the mediastinum to shift toward the dependent lung, decreasing ventilation (Tarhan and Moffit, 1973). This can be prevented by intermittent positive-pressure ventilation, which maintains airway and alveolar pressures above atmospheric (Peltola, 1983).

When the chest is open, pulmonary blood flow remains the same as in the closed chest position between the dependent lung and the nondependent lung. However, ventilation can no longer be spontaneous and must be accomplished by positive-pressure ventilation. Opening of the chest wall and pleural space will affect the distribution of the positive-pressure ventilation and perfusion (Kaplan, 1983). If the upper lung is no longer restricted by the chest wall, it will easily be overventilated (Kaplan, 1983). Conversely, the dependent lung continues to be poorly ventilated and overperfused (Wuff and Aulin, 1972).

It must be emphasized that spontaneous breathing during open-chest surgery can cause a mediastinal shift. With the chest open, atmospheric pressure in the chest cavity on the nondependent lung exceeds the negative pressure in the dependent hemithorax, causing an imbalance of the pressure in the mediastinum (Kaplan, 1983). This condition is augmented with inspiration and reversed with expiration (Fig. 28–49). The V_T in the dependent lung is decreased by an amount equal to the inspiratory displacement caused by mediastinal movement (Kaplan, 1983).

Technique. The most common way of providing one-lung anesthesia is by way of the double-lumen endotracheal tube. The advantage of this method is that it is possible to ventilate either one or both lungs independently. One lumen reaches into one of the main bronchi, whereas the other descends only as far as the trachea. Leakage of gas during positive-pressure ventilation is prevented by a cuff placed above the shorter lumen. Separation of gas flow and infected material can be accomplished by use of a cuff placed above the longer lumen. The tubes most commonly used today are the Carlens, White, Bryce-Smith, and Robertshaw. The Carlens tube, the first double-lumen tube to be used, is designed for a left-sided intubation and a right thoracotomy.

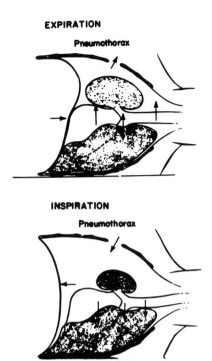

Figure 28–49. Schematic representation of mediastinal shift in the spontaneously breathing open-chested patient in the lateral decubitus position. During inspiration, negative pressure in the intact hemithorax causes the mediastinum to move downward. During expiration, relative positive pressure in the intact hemithorax causes the mediastinum to move upward. (*From Tarhan S, Muffitt EA: Surg Clin North Am 53:813, 1973.*)

It has a carinal hook for ensuring proper placement. It ranges in size from 35 to 37 French for females or young adults to 39 and 41 for males (Fig. 28–50).

The White tube is a modification of the Carlens and is used for right main bronchus intubation (left thoracotomy). The bronchial cuff is slotted to provide ventilation to the right upper lobe. It is available in 37, 39, and 41 French.

The Bryce-Smith also is a modification of the Carlens tube and can be used for intubation of right or left main bronchus. It does not have a carinal hook (Figure 28–51).

The Robertshaw tube is the most commonly used double-lumen endotracheal tube (Pappin, 1979). Because it has large lumens, airway resistance is minimized and suctioning is facilitated. It is available in both right- and left-sided tubes. There is no carinal hook (Fig. 28–52).

When isolation of the left lung is required, either a left- or right-sided tube may be used. If a right-sided tube is used for left lung isolation, the right upper lobe may be inadequately ventilated if there is no opening in the endobronchial cuff to permit right upper lobe ventilation. Consequently, some practitioners prefer to use only left-sided tubes for left lung isolation. Generally speaking, it is advisable to intubate the bronchus of the dependent nonoperative lung (Kaplan, 1983).

Prior to insertion of a double-lumen tube, the cuffs and connections must be checked for proper performance. The tube and stylet must be adequately lubricated. If the

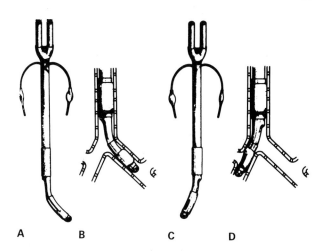

Figure 28–52. Left **(A)** and right **(C)** Robertshaw double-lumen endotracheal tubes; **(B)** and **(D)** show placement at the carina. On **C,** note the slotted endobronchial cuff, which has a relatively large proximal area for inflation to provide a better seal. (*From Miller RD: Anesthesia, 2nd ed, 1986. Courtesy of Churchill Livingstone.*)

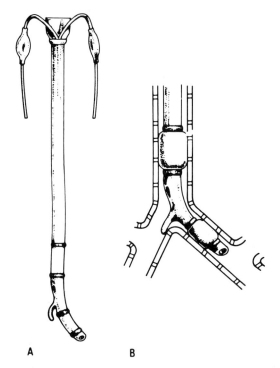

Figure 28–50. A. The Carlens double-lumen endotracheal tube; **B.** placement at the carina. (*From Miller RD: Anesthesia, 2nd ed, 1986. Courtesy of Churchill Livingstone.*)

Carlens or White tube is used, the carinal hooks should be down when inserted through the cords. Once through the cords, the hook should be rotated to pass through the glottis, then rotated 90 degrees to enter the appropriate bronchus. It is then advanced slowly until the hook engages the carina. Because carinal hooks can cause laryngeal trauma, these tubes must be inserted carefully.

The Robertshaw tube is passed with the distal curvature concave anteriorly, then rotated 90 degrees so that the proxi-

mal curve is concave anteriorly to allow for endobronchial intubation (Miller, 1981). Once resistance is met, passage of the tube should be stopped.

Proper positioning of the tube must be assessed; malposition is the most common cause of inadequate gas exchange.

Once the tube is inserted, both lungs should ventilate with inflation of either cuff. Slow inflation of the endobronchial cuff with the tracheal limb clamped confirms position in the appropriate bronchus.

With the tracheal cuff inflated, both lungs should ventilate. Next, one connecting tube should be clamped and the disappearance of breath sounds on that side noted. Breath sounds should be audible on the unclamped side. This procedure should then be repeated on the other side.

Once placement has been evaluated, the tube must be secured to avoid dislodgement during positioning of the patient. When the lateral decubitus position is assumed, the head must be kept in a neutral or slightly flexed position because head extension causes movement of the tube cephalad (Conrady et al, 1976).

Management of One-Lung Ventilation. Even though atelectasis of one lung is tolerated well in most instances, hypoxemia still occurs in some subjects. There are several steps that can reduce the incidence or degree of hypoxemia during one-lung anesthesia. First, two-lung ventilation should be maintained as long as possible. Once one-lung ventilation begins, a V_T of 8 to 10 ml/kg should be used and rate adjusted to maintain a Pco_2 of 40 mm Hg. High Fio_2 with frequent blood gas sampling is recommended.

If severe hypoxemia develops, down lung PEEP may be employed. Caution must be taken because even though PEEP may improve V:Q ratios in the down lung, it may also increase down lung pulmonary vascular resistance and shunt blood flow up to the nonventilated nondependent lung, resulting in no change or even a decrease in Pao_2 (Turhan and Lundborg, 1970).

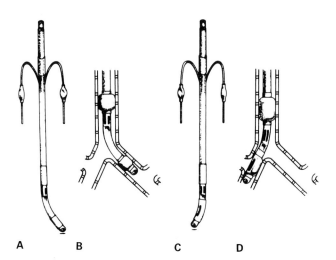

Figure 28–51. Left **(A)** and right **(C)** Bryce-Smith double-lumen endotracheal tubes; **(B)** and **(D)** placement at the carina. On **C,** note the slotted endobronchial cuff, which inflates primarily on the medial side. (*From Miller RD: Anesthesia, 2nd ed, 1986. Courtesy of Churchill Livingstone.*)

Complications to the Use of Double-Lumen Tubes. In addition to hypoxemia, other complications can occur with the use of double-lumen tubes. These include laryngitis, soft tissue injury, suturing of the tube to a pulmonary vessel, tracheobronchial laceration or rupture, and inability to deflate the nondependent lung (Miller, 1986; Kaplan, 1983). The development of such complications may be due to inadequate tube size, requiring overinflation of the bronchial cuff, malposition of the tip of the tube, or too rapid inflation of the distal cuff (Kaplan, 1983).

Anesthesia for Thoracic Procedures

Mediastinoscopy. Mediastinoscopy is a frequently performed diagnostic procedure used to determine the presence of lung tumors. During this procedure, a small incision is made in the right upper chest and the mediastinoscope tip is placed in the intrathoracic cavity. This can pose serious problems if the patient is breathing spontaneously. Because of the development of a negative intrathoracic pressure during inspiration, venous air embolism may occur. Controlled positive-pressure ventilation is indicated to minimize the risk of air embolism.

Another serious complication of this procedure is massive blood loss from accidental tear of a major vessel. Blood loss can be rapid and often not controllable by direct pressure on the bleeding site, necessitating a thoracotomy. Should hemorrhage originate from a superior vena cava tear, intravascular volume replacement and drug therapy may be lost in the surgical field unless these drugs are administered via a peripheral intravenous line placed in the lower extremity (Roberts and Gessen, 1979). During biopsy, the mediastinoscope can exert pressure on the innominate artery, causing a diminished flow to the right carotid and right subclavian arteries. A transient hemiparesis may occur. To prevent occlusion of the innominate, blood pressure should be measured in the left arm and the right radial artery pulse be monitored closely during this procedure. Some clinicians encourage the placement of a blood pressure cuff on both arms to rapidly assess compression of the innominate.

Pneumothorax is also a potential problem that usually occurs postoperatively. It usually does not require a chest tube, provided respiratory compromise is not evident.

Vagal stimulation and pressure on vessels may cause a sudden change in pulse or pressure and may be alleviated by repositioning of the mediastinoscope or by the use of an anticholinergic.

Bronchoscopy. Bronchoscopy, either rigid or flexible, is a valuable diagnostic tool and, in most instances, can be performed under local anesthesia. The most common complications are bronchospasm, pneumothorax, or hemorrhage. If the hemorrhage is severe, the patient should be placed in the lateral decubitus position with the bleeding side down to avoid bleeding into the opposite lung. A double-lumen tube may be necessary to occlude the bleeding bronchus and resection instituted if bleeding is not controlled by tamponade.

Tracheostomy. Indications for tracheostomy include (1) upper airway obstruction, (2) access for tracheal toilet, (3) administration of positive-pressure ventilation, and (4) airway protection from aspiration of gastric contents (Kaplan, 1983). Tracheostomy is usually performed under local anesthesia with some sedation. These patients are usually intubated and it is the responsibility of the anesthesia team to slowly withdraw the endotracheal tube so that the tracheostomy tube may be inserted. The most common complications include hemorrhage and failure to cannulate the trachea. If a tracheostomy is necessary, it should be performed between the second and third tracheal rings. Pulsation of a tracheostomy tube indicates pressure on the innominate artery; erosion can occur if the tube is not repositioned.

Lobectomy. The anesthetic considerations for a lobectomy are centered around problems that are incurred by insertion of a double-lumen tube and by assumption of the lateral decubitus position. The right upper lobe is most commonly resected followed by the left upper lobe (Kaplan, 1983).

The procedure for resection of the right upper lobe will be described (Fig. 28–53). A posterolateral thoracotomy incision is made and the pleural cavity is entered via the fourth intercostal space. The fifth rib may or may not be resected. The arterial supply to the lobe is located and ligated. The superior pulmonary vein, which drains the upper lobe, is divided and ligated cautiously so as not to interfere with drainage from the middle lobe. The posterior ascending artery (which supplies the posterior segment of the lobe) is located and ligated; then the upper lobe bronchus is isolated and divided. Care is taken to close the bronchial stump completely. At this time, a complete closure is confirmed by adding saline to the area and by having the anesthetist apply 20 to 30 cmH_2O pressure (Sabiston and Spencer, 1976). Absence of air bubbles ensures a secure closure. Once the lobe is removed, the middle and lower lobes are inflated and air leaks are looked for once again. Two chest tubes are inserted into the pleural cavity and connected to water seal drainage.

Provided that the patient is in good general health, this procedure is usually well tolerated. Intraoperative arrythmias in the form of supraventricular rhythms such as atrial fibrillation and flutter are frequent during major pulmonary resections (5 to 15 percent) (Mowry and Reynold, 1964; Shields and Ujike, 1968; Kaplan, 1983).

When a lobe of a lung is resected, a portion of the total alveolar, bronchial, and vascular mass is removed and an overinflation of the contralateral as well as the remaining ipsilateral lung occurs. There is increased perfusion to the remaining lung tissue. Although there is an increase in the ratio of dead space to total lung volume, a decrease of dead space occurs in respect to V_T. There is a loss of membrane diffusion capacity and overventilation and underperfusion of remaining lung tissue (Shields and Ujike, 1968).

Pneumonectomy. Patients undergoing pneumonectomy endure a high degree of surgical stress. This procedure should be performed in patients with sufficient cardiopulmonary reserve (Kaplan, 1983).

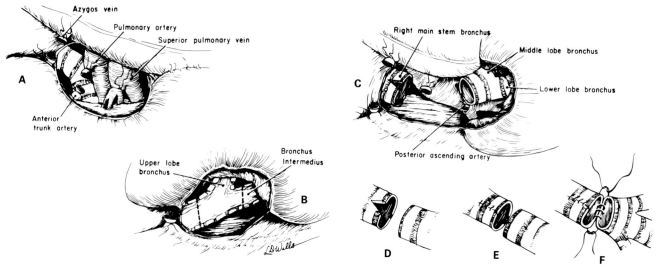

Figure 28–53. Schematic illustrations of steps of right upper lobectomy and sleeve resection of adjacent main stem bronchus. (*From Shields TW: General Thoracic Surgery, 1972. Courtesy of Lea & Febiger, Philadelphia.*)

Total removal of the lung is indicated for bronchial carcinoma, multiple lung abscesses, or extensive bronchiectasis. There are three positions that may be employed to facilitate this procedure: lateral, posterior, or anterior. The lateral position, using a posterolateral incision, in which the fifth rib is resected, provides the best access to the hilum of the lung (Sabiston and Spencer, 1976).

After the pleural space is entered, all adhesions are lysed, freeing the lung from the chest wall. The pulmonary artery is isolated, divided, and controlled. Next, the superior and then inferior veins are dissected and controlled. The main-stem bronchus is freed up to its junction with the trachea. A clamp is placed distal to the junction and the bronchus is divided above the clamp. The bronchial stump is then closed. After closure, the stump is covered with a flap of adjacent tissue to help prevent leak from the stump (Fig. 28–54). Positive pressure (30 cmH$_2$0) is applied to the lung to test the bronchial stump suture line (Sabiston and Spencer, 1976).

Problems in the intraoperative period center on operative exposure, methods of controlling bronchial closure, and hemostasis. Proper closure of the bronchial stump is extremely important to avoid bronchopleural fistula and infection.

The incidence of dysrhythmias is higher than with lobectomies (25 to 40 percent) (Kaplan, 1983).

Following pneumonectomy, the pulmonary artery and right ventricular pressures rise temporarily and a transient change in cardiac output occurs. In addition, the depth and rate of breathing increases. An increase in the ratio of the V$_T$ to FRC leads to an improved mixing of inspired gases. Compliance is reduced. Once the remaining lung adjusts to the new volume, it hyperinflates, resulting in a 10 to 30 percent increase in vital and total capacities (Shields and Ujike, 1968). The pulmonary artery pressure may be normal at rest or during mild exercise because a normal lung can adjust to double its blood flow. But with moderate or strenuous exercise, the pulmonary artery pressure increases.

If the remaining lung is diseased, the FRC and V$_T$ are decreased. This capacity is determined by the expansibility of the remaining vascular bed, and when the limit of the bed is reached or exceeded, persistent pulmonary hypertension occurs with the development of cor pulmonale (Shields and Ujike, 1968).

ESOPHAGEAL SURGERY

Patients with esophageal tumors or strictures are usually debilitated because of dysphagia with both solids and liquids. In addition, they are prone to regurgitation and aspiration during the induction of anesthesia. Poor nutritional status produces metabolic changes that can be problem-

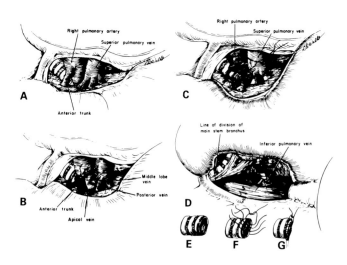

Figure 28–54. A to **C.** Schematic illustrations of isolation, control, and division of vascular structures of the right lung during pneumonectomy. **D** to **G.** Division of main-stem bronchus and its closure with the use of nonabsorbable sutures. (*From Shields TW: General Thoracic Surgery, 1972. Courtesy of Lea & Febiger, Philadelphia.*)

provoking for the anesthetist. These include dehydration and hypovolemia, which lead to hypotension, hypoalbuminemia resulting from decreased protein intake, which will affect the degree of drug binding, and reduction of hemoglobin and electrolytes, resulting in shifts in the oxyhemoglobin curve and cardiac dysrhythmias respectively (Kaplan, 1983). These abnormal values should be corrected preoperatively.

General anesthesia administered to these patients should be approached as if the patient had a full stomach. Patients with large hiatal hernias or large esophageal tumors should be intubated awake or be induced by rapid sequence.

The location of the tumor will determine the type of incision and the type of endotracheal tube. Tumors of the upper or lower third of the esophagus can be reached without thoracotomy incisions and can be managed with standard endotracheal tube. Midthoracic esophageal tumors must be approached by thoracotomy (Kaplan, 1983), and use of a double-lumen tube provides optimal exposure for the surgeon.

Intraoperative complications include hypotension from blood loss or from inferior vena caval obstruction during the dissection of the lower end of the esophagus. The carotid sinus reflex can be stimulated, causing bradycardia and hypotension, and the trachea may be ruptured during midesophageal resection (Kaplan, 1983). If tracheal rupture occurs, endobronchial intubation is necessary to provide ease of access to the trachea for repair. If an endotracheal tube is in place, it can be pushed down into the trachea to provide an endobronchial intubation until the repair is complete (Kaplan, 1983).

BRONCHOPLEURAL FISTULA

The occurrence of a bronchopleural fistula may be due to a ruptured lung abscess or bulla, a carcinomatous erosion, suture line separation after pulmonary resection, or trauma. The most common occurrence is after pulmonary resection for carcinoma (Kaplan, 1983).

A bronchopleural fistula interrupts air flow in the lung by providing an alternate pathway in which air bypasses the lungs. A gas loss across the bronchopleural fistula develops. This abnormal external communication may result in contamination of the lung, loss of air, or development of a tension pneumothorax during positive-pressure ventilation (Kaplan, 1983).

Treatment is aimed at reducing the flow of gas over the fistula, thereby promoting healing. If the lung is intact on the affected side, an effort is made to expand the lung fully and eliminate the gas in the pleural space. This is first attempted by a chest tube with negative pressure. Once the chest tube is inserted, hypoventilation usually occurs because of loss of V_T through the fistula (Kaplan, 1983). An increase in negative pressure or the application of positive pressure serves only to worsen the condition by increased flow across the fistula, and a reduction in rate and V_T is recommended (Kaplan, 1983). If the ventilatory status does not improve, selective endobronchial intubation and differential treatment of the lungs may permit diminution or cessation of flow across the bronchopleural fistula on the affected side while promoting adequate support of ventilation on the unaffected side (Miller, 1981; Kaplan, 1983).

Insertion of this long-term endobronchial tube is usually performed under local anesthesia if the physical status of the patient is poor or, if tolerated, under general anesthesia, spontaneously breathing, with the head-up position (Miller, 1981).

Recently, high frequency positive-pressure ventilation (driving pressure 35 psi, rate 115 breaths/min, inspiratory: expiratory ratio 1:2, gas flow 15 L/min) has been successfully used to provide adequate oxygenation and carbon dioxide removal in a patient with a large bronchopleural fistula (Carlon et al, 1980).

Aspiration presents a major risk to these patients. Sudden drainage of pus, with contamination of the healthy lung, can cause severe ventilatory problems or even death. The patient should be transported in the sitting position lying toward the affected side to avoid spillage into the contralateral lung. Bronchoscopy before intubation is recommended to analyze the degree of impairment or to delineate problems with intubation. Surgery is performed with the patient in the lateral position with the contaminated lung down. The pleural space should be aspirated as completely as possible.

BRONCHOPULMONARY LAVAGE

The technique of bronchopulmonary lavage is used to remove the lipoproteinacious material from the alveoli of patients with pulmonary alveolar proteinosis (Busque, 1977).

Lung lavage is performed under general anesthesia with the use of a double-lumen tube. Mild sedation can be used as a premedicant followed by oxygen by mask to avoid hypoxemia. Volatile inhalation anesthetic agents that do not induce bronchoconstriction are recommended. Muscle relaxation should be maintained to prevent coughing during the procedure. The double-lumen tube should be a left lung Robertshaw, which is a clear plastic, high-volume, low-pressure tube (Kaplan, 1983). A left lung tube is desirable because the cuff inflates symmetrically, providing a secure seal, whereas the right lung cuff inflates asymmetrically to avoid obstruction of the right upper lobe (Kaplan, 1983). Appropriate placement is absolutely essential to ensure separation of the lungs. The cuff must be inflated to a pressure high enough to withstand the peak inspiratory pressure and lavage pressures (the left endobronchial lumen should just begin to invaginate) (Miller, 1981; Kaplan, 1983). A fiberoptic bronchoscopy and chest x-ray should be performed to assess placement.

Once the endobronchial tube is inserted, a spirometer can be placed in the expiratory limb to measure V_T. A volume ventilator should be used to deliver high inflation pressure to noncompliant lungs (10 to 15 ml/kg). Prelavage compliance of both lungs and then each lung separately should be recorded (Kaplan, 1983).

Bilateral lung involvement is common, and lavage should be performed on the most severely affected lung first so that gas exchange can be provided from the less affected lung. The procedure takes several hours, and it is recommended that these patients be placed on a warming blanket to prevent hypothermia from lavage fluid temperature.

Baseline arterial gases and frequent intraoperative values should be drawn to monitor oxygenation. The lung to be treated should not be ventilated for several minutes before lavage to allow complete oxygen extraction and to augment the effectiveness of lavage (Miller, 1986).

Warm saline, 500 to 1000 ml, is used as the lavage fluid and is instilled by gravity from a height of 30 cm above the midaxillary line (Kaplan, 1983). After the lavage fluid ceases to flow, it is drained by a line to a collection bottle 20 cm below the midaxillary line (Kaplan, 1983). A total of 10 to 20 L of lavage fluid is generally used. During lavage, the fluid infusion pressure exceeds pulmonary pressure, causing nonventilated lavaged lung blood flow to be diverted to the ventilated lung (Rogers and Tantam, 1970; Rogers et al, 1972). As the lung drains, the pulmonary artery pressure exceeds the lavaged lung alveolar pressure and lavaged lung blood flow, which is transpulmonary shunt flow, is reestablished (Rogers and Tantam, 1970; Rogers et al, 1972). Thus, the degree of hypoxemia is greatest during lung drainage and gases should be monitored carefully during this time (Rogers and Tantam, 1970; Rogers et al, 1972; Busque, 1977; Miller, 1986). The nonaffected lung should be auscultated frequently to ensure that the lungs are still separated. The presence of air bubbles in the drainage fluid may represent a leak. The volume of fluid introduced into the lung should equal that of the drainage. If not, the presence of a leak should be suspected.

The insertion of a pulmonary artery catheter is strongly recommended. If the tip of the catheter is located in the pulmonary artery of the lung being lavaged, inflation of the balloon during lung drainage will divert blood flow away from the nonventilated lung and improve oxygenation (Alfey et al, 1980).

Once lavage is completed, the lung should be suctioned and positive pressure applied to reexpand alveoli (15 to 20 ml/kg) and chest wall percussion begun to improve lung compliance. This procedure is repeated until the compliance returns to the prelavage value. Muscle relaxation should be maintained until this process is completed. The patient is extubated if blood gases are normal and peak inspiratory force is greater than −20 cmH$_2$O. If not, an endotracheal tube should replace the endobronchial tube and the patient placed on PEEP or positive airway pressure (CPAP) with intermittent mandatory ventilation (IMV) (Kaplan, 1983).

TRACHEAL RESECTION

Lesions of the trachea may be congenital, neoplastic, or traumatic. Traumatic injuries may be the result of direct injury or from endotracheal or tracheostomy tubes. Lesions may also result from infections.

The clinical symptoms generally consist of dyspnea, especially with effort, wheezing, which may present as frank stridor, difficulty in clearing secretions, and eventually airway obstruction from inability to clear mucus or from tumor enlargement (Grillo, 1973; Kaplan, 1983).

A careful history is important to the diagnosis of these lesions because they often go undetected until the severe stages of respiratory obstruction develop. Symptoms are frequently inappropriately considered as an advancement of a preexisting cardiopulmonary problem. Or, frequently,

this process is misdiagnosed as asthma and not properly assessed until the routine corrective measures for asthma fail.

The existence of a tracheal lesion is detected by pulmonary function tests and radiologic study. Bronchoscopy should be deferred until the time of surgery to avoid precipitation of airway obstruction secondary to edema or hemorrhage (Kaplan, 1983).

Preoperative Evaluation and Preparation

The anatomic structure of the upper airway should be analyzed carefully, with attention to jaw motion or problems associated with mask fits to prevent unnecessary episodes of hypoxia.

Baseline blood gases can be drawn, although they are seldom abnormal in the presence of pure airway stenosis (Kaplan, 1983).

The use of premedicants is controversial. There are some concerns that sedative and drying agents may augment respiratory difficulty. These patients may be treated with steroids to reduce edema, and administration should be continued intraoperatively.

Four approaches have been used to provide adequate ventilation during tracheal resection. These include standard orotracheal intubation, insertion of a tube into the opened trachea distal to the area of resection, jet ventilation through the stenotic area, and cardiopulmonary bypass (Miller, 1986).

Routine monitoring measures should be employed. Arterial catheters should be placed in the left radial artery because the right artery pulse is often lost by compression or ligation of the innominate artery, which crosses the trachea (Kaplan, 1983).

Induction and Maintenance

Routine induction techniques can be employed in those patients with minimal airway obstruction. If the obstruction is severe, however, a slow inhalation induction should be used. Muscle relaxants should be avoided because a successful intubation may not be readily accomplished. Inhalation should proceed until it is determined that laryngoscopy can be performed without undue stress on the patient. The larynx should be anesthetized with a topical spray and bronchoscopy performed. Careful analysis of the lesion must be made at this time. Its exact location and size should be determined. Lesions involving the upper third of the trachea, especially those in the subglottic area, pose special problems with placement because of cuff position. A lesion that is located high in the airway, where the tube cannot be passed through the lesion because of a limited opening, will not allow the cuff to pass below the cords and results in inability to attain a complete seal of the airway. Lesions in the mid and lower thirds of the trachea are less problematic with respect to position but must be considered in view of the need to pass the tube through the lesion itself to maintain adequate ventilation until the trachea is resected or dilated (Kaplan, 1983). The bronchoscopy and intubation must be as gentle as possible so as not to cause serious bleeding or dislodgement of tumor, resulting in further obstruction. The inhalation agent of choice and oxygen are used as maintenance agents. Muscle relaxants should be avoided. Nitrous oxide may be used if arterial gases are within normal limits.

The location of the lesion will necessitate special anesthetic interventions during surgical reconstruction. For lesions of the upper half of the trachea, ventilation can be managed by one of two means. A standard endotracheal tube can be inserted above the lesion and is then advanced through the stenosis during resection. Second, intubation can be performed proximal to the lesion and then the surgeon can insert an additional endotracheal tube into the open trachea distal to the site of the lesion, requiring an additional anesthesia machine (Fig. 28–55) (Geffin, 1969; Bayan and Privitera, 1976). Anesthetic considerations for upper airway lesions include: (1) in those patients who are not intubated through the lesion, release of the supporting structure of the trachea may result in complete airway obstruction; (2) if nitrous oxide is being used, it should be discontinued at the time of the resection; (3) when anastomosis of the trachea begins, the endotracheal tube cuff should be deflated so that it is not damaged by the surgical needle; (4) flexion of the head is required for tracheal approximation, and care must be taken so as not to advance the endotracheal tube into the right main-stem bronchus; and (5) with the patient spontaneously breathing, extubation should proceed in the surgical suite so that reintubation, if necessary, takes place in a controlled environment (Grillo, 1973; Ellis et al, 1976; Kaplan, 1983).

Reconstruction of the lower trachea or carinal reconstruction is facilitated by a right thoracotomy incision and may require an endobronchial intubation if there is not enough distance between the tracheal lesion and the carina (Fig. 28–56) (Bayan and Privitera, 1976; Miller, 1986). Figure 28–57 demonstrates the surgical approach and airway management for carinal lesions. Anesthetic considerations for reconstruction of the lower trachea include: (1) the endotracheal tube must be long enough to enter the main-stem bronchus; (2) positive-pressure ventilation or high inspired oxygen concentrations are required to provide additional oxygen to compensate for periods of obstruction or tube

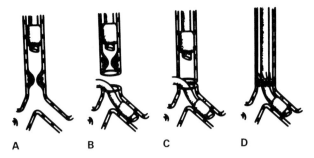

Figure 28–56. Airway management and surgical procedure for resection of a low tracheal lesion. **A.** Initial intubation above the lesion; **B.** endobronchial intubation distal to the lesion after the trachea has been opened; **C.** placement of sutures for the posterior anastomosis; **D.** the endobronchial tube has been removed and the original endotracheal tube advanced distal to the anterior anastomosis into an endobronchial position. (*From Geffin B, Bland J, Grillo HC: Anesth Analg 48:884, 1969.*)

displacement; (3) left main-stem intubation is necessary to provide adequate oxygenation once the trachea is divided, because the tracheal stump is short and cannot hold the endotracheal tube cuff, making it extremely difficult to ventilate both lungs; (4) additional right main-stem intubation may be necessary if adequate ventilation cannot be maintained with one-lung ventilation; this requires a second gas machine and sterile tubings to provide positive pressure to the independent lung; (5) once the repair has been established, an endotracheal tube can be passed through the anastomotic site and endobronchial tubes removed; (6) extubation is dependent on whether or not preexisting lung disease is present; and (7) frequent blood gas analysis is mandatory (Grillo, 1973; Bayan and Privitera, 1976; Ellis et al, 1976; Kaplan, 1983).

In addition to the above-mentioned techniques, jet (high-flow) ventilation through small-bore endotracheal catheters has been used (Lee and English, 1974). This technique appears to ventilate adequately, while providing little interference from the surgical standpoint because of the small tube size. Carinal resections have also been managed

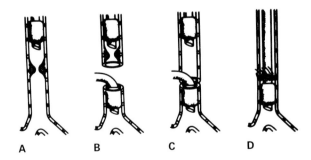

Figure 28–55. Airway management and surgical procedure for resection of a high tracheal lesion. **A.** Initial intubation above the lesion; **B.** second endotracheal intubation distal to the lesion after the trachea has been opened; **C.** placement of sutures for the posterior anastomosis; **D.** the second endotracheal tube has been removed and the original endotracheal tube advanced distal to the anterior anastomosis. (*From Geffin B, Bland J, Grillo HC: Anesth Analg 48:884, 1969.*)

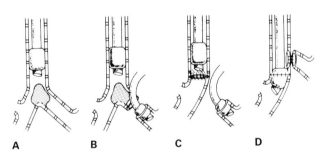

Figure 28–57. Airway management and surgical procedure for resection of a carinal lesion. **A.** Initial intubation above the lesion; **B.** left endobronchial intubation distal to the lesion after the left main-stem bronchus has been severed; **C.** the trachea is anastomosed to the right of main-stem bronchus; **D.** the left endobronchial tube has been removed to allow anastomosis between the trachea and left main-stem bronchus. Ventilation during **D** is accomplished via the original endotracheal tube. (*From Geffin B, Bland J, Grillo HC: Anesth Analg 48:884, 1969.*)

by means of cardiopulmonary bypass, but the risk of intra-pulmonary hemorrhage from heparinization limits its use (Geffin et al, 1969).

REFERENCES

Alfrey DD, Zamost BG, Benumof JL: Unilateral lung lavage; manipulation of pulmonary blood flow. Anesthesiology 53:5381, 1980.

Arfan A: Prosthetic cardiac valves—1983. Conn Med 47:10,619–625, 1983.

Ayres SM: Cigarette smoking and lung diseases: An update. Basics Respir Dis 3(5):1–6, 1975.

Balasoraswathi K, Glisson SN, et al: Haemodynamic and catecholamine response to isoflurane anesthesia in patients undergoing coronary artery surgery. Can Anesth Soc J 29:533–538, 1982.

Baraka A, Harrison T, Kacchachi T: Catecholamine levels after ketamine anesthesia in man. Anes Analg 52:198–200, 1973.

Barlett RH, Drinker PA, et al: Mechanical devices for cardiopulmonary assistance. Adv Cardiol 1971.

Barlett RH, Tony SW, et al: Hematologic response to prolonged extracorporeal circulation with microporous membrane devices. Trans Am Soc Artif Intern Organs 5:238, 1959.

Barry KG, Berman AR: The acute effect of intravenous infusion of mannitol on blood and plasma volume. N Engl J Med 264:1085, 1961.

Bayan PC, Privitera PA: Resection of stenotic trachea: A case presentation. Anes Analg 55:191, 1976.

Benumoff JL: Hypoxic pulmonary vasoconstriction and sodium nitroprusside infusion. Anesthesiology 50:481–483, 1979.

Benumoff JL, Mathers JM: Inhibition of hypoxic pulmonary vasoconstriction by decreased PVO_2: A new indirect mechanism. J Appl Physiol 51:871–874, 1981.

Benumoff JL Pirlo A: Cyclic hypoxic pulmonary vasoconstriction induced by concomitant carbon dioxide changes. J Appl Physiol 41:446–469, 1976.

Benumoff JL, Wahrenbock EA: Local effects of anesthetics on regional hypoxic pulmonary vasoconstriction. Anesthesiology 43:525–532, 1975.

Berne RM, Levy MN: Cardiovascular Physiology, 3rd ed. St. Louis, Mosby, 1977.

Bohr D: The Pulmonary hypoxic response. Chest 71:244–246, 1977.

Braunwald E: A Textbook of Cardiovascular Medicine. Philadelphia, Saunders, 1980.

Brewster D: Surgical management of renovascular disease. Harvard post-graduate course in vascular surgery. June, 1984.

Buist AS, Sexton GV, et al: The effects of smoking cessation and modification on lung function. Am J Respir Dis 114:115–122, 1976.

Bull BS, Hyse WM, et al: Heparin therapy during extracorporeal circulation. J Thorac Cardiovasc Surg 69:685–689, 1975.

Busque L: Pulmonary lavage in the treatment of alveolar proteinosis. Can Anaes Soc J 24:380, 1977.

Butler J, Caro CG, et al: Physiologic factors affecting airway resistance in normal subjects and in patients with COPD. J Clin Invest 39:584–591, 1960.

Carlon GC, Ray C, Jr, et al: High frequency positive pressure ventilation in management of a patient with bronchopleural fistula. Anesthesiology 52:160, 1980.

Chung EK: Artificial Cardiac Pacing: A Practical Approach. Baltimore, William & Wilkins, 1978.

Conrady PA, Goodman RA, et al: Alteration of endotracheal tube position: Flexion and extension of the neck. Crit Care Med 4:8, 1976.

Cooley DA, Norman JC: Techniques in Cardiac Surgery. Houston, Texas Medical Press, 1975.

Crawford ES, Cohen ED: Acute aneurysm: A multifocal disease. Arch Surg 117:1393, 1982.

Crawford ES, Saleh SA: Operative Techniques in Vascular Surgery. Orlando, Fla., Grune & Stratton, 1980.

Crawford ES, Saleh SA, et al: Infrarenal abdominal aortic aneurysm: Factors influencing survival after operation performed over a 25-year period. Ann Surg 193:699, 1981.

Davis JM, Lotto IP, et al: Effect of stopping smoking for 48 hours on oxygen availability from the blood: A study of pregnant women. Br J Med 2:355, 1979.

DeBakey ME, Crawford ES, et al: Cerebral arterial insufficiency. One- to eleven-year results following arterial reconstruction operation. Ann Surg 161:921, 1965.

Delaney TJ, Kistner JR, et al: Myocardial function during halothane and enflurane anesthesia in patients with coronary artery disease. Anesth Analg 59:240–244, 1980.

de Lange S., et al: Alfentanil-oxygen anesthesia for coronary artery surgery. Br J Anaesth 53:1291–1295, 1981.

Dellsperger KC, Wieting DW, et al: Regurgitation of prosthetic heart valves. Dependence on heart rate and cardiac output. Am J Cardiol 51:321–327, 1983.

Dewson B, Michenfelder JD, et al: Effects of ketamine on canine cerebral blood flow and metabolism modification by prior administration of thiopental. Anesth Analg 50:443, 1971.

Dorsen WJ, Larsen KG, et al: Oxygen transfer of blood: Data and theory. Trans Am Soc Artif Intern Organs 17:309, 1971.

Duncan SE, Edwards WH, et al: Caution regarding autotransfusion. Surgery 76:1024–1030, 1974.

Duncan SE, Klebanoff G, et al: A clinical experience with intraoperative autotransfusion. Ann Surg 180:296–304, 1974.

Dunn J, Kirsch MN, et al: Hemodynamic, metabolic and hematologic effects of pulsatile cardiopulmonary bypass. J Thorac Cardiovasc Surg 68:138, 1974.

Earley LE, Bartoli E, et al: Sodium metabolism. Clinical disorder of fluid and electrolyte metabolism, 2nd ed. New York, McGraw-Hill, 1972.

Eckenoff JE, Helrich M: The effect of narcotics, thiopental and nitrous oxide upon respiration and respiratory response to hypercarbia. Anesthesiology 19:240–253, 1958.

Eger EI: Cardiovascular effects of inhalation anesthesia. American Society of Anesthesiologists Annual Refresher Course Lectures, Atlanta, Ga., 1983.

Ellis RH, Hinds CJ, Gladd LT: Management of anesthesia during tracheal resection and reconstruction. Anesthesia 31:1076–1080, 1976.

Engeilman RM, Levitsky S: Textbook of Clinical Cardiology. New York, Futura Pub., 1981.

Epler GR, McLaud TC, et al: Normal chest roentgenograms in chronic diffuse infiltrative lung disease. N Engl J Med 298:934, 1978.

Ferrans VJ, Boyce SW, et al: Infection of glutaraldehyde preserved porcine valve hetero grafts. Am J Cardiol 43:1123–1136, 1979.

Finlayson D: Pharmacology for the anesthesiologist, 16th Annual Post-graduate Course: Therapeutic problems in respiratory and intensive care of critically ill patients. Atlanta, 1980.

Flynn PJ, Hughes R: The use of atracurium in cardiopulmonary bypass with induced hypothermia. Anesthesiology 59, 1983.

Geffin B, Bland J, Grillo HC: Anesthetic management of tracheal resection and reconstruction. Anes Analg 48:884, 1969.

Gelb AW, Knell RL: Subanesthetic halothane: Its effects on regulation of ventilation and relevance to recovery room. Canad Anaesth Soc J 25:488–494, 1978.

Gilboney GS: Ventricular septal defect. Heart Lung 12:3, 1983.

Gooding JM, Demick AR, et al: A physiologic analysis of cardiopulmonary responses to ketamine anesthetic in noncardiac patients. Anes Analg 56:813–816, 1977.

Goodman LS, Gilman A: The Pharmacological Basis of Therapeutics, 7th ed. New York, Macmillan, 1985.

Goudsouzian NG, Karamanian A: Physiology for the Anesthesiologist, 2nd ed. New York, Appleton-Century-Crofts, 1984.

Grant JL, Naylor RW, Crandall WB: Bronchial ademona resection with relief of hypoxic pulmonary vasoconstriction. Chest 77:446–449, 1980.

Gray H: Anatomy of the Human Body, 29th ed. Goss CM (ed.). Philadelphia, Lea & Febiger, 1973.

Grillo HC: Resection of the trachea. Experience in 100 consecutive cases. Thorax 28:667–679, 1973.

Guyton A: Human Physiology and Mechanics of Disease, 3rd ed. Philadelphia, Saunders, 1982.

Hammond GL, Barley WW: Bubble mechanics in oxygen transfer. J Thorac Cardiovasc Surg 68:138, 1974.

Henry WL, Bonon RO, et al: Observation on the optimum time for operative intervention for aortic regurgitation: I. Evaluation of the results of aortic valve replacement in asymptomatic patients. Circulation 61:471–483, 1980.

Hickey RF, Fourcader HE, et al: The effects of ether, halothane and forane on apneic thresholds in man. Anesthesiology 35:32–37, 1971.

Hilfiker O, Larsen R, et al: Myocardial blood flow and oxygen consumption during halothane-nitrous oxide anesthesia for coronary revascularization. Br J Anaesth 55:927–931, 1983.

Hug CC, Jr.: The pharmakokinetics of fentanyl. Janssen Pharmaceutical, 1981.

Hurst JW, Logue RB: The Heart, 2nd ed. New York, McGraw-Hill, 1970.

Isselbacher KJ, Raymond DA, et al: Harrison's Principle of Internal Medicine, 9th ed. New York, McGraw-Hill, 1980.

Jamison WRE, Turnball KW, et al: Continuous monitoring of mixed venous oxygen saturation in cardiac surgery. Can J Surg 25:538–543, 1982.

Jones P: Cardiac Pacing: Continuing Education in Cardiovascular Nursing. East Norwalk, Conn: Appleton-Century-Crofts, 1980.

Kaplan JA: Cardiac Anesthesia. New York, Grune & Stratton, 1979.

Kaplan J: Cardiac Anesthesia: Cardiovascular Pharmacology. New York, Grune & Stratton, 1983, Vol. 2.

Kaplan J: Thoracic Surgery. New York, Churchill Livingstone, 1983.

Kaplan JA, Jones EL: Vasodilator therapy during coronary artery surgery: comparison of nitroglycerin and nitroprusside. J Thorac Cardiovasc Surg 77:301–309, 1979.

Katz J, Benumoff J, et al: Anesthesia and Uncommon Diseases, 2nd ed. Philadelphia, Saunders, 1981.

Kerr JH, Smith AC, et al: Observations during endobronchial anesthesia II oxygenation. Br J Anaesth 46:84, 1974.

Knell RL, Manninen PH, Clement J: Ventilation and chemoreflexes during enflurane sedation and anesthesia in man. Canad Anaesth Soc J 26:353–360, 1979.

Lappas DG, Powel WJ, Jr, et al: Cardiac dysfunction in the perioperative period: pathophysiology, diagnosis and treatment. Anesthesiology 47:117–137, 1977.

Larrieu HJ: Current status of coronary bypass. Bol Asoc Med PR 10:473–478, Oct. 1981.

Lee P, English ICW: Management of anesthesia during tracheal resection. Anesthesia 29:305, 1974.

Lunn JK, Dannemiller FJ, et al: Cardiovascular responses to clamping of the aorta during epidural and general anesthesia. Anesth Analg 58:372–376, 1979.

Marshall BE, Wyche MQ, Jr: Hypoxemia during and after anesthesia. Anesthesiology 37:178–209, 1972.

McClung JA, Stein JH, et al: Prosthetic heart valves: A review. Prog Cardiovasc Dis 26(3):237–270, 1983.

Merin RG: The effects of anesthetics and anesthetic adjuvants on the heart. Con Anes Prac 2:1–18, 1980.

Miller RD (ed): Anesthesia, 2nd ed. New York, Churchill Livingstone, 1986.

Moore WS (ed.): Vascular Surgery: A Comprehensive Review. Orlando, Fla., Grune & Stratton, 1983.

Morris GC, Jr., DeBakey ME: Renal arterial hypertension. Cardiovascular disorders. Philadelphia, Davis, 1968.

Mowry F, Reynold E: Cardiac rhythm disturbances complicating resectional surgery of the lung. Ann Intern Med 61:688, 1964.

Murphy FL, Kennell EM, et al: The effects of enflurane, isoflurane, and halothane on cerebral blood flow and metabolism in man. Annual Meeting American Society of Anesthesiologists, Washington, D.C. Oct. 12–16, 1974. Abstracts, 61–62.

Nadel JA: Autonomic control of airway smooth muscle and airway secretions. Am Rev Respir Dis 115:117–126, 1977.

Naples J: Management of ventricular dysfunction. Presented at Baylor College of Medicine Anesthesia and Surgery for Ischemic Heart Disease, Houston, Tex., Nov. 1981.

Newhouse M, Sanchis J, Burnstock J: Lung defense mechanism. N Engl J Med 295:990–998, 1045–1052, 1976.

Nunn J: Applied Respiratory Physiology. London, Butterworth, 1969.

Orkin FK, Cooperman LH: Complications in Anesthesiology. Philadelphia: Lippincott 1983.

Oschner JL, Mills NH: Coronary Artery Surgery. Philadelphia, Lea & Febiger, 1978.

Packer M, Legemtel JH: Physiological and pharmacological determinants of vasodilator response. A conceptual framework for rational drug therapy for chronic heart failure. Prog Cardiovasc Dis 24(9):275–292, 1982.

Pappin JC: The current practice of endobronchial intubation. Anesthesia 34:59, 1979.

Paulson DB: Cerebral apoplexy (stroke) pathenogenesis, pathophysiology, and therapy as illustrated by regional blood flow measurement in the brain. Stroke 2:327, 1971.

Peltola K, Central haemodynamics and oxygenation during thoracic anesthesia. Acta Anesthesiol Scand 77:1–51, 1983.

Phillips RE: Cardiovascular therapy: A systemic approach to circulation. Philadelphia, Saunders, 1979, Vol. 1.

Pierce EC: Extracorporeal Circulation for Open Heart Surgery. Springfield, Ill., Chas C Thomas, 1969.

Pierce EC, Lamberstein CJ, et al: Cerebral circulation and metabolism during thiopental anesthesia and hyperventilation in man. J Clin Invest 41:1164, 1962.

Reiz S: Effects of enflurane-nitrous oxide anesthesia and surgical stimulation on regional coronary hemodynamics in a patient with LAD bypass. Acta Anaesthesiol Scand 417–420, 1983.

Rheder K, Wenthe FM, Sessler AD: Function of each lung during mechanical ventilation with Zeep and with Peep in man anesthetized with thiopental-meperidine. Anesthesiology 39:597–606, 1973.

Roberts JT, Gessen AJ: Management of complications encountered during anesthesia for mediastinoscopy. Anesthesiology Review 6:31, 1979.

Rogers RM, Szidan JP, et al: Hemodynamic response of the circulation to bronchopulmonary lavage in man. N Engl J Med 296:1230, 1972.

Rogers RM, Tantam KR: Bronchopulmonary lavage. A new approach to old problems. Med Clin North Am 54:755, 1970.

Sabawala P, Strong J, et al: Surgery of the aorta and its branches. Anesthesiology 33:229–259, 1970.

Sabiston DC, Spencer FC: Gibbon's Surgery of the Chest, 3rd ed. Philadelphia, Saunders, 1976.

Shapiro BA, Harrison RA, Trout CA: Clinical Application of Respiratory Care. Chicago, Yearbook Med Pub, 1975.

Sheffer L, Steffenson JL, Birch AA: Nitrous oxide induces diffusion hypoxia in patients breathing spontaneously. Anesthesiology 37:436–439, 1972.

Shields TW, Ujike G: Digitalization for prevention of arrythmias following pulmonary surgery. Gynecology and Obstetrics 126:743, 1968.

Smith HC, Frye RL, et al: Does coronary bypass surgery have a favorable influence on the quality of life? Cardiovasc Clin 13:253–264, 1983.

Smith JJ, Kampine JP: Circulatory Physiology. Baltimore, Williams & Wilkins, 1980.

Stalnecker MC, Surratt PM, Chandler JG: Changes in respiratory function following small bowel bypass for obesity. Surgery 87:645–651, 1980.

Stanley TH, de Lange S: Propranolol therapy for heart disease. Can Anaesth Soc J 29(4):319–324, 1982.

Stanley TH, Isern AJ: Periodic mixed venous oxygen tension analysis as a measure of the adequacy of perfusion during and after cardiopulmonary bypass. Can Anaesth Soc J 21:454, 1979.

Stoelting RK, Eger EI: Additional explanation for the second effect: A concentrating effect. Anesthesiology 30:273–277, 1969.

Szelagyi DE, Elliot JP, et al: Clinical fate of the patient with asymptomatic abdominal aortic aneurysm and unfit for surgical treatment. Arch Surg 104:600, 1972.

Tarhan S, Moffit EA: Principles of thoracic anesthesia. Symposium on surgery of the chest. Surg Clin North Am 53:813–826, 1973.

Tinker J: What the anesthesiologist should know about cardiopulmonary bypass. Annual Meeting American Society of Anesthesiologists. Atlanta, Ga., 1983.

Torda TA, McCullock CH, et al: Pulmonary venous admixture during one-lung anesthesia. The effect of inhaled oxygen tension and respiration rate. Anesthesiology 29:272, 1974.

Turhan S, Lundborg RO: Effects of increased expiratory pressure on blood gas tensions and pulmonary shunting during thoracotomy with use of the Carlens catheter. Can Anaesth Soc J 17:4, 1970.

Vanden Belt RJ, Ronan JA, et al: Cardiology: A Clinical Approach. Chicago, Yearbook Med Pub, 1979.

Wallace NE, Sadove MS: Halothane. Philadelphia, Davis, 1962.

Weinreich AI, Silvay G, Lumb PD: Continuous ketamine infusion for one-lung anaesthesia. Canad Anaesth Soc J 27:485–490, 1980.

West JB: Respiratory Physiology. Baltimore, William & Wilkins, 1974.

West JB: Ventilation/Blood Flow and Gas Exchange, 3rd ed. Oxford, Blackwell, 1977.

Wilson R: Principles and Techniques of Critical Care. Upjohn Company, 1976.

Wuff KE, Aulin I: The regional lung function in the lateral decubitus position during anesthesia and operation. Acta Anaesthesiol Scand 16:185–205, 1972.

Wylie WD, Churchill-Davidson HC: A Practice of Anesthesia, 3rd ed. Chicago, Yearbook Med Pub, 1972.

Yacoub O, Doell D, et al: Depression of hypoxic ventilatory response by nitrous oxide. Anesthesiology 45:385–389, 1976.

Zarslow MA, Benumof JL, Trousdale FR: Hypoxic pulmonary vasoconstriction and the size of the hypoxic compartment. Anesthesiology 35:A379, 1981.

Ziment I: The pharmacology of airway dilators. Respir Care 19:51, 1974.

29

Geriatric Anesthesia

Wynne R. Waugaman and Benjamin M. Rigor

Aging is a complex of phenomena, partly exogenous and partly endogenous, in which physiologic and pathologic processes are often inextricably mixed. Since World War II, our society has undergone profound changes, including rapid growth and greater sophistication in the delivery and technology of medicine. As a result, we are presented daily with larger numbers of patients who have lived longer and survived the physiologic effects of age and disease, only to require extensive surgery.

As the aged population increases, so will the incidence of Alzheimer's disease. The impact of this age factor is significant since demographic trends illustrate that the population susceptible to Alzheimer's disease is increasing rapidly. The risk for developing Alzheimer's disease in those who survive to 80 years of age is 20%.

The risk of surgery for many elderly patients is complicated by chronic disease processes. The reported incidence of the most prevalent diseases among the aged is osteoarthritis (78 percent), hypertension (40 percent), heart disease (40 percent), and diabetes mellitus (4 percent).

When adequately prepared, elderly people can tolerate many types of operations as well as young people. However, in the case of extensive major operations, the mortality rate for the aged may be four to eight times higher than for young patients. Patients over 70 years of age have an overall elective surgery mortality under 5 percent compared with nearly 10 percent for emergency surgery, with variations depending on anatomic site and development of complications. At least 2 percent of this mortality can be attributed to anesthesia. It has been reported that more than 100,000 patients over the age of 65 die postoperatively each year.

The success of anesthesia and surgery with these patients in part depends upon the nurse anesthetist's knowledge of physiologic alterations caused by the aging process and of the possible effects of anesthetics and adjuvant and supportive drugs on the aged. Although age alone does not preclude surgery, it is apparent that the anesthetic management of the aged is influenced by the frequency and severity of degenerative diseases and chronic illnesses.

ANESTHETIC IMPLICATIONS OF PHYSIOLOGIC ALTERATIONS IN THE AGED

The geriatric patient differs little from the young patient, even when the physiologic aspects of aging are considered, because, in general, neither group tolerates a prolonged anesthetic or extensive surgery. One can say, however, that the margin of safety and capacity for compensation are reduced appreciably at the extreme ages of life. The influence of age on the risks of anesthesia and surgery is determined by the type of associated disease and dysfunction. However, separating the effects of aging from those of degenerative disease processes is often difficult.

The aging process is not only a function of chronologic age. Organs and organ systems do not regress at the same rate and speed; thus patients must be assessed individually. Organ function declines 1 percent per year of the functional capacity present at age 30 (Fig. 29-1). These physiologic changes from aging often interfere with the uptake, distribution, biotransformation, and elimination of anesthetics. The significant physiologic alterations from the aging process and their implications in anesthetic management are discussed in the following sections.

General and Constitutional Changes

The elderly undergo a decrease in body fat and adipose tissue, which decreases their ability to retain body heat and in turn exposes them to hypothermia in the cool environment of the operating room.

Accurate determination of weight and weight changes is profoundly significant. Acute, sudden loss is usually due to loss of body water. Chronic loss is due to depletion of body stores of protein and fat. As a person ages, his or her body water naturally decreases. However, nutritional deficiencies may also occur in the elderly and are associated with a reduction in intracellular water and in total potassium. Hypovolemia, a natural consequence of this decrease

499

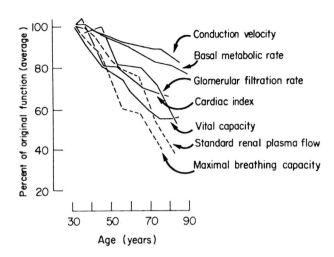

Figure 29–1. Changes in physiologic function with age in humans expressed as percentage of mean value at age 30 years. (*From Miller R: Anesthesia for the elderly. In Miller R (ed): Anesthesia, 2nd ed. New York, Churchill Livingstone, 1986.*)

in total body water, renders these persons vulnerable to hypotension during induction to anesthesia with potent intravenous agents such as sodium thiopental. Patients who are sedentary, bedridden, or immobilized for long periods are usually hypovolemic and will have more difficulty compensating for changes in circulatory physiology caused by altering their posture or position. Their lowered basal metabolic rate (hypothyroidlike state) reduces tolerance to increasing concentrations of premedication, anesthetic agents, postoperative sedatives, hypnotics, and analgesics.

Senile atrophy with collagen loss and decreased elasticity of tissue makes the skin more sensitive to trauma from tape and monitoring electrodes. When the patient is placed on the operating table, close attention must be paid to bony prominences and other areas sensitive to pressure. Arm boards should be padded properly and the patient's arms positioned comfortably. Care must be taken when a warming blanket is used because burns may occur more frequently in the elderly, particularly in those with peripheral vascular disease.

The airway of the geriatric patient presents several problems. There is a progressive decrease in reactivity of protective airway reflexes, such as coughing and swallowing, associated with age. The aged are often endentulous or have a few loose teeth remaining. These factors make an anesthetic mask fit tenuous and increase the likelihood of regurgitation of stomach contents with aspiration of vomitus into the lungs. Cervical osteoarthritis and laryngeal changes that accompany rheumatoid arthritis, as well as irregular dentition, often increase the difficulty of inserting an endotracheal tube into the trachea to maintain a proper airway and adequate ventilation of the lungs.

Cardiovascular System

Arteriosclerotic vascular changes and reduced myocardial reserve decrease cardiac output and stroke volume, prolong circulation time, and decrease perfusion of the vital organs

such as the brain, heart, liver, and kidneys. Heart rate also decreases during the aging process. When anesthesia is induced, these cardiac and vascular changes can cause diastrous consequences, such as hypotension, myocardial ischemia, or infarction, cerebral vascular accidents, and renal failure from decreased renal artery perfusion.

Coronary artery disease is prevalent in younger patients as well as geriatric patients. However, coronary obstructive lesions are seen more frequently in the elderly. It is important to remember that the patient with coronary disease is unable to significantly increase coronary flow. Therefore, preventive measures should be directed against increasing myocardial oxygen demand.

Rapid intravenous induction of potent short-acting barbiturates such as sodium thiopental or methohexital can provoke cardiovascular collapse as a result of poor compensatory hemodynamic response and inadequate cardiac function and blood volume.

A prolonged circulation time has profound implications for the intravenous agents. One can anticipate an induction time period of up to twice as long as would be expected in a younger individual. This prolonged circulation time not only prolongs the onset of action of succinylcholine but also decreases the tendency to fasciculate and increases the time during which pseudocholinesterase can act.

The age-related decrease in cardiac index provides a faster induction with volatile inhalation agents because of a more rapid rise in alveolar concentration. Hypotension may therefore appear sooner, especially in the patient who is hypovolemic.

Bradycardia in the aged is probably best treated with glycopyrrolate, as it does not cross the blood–brain barrier. This drug appears to be more desirable in the elderly than atropine.

The aging myocardium becomes thicker during both systole and diastole. There is a decrease in size and number of individual muscle fibers and an increase in fibrous and adipose tissue. Afterload increases with age. The elastic and muscular tissue in the arterial walls are replaced by fibrous tissue and calcium.

Peripheral vascular resistance increases with age to a greater degree than the decrease in cardiac output so the blood pressure increases. The most notable increase is generally the systolic pressure. Hypertension in the elderly may be considered to be above 160 systolic and 90 diastolic. These numbers may be acceptably increased as age increases.

The baroreceptor reflex is diminished during the aging process. There is less tachycardia to warn of hypovolemia, and less increase in vascular tone to maintain perfusion pressure.

Respiratory System

Significant respiratory changes that occur with aging include decreased breathing capacity, stiffening, and rigidity of air passages due to fibrosis, distension of peripheral air sacs, reduction of forced expiratory volume and forced vital capacity, decrease in diffusion properties, and an increase in closing volume. The consequence of these respiratory changes, especially in patients with chronic obstructive airway problems such as emphysema, predisposes the elderly to infection and collapse of airways in the early postoperative period. Changes in pulmonary dynamics also decrease or prolong uptake and distribution of less-soluble inhalation anesthetics.

After 65 the closing volume becomes greater than the functional residual capacity. There is airway closure with each breath and relatively decreased ventilation—perfusion resulting in shunting and a decrease in the Pa_{O_2} levels. An 80-year-old patient may have normal lungs but have a Pa_{O_2} of 75 torr. This level may be adequate to maintain the oxygen saturation of the blood, but a smaller margin of error exists for periods of hypoxia such as those created by airway obstruction or momentary apnea. This decrease in arterial oxygen tension due to age can be predicted by the equation, $Pa_{O_2} = 109 \text{ torr} - 0.43 \times \text{age (in years)}$. Other similar equations exist for the computation of expected Pa_{O_2}.

There is an increased risk of pulmonary embolism in the aged during the perioperative period, especially for operations conducted in the head-up position or for those involving prolonged immobility and bed rest. Miniheparinization, antiembolism stockings, and early ambulation may be helpful in reducing the incidence of pulmonary embolism.

Central and Peripheral Nervous Systems

The decreased requirement for both inhalation and intravenous anesthetics is related not only to circulatory and constitutional changes but also to decreased neuronal density. Decreased sensitivity to local anesthetic drugs was shown by Bromage (1978) to be due to changes such as alterations in vascular supply (arteriosclerosis), abnormal neural structures, and differences in the permeability coefficient of the drugs. The peripheral nerve changes that occur with aging are dimunition in size and in number of motor units.

Brain weight and number of neurons decrease with increased age. This causes the patient to become more sensitive to sedative and hypnotic drugs in terms of a more pronounced initial response and a prolonged recovery. There is also greater sensitivity to the toxic effects of anticholinergic agents such as atropine; doses that are normal for a young adult (0.4 to 0.8 mg) often cause psychosis in the elderly person.

Autoregulation of cerebral blood flow maintains flow independent of pressure until a critical mean pressure is reached; below this pressure a direct pressure–flow relationship is observed. This critical pressure may be raised in the elderly and in arteriosclerotic individuals. The anesthetist must be alert to avoid even a mild degree of hypotension in these patients.

Reduction in the dopaminergic receptors and postreceptor alterations (cell membrane, ion transport systems, etc.) occur during the aging process. Animal studies have shown that a reduction in total dietary intake of up to 40 percent causes no change in the number of dopaminergic receptors in the aged versus the young adult. Therefore one may predict that obesity further contributes to reduction in these receptors.

Hepatorenal System

The decrease in liver enzymes such as plasma pseudocholinesterase reduces the detoxification and elimination of ester-type local anesthetics such as procaine and tetracaine, muscle relaxants such as succinylcholine, and ganglionic blocking agents such as trimethaphan. Therefore, reduced dosages of these drugs are required. Poor or sluggish biotransformation and detoxification prolong and magnify the effects of anesthetics and other adjuvant or supportive drugs.

Changes in renal function due to aging influence other body physiology. Degenerative changes in renal circulation begin early. In fact, renal perfusion decreases by 1.5 percent per year, which means that there is a 40 to 50 percent decrease from ages 25 to 65. Reduction in plasma albumin and synthesis increases the levels of active drugs that are unbound to plasma proteins such as barbiturates, local anesthetics, and certain muscle relaxants. Glomerular filtration rate abruptly decreases after the age of 60, and effective renal plasma flow decreases 10 percent per decade. Creatinine clearance is the most sensitive indicator of renal function in the elderly. These hepatorenal changes not only reduce drug elimination but also raise, prolong, or sustain drug levels in blood and tissue.

Other Physiologic Changes Pertinent to Anesthesia

The aged patient has decreased capacity for thermal regulation, as shown by tests for regional cooling and homeostatic reaction to external temperature. Prolonged and extensive surgery with massive blood loss and exposed body cavities and organs induces hypothermia, which antagonizes the effect of nondepolarizing muscle relaxants such as d-tubocurarine or pancuronium bromide.

Although procedures preparing the large bowel for surgery have many attributes from the standpoint of reducing bowel flora, they have the disadvantage of disturbing the fluid and electrolyte balance. Cleansing enemas and cathartics cause significant losses of fluids containing quantities of sodium and potassium. There is also a loss of bicarbonate and chloride.

The frequently diminished renal function in the elderly may not permit prompt compensation for these abrupt body fluid and electrolyte shifts. Not only is adequate fluid needed, but additional sodium bicarbonate or sodium lactate is required to correct the hyperchloremic acidosis that may be caused by bowel preparation.

Because of a decrease in lean body mass, in the presence of drugs that are distributed primarily to this compartment, such as diazepam, the plasma levels are increased with a calculated dose and the half-life is increased.

Stress accentuates biologic differences between individuals, and there tends to be a wider variation among the elderly with regard to their responses to stress. The organic and physiologic alterations from aging decrease the rate of compensatory responses and recovery from the stress of anesthesia and surgery. This may be compounded by a decrease in adrenal–cortical secretions, also associated with the aging process.

Preoperative Evaluation and Preparation

All geriatric patients scheduled for elective surgery must have a preoperative visit from the anesthesiologist or anesthetist. Increased fear resulting from a previous unpleasant anesthesia experience may be alleviated by a pleasant preoperative experience. These fears and anxieties can provoke sympathetic nervous system responses and cardiac dysrhythmia during induction of anesthesia. Tactful and sympathetic visits allay apprehension, as well as give lasting, genuine reassurance.

After a review of the patient's chart and results of standard laboratory examinations, a physical examination is conducted with emphasis on the airway and airway problems, endocrine and metabolic signs of disease, and the stability of the hemodynamic components. The patient should be assessed with a simple tilt test. A positive result implies either hypovolemia or an unstable sympathetic nervous system.

The standard laboratory examinations must include a complete blood count, liver and renal function profile, electrolytes, chest x-ray, and electrocardiogram. Other examinations such as arterial blood gases, pulmonary function tests, blood coagulation profile, and highly specialized studies such as blood volume and urinary steriods should be ordered on an individual basis where indicated.

Elderly patients may take multiple drugs; therefore, a careful history of drug intake will reduce the incidence of undesirable drug interactions (Table 29–1). Prolonged intake of steriods in patients with arthritis or allergies indicates the possibility of adrenal insufficiency, necessitating an adjustment in this medication to compensate for the stress of anesthesia and surgery. Many medications should be continued up to the time of surgery, particularly the antihypertensive agents. One drug that requires preoperative withdrawal and substitution of another drug on an elective basis is clonidine. This drug may cause profound rebound hypertension if withdrawn suddenly. The drug should be withdrawn 2 to 3 weeks prior to elective surgery and substitution therapy made.

One of the most useful elements of the history is the patient's exercise tolerance. This will give the anesthetist an indication of cardiopulmonary reserve.

When assessing the anesthetic and operative risks, potential airway problems should be noted, as described earlier. Individuals with chronic obstructive pulmonary diseases or a smoking habit may require respiratory aerosol therapy, bronchial dilators, chest physical therapy, and antibiotic therapy for existing infections—for an appropriate length of time preoperatively. Correction or control of other associated medical problems such as diabetes, hypertension, angina, or congestive heart failure is mandatory. Elective surgery should be postponed if the medical conditions cannot be controlled or stabilized in time.

All possible complications, risks, and alternatives must be explained to the patient and family. The type of anesthetic management planned and the reason for the choice should be discussed with the patient, stressing that the patient's safety and welfare are the foremost considerations in this selection.

For certain patients with specific problems, useful and

TABLE 29–1. DRUGS AND ADVERSE EFFECTS AFTER CHRONIC INTAKE WITH POSSIBLE DRUG:DRUG INTERACTIONS IN THE AGED

Drug	Effect/Interaction
Digitalis	Hypokalemia, arrhythmias
Diuretics	Hypokalemia, arrhythmias
Alcohol dependence	Hepatic disease, chronic intake—decreased response to anesthetics
Sedatives, tranquillizers, barbiturates	Liver enzyme induction, need reduced dose of anesthetics following intake
Tricyclic antidepressants	Interface with myocardial conduction, arrhythmias after relaxant reversal. Discontinuation 48–72 hours preop probably advantageous
Echothiophate eyedrops	Pseudocholinesterase inhibition avoid or decrease succinylcholine
MAO inhibitors	Discontinue 10–14 days prior to surgery Hypotensive response with most anesthetics Hypertensive crisis with meperidine
Lithium carbonate	Atrial arrhythmias Muscle relaxant interaction
Antibiotics (streptymycin, gentamycin, neomycin)	Muscle relaxant interaction (prolonged response)
Quinidine	Muscle relaxant interaction
Aspirin	Bleeding and ulceration of gastrointestinal tract
Propranolol hydrochloride	Bradycardia and hypotension with potent halogenated anesthetic agents
Calcium-channel blockers	Interaction with beta blockers can lead to cardiac decompensation. Interaction with halogenated anesthetics at MAC may enhance drug effects

meaningful laboratory data such as blood volume, electrolytes, renal and hepatic functions, chest x-rays, electrocardiogram, arterial blood gases, and pulmonary function must be assessed thoroughly. The adequacy of blood volume and compensatory autonomic nervous system reflexes can be assessed by blood volume determinations using dye dilution studies. To assess forced expiratory volume and forced vital capacity, simplified pulmonary function tests can be done with a portable respirometer.

Invasive monitoring techniques such as right-sided heart, balloon-flotation catheterization (Swan–Ganz), and arterial catheterization for sampling may be indicated to assess the physiologic status of the patient for severe or extensive surgery. This invasive preoperative assessment may disclose serious physiologic abnormalities that require a delay in surgery or even cancellation of the procedure.

When gross physiologic decompensation is absent, the elderly patient may tolerate and demand effective premedication. Premedication should be prescribed to suit individual situations, but generally consists of a narcotic, a tranquilizer or hypnotic, an anticholinergic, or a combination of these. Doses should be reduced from a "normal adult dose" to ones suitable for an aged patient. Ideally, the patient should be premedicated 1 hour before being transported to the operating room so that the medication can achieve maximum effectiveness. Some controversy exists over the need for a narcotic as part of the preoperative medication routine in a patient who is not in pain. One must consider the consequences of producing respiratory depression in these patients.

ANESTHETIC MANAGEMENT

No shortcut anesthesia regimen can be used for the aged because their physiologic condition and its associated risks leave a very narrow margin of safety. The monitoring and surveillance of the aged must minimally include blood pressure, pulse, respiration, and temperature. In addition to standard noninvasive monitoring modes mentioned, monitoring of end tidal carbon dioxide concentration and oxygen saturation are particularly useful in assisting the anesthetist to maintain homeostasis intraoperatively. Invasive monitoring techniques such as central or peripheral arterial pressure, central venous pressure, and pulmonary artery pressure (Swan–Ganz catheter) are generally reserved for extensive surgery, where massive blood loss and fluid shifts are anticipated, and for patients with moderate-to-severe cardiopulmonary disease. Insertion of a urinary catheter for the monitoring of urinary output is helpful but may be contraindicated for patients with histories of multiple genitourinary infections or prostatic obstruction.

Temperature must be carefully monitored intraoperatively. Body temperature may decrease rapidly in the cool operating room environment. Preventive measures to maintain body heat include warming or hyperthermia blanket, warmed intravenous and irrigation fluids, a heated nebulizer, and reduction in total gas flows.

It is mandatory that the correction of abnormal physiologic parameters be confirmed, including blood volume in patients with chronic or acute hemorrhage, blood pressure stability and control in hypertensive patients taking diuretics and antihypertensive agents, and measurement of blood glucose levels in brittle diabetics prone to diabetic ketoacidosis. After prolonged diuretic therapy, the serum potassium level must be measured because electrolyte imbalance can cause fatal arrhythmias during anesthesia. Blood sugar determination by the glucose oxidase method (Dextrostix) is essential for patients who receive their maintenance insulin dose on the day of surgery and may be indicated for other insulin-dependent diabetics as well as for adult-onset diabetics prone to hypoglycemia.

The criteria for operability must take into account the possibility of partial-to-complete restoration of function, diminution of disability, alleviation of pain, and prolongation of life. Choice of anesthesia is based on the patient's condition, type of surgery, and the skills of the anesthesia care team and surgeon. The ideal anesthetic is one that can be controlled with very little effect on the already altered physiology. The anesthetic technique should be reversible so that, if complications arise, it can be discontinued abruptly and all vital functions may recover quickly.

GENERAL ANESTHESIA

General anesthesia includes intravenous and inhalation agents. In comparison to regional anesthesia, general anesthesia with insertion of an endotracheal tube has the advantages of better control of the airway and fast and smooth induction of anesthesia with unlimited duration, but it carries the hazard of aspiration of vomitus into the lungs, especially in patients with full stomachs.

Intravenous induction agents should be administered slowly in incremental doses so that the drug effect can develop completely and physiologic changes can be analyzed. Hypovolemia is common in the aged and, coupled with the reduced ability of the circulatory system to compensate for this, tends to make the induction of anesthesia with drugs such as thiopental potentially hazardous by producing poorly controlled swings in blood pressure and pulse. Hypertension and cardiac arrhythmias may occur if laryngoscopy is performed under light anesthesia. This is particularly dangerous to a patient with coronary insufficiency. Rapid, efficient laryngoscopy after intratracheal or intravenous treatment with lidocaine may help control the occurrence of arrhythmias during this procedure.

For many years, a balanced anesthetic technique—nitrous oxide, narcotic, tranquilizer, and muscle relaxant—was considered the safest for the aged patient. However, this technique has been reexamined and has been shown to cause myocardial or respiratory depression, or both (depending on which narcotic had been used). There is renewed interest in inhalation agents for anesthetic management of the aged, particularly with the introduction of isoflurane. It has been illustrated that, with age, the minimum alveolar concentration (MAC) in the lungs of inhaled agents progressively decreases (Fig. 29–2). Other investigators have made similar findings with different anesthetic agents when comparing MAC of inhalation agents with age. That is, age decreases the requirements for anesthesia with an inhalation agent.

Some of the effects of halogenated anesthetic agents on organs and organ systems include cerebral vasodilation with an increase in cerebral blood flow, early obtundation of laryngeal and phayngeal reflexes, respiratory depression, and depression of myocardial and vascular smooth muscles, which causes a decrease in systemic blood pressure, cardiac contractile force, cardiac output, total peripheral resistance, and whole body oxygen consumption. One should be aware of the incompatibility of halothane with exogenous and endogenous catecholamines, such as epinephrine, on a dose-related basis, resulting in cardiac arrhythmias. However, enflurane (and isoflurane) can be used in anesthetic management when a limited amount of exogenous epinephrine may be required to control capillary oozing. The ability of halogenated anesthetic agents to produce hepatorenal toxicity is related to the amount of biotransformation and the final or intermediate products of detoxification. This is possibly not a direct effect, but an indirect or autoimmune mechanism.

Inhalation agents have shown a higher incidence of

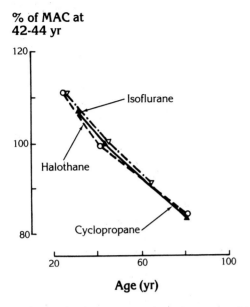

Figure 29–2. Anesthetic requirement (MAC) decreases with age. Values for MAC for nine groups of patients with mean ages ranging from 25 to 81 years are expressed as a percentage of MAC at 42 to 44 years for each agent. The parallelism of the slopes indicates similar responses. (*Reprinted with permission from the International Anesthesia Research Society. From Munson ES, Hoffman JC, Eger EI II: Use of cyclopropane to test generality of anesthetic requirement in the elderly. Anesth Analg 63:998–1000, 1984.*)

intraoperative hypotension and arrhythmias than intravenous agents. The intravenous or balanced anesthesia technique gives a smoother intraoperative course, but, reportedly, greater postoperative morbidity and mortality.

REGIONAL ANESTHESIA

Regional block or conduction anesthesia is ideal for surgery on the extremities and for many types of surgery below the level of the umbilicus. Because the aged may have degenerative nerve and vascular changes, their local anesthetic requirement is low, and incorporating drugs such as epinephrine to prolong nerve blocks is not recommended.

The obvious advantages of regional anesthetics are having a conscious patient and probably a better, faster recovery, with less likelihood of aspiration and other postoperative pulmonary complications.

The disadvantages of spinal or epidural anesthesia are that the sympathetic blockade can result in profound hypotension or cardiovascular collapse and that there may be technical difficulty with inserting the spinal needle into a patient with spinal arthritis or calcified ligaments.

Also, some patients tend to refuse this anesthetic technique in spite of its relative safety compared to general anesthesia. Many cling to unscientific traditional beliefs and fears that spinal anesthesia can cause paralysis, even though this complication is rare in this day and age.

Postoperative Evaluation and Management

Postoperative management includes proper monitoring of all vital signs and parameters, including fluid intake and output, adequacy of ventilation, and cardiac stability.

Among the most frequent postoperative complications are those that are pulmonary in nature. Prevention of these problems begins as soon as the operative procedure is completed. Tracheobronchial suctioning before removal of the endotracheal tube and oropharyngeal suctioning are basic methods for ensuring that ventilatory exchange is maintained in the immediate postoperative period. Often it is safer to leave the endotracheal tube in place after the operation until the patient reacts to its presence rather than to remove the endotracheal tube before the patient is conscious, is breathing adequately, and has regained control of all reflexes.

Despite preventive measures, tenacious sputum and atelectasis of the lung still may cause difficulties postoperatively. Forceful coughing must be encouraged and tracheal suctioning must be resorted to if coughing is ineffectual. Oxygen should be administered routinely through a high-flow mask; patients with chronic obstructive pulmonary disease who retain carbon dioxide should be provided with a Venturi type mask for the use of low concentrations of oxygen.

If the patient exhibits delirium in the recovery room, one should consider hypoxemia. If arterial blood gases are normal, 1 to 2 mg of physostigmine may be used to reverse the effect of anticholinergic toxicity if symptoms displayed are related to administration of anticholinergic drugs.

Hypothermia must be prevented in the early postoperative period. Shivering in response to hypothermia increases tissue oxygen demand by as much as 400 to 500 percent. This can initiate a cycle of increased minute volume and cardiac output. Unless cardiopulmonary compensation occurs, anerobic cellular metabolism will ensue, leading to severe metabolic acidosis. Postoperative hypothermia is more prolonged in the patient who has had regional anesthesia than in the one who has had general anesthesia.

Narcotics must be used with caution in older patients. The usual dosage may produce profound respiratory depression. For the majority of patients, a reduced analgesic dose will control pain and allay restlessness without having an adverse effect on respiratory or circulatory function.

The metabolic response to surgery in elderly patients is similar to what is seen in the younger age group, but certain important aspects particularly influence postoperative management and are especially important when cardiac or renal function is impaired. In the postoperative period, increased output of antidiuretic hormone by the posterior pituitary enhances reabsorption of water by the renal tubules and produces increased water retention. More adrenal hormones, principally aldosterone, are secreted and result in sodium retention. Basic fluid requirements, therefore, are limited to not more than 1000 ml (1 L) to cover insensible water losses and not more than 1500 ml to provide sufficient water for urine formation to excrete nitrogenous waste products. Not more than 500 ml of this should be isotonic sodium (normal saline solution). As soon as urinary output is ensured, potassium should be added to infused fluids, 40 to 60 mEq daily, to provide for potassium loss. Extrarenal losses of fluid, such as by gastric drainage, should be replaced by volume with appropriate solutions in addition to the quantities outlined.

After an operation, daily weighing is a valuable aid in determining hydration. Patients should be weighed at the same time each morning after voiding. After major surgery, weight loss should be anticipated. If weight loss does not occur by the third day, overhydration should be suspected and administration of fluids curtailed. Overzealous administration of fluids is a common cause of cardiac decompensation in the aged during the postoperative period.

Early ambulation and mobilization should be encouraged to prevent clot formation in the lower extremities and pelvic vessels. Pulmonary embolism is a complication that frequently occurs in the aged, particularly if there is no ambulation early in the postoperative period or if patients are not encouraged to wear antiembolism stockings. The goal for these patients is early rehabilitation and return to community activities and functions.

ALZHEIMER'S DISEASE

Alzheimer's disease or senile dementia of the Alzheimer's type (SDAT) is a complex degenerative process involving selective neuronal pathways. To date, no risk factors have been identified directly with the development of Alzheimer's disease although familial tendency seems to exist. Advanced chronological age itself appears to be the only factor directly related to the development of this disorder.

Because people are living longer, more elderly people may be faced with the prospect of elective or emergency surgery. Therefore, the number of patients with Alzheimer's disease undergoing surgery will continue to increase. Significant cognitive impairment is a cardinal sign of the disease and may not be a function of the aging process. Other symptoms of Alzheimer's disease are variable, but the patient may present a good state of physical health or have a health status compromised by other concurrent chronic disease processes. The overall physical condition of the Alzheimer patient should be a primary factor when considering outpatient, ambulatory, or inpatient surgery.

Cognitive impairment in the patient with Alzheimer's disease may include memory loss and reduced ability to concentrate. These factors make it difficult to take an accurate history from the patient. A close family member or guardian should be queried regarding the patient's past and current medical and surgical history including drug therapy. Patients with Alzheimer's disease may be taking a cadre of medications to modify behavioral changes such as aggressiveness, anxiety, depression, agitation, insomnia, and paranoia which may have resulted from the disease process. These patients are extremely sensitive to the effects of all medications and generally require reduced dosages to achieve the desired effect. The Alzheimer patient should be observed carefully for any side effects from medications, those taken preoperatively and those taken for concurrent chronic disease processes.

Any directions that the patient will be expected to follow should be written down for the patient in clear and concise terms. The written word is very helpful to reinforce any preoperative and postoperative instructions for the patient with Alzheimer's disease.

In all discussions with the patient regarding the upcoming surgery, the day and time of surgery should be mentioned. This will assist the patient to remain oriented to time and place. If the patient will be moved to a new unit or require special care postoperatively, the patient and family should be apprised of this preoperatively if feasible. The family should be involved as much as possible in the plans for postoperative care. In some cases, private duty nurses or family members may plan to stay with the patient postoperatively. If the quality of care the patient requires can be provided in this manner, this may be optimal for the patient with Alzheimer's disease. Because of the difficulty with orientation to time and place exhibited by these patients, the routines of specialty care units may add to their cognitive difficulties. The continuity of care provided by supportive family members and nurses familiar to the patient reinforce the patient's orientation to time and place. The charge nurse of the patient care unit should make every effort to assign a small number of nurses to care for the patient with Alzheimer's disease. The consistency of caregivers will provide stability for the patient during the hospital stay.

Patients with Alzheimer's disease requiring emergency surgery need special preoperative consideration. Explanations to the family and patient and an accurate accounting of the patient's history, particularly of drug therapy, are crucial. The number of individuals making a preoperative assessment of the patient should be kept to a minimum to reduce the degree of confusion associated with many new faces.

The same physical preparation should be made for Alzheimer's patients as for other elderly patients. A patient in the late stages of Alzheimer's disease may exhibit agitation and combative behavior. Restraint of the patient may be necessary to prevent accidental or self-inflicted injury.

Preoperative medication administered to these patients should be minimal since the patient may exhibit an exaggerated or untoward response to the medication which will make communication with and cooperation by the patient more difficult. Patients with Alzheimer's disease may be very sensitive to the depressant effects of hypnotics and narcotics since they generally are taking tranquilizers of some type. If a narcotic or sedative is administered preoperatively, the patient should be carefully monitored and observed for signs of respiratory depression. Administration of these drugs further depresses airway reflexes which increases the risk of passive regurgitation and aspiration of gastric contents. Vital signs must be monitored as these patients also may be sensitive to cardiovascular side effects such as hypotension from any narcotic or sedative preoperative medications administered.

Since the cholinergic system of these individuals has been shown to be impaired, anticholinergics such as atropine and scopolamine should be avoided. The use of these drugs could lead to an exacerbation of behavioral symptoms. The use of preoperative medication should be reserved for those instances when the patient requires analgesia or treatment of agitation. Patient rapport and understanding often serve as the most effective form of "preoperative medication."

Most patients with Alzheimer's disease will have their surgery performed under general anesthesia. Because of their difficulty with mentation and lack of understanding or cooperation, these patients generally are not good candidates for regional or local anesthesia except in the very early stages of the disease process when cognitive abilities are well maintained.

Delayed recovery from anesthesia is not uncommon in these patients. Therefore, prolonged observation of the patient will be required in the postanesthesia care unit as well as in the patient care unit. Every effort should be made intraoperatively and postoperatively to keep the patient normothermic. Hypothermia can delay recovery from anesthesia. Confusion in the postoperative phase has been attributed to low body temperature and inadequate hydration.

Preserving optimum body temperature and maintaining adequate hydration will help reduce the incidence of confusion postoperatively in patients with Alzheimer's disease. Outpatients should be apprised preoperatively by the surgeon and/or anesthetist of the prospect of hospital admission overnight following surgery should their recovery be delayed. Some patients have shown temporary improvement in their cognitive abilities due to administration of physostigmine anticholinesterase. The long term effects of the use of physostigmine as part of the treatment regime in Alzheimer's disease still is under investigation.

Postoperative medication for analgesia or sedation should be administered cautiously. These patients generally require reduced dosages of analgesics and sedatives or tranquilizers in the postoperative period. If narcotic analgesics and tranquilizers were administered intraoperatively, none may be required in the immediate postoperative period. When analgesics and/or tranquilizers are administered postoperatively, vital signs must be monitored closely. The patient should be well hydrated.

Postoperatively, the patient must be encouraged to orient to time and place. A family member should be involved in the postoperative care as soon as possible. The presence of a family member will assist the patient to become oriented to time and place more quickly in the unfamiliar hospital environment. Some elderly patients exhibit confusion following a local or general anesthetic and the type of anesthetic technique employed appears to have little effect on whether the patient becomes confused in the postoperative phase. Therefore, reinforcement to time and place and answering of all questions will assist the patient in his/her cognitive processes.

SUMMARY

The field of anesthesia for the aged or geriatric patient is very broad. This chapter has presented only a brief summary of the major points, issues, and physiologic alterations from the aging process that influence anesthetic management.

Information gained through studying our expanding life spans, coupled with increased technology and research in gerontology, will enhance our skill in anesthetic management of the aged.

REFERENCES

Bender A: Pharmacodynamic principles of drug therapy on the aged. J Am Geriatr Soc 22:296–303, 1974.

Bromage P: Epidural Analgesia. Philadelphia, Saunders, 1978.

Chadwick D: Reducing anesthetic risks for the geriatric surgical patient. Geriatrics 108–112, May 1973.

Cole W: Medical differences between the young and the aged. J Am Geriatr Soc 18:589, 1970.

DelGuercio L, Cohn J: Monitoring operative risk in the elderly. JAMA 243:1350–1355, 1980.

Drachman DA, Leavitt J: Human memory and the cholinergic system. A relationship to aging? Arch Neurol 30:113–121, 1974.

Ellison N: Problems in geriatric anesthesia. Surg Clin North Am 55:929–945, 1975.

Glenn F: Pre- and postoperative management of elderly surgical patients. J Am Geriatr Soc 21:385–395, 1973.

Gordon J: Planning a safe anesthesia for the elderly patient. Geriatrics 69–72, May 1977.

Gregory G: The relationship between age and halothane requirements in man. Anesthesiology 30:488, 1969.

Janis K: Anesthesia for the geriatric patient. In 1978 Annual Refresher Course Lectures. American Society of Anesthesiologists, Section 115: 1–11.

Jegarthesan S, Whitehill J: Surgery in the elderly. Postgrad Med 211–215, April 1971.

Jung D, et al: Thiopental disposition as a function of age in female patients undergoing surgery. Anesthesiology 56:263–268, 1982.

Kahunen U, Jönn, G: A comparison of memory function following local and general anesthesia for extraction of senile cataracts. Acta Anaesth Scand 26:291–296, 1982.

Lasagna L: Drug effects as modified by aging. J Chron Dis 3:567–574, 1956.

Miller R: Anesthesia for the elderly. In Miller R (ed): Anesthesia (2nd ed). New York, Churchill-Livingstone, 1986.

Munson ES, Hoffman JC, Eger EI II: Use of cyclopropane to test generality of anesthetic requirement in the elderly. Anesth Analg 63:998–1000, 1984.

Nagley SJ: Predicting and preventing confusion in your patients. J Gerontol Nurs 12:27–31, 1986.

Peters BH, Levin HS: Effects of physostigmine and lecithin on memory in Alzheimer's disease. Ann Neurol 6:219–221, 1979.

Pontoppidan H, Beeker H: Progressive loss of protective reflexes in the airway with the advance of age. JAMA 174:2209–2213, 1960.

Portzer M: Geriatric cardiovascular problems. J Am Assoc Nurse Anesth 690–718, Dec 1976.

Rees DI, Gaines GY III: Anesthetic considerations for patients with Alzheimer's disease. Tex Med 81:45–48, 1985.

Rigor BM, Waugaman WR: Anesthesia and the aged. Generations 8:38–41, 1983.

Roy R: Aging and Anesthesia. Curr Rev Clin Anesth 3:74–79, 1982.

Saunders R: Anesthesia and the Geriatric Patient. Otolaryngol Clin North Am 15:395–402, 1982.

Stefánsson T, Wickström I, Haljäme H: Cardiovascular and metabolic effects of halothane and enflurane anesthesia in the geriatric patient. Acta Anaesth Scand 26:378–385, 1982.

Tarhan S, Moffit EA, Sessler AD, Douglas WW, Taylor WF: Risk of anesthesia and surgery in patients with chronic bronchitis and chronic obstructive pulmonary disease. Surgery 74:720–726, 1973.

Vaughan MS, Vaughan RW, Cork RC: Postoperative hypothermia in adults: Relationship of age, anesthesia and shivering to rewarming. Anesth Analg 60:746–751, 1981.

30

Outpatient Anesthesia

G. D. Allen

Outpatient anesthesia may be performed in a hospital-based satellite, a special area of a hospital, an outpatient surgical unit, or in facilities provided in free-standing outpatient surgical clinics. They have an enviable safety record—in their 1978 report, the Free-standing Ambulatory Surgical Association for the 3-year period through 1978 recorded only 1 death in 283,658 cases, with a hospitalization rate of 0.007 percent. Outpatient anesthesia also involves general anesthetics given in office facilities. Approximately 5 million anesthetics per year, that is, a quarter of all general anesthetics administered in the United States, are given in dental offices, with a record of only 1 death in 860,000 patients. In addition, general anesthesia is given in the offices of plastic surgeons, urologists, ear, nose and throat surgeons, and dermatologists. Many of these general anesthetics are euphemistically called "sedative techniques" and fatalities have occurred. These patients deserve no less careful anesthetic consideration than those in a hospital or surgical clinic. The recent upsurge in outpatient anesthesia does not indicate an innovation in patient care, for the concept of a free-standing clinic was developed in 1919 by Waters and described in "The Downtown Anesthesia Clinic."

Up to 40 percent of surgery can be performed on an outpatient basis, and enthusiastic pursuit of the concept will promote further expansion of outpatient anesthesia. The financial necessity of outpatient anesthesia is a further imperative for selection of this mode of patient care. It is possible to save 40 to 50 percent of the expenses of a surgical procedure by having the surgery performed on an outpatient basis. There is a need to utilize a fixed procedure fee in order to demonstrate a saving rather than charge for time plus procedure. Hospital antagonism to outpatient anesthesia has not yet receded due to an overabundance of hospital beds while total commitment to outpatient anesthesia has not yet been accorded by all insurance carriers, but even now many insurers pay for outpatient general anesthesia or sedation for dentistry.

The administration of the outpatient anesthesia facility is the most critical feature. The significance of the administrative aspects of outpatient anesthesia can be noted in the publication of the Journal of Ambulatory Care Management. Recognition by the Joint Commission on Accredita-

tion of Hospitals (JCAH) is another significant milestone in the development of an outpatient anesthetic. Checklists of requirements to meet this accreditation are published. Without a well-organized administrative setup, outpatient anesthesia cannot succeed. The anesthetist must have a significant input into developing the guidelines for the administration of outpatient anesthesia.

The hospital outpatient facility should be in a separate location from the routine hospital inpatient surgical units. The importance of a separate waiting area from the discharge area must be emphasized, and a circular pattern of patient flow provides the smoothest form of organization. The recovery room should be provided with a changing area, and again the separation of waiting and recovery areas must be emphasized. A free-standing ambulatory anesthesia clinic should have firm and defined arrangements for the admission of patients for whom hospital admission is considered essential. The arrangements should be organized prior to the development of a problem. The provision of suitable parking areas and collection points is essential.

Patient acceptance of outpatient anesthesia is evident from the available data. Between 93 and 96 percent of patients reacted favorably to the concept of outpatient anesthesia, and between 87 and 91 percent of the patients indicated they would repeat the experience. Frequently, patient rejection of outpatient anesthesia experience is related to sociologic problems of handling the difficult child, or prolonged nausea and vomiting. Many patients, particularly those who suffered nausea and vomiting will attribute their unfortunate experience to the outpatient anesthetic. As noted in Table 30–1, the incidence of nausea and vomiting well exceeds that of the usual minimal 5 percent of patients for whom it is impossible to eliminate nausea and vomiting.

PREOPERATIVE PREPARATION

For outpatient anesthesia, this area is the most significant and will determine the successful outcome of any unit.

Patient Selection

Patients must agree with the concept of outpatient anesthesia and consider it to be the most ideal for them. Insurance must be reviewed and found to provide a fee for outpatient

508 VI: ANESTHESIA AND THE SUBSPECIALTIES

TABLE 30–1. PERCENTAGE COMPLICATIONS[a]

Nausea and vomiting	12–25
Headache	13–50
Sore throat	25–40
Muscle pain	12–25
TMJ pain	4
Drowsiness	30

[a] The common complications of outpatient anesthesia are all not particularly related to the outpatient setting. Women are more likely to suffer complications, and the greater the length of operation (20 minutes) the more frequent the complications.

surgical intervention. Social factors are of considerable importance. A lack of adequate home care for the patient in the immediate postoperative period would militate against an outpatient procedure. It has been suggested that the outpatient should reside within 1 hour's distance from the operative facility. This is usually considered driving time and not, as has been interpreted by some, flying time. Arrangements can frequently be made for the patient to remain at an adjacent motel for 24 hours following the procedure. This can still be an economical and more comfortable experience than being admitted to a hospital.

The experiences of the SurgiCenter in Phoenix indicate that the most common age group for acceptance of outpatient anesthesia is between 15 and 45 years, and only a very small percentage of patients (3.5 percent) are over 65. This has not been the experience at UCLA, where many of the outpatients undergo treatment for urologic problems, resulting in a larger proportion of the elderly patients receiving outpatient anesthesia. The age factor does, however, again emphasize the health of the outpatient. In reviewing the patients selected for outpatient anesthesia, it is usually considered they be Physical Status ASA 1 or 2. If they have another complicating disease, it must be controlled. There are exceptions to this rule, and many physical status ASA 3 patients are operated on in outpatient clinics for the unique benefits that outpatient anesthesia will provide for this type of patient. Thus, patients with leukemia or cystic fibrosis or on immunosuppressant drugs, where it is important to avoid contact with hospital bacteria, would benefit from outpatient anesthesia.

Surgical Preference

The desire of the surgeon to operate in an outpatient facility must be considered. The surgeon will be involved in more than just the operative procedure and will in part be responsible for the postoperative care of the patient. Although the anesthesiologist bears some responsibility in the care of the postoperative patient, the complications of outpatient surgery requiring admission are usually surgical, and thus the responsibility of the surgeon (Table 30–2). The operation should be of a superficial nature, and the duration preferably from 5 to 90 minutes. The critical surgical factor, which precludes using an outpatient anesthetic facility, is the presence or absence of postoperative bleeding. Any suggestion that this might occur would indicate a day-stay facility with overnight admission rather than use of an outpatient center. Naturally not all surgeons agree with the concept of outpa-

tient anesthesia and surgery; in particular, some surgical procedures are contraindicated. However, the potential range of operations performed spreads across the spectrum of surgery. The complications are related to the surgical practice and to the patient's acceptance and tolerance of the intended procedure. The thoracentesis may have extremely severe postoperative pain. The breast cyst, if malignant, may require instant radical mastectomy. The skin graft may require extensive postoperative care for immobility, while for the most common of all outpatient operations, the D & C, bleeding may present a problem. A herniorrhaphy has been suggested as unsuitable for an outpatient setting, as it requires the patient to lie immobile in bed, while a vasectomy, if done on an outpatient basis, can pose problems with postoperative hemorrhage. The immobility required after some orthopedic operations could mitigate outpatient anesthesia, and for many of the ear, nose, and throat operations, bleeding is an ever present hazard. The pain associated with the anal fissure or hemorrhoidectomy may be a contraindication to outpatient care, while operations on the eye muscles have a high incidence of postoperative nausea and vomiting, an indication for inpatient care where the distress for a patient is a major factor. Although all those types of surgery may be performed on outpatients, the postoperative care and complications must be considered.

Documentation

The instructions to the patient can be given by the surgeon during the initial discussion with the patient when outpatient surgical care is considered. If an outpatient anesthesia screening clinic is used, then documentation can be given at that time. A standard history form is of value, as screening can be performed rapidly and pertinent points reviewed. Initial evaluation of the patient will be rapidly performed by either the surgeon or anesthesiologist and the chance of omission be reviewed. Preoperative instructions should be given at this time and should indicate that under no circumstance will a patient be discharged except to a responsible adult and that arrangements should be made for the postoperative care of the patient. The postoperative care instructions must be given at this point rather than following the procedure. The importance of not taking food or drink by mouth, except as ordered by the physician, is important. Patients should be alerted to call prior to their procedure if there is any change in physical condition such as the development of acute respiratory infections.

Instructions for postoperative care should include a warning to avoid consumption of alcohol on the night before the procedure and driving or operating of machinery the

TABLE 30–2. MAJOR MORBIDITY[a]

Hypotension
Arrhythmia
Hemorrhage
Hypoventilation
Extended surgery

[a] The major problems that occur in outpatient anesthesia are usually surgical problems. Hypoventilation will not occur with alert anesthetists, and arrhythmias are not necessarily related to outpatient anesthesia.

day of the procedure. An admonition not to make any significant and important decisions until a period of 24 hours has elapsed following the anesthetic is important. Patients must be advised if the anesthetic given is likely to delay return of full mental faculties for more than 24 hours. Finally, a checklist for the patient should indicate capped teeth, partial or full dentures, wigs and false eyelashes, and particularly regarding premedication, contact lenses. A copy of the history and instructions signed by the patient or guardian should be retained in the chart as useful medico-legal documents.

Physical Evaluation

The concept of an anesthetic outpatient screening clinic has been noted. It is probably an unnecessary expense and visit for the patient. In a properly organized outpatient facility, review of the patient can be performed adequately the day of surgery, provided the instructions given at the initial examination have been followed. For a review of the history and physical, the anesthesiologist is adequately trained, and there is little need to have a detailed physical examination performed on the patient by an internist prior to administration of an outpatient anesthetic. A recent study indicated that a short checklist of important factors in the history, together with an end of the bed evaluation that looked for cyanosis, clubbing, dyspnea, and head and neck abnormalities, was able to successfully evaluate 96 percent of the patients presenting for anesthesia. This is not to suggest that a private physician should not perform an adequate physical examination, but the standard screenings performed by the anesthetist and the surgeon are more than sufficient to provide for an adequate physical evaluation of the patient prior to anesthesia. A standard form for completion is of value so that nothing is forgotten and to expedite the evaluation. The requirement of electrocardiogram and chest x-ray in asymptomatic patients is dependent on the facility. Some facilities require that there be a chest x-ray in patients over 30 years of age and an electrocardiogram in patients over 45 years of age. A recent evaluation of the cost effectiveness of routine laboratory tests in asymptomatic patients prior to anesthesia indicated that the only truly cost-effective laboratory test was an examination of the hemoglobin or urine. A hemoglobin or hematocrit is essential, and a simple urine dip stick will detect any problem. It has been reported that 0.8 percent of asymptomatic patients had hemoglobins of less than 10 g/100 ml, 0.7 percent had glycosuria, and 5 percent had indications of urinary tract infection. In 1000 presurgical asymptomatic patients, the total cost for a positive urine or hemoglobin was $400, in contrast to $500,000 for a chest x-ray. Unless there is any pressing need to perform chest x-rays, electrocardiograms, and further lab work for the benefits of the local requirements of hospitals, they are best avoided.

Premedication

Premedication is best avoided in outpatient anesthesia. The use of an opiate in the premedication will delay recovery; in the patient who may be mobile fairly soon after the operative procedure it will induce nausea and vomiting. In addition, the unnecessary additional injection of the standard intramuscular premedication adds to the discomfort of the patient. If, as some authorities believe necessary, an anticholinergic drug is to be given, oral forms of atropine should be used, as they are equally effective. In this regard oral cimetidine 300 mg has been shown to effectively reduce gastric fluid pH and volume in outpatients and might be a useful premedication.

Studies of secobarbital and propiomazine indicated recovery within 90 minutes of their intravenous administration. If the secobarbital was administered orally, then recovery was delayed a further 45 minutes, further support for the avoidance of premedication. As the majority of patients will receive intravenous induction of anesthesia, or if regional anesthesia will still require an open vein throughout the procedure, then use of intravenous preoperative sedation is indicated.

Diazepam produces good amnesia and sedation, but there have been reports of delayed effects due to metabolites up to 48 hours postoperatively. Lorazepam is a very good amnesic if given 45 minutes before the procedure but in moderate dosage produces little sedation. Midazolam will probably prove to be the most satisfactory benzodiazapine for intravenous premedication, as recovery and absence of delayed effects are evident. It can act for up to 6 hours. Intravenous pentobarbital has a well-established record of producing good sedation. If a narcotic is to be administered prior to the procedure, pentobarbital decreases the incidence of nausea with intravenous narcotics. The sedative technique of pentobarbital, meperidine, and scopolamine in the Loma Linda University, or Jorgensen Technique, provides good supplemental sedation for regional anesthesia in anxious patients. This technique does delay recovery, and selection of sedation for outpatient premedication should be made with the penalty of delayed recovery in mind. Hypnosis is an excellent adjunct for outpatient anesthesia, and even a short amount of time spent in inducing a hypnotic state in a patient benefits smooth induction. A technique for rapid hypnotic induction has been introduced by Barber.

Pediatric Factors

An anxious parent, or one with inadequate home facilities, obviously is not a candidate to care for a child following a surgical procedure. This is unfortunate, however, as there are many positive factors in the use of outpatient anesthesia in pediatric practice. The anxiety exhibited by the patient is reduced, and the separation is less traumatic if it is for a short time. Nosocomial infections are greatly reduced in the outpatient population. The outpatient will generally only contact 9 people, but an inpatient is contacted by 27 people while in the hospital. A 17 percent infection rate in a hospital surgical practice was reduced 50 to 70 percent by utilizing outpatient surgery. These reductions in infections are the indications for performing outpatient anesthesia on pediatric patients of ASA Class 3.

The reduction in infection of outpatient anesthesia is well worth the additional problems. The timing of the operation and the reduction of food intake are significant in children; naturally, the earlier the operation the better. A pediatric study noted that the plasma glucose level in a group of children under 5 years of age was 46 mg/100 ml for inpatients and 88.5 mg/100 ml for outpatients. This could be attributed to a less restricted fluid intake, or possibly to the increased activity of the patient prior to outpatient treatment. Care should be taken, as the hospital is a strange place with strange people, and every consideration be given to making a patient's stay beneficial. Postoperative admission rates for complications in pediatric outpatient anesthetic practice have ranged from 0.1 to 2 percent, a most acceptable level. Pediatric outpatient anesthesia has been found acceptable with only two features unique to children, a noticeable increase in postoperative anorexia, and an increased incidence of bad dreams.

In premedication of the pediatric patient, much has been made of the use of a solution of rectal methohexital 20 mg/kg or thiopental paste 40 mg/kg. Experiences of these drugs vary, and the latter is the author's personal preference, having had minimal success with rectal methohexital. Delayed recovery is a major factor in rejecting this form of *induction* of anesthesia, not premedication. The absence of unnecessary injections in children is a factor in selecting or rejecting premedication in children.

INTRAOPERATIVE TECHNIQUES

The timing of the admission of the patient to the surgical clinic is significant. The habit of having the patient arrive early and await the surgeon's or anesthetist's pleasure must be avoided. With limited operations of predetermined length, a firm schedule can be developed and the patient need not arrive unnecessarily early. This is the major advantage of having a separate outpatient surgical unit, rather than attempting to fit the outpatient into the general surgical scheduling. There are definite physiologic changes that relate to the duration of the wait prior to anesthesia. Interpretation of the significance of these changes may vary, but it is important that the peripheral vascular tone be preserved prior to the introduction of agents (anesthetics) that will cause vasodilation. Peripheral resistance falls and the patient becomes less able to initiate changes in response to vasodilator drugs (Figs. 30–1A and B).

Balanced Anesthesia

All forms of anesthesia currently administered can be considered balanced anesthesia, the object of which is to achieve minimal physiologic change with the earliest recovery. As outpatient anesthesia puts a premium on minimal cardiorespiratory change, together with early recovery, balanced anesthesia is obviously indicated. It may be achieved with any combination of sedatives, analgesics, and relaxants. The use of a narcotic in the premedication in anything other than a minimal dose to produce euphoria is thus not indicated. Studies of minimum alveolar concentration (MAC) have shown narcotic produces little reduction in the minimum anesthetic concentration required for other subsequent anesthetic agents and in addition delays recovery.

Sedation

Delay in recovery with sedation is common, and therefore its use must be carefully tempered with the appreciation that intravenous or inhalation sedation might delay recovery. Inhalation sedation with 20 to 40 percent nitrous oxide in oxygen produces minimal cardiorespiratory change, with almost instant recovery of all the patient's faculties at the conclusion of a procedure. Studies have shown complete return of full faculties after breathing room air for 5 minutes. Thus, patient comfort and balanced anesthesia can be achieved with minimal upset by the use of nitrous oxide–oxygen sedation. In addition, 25 percent nitrous oxide will produce analgesia equivalent to 10 mg of morphine. A personal practice in the majority of regional anesthetics is to supplement with nitrous oxide–oxygen sedation if the patient desires to have a lack of awareness of the surroundings. Alternate techniques of sedation may be diazepam, pentobarbital, the Jorgenson Technique, or the use of incremental doses or continuous infusion of thiopental or methohexital. The short-acting intravenous anesthetics will produce greater changes than the sedatives but are frequently used to supplement regional anesthetics. There is some confusion with regard to sedation or anesthesia. If a combination of fentanyl and droperidol (Innovar) is used, then it should

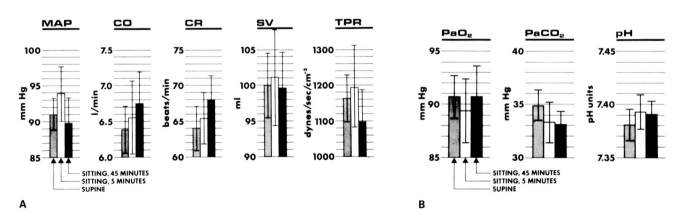

Figure 30–1. A and **B.** In a group of patients studied prior to oral surgery, the cardiorespiratory changes noted with a rest period prior to surgery are not necessarily beneficial. The rise in cardiac output and fall in peripheral resistance could be evidence of anxiety. The means and standard deviation are shown.

be appreciated that droperidol has an action of 6 hours, and this makes it totally unsuitable for outpatient use.

Regional Anesthesia

Regional anesthesia is frequently considered to be the most suitable form of outpatient anesthesia, as only the area to be operated on is anesthetized. However, in the true concept of balanced anesthesia, patient comfort is an important aspect and, thus, sedation must be considered a necessary component. The many and varied experiences with a regional anesthetic have resulted in some agreement regarding those that are unsuitable for outpatient use. The list varies if consideration of their use in pain clinics is included.

Early ambulation, a feature of outpatient anesthesia, is a precipitating factor in problems arising from the use of some regional techniques in an outpatient setting. Subarachnoid blocks would seem generally to be contraindicated in outpatient use. Early ambulation following a subarachnoid block is one of the most frequent causes of headache and should thus be avoided in an outpatient setting. The incidence of pneumothorax following a supraclavicular block or stellate ganglion block on an outpatient basis procedure is much greater if the patient is extremely active following these blocks. Perforation of the apex of the lung will not result in a pneumothorax unless vigorous breathing turns the puncture into a tear, and thus it is better to reserve the supraclavicular nerve block for inpatient procedures. The stellate ganglion block is commonly employed in pain clinic patients on a recurring basis, but these patients are less active. However, warnings as regards the extent of exercise following the use of such a block must be given.

One aspect that differs from inpatient anesthesia is that in preparation of the patient, antiseptics that would stain clothing should be avoided. In selection of an agent consideration should be given to the avoidance of including epinephrine in the solution and the advisability of using bupivacaine, because of its prolonged activity.

Other techniques of regional anesthesia advocated are pudendal, perianal, axillary, and the trigeminal blocks, all of which are suitably performed in an outpatient setting. The IV regional (Bier) block is a most suitable form of an outpatient anesthesia. Major blocks such as the four-quadrant or sciatic–femoral block may be used for outpatient procedures, particularly in the pain clinic, as may intercostal nerve blocks. Again, if precautions are not taken with the intercostal nerve block, pneumothorax may be produced. Lumbar and splanchnic nerve blocks can be performed in the correct setting for diagnostic and therapeutic purposes. Provided patient follow-up is adequate, the patient can be discharged the same day.

General Anesthesia

Induction. Various forms of induction of outpatient general anesthesia can be considered. Ketamine, which appears to be a particularly suitable agent for intramuscular induction in children, has been found to pose other problems (Table 30–3). Recovery may be prolonged, but this can be taken into account in the scheduling of the patient. Induc-

TABLE 30–3. PERCENTAGE CHANGE CARDIAC RATE[a]

Atropine	30
Hydroxyzine, alphaprodine, methohexital	14
Thiopental	25
Diazepam	31
Methohexital	45
Ketamine	82

[a] Studies in outpatients show changes of rate subsequent to administration of various medications is indicated. The changes in cardiac rate may be considered as arrhythmias. With methohexital and ketamine, particularly in the elderly with a fixed cardiac output, the rate alone could cause problems.

tion can be performed as indicated previously with a rectal barbiturate. Intravenous induction of anesthesia with 1 mg/kg of methohexital, or 3 mg/kg of thiopental, is the most satisfactory form of outpatient anesthetic induction. Methohexital allows for earlier recovery, although it produces more dramatic cardiovascular changes, a fall in peripheral resistance with compensatory increases in heart rate (Table 30–4). Intravenous etomidate 0.4 mg/kg is also available for induction of anesthesia, but it has the disadvantage of frequently causing venous thrombosis, pain on injection, and myoclonus. Ketamine 1 mg/kg can be used but delays recovery. All these IV induction agents can be used as supplements to nitrous oxide–oxygen for maintenance of anesthesia. Recovery is most rapid, and cardiorespiratory effects least, with etomidate. However, venous thrombosis and myoclonus are very real complications.

The use of inhalation induction with nitrous oxide–oxygen in combination with halothane or enflurane or isoflurane is a satisfactory technique in outpatients. In one study, it was shown that induction with nitrous oxide–oxygen/halothane occupied only 1 minute and for the majority of patients was not an unpleasant experience. Certainly in children, it is a frequent form of induction prior to the insertion of an intravenous cannulae. Halothane is the preferred supplement over isoflurane, as it is not pungent. Despite the physical characteristics of enflurane indicating more rapid induction, this, particularly in children, has not been confirmed by clinical experience.

Maintenance. Maintenance of anesthesia is preferable with nitrous oxide–oxygen/enflurane, isofluorane, or halothane. Ventricular arrhythmias are common with halothane in the unmedicated patient but are worsened with addition of atropine (Table 30–5). The arrhythmias are frequently

TABLE 30–4. RECOVERY[a]

	Sodium Thiopental	Methohexital
Verbal command	8.5 min	4.5 min
Wakening	30 min	20 min
Face–hand test	40 min	30 min
Driving reactor	21 min	14 min
EEG	24 hr	24 hr

[a] The duration of recovery with thiopental and methohexital single doses is related to various assessments of recovery. The electroencephalogram may not return to normal for 24 hours.

TABLE 30–5. PERCENTAGE VENTRICULAR ARRHYTHMIA[a]

N₂O Halothane	25
+Thiopental	10
+Thiopental and Atropine	20
+Propranolol	0

[a] Ventricular arrhythmias are related to catecholamine release in light anesthesia, worsened by the addition of atropine.

of ventricular nature. The use of short-acting narcotics such as fentanyl together with nitrous oxide–oxygen have been suggested for maintenance of outpatient anesthesia. The argument is that reversal of narcotic can be achieved at the conclusion of this procedure by the administration of naloxone. However, the time course of naloxone is different from that of the narcotic administered. In evaluating recovery, it was found that although recovery from a volatile agent was significantly more rapid in the period ½ to 1 hour postoperatively, after 1 hour the recovery rates with the narcotic and volatile agent were the same. Although fentanyl or alfentanil will decrease the amount of thiopental needed for general anesthesia, the incidence of apnea is greater than if thiopental alone is used as a supplement for nitrous oxide–oxygen. Ventilation with a mask can inflate the stomach, increasing the incidence of nausea and vomiting. Vomiting is also a frequent concomitant of overdose with naloxone, as there is total reversal of the analgesia produced. Generally, the administration of nitrous oxide–oxygen/halothane or isoflurane for maintenance of anesthesia has been found to be most satisfactory.

The use of an endotracheal tube is dependent on the surgery rather than the anesthetic, as it will frequently require the administration of a muscle relaxant, an added complication for the anesthetic. The use of an endotracheal tube is advisable if intraoperative regurgitation is a problem, although postoperative regurgitation and aspiration in the recovery room are more frequent when an endotracheal tube has been utilized. If a muscle relaxant is required throughout a procedure, as in tubal ligation, then endotracheal intubation is essential. Ventilation without a tube may inflate the stomach, resulting in postoperative nausea and vomiting. A good guideline for duration in this respect is that up to 2 hours of placement of an endotracheal tube results in microscopic damage of the trachea, whereas 6 hours produces macroscopic damage to the tracheal wall.

Muscle relaxants are frequently employed in outpatient surgical practice, and the use of intravenous drip with succinylcholine is considered by many to be an extremely satisfactory means of developing relaxation in balanced anesthesia. There are potential problems in the population in using succinylcholine, although these are usually only manifested in prolonged administration. However, the incidence of abnormal pseudocholinesterase is considered to be 1 in 3000, and the chances of prolonged apnea are considerable. If nondepolarizing relaxants are used in outpatient anesthesia, as for example in laparoscopy, the more recently introduced agents atracurium and vecuronium are preferable.

The concept of a minor anesthetic, wherein an anesthetic is used for a procedure taking less than 1 hour, is well substantiated in outpatient anesthesia. Outpatient ton-

sillectomy, in 1969, had a zero mortality in 40,000 patients, when these patients were not subject to endotracheal intubation, and the procedure was brief. If indeed the experiences of the SurgiCenter are noted, only 11 percent of their operations exceeded 1 hour. The shorter the operation, the fewer the physiologic effects. A short general anesthetic causes acute changes in renal hemodynamics related to a decrease in the mean arterial pressure. The changes are rapidly reversed and appear to be related to the effect on the afferent arteriolar circulation. General anesthesia lasting more than 60 minutes appears to cause efferent arteriolar vasoconstriction, with subsequent changes in the filtration factor. Anesthetics studied were methohexital/nitrous oxide, methohexital/nitrous oxide/halothane, thiopental/nitrous oxide/methoxyflurane, atropine/thiopental/nitrous oxide/methoxyflurane, and atropine/thiopental/nitrous oxide/halothane. The agent that appeared to cause least change in renal function was methoxyflurane (Fig. 30–2). To paraphrase R. T. Morris in "Fifty Years as a Surgeon," published in 1935, no matter what one does in the first 15 minutes, it is all right, whereas after one hour, it is bad. Anesthesia has progressed since 1935, but brief anesthetics produced minimal effects.

Monitoring. The use of a precordial stethoscope, temperature probe, and blood pressure monitor is considered essential. The use of an electrocardiogram does, however, add another dimension to monitoring of the outpatient. Ventricular fibrillation in the healthy patient who is administered outpatient anesthesia is an unexpected, but life-threatening hazard. The electrocardiogram detects this instantly. The placement of self-adherent electrodes is convenient and does not add time to the operative procedure. Certainly the placement of the blood pressure cuff involves equally as little time. Other monitors are really of little value in

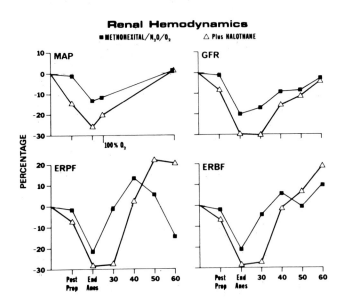

Figure 30–2. The renal effects related to mean arterial blood pressure in a brief outpatient anesthetic are illustrated. In brief anesthesia the renal changes parallel effects in mean arterial blood pressure. (*From Everett GB, Allen GD, et al: Renal hemodynamic effect of general anesthesia in outpatients. Anesth Analg 52:470, 1973.*)

these brief operations, in which minimal physiologic change is produced.

POSTOPERATIVE PATIENT CARE

The recovery room must be staffed by competent nurses who will be alert to the problems of aspiration, vomiting, or delayed recovery. A routine check of blood pressure and other vital signs until recovery is evident should be carried out. The duration of stay will be dependent upon the surgical procedure and the duration of the anesthetic—the longer the operation, the longer the recovery. In many instances, if an endotracheal tube has been placed, particularly in children, retention of the patient within the recovery room facility for 2 hours is considered desirable. If analgesia is required, then brief-acting narcotics such as fentanyl are indicated, and the patient should be detained until the respiratory depression of the analgesic has dissipated. If parenteral morphine is given, vomiting is a problem and parenteral narcotics should be avoided, if possible. Other potential analgesics are aspirin rectal suppositories; if oral medication can be taken, then aspirin and codeine combinations are the most efficacious.

Discharge criteria are important. It is already assumed that the necessary instructions were given to the patient preoperatively, and therefore it only remains for the patient to be assessed for what may be called street fitness. Much disagreement has arisen over this definition, because it has been demonstrated that intravenous barbiturates, such as thiopental, will produce electroencephalographic changes up to 24 hours postoperatively, whereas active metabolites of diazepam have been found in plasma more than 48 hours after administration. However, street fitness indicates whether or not the patient is able to be discharged. There are many available tests; a simple one is the face–hand test (Fig. 30–3). There are demonstrable differences in recovery with various anesthetic techniques. In comparing thiopental and methohexital induction of anesthesia, recovery as determined by the face–hand test was different (Table 30–4). These tests alone are not necessarily indications of patient fitness and should be taken in combination with other vital signs. The acceptable international standard of drug effect is the effect of alcohol on driving performance. Driving a car involves observation, judgment, and motor performance, possibly a complete psychomotor test. To achieve general acceptance by the judiciary, recovery from drug sedation would be best related to the effects of alcohol on driving performance. This has been seen with tests using the driving simulator to assess recovery from methohexital. There have been other psychosedation tests, but all are complex. The simple alcoholic evaluation tests have been the finger–nose test, the Romberg test, and "walking the line," all of which can be readily performed in an evaluation for street fitness. The car simulator is more involved, as is the use of body sway, the Maddox rod to determine eye occular balance, or a more recent development, the Phystester developed by General Motors. An additional new development has been the force control stick. These instruments were developed to eliminate the drunk driver from the road, and all have application in assessment of recovery from outpatient sedation. The critical flicker fusion

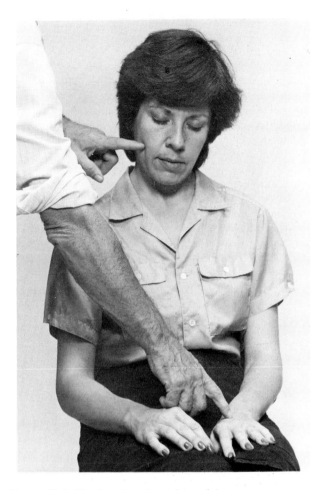

Figure 30–3. The face–hand test is useful to assess recovery from anesthesia or sedation. Due to facial dominance, extinction occurs in the sedated patient, when cheek and contralateral dorsum of hand are touched simultaneously. The patient will only notice touching of the cheek when recovery is complete.

and the face–hand test were utilized in a recent study to assess recovery from sedation. Both tests are equally accurate and simpler to perform than the Trieger gestalt test.

Some assessment or score is of value, in the assessment of recovery from outpatient anesthesia. It will not be an absolute indication but is a repeatable measure of recovery from the agents used. Complete recovery is often considered to occur at least 48 hours after introduction of the agent. The metabolism of halothane and enflurane produces metabolites that are present for some considerable time postoperatively and account for the hangover noted by some patients. In reviewing the postoperative morbidity of outpatients, changes up to and in excess of 5 days after the operation were noted in a few patients. Nonetheless, the essential feature of the assessment in the recovery is the ability of the patient to be discharged from that recovery room, *in the care of a responsible adult.*

COMPLICATIONS

The percentages of complications are shown in Table 30–1. They are significant. It behooves the anesthetist to avoid, if possible, problems such as nausea and vomiting, the headache associated with halothane outpatient anesthesia, and the additional special problems of pediatric patients. Low-dose droperidol (less than 1 mg) has been recommended to reduce the incidence of nausea and vomiting postoperatively; it is not, however, a drug that is recommended for use in outpatients. Admittance to hospital is rare, but must be made available and, if necessary, should be undertaken without hesitation. Major morbidity has been attributed to hypotension, arrhythmia, hemorrhage, hypoventilation, and extended surgery. Although complications occur, they are generally unrelated to the outpatient setting. Other complications relate to the amount of sedation the patient receives and the ability to concentrate on tasks. In some individuals, the response to sedation may necessitate a delay in returning to work; this individual response should be noted in discussions with the patient prior to the procedure. Temporomandibular joint pain is probably related to anterior dislocation of the jaw in an attempt to maintain an airway. In one study, convulsions in a few outpatients were noted. No mention was made of the agent, nor if pyrexia was a feature.

Compliance with instructions is variable in outpatients. Written instructions and verbal communication with an individual responsible for the patient regarding instructions are essential. The ambulatory surgery unit should contact patients for follow-up.

CONCLUSION

Anesthesia for the outpatient is similar to that for the inpatient, the object being to achieve balanced anesthesia. There is an emphasis on early recovery and minimal cardiorespiratory and other physiologic disturbances. The equipment for the administration of anesthesia and monitoring should be identical to that available for the inpatient, and there should be no compromise in the care or preoperative evaluation of the outpatient. The object is to provide a smooth and more economical means of patient care without the disruption or separation for either adult or child from their home environment. There are enumerable other benefits, such as the avoidance of nosocomial infections, and perhaps the emphasis on the brevity of the operation will result in less trauma to the patient than would occur in the more leisurely setting of the main operating suite.

Patient acceptance is generally good, in both pediatric and adult populations. A frequent cause for rejecting the opportunity to repeat the outpatient experience is that of the stress of patient care for the parent. A warning that

there may be a delay in returning to work should be given to all patients. Delays in return to work vary, from 5.4 percent of patients being unable to work the day after anesthesia to 9 percent who required more than 5 days away from work.

BIBLIOGRAPHY

Accreditation Manual for Ambulatory Health Care. Chicago, Joint Commission on Accreditation of Hospitals, 1978.

Allen GD: Minor anesthesia. J Oral Surg 31:330–335, 1973.

Barber J: Rapid induction analgesia procedure. In Allen GD (ed): Dental Anesthesia and Analgesia, 3rd ed. Baltimore, Williams & Wilkins, 1984, p 41.

Chiang TM, Sukis AE, Ross DE: Tonsillectomy performed on an outpatient basis. Report of a series of 40,000 cases performed without a death. Arch Otolaryngol 88:207–310, 1968.

Cohen DD, Dillon JB: Anesthesia for outpatient surgery. JAMA 196:1114–1116, 1966.

Davis JE: Ambulatory surgical care: Basic concept and review of 1000 patients. Surgery 73:483–485, 1973.

Dechéne J: Alfentanil as an adjunct to thiopentone and nitrous oxide in short surgical procedures. Can Anaesth Soc J 32:346, 1985.

Doenicke A, Kugler J, Laub M: Evaluation of recovery and "street fitness" by EEG and psychodiagnostic tests after anesthesia. Can Anaesth Soc J 14:567–583, 1967.

Erbstoeszer M: Ambulatory Surgery Criteria Standards Monograph. Prepared for the Health Resources Administration, Department of HEW, Rockville, MD, Contract No. HRA 106–74–56.

Fahy A, Marchall M: Postanaesthetic morbidity in outpatients. Br J Anaesth 41:433–438, 1969.

Ford JL, Reed WA: The surgicenter—An innovation in the delivery and cost of medical care. Arizona Med 26:801–804, 1969.

Fragen RJ, Shanks CA: Neuromuscular recovery after laparoscopy. Anesth Analg 63:51, 1984.

Katz RL, Stirt J, Murray AL, et al: Neuromuscular effects of atracurium in man. Anesth Analg 61:730, 1982.

Manchikanti L, Roush JR: Effect of pre anesthetic glycopyrrolate and cimetidine on gastric fluid ph and volume in outpatients. Anesth Analg 63:40, 1984.

Mehta MP, Dillman JB, Sherman BM, et al: Etomidate anesthesia inhibits the cortisol response to surgical stress. Acta Anaesthesiol Scand 29:486, 1985.

Nathanson BN: Ambulatory abortion, experience with 26,000 cases (July 1, 1970 to August 1, 1971). N Engl J Med 286:403–407, 1972.

Natof HE: Complications associated with ambulatory surgery. JAMA 244:1116–1118, 1980.

Rubin A, Allen GD, Everett GB: Induction of general anesthesia with diazepam or thiopental: A comparison of the cardiorespiratory effects. Anesth Prog 25:39–44, 1978.

31

Anesthesia for the Trauma Patient

Karen L. Zaglaniczny

The impact of trauma on health care has increased significantly over the past years. Statistics indicate that trauma is the third leading cause of death in the United States, surpassed only by heart disease and cancer. It is the leading cause of death in the first three decades of life.

Recent advances in emergency medical care have greatly improved survival rates. Rapid evaluation and aggressive resuscitation measures by a competent trauma health care team can be initiated upon the patient's arrival to the emergency room. Survival depends upon age, prior health status, extent of injury, and the rapidity with which adequate therapy is instituted.

Traumatic injuries can result from motor vehicle accidents, knives, guns, hatchets, and other objects. The insult may result in single or multiple organ damage. The type and severity of injury will determine guidelines for initial and subsequent management. Priorities of trauma management include securing of a patent airway and support of the circulation.

This chapter focuses on the general guidelines for optimal management of a trauma patient. Effective interaction with trauma team members is essential to facilitate the anesthetic process.

PHYSIOLOGIC RESPONSE TO TRAUMA

The physiologic responses that occur following a traumatic insult are adaptive mechanisms of the neuroendocrine and cardiovascular systems. The neuroendocrine responses are as follows:

1. Activation of the autonomic nervous system with release of endogenous catecholamines.
2. Renin–angiotensin–aldosterone secretion.
3. Antidiuretic hormone (ADH) secretion.
4. Stimulation of adrenocorticotropic hormone (ACTH) activity.

The cardiovascular system responds by attempting to maintain adequate perfusion to the vital organs. The degree of response is proportional to the amount of hemorrhage and area of injury, and, if inadequately treated, cardiovascu-

lar collapse occurs. A 10 to 15 percent loss of circulating blood volume can be tolerated by most patients. The blood pressure is normal with slight elevation of the heart rate. Intravascular volume can be restored with fluid therapy.

A 20 to 25 percent loss of circulating blood volume results in a decrease in cardiac output, hypotension, and tachycardia. Peripheral vascular resistance increases in an attempt to restore an effective circulating volume. Fluid and blood therapy are required to regain hemodynamic stability.

Losses of greater than 30 percent of vascular volume produce an acute insult on major organ systems. Myocardial, cerebral, and renal function are endangered by the presence of persistent hypotension and shock states. Aggressive treatment with fluid and blood therapy, correction of acid–base and electrolyte abnormalities, and control of hemorrhage are goals of treatment. The pathophysiologic events of hemorrhagic shock are described in Figure 31–1.

Initial stabilization of the patient occurs in the emergency room. If life-threatening hemorrhage is imminent, the severely injured patient may be quickly transported to the operating room for immediate surgical intervention and resuscitation.

PREOPERATIVE ASSESSMENT

Preoperative evaluation of the trauma patient may be limited by the urgency of the impending surgery and condition of the patient. The anesthetist should perform a rapid comprehensive assessment and examination of the patient. Further information can be obtained from the patient's chart, relatives, and surgeon.

The history and physical examination should include the following information:

1. Preexisting diseases
2. Current medications
3. Allergies
4. Previous anesthetic experience
5. Recent fluid and food intake
6. Alcohol ingestion
7. Extent of traumatic injury

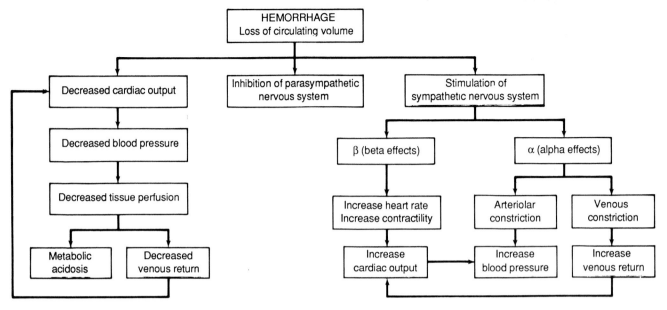

Figure 31–1. Pathophysiologic events of hemorrhagic shock.

Preexisting Disease

Trauma patients with major systemic preexisting disease have an approximate 10 percent increase in mortality rate. It is essential to determine the existence and severity of any major disease process. A systems approach assists in rapid evaluation of the patient (Table 31–1).

Current Medications

It is important to ascertain whether the trauma patient is taking any medications that might influence the course of the anesthetic. The time and dosage of most recent drug intake should be identified. The drug addict may exhibit signs of excitability or depression depending upon the drug ingested. If the patient has been an intravenous drug abuser for a significant length of time, there may be a problem in securing adequate intravenous lines. Insertion of internal jugular, subclavian, or venous cutdown catheters may be necessary prior to surgery.

Allergies

The patient is questioned for known allergies pertinent to the administration of anesthesia. These can include drugs and other substances such as iodine or intravenous x-ray dyes.

Previous Anesthetic Experiences

The date, type, and course of past anesthetic experiences are recorded. A familial history of previous anesthesia administration is also noted.

Recent Food and Fluid Intake

All trauma patients are assumed to have a full stomach. Gastric emptying ceases or is greatly diminished at the time of injury. The type and amount of recent food intake

as well as the presence of nausea or vomiting should be determined. A nasogastric tube may be in place to remove secretions but it will not remove large particles of food. It is postulated that the nasogastric tube may create a "Wick effect" during the induction of anesthesia. This term refers to the continued opening of gastroesophageal sphincter, allowing gastric secretions to drain into the oropharynx and possibly the trachea. Some authorities recommend the administration of preoperative antacids to reduce the acidity and volume of the gastric contents, but this practice is not universally accepted. The hazards associated with regurgitation and aspiration of gastric contents are always present in the trauma patient. Aspiration pneumonitis can occur with as little as 0.4 ml/kg of gastric fluid with a pH of less than 2.5. All appropriate measures must be utilized to reduce the risk of aspiration during the induction of anesthesia. These include an awake intubation or rapid sequence induction and cricoesophageal pressure.

ALCOHOL INGESTION. The intoxicated trauma patient may be uncooperative and combative. The blood alcohol level should be determined if possible. The depressant effects of alcohol on the respiratory, cardiovascular, neurologic and metabolic systems will be potentiated by anesthetic agents.

Extent of Injury

The severity of injury should be determined and evaluated. Episodes and duration of hypotension and estimation of initial blood loss should be noted. The amount of blood and fluid therapy used for initial emergency room resuscitation provides a guide for further replacement.

The chart can provide valuable information if the patient is unable to respond to questions. When available, laboratory data may include hemoglobin, hematocrit, electrolytes, blood urea nitrogen, creatinine, glucose, blood alcohol level, and urinalysis. Radiographic studies and an

TABLE 31–1. SYSTEMS REVIEW

Systems	Major Disease	Assessment/History
1. Respiratory	a. COPD b. Asthma c. Bronchitis	a. Respiratory rate and rhythm b. Chest expansion c. Patency of airway d. Smoking e. Chest x-ray f. Arterial blood gases
2. Cardiovascular	a. Coronary artery disease b. Myocardial infarction c. Hypertension d. Congestive heart failure e. Peripheral vascular disease	a. Range of blood pressure b. Episodes hypotension c. Pulse rate d. Jugular vein distention e. ECG f. Cardiac reserve g. Incidence of angina
3. Neurologic	a. Stroke b. TIA c. Seizures d. Head injury e. Skull fracture	a. Level of consciousness b. Pupil size and reaction c. Movement of extremities
4. Metabolic	a. Diabetes b. Hepatitis c. Pancreatitis	a. Jaundice b. Hypoglycemia–hyperglycemia c. Lab value—enzymes, blood sugar
5. Renal	a. Acute renal failure b. Chronic renal failure c. Glomerulornephritis	a. Urine output b. BUN, creatinine, electrolytes c. Urinalysis

electrocardiogram may also be helpful. All major trauma patients should be typed and cross-matched and there should be sufficient blood available for transfusion prior to the start of the surgical procedure.

The information obtained from the preoperative evaluation should be integrated with the patient status and discussed with the surgeon to formulate the optimal anesthetic plan. If the patient has sustained a life-threatening injury, little time will be available for chart review and patient assessment. For these patients, the anesthetist can consult with the surgeon and other health care team members to organize the priorities for management.

PREMEDICATION

Pharmacologic agents employed for routine premedication can exhibit profound cardiovascular and respiratory depressant effects in the trauma patient. The narcotics, barbiturates, and other hypnosedatives should be used judiciously or not at all to avoid undesirable effects. Anticholinergic agents such as atropine or glycopyrrolate may be administered to reduce secretions and suppress vagal reflexes. As stated previously, antacids may be used to raise gastric pH; the efficacy of this treatment is not absolute, however.

Intramuscular injection of any preoperative medication is avoided to prevent any possible delayed interactions with the anesthetics. All agents should be administered intravenously with cognizant monitoring of the patient.

PREPARATION OF ESSENTIAL EQUIPMENT

The operating room must be equipped with the necessary drugs and supplies prior to the patient's arrival. Valuable time can be saved if equipment and supplies are readily available and functioning. Frequently, trauma centers will designate one or more operative suites that are always prepared for emergency patients.

All routine equipment must be functional, including the gas machine, electrocardiac monitor, anesthesia ventilator, oxygen analyzer, temperature monitor, blood pressure cuff, and suction apparatus. Drugs to be administered during anesthesia must be prepared and labeled. Other essential supplies such as endotracheal tubes, laryngoscope, precordial and esophageal stethoscopes, blood warmers, micropore filters, blood infusion pumps, and intravenous fluids must be available. A hypothermia/hyperthermia blanket is placed on the operating table. An arterial line and pressure transducer can be prepared and calibrated. An emergency cart with resuscitative drugs and defibrillator must be immediately available.

MONITORING

Monitoring of the trauma patient requires continuous clinical assessment and accurate interpretation of data obtained from available monitoring devices. Use of routine and specialized equipment complements the senses of the anesthetist to provide information concerning the patient.

Routine monitoring of the vital signs through the use of a blood pressure cuff, electrocardiograph, and precordial and esophageal stethoscope is immediately applied upon patient arrival to the operating room. Further information related to the major organ functions can be obtained from additional monitoring devices.

A direct intraarterial catheter will display continuous blood pressure reading. A 20- or 22-gauge nontapered catheter can be inserted into the radial artery and attached to the pressure monitoring apparatus. The arterial line also provides an accessible route to obtain blood samples for arterial gases and other laboratory determinations.

The central venous pressure (CVP) measurement is a reflection of the blood volume, venous tone, and right ventricular pressure. In trauma patients receiving large volume replacements, the CVP can be a valuable guide. Serial measurements are obtained and interpreted to determine the adequacy of volume replacement. The external jugular or internal jugular veins can be cannulated for CVP monitoring.

Urine output measurements from a Foley catheter are a guide for adequacy of (1) renal perfusion, (2) volume replacement, and (3) transfusion reactions. The urine output should be maintained at a minimum of 1 to 2 ml/kg/hr.

The temperature is continuously monitored through an esophageal stethoscope or other available route. Trauma patients can be rapidly cooled through large incisions, cold operating rooms, the effect of anesthetic agents, and the administration of blood. A warming blanket will help maintain body temperature. Inspired gases can be warmed and humidified to provide additional heat.

Pulmonary artery pressure monitoring can provide information about left heart function. The pulmonary artery pressure (PAP), pulmonary capillary wedge pressure (PCWP), and cardiac output are measured via a pulmonary artery (Swan–Ganz) catheter. It is not a routine procedure to insert pulmonary artery catheters in trauma patients because of the time and specialized equipment required. The pulmonary artery catheter can be inserted postoperatively in critically injured patients for serial hemodynamic measurements.

Respiratory status is monitored for adequacy of ventilation and respiratory dysfunction. A precordial or esophageal stethoscope allows continuous assessment of the breath sounds. Observation of the inspiratory pressure will reflect changes in the compliance. Arterial blood gas determinations provide information about acid–base, arterial oxygenation, and adequacy of ventilation.

Serial determinations of laboratory values provide useful data related to blood replacement, electrolyte, and acid–base status. Arterial blood gases, hemoglobin, hematocrit, and electrolytes should be measured and correlated to the clinical status. Coagulation studies are measured in patients receiving large volumes of blood (ten or more units).

All of the information obtained must be integrated with the clinical assessment of the patient. One must not depend on the monitoring apparatus alone but must incorporate the anesthetist's own assessment skills to recognize and correct problems. Prompt interventions must be initiated to prevent a deterioration of the patient's condition.

INDUCTION

Choice of induction technique will depend upon the hemodynamic status and area of traumatic injury. Anesthetic guidelines for specific areas of injury are discussed later in this chapter. The most important consideration is airway management. The risks of regurgitation and aspiration in the trauma patient dictate the use of an awake intubation or rapid sequence induction. The technique that is safest for the patient and most familiar to the anesthetist should be chosen.

Awake intubation is considered the best approach in the cooperative patient and patients with severe maxillofacial or neck trauma. This technique should not be used in the patients who have neurologic or penetrating eye injuries. Guidelines for the awake intubation technique are as follows:

1. Administer a topical vasoconstrictor nasally for a nasal intubation.
2. Administer local anesthetic topically into oral cavity.
3. Supplement low dose of intravenous agents if patient is hemodynamically stable.
4. Proceed with technique of nasal or oral intubation.
5. Inflate the cuff.
6. Auscultate breath sounds.
7. Administer induction agent.

A rapid-sequence induction is employed in the intoxicated, confused, restless, or uncooperative trauma patient. Guidelines for this technique are as follows:

1. Connect nasogastric tube to suction (if in place).
2. Preoxygenate for 3 to 5 minutes with mask.
3. Administer a small dose of nondepolarizing muscle relaxant—curare 3 mg, vecuronium 0.5 to 1.0 mg, or pancuronium 0.5 to 1.0 mg—intravenously 3 minutes prior to succinylcholine to minimize fasiculations.
4. Intravenously administer the induction agent—ketamine 0.25 to 0.75 mg/kg, thiopental 2 to 3 mg/kg, diazepam 0.1 to 0.2 mg/kg, or midazolam 0.05 to 1.5 mg/kg.
5. Immediately follow with succinylcholine 1–2 mg/kg intravenously.
6. Cricoesophageal pressure may be applied immediately after loss of consciousness and is continued until the cuff is inflated.
7. Do not ventilate.
8. Intubate the trachea.
9. Inflate the cuff.
10. Ventilate.
11. Check breath sounds.

If the initial attempt at intubation is unsuccessful, gently ventilate with the mask while maintaining light cricoesophageal pressure and proceed with laryngoscopy.

The choice of induction agent depends upon the hemodynamic status of the patient. In some trauma patients the blood pressure may be falsely elevated due to restlessness, pain, or anxiety and a large dose of an induction agent may induce a precipitous fall in blood pressure. Thiopental in a reduced dose of 2 to 3 mg/kg intravenously may be used. Ketamine 0.25 to 0.75 mg/kg intravenously is frequently administered in patients with shock or hypotension. Diazepam 0.1 to 0.2 mg/kg or midazolam 0.05 to 0.15 mg/kg intravenously are other agents that may be considered in patients with cardiovascular instability. However, untoward side effects may occur. Several new intravenous induction agents, currently under investigation, may be beneficial to these patients.

ANESTHETIC MANAGEMENT

Immediately after the induction, hemodynamic stability is assessed prior to the introduction of additional anesthetic agents. Two general principles are considered for optimal management. First, resuscitate the patient with fluid and blood therapy, and then carefully titrate anesthesia according to need. Second, administer minimal amounts of anesthetic agents until the severity of the injury is determined and cardiovascular stability is present.

The severely injured patient will require the administration of oxygen, blood, fluids, and a nondepolarizing muscle relaxant, such as pancuronium or vecuronium. As soon as cardiovascular stability is restored other general anesthetic agents can be administered.

The inhalational agents isoflurane, enflurane, and halothane have several advantages in the trauma patient. Low concentrations (0.25 to 0.5 percent) can be slowly introduced, permitting careful observation of their hemodynamic effect. If the blood pressure falls, the agent can be easily eliminated. A high inspired oxygen concentration can be delivered with these agents.

Nitrous oxide (N_2O) has depressant effects in the hypotensive or hypovolemic patient. Low concentrations can be titrated and the hemodynamic effect observed. Adequate oxygenation must be ensured prior to the introduction of this agent.

The narcotics, tranquilizers, and ketamine can be administered in small incremental intravenous dosages. Muscle relaxants are usually used as adjunct agents to provide optimal relaxation. Pancuronium is most commonly selected for trauma, due to its minimal cardiovascular depressant effects.

A concern in trauma anesthesia is patient recall. This concept is usually false when dealing with the injured patient who has experienced shock. The priorities of anesthesia management are to ensure adequate oxygenation and restore hemodynamic stability before the administration of anesthetic agents.

MAJOR PROBLEMS

Major problems that may be encountered during the anesthetic management of the trauma patient include persistent hypotension, cardiovascular collapse and pulmonary edema. If the patient cannot be adequately resuscitated with blood and fluid therapy adjunct cardiovascular drugs are carefully administered (Table 31–2). Vasopressors can increase the blood pressure transiently but can also increase the severity of tissue acidosis. These drugs should not be used routinely to treat hypotension, but only as a last resort effort. Inotropic agents can be used to restore perfusion and aid myocardial contractility.

Pulmonary edema can result from massive infusion of fluids and blood. Prompt recognition and aggressive treatment is imperative to maintain adequate oxygenation and effective ventilation. Symptoms during anesthesia of pulmonary edema include rales, increased airway pressure, and large amounts of secretions. Treatment includes frequent suctioning, restriction of fluids, and possible low dosages of diuretics and cardiac glycosides.

FLUID MANAGEMENT

Guidelines for fluid and blood replacement therapy are correlated to the severity of the injury and amount of blood loss. The goals of volume therapy are to restore circulating blood volume, maintain adequate oxygen delivery to all tissues and ensure hemodynamic stability.

The physiologic responses to acute blood loss include alterations in cell membrane stability and transcapillary fluid shifts. Body fluids from the interstitial space replace those lost from the plasma space. Therefore, expansion of both the plasma and interstitial fluid space is required. Initial resuscitation begins with the infusion of balanced electrolyte solutions until blood components are available. It is essential to secure at least two large-bore (14 to 16 gauge) intravenous lines for rapid fluid administration because it is difficult to maintain adequate intravascular volume without them. The commercially available fluids include Polyonic, Isolyte, and Ringer's lactate. Advantages of balanced electrolyte solutions include physiologic components, availability, ease of administration, cost effectiveness, and long shelf life. Balanced electrolyte solutions with dextrose are not advocated since they may cause hyperglycemia and an osmotic diuresis. The plasma glucose level in trauma patients is elevated due to the injury and catecholamine release.

Monitoring of blood pressure, pulse pressure, heart rate, central venous pressure, pulmonary capillary wedge pressure, and urine output will guide volume replacement. Balanced electrolyte solutions are administered until hemodynamic stability is attained or until blood is available. Generally fluids are infused at a 3:1 ratio, that is, 3 ml of fluid for every 1 ml of blood loss. Clinical judgment individualizes volume therapy for the different types of trauma.

Blood therapy is initiated when the hematocrit is less than 30 percent or in the presence of obvious large losses of blood. Replacement should be with blood products that have been typed and cross-matched if possible. Cases of extreme emergency may warrant the infusion of type-specific or low-titer O negative non-cross-matched blood.

Recent trends in blood banking now advocate component therapy rather than whole blood administration. Whole blood when available is indicated for transfusion in massive trauma. Component therapy with packed red blood cells and fresh frozen plasma may be administered to maintain a hemoglobin level of 10 mg/100 ml or hematocrit of 30 percent.

One unit of packed red blood cells has an oxygen carrying capacity that is similar to 1 unit of whole blood. The hematocrit of each unit is 60 to 70 percent. Each unit may

TABLE 31–2. ADJUNCT CARDIOVASCULAR DRUGS

1. Dopamine (250 mg/500 ml)
2. Dobutamine (250 mg/500 ml)
3. Isoproterenol (2 mg/500 ml)
4. Epinephrine (1 mg/250 ml)
5. Phenylephrine (10 mg/250 ml)
6. Atropine sulfate (0.6 to 1 mg)
7. Calcium chloride (1 g)
8. Digitalis (0.25 to 1.0 mg)

be diluted with 100 to 200 ml of intravenous solution to facilitate rapid infusion. One unit of fresh frozen plasma is administered for every 4 to 6 units of packed red cells. Fresh frozen plasma contains all of the clotting factors except platelets and factors V and VIII. Platelets can be transfused if the platelet count is below 65,000 per mm^3. Controversy exists as to whether platelets are indicated in trauma patients.

Several storage and delivery problems can arise during blood administration. Changes in stored blood are listed in Table 31–3. The longer the blood is stored, the greater the accumulation of cellular debris, which may cause microemboli to be deposited in the respiratory system, leading to respiratory dysfunction. All blood must be warmed prior to administration in order to minimize hypothermia and arrythmias. Micropore blood filters will remove aggregates in stored blood.

Controversy about the administration of sodium bicarbonate and calcium chloride exists. These drugs should not be administered routinely. Frequent arterial blood gas determinations can guide sodium bicarbonate replacement to correct any metabolic acidosis. A guideline for calculation of bicarbonate replacement is patient weight in kilograms times base deficit times 0.3. One-half of two-thirds of the calculated dose is given intravenously and the arterial blood gases are repeated.

The ionized calcium levels may be dramatically lowered during transfusion. No conclusive data are available to support or disprove the use of calcium supplementation in trauma patients. Calcium chloride 1 g IV slowly can be administered to the severely injured patient for its inotropic effect.

Transfusion reactions can occur in any patient receiving blood. Prompt recognition and treatment is important. The clinical symptoms and treatment of allergic and hemolytic transfusion reactions are listed in Table 31–4.

Volume therapy requires close monitoring of the patient's blood pressure, pulse, urine output, central venous pressure, and pulmonary capillary wedge pressure. Effective communication with the surgeon and other health care team members will facilitate prompt volume restoration and hemodynamic stability. Blood components and balanced electrolyte solutions must be readily available and administered in proper amounts to avoid pathologic alterations in organ functions.

TABLE 31–3. CHANGE IN STORED BLOOD

	Normal Blood	Bank Blood
1. pH	7.40	6.65
2. Hct (%)	45	41
3. K$^+$ (mEq/L)	4.5	7–30
4. Ca^{2+} (mg/100 ml)	5	0.5
5. Na$^+$ (mEq/L)	140	170
6. O$_2$ saturation (%)	98	35
7. Pco$_2$ (mm Hg)	40	191
8. Platelets (mm^3)	230,000	0
9. Factors V, VII (%)	100	50
10. Temperature (C)	37.5	4–6

TABLE 31–4. TRANSFUSION REACTIONS

A. Hemolytic Reactions
  1. Clinical symptoms
    a. Hypotension
    b. Tachycardia
    c. Hemoglobinuria
    d. Oozing at operative site
    e. Increase in temperature
  2. Treatment
    a. Stop transfusion
    b. Administer fluids
    c. Administer diuretics
    d. Administer bicarbonate
    e. Administer steroids
    f. Support of hemodynamic status
B. Allergic Reactions
  1. Clinical symptoms
    a. Laryngeal edema
    b. Bronchospasm
    c. Urticaria
    d. Hives
  2. Treatment
    a. Stop transfusion
    b. Administer an antihistamine
    c. Administer bronchodilator
    d. Administer steroids

SPECIFIC AREAS OF INJURY

The major areas of injury are discussed, with focus on the anesthetic guidelines for each type of patient. All patients require the same priorities of management—airway and cardiovascular stabilization—regardless of the type of injury.

Thoracic Trauma

Statistics indicate that 25 to 30 percent of all injuries involve the thorax. Injuries can include damage to the heart, lung, diaphragm, and great vessels. Major problems that can result from thoracic injuries are pneumothorax, hemothorax, flail chest, and cardiac tamponade.

Pneumothorax is the accumulation of air within the pleural cavity. Intrapleural pressure is increased, resulting in collapse of lung tissue on the affected side and decreased effective ventilation. Venous return is diminished by a mediastinal shift and the effects of positive pressure. The most common clinical signs include respiratory distress and the absence of breath sounds on the affected side. Subcutaneous emphysema and a deviated trachea may also be present. Treatment includes insertion of a chest tube if the pneumothorax is greater than 10 percent. Under anesthesia a pneumothorax can be detected by an increased airway pressure, low compliance, absence of breath sounds, hypotension, and low arterial blood oxygen content. If a tension pneumothorax is present, a chest tube or large-bore needle should be immediately inserted into the second or third intercostal space in the midclavicular line. Adequate reexpansion of the lung and ventilation are observed. A chest x-ray is performed postoperatively.

Hemothorax is the accumulation of blood in the pleural cavity as a result of injury to the great vessels or thoracic organs. The clinical signs are similar to those of pneumothorax, although if blood loss is significant, rapid deterioration of vital signs may occur. Treatment includes insertion of a chest tube, close monitoring of chest tube drainage, and institution of resuscitation measures. Assessment of the amount of blood loss in the chest drainage tube and hemodynamic stability are important prior to the selection of anesthesia techniques.

Flail chest results from two segmental fractures in each of three adjacent ribs. The injured segment causes paradoxical movement of the chest wall, leading to ventilation–perfusion abnormalities. Treatment includes maintenance of effective ventilation, stabilization of the flail segment, and administration of pain medication.

Cardiac tamponade is the rapid accumulation of blood in the pericardial sac. The rate and amount of blood accumulation will determine the pathophysiologic response. The increase in intrapericardial pressure causes impairment of diastolic ventricular filling and reduces cardiac output. The heart rate and peripheral vascular resistance increase as compensatory mechanisms. However, as the intrapericardial pressure continues to increase, cardiovascular collapse ensues. Clinical symptoms include increased central venous pressure, jugular vein distention, pulsus paradoxus, muffled heart sounds, tachycardia, and hypotension. Treatment involves cardiovascular support, pericardiocentesis, and, possibly, thoracotomy. Anesthetic management of the patient consists of careful titration of anesthetic induction agents. Ketamine (0.25 to 0.75 mg/kg) is usually the agent of choice for a rapid-sequence induction. The surgeon must be ready to immediately perform a thoracotomy if cardiac arrest occurs during the induction. Once the tamponade is released, and cardiovascular stability returns, further anesthetic agents may be administered.

Cardiac contusions should be suspected in the patient with blunt chest injuries. The most common presenting symptom is arrhythmias. The electrocardiogram may not initially reflect evidence of myocardial damage. Anesthetic consideration for these patients includes prevention of myocardial depression and close monitoring of heart rate and rhythm.

Thoracic aortic injuries are associated with significant mortality rates. The primary goal of anesthetic management is to maintain cardiovascular stability until the surgeon can repair the injured area. Large amounts of blood and fluid should be administered to maintain an effective vascular volume and perfusion pressure.

One-lung anesthesia may be required to aid in control of bleeding and surgical exploration of the thoracic injury. Endobronchial intubation with a Carlens or Robertshaw tube can be performed using a rapid-sequence induction technique. Close monitoring of the adequacy of ventilation and oxygenation is imperative, as is maintenance of hemodynamic stability. Knowledge of the physiologic alterations induced by one-lung anesthesia is mandatory. Any patient with significant lung injury should be mechanically ventilated postoperatively until adequate respiratory function is restored.

Abdominal Trauma

Blunt or penetrating abdominal injuries can cause single or multiple organ damage. Most injuries involve the liver, spleen, or small intestine. In severe injuries, bleeding into the abdominal cavity occurs, causing a tense, distended abdomen and creating a tamponade. Symptoms of hemorrhagic shock can be present, requiring aggressive resuscitation with blood and fluid therapy and immediate surgical intervention.

A rapid-sequence induction is followed by the administration of minimal depressant agents until the extent of injury is determined and the bleeding is controlled. When the abdomen is opened, a precipitous drop in blood pressure can occur from the release of the tamponade. The anesthetist must be prepared to immediately infuse large volumes of fluid and blood to maintain an adequate perfusion pressure. Further management guidelines include accurate assessment of blood loss, correction of acid–base abnormalities, and careful titration of anesthetic agents.

Maxillofacial Injuries

Over 72 percent of persons involved in motor vehicle accidents sustain injury to the head and neck area. Other sources of injury are gunshot and stab wounds. The most important priority for successful management is to establish a patient airway. Depending upon the severity and nature of the injury, endotracheal intubation or tracheostomy is performed. Endotracheal intubation may be accomplished in several ways, awake oral or nasal, asleep oral or nasal, or by the use of a fiberoptic bronchoscope. The choice of technique will depend upon the area and severity of injury. Direct visualization of oropharyngeal structures may be necessary in the presence of large amounts of bleeding or complex facial fractures. Nasal intubation is avoided in any patient with suspected communicating facial and neurologic injury. Consideration of cervical spine injury warrants neck stabilization and immobilization during intubation. Control of bleeding, cardiovascular support, and elevation of injuries are other goals of initial management.

The patient transported to the operating room for surgical exploration must be carefully assessed to determine the extent of airway difficulty caused by the injury. Prior planning of airway management prevents catastrophic situations such as inability to ventilate or intubate, leading to episodes of hypoxia. If a question arises as to whether successful asleep intubation can be accomplished, an awake intubation or tracheostomy is performed. Following surgical explorations of the injury, the patient is closely observed and carefully assessed prior to extubation.

Management of the trauma patient who has sustained an ocular injury poses several conflicting problems. Prevention of increase in intraocular pressure and guarding against aspiration are the goals of management. A rapid-sequence intravenous induction with vecuronium or pancuronium 0.10 to 0.15 mg/kg, thiopental 3 to 5 mg/kg, and lidocaine 1 to 1.5 mg/kg is advocated by many practitioners. Other authorities recommend the following technique; pretreatment with a nondepolarizing muscle relaxant, thiopental 3 to 5 mg/kg and succinylcholine 1.5 mg/kg intravenously.

Conflicting reports exist as to whether succinylcholine does increase intraocular pressure during induction. Ketamine should be avoided in these patients. Awareness of the factors that may raise intraocular pressure is essential. These factors include light planes of anesthesia, hypertension, and coughing. Emergence and extubation are potentially difficult because of the conflicting desire to have the patient fully awake to guard against aspiration and yet in a plane of anesthesia deep enough to prevent coughing on the endotracheal tube. Establishment of priorities will guide individual judgment.

Head Trauma

Successful anesthetic management of the patient with acute head injuries incorporates the basic principles of neuroanesthesia and trauma. Priorities include airway patency, cardiovascular support, and measures to decrease intracranial pressure. Endotracheal intubation and hyperventilation are usually initiated in the emergency room. Once the patient is transported to the operating room, essential monitoring is applied, and controlled hyperventilation is continued.

If the patient is not intubated prior to surgery, a rapid-sequence intravenous induction with thiopental 3 to 5 mg/kg, vecuronium or pancuronium 0.10 to 0.15 mg/kg, or succinycholine 1.5 mg/kg and lidocaine 1 to 2 mg/kg is advocated. Controversy exists regarding the use of succinylcholine in head trauma, but the prior administration of a low-dose, nondepolarizing muscle relaxant and high dose of thiopental aids in preventing any increase in intracranial pressure. Ketamine is avoided. Further anesthetic agents and fluid and blood replacement are titrated depending upon hemodynamic stability. Controlled ventilation is used to maintain a $Paco_2$ of 25 to 30 torr. Postoperatively, management depends upon the severity of intracranial injury and the overall status of the patient.

MULTIPLE INJURIES

The trauma patient who has sustained multiple organ injuries presents an anesthetic challenge. Multiple injuries most frequently include head trauma, with major abdominal or thoracic organ involvement. Initial management focuses on prompt recognition and accurate diagnosis of all injuries. Adequate oxygenation and stabilization of the blood pressure are of the utmost importance. Priorities are then established to maintain adequate support of the major organ systems.

Anesthetic guidelines follow those already mentioned in the previous discussion.

POSTOPERATIVE CONSIDERATIONS

Close observation of major system function continues in the postoperative period. Mechanical ventilation is indicated for any patient who has sustained life-threatening injuries. Assessment of the patient's respiratory function is essential prior to extubation. Hemodynamic stability is monitored with proper fluid, blood, and drug therapy instituted as needed. Serial laboratory determinations are evaluated. Effective communication with the surgical staff and recovery room personnel is essential to promote optimal postoperative care of the trauma patient.

BIBLIOGRAPHY

Alexander W: Early Care of the Injured Patient. Philadelphia, Saunders, 1982.

Altura BM, Lefer AM, Schumer W: Handbook of Shock and Trauma. Volume 1: Basic Science. New York; Raven, 1983.

Bevan DR: Metabolic response to anesthesia, surgery, and trauma. In Gray TC, Utting JE, Nunn JF (eds): General Anesthesia, 4th ed. London, Butterworth, 1974, vol 2, pp 1017–1036.

Buchanan EC: Blood and blood substitutes for treating hemorrhagic shock. Am J Pharm 34:631–636, 1977.

Finucane BT: Thoracic trauma. In Kaplan JA (ed): Thoracic Anesthesia. New York, Churchill Livingstone, 1983, pp 475–504.

Giesecke AH: Anesthesia for trauma surgery. In Miller RD (ed): Anesthesia. New York, Churchill-Livingstone, 1981, vol II, pp 1247–1263.

Inglesee-Bieber M, Slaby AE: Serum alcohol levels and the incidence of trauma. In Galanter M (ed): Currents in Alcoholism. New York, Grune & Stratton, 1982, pp 269–281.

Karrel R, Shaffer MA: Emergency diagnosis, resuscitation and treatment of acute penetrating cardiac trauma. Ann Emerg Med 11: 504–517, 1982.

Lucas CE, Ledgerwood AM: The fluid problem in the critically ill. Surg Clin North Am 63(2):439–454, 1983.

Mandless J: Perioperative care: Emergency anesthesia. Br J Hosp Med 19:437–443, 1978.

Owens WD, Cobb ML: Anesthetic management of the trauma victim. In Zuidema GD, Rutherford RB, Ballinger WF (eds): The Management of Trauma. Philadelphia, Saunders, 1979, pp 102–113.

Swan KG, Swan RC: Gunshot Wounds: Pathophysiology and Management. Littleton, MA, PSG, 1980.

Trunkey DD (ed): Symposium on trauma. Surg Clin North Am 621(1), 1982.

Walters FJM, Nott MR: The hazards of anesthesia in the injured patient. Br J Anesth 49:707–720, 1977.

Worth MH: Principles and Practice of Trauma Care. Baltimore, Williams & Wilkins, 1982.

Zimmerman BL: Uncommon problems in acute trauma. In Katz J, Benuof J, Kadis LB (eds): Anesthesia and Uncommon Diseases Pathophysiological and Clinical Correlations. Philadelphia, Saunders, 1981, pp 635–671.

32

Current Practices in Neuroanesthesia

Barbara Shwiry

New diagnostic and monitoring techniques have improved the results obtained by operative intervention in patients with neurologic disease. The introduction of computerized tomography (CT) and magnetic resonance imaging (MRI) provided rapid initial identification of pharmacologically or surgically treatable lesions such as tumors, abscesses, hematomas, and edema. These new imaging modalities spare patients significant hazards that previously resulted from delayed diagnosis, mechanical complications, and expansion of residual ventricular air from pneumoencephalography by nitrous oxide (N_2O) administration. Electrophysiologic monitoring of the brain with electroencephalogram (EEG) and multimodality evoked potentials readily detects abnormal neuronal function in the presence of ischemia. In selected cases, intracranial pressure (ICP) monitoring has also proved to be an essential guide to the initiation and effectiveness of therapy, as well as a prognostic indicator of outcome, especially after head trauma.

Expanded care of comatose patients and the introduction of barbiturates for control of intracranial hypertension and protection against ischemic injury have necessitated the institution of unique life-support measures in a setting oriented to the central nervous system (CNS)—the neurologic intensive care unit. This specialized attention is initiated before surgery and continues into the postoperative period, since ICP, cerebral blood flow (CBF), and the formation of edema are affected by alteration of arterial blood pressure, central venous pressure (CVP), inspiratory airway pressure, arterial oxygen (Pa_{O_2}) and carbon dioxide (Pa_{CO_2}) tension, and hydrogen ion concentration (pH). Close attention to cardiopulmonary dynamics in patients with poor intracranial compliance will significantly improve survival. Consideration of the effect of cardiopulmonary parameters and pharmacokinetics on intracranial dynamics in this specialized intensive care environment, in conjunction with new diagnostic and monitoring techniques, has contributed greatly to improved management and outcome of the neurosurgical patient.

CEREBRAL PHYSIOLOGY

Global CBF, total volume of blood passing through the brain, is 44 to 50 ml/100 g/minute in adult humans. CBF is sensitive to a variety of chemical, myogenic, and neuro-genic factors and is closely related to the cerebral metabolic requirement for oxygen (CMR_{O_2}).

Although global CBF is stable, alterations in regional CBF (rCBF) occur frequently and rapidly, varying from 20 to 80 ml/100 g/minute. At regional levels, variations in activity produce increased O_2 demand, which is met by increased supply to the specific areas of activity. Since the number of brain cells involved in such shifts in rCBF is small compared with total brain mass, global CBF does not change. However, such CMR_{O_2}-related changes in rCBF are vital to neuronal function, and regional ischemia can quickly cause marked neurologic deficits. The regulation of rCBF is thought to be mediated by local changes in pH, increased extracellular concentration of hydrogen and potassium, and decreased extracellular calcium. In situations where cortical activity is depressed, such as barbiturate anesthesia or hypothermia, rCBF remains under metabolic influence—that is, the reduction in CBF parallels the reduction in CMR_{O_2}. In certain situations, such as in brain injury or when inhalational anesthetics are used, there may be an uncoupling of the CMR_{O_2}/CBF relationship, and a relative hyperemia is observed.

Myogenic regulation of CBF—that is, autoregulation, is a control process by which normal CBF is maintained relatively constant over a wide range of arterial pressures, provided systemic arterial pressure (SAP) changes relatively slowly. Autoregulation is thought to be a stretch receptor response of arteriolar smooth muscle by which distension of the vessel due to increased SAP induces cerebral arteriolar constriction in a negative feedback loop, with subsequent decreased flow into the capillaries. Decreased SAP reduces cerebral arteriolar muscle tone, causing capillaries to dilate in order to augment the flow.

Autoregulation normally functions over a mean arterial pressure (MAP) range of 50 to 150 mm Hg in normotensive patients. Autoregulation begins to fall at an MAP of 50 mm Hg. As MAP falls below this level, flow becomes dependent on pressure, and progressive cerebral ischemia ensues. If the MAP exceeds 150 mm Hg, the high flow at this pressure overwhelms the arteriolar constrictor response, injuring the endothelial cells of the capillary bed (the blood–brain barrier) and impairing their normal semipermeability.

The resultant increase in transudation of fluid and protein across damaged capillaries and into the cerebral extracellular spaces will produce edema.

In chronic arterial hypertension of more than 2 to 3 months' duration, the autoregulatory curve is displaced to the right. Cerebral vessels adapt to higher pressure levels, and upper and lower limits of autoregulation are increased.

In awake patients with hypertension (MAP between 125 and 180 mm Hg), the lower limits of autoregulation are 90 to 125 mm Hg. In these patients, clinical signs of cerebral ischemia occurred when the MAP ranged from 35 to 80 mm Hg.

Impairment of autoregulation may result from hypoxia, ischemia, acidosis, volatile anesthetics, and trauma. Impaired autoregulation can cause cerebral vasomotor paralysis, which leaves the arterioles in a state of dilatation and renders the capillary bed vulnerable to hypertensive insult or ischemia.

Cerebral perfusion pressure (CPP) is an estimate of the pressure gradient between the internal carotid artery and the subarachnoid veins—that is, the pressure gradient across the entire brain. CPP is equal to the difference between the MAP and the ICP (CPP = MAP − ICP). In functioning autoregulation, CPP ranges from 85 to 95 mm Hg. CPP may be narrowed by either a fall in MAP or an increase in ICP.

The chemical determinants (acid–base) of CBF operate primarily through the effect of $Paco_2$ on the pH of interstitial fluid. The blood–brain barrier is permeable to CO_2 and essentially impermeable to bicarbonate; therefore, Pco_2 of cerebrospinal fluid (CSF) is largely determined by $Paco_2$; bicarbonate concentration is controlled by cerebral metabolic processes. Bicarbonate and Pco_2 are primary determinants of environmental pH, to which arterial smooth muscle is extremely responsive. Variations of $Paco_2$ from 20 to 80 mm Hg produce direct 2 percent changes in CBF for every 1 mm Hg change in $Paco_2$ (Fig. 32–1). Hypercapnia causes periarteriolar acidosis and marked cerebral vasodilation, thereby increasing cerebral blood volume (CBV) and CBF. Hypocapnia-induced periarteriolar alkalosis causes constriction of the cerebral vessels, thus decreasing CBF and CBV. In patients with intracranial hypertension, hyperventilation is a useful therapeutic maneuver.

Marked hypoxia (Pao_2 less than 50 mm Hg) causes progressive brain tissue lactic acidosis, which has a potent dilatory effect on arterioles. Marked hypoxia significantly increases CBF and is capable of overriding hypocarbia.

Neurogenic control through autonomic innervation of the cerebral vessels plays a relatively minor role in determining arteriolar tonus. Sympathetic innervation to the larger cerebral arteries and arterioles is derived from the superior cervical ganglion. Parasympathetic innervation is from the greater petrosal branch of the facial nerve. Maximum autonomic stimulation alters CBF by 5 to 10 percent. The major contribution of neurogenic influence of CBF is seen during hemorrhagic or hypovolemic hypotension, which is accompanied by an adrenergic vasoconstrictor response. In the brain, this sympathetic vasoconstriction is superimposed on myogenic vasoconstriction, thus tending to produce maximum vasoconstriction at a higher MAP. Under these circumstances, autoregulation fails at a higher threshold (as in chronic hypertension). Controlled hypotension does not appear to induce the sympathetic vasoconstrictor response seen with hemorrhagic shock and is better tolerated than hemorrhagic shock, since less cerebral lactic acidosis occurs.

High flow in excess of metabolic need, referred to as luxury perfusion, results from a condition of vasomotor paralysis of vessels in tissue surrounding ischemic or infarcted areas and brain tumors. The low pH due to the accumulation of lactic acid or other acid metabolites is the main factor responsible for the loss of normal vascular responsiveness. Should hypercapnia now cause a dilatation of surrounding responsive arterioles, blood may be directed away from the zone of vasomotor paralysis (the "steal" phenomenon) to normal areas, because the affected arterioles cannot dilate further. Conversely, hypocarbic vasoconstriction of normal vessels can direct yet more blood into the bed of paralyzed, maximally dilated vessels, which do not constrict in response to hypocarbia (the inverse steal or "Robin Hood" phenomenon).

Physiologic control of CBF is, in summary, a multifactorial system in which the cerebral arterioles respond with varying intensity to a variety of stimuli, including the following: (1) The acid–base or chemical determinants of arteriolar tonus operate primarily through the effect of $Paco_2$ on the pH of interstitial fluid and through the production of lactic acidosis when the brain functions in a hypoxic milieu (Pao_2 less than 50 mm Hg). Acidosis, whether secondary to hypercarbia or ischemia, has a potent dilatory effect on arterioles. (2) Autoregulation, the property inherent in arteriolar smooth muscle, causes constriction in response to stretch forces. (3) The cerebral metabolic rate determines arteriolar tonus by a yet undefined mechanism. (4) Neurologic control through autonomic innervation of the cerebral vessels plays a relatively minor role in determining arteriolar tonus. Each determinant of CBF has a characteristic response curve (see Fig. 32–1).

INTRACRANIAL PRESSURE

The intracranial contents—including the brain, its associated intra- and extracellular water, CSF, blood, and meninges—generate an ICP of 8 to 12 mm Hg. Since the skull is relatively rigid, a change in volume of one of the intracra-

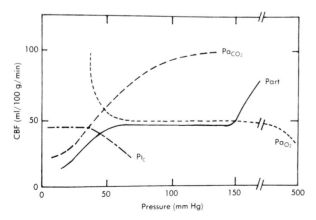

Figure 32–1. Variation of CBF with changes in SAP, $Paco_2$, Pao_2, and ICP (PI_c). "Part" shows limits of autoregulation. (*Reprinted with permission, Shapiro HM: Anesthesiology 43:445, 1975.*)

nial constituents must be accompanied by a reciprocal change in one of the other constituents if increased ICP is to be avoided. When the increase in the volume of one of the intracranial constituents is not accompanied by a reciprocal decrease in the volume of another, the craniospinal compartment is said to be noncompliant, or "tight." A "slack," or compliant, brain is associated with reciprocal volume change. Intracranial compliance permits limited expansion of intracranial volume without an increase in ICP or production of symptoms. Patients with low compliance poorly tolerate further increases in intracranial volume (Fig. 32–2). Initially, spatial compensation is accomplished by shift of CSF into the distensible subarachnoid space, increased absorption of CSF across the arachnoid villi, and translocation of intracranial blood volume to the rest of the body due to the pressure exerted on the thin-walled cerebral veins. As much as 1 ml of CSF per minute can be expressed from the cranial space in the presence of increased pressure. If rapid spatial compensation were not possible, rapid expansion of even the smallest mass would be incompatible with life.

When the ability of CSF to act as the ICP buffer has been exhausted and further spatial compensation cannot be achieved by reduction in intracranial blood volume, displacement of brain structures through midline shifts and herniation (Fig. 32–3), collapse of CSF cisterns, and compression of the arachnoid villi occur.

The management of intracranial hypertension is aimed at reduction of the intracranial volume and improving cerebral perfusion and energy supply and demand. Hyperosmolar diuretics (mannitol and glycerol), systemic diuretics (furosemide and ethacrynic acid), corticosteroids, appropriate respiratory care including hyperventilation, barbiturates, sedatives, muscle relaxants, hypothermia, CSF diversion, and surgical decompression play a significant role in the management of patients with neurologic disease and increased ICP.

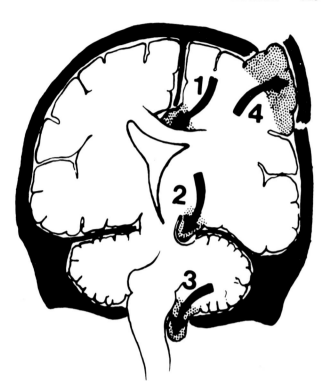

Figure 32–3. Areas of potential brain herniation: (1) cingulate, (2) temporal (uncal), (3) cerebellar, (4) transclival (postoperative or traumatic). Intracranial component (ICP) normally comprises the meninges, brain tissue, intra- and extracellular water, blood, and CSF. Intracranial masses (tumor, hematoma, or abscess) and edema expand these components and increase ICP. (*Reprinted with permission from Fishman RA: Brain edema. N Engl J Med 293:706–711, 1975.*)

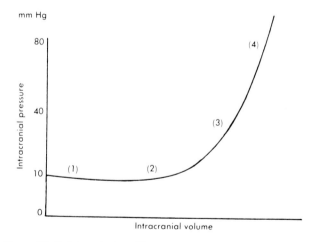

Figure 32–2. Interrelation of intracranial volume and intracranial pressure (ICP) within the closed cranium. As volume expands progressively, compliance is reduced so that each increment in volume (points 1, 2, 3) causes a more marked rise in ICP. When ICP is already elevated (point 3), even a small increase in intracranial volume may cause ICP values to surge tremendously (point 4). (*Adapted with permission from Shapiro HM: Anesthesiology 43:445, 1975.*)

AIRWAY MANAGEMENT

Maintaining an adequate airway is critical in the care of neurosurgical patients. Airway obstruction must be alleviated because the increased intrathoracic pressure will exacerbate intracranial hypertension. By preventing adequate oxygenation, airway obstruction also causes secondary damage to the brain, compounding the initial biomechanical disruption from trauma or operation. In the presence of obstruction, accumulation of CO_2 dilates cerebral vessels and increases CBF and CBV. Both improved oxygenation and adequate ventilation are achieved by airway control.

The decision to intubate a comatose patient depends on the depth of coma. When there is airway obstruction, loss of reflexes, or inability to clear secretions, the patient should be intubated in order to ensure oxygenation and prevent aspiration. If the patient exhibits purposeful movements in response to a painful stimulus, the protective reflexes are probably intact. Rather than immediate intubation, close observation may be indicated—bearing in mind that the patient's neurologic status is dynamic and may deteriorate precipitously at any time.

There are potential difficulties with airway management and intubation in patients with cervical spinal fractures, cervical spine fixation, head and neck trauma, and impaired mandibular motion. The necessity of avoiding flexion and extension of the neck may make airway maintenance impossible after an anesthetic-induced loss of muscle tone. For this reason, intubation is accomplished with the patient awake or mildly sedated.

Awake tracheal intubation may be facilitated by local anesthetic blockage of the upper airway by topical application of local anesthesia to the nose and mouth, to the trachea via cricothyroid puncture, and to the larynx via the bilateral superior laryngeal nerve block. Lidocaine is the most reasonable choice of anesthetic, considering the beneficial effects of this drug in patients with head injury. An absolute contraindication to the technique is the patient with a full stomach because of the risk of aspiration of gastric contents through the anesthetized larynx. In addition, infection or tumor in the area of the block would be a contraindication to its use.

When this technique was used in patients already intubated and requiring ventilatory support, the discomfort of the tube was decreased by the block. Although the duration of action of lidocaine is only 90 minutes, there appeared to be an obtunded laryngeal reflex, which outlasted the duration of nerve block. Lidocaine, administered intravenously (1 mg/kg), may be substituted for the transtracheal method. A complete description of the technique has recently been reviewed by Shwiry, Josephs, Gotta, and Sullivan (1984).

Patients who cough and strain on the endotracheal tube despite local anesthesia require sedation to prevent elevation of ICP and deficits in rCBF. In ventilated patients, muscle relaxation may be required as poor synchronization with the ventilation and inadequate muscle relaxation may also raise ICP.

Damage to the respiratory center or to the ninth, tenth, and twelfth cranial nerves from trauma or during posterior fossa exploration may cause central impairment of respiration. The possibility of operative trauma requires cautious assessment of airway and swallowing after extubation and during the first feeding. Complete inability to cough or swallow effectively may necessitate tracheostomy, but patients eventually compensate for unilateral paralysis of the vagus nerve.

Dissection or hemorrhage in the area of the posterior fossa can directly compress the respiratory center. Perifocal edema associated with tumor, trauma, or surgery may increase ICP, causing brain stem compression. Compression impairs pharyngeal reflexes and may lead to airway obstruction. Such occurrences may be preceded by a period of ataxic respiration, especially after an interval of wakefulness and adequate spontaneous ventilation. Prompt reintubation and mechanical hyperventilation are indicated, especially since hyperventilation can reduce brain volume and control edema formation. CT scan or MR imaging will identify surgically removable hematomas.

Whenever any respiratory treatment modality is instituted in the neurosurgical patient, the possible effects on CBF, CPP, and ICP must be taken into consideration. Tracheal suctioning during tracheal toilet will significantly increase ICP by producing an arousal response or, in the apneic patient, by causing accumulation of CO_2. The arousal response can be mitigated by prior sedation with intravenous (IV) lidocaine followed by instillation of lidocaine in the tube.

Moving the head to the left or right can increase ICP by altering cerebral venous outflow. It is therefore advisable to avoid rotation of the head during tracheal suctioning and transport of patients. Elevation of the head to 30 degrees above the horizontal helps to control ICP, since this facilitates cerebral venous and CSF drainage. The 30-degree head-up position is helpful in counteracting the elevation of ICP produced by positive end-expiratory pressure (PEEP). Repeated lowering of the head of the bed for tracheal suctioning or measurement of CVP or pulmonary capillary wedge pressure (PCWP) must be minimized.

Mechanical positive-pressure ventilation significantly affects CBF, CPP, and ICP. Controlled mechanical ventilation (CMV) eliminates the negative intrathoracic pressure of normal inspiration, thus decreasing venous return. If this reduction in preload is superimposed on preexisting hypovolemia, arterial hypotension may quickly follow institution of CMV and significantly affect CBF, especially in the presence of increased ICP. In addition, the intrathoracic positive pressure generated during the inspiratory phase of CMV is transmitted to the great veins and contributes to increasing ICP by increasing CVP. Maintenance of normovolemia and the 30-degree head-up position improve central venous outflow and are therefore indicated during CMV.

The use of PEEP for treatment of refractory hypoxemia with increased intrapulmonary shunt and decreased functional residual capacity produces similar cardiovascular changes that may elevate ICP. PEEP should be instituted at low pressures and decreased gradually as oxygenation improves, since sudden reductions may increase cardiac output, causing an increase in CBF and ICP.

Intermittent mandatory ventilation (IMV) is a useful technique for supplying supplemental ventilation to the spontaneously breathing patient who requires assistance to maintain an acceptable $Paco_2$. IMV permits the patient to breathe at his or her own rate while receiving a "machine breath" every 6 to 15 seconds. This mode reduces the risk of hypotension or decreased cardiac output in the presence of increased ICP. Modern ventilators have internal IMV circuits with mandatory breath cycles timed so that breaths occur at the beginning of the spontaneous inspirations. This is referred to as synchronized IMV. If spontaneous ventilation is borderline, IMV will decrease the work of breathing, thus providing a useful alternative to the combination of CMV plus sedation in the patient who tolerates the ventilator poorly.

Controlled, or therapeutic, hyperventilation is a major nonoperative technique for decreasing ICP. Reduction of $Paco_2$ to 25 to 30 mm Hg constricts cerebral vessels and decreases CBF, CBV, and ICP with minimal risk of cerebral ischemia. CBF and CSF pH normalize after a few days of hypocarbia, therefore this technique may have diminished effect as its use is prolonged. Although the duration of ICP reduction may be limited, there is little doubt about the acute effectiveness of hyperventilation in decreasing ICP. A $Paco_2$ less than 20 mm Hg may be associated with ischemia due to extreme cerebral vasoconstriction. The ideal level of hypocarbia is difficult to define, since variations in CBF are not usually monitored. However, if the patient hyperventilates spontaneously, ventilator assistance should be adjusted to maintain the spontaneously achieved level of hypocarbia.

Hyperventilation is most effective as an acute, short-term means of reducing ICP and in practice is often combined with the administration of steroids, diuretics, and occasionally barbiturates.

Diuretics

Osmotherapy is a mainstay in the treatment of increased ICP in the presence of brain edema. Interstitial water in normal brain tissue is transposed to the intravascular compartment by creation of an osmotic gradient. The hypertonicity also results from the hypernatremia secondary to hypotonic losses during osmotic diuresis.

Reductions in ICP of greater than 10 percent can be obtained by osmotherapy. Following osmotic intervention, ICP returns to the pretreatment level within 45 minutes to 11 hours. However, rebound of ICP to higher than pretreatment level can occur with all osmotic drugs. There are several mechanisms that may be responsible for this rebound phenomenon. Diffusion of the osmotic agent into brain interstitial space and CSF causes the interstitial osmolarity to be higher than the plasma level as the osmotic agent is excreted renally. Disruption of the blood–brain barrier following trauma also permits rapid diffusion of the osmotic agent into the interstitial space. Brain cells generate their own osmotic molecules as well, and these in part balance the osmotic gradient, favoring cellular dehydration. The identity of these molecules is not clear, but some appear to be amino acids, which constitute up to 50 percent of the intracellular solute 7 days after the induction of experimental hypernatremic hyperosmolarity. The significance of these idiogenic osmoles in blunting acute osmotherapeutic maneuvers is probably not great, but they do appear to reduce the effectiveness of chronic or long-term administration of hyperosmolar drugs.

Mannitol, a naturally occurring polyhydric alcohol originally obtained from the manna plant, is the most widely used osmotic diuretic. Its molecular weight (MW) is 182.17. Mannitol is not metabolized and is not reabsorbed by the renal tubules. The usual IV dose of mannitol is 0.25 to 1.5 mg/kg administered as an infusion over 15 to 30 minutes. Onset of action begins within 20 minutes, is maximal between 1 and 2 hours, and wears off in 6 hours. Needle-like crystals of the drug may precipitate with cool storage and must be dissolved by heating before use.

Rapid administration of mannitol expands circulatory volume and may precipitate left ventricular failure, especially in patients with preexisting cardiovascular disease. This acute volume expansion, coupled with hypertonic cerebral vasodilation and increased CBF, increases ICP. Therefore, osmodiuretics should be administered slowly to patients with increased ICP. Increased CBF may be beneficial in those patients with ischemic cerebrovascular disease. However, osmotherapy is relatively contraindicated in patients with cerebrovascular lesions such as aneurysms and arteriovenous malfunction. It must be used with caution in elderly patients, in whom sudden shrinkage of brain mass can cause rupture of bridging veins and subsequent

intracranial hemorrhage. Also, if intracranial bleeding is suspected, shrinkage of brain tissue, which may have been acting as a tamponade, may cause expansion of the hematoma. Repeated or long-term administration of mannitol induces electrolyte imbalance (hyponatremia and hypokalemia) and hyperosmolar states (greater than 320 mOsm) above the therapeutic level, beyond which neurologic and renal dysfunction may occur. Mannitol also increases cerebral edema and ICP because it is able, in the presence of extensive breakdown of the blood–brain barrier, to diffuse into brain tissue and reverse the osmotic gradient.

Several techniques have been suggested to reduce the undesirable effects of mannitol osmotherapy. Lower dose ranges of 0.25 to 0.5 g/kg reduce the risk of acute expansion of intravascular volume and induction of intersititial hyperosmolarity. Such doses have been shown to produce as much reduction in ICP as larger doses, although the effect is shorter in duration. The administration of furosemide (1 mg/kg) before or with mannitol may reduce the incidence and severity of the rebound effects on ICP. Rebound elevations of ICP may also be minimized by restricting fluid replacement to one-half to two-thirds the volume of urine produced by the osmotic diuresis.

Urea is a smaller molecule (MW 60.06) that diffuses through tissues more rapidly and has a short duration of action and a purportedly greater rebound effect. Glycerol may have advantages over mannitol or urea, since 80 percent is metabolized by the liver, thereby reducing the potential for rebound. Glycerol should be infused initially at 5 mg/kg/minute for 30 minutes and then at 3 mg/kg/minute for the next 90 minutes. However, experiments with rat brains suggest that glycerol may exacerbate ischemic cerebral edema.

The loop diuretics, furosemide (Lasix) and ethacrynic acid (Edecrin), have been used to control brain edema associated with tumor and head injury. Furosemide has recently been used for reduction of ICP in patients with aneurysmal subarachnoid hemorrhage (Samson, Reyes 1982).

The diuretic effect of furosemide is due to inhibition of sodium absorption in the proximal and distal tubules and in the loop of Henle. Furosemide effects a reduction in ICP by systemic diuresis, relaxation of capacitance vessels, inhibition of astroglial chloride and water transport, and reducing CSF production through carbonic anhydrase inhibition. Furosemide reduces ICP without significant osmolar or electrolyte change and can be given as a primary (1 mg/kg) or adjuvant (0.15 to 0.30 mg/kg) diuretic.

Furosemide may be considered as a substitute for mannitol in neurosurgery in those patients presenting with increased ICP, an altered blood–brain barrier, or increased pulmonary water content, and for those patients who have preexisting cardiac and electrolyte abnormalities.

Diuretic therapy is monitored by appropriate determination of serum and urine osmolarity and electrolytes, especially during chronic administration. Ideally, ICP should be measured to ascertain the effectiveness of treatment and adjust the dose and frequency of diuretic administration.

Steroids

Galilich and colleagues introduced the use of steroids for reduction of edema associated with brain tumors in 1961.

The effect of steroids is presumably due to their ability to stabilize membranes, inhibit lysosomal enzyme release, and scavenge free radicals. The effectiveness of steroids. particularly dexamethasone and methylprednisolone, in decreasing the vasogenic edema associated with brain tumor and abscess is undisputed. With increase of intracranial compliance, the level of consciousness frequently improves and neurologic deficits resolve before ICP is reduced. Operative and postoperative cerebral edema is also reduced by steroids.

Steroids appear to be less effective in treating cytotoxic edema associated with ischemia, hypo-osmolality, asphyxia, and hypoxia. The results of steroid therapy for experimental and clinical ischemic cerebral edema are inconclusive. Membrane stabilization may not, however, be crucial to the effect of steroids in reducing cerebral edema, because accumulation of water in ischemic cerebral edema peaks before significant alteration in the permeability of the blood–brain barrier occurs. Clinical use of steroids for control of ischemic cerebral edema has met with varying success. Patten and colleagues gave dexamethasone or placebo to patients with acute strokes in a double-blind, randomized, prospective study and found that the treated group improved but the placebo group deteriorated. Other investigators observed no improvement in either survival or neurologic function with steroid treatment.

The role of steroids in the treatment of patients with head injury remains controversial. Although steroids in low doses (dexamethasone, 10 mg IV initially, followed by 4 mg every 6 hours) have been ineffective, a recent randomized, double-blind, prospective trial indicated that therapy with steroids in high doses (0.5 to 15 mg/kg) may improve the quality of life as well as prolong survival after craniocerebral trauma. Patients with severe structural derangement die early, however, despite treatment with steroids.

Attempts to determine the efficacy of steroids in reducing edema following head injury may be complicated by the fact that the initial brain swelling following trauma is due to vascular engorgement from an increase in CBF rather than to formation of edema. The increase in ICP as a result of this augmentation of CBV may actually serve to counteract edema formation. CT scans of patients with head injury substantiate an initial absence of edema, the increased density suggesting blood rather than water. This may explain the lack of early response to steroid therapy in patients with head trauma. However, resolution of subsequently formed edema is enhanced by a reduction in ICP, which facilitates bulk flow of edema fluid from the interstitium to the ventricles.

Hypothermia

There are few situations in which induced hypothermia may be considered. Fever reduction is the most common situation requiring hypothermic techniques. Hyperthermia increases CBF and CMR_{O_2} by 7 percent per degree of elevation over 37C. Operations on cerebral vessels that may cause prolonged cerebral ischemia are another indication for induced hypothermia if vascular pathology is severe. (This is considered in more detail in the discussion on aneurysms.) Hypothermia would be used in conjunction with deliberate circulatory arrest. Cerebral metabolism is reduced 7 percent for each degree of decrease below 37C. CBF and, therefore, ICP are also reduced. Slowing of cerebral edema formation, decreased inflammatory reaction to injury, and decreased CSF secretion may also occur. Among the complications of induced hypothermia are cardiac arrythmias (less than 30C) and shivering during cooling and rewarming, which increases CMR_{O_2} by 50 to 200 percent. Decreased cardiac output, increased blood viscosity, and immobilization may predispose the patient to venous thrombosis and subsequent embolism. If continued through the postoperative period, temperature suppression, especially with steroid therapy, will mask signs of infection.

CSF Diversion

When intracranial CSF pathways are obstructed, shunts are inserted to reduce ICP by providing a low-resistance pathway for CSF. Ventriculoperitoneal shunts are most commonly used; ventriculoatrial shunts are avoided because of the risk of introducing an infection into the heart. Direct ventricular tap or spinal subarachnoid catheter placement may be instituted intraoperatively to relieve brain tension prior to dural opening and to increase operative space.

Surgical Decompression

Internal and external surgical decompression may be done for uncontrollable brain swelling, especially in patients with severe craniocerebral trauma. Internal decompression involves removal of intracranial tissue. This will decrease ICP and reduce midline shift, brain herniation, and brain stem displacement. External decompression involves removal of part of the skull, usually for evacuation of epidural or subdural hematomas. External decompression can actually increase brain tissue distortion and neurologic deterioration. Decompressive surgery is generally considered a last resort for persistent intractable cerebral edema.

Neurodiagnostic Techniques

Neurodiagnostic techniques include MR imaging, positron emission tomography (PET), CT, cerebral angiography, pneumoencephalography, ventriculography, and myelography.

Neurodiagnostics are frequently performed without assistance from anesthesia. However, there are certain situations when monitored anesthesia care or general anesthesia may be required. Testing in pediatric, elderly, debilitated, uncooperative, and decompensating or severely injured patients may best be done under conscious sedation or general anesthesia. The principles of neuroanesthesia should be maintained throughout all procedures. Careful, continuous observation of vital signs and respiration is mandatory, especially when conscious sedation is used. Technical difficulties may arise as a result of inadequate facilities in diagnostic suites to accommodate anesthesia equipment. Anesthesia and monitoring systems often must be transported to the diagnostic area. The environment is often dark, impairing assessment of the patient's skin color and respiration and making it difficult to read the dials and numeric displays on equipment. Air flow turnover may be inadequate, thereby increasing the levels of gases in the environment. Proper maintenance and function of the diagnostic equipment require that the suite be maintained at a temperature of 60 to 65F. Control of body temperature, especially in babies, small children, and the elderly, is an important consideration.

Radiopaque iodine-containing contrast media may be injected into arteries, veins, or CSF spaces. Careful observation during injection of these dyes is necessary, as they can cause allergic reactions ranging from mild skin rashes to anaphylactic shock. Seizures and cardiovascular reactions may also occur. A burning sensation and flushing during injection are fairly common reactions during angiography.

If the patient has a history of allergy to iodine, steroids should be given several hours before the study and diphenhydramine hydrochloride (Benadryl) administered immediately before the contrast dye is given.

Gas Studies

Pneumoencephalography and ventriculography, rarely used today, involve the incremental removal of up to 70 ml of CSF and replacing that volume with air, O_2, or N_2O injected into the spinal subarachnoid space or directly into the ventricles. The patient is securely positioned in a special chair that allows a variety of positions and complete somersaulting to aide passage of the gas through the ventricles and subarachnoid space. Usually, mild sedation and local anesthesia are sufficient for gas encephalography. When general anesthesia is required, care must be taken to support the patient's head. A spiral embedded tube may be used to prevent kinking of the endotracheal tube with position changes. If N_2O is used as the contrast agent, then it may be incorporated into the anesthetic technique. If air or O_2 is used, N_2O is not recommended as it will rapidly equilibrate into the gas-filled ventricle or subarachnoid space and add unmeasurably to the intracranial volume. Air embolus is a distinct possibility especially if the patient has a patent ventricle-to-atrial CSF shunt. N_2O is reabsorbed from the ventricles and subarachnoid space in about 1 hour. Air takes approximately 1 week for complete reabsorption. For this reason, general anesthesia planned within 1 week after gas studies should avoid N_2O unless complete reabsorption of the N_2O is confirmed by skull roentgenogram.

Poststudy headache, nausea, and vomiting are usually due to air remaining in the ventricles. Appropriate analgesics and antiemetics can provide comfort to the patient until the air is completely reabsorbed. Occasionally, the nausea and vomiting are due to postural hypotension and may be relieved by maintenance of a normal MAP and Trendelenburg's position.

Myelography

Myelograms are usually performed under local anesthesia, possibly with mild sedation. If general anesthesia is necessary, consideration must be given to the fact that lumbar and cervical myelography is usually done in the prone position. Cervical myelography may involve hyperexten-

sion and flexion of the neck. Complications of myelography are due to the use of contrast media and may include local infection at the site of needle puncture, bacterial or aseptic meningitis, venous extravasation of contrast media, headache, adhesive arachnoiditis, and allergic reaction.

Iophendylate (Pantopaque) is an oil-based contrast medium, and as such it is nonabsorbable and must be removed after the study.

Metrizamide (Amipaque) is a water-soluble, iodinated contrast material. Its benefits include decreased incidence of headache (if the patient is well hydrated premyelography), nausea, vomiting, hypotension, arachnoiditis, and seizures. Metrizamide does not need to be withdrawn after the study because it is quickly diluted by the CSF and absorbed into the bloodstream. For this very reason, studies must be completed in a much shorter period of time. A major drawback of metrizamide is that it cannot be used in patients receiving medications that lower the seizure threshold. These drugs include phenothiazines, monoamine oxidase inhibitors, antihistamines, tricyclic antidepressants, CNS stimulants, and psychoactive drugs (analeptics, major tranquilizers, and antipsychotic drugs). The synergistic action between metrizamide and any of these drugs can precipitate epileptic seizures. These medications should be discontinued 24 hours prior to the study. Clearly, since antihistamines cannot be used, metrizamide must be avoided in patients with a history of allergy to iodinated compounds.

CT scan is a noninvasive technique that gives an anatomic depiction of a transverse section of the head. The scanning device rotates around the patient's head in a 180-degree arc. The anatomic images are depicted on a cathode ray screen and can be processed as a hard-copy x-ray film. Anatomic and pathologic structures are differentiated by density. The lower the density of the substance, the darker the shade. Abnormalities can be identified by differences in density or by displacement of normal structures. Contrast media may be used for greater differentiation. Radiation exposure to the patient in the area being scanned is approximately equal to that received with conventional skull x-ray per half-hour scan. Skin dose to the anesthetist is many times less than that. Anesthesia or IV sedation may be required when patient movement threatens to invalidate the scan.

MR imaging is a painless, noninvasive technique that uses magnetic fields and radio-frequency pulses for the production of its images. MR imaging is superior to CT scan in differentiating between white and gray matter; displaying images in sagittal, coronal, or axial planes with equal ease; reflecting the chemical environment as well as the elemental structure of tissue; and in visualization of the posterior fossa. To date, MR imaging is available in only a few centers throughout the United States. Accordingly, there have been no reported experiences of anesthetic management of patients undergoing MR imaging. Since the diagnostic procedure is so similar to the procedure for obtaining CT scan, it is reasonable to assume that the indications for anesthetic intervention during MR imaging would be the same as those for CT scan. However, MR imaging poses a unique problem for anesthetic equipment in that anything affected by or that would affect a magnetic field would be affected by the MR unit. All anesthetic equipment within 20 feet of the unit must be nonmagnetic. So far, no adverse effects to personnel of magnetism or radio-frequency fields have been identified.

PET uses radiation emitted as a consequence of radioactive decay to reconstruct an image or to produce spatially identified digital data. This device is used primarily for in vivo study of cerebral metabolic activity and drug interactions. Unless anesthetic agents are the materials under study, no anesthetic intervention should be required.

ANESTHETIC MANAGEMENT

Preoperative Evaluation

The preoperative anesthetic visit includes evaluation of the general medical condition and intracranial tension. Assessment should be made of any peripheral sequelae associated with the intracranial lesion. In the case of traumatic head injury, careful examination should be made for multiple injuries, especially those of the chest and abdomen. Those patients exhibiting altered states of consciousness should be examined for aspiration pneumonitis; chest x-ray and arterial blood gases can provide valuable information. Assessment of intravascular volume and electrolyte balance is essential, especially in those patients treated with diuretics. Patients with lesions of the pituitary should be evaluated for endocrine abnormalities.

The state of intracranial tension determines the use of premedicants. In all cases, those drugs that cause respiratory depression, hypotension, nausea, vomiting, or significant alteration in consciousness should be avoided. These include narcotics, butyrophenones (droperidol), and, in the case of cerebral aneurysms, atropine because of the increased heart rate and MAP. Glycopyrrolate may be used to protect against excessive secretions and vagal reflexes. Hydroxyzine (Vistaril) or diazepam may be used to sedate awake, anxious patients. Hydroxyzine has antiemetic and sedative affects with little effect on ICP. Diazepam has amnestic, antiseizure activity and decreases CBF with minimal effect on the cardiorespiratory system. Obviously lethargic, obtunded patients need no premedication.

Monitoring

Close monitoring during neurosurgical procedures affords opportunity for prompt identification of potential complications such as increased ICP, extensive blood loss, venous air embolism, cardiac arrhythmias, fluctuations in blood pressure, pulmonary abnormalities, and increased urine output.

Monitoring of intraarterial blood pressure provides essential beat-to-beat information. It should be instituted prior to induction whenever possible and maintained through the postanesthetic period. Arteries suitable for short-term cannulation are the radial, brachial, axillary, and dorsal artery of the foot. Before an arterial catheter is placed, collateral circulation should be ascertained. This may be done by palpation or Doppler. Prior to cannulation of the radial artery, in a patient who is able to cooperate, patency of the palmar arch may be determined by a modified Allen's

test. The hazards of arterial cannulation include proximal artery thrombosis and thrombotic and air emboli. The arterial transducer should be zeroed at the highest point of the skull to accurately assess CPP.

Maintaining appropriate anesthetic depth and adequate muscle relaxation is necessary to prevent straining and coughing, especially while the dura is open. A peripheral nerve stimulator (PNS) will help to assess the extent of muscle paralysis, and supplemental doses of muscle relaxant may then be given in order to prevent movement during microdissection of vital structures.

Measurement of urinary output provides an indication of intravascular volume. Knowledge of the exact urinary output is important after administration of osmotic and loop diuretics and in patients with diabetes insipidus or abnormalities of antidiuretic hormone secretion. Decreased urinary output during induced hypotension may indicate decreased renal perfusion and the need to increase blood pressure.

Body temperature is measured by an esophageal or nasopharyngeal thermistor. Rectal temperature does not reflect core temperatures as well as esophageal temperature, especially during hypothermia. Body temperature can be raised intraoperatively by warmed blankets, increased ambient temperature, warmed IV solutions, and decreased flow of anesthetic gas. Chlorpromazine is an effective antipyretic and will prevent shivering by hypothalamic suppression. Muscle relaxants also prevent shivering.

Changes in breath sounds and heart rate and rhythm can be detected by the precordial or esophageal stethoscope.

The electrocardiogram (ECG) is monitored continuously. Posterior fossa dissection and venous air embolism frequently produce bradycardia and arrhythmias. Myocardial ischemia, if present, will be demonstrated in the precordial leads.

The pulse oximeter is a noninvasive technique that continuously and accurately measures arterial oxygen saturation from the pulse at the tip of the finger. In addition to its intraoperative application, this monitor is useful during the immediate postanesthetic period to provide early warning of hypoxemia.

Mass spectrometry provides highly accurate breath-by-breath analysis of all respiratory and anesthetic gases to an accuracy of 0.1 percent of measured value. The most commonly used mass spectrometer in the United States is a multiple-site, or shared, system. A single mass spectrometer unit is used to sample gases from as many as 30 locations, each one equipped with a gas sample outlet and an in-room computer. When the system is shared, there is a delay between samples from each unit as the other units are being sampled in turn. If all 30 are in use, there will be a 5-minute delay between each sample on a given unit. For these reasons, when continuous end-tidal CO_2 (ET_{CO_2}) detection is desired, a separate monitor should be used unless sampling delay is less than 1 minute. Likewise, when more than six sites are used, a separate O_2 analyzer should be used.

Noninvase electrophysiologic monitoring of the CNS is accomplished with the intraoperative use of the EEG and with evoked potentials.

The EEG is useful for detection of compromised cerebral

perfusion or oxygenation and drug effects during anesthesia.

Evoked potentials can be used to monitor a sensory pathway at risk during neurosurgical manipulation. Application of a stimulus to a peripheral nerve elicits voltage changes in the EEG. If the stimulus applied to one part of the nervous system elicits a recordable response in another part of the nervous system, then one can assume that the pathway between stimulus and response is functioning properly.

The most frequently used evoked potential is somatosensory evoked potential monitoring, which is used during procedures on the spine, spinal cord, or vasculature.

Brainstem auditory evoked responses (i.e., potentials) are used to monitor function of the auditory pathway between the eighth cranial nerve and the brainstem. Surgical retraction and manipulation of structures in the posterior fossa can impede impulse transmission along this pathway.

Visual evoked responses monitored in the operating room use flash stimulation through opaque goggles over closed eyes. Monitoring of visual evoked responses is useful for surgery on the anterior vasculature, sphenoid wing, optic chiasm, pituitary, and occipital poles.

Functional areas of the brain can be localized using sensory evoked potentials recorded from the surface of the brain or from deeper within the tissue with probes. Cortical evoked potentials are sensitive to global insults such as hypoxia or anesthetic overdose.

Intraoperative application of these monitors requires considerable technical and interpretive expertise. Much progress has been made in equipment design and adaptability to the operating room, although some of the smaller units, such as the cerebral function monitor, offer convenience and ease of interpretation but at the expense of sacrificing much information.

During operations in which the level of the wound is 5 cm or more higher than the right heart, a negative pressure is created in the venous system and air entrapment is a major hazard. This is a complication most often encountered when the patient is in the sitting position but may also occur with the patient in the lateral, supine, or prone positions. Right atrial catheterization and special monitoring techniques including those just described are required for the detection and treatment of venous air emboli.

A right atrial catheter is essential for aspiration of venous air emboli and may be introduced through the basilic, subclavian, or internal or external jugular vein. Position of the catheter is verified in the operating room with the patient in as close to final position as possible. Verification is made by transduced pressure tracing or chest x-ray or by the P-wave configuration on ECG. This is accomplished by connecting the saline-filled catheter to the V lead of the ECG by means of a metal stopcock, converting the catheter into an ECG lead. Characteristic ECG changes are observed as the catheter is advanced into the right atrium. A biphasic P wave indicates that the catheter tip is in proper position. Caution must be exercised that faulty equipment is not connected to the patient, as the catheter can now act as an electroconductor directly into the heart. Recent studies (Albin, 1981) indicate that optimal position of the catheter tip is at the junction of the superior vena cava

and the right atrium. In addition, a multiorificed catheter allowed for maximal air aspiration and eliminated the possibility of suction adhesion to the chamber wall, and efficiency of the catheter was not as severely compromised by clot formation.

The precordial Doppler is still the device most relied on for detection of venous air emboli. The Doppler is placed over the right atrium, from the fourth through sixth intercostal spaces, to the right of the sternum. Correct positioning of the Doppler in relation to the tip of the central venous catheter is ascertained by injecting a 10-ml bolus of crystalloid solution through the catheter. The immediately resultant turbulence and micro air bubbles generate sounds similar to those of air in the right heart. It should be noted that some studies have found that the turbulent heart sounds generated by saline injection through the catheter were produced even when the catheter was withdrawn up to 30 cm. However, it was also noted that the further away the catheter was from the right atrium, the greater the time lag between the injection of saline and the turbulent Doppler sounds. Also, the Doppler may not be as effective in patients who have distortion in intrathoracic structure, as with scoliosis or following pneumonectomy. A transesophageal Doppler, so far successful in animal experiments, would attenuate any problem of precordial Doppler positioning. Transesophageal echocardiography can detect air bubbles, provide a visualization of air in the right and left heart, and detect paradoxical air emboli.

The Doppler is usually used in conjunction with an $ETco_2$ analyzer, mass spectrometer, or a Swan-Ganz catheter. The $ETco_2$ analyzer is a noninvasive device that attaches between the endotracheal tube and the breathing circuit. During normal ventilation–perfusion, the $ETco_2$ is directly proportional to the $Paco_2$. Balloon-tipped, flow-directed thermodilution catheters for measuring pulmonary artery pressure (PAP) and PCWP and computing cardiac output are helpful for detecting venous air emboli, obtaining a reliable measurement of intravascular volume, and monitoring patients with severe myocardial dysfunction. In addition to monitoring left ventricular function and fluid status, pulmonary artery catheters provide blood samples for determining mixed venous O_2 content (Pvo_2). An acute increase in PAP suggests air embolus. An increase in Pvo_2 at a low MAP indicates impaired tissue perfusion and decreased O_2 extraction.

ICP is monitored by inserting a subdural screw, an epidural fiberoptic transducer or cup catheter, or an intraventricular catheter. (Fig. 32–4). An increase in the incidence of infection occurs when the dura is punctured. Besides infection, hazards of ICP monitoring include nerve tissue damage and hematoma formation. This is especially seen with the use of intraventricular catheters in patients in whom brain tissue distortion alters position of vital structures and ventricles. However, an intraventricular catheter has the advantage of permitting CSF drainage, thus directly decreasing ICP. With all forms of monitors, distorted ICP readings occur if the brain herniates against the monitor.

A normal ICP is a pulsatile pressure that varies with cardiac impulse and respiration. Normal ICP has been described (Lundberg 1972) as less than 10 mm Hg, slightly increased as 11 to 20 mm Hg, moderately increased as 21

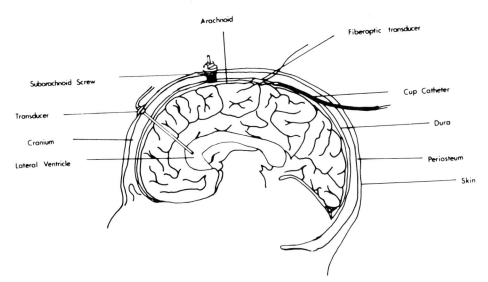

Figure 32–4. Monitoring of ICP. For the epidural technique, a cup catheter or fiberoptic transducer is inserted into the epidural space. For the subdural technique, a screw is inserted into the subdural space. CSF can be aspirated from an intraventricular center. (*From Shapiro HM: Neurosurgical and intercranial anesthesia hypertension. In Miller RD (ed): Anesthesia, Vol. 2, 2nd ed. New York, Churchill Livingstone, 1986.*)

to 40 mm Hg, and severely increased as greater than 40 mm Hg. At pressures greater than 40 mm Hg, compromise of cerebral perfusion begins to occur. ICP can be normal in the presence of an intracranial mass. However, compliance can be significantly decreased. Compliance can be evaluated by injecting 1 ml of saline through the intraventricular catheter, the subdural screw, or the epidural transducer and noting the resultant rise in ICP (volume–pressure response) (see Fig. 32–2). If an increase greater than 2 mm Hg occurs, compliance is impaired and care must be taken to avoid further increase in intracranial content. Treatment is indicated when ICP reaches 20 mm Hg. Severe elevation of ICP to 40 to 50 mm Hg for more than 4 to 8 minutes is associated with significantly increased morbidity and mortality.

In studies of neurosurgical patients with a wide variety of intracranial pathology (excluding craniocerebral trauma), three distinct, spontaneous pressure wave fluctuations were noted: A waves, which are high-amplitude plateau waves; B waves, which are small-amplitude nonplateau, 1-minute waves; and C waves, which are small-amplitude, 6-minute waves. B and C waves were of limited clinical usefulness. B waves were associated with but not precursors of Cheyne–Stokes respirations. C waves were associated with blood pressure waves. Both B and C waves were associated with natural and pathologic depression in level of consciousness.

A waves—plateau waves—were clinically significant. They varied in amplitude and duration. Plateau waves occurred with elevations of ICP greater than 20 mm Hg and were frequently associated with overt symptoms of increased ICP (Fig. 32–5).

Positioning

The sitting position affords excellent surgical access and reduces bleeding and ICP by gravitational drainage of blood and CSF from the cranium. The disadvantages of the sitting position include an increased incidence of venous air embolism, hypotension due to peripheral pooling of blood, impaired venous return, and decreased cardiac output—

especially in elderly, debilitated, or dehydrated patients. Cerebral ischemia may go undetected, since blood pressure at the level of the brain is 2 mm Hg less for every inch the head is elevated above the heart. The transducer is therefore placed at the level of the head. For patients in poor physical condition, the lateral decubitus or prone position is appropriate.

In the correct sitting position, the back forms a 60-degree angle with the horizontal, the hips are flexed, and the knees are elevated to heart level to facilitate venous return. Postural hypotension accompanying position change is minimized by ensuring an adequate circulating blood volume, by wrapping the legs with elastic bandages, and by moving the patient to the sitting position gradually, while blood pressure and heart rate are continuously monitored. The patient's head is supported in a three-point pin head-holder. To avoid pressure necrosis of the skin, increase in ICP, and ischemic damage to the cervical spinal cord, flexion of the neck must leave at least 2 cm between the mandible and sternum at the peak of inspiration. A soft bite-block is recommended instead of an oropharyngeal airway in order to avoid obstruction of venous and lymphatic drainage by compression of oral soft tissue.

The lateral decubitus position offers wide exposure of the lateral posterior fossa structures and the temporal region. To prevent jugular compression, increased venous bleeding, and elevated ICP, excessive lateral flexion of the head on the dependent shoulder is avoided. Pillows or blankets cushion the arms and legs, and the feet rest on foam pads. Inserting a roll of toweling through the dependent axilla protects the brachial plexus from compression injury. In addition, the adequacy of circulation is tested by transducing or palpating the radial pulse in the downside arm.

The prone position provides access to midline and lateral structures. Venous air embolism is less likely in this position. To ensure adequate gas exchange and decrease vena caval compression, ventilation is controlled and bolsters are placed under the patient on each side from shoulder to shoulder.

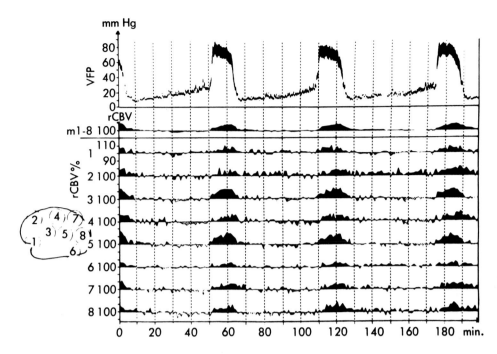

Figure 32–5. Recordings showing that plateau (A) waves are associated with a simultaneous increase in CBV. The increase in CBV is thought to be the etiology of the plateau wave. (*Reprinted with permission from Risberg J, Lundberg N, Ingrav DM: J Neurosurg 31:303, 1969.*)

Anesthetic Pharmacology and Technique

The objective in anesthetizing patients for neurosurgical procedures is to facilitate recovery with minimal neurologic deficit. Of utmost importance is the maintenance of CPP in the presence of disordered autoregulation, impaired response to changes in $Paco_2$, abnormal rCBF, and decreased intracranial compliance. Selection of anesthetic techniques is governed by the anesthetic drugs' effects on CBF, CBV, cerebral compliance, ICP, and $CMRo_2$. The inhalation anesthetics halothane, enflurane, and isoflurane decrease cerebral vascular resistance, causing vascular dilatation, dose-dependent impairment of autoregulation, and increases in CBF, CBV, and ICP; $CMRo_2$ is decreased. Halothane at 0.5 MAC causes minimal disturbance; at 1.6 MAC CBF triples. Enflurane and isoflurane at 1.6 MAC doubles CBF (Fig. 32–6). The resultant rise in ICP due to an impairment of autoregulation during an anesthetic-induced reduction in MAP can severely compromise CPP and cause focal or generalized ischemia or even brain herniation. Since CO_2 responsiveness is retained with all three inhalation anesthetics, the elevation in ICP as occurs with these agents may be attenuated by prior hyperventilation and barbiturates. However, there are reports of an increase in ICP despite hypocarbia and barbiturates. This may be due to the impairment of vascular CO_2 responsiveness that accompanies extensive intracranial disease. (However much CO_2 responsiveness remains will be retained; but this may be of little value in severely damaged tissue.)

Additionally, halothane has been found to alter brain water and electrolyte distribution and permeability of the blood–brain barrier, thus contributing to the formation of cerebral edema. Enflurane has been associated with convulsant activity as noted by EEG, especially during deep anesthesia combined with hypocarbia. If an inhalational anesthetic is to be used, low-dose isoflurane combined with hypocarbia would be the most rational choice. In a study

involving normotensive, normocarbic subjects, CBF did not increase up to 1.0 MAC. At 1.1 MAC, CBF did increase, and at 1.5 to 2.0 MAC, alterations in autoregulation occurred.

In animals, comparative studies indicate that increases in ICP and edema were greatest with the inhalation anesthetics and least with barbiturate and neurolept anesthetics. Furthermore, an acute rise in blood pressure has been shown to cause more damage to the blood–brain barrier in animals anesthetized with inhalation agents than those given thiopental.

N_2O, when used with O_2 only, will increase CBV and

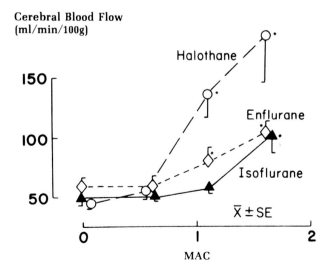

Figure 32–6. Measurement of CBF in volunteers receiving various levels of MAC for halothane, enflurane, and isoflurane. $Paco_2$ and MAP were kept at normal levels. (*From Eger EI II: Isoflurane: A compendium and reference, 1981. Reprinted with permission of Anaquest, BOC, Madison, WI.*)

ICP by cerebral dilation. The cerebral vasoconstrictive effects of hyperventilation, barbiturates, and narcotics will counteract the dilatory effect of N_2O when used concomitantly. Of interest is a very recent study and literature review (Hartung and Cottrell, 1987) comparing the effective cerebral protective effect of barbiturates with and without simultaneous N_2O administration in hypoxic and anoxic mice. Their findings strongly indicate that N_2O offsets thiopental's protective effect during hypoxia and significantly diminishes that effect during anoxia.

Barbiturates are potent cerebral vasoconstrictors. As such, they increase cerebrovascular resistance (CVR) and reduce $CMRO_2$, CBF, CBV, and ICP. The reduction in $CMRO_2$ parallels the reduction in CBF. Because of these effects, thipoental is a drug of choice for patients with poor cerebral compliance. In addition, barbiturates may improve operative results following temporary periods of focal ischemia, such as before clip ligation of aneurysm.

Etomidate decreases CBF, $CMRO_2$, and ICP; CO_2 reactivity is maintained. The minimal cardiovascular effects of this agent result in an unchanged or mildly increased CPP. Major objections to the use of this agent are the reportedly high incidence of nonpurposeful movements and thrombophlebitis.

Midazolam maleate, a water-soluble benzodiazepine, has been shown to maintain better hemodynamic stability than thiopental when administered to patients with intracranial mass lesions. In these patients, MAP was better maintained and CPP did not decrease, as compared with similar patients anesthetized with thiopental.

Total muscle relaxation, narcosis, and sedation are essential for prevention of increased ICP associated with laryngoscopy, intubation, and other noxious stimuli.

Since ICP changes are insignificant following its use, pancuronium bromide 0.06 to 0.1 mg/kg, has been the muscle relaxant of choice for intubation and maintenance. The mild supraventricular tachycardia seen with pancuronium is due to vagolysis and has no effect on systemic pressure or ICP. Pancuronium, 0.15 to 0.20 mg/kg, may be used for patients requiring rapid-sequence induction, since onset is as rapid as with succinylcholine. Tubocurarine, because of its histamine-releasing property, causes transient decreases in MAP and CPP and increases in CBF, CBV, and ICP.

Among the intermediate acting nondepolarizing muscle relaxants, atracurium is not recommended for use in neurosurgical patients because of its potential for releasing histamine. Vecuronium is a safe alternative to pancuronium. Vecuronium has a shorter onset and duration of action than pancuronium and maintains hemodynamic and intracranial stability. Doses of 0.07 to 0.10 mg/kg provide complete muscle relaxation. Vecuronium may also be used for intubation or in patients requiring rapid-sequence induction. A small, subparalyzing primary dose of 0.01 mg/kg 4 minutes prior to the intubating dose of 0.07 to 0.15 mg/kg will allow safe intubating within 90 seconds.

Succinylcholine has been noted to increase ICP regardless of whether or not the patient fasciculates (Fig. 32–7). The increased ICP is attributed to sympathetic stimulation and increased serum norepinephrine. Succinylcholine is contraindicated in paretic or paralyzed patients who have denervated muscle or are chronically immobilized, because denervated and atrophied muscle releases potassium and there is a potential for cardiac arrest. A case study (Stevenson and Birch, 1979) describes succinylcholine-induced hyperkalemia with life-threatening cardiac arrhythmias in a patient with closed head injury without peripheral paresis or paralysis. In-depth investigations are being conducted to determine the safety of succinylcholine in neurosurgical patients.

The narcotics morphine, meperidine, fentanyl, and sufentanil maintain CO_2 responsiveness and autoregulation. In addition, formation of edema in response to injury is reduced. The mild cardiovascular changes associated with narcotics are primarily due to bradycardia and venous dilatation, which produce a mild decrease in MAP. Morphine and meperidine cause dose-dependent, parallel decreases in CBF and $CMRO_2$. Since ICP decreases more than MAP,

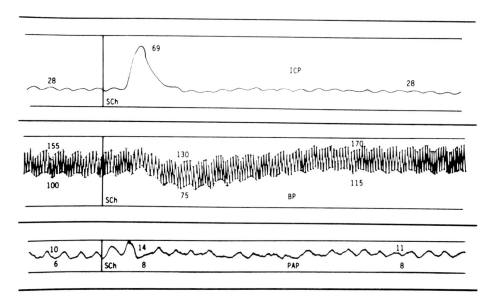

Figure 32–7. Tracing of ICP, blood pressure (BP), pulmonary arterial pressure (PAP) for approximately 100 sec. Vertical line = injection of succinylcholine (Sch) (1.5 mg/kg; from cat #10, initial ICP increased). (*Reprinted with permission from Cottrell JE et al: Anesth Analg 62:1006–1009, 1983.*)

CPP is increased. Fentanyl decreases CBF, with less of a decrease in $CMRO_2$.

Because of its alpha-adrenergic blocking effect, droperidol may decrease MAP and increase CPP with little effect on CBF and $CMRO_2$. Reactivity to CO_2 is maintained with droperidol. The effects on autoregulation have not been determined. The combination of droperidol and fentanyl (Innovar) was not associated with significant change in CBF or $CMRO_2$ in human subjects.

Diazepam and lorazepam reduce CBF and $CMRO_2$, with little or no effect on the cardiovascular system.

Droperidol, diazepam, and lorazepam might best be used in small doses, since CNS depression persists for many hours and may mask signs of intracranial events.

Ketamine is not recommended for neurosurgical patients. Ketamine causes profound cerebral vasodilation and greatly increases CNS activity. Table 32–1 describes effects of anesthetic agents on intracranial dynamics.

Increases in ICP associated with endotracheal intubation and other noxious stimuli may be attenuated or prevented by IV lidocaine (1.5 mg/kg) 1 minute prior to stimulation. Although equipotent doses of thiopental are as effective to control intracranial hypertension, SAP would also be reduced. Lidocaine may prevent increases in ICP without cardiovascular depression. A reduction in MAP may compromise cerebral perfusion in patients with intracranial hypertension and systemic hypotension.

Fluid Management

Patients who are undergoing elective neurosurgical procedures and who show no evidence of increased ICP will generally have a normal intravascular volume. Skin turgor, moistness of mucous membranes, and urine output will help determine the volume status of these patients. How

ever, many neurosurgical patients will present with depleted intravascular volume due to aggressive diuretic therapy, restriction of IV fluids, and abnormalities of antidiuretic hormone release. Poor oral intake may be due to deliberate restriction, decreasing level of consciousness, or nausea and vomiting from increased ICP. In the otherwise healthy accident victim, hypovolemia may be masked by a compensating vascular system and by arterial hypertension, which often occurs with intracranial damage. Traumatic head injury is often associated with peripheral injury. Blood loss from 500 to 1500 ml may be sequestered, for example, in the retroperitoneum or following femoral fracture. Blood loss from open wounds tends to be underestimated. In all of these patients, an adequate circulating blood volume is necessary to prevent severe hypotension on induction. Measurement of CVP or PCWP may be the best approach to rational fluid therapy. Overhydration must be avoided; it can rapidly lead to cerebral edema since the blood–brain barrier is disrupted by trauma and surgery.

Unless there are signs or symptoms of hypovolemia, it is not necessary to replace overnight losses. Maintenance fluids consist of Ringer's lactate or other balanced salt solution given at a rate of 1.0 to 1.5 ml/kg/hour. Volume replacement is done with Ringer's lactate, 5 percent albumin, or blood. Whenever possible, blood loss should be replaced with blood. Rapid volume expansion with isotonic salt solution should be avoided, as this can elevate ICP. Large volumes of dextrose solutions should also be avoided because the free water of the solution plus the water of oxidation of the glucose will contribute to cerebral edema formation. Although hypertonic dextrose solutions will initially decrease ICP, there will be a rebound increase in ICP from glucose metabolism. In addition, there is evidence that cerebral ischemia may be worsened by higher than normal serum glucose levels. The use of albumin is controversial.

TABLE 32–1. EFFECTS OF ANESTHETIC AGENTS ON INTRACRANIAL DYNAMICS[a]

Agent	CBF	CMRo₂	ICP	CPP
Halothane	↑↑	↓	↑	↓
Enflurane	↑	↓	↑	↓
Isoflurane	↑	↓	↑	↓
Nitrous oxide	↑	↓	↑	↓
Nitrous oxide with thiopental for narcotics	↓	↑↓	↑	↓
Ketamine	↑↑↑	↑	↑↑↑	↓
Morphine with hypocarbia	↓	↓	↓	↑
Meperidine with hypocarbia	↓	↓	↓	↑
Fentanyl	↓	↓	↓	↑
Droperidol	↓	↓	↓	sl ↓
Innovar	↓	↓	↓	↑
Diazepam	↓	↓	↓	↑
Thiopental	↓↓	↓↓	↓↓	↑
Midazolam	↓	↓	↓	↑
Etomidate	↓	↓	↓	sl
Lidocaine	↓	↓	↓	↑
Succinylcholine	Z	Z	? ↑	Z
d-Tubocurarine	↑	NC	↑	
Pancuronium	NC	NC	NC	NC
Vecuronium (Norcuron)	Z	Z	NC	NC
Atracurium	?	Z	NC	NC

[a] sl = slightly; NC = no change; Z = effects of agent on these parameters have not been established (compiled from various sources).

A disrupted blood–brain barrier is highly permeable to most fluids, including albumin. Experimentally, when the plasma concentration of albumin fell, the albumin in brain tissue remained elevated. This creates an osmotic gradient favoring cerebral edema. Other fluids are more easily mobilized from the interstitial space than is albumin.

Inadequate fluid volume is indicated by tachycardia, hypotension, sensitivity to vasodilators or inhalational anesthetics, and an inspiratory–expiratory variation in blood pressure when peak expiratory pressure exceeds 20 mm Hg. If CVP is being monitored, a pressure of 0 to 2 mm Hg is acceptable if all other parameters are stable.

In the patient undergoing surgery for cerebral aneurysm, an especially careful fluid balance is required. Aneurysm rupture can occur as a result of overhydration and hypertension. Deliberate hypotension is often required immediately prior to clip ligation of the aneurysm. A decreased circulating volume may make the response to vasodilators unpredictable. Most neurosurgeons believe that, after ligation of the aneurysm, volume replacement and mildly increased blood pressure (about 10 percent above normal) will reduce the risk of vasospasm. A CVP of 12 mm Hg or a PCWP of 18 mm Hg is considered optimal.

Arterial blood gases, hematocrit, and serum potassium, chloride, sodium, and glucose should be frequently assessed intra- and postoperatively.

Induction of Anesthesia

Implementing the principles of neurophysiology and the effects of anesthetic agents on intracranial dynamics, an anesthetic plan is devised for each patient.

Noninvasive monitoring applies to all patients regardless of pathology and should be applied prior to induction. These include blood pressure cuff, modified V_5 ECG, PCS, PNS, pulse oximetry, $ETco_2$, and mass spectrometry. Ideally, invasive monitors (arterial line, CVP, pulmonary artery (PA) catheter, EEG, evoked potential) should also be placed prior to induction. However, in the overly anxious patient it may be wiser to wait until the patient has been sedated or anesthetized.

Induction of anesthesia should proceed smoothly and carefully. The patient should be preoxygenated with 100 percent O_2 via face mask, which may be held to the side for patient comfort. Sedation with small amounts of benzodiazepines or butyrophenones and incremental narcotic are guided by vital signs. Prior sedation allows for smaller induction doses of thiopental. Once the patient is induced and the airway secure, muscle relaxant may be given. Although succinylcholine is certainly not contraindicated, intubation with vecuronium or pancuronium is a safe alternative. Systemic and intracranial hypertension during laryngoscopy and intubation are prevented by additional thiopental or narcotic and IV lidocaine 1 minute prior to laryngoscopy. Lidocaine spray may also be applied topically to the larynx and trachea. An armored or spiral embedded endotracheal tube (anode tube) may be used if positioning requires extreme rotation or flexion of the head. Care must be taken to secure all endotracheal tube connections, since the patient's airway may be out of view and repositioning of the head during surgery can cause disconnection or accidental extubation.

Anesthesia is maintained with continuous administration of N_2O, O_2, and intermittent doses of narcotic, muscle relaxant, and barbiturate. Lidocaine may be used to prevent an increase in ICP from noxious stimuli without altering cardiovascular parameters. Intubation, application of the head pins, drilling through bone, and insertion of the Gigli's saw guide are highly stimulating and can cause significant elevation of ICP. Lidocaine has been shown to prevent or attenuate the response to these maneuvers. Low concentrations of isoflurane or trimethaphan (Arfonad) may be used as necessary to control blood pressure. After adequate depth of anesthesia is established, ventilation is adjusted to keep the arterial $Paco_2$ between 25 and 30 mm Hg. Although the rate, rhythm, and depth of spontaneous respiration have been used to assess brain stem integrity intraoperatively, blood pressure and cardiac rate and rhythm are sufficiently sensitive and their control centers are sufficiently close to respiratory areas to indicate compromise of respiratory centers during controlled ventilation.

Smooth emergence from anesthesia requires that the patient neither cough nor strain on the endotracheal tube, as systemic pressure and ICP will rise and endanger hemostasis. IV lidocaine may be used to prevent an increase in ICP associated with endotracheal stimulation during emergence. Muscle relaxation is reversed with anticholinesterase and parasympatholytic drugs. Stable, responsive patients with adequate spontaneous respiration are extubated in the operating room. Naloxone may be used in small doses (0.1 to 0.4 mg) for the treatment of persistent respiratory depression after reversal of muscle relaxation and reaccumulation of CO_2 to the normal level. Narcotic reversal should be avoided if increased MAP is undesirable. Patients to be ventilated postoperatively because of trauma, cerebral edema, or poor preoperative status remain asleep and paralyzed.

Portable ECG and blood pressure monitoring equipment accompany the patient from the operating suite to the recovery room, where complete monitoring is continued. Except in cerebral vascular surgery, hypocarbia is maintained during the immediate postoperative period. Adequately reversed, extubated patients frequently spontaneously hyperventilate. Laboratory tests, including determinations of arterial blood gases, complete blood count, glucose, serum electrolytes and osmolality, and urine specific gravity, as well as a chest roentgenogram and an ECG, are performed in the recovery room as soon as the patient's vital signs have stabilized. Unless otherwise contraindicated, the patient is maintained in a semi-Fowler's position.

Intraoperative Problems

Cardiovascular instability during surgery can result from drug administration, insufficient intravascular volume, hypoxia, hypercarbia, or surgical manipulation. Hypotension may be secondary to drugs or surgical manipulation or hypovolemia following dye studies, bed rest, subarachnoid hemorrhage, inadequate oral intake, diuresis, or operative blood loss.

Hypertension occurs with light anesthesia or with surgical manipulation and retraction of the brain stem and cranial nerves. Beta-blockade with propranolol hydrochloride (Inderal) may be used to treat hypertension with tachycardia that is not associated with surgical manipulation and that does not respond to deepening anesthesia. Propranolol must be used cautiously: 0.1-mg increments every 2 minutes until a response is elicited. This intervention can also cause bradycardia, tachycardia, and arrhythmias. Other antihypertensive therapy is discussed in that section. Other neurosurgical procedures associated with cardiac arrhythmias include orbital decompression, carotid ligation, sudden intracranial decompression, and manipulation of the vagus and trigeminal nerves. The perturbations caused by surgical manipulation usually resolve with cessation of stimulation and deepened anesthesia. If persistent stimulation of the brain stem or cranial nerves is necessary because of the location of the lesion and deepened anesthesia does not ameliorate the response to stimulation, the surgeons can apply local anesthetic directly to the area. Small amounts of IV atropine may be used to block persistent vagal stimulation.

Venous Air Embolism

Venous air embolism can occur whenever a gradient of 5 cm or more exists between the wound and the right side of the heart. Although the incidence of air embolism is 25 to 35 percent among patients operated in the sitting position, air has also entered during operations in the lateral, supine, and prone positions. One study found that air was entrained most often (78.7 percent of cases) during the early part of the operation, when the bone flap was being elevated and the dura opened; less frequently (18.0 percent) during the conclusion part of the operation; and least frequently (3.3 percent) during the surgery. The head pin site may also be a source of entrained air. This may be prevented by wrapping the pins and covering the site with petrolatum (Vaseline) gauze after insertion of the pins.

Pathophysiologic effects of entrained air include hypotension, arrhythmias, hypercarbia, hypoxia (secondary to reflex bronchoconstriction and pulmonary edema), and asystole. These sequelae follow accumulation of more than 50 ml of air because of obstruction of right ventricular and pulmonary arterial outflow, which increases PAP, PCWP, and Pa_{CO_2}, and decreases cardiac output, Pa_{O_2}, and ET_{CO_2}. Paradoxical air emboli may occur in which air passes directly through the pulmonary circulation or through right-to-left intracardiac shunts to reach the coronary and cerebral circulation. Death in these instances results from air occlusion of coronary arteries and ventricular fibrillation.

Early diagnosis of air embolism is essential to successful treatment. The mass spectrometer and Doppler ultrasonic unit are the most sensitive methods for detection of air embolism. Air is "heard" because the air–blood interface is a much better acoustical reflector than blood alone, producing a noise of characteristic frequency. The mass spectrometer is reportedly as sensitive as the Doppler in detecting small quantities of air. In fact, identification by mass spectometer was 30 to 90 seconds sooner than by Doppler. In addition to monitoring ET_{CO_2}, a measurement of ET_{N_2} indicates air entrained from surgical sites or IV access. Sources of Fi_{N_2} are mechanical failure such as leaks in ventilators, connecting tubing, partial endotracheal tube disconnections, and mask fit. Table 32–2 summarizes the cardiopulmonary changes associated with air emboli.

TABLE 32–2. HEMODYNAMIC CHANGES OCCURRING WITH AIR EMBOLI

Parameter	Change
PAP[a]	Increases
PCWP	Increases
CVP	Increases
Cardiac output	Decreases
ECG	Arrythmias
MAP[b]	Decreases
Paco$_2$	Increases
Pao$_2$[b]	Decreases
ETco$_2$	Decreases
ETN$_2$	Measureable
Doppler sounds	Turbulent
Cyanosis[b]	Present
Neck vein congestion[b]	May Occur

[a] PAP increases in proportion to the volume of air embolized and corresponds to the change in ETco$_2$.
[b] These relatively late-occurring changes precede cardiovascular collapse.

As soon as a change in Doppler signal or monitored parameters occurs, N_2O is turned off and ventilation continued with 1.0 fraction of inspired oxygen (Fi_{O_2}) in order to avoid increasing the size of embolic bubbles. The anesthetist aspirates the right atrial catheter while the surgeon occludes possible sites of air entry by irrigating the wound with saline and waxing the bone edges. (The proximal and distal lumens on the Swan-Ganz catheter are too narrow to adequately aspirate air. If a pulmonary artery catheter is used, a separate, large-bore right atrial catheter should also be placed to allow optimal aspiration of air). The anesthetist performs a Valsalva maneuver and adds PEEP to demonstrate bleeding points and reduce negative pressure in the venous sinuses. Pulmonary artery or ET_{CO_2} measurements aid in calculating the amount of air and the duration of its presence in the pulmonary vasculature. No change in PAP or ET_{CO_2} with reintroduction of N_2O indicates resolution of the air and safe continuation of surgery. Massive air embolism or inability to arrest air entry necessitates placement of the wound at or below heart level and termination of the operation.

Immediate Postoperative Problems

Neurosurgical patients frequently exhibit hypertension in the recovery room, particularly after neurovascular and posterior fossa procedures. Although this usually resolves within 12 hours after surgery, the danger of hematoma formation or hemorrhagic infarction requires that hypertension be treated immediately. When analgesics in small doses are not effective, sodium nitroprusside (SNP), nitroglycerin, trimethaphan, labetalol, or propranolol is indicated for rapid control. All of these agents are included in the discussion on deliberate hypotension.

Needless to say, postoperative direct arterial monitoring is imperative. Hypertension with tachycardia that is not caused by respiratory difficulty or pain may be treated with increments of propranolol. Both atrial and ventricular ectopic beats occur with increased frequency in the first 24 hours after surgery, requiring continuation of ECG monitoring. Elevation of temperature in the immediate postoperative period is usually due to blood irritation of the meninges.

Deliberate Hypotension and Antihypertensive Therapy

During neurosurgical procedures, blood pressure is reduced to treat hypertension and to facilitate clipping of aneurysms and resection of arteriovenous malformation (AVM) and vascular tumors (meningiomas and hemangioendotheliomas). In addition, pharmacologically decreasing MAP reduces blood loss and, by affording better surgical conditions, decreases operative time. Adjuvant techniques to complement the primary action of the hypotensive drug and aid in achieving precise blood pressure control include alterations of position or airway pressure or addition of other vasoactive drugs.

Ideally, induction of hypotension should decrease CPP without significantly reducing CBF. This is accomplished by maintaining a normal circulating blood volume and cardiac output as CVR falls. Increased intrapulmonary shunting accompanies the use of vasodilators. In order to avoid ischemia, it is critical to ensure adequate Pao$_2$ during a reduction in CPP. Hypocarbia to 30 mm Hg when MAP is less than 50 mm Hg in normotensive patients produces ischemia. It is best to maintain a Paco$_2$ of 35 to 40 mm Hg when inducing hypotension. In most patients, MAP may be safely reduced to 50 mm Hg without causing ischemic depletion of brain energy substances or accumulation of acid metabolites. Higher pressure levels are required in patients with chronic arterial hypertension, altered autoregulation in brain regions compressed by masses, and in those receiving trimethaphan. In chronic arterial hypertension, the lower limits of autoregulation are shifted to the right, which means that higher MAP is necessary to prevent ischemia. Unless EEG and CBF are monitored, it is difficult to determine the level to which MAP may be safely reduced. A 50 percent decrease in MAP was tolerated in an experiment involving hypertensive and normotensive animals. In humans, MAP is usually not decreased more than 30 percent.

In addition to disturbances of the blood–brain barrier and of autoregulation, patients in the acute phase of subarachnoid hemorrhage may also present with cardiopulmonary problems and decreased blood volume. Recent myocardial infarction (within 6 months) is an absolute contraindication to induced hypotension. A history of cardiac, pulmonary, renal, or hepatic disease is a relative contraindication. At the very least, continuous intraarterial MAP monitoring and frequent analysis of PAo$_2$, Pvo$_2$, and Paco$_2$ or ETco$_2$ are necessary whenever MAP is manipulated. Those agents most frequently used to alter blood pressure will now be reviewed.

SNP is currently the most widely used hypotensive drug because it is easy to control and short in its duration of action. Despite the reduction in blood pressure, primarily due to decreased afterload, CBF continues to be adequate since CVR is reduced while cardiac output remains near normal. This arteriolar dilatation increases CBV and ICP, especially in patients who have impaired intracranial compliance. For this reason, SNP is not administered until the dura is opened or until compliance has improved.

SNP is supplied in amber vials containing 50 mg of SNP dehydrate. SNP should be dissolved in 5 percent dextrose and water (D$_5$W); 50 mg/250 ml D$_5$W gives a concentration of 200 μg/ml; 50 mg/500 ml gives 100 μg/ml; 50 mg/1000 ml gives 50 μg/ml. In solution, SNP is photosensitive and should be protected from light by wrapping the solution container and tubing in aluminum foil. Once in solution, SNP is stable for no more than 4 hours. Infusion is begun at 0.2 to 1.0 μg/kg/minute and titrated to 10 μg/kg/minute to maintain the desired MAP. It is easiest and most accurate to use a volumetric pump to administer SNP. Onset is within 30 seconds; duration is 2 to 4 minutes. If an infusion of 10 μg/kg for 10 to 15 minutes does not provide an adequate reduction in blood pressure, SNP should be discontinued and another agent substituted. SNP should be used with caution in patients with hepatic or renal insufficiency. The hepatic enzyme rhodanese mediates the conversion of cyanide to thiocyanate. Thiocyanate is excreted by the kidneys. Diseased kidneys may also have a greater secretion of renin. The adverse effects associated with SNP administration include increased ICP, rebound hypertension, cyanide and thiocyanate toxicity, hypothyroidism, and blood coagulation abnormalities.

Rebound hypertension occurs following abrupt discontinuance of SNP. It is especially dangerous in patients with neurovascular disorders, since the upper limits of autoregulation may be exceeded and formation of cerebral edema enhanced. Rebound hypertension results from increased plasma renin activity, possibly because of renal artery dilation or renal ischemia. Renin has a plasma half-life of 30 minutes, SNP has a biologic half-life of 2 minutes. Discontinuing SNP over 30 to 60 minutes or administration of propranolol, 20 mg po preoperatively, or small amounts IV intraoperatively may be effective in preventing rebound hypertension because it decreases renin release.

The major disadvantage of SNP is the toxicity caused by its metabolic decomposition to cyanide (Fig. 32–8). Cyanide reacts in mitochondria to form a cyanide–cytochrome oxidase complex that inhibits cellular respiration and produces cellular hypoxia. Signs of toxicity include tachyphylaxis, tachycardia, metabolic acidosis, and cardiovascular collapse. The total amount of SNP administered should not exceed 0.7 μg/kg over 2 to 3 hours, since the blood cyanide level correlates directly with the total dose. Administration of IV hydroxocobalamin together with SNP will decrease the blood cyanide concentration. Thiosulfate also decreases blood cyanide by increasing urinary excretion of thiocyanate. If the patient develops acidosis or tachyphylaxis, SNP should be discontinued and another hypotensive drug substituted.

Thiocyanate inhibits uptake and binding of iodine by the thyroid, thus hypothyroidism can be induced.

Blood coagulopathies may occur after SNP-induced platelet disintegration and inhibition of platelet aggregation.

Nitroglycerin acts primarily by relaxing capacitance vessels—that is, by decreasing preload, which decreases venous return, stroke volume, and MAP. Since nitroglycerin reduces MAP by acting on the peripheral circulation, there is no direct effect on the normal heart. Nitroglycerin has a short duration of action, is easy to control, and does not cause tachyphylaxis, production of toxic metabolites, or rebound hypertension. However, ICP increases as blood accumulates and pools in the cranium faster than it can

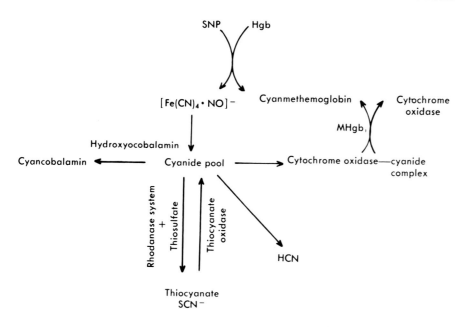

Figure 32–8. Biotransformation of SNP. Hemoglobin, Hgb; methemoglobin, MHgb; thiocyanate, SCN; hydrogen cyanide, HCN. (*Reprinted with permission from Cottrell JE, Van Aken H, Gupta B, Turndorf H: Induced hypertension. In Cottrell JE, Turndorf H (eds): Anesthesia and Neurosurgery, 2nd ed. St. Louis, Mosby, 1986, p. 421.*)

exit through the rigid venous channels. As with SNP, nitroglycerin should not be administered to patients with intracranial hypertension until the dura is opened or intracranial compliance has improved. Nitroglycerin may fail to induce adequate hypotension in younger patients, especially those under balanced narcotic anesthesia, necessitating the use of alternate drugs. Parenteral nitroglycerin (Tridil) is absorbed by polyvinylchloride solution bags and IV administration sets. The amount of drug absorbed and, therefore, the amount actually administered to the patient cannot be calculated. Tridil should be diluted in *glass* containers of D_5W or 0.9 percent sodium chloride and administered through the nonabsorbant tubing supplied with Tridil. When diluted in glass containers, the solution is stable for up to 48 hours at room temperature and 7 days under refrigeration. Nitroglycerin is not light sensitive.

Administration should be made with a volumetric pump. Infusion should start with 1 to 2 µg/kg/minute and titrated for desired MAP levels. Nitroglycerin has a biologic half-life of 1 to 4 minutes. Adverse reactions including severe tachycardia or paradoxical bradycardia are rare. Toxic effects have not been described. Nitroglycerin should be used with caution in patients with hepatic or renal disease, as the drug is metabolized by the liver and excreted by the kidneys.

Pentolinium (Ansolysen) and trimethaphan induce hypotension by occupying sympathetic and parasympathetic ganglionic receptor sites and stabilizing the postsynaptic membrane against acetylcholine. Depression of parasympathetic activity causes tachycardia, mydriasis, cycloplegia, decreased gastrointestinal tone and motility, and urinary retention.

In addition to ganglionic blockade, trimethaphan decreases MAP by histamine release and direct vasodilatation. Because it is rapidly inactivated by plasma cholinesterase and excreted by the kidneys, trimethaphan has a short duration of action. It is easy to control and does not increase ICP, because autoregulation remains intact as MAP decreases. Trimethaphan should probably be used to treat intraoperative hypertension that occurs before the dura is opened and should be avoided when hypotension to MAP of 50 mm Hg is required. At a MAP of 50 mm Hg, the drug has direct cerebral toxic effects. Signs of this include burst suppression, slowing, high-voltage waves on EEG, and elevation of brain lactate levels (indicating glycolysis). Tachyphylaxis, histamine-induced bronchospasm, and myoneural blockade have been associated with the use of trimethaphan. At high doses or after prolonged use (several hours), cycloplegia (fixed, dilated pupils) can occur, possibly interfering with postoperative neurologic assessment. Trimethaphan can be diluted in D_5W and, at room temperature, is stable in solution for 24 hours. It is not light sensitive. Infusion through a volumetric pump should be started at 30 to 50 µg/kg/minute and titrated to the desired MAP.

Pentolinium is currently not available in the United States.

Hydralazine hydrochloride (Apresoline) is a direct-acting, predominantly arteriolar vasodilator. Diastolic pressure is usually decreased more than systolic. Heart rate, stroke volume, and cardiac output are increased. Tachycardia following hydralazine is often significant. Unless the drop in MAP is severe, CBF is increased. Hydralazine is best used in neurosurgical patients after intracranial compliance has improved. Parenteral hydralazine may be given without dilution. Onset of action is within 10 to 20 minutes. Although 20 to 40 mg is the recommended dose, our experience has been that much smaller doses are usually adequate. Control of hypertension can be accomplished with 5 mg IV every 20 minutes until effect; this may be followed by 10 to 20 mg IM.

Administered in high concentration, the volatile anesthetics produce hypotension by causing myocardial depression and direct vasodilation. Since these agents also decrease CVR and raise CBF, ICP will be increased, cerebral perfusion reduced, and the likelihood of edema formation enhanced. Therefore, the volatile anesthetics should be avoided for induction of hypotension during neurosurgical procedures.

Labetalol is a partial antagonist at both alpha and beta adrenoreceptors. In humans, the beta-blocking properties are greater than those of the alpha receptors. Due to its combined blocking effect, labetalol reduces MAP by reducing peripheral vascular resistance while preventing a reflex increase in heart rate or cardiac output. When combined with halothane, labetalol produced profound hypotension. Experimentally, when labetalol was used during neuroleptanesthesia, a maximum decrease in MAP of 30 percent was produced. Increasing the dosage of labetalol did not produce any further reduction in MAP.

Labetalol may best be used immediately prior to induction and on emergence. Labetalol, when given in a dose of 0.3 to 0.6 mg/kg IV bolus or continuous infusion prior to induction, prevents the pressure response of laryngoscopy and intubation. Hypertension during emergence and in the postoperative period may be prevented or treated with IV labetalol. Attention must be paid to blood loss, since under labetalol the usual reactions do not appear. Labetalol is contraindicated in patients with atrioventricular block, heart failure, hypovolemia, and bradycardia. Because the beta-blocking property of labetalol is not cardioselective, it should be avoided in patients with obstructive pulmonary disease.

Ionic channel blockers ("slow" sodium and calcium channels) have been the object of intensive investigation over the past decade. Calcium and sodium are involved in a vast array of physiologic processes including muscle contraction. Calcium plays an especially significant role in the membrane excitation in the sinus node, atrioventricular node, and in myocardial cells. Compared with skeletal muscle, cardiac and vascular smooth muscle have relatively small amounts of endoplasmic calcium and, therefore, are more dependent on calcium influx. Blocking calcium channels can interfere with the cardiac electrical pathway, inhibit myocardial contractility, and cause vasodilatation. Verapamil and nifedipine are two of the most widely used calcium channel blockers. Verapamil is primarily an antiarrythmic. It has significant negative inotropic effect because of its depression of sinus and atrioventricular node conduction. Nifedipine produces potent vasodilatation, apparently without depressing the myocardium or interfering with sinus and atrioventricular node conduction. The calcium channel blockers require further investigation to determine if they are useful agents to induce hypotension in neurosurgical patients. Nifedipine, verapamil, and diltiazem increased ICP in animal studies. Diltiazem produced life-threatening arrythmias when given in doses to produce hypotension. Table 32–3 reviews the most common agents used for deliberate hypotension.

MANAGEMENT OF SPECIFIC NEUROLOGIC DISORDERS

Head trauma is a problem of large proportion in all industrialized countries. In the United States each year, more than 600,000 people sustain epidural or subdural hematoma or cerebral laceration. Deaths from vehicular accidents involving head injuries number 33,000 annually. Since 50 percent of these deaths from head injury occur within the first 2 hours, optimal management requires effective emergency treatment at the site of the accident and rapid transport to hospitals where appropriate care is available. Highly trained, mobile paramedical personnel capable of establishing an airway and performing resuscitation and ongoing life support while in radio communication with a hospital-based physician are crucial in the effort to reduce immediate mortality. The initial management of acutely injured and decompensating patients is aimed at rapid reduction of the intracranial volume to decrease ICP, improvement of cerebral perfusion, and balancing energy supply and demand. In addition, the systemic effects produced by brain shift and distortion may be corrected.

Aggressive management with hyperventilation, dehydrating agents, and sedatives has been effective in reversing impending herniation. In addition to this therapy, steroids, muscle relaxants, and, in certain cases, barbiturates in conjunction with ICP monitoring can significantly improve the prognosis of patients with head injury.

Frequently, these patients spontaneously hyperventilate and may be hypertensive. Hyperventilation is apparently centrally induced by the acidic cerebral metabolites that accumulate in the area of injury (and are probably distributed by CSF flow). Cerebral vascular reactivity to P_{CO_2} may be impaired in areas of injury; however, reactivity should remain in the surrounding tissue. Hyperventilation

TABLE 32–3. DELIBERATE HYPOTENSION—ADMINISTRATION AND HEMODYNAMIC AND TOXIC EFFECTS OF THE MOST COMMONLY USED AGENTS

Drug	Dosage	Onset/Duration	CO	PCWP	SVR	CVR	CBF	ICP	CPP	Toxic Effects
Trimethaphan	2–4 mg/min; titrate to desired MAP	1–2 min/4–8 min	↓	↓	↓	0	0	0	0	Direct cerebral toxicity (MAP < 50 mm Hg)
Nitroprusside[a]	0.2–1.0 μg/kg/min; titrate to 10 μg/kg/min; max 0.7 μg/kg over 3–4 hours	30 sec/2–4/min	0	↓	↓	↓	↑	↑	↓	Cyanide toxicity rebound hypertension, ↓ Pao₂
Nitroglycerin[a]	2.4–5.0 μg/kg/min; titrate to desired MAP	1–2 min/10 min	0	↓	↓	↓	↑	↑	↓	↓ Pao₂

↑ = increase; ↓ = decrease; 0 = no change; CO = cardiac output.
[a] Should not be used until the dura is open or measures have been taken to improve intracranial compliance. (Compiled from various sources.)

will stimulate restoration of normal cerebral pH, thereby limiting the development of secondary injury due to acidosis and hypoxia, and will aid in the preservation of viable brain tissue. In addition, hyperventilation may provide time for corticosteroids to take effect.

Hypertension in acute, decompensating head injury is a compensatory mechanism to maintain CPP. Attempts to decrease MAP should not be instituted until medical or surgical measures to decrease ICP and improve compliance have been effective. Often the MAP will decrease spontaneously as compliance improves. If the MAP remains elevated despite reduction in ICP and improvement in compliance, then one of the antihypertensive agents previously mentioned should be considered.

Temperature control is essential in all patients with head injury. Hyperthermia may result from blood in the subarachnoid space, especially in the area of the posterior fossa. The effects of and treatment for hyper- and hypothermia have been discussed.

Depressed skull fractures and acute epidural, subdural, and intracerebral hematomas frequently require craniotomy. Chronic subdural hematomas are often evacuated through burr holes. Occasionally, cerebral contusion may require removal of contused brain tissue and subtemporal decompression.

The majority of patients who undergo surgical procedures are unconscious preoperatively and usually remain so postoperatively. Their stay in the recovery room before transfer to a neurologic intensive care unit will often be short. Their treatment involves a coordinated approach to respiratory care, maintenance of hemodynamic stability and fluid and electrolyte balance, as well as specific measures to control CBF and ICP.

Removal of an acute subdural hematoma is frequently followed by significant postoperative elevation of ICP. ICP monitoring and one or more of the treatment modalities to reduce ICP should be continued during the recovery period, if not previously instituted. Recent data suggest that, by effective use of techniques for control of ICP, mortality due to severe head injury can be reduced from 70 percent to 30 percent in adults and to as low as 7 percent in children.

Traumatically injured patients should always be evaluated for concomitant head injury; conversely, patients with obvious head injury should be carefully evaluated for other injuries, especially those of the spinal column, chest, and abdomen.

Cerebrovascular Disease

Carotid Endarterectomy. Carotid endarterectomy for stenosis or ulcerated plaques of the internal carotid artery may be performed under regional or general anesthesia. Regional anesthesia affords the advantage of an awake patient, facilitating intraoperative monitoring of the neurologic state. Changes in mental status and the occurrence of aphasia, paresis, or loss of consciousness can be observed immediately. General anesthesia affords superior physiologic control, especially in the maintenance of acceptable levels of arterial blood gases, and limits patients' discomfort and anxiety and problems with aspiration. Many of the patients

have coronary artery disease, and in these patients anxiety and the attendant rise in rate-pressure product may increase the likelihood of their developing myocardial ischemia or infarction intraoperatively. A precordial ECG will reflect myocardial ischemia.

Anesthetic agents and techniques that will maintain blood pressure and CPP are chosen. It is most desirable to decrease CMR_{O_2} while maintaining CBF, without hypotension and myocardial ischemia in these patients. Induction and intubation should be slow and smooth, without hypertension or tachycardia. Inhalation agents, which decrease CMR_{O_2} and increase CBF, may be preferable to neuroleptanesthesia, which generally produces a parallel reduction in CMR_{O_2} and CBF. Blood pressure should be kept at or slightly above (approximately 10 percent) normal levels. Normocarbia should be maintained. Intraoperative bradycardia and hypotension may be due to surgical manipulation at the carotid bifurcation. This response can be treated with IV atropine or by local infiltration with 1 percent lidocaine. Emergence should be smooth and prompt to allow assessment of neurologic studies. Special monitoring includes an electrophysiologic reflection of brain function, such as EEG. Stump pressures and jugular bulb O_2 tension do not correlate well with the development of postoperative neurologic deficits.

Direct blood pressure monitoring by intraarterial catheter is continued during transfer from the operating room and in the recovery room. Hyper- or hypotensive episodes occur in 40 percent of patients in the immediate postoperative period. Hypotension may result from temporary impairment of carotid sinus baroreceptor reflexes. Since these patients are unable to raise their pressure, any fall must be treated promptly to prevent ischemic insult to the brain. Therapy includes placing the patient in the supine or Trendelenburg position and administering crystalloid or colloid solution if the CVP is low or vasopressors if the response to volume loading is inadequate.

Hypertension in the 12 to 24 hours following surgery may reflect a transient increase in sympathetic tone, as occurs following posterior fossa procedures. Loss of cerebral autoregulation, cerebral edema, and stroke may ensue. If the blood pressure is moderately elevated (10 to 15 percent above preoperative level), IV chlorpromazine, 1 to 5 mg, blocks adrenergic receptor sites and may be adequate for control. Repeat doses of 2.5 to 5.0 mg IV may be given every 4 to 6 hours as needed. Marked blood pressure elevation (greater than 25 percent above preoperative levels) will often be best managed by IV infusion of short-acting vasodilators such as SNP, trimethaphan, or nitroglycerin.

Carotid body function may be affected after bilateral carotid endarterectomy, with the loss of the normal cardiorespiratory response to hypoxia, including increase in pulse, blood pressure, and ventilation. These patients may experience severe hypoxia without ventilatory or circulatory response. When conditions known to provoke hypoxemia emerge, the potential loss of carotid body function can be averted by means of adequate supplemental oxygen, blood gas monitoring, and close observation.

An uncommon but potentially catastrophic cause of acute respiratory distress following carotid endarterectomy is tracheal compression by cervical hematoma, which requires immediate evacuation. Other causes of acute respiratory distress following carotid endarterectomy are tension pneumothorax and vocal cord paralysis.

Intra- or postoperative acute myocardial infarction is reported to be the second most frequent cause of morbidity and death after carotid endarterectomy. A recent study found that, following 683 procedures for carotid endarterectomy, 2.3 percent of patients developed an acute myocardial infarction within 72 hours. Mortality rates ranging from 9.6 to 16 percent have been reported for patients with a history of heart disease who undergo carotid endarterectomy. Preexisting cardiovascular disease appears to be the major predisposing factor; and for such patients, intraoperative administration of vasopressors during clamping of the carotid artery increases the incidence of acute myocardial infarction. The use of intracarotid shunts, rather than induced hypertension, has been recommended when carotid clamping is not tolerated. A 12-lead ECG taken in the recovery room should be compared with the preoperative ECG. The precordial ECG is monitored postoperatively, and appropriate therapy (i.e., nitroglycerin) is instituted if ischemia occurs.

EC-IC Cerebral Revascularization.

Blood flow to ischemic areas of the brain in patients with cerebrovascular insufficiency secondary to occlusion distal to the cervical portion of the internal carotid artery is restored by creation of microvascular extracranial-to-intracranial (EC-IC) anastomoses. Donaghy and Yasargil first described the anastomosis of the anterior circulation between the superficial temporal artery (STA) and the middle cerebral artery (MCA). Connections are also created posteriorly between the occipital artery and the posterior inferior cerebellar artery.

Continuing refinements in microsurgical technique and the use of the operating microscope have enhanced the success of these procedures. The anastomosis should create a gentle angulation between the parent vessel (STA) and the recipient (MCA), orienting the flow to minimize turbulence. Heparin may or may not be used. Long-term patency rates of greater than 90 percent have been reported, with an operative mortality of 1.7 percent.

Although patients with a local, relative reduction in CBF benefit most from EC-IC bypass, it is not clear whether the increase in CBF after EC-IC bypass will prevent infarction in the acutely ischemic cortex. Crowell demonstrated neurologic improvement in animals with an STA anastomosis 2 hours after ligation of the MCA and concluded that STA-MCA bypass could be beneficial in some cases of acute cerebral ischemia, provided that perfusion is restored shortly after the development of symptoms. However, others have demonstrated exacerbation of edema and further clinical deterioration in dogs despite bypass within 24 hours after the onset of ischemia. Likewise, in patients with acute occlusion, bypass restores flow but is detrimental clinically. Acute cerebral revascularization may thus be harmful for patients with large infarctions but is of potential benefit to those with smaller ones.

Patients selected for EC-IC bypass are typically in the sixth decade of life, and males predominate. They frequently have a number of risk factors for stroke and heart disease, including a history of transient ischemic attacks or of partially completed stroke, hypotension, smoking, previous vascular surgery, and associated pulmonary or renal disease.

Monitoring during EC-IC anastomosis is the same as for other craniotomies and includes ECG, CVP, intraarterial catheter, esophageal thermistor, and urinary catheter. Blood pressure is maintained at normal to mildly elevated levels to ensure cerebral perfusion and to prevent thrombosis. Since the procedure is actually superficial and is performed through a small craniotomy, reduction of brain volume with hyperventilation or osmotic diuretics is not indicated. Ventilation is adjusted to keep the Pa_{CO_2} between 35 and 40 mm Hg. Minimal movement of the brain during respiratory excursions is achieved by the use of low tidal volumes and increased rate.

An anesthetic technique is indicated that will maintain CPP, limit cerebral oxygen requirement, sustain systemic arterial pressure, and render the patient awake and responsive at the conclusion of the operation to permit immediate assessment of neurologic status. The CMR_{O_2} is reduced by either barbiturates or inhaled agents. Since barbiturates constrict cerebral arteries, low-dose inhalation agents may be advantageous in that they provide a measure of vasodilatation. There is evidence that halothane exacerbates infarction in areas previously rendered ischemic. Furthermore, halothane may have a direct and possibly deleterious effect on the blood-brain barrier, since clearance of umbelliferone, a fat-soluble indicator, is apparently not affected by barbiturate anesthesia but is changed by deep halothane anesthesia. Since results of both in vitro and in vivo studies suggest a toxic metabolic effect of halothane at concentrations greater than 2.0 percent, the combination of thiopental and a narcotic with halothane, enflurane, or isoflurane is appropriate, as this will provide analgesia while permitting reduction of the concentration of inhaled agent.

The prime concern in postoperative care of patients after EC-IC bypass is augmentation of blood flow through the new anastomosis by maintaining blood pressure in the high normal range and expanding intravascular volume by administration of colloid or low-molecular-weight dextran at 50 to 100 ml/hour. Neurologic assessment should be performed frequently.

Aneurysms

Cerebral aneurysms are abnormal, localized dilatations of the arteries within the skull. They are classified as congenital (berry), mycotic, traumatic, dissecting, neoplastic, and arteriosclerotic. Rupture of an intracranial aneurysm is one the leading causes of subarachnoid hemorrhage (SAH).

The signs and symptoms of intracranial aneurysms are usually those of SAH or of an intracranial mass. The presence of blood after SAH impairs consciousness and produces signs of meningeal irritation (headache, meningismus, photophobia). Patients may present with convulsions, nausea, vomiting, dizziness, paresthesia or paralysis, alterations in consciousness, or neurogenic pulmonary edema. Signs such as cranial nerve paresis or impairment of brain stem function may result from direct pressure of the aneurysm on adjacent neural structures. Neurologic dysfunction may also occur as a result of an elevation of ICP due to disruption of the brain parenchyma by an associated hematoma, by cerebral vasospasm or infarction, or by the mass effect of the aneurysm itself.

The diagnosis of a cerebral aneurysm is based on the clinical history, general physical and neurologic examinations, examination of CSF obtained via lumbar puncture, CT, and complete angiographic studies. The most important guide to the individual patient's diagnosis and prospect for ultimate recovery is the clinical condition (Table 32–4—the Hunt Classification) at the time therapy is initiated.

The natural history of the untreated intracranial aneurysm is such that the mortality rate during the first week after the initial SAH is 27 percent, and 49 percent during the first month. Ninety percent of the patients who die within 72 hours after SAH have an associated intracerebral, intracerebellar, or subdural hematoma. Rebleeding occurs within 1 month after the first SAH in 23 percent of cases. There is, however, a 40 percent mortality rate during the first year after the rupture of a single aneurysm. The mortality from the second SAH approaches 78 percent. The risk of rebleeding is greatest during the first 24 hours after SAH and declines to 37 percent annually.

Preoperative management of patients after SAH is directed toward minimizing complications, preventing rebleeding, and facilitating recovery from the initial insult. The patient is monitored closely in a tranquil environment. The treatment regimen includes complete bed rest, sedation, analgesia, administration of corticosteroids to reduce cerebral edema, maintenance of normal fluid and electrolyte balance, and attention to respiratory function. Blood pressure is maintained at the patient's high normal range to minimize ischemia from vasospasm. Epsilon-aminocaproic acid (Amicar) has been extensively studied to determine its effectiveness in preventing recurrent SAH from ruptured cerebral aneurysms. Clinical reports to date have been contradictory and inconclusive. Some have reported as high as an 88 percent incidence of rebleeding among those patients treated with epsilon-aminocaproic acid. No obvious difference was noted between the control group and the treated group in one study at the time of surgery in regard to adhesions, firmness of the aneurysmal sac, or difficulty in dissection. Although some reports reveal no significant complications associated with the administration of epsilon-aminocaproic acid, Hugenholtz and Elgie (1982) noted a number of complications in patients treated with epsilon-

aminocaproic acid, including pulmonary embolus and venous thrombosis. Operatively, they noted unusually tenacious adherence of the clot to the aneurysmal sac and its surroundings. Further studies, double-blinded, randomized, and with objective documentation of rebleeding, are necessary before the efficacy of this drug in preventing recurrent SAH can be proved.

The timing of surgery is an important factor in determining prognosis, but the optimal interval has not yet been established. Classically, surgery is delayed 1 to 3 weeks after a bleed. It is hoped that during that time the patient will recover from the acute effects of SAH, which include disrupted autoregulation and edema, and thus allow for optimal surgical conditions. However, the risk of rebleeding and clinically significant ischemia from vasospasm is high. Most damage from rebleeding occurs 1 to 2 weeks after SAH. Treatment of vasospasm includes mildly increased circulatory volume and moderate hypertension. In the patient with an unclipped aneurysm, this treatment can significantly increase the risk of rebleeding. The highest incidence of vasospasm seems to occur within 5 to 9 days after SAH.

Management of patients from the time of SAH until surgery is the same for both the early and late groups. However, the complications from medical treatment and prolonged bed rest were noted with greater frequency in the late group.

In both groups, surgery is scheduled after demonstration of the absence of vasospasm on the preoperative angiogram and no infarction with mass effect on CT scan. Vasospasm at the time of surgery would contraindicate the use of profound arterial hypotension. Vasospasm plus hypotension can produce severe ischemia and possibly infarct. Mass effect on CT scan would illustrate less than optimal surgical conditions, as the brain would be edematous and vital structures distorted and shifted. Unless the situation is life-threatening, the presence of vasospasm and its mass effect requires postponement of surgery.

Some institutions do not perform preoperative angiography because they believe the degree of spasm does not correlate well with the clinical picture. Instead, they will take the patient to the operating room and induce hypotension with the patient awake. If a neurologic deficit develops (aphasia, hemiparesis, etc.), the MAP is increased to normal levels, resolution of the deficit demonstrated, and surgery postponed for several days. If no deficit develops, the pressure is allowed to return to normal values, the patient is induced, and surgery may commence.

Many surgeons do not operate on stuporous patients who have hemiparesis, decerebrate rigidity, or vegetative disturbances, except those who have a life-threatening intracerebral hematoma. The mortality rate for operations to remove such hematomas is high, and prognosis is poor. Although many patients with intracranial hematomas can be stabilized so that their surgery for clot evacuation and aneurysm clip ligation can be performed electively, the decision to perform evacuation of a hematoma is based on the rapidity of neurologic deterioration, the location and size of the hematoma, anatomic characteristics of the aneurysm, and the patient's age and clinical grade. Important considerations for these patients are maintenance of blood pressure and intravascular volume and improvement of

TABLE 32–4. THE HUNT CLASSIFICATION

Grade 0	Unruptured
Grade 1	Asymptomatic or minimal headache, slight nuchal rigidity
Grade 1A	Stable, residual neurologic deficit, past the period of further cerebral reaction
Grade 2	Moderate to severe headache, nuchal rigidity no deficit except palsy of cranial nerve III
Grade 3	Drowsiness, confusion, mild focal deficit
Grade 4	Stupor, hemiparesis
Grade 5	Deep coma, decerebrate rigidity, moribund

Prognosis after SAH is closely related to the patient's initial condition. The Hunt Classification is one of the systems that is used to grade patients on admission and that allows for comparison among various studies.

intracranial compliance. Since aneurysms are space-occupying lesions, their effect on intracranial compliance must also be recognized in these situations.

Surgical treatment of aneurysms has been refined considerably by the development of microsurgical instrumentation and techniques that permit small exposure and precise dissection, minimize retraction and consequent trauma to the brain, and prevent premature aneurysmal rupture. Clipping of the neck of the aneurysm is the treatment of choice in the majority of cases. Large aneurysms and those with anatomic features that preclude safe clip ligation of the neck may be reinforced with muslin. This causes intense scarring, which in time strengthens the wall of the aneurysm. "Giant" aneurysms are treated by induction of a thrombus by direct or stereotactic insertion of a fine wire through the aneurysm wall to reduce the risk of recurrent hemorrhage or pressure-induced neurologic deficit. The only definitive therapy, however, is clip ligation. Therefore, the same precautions necessary to prevent aneurysmal rupture during induction of anesthesia are indicated during emergence from anesthesia after the aneurysm has been clipped.

Cerebral Vasospasm. Vasospasm is the clinical syndrome of neurologic deterioration that follows rupture or attempted surgical treatment of a narrowing of the cerebral arteries—focal, segmental, or diffuse—involving vessels either near to or distant from the presumed site of aneurysmal rupture. This arterial narrowing results in impaired cerebral perfusion and secondary infarction of the brain. The correlation between neurologic deterioration and angiographic evidence of vasospasm is questionable.

Rarely detected until 2 to 3 days after SAH, vasospasm may remain severe for 2 to 4 weeks. Surgery is frequently postponed until there is clinical and angiographic evidence that the spasm has resolved. Vasospasm also occurs postoperatively, either immediately or after 3 or 4 days of satisfactory progress.

The incidence of radiographically indicated vasospasm following SAH from aneurysmal rupture has been correlated with the location of the aneurysm, the number and severity of hemorrhages, catecholamine levels in blood and urine, blood white cell count, ECG abnormalities (Q waves, elevated ST segments, peaked T waves, short PR interval, large U waves, QT prolongation), and operative employment of hypothermia.

The etiology of vasospasm remains a puzzlement, especially since there are two phases: (1) early spasm, which is of brief duration, and (2) delayed, or recurrent, spasm, which develops 3 to 7 days after hemorrhage and is usually responsible for ischemic damage to the brain. This recurrent spasm is more intense, involves vessels far from the site of rupture, and may last for days or weeks. Direct trauma to vessels or mechanical distortion or displacement produces localized, short-lasting spasm. Extravasated blood itself produces severe vasospasm. The products of hemoglobin breakdown have been implicated in the process. Platelets too are spasmogenic because of their high serotonin content. Concentrations of serotonin similar to those in the CSF of patients after SAH are capable of producing vascular muscle contraction in vitro. Prostaglandins have also been implicated in the development of vasospasm.

Synthesized by platelets and brain tissue as a response to injury, prostaglandins modify CBF by affecting the action of adenylate cyclase in the synthesis of cyclic adenosine monophosphate (cAMP), which mediates the relaxation of vascular smooth muscle.

The variety of therapeutic efforts directed toward alleviating vasospasm reflects their limited success (Table 32–5). Physiologic measures include elevation of blood pressure and expansion of intravascular volume. This approach is based on demonstration of a passive increase in rCBF following hypertension in the ischemic hemispheres of animals with vasospasm. Because of the risk of rebleeding, both hypertension and hypervolemia are used cautiously in the period preceding surgical correction by clip ligation. However, patients with aneurysms frequently receive intraoperative transfusions, despite unremarkable blood loss, to augment intravascular volume and prevent vasospasm.

Most of the drugs known to dilate cerebral vessels produce significant systemic hypotension before cerebrovascular relaxation occurs. As a direct smooth-muscle relaxant, SNP has been used in combination with dopamine to achieve relief of spasm without causing systemic hypotension. The alpha-adrenergic antagonists phentolamine and phenoxybenzamine reduce or abolish spasm only when applied topically; the results after intracarotid and IV administration are disappointing. The beta-adrenergic agonist isoproterenol produces vasodilatation through stimulation of adenylate cyclase, which activates phosphorylase by means of cAMP, resulting in increased calcium permeability and, consequently, relaxation. Isoproterenol, in combination with lidocaine to counteract ventricular irritability, has produced encouraging results.

Inhibition of phosphodiesterase, which degrades cAMP, would allow cAMP to accumulate and thus promote vascular smooth muscle relaxation. The xanthine derivatives aminophylline and theophylline are potent phosphodiesterase inhibitors that, in combination with isoproterenol, have produced clinical improvement in patients with vasospasm.

Reserpine releases serotonin and catecholamines from

TABLE 32–5. VASOSPASM TREATMENT MODALITIES

Augmentation of blood pressure and intravascular volume

Vasodilatation and blood pressure support
     Sodium nitroprusside
     Dopamine

Topical alpha antagonism
     Phentolamine
     Phenoxybenzamine

Beta agonism and antiarrhythmics
     Isoproterenol
     Lidocaine

Phosphodiesterase inhibition
     Aminophylline
     Theophylline

Serotonin and catecholamine reduction
     Reserpine
     Kanamycin

Calcium entry blocking drugs
     Nimodipine[a]

[a] Of the various pharmacologic methods used to treat vasospasm, nimodipine is the most recent addition and is presently under investigation.

storage vesicles of presynaptic terminals and platelets, exposing them to metabolic degradation by cytoplasmic monoamine oxidase. Reserpine also inhibits phosphodiesterase activity, preventing deactivation of cAMP. Both reserpine and kanamycin lower serotonin blood levels and, administered in combination, have been successful in the prophylaxis of experimental vasospasm but not in the treatment of clinical vasospasm.

Anesthetic Consideration. Preoperative evaluation is the same for these patients as for any other neurosurgical patient. In view of the potentially disastrous effects of vasospasm and hypo- or hypertension, careful assessment of extravascular volume is essential. Antihypertensive agents or vasopressors should be continued up until the time of surgery. Preoperative medication may be given according to patient status. Hemodynamic monitoring should be continuously monitored from the time the patient arrives in the operating suite. Direct arterial monitoring is essential. Balloon-tipped, flow-directed thermodilution may be valuable in these patients for monitoring myocardial function and providing a reliable indicator of intravascular function. Obviously, ECG (V_5), temperature probe, peripheral nerve stimulator, Foley catheter, and esophageal stethoscope are required. If the patient is to be in a sitting position, a precordial Doppler, central venous line, and $ETCO_2$ analyzer (in the absence of pulmonary artery catheter) are essential.

The selection of anesthetic agents is governed by the patient's overall status, with consideration given to avoid extreme changes in blood pressure and provide improvement in cerebral oxygenation and cerebral protection in the event of focal ischemia. For these purposes, a balanced narcotic technique as previously described would be a wise choice.

Osmotic dehydrating agents may be avoided during aneurysm surgery or used in smaller doses in conjunction with spinal drainage. Spinal drainage of CSF may be used to produce a slack, easily retractable brain and thus improve operating conditions. Spinal drainage is accomplished with indwelling subarachnoid catheters or malleable needles inserted through the lumbar 3–4 or 4–5 interspace. Usually two catheters or needles are placed; in case of occlusion of one, the other is available. Care must be taken to avoid excessive loss of CSF on lumbar puncture, as the sudden decrease in pressure can cause hemorrhage or herniation. The needles or catheter may be attached to a transducer to monitor lumbar CSF pressure. Usually the catheters or needles are attached to a calibrated drip chamber receptacle and clamped *closed*. Drainage is not begun until the dura is opened to prevent the development of pressure gradients across the brain. Cerebrospinal flow should be drained slowly; approximately 5 ml/minute may be drained passively. As much as 150 ml may be withdrawn, as required for adequate surgical exposure. Drainage is stopped when dural closure begins, and the catheters or needles are withdrawn at the end of the case.

During anesthetic maintenance, arterial blood gases are monitored frequently to maintain a $PaCO_2$ at the patient's preoperative level. If hypocarbia is necessary to allow dissection, normocarbia is restored before controlled hypotension is induced. The combined effects of vasoconstriction and hypotension can cause severe ischemia and infarct.

Fluids (lactated Ringer's) are given to replace urine loss and maintain hourly requirements. Packed cells or whole blood is given to replace blood loss. An additional one or two units of blood may be given to augment intravascular volume and counteract vasospasm after ligation of the aneurysm. MAP is maintained at the patient's high normal range. Controlled hypotension is frequently used to decrease blood loss and operative time and to facilitate dissection and clipping of the aneurysm. Normotensive patients can usually tolerate a reduction in MAP to 50 mm Hg (at normocarbia). Chronically hypertensive patients have higher limits of autoregulation and do not tolerate a reduction as low as normotensive patients. A 30 percent reduction in MAP is usually tolerated. ECG and urine output should be carefully monitored for signs of ischemia or decreased renal blood flow. Controlled hypotension can be achieved with SNP, nitroglycerine, or trimethaphan in the manner previously described.

Hypothermia may be used during clip ligation of aneurysms. The brain can tolerate complete ischemia for 4 minutes at 38C, 8 minutes at 30C, 16 minutes at 22C, and more than 30 minutes at 16C. There are few deleterious systemic effects of hypothermia when body temperature remains above 30C. Liver, kidney, and endocrine function are decreased during hypothermia but return to normal within 24 hours after rewarming. The action of narcotics and muscle relaxants is prolonged with hypothermia.

Hypothermia does not produce significant metabolic alteration unless there is shivering, poor tissue perfusion, or prolonged circulatory arrest. Shivering may be accompanied by anaerobic metabolism, progressive metabolic acidosis, and cardiac depression. As temperature decreases, there is an increase in CO_2 solubility, pH, and CO_2-combining power and a decrease in buffer capacity. Maintaining levels of hypocarbia appropriate to the normothermic patient will result in progressive respiratory alkalosis. The increased pH and lower temperature combine to produce a leftward shift in the oxygen-hemoglobin disassociation curve and a greater affinity of oxygen. A decrease in $PaCO_2$ is required as body temperature falls to preserve a constant relative alkalinity. This will maintain CO_2 stores of blood and tissue at a constant level. In practice, it means that the pulmonary ventilation should be kept at or near the euthermic setting as the body is cooled. The $PaCO_2$ decreases as the metabolic rate diminishes, but acid-base balance remains normal in blood as well as tissues because of the relative increase in ventilation.

The desired temperature is attained by surface cooling with blankets that circulate cold liquid. The blanket controls are turned back to the warm mode when the esophageal temperature falls to 33C, because the temperature will drift downward another 2 to 3C. Extracorporeal circulation is required to achieve profound hypothermia.

Emergence must be smooth, as described for all neurosurgical patients, following the same criteria for extubation.

Arteriovenous Malformations

In patients with AVM, there may be, in addition to the mass effect from the lesion itself and associated hematomas, a steal phenomenon in which blood is shunted away from healthy brain to the AVM, resulting in neurologic deficit.

To avoid exacerbating this phenomenon, maintenance of blood pressure during anesthesia is critical. The size of the AVM and the flow through its feeding arteries may be decreased by selective preoperative embolization with particulate matter or rapidly polymerizing glue. During this procedure, patients are sedated yet awake to permit frequent neurologic evaluation. Although surgical resection is facilitated and blood loss reduced by neuroradiologic vascular occlusion, intracranial hemorrhage and stroke are potential complications.

Considerations in Pediatric Neuroanesthesia

With a few differences, the principles of neuroanesthetic technique for adult patients apply to the pediatric population. These differences are related to the anatomic, physiologic, and pharmacokinetic characteristics common to premature babies, neonates, infants, and children. For a complete discussion on pediatric anesthesia, refer to the appropriate sections of this book. Our discussion will focus on some of the more pertinent neurologic differences in children.

Premature babies are classified as those born less than 37 weeks after conception. Low-birth-weight babies are those who weigh less than 2500 g at birth. Any alterations in response typical of the full-term, normal-birth-weight baby will be increasingly obvious with greater deficits of age and weight.

Cerebral vasculature and the CNS are very immature in premature babies. Intracranial hemorrhage, subependymal and intraventricular, occur in 40 to 50 percent of sick premature infants. There is an increased incidence of intracranial hemorrhage with stress from such causes as traumatic delivery, hypoxia, and struggling. Aggressive correction of metabolic acidosis with sodium bicarbonate may cause hyperosmolarity and may lead to intracranial hemorrhage. For this reason, bicarbonate administration should be done very slowly and cautiously, perhaps in less than the calculated dosage. These children are also subject to seizure and apneic spells.

Autoregulation is often absent in the premature baby but present in the neonate. The blood-brain barrier, if present, is certainly immature. Cerebral vessels are immature; tone, CVR, and responsiveness to $Paco_2$ are decreased. Considering the lower MAP, CPP is also much lower in proportion to the age and weight of the child. $CMRo_2$ is 5 to 6 ml/100 g of brain tissue per minute and gradually increases to adult levels. In general, physiologic functions reach adult levels by 1 year of age. Intracranial hypertension is usually not a problem in neonates and infants, owing to the open sutures and fontanels. The exception would be those infants born with craniosynostosis and severe hydrocephalus. The posterior and coronal fontanels close by 3 months of age, the anterior fontanel by 18 months. The sutures (sagittal, coronal, lambdoidal) usually close by 1 year.

One of the most frequent situations requiring surgery in pediatric neurologic patients is hydrocephalus. Hydrocephalus refers to a group of conditions characterized by enlarged ventricles usually secondary to a blockage of the normal CSF circulation or failure of the normal CSF reabsorption process. ICP is normal or raised depending on the pathology of the hydrocephalus.

Hydrocephalus is usually categorized as communicating or noncommunicating. In communicating hydrocephalus, the obstruction is distal to the fourth ventricle outlets, or at the arachnoid villi, or within the arachnoid surface over the brain. Communicating hydrocephalus may be caused by adhesions or obstruction of basilar or surface subarachnoid space (e.g., hemorrhage, infection, meningitis), development failure of arachnoid villa, or overproduction of CSF from choroid plexus papilloma.

Noncommunicating hydrocephalus is an intraventricular obstruction, usually where the pathways are narrow. Noncommunicating hydrocephalus may be caused by aqueductal (between the third and fourth ventricle) maldevelopment-stenosis, atresia, mass lesion obstruction, hemorrhage, infection, arachnoiditis, or Dandy-Walker syndrome.

Ideal management of hydrocephalus is removal of the cause, although this is not always possible. CSF shunting—ventriculoatrial or, more commonly and with less hazard, ventriculoperitoneal—is the mainstay of therapy. General anesthesia is usually required for insertion of these shunts, and, in addition to routine pediatric anesthetic considerations, specific consideration must be given to the cause of the hydrocephalus.

Various birth defects of the CNS may bring the neonate to the operating room within the first hours or days of life. Systemic complications are often associated with the neurologic defect. Cerebrovascular defects such as vein of Galen aneurysms may present with congestive heart failure, high-output failure, and cranial bruits. Spina bifida is a developmental defect of the vertebrae in which the canal fails to close normally. The defect may be limited to bony malformation (spina bifida occulta) or may include herniation of the meninges (meningocele) and nerve roots and spinal cord (myelomeningocele). Neurologic and systemic symptoms are associated with the spinal cord level involved. Meningitis is always a threat with meningocele and myelomeningocele. These same defects may occur over the cranium. Cranium bifidum is a defect of fusion of the cranial bone. Meningoceles and encephalocele (protrusion of meninges and brain tissue) may accompany cranium bifidum. Meningoceles, myelomeningocele, and encephalocele usually require excision of the sac and its contents, with dural closure very early in life. If large amounts of nervous tissue are present in the sac, normal developmental prognosis is usually poor. Hydrocephalus commonly occurs with many of these conditions or follows surgical closure of the sac.

Craniosynostosis involves premature closure of the sutures with malformation of the skull and may produce secondary effects on the brain and eyes. This defect may be present at birth or may not be evident until the child is a few months old. Correction of craniosynostosis is usually performed during the first few months of life. If there are no other CNS defects, outcome is usually very good, with no retardation or neurologic deficit. On occasion, correction of craniosynostosis is purely for cosmetic reasons; the patient has progressed through a normal developmental state. A major anesthetic concern during correction of this defect is the large blood loss that occurs because of the removal of large amounts of cranial bone. Blood loss is carefully measured and replaced milliliter-for-milliliter from the start of the case.

Arnold-Chiari malformation is a congenital defect involving projection of the medulla and cerebellum through the foramen magnum and into the cervical spinal canal. It is thought to develop during fetal life, with fixation of the lower spinal cord or nerve roots exerting a downward pull on the upper cervical cord and brain stem. It may be associated with spina bifida, hydrocephalus, and other defects of bone, meninges, and nervous tissue. Treatment during infancy, childhood, or early adulthood involves decompression of the posterior fossa and, on occasion, correction of hydrocephalus. In older children and adults, pheochromocytoma occasionally coincides with Arnold-Chiari malformation and must be ruled out before surgery is scheduled.

Platybasia is a deformity of the occipital bone and upper cervical spine. Compression of the medulla and obstruction of the subarachnoid space and hydrocephalus occur. Treatment involves decompression of the foramen magnum, freeing of adhesions, and possibly amputation of cerebellar tonsils.

Tumor, infection, and head trauma tend to occur more in older than younger children. Tumors in older children have a tendency to present in the posterior fossa.

Anesthetic management is based on the child's age, weight, clinical status, and surgical lesion. All indications for drug selection and monitoring for adults apply to children as well. Perhaps the most difficult and controversial aspect is induction of anesthesia in young children. Although an inhalational induction may appear outwardly smooth, the effects of these agents on ICP can be just as detrimental in children as they are in adults. In a well-sedated child, it may be possible to start an IV route without much ado and proceed with a balanced narcotic anesthetic. Rectal thiopental (Pentothal) may offer a safe alternative to preoperative sedation on the child in whom intracranial compliance may be compromised. Thiopental, 25 to 30 mg/kg, either the solution or a suppository, may be given rectally in the operating suite to sedate the child, then an IV may be started. Preoperative colon evacuation may minimize the problems of unpredictable absorption of the drug and evacuation after administration of the drug.

Pancuronium bromide (Pavulon) should be used with caution in the sick premature child. The combination of increased heart rate and increased MAP from light anesthesia may stress the delicate intracranial vessels and cause hemorrhage. Vecuronium may be a safer alternative for muscle relaxation.

Temperature control is particularly important in neonates and infants. Hypothalamic temperature regulation does not mature until about 6 months of age.

CONCLUSION

Perioperative and anesthetic management significantly affect the prognosis of the patient undergoing a neurosurgical procedure. Because the interaction between pharmacologic and mechanical maneuvers and intracranial pathophysiology is critical in determining the results of therapeutic intervention, we have reviewed these relationships in the context of the anesthetic care of the neurosurgical patient.

The recent advances in neuroanesthesia have contributed significantly to the greater safety and success of neurosurgical procedures. Improved understanding of the intracranial effects of pharmacologic and mechanical intervention during anesthesia and intensive care has diminished secondary traumatic and operative neurologic injury by providing a means for enhancement of cerebral perfusion and for reduction of cerebral edema. Sophisticated developments in the practice of neurosurgery have been fostered also by parallel progress in the technology of monitoring, neuroradiology, and the surgical microscope. It is these technical and conceptual refinements that have enabled neurosurgeons and neuroanesthesiologists to undertake more intricate operations and achieve decreased mortality and improved results.

Acknowledgments. The author wishes to express her appreciation to Dr. Joseph P. Griffin, Dr. James E. Cottrell, and Dr. Philippa Newfield for their assistance in the preparation of this chapter. Special thanks go to Ellen Jackson for manuscript preparation.

BIBLIOGRAPHY

Adams RW, Cucchiara RF, et al: Isoflurane and cerebrospinal fluid pressure in neurosurgical patients. Anesthesiology 54:97–99, 1981.

Adams RW, Gronert GA, et al: Halothane, hypocapnia, and cerebrospinal fluid pressure in neurosurgery. Anesthesiology 37:510–517, 1972.

Albin MS: Spinal cord injuries—anesthetic and clinical considerations. Proc Symp Neuroanesthesia. San Antonio, Texas, 1981, pp 1–11.

Albin MS: Resuscitation of the spinal cord. Criti Care Med 6:170, 1978.

Albin MS, Babinski M, et al: Anesthetic management of posterior fossa surgery in the sitting position. Acta Anaesthesiol Scand 20:117–128, 1976.

Alexander SC, Lassen NA: Cerebral circulatory response to acute brain disease. Implications for anesthetic practice. Anesthesiology 32:60, 1970.

Artu AA, Steen PA, Michenfelder JD: Cerebral metabolic effects of naloxone. Abstracts of Scientific Papers Annual Meeting of American Society of Anesthesiologists, 1979.

Basta SA, Savarese JJ: Comparative histamine-releasing properties of vecuronium, atracurium, tubocurarine and metocurine. Clinical Experience with Norcuron. Excerpta Medica Current Clinical Practice Series 11:183–184, 1983.

Bedford RF, Marshall WK, et al: Cardiac catheters for diagnosis and treatment of venous air emboli. J Neurosurg 55:610–614, 1981.

Bedford RF, Persing JA, et al: Lidocaine or thiopental for rapid control of intracranial hypertension. Anesth Analg 59:435–437, 1980.

Bedford RF, Winn HR, et al: Lidocaine prevents increased ICP after endotracheal intubation. Intracranial Pressure. IV. New York, Springer-Verlag (in press).

Bourke RS, Kimelburg HK, et al: Studies on the formation of the astroglial swelling and its inhibition by clinically useful agents. In Neural Trauma, Popp AJ, Bourke RS, Nelson LB, et al. (eds): Seminars in Neurological Surgery. New York, Raven Press, 1979.

Brown EM, Krishnaprasas D, Smiler BG: Pancuronium for rapid induction technique for tracheal intubation. Can Anaesth Soc J 26:489, 1979.

Bynegin L, Albin MS, et al: Positioning the right atrial catheter: A model for reappraisal. Anesthesiology 55:343–348, 1981.

Burrows G: On disorders of cerebral circulation and on the connection between affections of the brain and diseases of the heart. London, Longman, 1846.

Chen K, Rose CL, Clowes GH: Comparative values of several antidotes in cyanide poisoning. Am J Med Sci 188:767–787, 1934.

Chestnut JS, Albin MS, Gonzalez-Abola E, et al: Clinical evaluation of intravenous nitroglycerin for neurosurgery. J Neurosurg 48:704–711, 1978.

Christensen MS, Hoedt-Rasmussen K, Lassen NA: Cerebral vasodilatation by halothane anaesthesia in man and its potentiation by hypotension and hypercapnia. Br J Anaesth 39:927–934, 1967.

Cotev S, Shalit MN: Effects of diazepam on cerebral blood flow and oxygen uptake after head injuries. Anesthesiology 43:117, 1975.

Cottrell JE: Considerations for intraoperative fluid replacement in the neurosurgical patient. For the American Association of Neurological Surgeons. Breakfast Panel, 1981.

Cottrell JE, Casthely P, Brodie JD, et al: Prevention of nitroprusside-induced cyanide toxicity with hydroxocobalamin. N Engl J Med 298:809–811, 1978.

Cottrell JE, Giffin JP, Hartung J, et al: Intracranial pressure during nifedipine-induced hypotension in cats. Anesth Analg 62:245, 1983.

Cottrell JE, Giffin JP, Hartung J, et al: Succinylcholine and intracranial pressure in cats. ASA Abstracts, 1981 Annual Meeting.

Cottrell JE, Giffin JP, Lim K, Milhorat T, Stein S, Shwiry B: Intracranial pressure, mean arterial pressure, and heart rate following midazolam or thiopental in humans with intracranial masses. ABA Abstracts, 1982 Annual Meeting.

Cottrell JE, Gupta B, et al: Intracranial pressure during nitroglycerin induced hypotension. J Neurosurg 53:309–311, 1980.

Cottrell JE, Van Aken H, Gupta B, Turndorf H: Induced hypotension. In Cottrell JE, Turndorf H (eds): Anesthesiology and Neurosurgery, 2nd ed. St. Louis, Mosby, 1986, p. 421.

Cottrell JE, Hartung J, Giffin JP, et al: Intracranial and hemodynamic changes after succinylcholine administration in cats. Anesth Analg 62:1006–1009, 1983.

Cottrell JE, Illner P, Kittay MS, et al: Rebound hypertension after sodium nitroprusside-induced hypotension. Clin Pharmacol Ther 27:32–37, 1980.

Cottrell JE, Newfield P: Anesthetic considerations for neurovascular surgery. In Flamm E, Fine J (eds): Neurovascular Surgery. New York, Springer-Verlag (in press).

Cottrell JE, Patek K, et al: Intracranial pressure changes induced by sodium nitroprusside in patients' intracranial mass lesions. J Neurosurg 48:329–331, 1978.

Cottrell JE, Patel KP, et al: Cerebrospinal fluid cyanide after nitroprusside. Can Anaesth Soc J 28:228, 1981.

Cottrell JE, Patel K, et al: Nitroprusside tachyphylaxis without acidosis. Anesthesiology 49:141–142, 1978.

Cottrell JE, Patel K, et al: Intracranial pressure changes induced by sodium nitroprusside in patients with intracranial mass lesions. J Neurosurg 48:329–331, 1978.

Cottrell JE, Robustelli A, et al: Furosemide- and mannitol-induced changes in intracranial pressure and serum osmolality and electrolytes. Anesthesiology 47:28–30, 1977.

Cottrell JE, Robustelli A, et al: Furosemide and mannitol-induced changes in intracranial pressure and serum osmolality and electrolytes. Anesthesiology 47:28–30, 1977.

Cottrell JE, Turndorf H: Intravenous nitroglycerin. Am Heart J 96:550–553, 1978.

Cutler RWP, et al: Formation and absorption of cerebrospinal fluid in man. Brain 91:707, 1968.

Dahlgren BE, Gordon E, Steiner L: Evaluation of controlled hypotension during surgery for intracranial arterial aneurysms. Progress in Anesthesiology. New York, Excerpta Medica, 1970, p. 1232.

Davies DW, Greiss L, et al: Sodium nitroprusside in children: Observations on metabolism during normal and abnormal responses. Can Anaesth Soc J 22:553–560, 1975.

Davies DW, Kadar D, et al: A sudden death associated with the use of sodium nitroprusside for induction of hypotension during anesthesia. Can Anaesth Soc J 22:547–552, 1975.

Donegan M, Bedford RF, Dacey R: IV lidocaine for prevention of intracranial hypertension. Anesthesiology 51:S201, 1979.

Durham CF, Harrison TS: The surgical anatomy of the superior laryngeal nerve. Surg Gynecol Obstet 118:38, 1964.

Estilo AE, Cottrell JE: Hemodynamic and catecholamine changes after administration of naloxone. Anesth Analg 61:349–353, 1982.

Fahmy NR: Nitroglycerin as a hypotensive drug during general anesthesia. Anesthesiology 49:17–20, 1978.

Fitch W: Anaesthesia for carotid artery surgery. Br J Anaesth 48:791–796, 1976.

Fitch W, Barker J, et al: The influence of neuroleptanalgesic drugs on cerebrospinal fluid pressure. Br J Anaesth 41:800–806, 1969.

Fitch W, McDowall DG: Hazards of anesthesia in patients with intracranial space-occupying lesions. Int Anesthesiol Clin 7:639–662, 1969.

Fitch W, McDowall DG: Effect of halothane on intracranial pressure gradients in the presence of space-occupying lesions. Br J Anaesth 43:904–911, 1971.

Forster A, Van Horn K, et al: Influence of anesthetic agents on blood-brain barrier function during acute hypertension. Acta Neurol Scand [Suppl] 64:60–63, 1977.

Frost EAM, Tabuddor K, et al: Efficacy of induced barbiturate coma in control of intracranial hypertension. Anesthesiology 8:10, 1981.

Furuya H, Suzuki T, et al: Detection of air embolism by transesophageal echocardiography. Anesthesiology 58:124, 1983.

Gagnon RL, Marsh ML, et al: Intracranial hypertension caused by nitroglycerin. Anesthesiology 51:86, 1979.

Gandhi P, Cottrell JE, et al: Deliberate hypotension with labetalol in neurological patients (Abstract). Anesthesiology 59(3A):360, 1983.

Giffin JP: Anesthetic management of acute spinal cord injured patients. Proc Workshop Neurosurg Anesth—The Spinal Cord, New York, May, 1982.

Giffin JP, Hartung J, et al: Effect of vecuronium on intracranial pressure, mean arterial pressure, and heart rate in cats. Br J Anaesth 58:441–443, 1986.

Goodman LS, Gilman A: The Pharmacological Basis of Therapeutics, 7th ed. New York, Macmillan, 1985, p. 215.

Gordon E: The technique of reduction of the intracranial pressure. In Gordon E (ed): A Basis and Practice of Neuroanesthesia. New York, Excerpta Medica, 1975, Vol. 2, pp. 209–218.

Gotta AW, Sullivan CA: Anesthesia of the upper airway using topical anesthetic and superior laryngeal nerve block. Br J Anaesth 53:1055–1058, 1981.

Grundy BL: Electrophysiologic monitoring: Electroencephalography and evoked potentials. In Newfield P, Cottrell JE (eds): Handbook of Neuroanesthesia: Clinical and Physiologic Essentials. Boston, Little, Brown, 1983, pp. 28–59.

Gupta B, Cottrell JE, et al: Nitroglycerin raises intracranial pressure. J Neurosurg 1979.

Hamill JF, Bedford RF, et al: Lidocaine before endotracheal intubation: Intravenous or laryngotracheal? Anesthesiology 55:578, 1981.

Harp RJ, Hagerdal M: Brain oxygen consumption. In Cottrell JE, Turndorf H (eds): Anesthesia and Neurosurgery. St. Louis, Mosby, 1980, pp. 25–36.

Harp JR, Wollman H: Cerebral metabolic effects of hyperventilation and deliberate hypotension. Br J Anaesth 45:256, 1973.

Hartung J, Cottrell JE: Nitrous oxide reduced thiopental-induced prolongation of survival in hypoxic and anoxic mice. Anesth Analg 66:47–52, 1987.

Henriksen HT, Jorgensen PB: The effect of nitrous oxide on intracranial pressure in patients with intracranial disorders. Br J Anesth 45:486, 1973.

Hochwald G: Cerebrospinal fluid mechanisms. In Cottrell JE, Turndorf H (eds): Anesthesia and Neurosurgery. St. Louis, C.V. Mosby, 1980, pp. 37–53.

Hoff JT, Smith AL, et al: Barbiturate protection from cerebral infarction in primates. Stroke 6:28–33, 1975.

Javid M, Gilboe D, Cesario T: The rebound phenomenon and hypertonic solutions. J Neurosurg 21:1059–1066, 1964.

Jennett WB, Barker J, et al: Effects of anaesthesia on intracranial pressure in patients with space-occupying lesions. Lancet 1:61–64, 1969.

Jennett WB, McDowall DG, Barker J: The effect of halothane on intracranial pressure in cerebral tumors: Report of two cases. J Neurosurg 26:270–274, 1967.

Jones TH, Chiappa KH, et al: EEG monitoring for induced hypotension for surgery of intracranial aneurysms. Stroke 10:292, 1979.

Kelly PJ, Gorten RJ, et al: Cerebral perfusion, vascular spasm, and outcome in patients with ruptured intracranial aneurysms. J Neurosurg 47:44–49, 1977.

Kerber C: Intracranial cyanoacrylate: A new catheter therapy for arteriovenous malformation. Invest Radiol 10:536–538, 1975.

Lall NG, Jain AP: Circulatory and respiratory disturbances during posterior fossa surgery. Br J Anaesth 41:447–449, 1969.

Langfitt TW: Increased intracranial pressure. In Youmans JR (ed): Neurological Surgery. Philadelphia, Saunders, 1973, pp. 496–506.

Lassen NA: Cerebral blood flow and oxygen consumption in man. Physiol Rev 39:183–235, 1959.

Lassen NA: Cerebral and spinal cord blood flow. In Cottrell JE, Turndorf H (eds): Anesthesia and Neurosurgery. St. Louis, Mosby, 1980, pp. 1–24.

Lassen NA, Tweed WA: A basis and practice of neuroanesthesia. In Gordon E (ed): Monographs in Anesthesiology. New York, Elsevier, 1975, Vol. 2, pp. 113–133.

Latchlaw RE, Gold LHA: Polyvinyl foam embolization of vascular and neoplastic lesions of the head, neck, and spine. Radiology 131:669–679, 1979.

Lewelt W, Moszynski K, Kozniewska H: Effects of depolarizing, nondepolarizing muscle relaxants and intubation on the ventricular fluid pressure. In Beks JW, Bosch DA, Brock M (eds). Intracranial Pressure. New York, Springer-Verlag, 1976, pp. 215–218.

Lundberg N: Monitoring of the intracranial pressure. In Critchley M, O'Leary JL, Jeannett B (eds): Scientific Foundations of Neurology, Philadelphia, Davis, 1972, pp. 356–371.

Lundberg N, et al: Non-operative management of intracranial hypertension. In Krayenbuhl H (ed): Advances and Technical Standard in Neurosurgery. New York, Springer-Verlag, 1974, Vol. 1, pp. 1–59.

MacCarthy E, Bloomfield SS: Labetalol: A review of its pharmacology, pharmacokinetics, clinical uses and adverse effects. Pharmacotherapy 3:193–219, 1983.

McDowall DG: The influence of anesthetic drugs and techniques on intracranial pressure. In Gordon E (ed): A Basic Practice of Neuroanesthesia., New York, Excerpta Medica, 1975, Vol. 2, pp. 135–170.

McDowall DG: The effects of clinical concentrations of halothane on the blood flow and oxygen uptake of the cerebral cortex. Br J Anaesth 39:186–196, 1967.

McDowall DG, Barker J, Jennett WB: Cerebrospinal fluid pressure measurements during anesthesia. Anesthesia 21:189–201, 1966.

McKay RD, Sundt TM, Michenfelder JD, et al: Internal carotid artery stump pressure and cerebral blood flow during carotid endarterectomy: Modification by halothane, enflurane, and Innovar. Anesthesiology 45:390–399, 1976.

McQueen JD, Jeanes LD: Dehydration and rehydration of the brain with hypertonic urea and mannitol. J Neurosurg 21:118–128, 1964.

Maroon JC, Goodman JM, et al: Detection of minute venous air emboli with ultrasound. Surg Gynecol Obstet 127:1236–1238, 1964.

Marsh ML, Dunlap BJ, et al: Succinyl-intracranial pressure effects in neurosurgical patients (Abstract). Anesth Analg 59:550–551, 1980.

Marshall WK, Bedford RF: Use of a pulmonary artery catheter for detection and treatment of venous air embolism. Anesthesiology 52:131, 1980.

Mehta P, Mehta J, Miale TD: Nitroprusside lowers platelet count (Letter). N Engl J Med 299:1134, 1978.

Michenfelder JD, Theye RA: Canine systemic and cerebral effects of hypotension induced by hemorrhage, trimethaphan, halothane, or nitroprusside. Anesthesiology 46:188–195, 1977.

Michenfelder JD, Tinker JH: Cyanide toxicity and thiosulfate protection during chronic administration of sodium nitroprusside in the dog. Anesthesiology 47:441–448, 1977.

Michenfelder JD, Theye RA: Effects of fentanyl, droperidol, and Innovar on canine cerebral metabolism and blood flow. Br J Anaesth 43:630–636, 1971.

Milhorat TH: Structure and function of the choroid plexus and other sites of cerebrospinal fluid formation. Int Rev Cytol 47:225, 1976.

Miller RD, Savarese JJ: Pharmacology of muscle relaxants, their antagonists, and monitoring of neuromuscular function. In Miller RD (ed): Anesthesia. New York, Churchill Livingstone, 1986, pp. 889–944.

Miller RD, Tausk HC: Prolonged anesthesia associated with hypotension induced by trimethaphan (Arfonad). Anesthesiol Rev 1:36–37, 1974.

Misfeldt BB, Jorgensen PB, Rishos M: The effect of nitrous oxide and halothane upon the intracranial pressure in hypocapnic patients with intracranial disorders. Br J Anaesth 46:853–858, 1974.

Monroe A: Observations on the structure and functions of the nervous system. Edinburgh, Creech & Johnson, 1983.

Morita H, Nemoto EM, et al: Brain blood flow autoregulation and metabolism during halothane anesthesia in monkeys. Am J Physiol 233:H670–H676, 1977.

Munson ES, Merrick HC: Effect of nitrous oxide on venous air embolism. Anesthesiology 27:783–787, 1966.

Munson ES, Paul WL, et al: Early detection of venous air embolism using a Swan-Ganz catheter. Anesthesiology 42:223–226, 1975.

Murphy FL Jr, Kennell EM, et al: The effects of enflurane, isoflurane, and halothane on cerebral blood flow and metabolism in man. Abstracts of Scientific Papers. Annu Meet Am Soc Anesthesiol, 1974, pp. 61–62.

Needleman P, Jakschik B, Johnson EM, Jr: Sulfhydryl requirement for requirement of relaxation of vascular smooth muscle. J Pharmacol Exp Ther 187:324–331, 1973.

Neigh JL, Garman JK, Harp JR: The electroencephalographic pattern during anesthesia with Ethrane: Effects of depth of anesthesia, $PaCO_2$ and nitrous oxide. Anesthesiology 35:482–487, 1971.

Pierce EC Jr, Lambertsen CJ, Deutsch S, Chase PE, Linde HW, Dripps RD, Price HL: Cerebral circulation and metabolism during thiopental anesthesia and hyperventilation in man. J Clin Invest 41:1664–1671, 1962.

Pleiderer T: Na^+ nitroprusside, a very potent platelet disaggregating substance. Acta Univ Carol, 53:147–150, 1972.

Pollay M: Formation of cerebrospinal fluid: Relation of studies of isolated choroid plexus to the standing gradient hypothesis. J Neurosurg 42:665–673, 1975.

Posner MA, Tobey RE, McElroy H: Hydroxocobalamin therapy of cyanide intoxication in guinea pigs. Anesthesiology 44:157–160, 1976.

Reves JG, Kissin I, et al: Calcium entry blockers: Uses and implications for anesthesiologists. Anesthesiology 57:504–518, 1982.

Rich NM, Hobson RW: Carotid endarterectomy under regional anaesthesia. Am Surg 41:253–259, 1975.

Roberts BE, Smith PH: Hazards of mannitol infusions. Lancet 2:421, 422, 1966.

Rockoff MA, Marshall LF, Shaprio HM: High-dose barbiturate therapy in humans: A clinical review of 60 patients. Ann Neurol 6:194–199, 1979.

Rogers MC, Hamburger C, et al: Intracranial pressure in the cat during nitroglycerin-induced hypotension. Anesthesiology 51:227–229, 1979.

Rottenberg DA, Posner JB: Intracranial pressure control. In Cottrell JE, Turndorf H (eds): Anesthesia and Neurosurgery. St. Louis, Mosby, 1980, pp. 89–113.

Rueger RS: The superior laryngeal nerve and the interarytenoid muscle in humans: An anatomical study. Laryngoscope 82:2008, 1972.

Saidman LJ, Eger El II: Change in cerebrospinal fluid pressure during pneumoencephalography under nitrous oxide anesthesia. Anesthesiology 26:67–71, 1965.

Samuels SI: Anesthesia for supratentorial tumor. In Cottrell JE, Turndorf H (eds): Anesthesia and Neurosurgery. St. Louis, Mosby, 1980, pp. 150–167.

Shenkin NA, Bouzarth WF: Clinical methods of reducing intracranial pressure. Role of the cerebral circulation. N Engl J Med 282:1465, 1970.

Schettini A, Furniss WM: Brain water and electrolyte distribution during the inhalation of halothane. Br J Anesth 51:1117, 1979.

Schettini A, Mahig J: Comparative intracranial dynamic responses in dogs to three halogenated anesthetics. Abstracts of Scientific Papers. Annu Meet Am Soc Anesthesiol 1973, pp. 123–124.

Shapiro HM: Intracranial hypertension: Therapeutic and anesthetic considerations. Anesthesiology 43:445–471, 1975.

Shapiro HM, Ardinio SJ: Neurosurgical anesthesia. Surg Clin North Am 55:913–927, 1975.

Shapiro HM, Galindo A, et al: Rapid intra-operative reduction of intracranial hypertension with thiopentone. Br J Anaesth 45:1057–1062, 1973.

Shapiro HM, Wyte SR, Harris AB: Ketamine anesthesia in patients with intracranial pathology. Br J Anaesth 44:1200, 1972.

Shapiro HM, Wyte SR, et al: Acute intraoperative intracranial hypertension in neurosurgical patients: Mechanical and pharmacologic factors. Anesthesiology 37:399–405, 1972.

Shapiro HM, Yoachim J, Marshall LF: Nitrous oxide challenge for detection of residual intravascular pulmonary gas following venous air embolism. Anesth Analg 61:304, 1982.

Shwiry B, Josephs S, Sullivan CA, Gotta AW: A method of intubation for cervical spine injured patients. ANAJ 51:403–405.

Siesjo BK, Norberg K, et al: Hypoxia and cerebral metabolism. In Gordon E (ed): A Basis and Practice of Neuroanesthesia: Monographs in Anesthesiology. New York, Elsevier, 1975, Vol. 2, pp. 47–83.

Smith, AL, Marque JJ: Anesthetics and cerebral edema. Anesthesiology 45:64–72, 1970.

Smith AL, Wollman H: Cerebral blood flow and metabolism. Anesthesiology 36:378–400, 1972.

Smith RD, Kruszyna H: Nitroprusside produces cyanide poisoning via a reaction with hemoglobin. J Pharmacol Exp Ther 191:557–563, 1974.

Steffey EP, Gauger GE, Eger El II: Cardiovascular effects of venous air embolism during air and oxygen breathing. Anesth Analg 53:599–604, 1974.

Stevenson PH, Birch AA: Succinylcholine-induced hyperkalemia in a patient with a closed head injury. Anesthesiology 51:89–90, 1979.

Stone WA, Beach TP, Hamelberg W: Succinylcholine—danger in the spinal-cord-injured patient. Anesthesiology 32:168–169, 1970.

Stoyka WW, Schutz H: The cerebral response to sodium nitroprusside and trimethaphan controlled hypotension. Can Anaesth Soc J 22:275–283, 1975.

Strandgaard S, MacKenzie ET, et al: Upper limits of autoregulation of cerebral blood flow in the baboon. Circ Res 34:435–440, 1974.

Strandgaard S, Oleson J, Skinhoj E, et al: Autoregulation of brain circulation in severe arterial hypertension. Br Med J 1:507–510, 1973.

Stullken EH Jr, Sokoll MS: Anesthesia and subarachnoid intracranial pressure. Anesth Analg 54:494–500, 1975.

Swan HJC, Ganz W, Forrester J, et al: Catheterization of the heart in man with use of a flow-directed balloon-tipped catheter. N Engl J Med 283:447–451, 1970.

Todd MM, Hehls DG, Drummond JC, Spetzler RF, Thompson R, Johnson P: A comparison of the protective effects of isoflurane and thiopental in a primate model of temporary focal cerebral ischemia. ASA Abstracts A412:63, 1985.

Van Aken H, Fitch W, Brussel T, Graham DI: The influence of isoflurane-induced hypotension on cerebral blood flow and cerebral autoregulation in baboons. ASA Abstract A394:63, 1985.

Weiss MH, Wertman N, et al: The influence of myoneural blockers on intracranial dynamics. Bull Los Angeles Neurol Soc 42:1–7, 1977.

Windle WF: The spinal cord and its reaction to traumatic injury. New York, Dekker, 1980, p. 69.

33

Anesthesia for Nose and Throat, Head and Neck, and Oral and Maxillofacial Surgery

Joel M. Weaver and Paul B. Oppenheimer

PREOPERATIVE EVALUATION

Preoperative evaluation of patients for nose–throat, head and neck, and oral and maxillofacial surgery is performed in the usual manner, with particular emphasis placed on the airway. Conditions such as nasal polyps, maxillary and/or mandibular fractures, tumors, trismus, hemorrhage, edema, retrognathia, and previous neck radiation and surgery may cause the anesthetist unusual difficulty in establishing and securing a patent airway. Additionally, because the airway is the common focus of attention of both the anesthetist and the surgeon, cooperation is essential for the safe anesthetic management of the patient.

Patients undergoing head and neck cancer surgery usually have chronic bronchitis, obstructive pulmonary disease, and emphysema. Preoperative evaluation of pulmonary status with arterial blood gas analysis and pulmonary function testing can help the anesthetist make decisions on appropriate anesthetic techniques and monitoring devices for such patients.

The patient should be examined for ability to open the mouth and for neck mobility. A normal distance between upper and lower incisor teeth is 35 mm for adult women and 40 mm for adult men. Patients with limited opening should be further evaluated and consultation with the surgeon is suggested to determine the etiology. An awake intubation may be necessary if a mechanical problem such as a depressed zygomatic arch fracture limits mandibular opening. Previous radiation therapy to the neck may decrease the mobility of soft tissues and certain anatomic structures, making laryngoscopy and intubation difficult. Likewise a previous cervical spine fusion or neck arthritis may also cause a decrease in neck mobility.

PATIENT POSITIONING

The head is placed in the "sniffing position" prior to induction and intubation. A 1-L intravenous fluid bag wrapped in a pillowcase or folded sheets placed under the occiput may facilitate this maneuver. Extension at the atlanto-occipital joint and flexion of the cervical spine helps to properly align the airway structures. Proper positioning prior to the initiation of surgery is important to avoid strain on the neck, particularly when the head is turned to one side or when a shoulder-roll is used to hyperextend the neck for laryngeal or thyroid surgery. Pressure points such as the elbows and heels should be padded, and a pillow should be placed under the knees. For nasal, maxillary, or sinus surgery, placing the patient at a 15- to 20-degree head-up tilt may help decrease bleeding when used in conjunction with other local methods such as topical cocaine or epinephrine. The eyes should be protected not only from dryness during anesthesia, but also from inadvertent damage from the surgeon as he or she operates near them. Lubrication with a bland ointment and taping of the lids is recommended in most instances.

Frequently the anesthetist assumes a position that is remote to the surgical site, where direct access to the airway is difficult or impossible. Problems such as a disconnection or kinking of the endotracheal tube must be anticipated and should be immediately recognized by the anesthetist, who continuously monitors breath sounds with an esophageal or precordial stethoscope and observes for proper chest expansion.

MONITORING

The standard monitoring devices used in these types of surgeries include blood pressure cuff, temperature probe, ECG monitor, and either a precordial or esophageal stethoscope. If possible, the patient's hand should be readily available to the anesthetist to permit palpation of the pulse, observation of the nail beds, and arterial blood sampling. Breath-by-breath analysis of end-expiratory CO_2 and transcutaneous oxygen and carbon dioxide monitoring provide useful information of ventilatory status, although hypotension or hypothermia may decrease the accuracy of the transcutaneous oxygen monitor. The pulse oximeter, which measures oxygen saturation noninvasively, has also become popular in recent years. Medically compromised patients or those undergoing exceptionally extensive surgical procedures may benefit from arterial cannulation for direct blood pressure and blood gas monitoring, central venous pressure monitoring, and pulmonary artery catheterization. Urinary catheterization is necessary for procedures longer than 4 hours or when monitoring urinary output is desirable.

CHOICE OF ANESTHETIC

Although there are many variables to consider in choosing a particular anesthetic technique, several generalities can be made. A rapid, smooth, and reasonably pleasant induction with O_2–N_2O–halothane is most often used for children. Patients with oral, pharyngeal, or laryngeal carcinomas usually have significant smoking histories, which may indicate the use of halothane or other volatile agents to dilate bronchioles and permit the delivery of high concentrations of oxygen. Limited cardiac reserve in some patients may indicate a nitrous oxide–oxygen–narcotic (fentanyl or morphine) anesthetic to maintain adequate cardiac output. Patients without significant cardiorespiratory disease who may be expected to experience considerable blood loss may benefit from intentional hypotensive anesthesia, utilizing deep halothane, nitroprusside, nitroglycerin, or ganglionic blockade techniques.

ESTABLISHING A PATENT AIRWAY

For adult patients who are deemed unlikely to present the anesthetist with a difficult airway problem, a barbiturate induction following preoxygenation and succinylcholine relaxation is generally utilized for endotracheal intubation. However, occasionally unexpected difficulty is encountered and the anesthetist must be fully prepared both mentally and technically to properly gain control of the airway. Various sizes and types of face masks, laryngoscope blades, endotracheal tubes, oral and nasal airways, stilets, and a functioning suction are mandatory. If nasal intubation is planned, an acute-angle metal adapter should be inserted in the tube as a connector to anesthesia tubing to maintain a low profile on the forehead. A nasal tube custom-trimmed to appropriate length and use of the acute angle connector will help prevent ischemia and necrosis of the tip of the nose. A nasal Rae tube which is pre-bent as it exits the nose and crosses the forehead is also available.

Awake Oral Intubation

In patients who seem likely candidates for difficult intubation or for whom anesthesia prior to intubation may be dangerous, awake oral intubation is one alternative. After an intravenous infusion has been established, light sedation with diazepam may be helpful to gain patient cooperation. Careful explanation of the necessity of the procedure and the steps involved will greatly enhance its smoothness and markedly decrease the amount of diazepam that might otherwise be necessary.

The oral cavity and oral pharynx should be sprayed with 4 percent lidocaine, and after several minutes a laryngoscope is partially inserted to retract the tongue. The posterior pharynx is sprayed repeatedly until the laryngoscope can be fully inserted without patient discomfort. A glossopharyngeal nerve block at the posterior tonsillar pillar may be attempted bilaterally to inhibit gagging as an alternative or in addition to topical spray. Finally, the larynx and laryngopharynx are sprayed. While the patient is holding his or her breath after a full inspiration, 2 or 3 ml of 4 percent lidocaine is instilled into the trachea via a 20-gauge needle through the cricothyroid membrane. The violent coughing that results will spread the lidocaine and anesthetize the trachea and larynx. After 2 minutes' direct laryngoscopy is accomplished, and with the patient panting like a dog to help maintain an open glottis, the endotracheal tube is inserted and the cuff inflated. Induction of anesthesia may proceed as soon as the tube is checked for proper position and is secured.

Awake Nasotracheal Intubation

Awake nasotracheal intubation can be used as an alternative to awake oral intubation. It is usually better tolerated, particularly when accomplished blindly without the use of the laryngoscope. The same local anesthetic procedures used in the awake oral technique are used for the awake nasal intubation so that direct laryngoscopy can be accomplished if needed. Additionally 4 percent cocaine is sprayed into each nostril while the patient sniffs it in. The spray is more likely to spread throughout the entire surface of the nasal mucosa than when applied with cotton applicators. Widespread vasoconstriction and subsequent shrinkage of nasal mucosal membranes will decrease the incidence and severity of nasal hemorrhage. A soft nasopharyngeal tube thickly coated with lidocaine ointment is gently inserted into the nostril that appears to be more patent or through which the patient feels he or she can best breathe. If there is no preference, the right side should be attempted first since the smooth bevel on most tubes would then slide along the nasal septum and would result in reduced frequency of turbinate or other nasal damage. If any resistance to passage of this tube is encountered, the anesthetist should not hesitate to try the opposite side. The nasopharyngeal tube not only helps apply more topical anesthetic to the exact areas where the endotracheal tube will pass but also provides insight into the patency of the passageway.

The maxillary division of the trigeminal nerve may also be blocked to provide profound anesthesia in the middle and posterior portions of the nasal passage. A 25-gauge, 1½-inch needle is inserted into the anterior palatine foramen and up the greater palatine canal, and 4 ml of 2 percent lidocaine is injected. The maxillary nerve block may also be attempted extraorally with the use of a 4-inch needle. It is inserted beneath the midpoint of the zygomatic arch and passes through skin, subcutaneous tissue, masseter and lateral pterygoid muscles, and finally through the pterygomaxillary fissure into the pterygomaxillary fossa. These procedures, also called a second division nerve block, or V-2 block, are explained in detail in dental anesthesia texts.

The nasoendotracheal tube is then lubricated and the tip is softened by the anesthetist's warm hand or by immersion in warm water for several minutes. Sterility during this process can be easily maintained if the tube is placed back in its sterile wrapper while warming. After the naso-pharyngeal tube is removed, the nasoendotracheal tube is inserted in the same manner and direction. The tube is twisted slightly so that the tip is directed toward the midline. With the patient's head elevated at the occiput into the sniffing position, the tube is slowly advanced while the anesthetist listens for breath sounds. The disappearance of breath sounds indicates that the tube has passed beyond the glottis and is in the esophagus, the vallecula, or piriform recess. The appearance of a bulge on either side of the neck produced by the tube may often be observed. The tube must be withdrawn at least 2 inches to clear the aryepi-glottic fold and is slightly twisted toward the midline again, then slowly advanced. If the tube is posterior to the glottis and advances into the esophagus, no bulge will appear. The head should be further extended so that the tip of the tube moves more anteriorly. Flexion of the head will allow the tip to move posteriorly if it is projecting too far anteriorly. As the tube approximates the glottis, the breath sounds increase in volume and pitch and the tube is ad-vanced into the trachea. If these techniques are not success-ful, direct laryngoscopy and manipulation of the tube with McGill forceps may be necessary.

Occasionally, the curve of the tube is such that the tip of the bevel may catch on the anterior commissure of the glottis. If excessive force is used to advance the tube, tracheal damage can result. By simply rotating the tube in a full circle while applying gentle forward pressure, the angulation of the tube will change, and it will easily advance unless tracheal stenosis or other pathology exists.

Nasal Intubation During General Anesthesia

Nasal intubation is necessary for many oral surgical proce-dures. The vast majority of these nasal intubations can be accomplished safely and comfortably after induction of gen-eral anesthesia.

Cocaine nasal spray and a well-lubricated, presoftened endotracheal tube of proper diameter (7.0 mm inner diame-ter and 27 cm in length for an average adult) are essential for an atraumatic procedure. The patient may be intubated under deep halothane anesthesia with spontaneous respira-tion or may be induced with a barbiturate, relaxed with succinylcholine, and intubated blindly or with direct laryn-goscopy. The technique of blind intubation in the paralyzed patient utilizes observation or palpation of the tube in the neck instead of listening for breath sounds to guide the tube. In either case, if intubation is not accomplished within a reasonable amount of time, the tube may be partially withdrawn and positive pressure ventilation accomplished by using it as a nasopharyngeal airway after the mouth and opposite nostril are closed. If ventilation is not satisfac-tory, the nasal tube should be removed and a full face mask applied for proper ventilation prior to a second nasal attempt.

Nasal intubation in the anesthetized, paralyzed patient utilizing direct laryngoscopy involves a combination of twisting the tube to orient it in the midline and flexion or extension of the head to move the tip in the proper anterior–

posterior position. McGill forceps may also be used to grasp the tube and place it into the glottis.

Nasal Intubation with the Fiberoptic Laryngoscope

The use of the flexible fiberoptic laryngoscope is particularly useful in the patient who for one reason or another has not been able to be intubated by some other method. Some anesthetists feel that it is the method of choice for awake nasal intubation. In addition to the advantage of directly viewing the patient's airway anatomy, the anesthetist can control the position of the tip of this device by rotating a knob for antero-posterior movement or by rotating the entire apparatus for side-to-side motion. Once the flexible tip is positioned in the trachea, the endotracheal tube is advanced over it in the same manner as a stylet is used in advancing an oral tube.

For successful use of the flexible fiberoptic laryngo-scope, great attention to detail is very important. Most of these devices necessitate the use of endotracheal tubes that may be rather large for some patients, and they make the tube more rigid. This increases the chances for bleeding during insertion through the nose, particularly if the patient has not been sprayed with cocaine. The blood will cover the optical portion of the tip and interfere with the view. Premedication with drying agents such as atropine, antihis-tamines, and meperidine will help prevent accumulation of secretions on it. Antifogging solution may be applied to the tip to aid visualization.

Retrograde Intubation

When all other methods of intubation fail, the retrograde technique is usually successful. A convenient method is to introduce an epidural catheter through a needle placed through the cricothyroid membrane. The catheter is ad-vanced through the larynx and into the mouth (or nasal passage). A suitable endotracheal tube is then passed over the catheter and into the trachea. The catheter is then re-moved from the neck and the tube advanced into proper position. Although the performance of retrograde intuba-tion may produce complications, e.g., tracheal damage, bleeding, infection, or false passage, it may be a safer alter-native to elective or emergency tracheostomy.

Cricothyroidotomy

When endotracheal intubation cannot be accomplished and an acute respiratory emergency requires immediate ventila-tion, a cricothyroidotomy with insertion of a small endotra-cheal tube may be lifesaving. Advantages of the procedure include ease and rapidity and a lower complication rate than a "rapid" emergency tracheostomy. A horizontal inci-sion through skin, subcutaneous tissue, fascia and cricothy-roid ligament, and membrane is made with a scalpel, and a small (4.0 to 5.0 mm) endotracheal tube is inserted into the trachea. To check for proper placement, light compres-sion of the chest will produce air flow from the tube and positive pressure ventilation can then be safely initiated.

An alternative procedure is to insert a 10-gauge catheter-over-needle through the cricothyroid membrane, removing the steel needle, and attaching the connector from a no. 3 endotracheal tube to the hub. Although such an airway is of small diameter, the insufflation of 100 percent oxygen may sustain life for a few minutes until a more permanent airway can be established under more controlled conditions.

Tracheostomy

Tracheostomy may be performed as an emergency or elective procedure under local anesthesia in the conscious patient or under general endotracheal anesthesia as an elective procedure. Conscious patients should be given oxygen and light sedation with verbal and tactile reassurance to decrease anxiety. For patients who are intubated, whether conscious or under general anesthesia, the anesthetist must usually back out the endotracheal tube to permit the surgeon to place the tracheostomy tube in the trachea. The endotracheal tube should not be entirely removed from the trachea until the surgeon and the anesthetist are satisfied that the patient is being properly ventilated via the new airway. If the surgeon is unable to properly insert the tracheostomy tube the anesthetist may need to advance the endotracheal tube past the surgical site to provide an adequate seal for ventilation. A postoperative chest film should be taken to rule out pneumomediastinum and pneumothorax.

INTRAOPERATIVE MAINTENANCE

When the anticipated duration of the surgery is at least 4 hours or when major blood loss is expected, additional preoperative preparation may include large-bore intravenous catheters, central venous pressure (CVP) measurement, intraarterial catheterization, urinary catheter, heating blanket, blood warmer units, and the use of humidified, heated, low-flow anesthetic gases. Head and neck cancer patients frequently have bronchitis and chronic obstructive pulmonary disease. Preoperative and intraoperative blood gas analysis as well as hematocrit and electrolyte data may be extremely useful. The necessity of positive end-expiratory pressure (PEEP) valves placed on the expiratory limb of the anesthetic circuit should also be anticipated for such cases if the anesthetic machine does not already have PEEP capability. Bronchodilators such as terbutaline 0.25 mg subcutaneously, aminophylline intravenously, or albuterol by spray mist into the endotracheal tube may improve compliance.

Blood loss is often difficult to judge in head and neck surgery. Surgical assistants must keep careful records of the amounts of irrigation fluid used, and sponges may need to be weighed to more accurately evaluate blood loss. Large volumes of blood may also be "hidden" in the drapes and on the floor. Tachycardia, hypotension, and reduced CVP and urine output signal the presence of hypovolemia, and corrective measures must be quickly accomplished. Close cooperation with the hospital's blood bank is essential to ensure that an adequate supply of blood products is readily available.

SPECIAL CONSIDERATIONS FOR INDIVIDUAL OPERATIONS

The following sections discuss the types of surgical procedures performed by surgeons in the head and neck region, and the special anesthetic considerations for each.

Facial Nerve Exploration and/or Reconstruction

The patient's head will be turned to the side, which may dislodge the endotracheal tube. Cloth tape that will not stretch should be used to secure the position of the oral endotracheal tube. Additional adhesive such as tincture of benzoin applied to the skin will help the tape stick more firmly. Tubes that are positioned with sharp bends will often collapse once they begin to warm and become soft. Sudden unexpected increases in airway resistance may not be due to light anesthesia or bronchospasm but rather to a kinked tube. Coiled-wire or armored tubes are often used in such instances.

Skeletal muscle relaxation is usually not required and may inhibit the surgeon's ability to identify the facial nerve with an electrical stimulator. If neuromuscular relaxation is a necessary component of the anesthetic, a peripheral nerve blockade monitor must be used to ensure that the surgeon's nerve stimulator can function properly.

Nasal Surgery

Although many types of nasal surgery are performed with local anesthesia and sedation, general anesthesia with oral intubation is quite popular. Major blood loss may occur and is difficult to quantify in the conscious patient who may swallow a considerable amount. A cuffed endotracheal tube and a moistened gauze posterior pharyngeal pack are essential during general anesthesia to help prevent aspiration, postoperative nausea, and vomiting of blood swallowed intraoperatively during light anesthesia. Anterior and occasionally posterior nasal packs are placed to control hemorrhage. The position and number of posterior packs must be known since they may become dislodged during recovery and cause respiratory obstruction. Since epinephrine is frequently used by the surgeon, the anesthetist must plan the anesthetic technique to include agents compatible with the amount of epinephrine used. For plastic reconstructive nasal surgery the endotracheal tube should be secured in such a manner that excessive pull on tissues does not cause distortion of the face. An oral pre-formed (Rae) tube or an armored tube should exit the mouth in the midline over the lower central incisor teeth and be secured with a short piece of tape to the chin. For additional security, the anesthesia circuit tubes may be taped to the patient's chest.

After an adequate oxygenation period, extubation is usually not performed until the patient can respond to verbal commands to ensure the return of protective reflexes. Since application of the full face mask may cause distortion of the unstable nose, it should not be used unless absolutely necessary. It is the responsibility of both the surgeon and the anesthetist to be sure that the pharyngeal pack is removed and the pharynx suctioned prior to extubation. A large suture placed through the pharyngeal pack and extending out of the oral cavity may act as a visual reminder that the pack is still in place.

The patient who arrives in surgery from the emergency room with continual uncontrollable epistaxis presents several special problems. Ligation of the internal maxillary artery under general anesthesia is often required. The patient is usually uncomfortable, nauseated, extremely tired, agitated, tachycardic, hypovolemic, and anemic. Because much of the blood has been swallowed, the patient should be induced by rapid-sequence induction after rehydration via a large-bore intravenous infusion line. Alternatively, an awake oral intubation may be attempted, but the increased stress to this patient may increase the amount of hemorrhage. A large induction dose of anesthetic may produce severe hypotension if peripheral vascular resistance falls despite attempts of preinduction hydration.

Laryngoscopy and Bronchoscopy

The anesthetic considerations for laryngoscopy and bronchoscopy vary with the anticipated duration of the procedure, the type of equipment used by the surgeon, and the physical status of the patient. If the procedure is only for a quick look lasting no more than 1 or 2 minutes, some anesthetists prefer a barbiturate induction and succinylcholine relaxation without insertion of an endotracheal tube or other means of ventilatory support. Hypoxia, hypercarbia, and arrhythmias may occur and have made this "apneic technique" somewhat archaic. The anesthetic is often a delicate balance between the surgeon's access requirements and proper ventilation. Laryngoscopy and bronchoscopy with ventilation is recommended.

Preoperative discussion with the surgeon and examination of x-rays may denote the size and location of the suspected pathology. Awake oral intubation by direct laryngoscopy may be necessary if the anesthetist suspects that the lesion might cause a soft tissue or ball-valve obstruction during relaxation and positive-pressure ventilation by mask. A patient who exhibits stridor and dyspnea with exertion is expected to require a smaller endotracheal tube if it is to pass beside the area of the lesion. Stridor and dyspnea at rest combined with use of accessory muscles of respiration, sternal retraction, and flaring of the nares are best managed with a tracheostomy under local anesthesia with or without light intravenous sedation prior to other procedures.

Laryngoscopy and bronchoscopy are frequently performed under general anesthesia with a small (5 or 6 mm) endotracheal tube that can be manipulated by the surgeon for surgical access. If the cuff must be deflated during bronchoscopy, increasing gas flows will generally compensate for the leak. Ventilating laryngoscopes and bronchoscopes are available that provide the patient with adequate gas exchange.

Complications of laryngoscopy and bronchoscopy include trauma to teeth if a mouth guard is not used; tracheal tear; pneumothorax, laryngeal and epiglottal edema; thick copious secretions; hemorrhage; accidental extubation during removal of the endoscope; and laryngospasm. The well-oxygenated patient should be extubated when awake to ensure the return of protective reflexes and muscular tone.

Provision should be made for immediate reintubation when necessary.

Postoperative stridor is not uncommon, particularly after a biopsy has been performed. The patient should be in a head-up position at approximately a 45-degree angle. Humidified oxygen should be delivered by face mask and the patient closely observed. Intravenous steroids and racemic epinephrine aerosol may be administered to decrease laryngeal edema. Thick copious secretions, bleeding, edema, and distorted anatomy may prevent reintubation if it is needed. Cricothyroidotomy or tracheostomy may be required.

Tonsillectomy and Adenoidectomy

Although adult patients are occasionally managed with local anesthesia and light sedation for tonsillectomy and adenoidectomy, such surgery is most often accomplished under endotracheal general anesthesia. Halothane–N_2O–O_2 inhalation induction followed by the insertion of an intravenous catheter for succinylcholine with oral intubation is the most common anesthetic technique for children, whereas thiopental induction, oxygen, nitrous oxide–narcotic–succinylcholine maintenance with an endotracheal tube is quite commonly used for adults. Extremely large tonsils, particularly those that are abscessed, may produce upper airway obstruction upon induction. Oral airways and endotracheal tubes must be inserted carefully since these enlarged tissues may be quite friable. Additionally, children between the ages of 5 and 12 are likely to have spontaneous shedding of deciduous teeth, which may be aspirated. Since reflex bradycardia and preventricular contractions during light halothane anesthesia are quite common during tonsillectomy, the ECG should be monitored closely. Bradycardia may be treated by cessation of surgery and administration of atropine. Hyperventilation, deepening the plane of anesthesia, and possible intravenous lidocaine are recommended for the treatment of ventricular ectopy.

The anesthetist must recognize that the surgeon may move the endotracheal tube during his or her manipulations so that either endobronchial intubation or extubation can result.

Considerable bleeding may occur in a relatively short period of time, resulting in tachycardia and hypotension. Blood loss, particularly in small children, should be carefully measured throughout the procedure. In healthy children a pale skin color due to peripheral vasoconstriction and tachycardia are early signs of hypovolemia whereas hypotension generally occurs later.

After surgery, the nose and throat should be carefully suctioned and the patient extubated when cough and swallowing reflexes return. Alternatively, in selected cases where bleeding is extremely well controlled, the patient may be extubated under deep halothane anesthesia. Children are placed in the lateral position with the head down to allow blood and other secretions to roll out the corner of the mouth.

Airway obstruction and continued bleeding are the two major problems of the recovery period. Airway obstruction generally responds to the usual methods of treatment, such as head position, humidified oxygen, and rarely oral airways. Bleeding may be treated with a head-up position after the patient is awake. Calming the patient with reassuring words and a gentle touch may also be helpful.

The anesthetist may need to reanesthetize the patient so that the surgeon can obtain control of a severely bleeding operative site. The patient should be regarded as having a full stomach due to excessive amounts of blood swallowed after the initial surgery. After preoxygenation, a rapid-sequence induction of a relatively small dose of intravenous thiopental plus succinylcholine with cricoid pressure is recommended only after rehydration with crystalloid or blood. It is critical for the anesthetist to consider that a hypovolemic, vasoconstricted patient may experience severe hypotension during the induction, particularly if a "usual" dose of thiopental is administered. High-volume suction should be readily available to facilitate intubation. A large-bore gastric tube should be inserted to evacuate swallowed blood and then removed prior to extubation.

Thyroidectomy and Parathyroidectomy

Hyperthyroidism or Graves' disease frequently produces symptoms of tachycardia, arrhythmias, nervousness, weight loss, peripheral vasodilation, and heat intolerance. Surgery is usually considered after treatment with propylthiouracil produces a drug-induced euthyroid state. Lack of control may predispose the patient to a thyroid storm during the manipulation associated with thyroid surgery. The tachyarrhythmias may be treated with 0.5-mg increments of intravenous propranolol. Postoperative stridor or obstruction following extubation may be caused by damage to one or both recurrent laryngeal nerves. Laryngoscopy should differentiate the subsequent vocal cord paralysis from laryngeal edema, tracheal compression from massive hematoma formation, or hypocalcemic tetany after inadvertent parathyroidectomy. Laryngeal edema may respond to vasoconstrictor (racemic epinephrine) nebulization, warmed moist oxygen mist, and steroids. A hematoma should be drained. Hypocalcemic tetany may be associated with hyperreflexia, muscle weakness, and low serum calcium levels. Slow and careful calcium replacement may be initiated by intravenous drip infusion until normal levels are reached. Reintubation in any of the aforementioned cases may be necessary.

Anesthesia considerations for parathyroid surgery differ from thyroid surgery only by the potential for high preoperative calcium levels, which may cause hypercontractibility of the heart and bradycardia. Proper medical management and recent laboratory analysis of calcium should be completed prior to parathyroid surgery.

Major Head and Neck Cancer Surgery

Extensive head and neck cancer surgery includes such procedures as supraglottic laryngectomy, total laryngectomy, pharyngectomy, radical neck dissection, mandibulectomy, maxillectomy with or without orbital exoneration, and tracheal resection.

Many of these patients have a history of alcohol or tobacco abuse, or both, and usually present with pulmonary and cardiovascular disease in addition to their cancer. Pre-

operative assessment may include pulmonary function tests, arterial blood gas analysis, chest radiographs, antibiotics for bronchitis, chest physiotherapy, and tomograms of the tumor or lesion. Previous surgery such as a supraglottic laryngectomy, radiation therapy, or a large friable tumor may cause difficulty for intubation or airway obstruction.

Anesthetic techniques that allow spontaneous assisted ventilation with high concentrations of oxygen may be an advantage during laryngectomy when a sterile spiral embedded (nonkinking) tube inserted into the transected trachea replaces the orotracheal tube. Controlled ventilation with or without PEEP may help prevent air embolism in more radical surgeries where large neck veins could be open. Sudden deterioration in vital signs accompanied by a millwheel murmur, pulmonary artery hypertension, and elevated CVP are pathognomonic for an air embolism. The patient should be turned in a left lateral position with the head down after the wound is packed with moistened gauze. Hyperventilation with 100 percent oxygen and symptomatic treatment to improve vital signs should be initiated until air can be aspirated from the right atrium.

Major blood loss should be anticipated, particularly for the longer, more radical procedures. A Foley catheter is necessary for procedures lasting 4 hours or more, when large volumes of fluid replacement are anticipated, or to monitor kidney perfusion and urinary output in patients with severe cardiovascular or renal impairment.

Pressure or manipulation of the carotid sinus may cause significant bradycardia. Immediate cessation of surgical stimulation followed by infiltration of the adventitia at the bifurcation of the carotid artery with a local anesthetic is recommended. Intravenous atropine may also be helpful if the bradycardia is severe or accompanied by hypotension.

Ligation of the internal jugular vein frequently produces cyanosis and edema of the face until alternative venous drainage develops. Postoperatively, the patient should be placed in a head-up position; diuretics with fluid restrictions may also be necessary. Cerebral edema is a potential complication in severe cases, and careful evaluation of neurologic signs and frequent temperature measurements should be performed. A temperature rise about 12 hours after surgery may indicate cerebral edema and anoxia from compression.

The CO_2 Laser and Surgical Applications

The word *laser* is an acronym for "Light Amplification by Stimulated Emissions of Radiation." Ordinary light radiates in all directions. The wavelengths interfere with each other and the energy density is low. A laser beam emits light waves that are parallel and coherent. These light waves undergo summation and create a beam of great intensity. There are no radiation hazards from the laser beam. Carbon dioxide lasers emit energy that is absorbed by any material or tissue that significantly absorbs heat. The surgical effect of the CO_2 laser results from the concentrated local absorption of heat. The major effect of the heat in living tissue is to almost instantly convert extra- and intracellular water to steam. The steam then expands explosively, separating and destroying the tissue's cells. In mucosal or respiratory epithelial tissue with a high water content (as in the upper airway) wound healing is excellent. Local edema is minimal, and there is no underlying tissue drainage. Other advantages are microscopic precision, a bloodless field, and complete sterility.

When surgery is contemplated in the upper airway, the known hazards and problems that existed prior to laser surgery are still present and must be considered. An obvious competition between the surgeon and anesthesiologist for control and space in the airway exists. A tumor may present as a pedunculated lesion that will obstruct the airway upon induction of anesthesia. It is common for a lesion to hemorrhage when traumatized by a laryngoscope blade or endotracheal tube. The resultant hemorrhage can produce ventilatory embarrassment or interfere with vision, making intubation more difficult. The lesion to be excised already may be causing clinically evident airway obstruction. Some patients with recurrent papillomas have an elective tracheostomy in place. Although an emergency tracheostomy is always a consideration, our experience indicates that endotracheal intubation by an experienced anesthesiologist or anesthetist usually provides the best and safest approach to management of the airway. Communication between the anesthesia care team and surgeon is necessary. A plan for tracheostomy must be in hand before induction of anesthesia. Of course, when a compromised airway is known to exist, the patient should receive no preanesthetic medication that would depress respiration or increase the viscosity of the respiratory tract secretions. Such medication may be given in the operating suite where equipment and personnel are immediately available should resuscitation become necessary. It also is preferable to schedule surgery for these patients as early in the day as possible.

When laser surgery on upper airway lesions is planned, the paramount problem is the hazard of fire. It is now well known that if the CO_2 laser beam strikes an unprotected portion of a rubber or plastic endotracheal tube it will burn. The polyvinylchloride (PVC) material produces an explosive fire that is generally contained in the subglottic area or upper trachea. Burning will proceed distally with a torchlike flame as the anesthesia gases pass through the fire and support combustion. Hot foreign bodies, including portions of the endotracheal tube or aluminum tape, may be blasted into the distal airway and here produce local areas of high-intensity burn. Flame may also pass proximally and burn the lips and face. The larynx may be burned by heat transmitted from the endotracheal tube. In addition, the fumes produced by burning PVC are very toxic to the respiratory epithelium. There is probably some loss of surfactant within the lung, which may lead to atelectasis. The endothelial and epithelial damage increases pulmonary capillary permeability and the potential for pulmonary edema at the alveolar level is coexistent with the loss of surfactant.

Since the anesthesia endotracheal tube must be in close proximity to the CO_2 laser beam, it is necessary to utilize measures that will diminish the probability of a calamitous fire in the patient's airway. Obviously no ideal has been found as yet because there are many options available. (See Fig. 33–1.)

Polyvinylchloride endotracheal tubes have been altered in ways to make them resistant to burning when contacted by the CO_2 laser beam. Some examples that have been

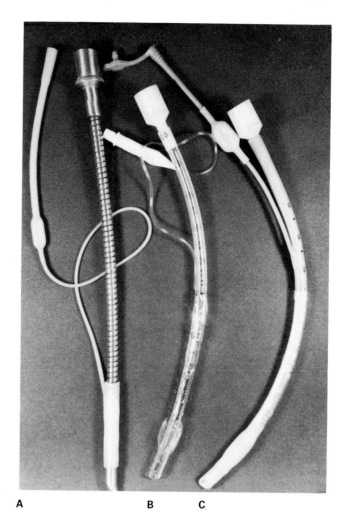

Figure 33–1. Three different types of tubes used for oropharyngeal laser surgery: **A.** Metal endotracheal tube with cuff. **B.** Red rubber endotracheal tube wrapped. **C.** Polyvinyl chloride endotracheal tube wrapped. All nonmetal tubes are wrapped with Radio Shack $\frac{1}{4}$-inch sensing foil.

used are wrapping them in muslin or aluminum foil or coating them with dental acrylic. The violent, explosive fire produced by ignition of a PVC endotracheal tube may lead to the conclusion that they should not be used in conjunction with CO_2 laser surgery of the aerodigestive tract. However, many institutions utilize this technique without any reported complications.

An alternative is the Norton tube. It is flexible stainless steel (V. Mueller Co., Chicago, Illinois). This tube is relatively nonabrasive, totally noncombustible, and reusable. The Norton tube comes close to an ideal solution but there is the problem of cuff exposure. The cuff sidearm extends proximally through the glottis where it is vulnerable to ignition. The surgeon, therefore, must pack it away with pledgets that have to be maintained in a moistened state at all times. One disadvantage is that there is less room available for surgery in an already crowded area, and the equipment is no longer noncombustible.

Another management of the airway during CO_2 laser surgery of the aerodigestive tract is to utilize a rubber endotracheal tube that has the cuff side arm integrated into the wall of the tube. The tube must be wrapped with aluminum foil (Realistic #100 44–1155 metallic sensing tape, Radio Shack) in the following manner:

1. To cover red rubber endotracheal tubes spray the tube area that is to be covered with an adhesive prior to wrapping to increase adhesion of the metallic tape.
2. Wind metallic tape (Cavitron P/N 100717 or Realistic #100 metallic sensing tape no. 44–1155) carefully around the endotracheal tube starting at its distal end or immediately proximal to the cuff. Cut a sharp bevel at the beginning of the tape (Fig. 33–2A) in order to eliminate any free edge that could cause the tape to unravel while it is in place.
3. Continue wrapping so that any portion of the tube that might be exposed to the laser is covered, generally at least 6 to 10 cm of the most distal portion of the tube. Take care to overlap the tape at least one third to one half its width at each consecutive turn and apply enough tension so that the tape does not buckle or wrinkle as it is wound (Fig. 33–2B) and there are no gaps in the wrapping.
4. After the tube has been satisfactorily wrapped, cut a sharp bevel at the end of the tape to eliminate

any possible starting point for unravelling the tape.
5. Wrapped tubes may be ethelene oxide sterilized, and the tubes may be prewrapped, sterilized, and stored for future use.
6. Inspect tubes before and after their use for possible damage or gaps in their reflector tape. If damage is observed during surgery, replace the tube immediately before continuing use of the laser.
7. Reduce intubation trauma with water-based lubricating jelly.

The selection of tape is critical. Lead tape is not acceptable. It is easily broken or melted and the vapors are toxic. There are reflective tapes available that are nonmetallic and may have the appearance of aluminum tape. They are usually mylar tapes with a thin evaporated aluminum film. Mylar tapes are reflective to light but they do not reflect CO_2 laser energy and therefore will burn. They should not be used for laser surgery. If there is any uncertainty, the tape should be tested for nonflammability with the laser. A water-based lubricating jelly may be used but lubricating with tap water is suggested. An oil-based ointment cannot be used as it could be ignited by a CO_2 laser pulse.

A smaller-than-usual endotracheal tube is used. This diminishes the possibility of mucosal trauma from the metallic wrapping. It is cuffed in adults and uncuffed in children.

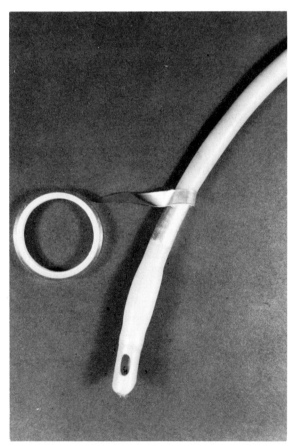

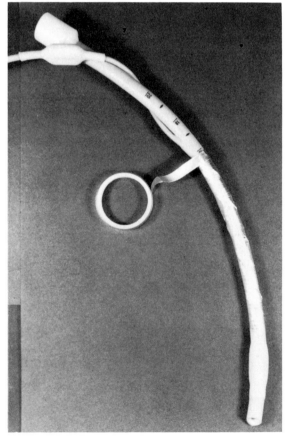

A   B

Figure 33–2. A and **B** illustrate the method for wrapping an endotracheal tube, red rubber, with Radio Shack ¼-inch sensing foil.

The size selected for the average adult is 5.0- to 6.0-mm inner diameter. The anesthesiologist or anesthetist will ultimately be stationed at the patient's side. For this reason, an angled connector is placed to avoid severe bending of the tube. The standard red rubber endotracheal tubes are known to kink and the angle connector obviates this problem.

Anesthesia is induced in a manner appropriate for the particular patient. Children are given nitrous oxide and oxygen with an increasing concentration of enflurane, isoflurane, or halothane. Succinylcholine is used to facilitate intubation. The tube is then moved to the patient's left lingual sulcus. The tube is secured with one piece of tape. This allows for rapid removal in the event of ignition. A second laryngoscopy is performed to be certain of tube placement. Only the protected portion of the tube can be observed rising from the glottis. In order to minimize exposure of the unwrapped cuff the surgeon should place wet pledgets in the subglottic area. To avoid aspiration of pledgets, strings, preferably of wire, are attached to the pledgets. It has also been advocated to fill the endotracheal tube cuff with water or saline. Ignition of the cuff then would release the fluid and squelch the fire. However, the endotracheal tube cuff can be inflated adequately with air.

The patient is allowed to recover from the intubation dose of succinylcholine. An infusion of 0.2 percent succinylcholine is started or an intermediate nondepolarizing agent is administered to ensure complete muscle relaxation during laser surgery. Any movement of the vocal cords or other structures could result in the CO_2 laser beam destroying tissue other than the lesions selected. If preferred an intermediate-acting, nondepolarizing drug may be employed as the muscle relaxant of choice. Anesthesia is maintained for the duration of the surgery. It has been widely accepted that reducing the inspired concentration of oxygen and replacing it with nitrous oxide does not diminish the hazard of endotracheal tube ignition because nitrous oxide supports combustion almost as well as oxygen. However, during in vitro laboratory experiments by Patel and Hicks, endotracheal tubes ignited with greater ease and there was more propagation of the flame as the oxygen concentration of an oxygen–nitrous oxide mixture was increased. Therefore a 30%:70% oxygen–nitrous oxide mixture is recommended.

With an admittedly small endotracheal tube in place and the patient rendered immobile with a muscle relaxant, the ventilation must be controlled manually until the operation is over and recovery from the muscle relaxation is satisfactory.

As may be expected after surgery on the vocal cords there is a predisposition to laryngospasm. For this reason ketamine probably should not be used because it tends to increase airway reflexes and laryngeal irritability.

A sign should be placed on the outside of the operating room door indicating that laser surgery is taking place inside. The CO_2 laser beam may be reflected from a metallic surface and change direction without losing any power. This presents a unique hazard to the patient and the operating room personnel. Significant injury to skin distant from the operating site is unlikely. However, the corneas of the eyes are very susceptible to injury by CO_2 laser reflexion. All operating room personnel must wear their own glasses or plain glass spectacles. Ophthalmic ointment is placed in both eyes of the patient and they are taped closed. All other tissues near the operative site are protected with moist gauze. Any pledgets and attached strings must be continuously moistened to avoid ignition with the CO_2 laser beam.

At the conclusion of surgery the patient is extubated. The integrity of the adhesive wrapping is confirmed. If any tape is missing, laryngoscopy and bronchoscopy are performed. Steroids have been advocated to prevent edema. Early postoperative laryngeal edema can occur and is usually manifested in the recovery room by inspiratory stridor and retractions. Humidified oxygen should be given routinely. Topical anesthesia of the larynx, prior to intubation, reduces the incidence of postoperative laryngospasm.

Ignition of the endotracheal tube may occur despite the best efforts to prevent it. The severity of the subsequent injury to the patient will depend on the reaction of the operating room team. Proper and timely management is needed. Following ignition the patient should be immediately extubated and ventilated with pure oxygen by mask. Anesthesia with a narcotic muscle relaxant should be continued to facilitate the necessary evaluation and management. A small endotracheal tube should be used to reintubate the patient.

The surgeon should perform a bronchoscopy and remove any remnants of the tube, tape, or other large foreign bodies. A flexible fiberoptic bronchoscope is then used to evaluate the distal airways and remove swollen particles of foreign matter. The larynx and pharynx should be examined and any shreds of tissue excised to prevent their being aspirated. A chest x-ray should be obtained as soon as possible.

In most cases it is necessary to perform a tracheostomy. High-humidity ventilation is maintained because mucous plugs may form and secretions may be aspirated. Immediate consultation with a pulmonologist is obtained. The needs of each patient will then vary with the extent of injury.

The advantages of CO_2 laser surgery on upper airway lesions make it a worthwhile mode of therapy. The severity of patient injury that may result from endotracheal tube ignition places a burden on the providers of anesthesia service to use a very careful anesthesia management.

Oral and Maxillofacial Trauma Surgery

Trauma to the face may produce fractures of the mandible, maxilla, zygoma, and associated structures. Additionally, skull fracture, intracranial hematoma, cervical spine injury, and laryngeal and tracheal damage may also be present. Preoperative assessment should include questioning about loss of consciousness, a neurologic examination, radiographs of the skull, cervical vertebrae, and chest, and identification of nasal secretions for possible cerebral spinal fluid leak.

The airway deserves careful examination. Upper airway obstruction may result from complete dislocation of the maxilla, blood, avulsed teeth, edema, and hematoma formation. Bilateral fracture of the necks of the mandibular condyles may allow the mandible and base of the tongue to drop posteriorly, causing airway obstruction. The tongue, mandible, maxilla, or all three, may need to be temporarily pulled forward until the airway can be stabilized. A towel clip placed through the body of the tongue may be a lifesaving method of pulling it forward to treat airway obstruction in such cases. Unless contraindicated by severe nasal damage, a nasoendotracheal tube is preferred, since the application of arch bars and intermaxillary fixation with wires or elastic bands is commonly used to stabilize maxillary and mandibular fractures. Laryngeal and tracheal damage may be recognized by noting hoarseness, inspiratory stridor, inspiratory retraction, and submucosal emphysema or hematoma.

Patients who are likely to have swallowed large amounts of blood should be considered to have full stomachs and induced accordingly. A pharyngeal gauze pack should be placed following intubation to absorb blood and secretions and to keep the laryngeal pharynx clear of bone fragments, broken teeth, and other debris. Removal of the pack prior to intermaxillary fixation is mandatory. Failure to remove the pack and subsequent extubation of the patient whose jaws are wired together may be a fatal error.

Mandibular fractures are often accompanied by trismus, and pain is frequently the limiting factor in the patient's inability to open normally. If the inability to open is caused by a mechanical obstruction such as a depressed zygomatic fracture impinging on the coronoid process of the mandible or in the presence of a full stomach, an awake nasal intubation is necessary. Otherwise induction of general anesthesia and nasotracheal intubation may proceed as usual. Direct laryngoscopy is not contraindicated in most mandibular fractures and will not normally further damage the fracture site, although some additional bleeding may occur.

Maxillary fractures are classified as LeFort I, II, or III, depending on the extent of the injury. A LeFort I fracture is a transverse fracture of the maxilla above the roots of the teeth. It produces a fracture segment that includes the alveolar process, portions of the maxillary sinus, the palate and lower portion of the pterygoid process of the sphenoid bone. It usually does not present the anesthetist with unusual problems. A LeFort II fracture involves the nasal bones, frontal process of the maxilla, lacrimal bones, inferior rim of the orbit, and the zygomaticomaxillary suture area. The lateral wall of the maxilla, the pterygoid plates, and the pterygomaxillary fossa are also included. A LeFort III fracture is synonymous with craniofacial dysjunction, which is the separation of the facial bones from their attachments to the cranium, including zygomaticofrontal, maxillofrontal, and nasofrontal sutures, orbital floors, ethmoid sinus, and sphenoid bones. Usually many other facial bones are also fractured. One side of the face may have one type of LeFort fracture and the other side may have another. A cerebrospinal fluid (CSF) leak may occur as a result of a dural tear in the cribriform area, and despite antibiotics given to prevent meningitis and surgical reduction of the fractures, some anesthetists prefer not to nasally intubate patients who have a CSF leak. A CSF leak, however, does not necessarily contraindicate a nasal intubation. LeFort II and III fractures may be associated with *severe* nasal damage, a contraindication to nasal intubation. If some doubt exists as to the extent of nasal damage, consultation with the surgeon and a very gentle attempt to pass a small,

lubricated, soft nasopharyngeal tube may be helpful. The nasopharyngeal tube may be used to guide a small nasogastric tube through it and into the oropharynx. The nasopharyngeal tube is removed over the nasogastric tube, which remains in the pharynx. The nasotracheal tube is then inserted through the nose using the nasogastric tube as a guide. Such a procedure may reduce the incidence of additional trauma and false passage. Obstruction to the passage of the nasopharyngeal tube or other evidence of *severe* nasal damage necessitates an oral intubation or tracheostomy. Occasionally oral intubation is chosen initially when patient cooperation is minimal. The nasal passages are then examined under general anesthesia and, if suitable, nasal intubation under direct vision is accomplished by removing the oral tube when the nasal tube is in close approximation to the glottis.

Nasal intubation should be through the naris on the side opposite from a unilateral maxillary fracture where packing the maxillary sinus and supporting the orbital floor with gauze is anticipated. For ease of removal the end of the gauze is often placed through a surgically made nasoantral fistula in the anterior portion of the nasal floor on the side of the fracture.

Massive bleeding that is difficult to isolate and control may occur as a result of massive midface trauma or upon attempts at reduction of these maxillary fractures. One or more large-bore intravenous lines and pressure bags or 50-ml syringes to facilitate rapid volume replacement should be immediately available. Bags of packed red cells may be prewarmed in water prior to being hung to facilitate rapid infusion, even when an in-line blood warmer is being used. A large nasogastric tube (18 gauge), which is less likely to clot off with blood, should be inserted prior to intermaxillary fixation and its position checked by auscultation of air in the stomach. If the tube is placed after fixation of the jaws it may curl in the pharynx and may even tie itself in a knot, which will prevent its removal through the nose.

Extubation of patients in intermaxillary fixation is most safely done when the patient is awake and is responsive to command. After a deep inspiration the tube is removed from the trachea. It may be used as a nasopharyngeal tube or may be entirely removed with suction tubing applied directly to the connector to clear the pharynx and nasal passage of blood and secretions. It may become difficult or impossible to remove the endotracheal tube if a pin, wire, or a Kirschner wire (which is drilled from a normal zygoma on one side through the nasal septum and through the fractured zygoma on the other side) pierces the tube and impales it. Extubation may be delayed for several days or more for patients with severe midface (LeFort III) fractures. When prolonged intubation is anticipated, a low-pressure, high-volume cuffed endotracheal tube should be chosen preoperatively.

Since breathing through the mouth is limited by the intermaxillary fixation and nasal breathing may be impaired by blood, edema, and the nasogastric tube, a soft nasopharyngeal tube may be helpful if increased respiratory effort is noted following extubation. This tube must be diligently cleaned every half hour because clotted blood and mucus may plug the patient's only major source of air. Postoperative restlessness and agitation must initially be regarded as signs of airway obstruction and not pain or anxiety until proven otherwise. Only then should the judicious use of tranquilizers or narcotics be considered. The nasogastric tube should be left on continuous low-pressure suction and irrigated frequently until the return is clear, an indication that hemorrhage has ceased. The time for its removal is somewhat arbitrary, depending on the type and extent of surgery, the patient's ability to tolerate it, the presence of nausea, the patient's ability to swallow, and the surgeon's judgment.

Elective Oral and Maxillofacial Surgery

The spectrum of elective oral and maxillofacial surgery includes dentoalveolar, soft-tissue, temporomandibular joint, augmentation of bony ridges and clefts, and orthognathic surgery. Incision and drainage of an abcess may be considered elective or semielective. These procedures can be managed with the patient in a semireclined position with the head and upper body at a 30-degree angle and the legs elevated and flexed at the knees. This position is particularly advantageous for minor procedures such as tooth extraction in the conscious, sedated patient who receives local anesthesia or the patient under general anesthesia where a nasal mask or nasopharyngeal tube and an oral gauze protective pack are used. When using the nasal mask, the anesthetist positions the head in the sniffing position, extends the mandible with the fingers, and holds the mask in place with thumb traction on the inhalation tubes. The Bain circuit, which is designed for spontaneous unassisted ventilation with relatively high gas flows, is ideal for this procedure. A nasopharyngeal tube may be placed under the mask for additional airway support or the nasopharyngeal tube may be connected directly to the anesthesia circuit with an acute-angle adapter. Proper positioning and support of the mandible by the anesthetist is necessary in either case.

Endotracheal intubation should be utilized if

1. Ventilation is inadequate during nonintubated cases.
2. The surgical procedure is prolonged or complicated.
3. The surgeon requests greater access to the head area with the anesthetist positioned to the side.
4. The anesthetist is inexperienced or uncomfortable without endotracheal control of the airway.

Nasotracheal intubation is most commonly used during major oral and maxillofacial surgery. Patients scheduled for temporomandibular joint surgery frequently have a mechanical limitation of jaw opening and may require awake nasal intubation. An anesthetic without skeletal muscle relaxant will permit the surgeon to electrically identify branches of the facial nerve during this extraoral procedure. Patients with a narrow palate frequently undergo rapid surgical expansion or palatal split procedures. Such patients will have narrow nasal passages, necessitating the use of small nasotracheal tubes or less frequently, an oral intubation. The nasal intubation should first be attempted through the naris opposite the side of the nasal septum along which the surgeon plans the palatal bone cut so that burs or chisels

are less likely to pierce the tube. Edentulous patients requiring bony augmentation of a pencil-thin mandible may sustain a fracture during forceful manipulation of the mandible during ventilation with a full-face mask or during intubation.

A LeFort I or II osteotomy for surgical repositioning of the maxilla may also expose the endotracheal tube to the hazard of inadvertent surgical puncture. Spontaneous assisted ventilation during this portion of the surgery is suggested should damage to the tube occur. If access to the damaged area exists, the tube can be taped or sutured. A long, large suture should be placed through the portion of the tube distal to the damage and extended through the nose onto the face. If the tube should break during extubation, the suture will permit retrieval of the distal portion. If absolutely necessary, the tube may be replaced after hemostasis is accomplished. After removal of the pharyngeal pack a small nasogastric tube or epidural catheter is inserted into the trachea through the damaged tube, which is then removed over it, and another endotracheal tube is guided into position.

Since the maxilla is richly supplied with blood, the surgeon may wish to infiltrate the area with 1:100,000 or 1:200,000 epinephrine. The anesthetist may choose anesthetic agents compatible with epinephrine or consider deliberate hypotensive anesthesia techniques such as deep halothane, nitroglycerin, or nitroprusside. Major bleeding may occur acutely as a result of downfracture of the maxilla or chiseling the pterygoid plates, possibly necessitating rapid replacement of volume through a large-bore intravenous line. A large nasogastric tube should be placed to help prevent nausea from blood swallowed during the recovery period. The patient should not be extubated until awake and responsive because intermaxillary fixation limits direct access to the airway.

A mandibular osteotomy may be a singular procedure or may be combined with maxillary surgery to treat either mandibular prognathia or retrognathia. Prognathic patients usually have a large tongue whereas retrognathic patients frequently have an anteriorly positioned larynx, which may make direct laryngoscopy and intubation difficult. The patient is placed in intermaxillary fixation intraoperatively and extubated when awake and responsive to commands. An anesthetic technique that permits smooth awakening will help prevent bucking and attempts to open the mouth. Patients who are informed of what to expect in the immediate postoperative period will be better prepared to accept the tubes and fixation appliances upon awakening. The anesthetist, recovery room nurses, and floor nursing personnel must also learn of the number and location of wires that may be used to fixate the mandible to the maxilla so that they may be cut if necessary for emergency access to the airway. Wire-cutting scissors should be taped to the head of the bed for immediate availability.

Incision and drainage of severe oral–facial infections is usually done under general anesthesia. Patients are normally febrile and severely dehydrated. Application of a full face mask prior to induction may cause excruciating pain. Trismus, large intraoral abcesses, and an elevated, swollen floor of the mouth may make ventilation or direct laryngoscopy impossible. Endotracheal tubes, oral airways, or the laryngoscope blade may cause massive intraoral drainage and aspiration of pus in the anesthetized patient. Consultation with the surgeon and examination of the patient for intraoral swelling makes awake nasal intubation the safest alternative in such situations. Tracheostomy under local anesthesia may be necessary in life-threatening cases such as Ludwig's angina if a nasal tube cannot be passed successfully.

SUMMARY

A complete preoperative evaluation of the patient's medical history, physical status, and extent of injury or disease, as well as an assessment of the controllability of the airway, are essential for the safe induction of anesthesia in head and neck surgeries of all types. Communication and close cooperation with the surgeon to establish a "game plan" is necessary. Diligent intraoperative monitoring of vital signs and functions and knowledge of the surgical procedures with attendant complications make these cases quite challenging even for the most experienced anesthetist. Finally, postoperative management of the patient with attention focused on the maintenance of a patent airway and adequate ventilation may avert serious complications during this period when there is a natural tendency to relax "now that the serious part of the operation is over." Careful attention to detail and conservative, often time-consuming, anesthetic management will increase the likelihood of both the anesthetist and the patient reaching their common goals.

REFERENCES

Baddour HM, Hubbard AM, Tilson HB: Maxillary nerve block used prior to awake nasal intubation. Anesth Prog 26:43–45, 1979.

Barton S, Williams J: Glossopharyngeal nerve block. Arch Otolaryngol 93:186, 1971.

Bennett EJ, Gundy EM, Patel KP: Visual signs in blind nasal intubation—a new technique. Anesth Rev 5:18, 1978.

Bennett RC: Monheim's Local Anesthesia and Pain Control in Dental Practice, 6th ed. St. Louis, Mosby, 1978.

Blane VF, Tremblay NAG: The complications of tracheal intubation: A new classification with a review of the literature. Anesth Analg 53:202–213, 1976.

Davies RM, Scott JG: Anesthesia for major oral and maxillofacial surgery. Br J Anesth 40:202, 1968.

Eckenhoff JE: Deliberate hypotension. Anesthesiology 48:87, 1978.

Gaisford JC, Hanna DC, Monheim LM: Endotracheal anesthesia complications associated with head and neck surgery. Plast Reconstr Surg 25:463–471, 1959.

Geffin B, Bland J, Grillo M: Anesthetic management of tracheal resection and reconstruction. Anesth Analog 48:884, 1969.

Hermens JM, Bennett MJ, Hirshman CA: Anesthesia for laser surgery. Anesth Analg 62:218–229, 1983.

Knill RL, Clement SL, et al: Assessment of two noninvasive monitors of arterial oxygenation in anesthetized man. Anesth Analg 61:582, 1982.

Kopman A, Wollman SB, Ross K, Surks SN: Awake endotracheal intubation. A review of 267 cases. Anesth Analg 54:323–327, 1975.

Lee C, Schwartz S, Mok MS: Difficult extubation due to transfixation of a nasotracheal tube by a Kirschner wire. Anesthesiology 46:427, 1977.

LeForte R (Translated by Dr. P. Tessier): Experimental study of fractures of the upper jaw. Plast Reconstr Surg 30:6, 1963.

Mason SL, Simpson GT, Mouney DF: Basic laser physics, laser soft tissue interaction and surgical applications of laser surgery. Ear Nose Throat J 61:485–489, 1982.

Norton ML: New endotracheal tube for laser surgery of the larynx. Ann Otol 87:554–557, 1978.

Norton ML, Simpson GT: Anesthesia management in laser surgery of the upper aerodigestive tract. Ear Nose Throat J 61:490–493, 1982.

Patel KF, Hicks JN: Prevention of fire hazards associated with the use of carbon dioxide lasers. Anesth Analg 60:885–888, 1981.

Raj PP, Forestner J, et al: Technics for fiberoptic laryngoscopy in anesthesia. Anesth Analg 53:708–714, 1974.

Schramm VL, Mattox DE, Stool SE: Acute management of laser ignited intratracheal explosion. Laryngoscope 91:1417–1426, 1981.

Schwartz HD, Bauer RA, Davis NJ, Guralnick WC: Ludwig's angina: Use of fiberoptic laryngoscope to avoid tracheostomy. J Oral Surg 32:608–611, 1974.

Snow JC, Kripke BJ, Strong MS, et al: Anesthesia for carbon dioxide laser microsurgery on the larynx and mouth. Anesth Analg 53:507–512, 1974.

Triplett W, Ondrey J, McDonald JS: The use of the fiberoptic laryngoscope for nasotracheal intubation—a case report. Anesth Prog 26:49, 1979.

Wainwright AC, Moody RA, Carruth JAS: Anesthetic safety with the carbon dioxide laser. Anesthesia 36:411–415, 1981.

34

Anesthesia for Ophthalmic Surgery

Paul B. Oppenheimer

The development of microscopic surgical techniques has contributed to the current trend toward use of general anesthesia for ophthalmic surgery. Improved general anesthesia techniques make possible sure control of the patient's pulse rate, blood pressure, hydration, and respiratory exchange; the patient under general anesthesia will not move or cough during a delicate microscopic procedure.

General anesthesia may be indicated for a child or for a patient who is uncooperative, emotionally unstable, extremely apprehensive, or psychotic. An emotionally stressful procedure such as enucleation or a long, uncomfortable surgery, such as repair of retinal detachment may be better performed with general anesthesia.

THE GERIATRIC PATIENT

The vast majority of patients presenting for elective ophthalmic surgery are 65 years of age or older. Although anesthesia for the geriatric patient improved greatly in the early 1980s, there are surgical risks specific to ophthamalic surgery. In ophthalmic anesthesia, exposure of the vitreous to the atmosphere presents the anesthetist with a particularly difficult problem. If the patient is allowed to buck, cough, or strain, there may be profound loss of the ocular contents, resulting in an eye to which sight cannot be restored. The anesthetist must know the basic physiology of the eye and the steps of the surgical procedure to understand when the hazard of loss of vitreous will be greatest; the anesthetist must control the depth of anesthesia to prevent unfavorable responses by the patient particularly during these time periods of increased surgical risk for loss of ocular contents.

The elderly ophthalmic patient rarely presents with an emergency; he or she has been admitted to the hospital for the saving (retinal detachment) or improving (cataract removal) of his or her vision. Because the operation is usually performed on the day after admission, there is time for only the most necessary medical evaluation.

It is preferable to have a consultation with the patient's attending physician. The anesthesia team should select the anesthetic technique, but the attending physician should give information about the patient's medical condition and provide guidance about the management of the patient's regular medications.

Virtually all the medications the patient was taking before admission should be continued until surgery, with the possible exception of diuretics. It is imperative that propranolol hydrochloride or other β-antagonists (ophthalmic solutions, which are effective β-antagonists, are widely used), digoxin, antihypertensives, hypoglycemic agents, and steroids not be discontinued for a long time before anesthesia. We try to make it a practice to administer the usual dose of propranolol hydrochloride on the day of surgery.

Elective surgery should be postponed in certain medical conditions, such as recent myocardial infarction, poorly controlled diabetes, and chronic lung disease. The latter is important because the ophthalmic patient should cough as little as possible.

Because many of the elderly are in compensated or borderline congestive heart failure and their kidneys may not be able to excrete electrolytes rapidly, an intravenous infusion of D_5W or lactated Ringer's solution with 5% dextrose must be started. Blood loss will be minimal, so the usual guidelines of fluid maintenance can be hedged toward the side of dehydration. Under certain circumstances, of course, the rate of infusion is increased. Monitors for electrocardiogram (ECG) and blood pressure are applied. Before induction, arrhythmias and hypertension are treated. With intubation, a bradycardia may decrease to a cardiac standstill or ventricular escape, so if the pulse rate is below 60 beats per minute, atropine sulfate (0.4 mg) is administered intravenously. Tachycardia should be avoided because it decreases coronary flow time and increases the oxygen requirements of myocardium. A pulse rate above 100 beats per minute may be treated with small doses of narcotic, depending on the clinical situation. If the results are not satisfactory, incremental dosages of propranolol hydrochloride (0.25 mg) are given intravenously. Patients exhibiting ventricular arrhythmias from more than one focus (coupling) should have their surgery postponed until a more extensive medical workup can be performed. Laboratory studies must be reviewed to be certain that the patient has not had a recent myocardial infarction, a digitalis (such as digoxin) intoxication, or another life-threatening situation. If the arrhythmia has a single focus, a bolus (1 mg) of propranolol hydrochloride is given. Persistence of an arrhythmia is treated with a bolus of lidocaine hydrochloride, 1 mg/kg of lean body weight, followed by an infusion of lidocaine hydrochloride (solution 0.2 percent).

Hypertension increases ventricular wall tension and results in a subsequent decrease in flow through the coronary arteries. Most of the commonly employed inhaled anesthetic agents are of themselves antihypertensive agents because they either depress the myocardium and/or dilate the peripheral vasculature. An inhalation agent administered by mask and 25- to 50-mg increments of thiopental sodium will promptly reduce the blood pressure to an acceptable level and facilitate the induction of anesthesia. The trachea should not be intubated under light anesthesia because this will produce a significant increase in circulating endogenous catecholamines, subsequently producing hypertension and ventricular arrhythmias. Fifty- to 100-mg doses of thiopental sodium are given until a total dose of 250 to 500 mg or an adequate sleep dose is achieved. The inhalation agent is continued at a low concentration, with frequent monitoring of blood pressure. This method may be time-consuming but is a gentle means of induction for a fragile elderly patient.

Laryngoscopy is performed, and the upper airway is sprayed with the standard lidocaine hydrochloride (400 mg) laryngotracheal anesthesia. An alternative to using a laryngotracheal topical anesthetic is to administer 1.5 mg/kg of lidocaine intravenously. Both procedures have been demonstrated to decrease significantly the cardiovascular response to endotracheal intubation. The lidocaine acts centrally to produce a decrease in airway reflexes. Because these patients will have assisted or controlled ventilation throughout the operation and will be extubated promptly at its conclusion, an endotracheal tube a full millimeter smaller in diameter than that ordinarily used for other types of surgery is chosen. One advantage of this technique is that less coughing can be expected in the immediate postoperative period. The tube is fixed in the usual manner, and all of the equipment is moved to the patient's side, giving the surgical team complete access to the head. The eye that is not to be operated on is taped securely, but generally no ointment is instilled; thus when the patient wakes in the recovery room, he or she will be able to see normally with the unprotected eye.

The most desirable general anesthetic technique appears to be an inhalation agent (such as halothane, enflurane, or isoflurane) supplemented with small doses of narcotic (such as meperidine hydrochloride or fentanyl) and thiopental sodium as the clinical situation dictates. This means of anesthesia delivery allows more control of anesthetic depth and patient well-being. The narcotic of choice is administered in small increments when the vital signs are stable and is titrated to achieve a respiratory rate of 8 to 10 per minute.

Unless the patient has an excessive response to the surgical preparation or incision, no more thiopental sodium should be needed following induction. Rather, the concentration of the inhalation agent is increased with careful monitoring until an appropriate anesthetic level is reached and spontaneous ventilation returns. When the patient's anesthetic state is satisfactory and as the operation progresses, the anesthetist observes the surgical procedure to ascertain when the vitreous may be exposed to the atmosphere. To assure hyporeflexion, an additional increment of thiopental sodium may be administered approximately 1 minute before this point in the procedure is reached. Thiopental sodium is an excellent hyporeflexive agent. Its effect peaks in just under a minute and it is effective for several minutes. If the vital signs are stable, a dose of 50 to 100 mg is considered to be safe and effective. This maneuver frequently will cause a short period of apnea, during which ventilation must be controlled. If the operation takes an unusually long time to complete or if the patient appears to be reacting by a decrease in compliance or increase in pulse rate or blood pressure, the dose of thiopental sodium may be repeated. It is important to achieve satisfactory spontaneous ventilation so the patient can be promptly extubated at the conclusion of surgery.

There are those few patients who cannot tolerate the recommended doses or the additional incremental doses of thiopental sodium. If, following the induction dose of thiopental sodium or when the anesthesia is deepened by increasing the concentration of inhalation agent, the blood pressure drifts down to an unacceptable level, the anesthetist may administer approximately one-third to one-half of the paralyzing dose of pancuronium bromide or 0.25 mg/kg atracurium besylate in order to permit a lighter plane of anesthesia to be utilized. Response and recovery from the muscle relaxant is monitored with a nerve stimulator. The small dose will usually allow for adequate spontaneous ventilation by the end of the operation. When the patient's ventilatory effort is not satisfactory, the muscle relaxant is easily reversed with atropine or glycopyrrolate and neostigmine or pyridostigmine. This technique provides for safe anesthesia and prevents patient movement during a critical period of the surgery.

Some patients will have to have pharmacologic intervention to increase blood pressure or pulse rate, or both. To treat hypotension, first lower the concentration of anesthetic, increase intravenous fluid flow rate, and administer 10-mg increments of mephentermine sulfate. This drug appears to have a good inotropic effect without apparent peripheral vasoconstriction. To increase the blood pressure and pulse, 5- to 10-mg increments of ephedrine sulfate are given. This drug has a potent inotropic and chronotropic effect. To increase the pulse rate alone, 0.4 mg of atropine sulfate may be administered intravenously.

Except for specific indications or contraindications, the choice of inhalation agent is unimportant. Halothane is selected for patients with bronchospastic disease. If the patient is known to have liver disease or ventricular arrhythmias or if epinephrine is going to be injected, enflurane or isoflurane may be used. It is common for the same patient to have the other eye operated on in the same week. There is no scientific reason not to repeat halothane, but for medicolegal considerations, it may be prudent to use a different agent for the second operation. If there is a medical indication, such as asthma, the use of halothane may be indicated for both operations.

A previous history of seizure activity precludes the use of enflurane. Because one of the metabolites of enflurane is inorganic fluoride ion and high levels of this ion may cause renal damage, some argue that enflurane should not be used in patients with renal disease. This determination is questionable, because the level of fluoride ion from enflurane metabolism is lower than any level known to cause renal problems when methoxyflurane was used. No difference in postoperative nausea and vomiting caused by the different agents in current use has been noted.

Ophthalmic surgery on patients with coronary artery disease has not been proved to be safer under local anesthesia than under general anesthesia. If those patients receiving local anesthesia were monitored as closely as those receiving general anesthesia, it would become obvious that the patients receiving local anesthesia also have a high incidence of sustained hypertension and arrhythmias. It has been our experience during the past 4 years that general anesthesia can be administered to more than 1000 patients with a documented previous myocardial infarction without incident. These patients had ophthalmic surgery and had a zero rate of perioperative reinfarction.

Postoperative recovery is rapid, and postoperative pain is minimal following ophthalmic surgery. An increased incidence of nausea and vomiting has been reported following eye muscle surgery. Those patients should receive an antiemetic intraoperatively or in the immediate postoperative period. All preoperative medications are resumed. The hospital stay is short. Most operations are done on an outpatient basis.

INTRAOCULAR PRESSURE

Intraocular pressure (IOP) is normally 10 to 22 mm Hg (torr). A pressure above 25 mm Hg is considered pathologic.

Many factors such as venous and arterial blood pressure, patient position, external pressure (e.g., from an anesthesia mask), intracranial pressure, coughing, straining, volatile anesthetics, muscle relaxants, and endotracheal intubation can influence IOP.

Succinylcholine

The transient muscle fasciculations that follow succinylcholine administration are considered to cause a rise in IOP by producing a sustained contracture of the extraocular muscles, thereby increasing the external pressure on the eye.

An increase in IOP occurs within the first minute, with an average peak increase to 6 to 8 mm Hg between 1 to 4 minutes and a return to control measurements by 5 to 7 minutes. This occurs whether succinylcholine is given as a single intravenous injection or as a continuous infusion. Patients with glaucoma do not appear to have an unusually exaggerated or prolonged increase in IOP.

Pretreatment with a small dose of nondepolarizing muscle relaxant or incremental doses of succinylcholine administered slowly appears to have no effect on controlling the rise in IOP.

Laryngoscopy and Endotracheal Intubation

IOP is substantially increased during routine intubation. Laryngoscopy and intubation are sympathetic stimuli and can cause rapid elevation of arterial blood pressure. A typical pressor response of 10 to 30 mm Hg can be minimized by ensuring sufficient depth of anesthesia at the time of intubation.

Various reports state that a paralyzing dose of curare or pancuronium bromide or intravenous lidocaine 1.5 mg/kg 90 seconds before laryngoscopy have been effective in attenuating the increase in IOP encountered with endotracheal intubation.

Another important aid is topical lidocaine (400 mg laryngotracheal spray) applied to the larynx and trachea.

Anesthetic Agents

Contrary to earlier data, ketamine appears to have no significant effect on IOP. It is not suitable for ophthalmic anesthesia, however, because it can produce blepharospasm and nystagmus.

Volatile inhalation agents are alleged to cause a decrease in IOP. More recent work has indicated that if adequate preoperative sedation is established before control IOP measurements are obtained, the inhalation agents will produce no change in IOP.

After vitrectomy, pressure must be maintained in the posterior chamber to keep the retina firmly against the sclera. To ensure that pressure in the posterior chamber does not diminish after termination of the procedure, any nitrous oxide used as a part of the anesthetic must be eliminated.

During cataract extraction, there is a vulnerable period during which an increase in IOP can have disastrous results. If the patient is allowed to buck, cough, or strain, there may be a profound loss of vitreous, iris prolapse, or explosive hemorrhage. The result will be an eye that is damaged beyond surgical repair.

Osmotic Diuretics

Osmotic diuretics increase plasma oncotic pressure relative to aqueous humor and produce an acute, although temporary, decrease in IOP. The most clinically useful agent for this purpose is mannitol, discussed later in this chapter.

DIABETES MELLITUS

Since Banting and Best's introduction of exogenous insulin for the treatment of diabetes mellitus, the length and often the quality of life of the diabetic patient have been improved. Along with this increased life span has come the necessity for dealing with complications of this multisystem disease that rarely were seen before 1923. Treatment of the ocular manifestations of long-standing diabetes mellitus has emerged in recent years as a new challenge for the ophthalmic surgeons.

The ophthalmic complications of diabetes are well known. Fortunately, the application of laser photocoagulation and the development of vitrectomy surgery have maintained visual function in many patients who would have otherwise become blind. Although patients whose ocular signs and symptoms can be treated reasonably effectively, the application of the treatment may be complicated by the disease in other organ systems. This makes management very difficult.

Diabetic Eye Changes

To understand the ocular changes in diabetes, it is helpful to place them on a continuum, with the basic pathologic condition being ischemia of the tissues of the eye. These changes are (1) cataract, (2) muscle palsy, (3) diabetic retinopathy, and (4) neovascular glaucoma.

Cataracts in these patients are identical histopathologically to cataracts in the nondiabetics. Although cataracts tend to occur in diabetics at an earlier age than in nondiabetics, surgical therapy is the same.

Most recent innovative therapy has been directed toward diabetic retinopathy, the leading cause of blindness in diabetics. The onset of diabetic retinopathy is apparently time related. It is usually not seen until 10 years after diagnosis of diabetes mellitus is made. It progresses from the early changes of microaneurysm formation, intraretinal hemorrhage, and retinal edema to the proliferative stage, neovascularization of the retina and optic nerve. The proliferative phases are complicated by vitreous hemorrhage and traction detachment. Vitrectomy, alone and in combination with scleral buckling, photocoagulation, lensectomy, and gas–fluid exchange, has been applied to treat these later stages of retinopathy; unfortunately, however, the functions of other organ systems are also deteriorating, increasing the surgical and anesthetic risk for these patients.

Neovascular glaucoma usually occurs in patients in the proliferative phase of retinopathy. This condition is very difficult to treat and control. Initially, drugs such as timolol maleate and diuretics are employed. The systemic effects of timolol maleate, a β-blocking agent, are discussed later in this chapter. The carbonic-anhydrase-inhibiting group of diuretics—acetazolamide, dichlorophenamide, methazolmide—is also used, and their systemic side effects are also discussed in another section. If medical therapy fails, surgical intervention may be attempted to control the process, although success has been limited. In these patients, the ophthalmologist must use drugs that may further compromise organ systems whose function is already reduced.

Anesthetic Management of the Diabetic Patient

Like management of the nondiabetic patient, anesthetic management of the diabetic patient includes a preoperative evaluation, plan of anesthetic, and postoperative care. With the diabetic patient, however, there are special problems that require extra diligence. The disease causes advanced arteriosclerosis in most patients, resulting in an increased rate of morbidity to two major organ systems during anesthesia and surgery: the heart and the kidneys. Myocardial infarction is approximately five to ten times more common in diabetics than in the general population. Renal disease commonly manifests as an infective process such as pyelo-

nephritis and often as nephrosclerosis subsequent to arteriosclerosis.

Ophthalmic surgery is usually elective, which leaves ample time to assess the medical history. The juvenile diabetic requires different management from the adult-onset diabetic, so the differentiation must be established initially. The history should include the duration of disease and means of control, with emphasis on insulin dosage and the patient's reaction to it.

After proper documentation of the patient's diabetic history, the review of systems should include a detailed workup for hypertension, angina pectoris, myocardial infarction, or heart failure. Inquire if a physician ever informed the patient of a myocardial infarction by interpretation of a random ECG strip. Silent infarction is common in the diabetic patient. Renal disease may be asymptomatic and can be assessed with a urinalysis and laboratory studies (serum creatinine and blood urea nitrogen). Vital preoperative laboratory studies to be completed for these patients include blood glucose and electrolytes, an ECG, and a chest x-ray. The serum potassium level should receive special attention because it may be depleted by osmotic diuresis. When insulin is administered, serum potassium may be further depleted by the shift of this ion into the cell. A low serum potassium level will cause an unstable myocardial membrane and produce life-threatening arrhythmias during anesthesia. The threat is more pronounced if the patient is digitalized.

The ECG may reveal a previous myocardial infarction, ischemia, or arrhythmias. The blood glucose gives a baseline for maintaining the blood glucose level between 150 and 250 mg/1000 ml. For the patient with adult-onset diabetes who has never required insulin therapy and has a satisfactory blood glucose level, no further attention is necessary during anesthesia for ophthalmic surgery.

The insulin-dependent diabetic presents more of a challenge. The patient may be using any one of a combination of insulin preparations. Regular (crystalline) insulin has an onset time of 15 minutes. It achieves maximum effect in 4 to 6 hours and has a duration of 6 to 8 hours. The intermediate insulins are insulin zinc (lente insulin) and isophane (NPH) insulin (Iletin). These have an onset of 3 hours, peak at 8 to 12 hours, and last for 18 to 24 hours. The long-lasting preparations are insulin zinc (ultralente insulin) and protamine zinc insulin (Iletin). These have an onset of 3 to 4 hours, peak at approximately 18 hours, and have a duration of 24 to 36 hours. The objective is to maintain a safe level of blood glucose to prevent damaging hypoglycemia, at the same time allowing for cellular glucose use to prevent ketoacidosis. The method of achieving this objective is, at present, controversial. Because ophthalmic surgery is of relatively short duration, the most widely accepted approach is to give one-half the patient's usual daily dose of intermediate-acting insulin in the morning. Glucose is given by intravenous infusion, 50 g every 8 hours until the patient is able to take food orally. If the operation is scheduled for later in the day, one-third of the usual daily dose is given in the morning. The blood glucose level should be determined preoperatively and again when the patient enters the recovery room.

If the surgical procedure takes longer than 3 hours,

the anesthetist may measure the blood glucose level in the operating room using Dextrostix® reagent strips. These are glucose-oxidase-impregnated paper strips that turn purple, the color developing according to the concentration of blood sugar. Outdated strips or a bottle that has been open longer than 2 months will give an unreliable reading. An intravenous bolus of 5 units of regular insulin may be given as needed to reduce blood glucose level during surgery. To increase the level, the rate of the intravenous glucose infusion is increased. Thus, during operations of long duration, the blood glucose level can be measured with the Dextrostix® method, intravenous insulin can be used to lower the blood glucose level, and an increased infusion rate can be used to increase the blood glucose level.

Most anesthetists prefer that patients with adult-onset diabetes controlled by oral medication omit their dose on the day of surgery. Although these patients usually have mild diabetes and are unlikely to experience ketosis, the stress of surgery may induce ketosis even in these patients. In these patients, insulin is required depending on the blood glucose level determination.

There are three commonly used oral hypoglycemic agents. Tolbutamide (Orinase) has a half-life of 5 hours and a duration of activity of 10 hours. Acetohexamide (Dymelor) has a half-life of 6 hours and a duration of activity of 12 to 24 hours. The third medication, chlorpropamide (Diabinese) requires special attention. This drug has a half-life of 35 hours and a duration of activity of 60 hours. It should be discontinued 48 hours preoperatively. The patient then can be managed as a mild diabetic who will probably not require insulin. If ketosis develops in the adult-onset patient, 5 units of isophane insulin or insulin zinc may be substituted for the oral agent and the patient managed on the day of surgery as previously described for the juvenile-onset diabetic patient.

Postoperatively, insulin dosage can be determined by a sliding scale depending on the degree of glycosuria. The Clinitest® method measures urine glucose, but, as with the Dextrostix® used to measure blood glucose, one must be certain that the tablets are not outdated. The following dosage is recommended every 6 to 8 hours:

Urine Glucose	Regular Insulin
1+	0
2+	5 units
3+	10 units
4+	15 units

It is important to remember that the correlation of glycosuria and blood glucose will vary from patient to patient. To adjust the sliding scale, several daily blood glucose determinations will be necessary.

The ophthalmic patient should be able to accept oral intake within a relatively short time after surgery. When oral intake is satisfactory, the patient may resume his or her usual means of diabetic control.

Studies investigating the hyperglycemic effects of anesthetic agents and their adjuncts—beginning with diethyl ether up to and including our newest agents—have proliferated. In fact, there is no agent or anesthetic technique employed at present that should be excluded or selected because of its effect on the blood glucose levels. The slight deviation from the ideal condition of mild hyperglycemia that may be caused by anesthesia is of no clinical consequence.

THE OCULOCARDIAC REFLEX

The oculocardiac reflex was first described in 1908. This term is used to designate a variety of cardiac arrhythmias that may result from manipulation of the eye. Traction of the extraocular muscles, especially the medial rectus; pressure on the globe; or traction on the conjunctiva and orbital structures stimulate the afferent component. Afferent impulses originate in the long and short ciliary nerves and subsequently traverse the ciliary ganglion, the ophthalmic division of the trigeminal nerve and trigeminal ganglion, to terminate in the main sensory nucleus of the trigeminal nerve near the fourth ventricle. The efferent limb is vagal and most often manifests in a 10 to 50 percent decrease in heart rate. Cardiac standstill, atrioventricular block, ventricular bigeminy, idioventricular rhythm, and junctional rhythm can also occur.

These arrhythmias are often going to occur during ophthalmic surgery. Since they range from benign to life-threatening situations, the anesthetist must have a regimen to deal with them.

Various methods to avoid the reflex have been recommended. Retrobulbar block is controversial because it can cause the oculocardiac reflex as well as protect against it. It also exposes the patient to hazards of hemorrhage and optic nerve injury. Preoperative atropine sulfate administered intramuscularly is not effective. Intravenous administration of atropine sulfate as surgery commences will prevent bradycardia but can cause or contribute to more serious arrhythmias.

If prophylactic measures are not an effective guard against the oculocardiac reflex, what is the best course of action? The patient must be continuously monitored with a precordial stethoscope and an ECG. At the first indication of an arrhythmia, the surgeon is asked to release all pressure or traction from the eye. The rhythm will usually return to normal within seconds. If a bradycardia persists, intravenous atropine sulfate is administered. The surgeon then is advised to continue, because the oculocardiac reflex fatigues rapidly at the level of the cardioinhibitory center. If the reflex recurs, intravenous atropine sulfate is administered again.

It is important to remember that hypoxia or hypercarbia, like any arrhythmia, can be an underlying cause of an oculocardiac reflex. Therefore, an assessment should be made of the patient's ventilatory status. Monitoring the rhythm, assessing ventilation, and rapidly responding to the initial reflex will lessen the chance of a life-threatening arrhythmia.

PHARMACOLOGY

Anesthetic agents can alter the patient's ocular physiology. Ophthalmic medications can alter the response to anesthesia. The drugs encountered most often during the interface of ophthalmic surgery and anesthesia will be discussed individually.

Timolol Maleate

Timolol maleate is a β-adrenergic blocking agent used topically for the treatment of chronic open-angle glaucoma, aphakic glaucoma, and secondary glaucoma. β-Adrenergic blocking agents have been shown to reduce IOP by reducing the production of aqueous humor by the ciliary body.

Systemic absorption of the drug does occur. Patients who receive timolol maleate should be treated anesthetically as if they were receiving propranolol hydrochloride. Extra caution is urged in patients with bronchospastic disease, heart block, bradycardia, or heart failure. The negative inotropic and chronotropic effects of anesthesia will compound those already produced by timolol maleate.

If a neuromuscular block is reversed with neostigmine methylsulfate, it may be difficult to increase a significant subsequent bradycardia with atropine sulfate in the presence of a negative chronotropic effect from timolol maleate. Therefore, neostigmine methylsulfate should be avoided in patients who are treated with timolol maleate and who are already exhibiting a bradycardia.

Acetylcholine Chloride

Acetylcholine chloride is used to produce a rapid miosis. When used topically as indicated, this drug does not produce significant cardiopulmonary effects. However, it may produce the same systemic effects as pilocarpine hydrochloride.

Pilocarpine Hydrochloride

By mimicking the action of acetylcholine chloride at the junction of parasympathetic nerve endings in the smooth muscle cells of ocular structures, pilocarpine hydrochloride causes the iris, ciliary body, and sphincter muscles to contract. The resulting miosis helps to open the trabecular meshwork in the anterior chamber angle of the eye. Fluid flows out more easily, reducing the IOP. Chronic use of pilocarpine hydrochloride may result in hypotension and bradycardia, bronchospasm, and increased bronchial secretions and salivation.

Echothiophate Iodide Ophthalmic Solution

Echothiophate iodide inactivates cholinesterase, allowing the action of acetylcholine chloride, or parasympathetic miosis. It also inhibits pseudocholinesterase, and this action has generated a controversy. Anesthetic and ophthalmic literature traditionally has described a decrease in pseudocholinesterase activity for up to 7 weeks after chronic echothiophate iodide therapy. The controversy is about whether patients should have surgery delayed for 7 weeks while they are withdrawn from echothiophate iodide therapy. Succinylcholine has been used in patients receiving chronic echothiophate iodide therapy in increasing doses up to 1 mg/kg. In these instances, the recovery time from succinylcholine may be 7 to 10 minutes, rather than the usual 3

to 5 minutes. Delay of surgery is thus not necessary, especially with the availability of immediate-acting nondepolarizing muscle relaxants.

Phenylephrine Hydrochloride (Neo-Synephrine Hydrochloride or AK-Dilate)

Ophthalmologists use phenylephrine hydrochloride topically to attain pupillary dilation. Systemic effects are rare after topical application, but constant surveillance of the blood pressure is mandatory. Reports of severe hypertension and even subarachnoid hemorrhage after instillation of phenylephrine hydrochloride ophthalmic solution have been cited. Children seem to be especially susceptible because of the effects of this potent vasopressor on their small vascular system. Therefore, the 2.5-percent solution is recommended for children.

Atropine Sulfate

Atropine sulfate may be administered preoperatively to prevent parasympathetic reflexes and to decrease oral secretions. Although some anesthesia care providers still maintain that preoperative atropine sulfate is contraindicated in glaucoma patients, this prohibition is most likely not valid. Atropine sulfate injected intramuscularly in the usual preoperative doses does not appear to affect the eye. Atropine sulfate premedication has no effect on IOP in either open- or closed-angle glaucoma. When 0.4 mg atropine sulfate is given to a 70-kg person, approximately 0.001 mg is absorbed by the eye.

Acetazolamide

Acetazolamide is a carbonic anhydrase inhibitor. It is used in acute glaucoma to depress the sodium pump process that is responsible for the secretion of aqueous humor. IOP is reduced correspondingly.

During the initial phase of treatment, acetazolamide produces a marked increase in potassium excretion, attributable to enhanced secretion in the distal nephron. Unfortunately, the cardiac instability and anesthetic implications related to a low plasma potassium are too well known. The patient population most likely to need this medication is middle-aged or older and may be using other drugs, such as digitalis, that further enhance the risk of electrolyte depletion. A patient receiving acetazolamide therapy should have the plasma electrolyte levels surveyed the night before the administration of anesthesia. If the serum potassium level is less than 3.0 mEq/L, the elective case should be cancelled until further evaluation studies can be conducted.

Osmotic Agents

The surgeon may require a decrease in the normal IOP during certain intervals of the procedure. Osmotic agents have been used to increase plasma oncotic pressure relative to aqueous humor. This produces an acute, temporary drop in the IOP, which may be advantageous when an opacified lens is removed and a new lens implanted.

After intravenous infusion of mannitol, maximum reduction of intraocular water occurs within 30 to 45 minutes, with a return to baseline levels in 5 to 6 hours. The subsequent diuresis may result in distension of the bladder, which may cause systemic hypertension under anesthesia and may necessitate placement of a urinary catheter. An osmotic diuretic also may be associated with an acute intravascular volume overload. Therefore, the anesthesia care team must evaluate the patient's cardiac status preoperatively and assess the patient's ability to tolerate a sudden increase in the circulating blood volume.

Intravenous urea will produce results similar to mannitol, but it is associated with tissue damage if extravasation occurs. Glycerol is nontoxic and is effective orally. Onset of action occurs within 10 minutes. The oncotic effect peaks at 30 minutes and lasts for 5 to 6 hours. The ocular hypotensive effect is less predictable than that of either mannitol or urea. Glycerol also increases the risk of aspiration because it may trap gastric fluid in the stomach. Isosorbide is another oral osmotic agent that is effective in lowering the IOP and is better tolerated than glycerol.

OPEN EYE—FULL STOMACH

The dilemma in dealing with a patient who has recently eaten and has sustained a severe laceration of the eye is a difficult one. There is no ideal anesthetic management of the problem. A sudden increase in IOP caused by intubation of the trachea or succinylcholine administration may lead to extrusion of ocular contents, including prolapse of the iris, lens, and vitreous. Aspiration of gastric contents will cause a Mendelson's syndrome with subsequent cardiopulmonary morbidity and even death. Striving toward prevention of one complication increases the risk of occurrence of the other. The possible loss of vision in the affected eye must be weighed against the possible loss of life. An awake intubation would safeguard the lungs and risk the eye. An increased dose of a nondepolarizing muscle relaxant would preserve the integrity of the eye but might leave the airway vulnerable for minutes before a smooth intubation could be performed. Postoperative mechanical ventilation also would be necessary. The solution lies between these two extremes.

First, consider that most of these injured patients are young and healthy. Some irreversible damage has already been done to the eye. Avoiding aspiration must be the dominating consideration, and at present, the classic "rapid sequence" induction and intubation is the most effective method.

We now know that "pretreatment" consisting of a nondepolarizing muscle relaxant prior to succinylcholine will decrease the intragastric pressure created by succinylcholine-induced fasciculations. It does little, however, to prevent the increased IOP produced by succinylcholine, which is 6 to 8 mm Hg after 1 to 4 minutes of administration. The patient has already experienced higher IOP since the injury because of pain, cough, transportation, Valsalva's maneuver, and a host of other reasons. The eye is already damaged, and a transient increase in pressure of 6 to 8 mm Hg is unlikely to have any influence on the final outcome. This increase in pressure will last only from 5 to 7 minutes. It should be mentioned that to prevent vomiting,

narcotics should not be used preoperatively. Administration of a small dose (1.25 mg) of droperidol may be useful to reduce the incidence of postoperative nausea and vomiting.

The patient is positioned on the operating table with a 30-degree head-up tilt. Oxygen is administered by mask, and care is taken not to apply pressure on the injured eye. One-fourth of the paralyzing dose of a nondepolarizing muscle relaxant is given. Three minutes are allowed to elapse. A sleep dose of barbiturate is given, followed immediately by an adequate paralyzing dose of up to twice the calculated amount of succinylcholine. An assistant applies cricoid pressure. When complete relaxation is apparent, a well-lubricated endotracheal tube is inserted and the cuff rapidly inflated. Administering a dosage of pancuronium bromide (0.15 mg/kg) or atracurium (0.5 mg/kg) or vecuronium (0.15 mg/kg) also may be a safe technique because this increased dosage may increase the onset of action of these drugs. Now the lungs are protected from aspiration of gastric contents, and little if any damage has been done to the injured eye. The anesthesia should be deepened immediately because bucking or coughing on the endotracheal tube can increase IOP as much as 30 to 50 mm Hg and cause significant detrimental changes to the affected eye.

Caution must be taken because people who receive an anesthetic with a full stomach may vomit on arousal rather than on induction. The endotracheal tube should be left in place with the cuff inflated until the patient is awake enough to protect the lower airway from aspiration of gastric contents.

LOCAL ANESTHESIA

Many types of ophthalmic surgery can be conducted under local anesthesia. A retrobulbar or peribulbar block accompanied by supplemental oxygen and sedation may be an appropriate alternative to general anesthesia. Patients receiving local anesthesia should be monitored utilizing all available parameters. An oxygen saturation monitor is particularly useful. The appropriateness of local anesthesia especially for the elderly must be carefully evaluated since many of these patients may be restless and unable to cooperate with the surgeon.

BIBLIOGRAPHY

Adams AP, Fordham RMM: General anesthesia in adults. Int Ophthalmol Clin 13:83, 1973.

Albert KGMM, Thomas DJB: The management of diabetes during surgery. Br J Anaesth 51:693, 1979.

Blichert-Toft M, et al: Influence of age on the endocrine metabolic response to surgery. Ann Surg 190:761–770, 1979.

Djokovic JL, Hedley-Whyte MD: Prediction of outcome of surgery and anesthesia in patients over 80. JAMA 242:2301, 1979.

Foulds WS: The changing pattern of eye surgery. Br J Anaesth 52:643–647, 1980.

Gordon JL: Planning a safe anesthesia for the elderly patient. Geriatrics 32:69, 1977.

Karhunen U, Jonn G: A comparison of memory function following local and general anaesthesia for extraction of senile cataract. Acta Anaesth Scand 26:291–296, 1982.

Miller R, Marlar K, Silvay G: Anesthesia for patients aged over 90 years. NY State J Med 77:1421, 1977.

Pender JW, Basso LV: Diseases of the endocrine system. In Katz J, Benumof J, Kadis LB (eds): Anesthesia and Uncommon Diseases: Pathophysiologic and Clinical Correlations. Philadelphia, Saunders, 1981, pp. 204–213.

Shiehy TW: Assessing the surgical risk in an elderly patient. Med Times 108:37, 1980.

Smith RB: Physiology and pharmacology of local anesthetics in ophthalmology and otolaryngology. Trans Pa Acad Ophthalmol Otolaryngol 29:157, 1976.

Vernon SA, Cheng H: Comparison between the complications of cataract surgery following local anaesthesia with short stay and general anaesthesia with a five-day hospitalisation. Br J Ophthalmol 69:360–363, 1985.

Weiss MF, Lesnick GJ: Surgery in the elderly: Attitudes and facts. Mt Sinai J Med (NY) 47:208–214, 1980.

Wylie WD, Churchill-Davidson HC: A Practice of Anesthesia, 5th ed. Philadelphia, Yearbook, 1984, pp. 1268–1274.

35

Regional Anesthesia

Francis Gerbasi

Regional anesthesia offers the patient a safe and effective alternative to general anesthesia for certain types of surgical and diagnostic procedures. It provides a relatively painfree state without necessitating a loss of consciousness.

Analgesia and motor blockade result from the interruption of nerve impulses before they reach and after they leave the spinal cord. This is accomplished by the administration of a local anesthetic solution at a specific site along the pathway of a nerve. Various types of regional anesthetics can be utilized and are designated according to the specific site of blockade (e.g., field blocks, specific nerve or plexus blocks, and ganglionic blocks).

This chapter discusses four major regional anesthetic techniques—spinal, epidural, brachial plexus, and intravenous regional anesthesia. The primary intent is to emphasize the administration process rather than to encompass all other related material. It is recommended that additional references be consulted along with supervised clinical experience prior to performing any of the regional anesthetics discussed.

PREOPERATIVE ASSESSMENT

The preoperative assessment of a patient about to undergo regional anesthesia should encompass three primary objectives:

1. Initially, an appropriate rapport should be established with the patient. The patient should understand the anesthetic procedure being considered, along with its advantages and possible complications. Usually, increased patient understanding will increase acceptance and facilitate the anesthetic and operative procedures.
2. Secondly, the preoperative evaluation period provides the ideal time to gain pertinent patient information. A thorough history and physical should be obtained, including information as to previous anesthetic experiences, allergies, drug therapy, and possible neurologic problems.

3. Finally, the proper anesthetic management is determined based upon the specific indications and contraindications for a given regional block in relation to the patient's condition and operative procedure.

SPINAL ANESTHESIA

A spinal anesthetic, or subarachnoid block, consists of the injection of a local anesthetic solution into the subarachnoid space, with resultant blockade of the spinal nerve roots. August Bier is credited with the first planned spinal anesthetic in 1898 but it was not until 1921, when Gaston Labat published an article dealing with eliminating the dangers of spinal anesthesia, that it became a relatively popular technique (Lund, 1983).

Advantages and Disadvantages

In selecting a subarachnoid block, as in the process of determining any anesthetic management, the anesthetist must consider the patient's emotional and physical makeup, and the needs of the surgeon.

Usually, spinal anesthesia is administered for surgical procedures performed on the lower abdomen, inguinal region, or lower extremities. It may, however, be used in certain situations for upper abdominal procedures. The degree of muscle relaxation and contraction of the bowel obtained with spinal anesthesia is unrivaled by any other anesthetic technique.

A subarachnoid block also presents certain disadvantages. The anesthetist must remember that the duration of anesthesia will be limited and that there is a statistical chance of failure associated with administration. The possibility of hypotension, resulting from sympathetic blockade, may present concerns, particularly in the patient who has preoperative hypovolemia. Also, the patient's airway and ventilation systems are not under direct control, as with general anesthesia.

Anatomy

A basic knowledge of the vertebral column and spinal cord and its surrounding structures is of the utmost importance to the anesthetist administering a spinal anesthetic. The following discussion highlights the main areas that directly relate to spinal anesthetic administration.

The vertebral column comprises four curves, two being concave anteriorly (thoracic and sacral curvature) and two being convex anteriorly (cervical and lumbar curvature). Prior to the administration of a spinal anesthetic, the lumbar curve is often modified by having the patient arch his or her back posteriorly. This modification facilitates spinal needle placement by opening the interspinous spaces. Kyphosis, scoliosis, and lordosis can represent variations in the natural spinal curvature and can make the administration of a spinal anesthetic difficult.

The initial placement of the spinal needle is determined by the specific relationship between the fourth lumbar vertebra and the top of the iliac crests. Based on the fact that these two structures lie at corresponding levels, each vertebra's location and respective interspaces can be determined. The most commonly utilized interspace is between the third and fourth lumbar vertebra. The interspaces between the second and third lumbar vertebra may also be used, but only with caution, because occasionally the spinal cord may extend to this level (Reimann and Anson, 1944; Macintosh, 1957).

To place a spinal needle in the subarachnoid space, the correct intervertebral space must be determined and the needle inserted at an appropriate angle. Each of the spinal vertebrae has a spinous process extending posteriorly. The direction in which these spinous processes extend determines, to a large extent, the angle at which the spinal needle must be inserted. The spinous process of the last four lumbar vertebrae, as compared to the other spinous processes, extends in a more horizontal plane. The spinal needle must be introduced parallel to this angle to reach the subarachnoid space (Fig. 35–1).

The subarachnoid space is contained within the vertebral canal. The vertebral canal runs vertically in the vertebral column and is bounded anteriorly by the bodies of the vertebrae and intervertebral discs. The vertebral canal is bounded posteriorly by the arch bearing the spinous process and the interspinous ligaments. The vertebral canal contains the spinal cord, spinal nerve roots, cerebrospinal fluid, and

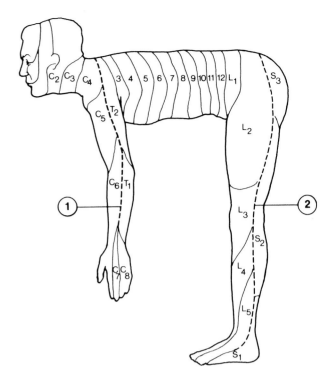

Figure 35–2. The dermatomes of the body indicating an orderly cranial to caudad sequence. Number 1 and number 2 indicate the axial lines around which the upper and lower extremities' dermatomes are distributed. (*From Foerster I: Brain 56:1, 1933. By permission of Oxford University.*)

membranes that enclose the spinal cord. Although some anatomic variations are seen, the spinal cord usually extends down the spinal canal to the level of the second lumbar vertebra. A spinal needle, therefore, *should not be inserted above the second lumbar vertebra* in order to prevent possible spinal cord damage.

If a midline approach is utilized, the spinal needle pierces various ligaments while being introduced into the subarachnoid space. These ligaments, in order of their penetration, are the supraspinous, interspinous, and ligamentum flavum. If a paramedian or lateral approach is used only the ligamentum flavum is pierced.

Spinal anesthesia results primarily from blockade of the spinal nerve roots. These spinal nerves originate from the spinal cord as the anterior and posterior roots. The nerve roots unite in the intervetebral foramen to form the spinal nerve, which then extends and divides into an anterior and posterior division supplying a specific area of the body, termed a dematome (Fig. 35–2).

Sympathetic nerve fibers run with the spinal nerves and supply various organs. Figure 35–3 indicates the sympathetic innervation corresponding to specific levels of the vertebral column. Primarily, due to the small size of the sympathetic fiber, one can anticipate the sympathetic impulses to be blocked approximately two spinal levels above the corresponding sensory block. Motor blockade usually occurs approximately two spinal levels below the sensory level (Freund et al, 1967). A decrease in blood pressure is often the result of sympathetic blockade and may indicate

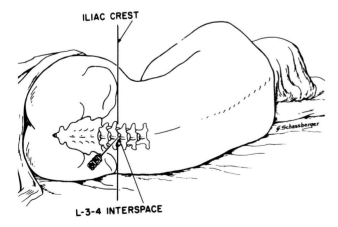

Figure 35–1. Anatomic orientation for spinal needle placement at the L3–L4 interspace. Note that the top of the iliac crest corresponds to the fourth lumbar vertebra.

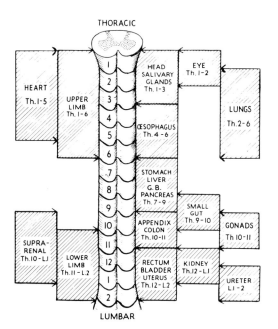

Figure 35–3. Spinal levels of sympathetic innervation. (*From Last RJ: Anatomy, Regional and Applied, 6th ed. Edinburgh, Churchill Livingstone, 1978.*)

a relatively high block if it occurs rapidly following spinal administration.

Indications and Contraindications

The indications and contraindications for a spinal anesthetic are listed in Table 35–1. Contraindications can be viewed on an absolute or relative basis. A spinal anesthetic should not be administered in the presence of an absolute contraindication. If a relative contraindication is present, one must weigh the advantages and disadvantages of the technique to arrive at the most appropriate anesthetic management.

TABLE 35–1. INDICATIONS AND CONTRAINDICATIONS OF SPINAL (SUBARACHNOID) ANESTHESIA

Indications
1. Procedures involving the lower abdomen and extremities
2. Obstetric procedures
3. Patient preference

Contraindications
Absolute
1. Anticoagulant therapy or coagulation abnormalities
2. Systemic or localized infection at puncture site
3. Allergy to anesthetic drug
4. Increased intracranial pressure
5. Presence of acute neurologic disease
6. Patient refusal
Relative
1. Chronic neurologic disorders
2. Backache
3. Headache
4. Psychological disorders

Generally, spinal anesthesia is indicated for lower abdominal procedures, such as transurethral prostatectomy or inguinal herniorrhaphy. It is particularly useful in a patient whose condition may be aggravated by a general anesthetic or in the patient who fears losing consciousness. Spinal anesthesia has been extremely useful in obstetrics for vaginal deliveries or cesarean sections, although epidural anesthesia presently is gaining preference.

Procedure

The following procedure describes the administration of a spinal anesthetic utilizing a 22-gauge spinal needle. This size of spinal needle can facilitate the procedure by providing relatively easy penetration of the tissues and aspiration of cerebrospinal fluid. However, a smaller-gauge needle (e.g., 25 gauge) may also be used and offers the advantage of a decreased incidence of postspinal headache (Greene, 1979).

The importance of adequate preparation prior to administration of a spinal anesthetic cannot be overstressed. Table 35–2 indicates some important points with respect to preparation and actual administration of the block.

As with any anesthetic technique this procedure should not be performed without the immediate availability of proper resuscitation equipment and medications. The anesthetist must remember that this is a sterile procedure; therefore, a sterile technique must be utilized. Also, in preparation the patient should receive a preload of fluid and

TABLE 35–2. IMPORTANT POINTS IN THE ADMINISTRATION OF A SPINAL (SUBARACHNOID) ANESTHETIC

I. PREPARATION
  A. Equipment
    1. Resuscitation equipment and medication immediately available
    2. Sterile gloves and prep solution
    3. Spinal anesthesia tray sterility verified and prepared for easy use
  B. Patient
    1. Explanation of procedure
    2. Vital signs obtained
    3. Appropriate position—sitting or lateral
      a. Back at edge of table
      b. Proper body alignment with support
      c. Knees and head flexed
      d. Patient relaxed
II. PERFORMANCE
  A. Landmarks identified
  B. Skin wheal raised at site
  C. Spinal needle insertion
    1. Spinal needle introduced—bevel parallel to dura fibers
    2. Needle advanced gently
    3. Frequent check for CSF
    4. Subarachnoid space identified
    5. Needle rotated 90 to 180 degrees
  D. Medication injected
    1. Needle stabilized—syringe attached
    2. Aspiration of CSF—medication injected
    3. Postinjection aspiration
  E. Needle and syringe assembly removed
  F. Patient repositioned

have blood pressure, pulse, and respirations measured and recorded.

One of the most important aspects in preparing to administer a spinal anesthetic is patient positioning. Proper positioning of the patient will ensure a good anatomic orientation and obtain maximum opening of the interspinous spaces. An assistant should be available at all times to help position and support the patient during the administration of a spinal anesthetic. I personally find that opening of the interspinous spaces can best be accomplished in the lateral position by having the patient "curl up" as much as possible and flex his or her back posteriorly. Anatomic orientation is best accomplished by having the patient assume a sitting position. This may be particularly useful in the obese patient. The utilization of a marking pen to indicate anatomic landmarks can also assist in maintaining good anatomic orientation.

There are many variations in skin preparation, each one being deemed the best by that particular individual. In general, one should prepare the skin by maintaining the standards of one's department and in accordance with sterile technique. Informing the patient of disinfectant solution application and impending needle insertion is particularly important in helping ensure against movement and will provide the patient with a more pleasant experience. Several sponges are used to remove the disinfectant solution and the area is draped to maintain sterility.

Presently, a number of spinal trays are commercially available and provide all the necessary syringes, needles, and medications to administer a subarachnoid block. The spinal tray may be prepared between application and removal of the disinfectant solution or prior to application of the solution. It should be prepared so that medications and needles can be obtained easily. The spinal tray is then placed on the side of dominance, which will facilitate maintaining the needle site with one hand while obtaining equipment with the other.

The medications are prepared using standard techniques to ensure proper identification of medications and sterility. Various agents may be used, including lidocaine, bupivacaine, procaine, and tetracaine. Table 35–3 provides dosages of tetracaine in relation to specific spinal levels. It should be noted that individual dosages may vary according to patient characteristics and operative requirements. The effect of gravity in relation to patient positioning is a very important factor in determining the spinal level achieved. If a hyperbaric spinal solution is desired, the local anesthetic agent should be mixed with 10 percent

dextrose in water solution. This may be done by combining equal volumes, on a milliliter basis, although individual variations of this ratio are often seen.

Utilizing the top of the iliac crest as a reference the fourth lumbar (L4) vertebra is located and the appropriate interspace determined. One should not go above the second lumbar vertebra. The step-by-step technique is indicated in Table 35–2. The spinal needle is introduced with the bevel parallel to the fibers of the dura, which run cephalad to caudad. This will decrease the number of transected dura fibers. As it is initially introduced, the spinal needle should be held securely; then two hands should be used to gently guide the needle inward. The anesthetist must maintain a firm understanding of the anatomic orientation during insertion. It is on this basis that one directs the needle into the subarachnoid space (Fig. 35–1).

The needle is advanced until a give or "pop" is elicited. The stylet is removed and a return of cerebrospinal fluid indicates entry into the subarachnoid space.

Occasionally, blood will be obtained upon stylet removal. Usually, this will clear after a few drops. If clearing does not occur, the needle may be repositioned until clear cerebrospinal fluid is obtained. *At no time should the agent be injected in the presence of a bloody tap or abnormally appearing cerebrospinal fluid.*

Rotating the needle 90 to 180 degrees after obtaining cerebrospinal fluid will help ensure appropriate needle placement. Then, while the needle is firmly supported, the syringe is attached. One should support the needle with one's hand, utilizing the patient's back to assist in stabilizing the spinal needle. This is a very crucial point in the technique. The importance of maintaining needle placement cannot be overstressed. Even a very slight movement may reposition the needle outside the subarachnoid space. Cerebrospinal fluid is then aspirated to confirm needle placement and the local anesthetic is injected. After injection, cerebrospinal fluid is again aspirated as an indication of efficacy and the needle/syringe assembly removed. The patient should then be repositioned according to the level desired.

Occasionally, a nerve fiber will be touched by the spinal needle, causing a temporary paresthesia that dissipates rapidly. The medication may be injected in this situation but *at no time should the local anesthetic agent be injected in the presence of persistent paresthesia.*

Management

Generally, a spinal anesthetic is administered to obtain a desired level of anesthesia. Specific factors that will influence the level obtained are (1) the specific gravity of the agent employed, (2) the volume injected, (3) the speed of injection, and (4) the patient's position immediately after administration.

Of these factors, patient positioning should be instituted immediately after injection. If a hyperbaric solution is utilized, the effect of gravity will move the medication to the lowest point of the vertebral column. If a unilateral block is desired, the patient should remain on the side to be anesthetized for approximately 5 minutes after administration. If the patient is supine, the table may be placed

TABLE 35–3. DOSAGES OF TETRACAINE NECESSARY TO ACHIEVE AN APPROPRIATE T10 ANESTHETIC LEVEL IN RELATION TO PATIENT'S HEIGHT[a]

Height (inches)	Dosage (mg)
60	10
66	12
72	14

[a] These dosages assume mixing with an equal volume, on a milliliter basis, of 10 percent dextrose–water. Please refer to text for factors that influence analgesic level achieved.

in a Trendelenberg position to increase the height of the block.

After the patient has been repositioned, the vital signs should be assessed and recorded every minute for the first 20 minutes, and then monitored every 5 minutes. Oxygen should be administered on a routine basis and significant hypotension should be treated with appropriate fluids and a vasopressor (e.g., ephedrine or mephentermine).

The patient's respirations must be closely monitored. Although an approximate fixing time of 20 minutes is expected with tetracaine, this may vary and the spinal level can rise, causing respiratory embarrassment.

The anesthetic level can be assessed, following administration, by using a large-gauge needle and touching the skin lightly to determine patient sensitivity (pinprick method). Characteristically, onset of the block proceeds in the following order: sympathetic blockade, superficial pain and temperature, motor and proprioception, and, finally, loss of sensation to touch and deep pressure. Therefore, a patient may feel the touch and pressure associated with disinfectant solution application, but is insensitive to pain.

Effective communication is essential at this time to alleviate anxiety and assess the patient's status. Symptoms of a high spinal, such as numbness in the hands or difficulty in breathing can be detected and the appropriate treatment initiated.

Duration of action will vary and depends on the dosage of agent employed, level of anesthesia, type of local anesthetic used, and the patient's age. If epinephrine or phenylephrine has been added, a clinically significant prolongation of regression of analgesia and anesthesia with tetracaine is seen (Armstrong et al, 1983).

Recovery is primarily due to diffusion and vascular absorption of the local anesthetic agent from the subarachnoid space (Green, 1983). Characteristically, nerve function will recover in reverse order of onset.

EPIDURAL ANESTHESIA

The injection of a local anesthetic agent into the posterior lumbar epidural space that surrounds the dural sac in the vertebral canal is termed epidural anesthesia or epidural block. In 1885, Corning produced the first epidural block and since that time various administration techniques have been developed. The following emphasizes the loss of resistance technique and indicates specific points of importance in its administration.

Advantages and Disadvantages

As compared to a subarachnoid block, epidural anesthesia offers distinct advantages. An epidural block has a slower onset of sympathetic blockade, which allows for compensatory vasoconstriction to occur. This may decrease the incidence of hypotension following administration. There is a greater number of agents available for an epidural block compared to a subarachnoid block, which allows the anesthetic to be tailored to the specific needs of the procedure. A distinct advantage is the absence of a postlumbar puncture headache as long as the dura has not been penetrated.

A disadvantage of the technique is its relative difficulty. *The technique requires careful administration and the importance of proper training and supervised experience cannot be overemphasized.*

Anatomy

An understanding of the anatomic relationships discussed earlier in regard to spinal anesthesia is also important in the administration of an epidural block.

The epidural space, which extends from the foramen magnum to the sacral hiatus, lies between the periosteal and investing layers of the dura. It is approximately 6 mm at its widest point and is bordered posteriorly by the ligamentum flavum (Ching, 1963). It contains the spinal nerve roots, blood vessels, and fatty areolar tissue.

The anterior and posterior spinal nerve roots pass through the epidural space, surrounded by a dural cuff, and then unite and exit through the intervertebral foramen. These nerves are characteristically less movable in the epidural space and, therefore, are vulnerable to needle trauma. It is postulated that an epidural anesthetic blocks the spinal nerves by a variety of pathways, including diffusion of the local anesthetic through arachnoid villi. The arachnoid villi are located in the dural cuff, which surrounds the nerve roots.

Another important feature of the epidural space is the demonstrable negative pressure that is encountered upon initial entry. This is believed to be caused by the transmission of negative thoracic pressure through the intervertebral foramina. The negative pressure may be utilized to locate and verify the epidural space and can promote the cephalad spread of a local anesthetic agent. An exception is noted in advanced pregnancy, where a positive epidural pressure is present (Moya and Smith, 1962).

Indications and Contraindications

Epidural anesthesia may be utilized for many types of operative and diagnostic procedures. Its popularity has increased in obstetrics due to its ability to provide a relatively painfree labor and analgesia for either cesarean or vaginal delivery.

Contraindications are similar to those associated with a subarachnoid block and are listed in Table 35–4.

Procedure

Initially, the procedure should be discussed with the patient and his or her consent obtained. Prior to administration, an intravenous cannula must be inserted and the appropriate fluid therapy initiated. The vital signs should be measured and recorded and standard resuscitation equipment should be immediately available to treat possible complications.

A standard commercial epidural tray will generally contain all the necessary equipment to administer the block, with the possible exception of the local anesthetic agent and the disinfectant solution.

A wide range of local anesthetic agents of various concentrations may be utilized. The proper selection depends on the characteristics of the block required. Some specific

TABLE 35–4. INDICATIONS AND CONTRAINDICATIONS OF EPIDURAL ANESTHESIA

Indications

1. Postoperative pain relief
2. Lower abdominal operative procedures
3. Normal- and high-risk obstetric procedures

Contraindications

Absolute

1. Anticoagulant therapy
2. Hypovolemia
3. Systemic or localized infection near needle puncture site
4. Increased intracranial pressure
5. Patient refusal

Relative

1. Inexperience with the technique
2. Active disease of CNS
3. Previous laminectomy

TABLE 35–6. IMPORTANT POINTS IN THE ADMINISTRATION OF AN EPIDURAL BLOCK—LOSS OF RESISTANCE TECHNIQUE[a]

I. PREPARATION
  A. Equipment
    1. Resuscitation equipment and medication immediately available.
    2. Sterile gloves and disinfectant solution.
    3. Epidural tray—sterility verified and prepared for easy use.
  B. Patient
    1. Explanation of procedure.
    2. Positioned appropriately.
II. PERFORMANCE
  A. Landmark identified—site selected.
  B. Disinfectant solution applied.
  C. Skin wheal raised at site.
  D. Skin pierced with 15-gauge needle.
  E. Epidural needle insertion.
    1. Epidural needle introduced.
    2. Advance gently.
    3. Increased resistance—remove stylet.
    4. Attach lubricated 5-ml glass syringe to needle—check resistance.
    5. Advance slowly, checking resistance.
    6. Epidural space identified—check for CSF or blood.
  F. Medication injection.
    1. Aspirate—introduce test dose—monitor for symptoms of spinal or toxic reaction.
    2. If negative, administer remaining dosage in incremental doses.
  G. Catheter insertion.
    1. After test dose, insert catheter 3 cm beyond needle tip.
    2. Remove needle.
    3. Tape catheter securely and attach syringe assembly.
  H. Reposition patient.

[a] Refer to text for additional information.

local anesthetic agents are indicated in Table 35–5, along with their respective dosages and approximate duration of action.

The patient is positioned and disinfectant solution applied utilizing a technique similar to that described for subarachnoid block administration. (Refer to Table 35–6 for important points in the administration of an epidural block.)

The appropriate interspace is identified according to the desired area being blocked. A skin wheal of local anesthetic is raised, followed by a secondary skin puncture with a 15-gauge needle. This helps prevent the epidural needle from removing a piece of epidermis, which could lead to a cyst formation.

Utilizing a midline approach, the anesthetist inserts an epidural needle in a median plane. The stylet must be firmly held in place during insertion to prevent possible tearing of the epidermis. Upon entry into the interspinous ligament, which is identified by increased resistance, the stylet is removed.

A well-lubricated air or normal saline filled 5-ml glass syringe is then attached and the feeling of resistance noted in the plunger. The needle is advanced a few millimeters at a time and the plunger retested. If no change in resistance is noted after continued advancement, the needle may be withdrawn and redirected. Penetration into the epidural space is identified when a distinct "pop" through the ligamentum flavum is noted associated with a loss of resistance to injection. At this point, if no paresthesia is present, the syringe is disconnected and viewed for cerebrospinal fluid or blood. If negative, a test dose of 2 to 3 ml is slowly administered and the patient is observed for signs of spinal anesthesia (Reisner et al, 1980) (e.g., numbness of the extremities); an additional 3 to 5 ml is then administered to test for intravascular injection (e.g., metallic taste, dizziness). If no adverse symptoms are noted, a loading dose is administered in incremental injections, and the needle removed. This is termed the "single administration" technique.

If cerebrospinal fluid is noted after removal of the stylet, one may elect to administer a spinal anesthetic at that time or utilize an adjacent space. Sixty milliliters of normal saline should then be administered in the epidural space at termination of the technique. This may help prevent a postlumbar puncture headache. If blood is present, the needle

TABLE 35–5. LOCAL ANESTHETIC AGENTS: CONCENTRATIONS AND APPROXIMATE DURATION OF EPIDURAL ANESTHESIA[a]

Agent	Concentrations (%)	mg/Segment	Duration (min)
2-Chloroprocaine	3	45	60
Lidocaine	2	31	46
Mepivacaine	2	31	60
Bupivacaine	0.5	7	170

[a] These dosages should be decreased in the elderly patient.

should be repositioned to ensure against intravascular injection.

Continuous epidural analgesia is obtained by insertion of a catheter through the epidural needle into the epidural space after administration of a test dose to verify needle position. Once the catheter has passed the tip of the needle, it is advanced approximately 3 cm. The needle is removed over the catheter and the catheter taped securely. *At no time must the catheter be removed from the needle after insertion due to the possibility of catheter shearing.* Prior to local anesthetic injection, catheter position should be verified by administration of a test dose to ensure that the catheter does not communicate with a blood vessel or cerebrospinal fluid. Repeat dosages of the local anesthetic agent may then be administered to maintain continuous analgesia. The repeat dosages should consist of a test dose, with aspiration before and after injection, followed by repeated fractional doses to obtain the refill dose (Covino et al, 1980).

Problems may be encountered associated with catheter placement, such as difficulty in advancement and unilateral analgesia. These may be corrected by various catheter and needle maneuvers, but at no time should the catheter be removed from the needle.

Management

Following administration the patient should be repositioned according to the procedure to be performed. In the parturient, the patient may be positioned on her left side, thus providing left lateral displacement during labor. If a lower extremity or abdominal procedure is to be performed, the patient can be placed in a supine position.

As with a spinal anesthetic, the patient's vital signs should be measured every minute for the first 20 minutes, and then monitored every 5 minutes.

The level of analgesia can be expected in approximately 20 minutes, although the time varies according to the agent employed. Generally, the shorter-acting local anesthetic agents (e.g., 2-chloroprocaine) have a faster onset than those of longer duration (e.g., bupivacaine). The level of analgesia can be determined by utilizing the pinprick technique that was previously discussed in relation to spinal anesthesia assessment.

After repositioning and initial assessment, the anesthetist must monitor the patient for possible complications such as hypotension, respiratory insufficiency, and toxic reactions throughout the procedure.

The epidural catheter is removed when analgesia is no longer required. At this time the catheter should be inspected to ensure complete removal and the findings should be documented in the patient's record.

BRACHIAL PLEXUS ANESTHESIA: AXILLARY APPROACH

The technique of blocking nerve impulses to and from the arm by injecting a local anesthetic solution into the group of nerves, or plexus, innervating the extremity is termed brachial plexus anesthesia.

Blocking of the brachial plexus can be performed in a variety of ways, for example, the subclavian, interscalene,

and axillary techniques. Each of these methods varies according to the approach utilized to reach the plexus and the extent to which the extremity is blocked (Lanz et al, 1983). Blockage of the brachial plexus by the axillary approach is discussed in the following section, with an emphasis on aspects involved in the administration process.

Advantages and Disadvantages

Brachial plexus anesthesia by the axillary approach has distinct advantages and disadvantages in comparison to the subclavian and interscalene techniques and to general anesthesia. The axillary approach has the advantage of being less disturbing to general body physiology than general anesthesia, which may be of special importance in the poor-risk patient. Postoperative nausea and vomiting are lessened and other complications of general anesthesia are avoided. As compared to the subclavian and interscalene techniques of blocking the brachial plexus, the axillary approach eliminates the risk of pneumothorax and thus is considered a safer technique. It is also impossible to block the phrenic, vagus, and recurrent laryngeal nerves or the stellate ganglia when this approach is utilized.

As with any anesthetic technique, the axillary approach has disadvantages. It has a prolonged onset time and produces less muscle paralysis in comparison to other approaches. Analgesia may be spotty and may be inadequate for surgery beyond the hand into the forearm. Complete anesthesia of the entire upper extremity is not possible, because the level of injection is made where the nerve fibers begin to leave the axillary sheath.

Anatomy

Understanding the distribution and anatomic location of the various nerve fibers supplying the arm is useful in administering an axillary block (Table 35–7). Based on this knowledge, the anesthetist can relate paresthesias elicited during needle insertion to the needle's anatomic orientation. This can help to ensure adequate analgesia to a particular area of the extremity.

The brachial plexus is an arrangement of nerve fibers supplying both sensory and motor nerve impulses to and from the arm. The nerve fibers originate from the fifth cervical vertebra (C5) through the first thoracic vertebra (T1) (Reese, 1977). The nerves leave their respective vertebral foramen and the nerve roots form three groups, termed the upper, middle, and lower trunks (Fig. 35–4). An extension of the prevertebral fascia surrounds the nerves as a multicompartmented sheath.

The upper trunk is formed by the fifth and sixth cervical

TABLE 35–7. THE MAJOR NERVES AND THEIR DISTRIBUTION IN THE ARM

Nerve	Area Supplied
Musculocutaneous	Brachial muscle
Medial	Lateral arm and thumb
Ulnar	Medial arm
Radial	Posterior arm and hand

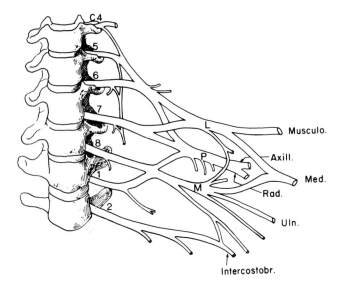

Figure 35-4. Depicts the nerve fibers composing the brachial plexus. The lateral (L), medial (M), and posterior (P) cords give rise to the musculocutaneous, axillary, median, radial, and ulnar nerves. C5–C7 also form the long thoracic nerve.

nerves. As the upper trunk progresses, it gives rise to the suprascapular and subclavicular nerves. The upper trunk then forms the lateral cord, which has two primary branches. One branch forms the musculocutaneous nerve and a second branch assists in forming the median nerve.

The lower trunk is formed by the eighth cervical and first thoracic nerves. The lower trunk progresses into the medial cord, which has two primary branches. One branch assists in forming the median nerve while a second branch forms the ulnar nerve.

The middle trunk is formed by the seventh cervical nerve. The middle trunk, along with a branch from the upper and lower trunks, forms the posterior cord. The posterior cord branches into the suprascapular, axillary, and radial nerves.

The intercostal brachial nerve, originating from the second thoracic vertebra (T2), is important due to its innervation of the proximal inner arm.

Indications and Contraindications

Axillary block of the brachial plexus is indicated for surgical procedures involving the arm and hand. It can be used to differentiate central and peripheral pain. The technique is useful for surgical procedures on patients with a full stomach, patients who fear losing consciousness, and patients with complicating conditions.

Axillary block is contraindicated in patients with active infections of the extremity due to lymphadenopathy. The block is also contraindicated in patients with coagulation disorders and in patients whose injury would prevent them from abducting the arm. The presence of a nerve injury may also be a contraindication because of legal implications. Difficulty should be anticipated in the markedly obese patient, whose axillary artery may be difficult to palpate.

Procedure

Proper preparation is very important. Table 35–8 offers a step-by-step approach for administration of an axillary block.

One should have all the necessary equipment available for resuscitation prior to proceeding with the block. If it is performed in the holding area, resuscitation equipment should be readily available. *At no time should this anesthetic technique be performed without equipment on hand for the treatment of complications.*

The specific local anesthetic agent used may vary and there is no one ideal agent. In deciding which agent to use, one must consider the duration of action needed and degree of block required. Also, one must consider the agent's potency, duration of action, toxic dosage, effective concentration, and the presence of allergies.

Table 35–9 provides a listing of commonly used agents, including their concentrations and approximate duration of action. Using a sufficient volume (40 to 50 ml) will help ensure adequate spreading of the agent, but the recommended toxic dose should not be exceeded. The use of epinephrine will prolong the action of shorter-acting agents but is of little such benefit to those of longer duration.

TABLE 35–8. IMPORTANT POINTS IN THE ADMINISTRATION OF A BRACHIAL PLEXUS BLOCK VIA THE AXILLARY APPROACH[a]

I. PREPARATION
  A. Equipment
    1. Resuscitation equipment and medication immediately available.
    2. Sterile gloves and disinfectant solution.
    3. Two 20-ml syringes, stopcock, extension, and B-beveled needle.
  B. Patient
    1. Explanation of procedure.
    2. Patient supine—arm abducted 90 degrees—Dorsum of hand by head.
    3. Anatomic landmarks noted.
    4. Disinfectant solution applied.
II. PERFORMANCE
  A. Identify landmarks—site selected.
  B. Skin wheal raised at site.
  C. Needle insertion.
    1. 22-gauge B-beveled needle inserted and advanced.
    2. Continuous aspiration performed while inserting needle.
    3. Needle enters sheath—"pop" felt.
    4. Parethesia elicited.
  D. Medication injected.
    1. Needle withdrawn slightly and digital pressure applied.
    2. Medication injected—symptoms of toxicity monitored.
    3. Medication in extension tubing left for T2 block.
  E. Needle withdrawn to subcutaneous tissue.
  F. Blockade of intercostal brachialis (T2)
    1. Needle advanced upward in axilla and medication injected.
    2. Needle advanced downward in axilla and medication injected.
  G. Needle removed and arm abducted with gentle massage of axilla.

[a] Refer to text for additional details on each point.

TABLE 35–9. VARIOUS ANESTHETIC AGENTS UTILIZED FOR BRACHIAL PLEXUS BLOCK–AXILLARY APPROACH, THEIR CONCENTRATIONS, AND APPROXIMATE DURATIONS OF ACTION

Agent	Concentrations (%)	Duration
Bupivacaine	0.5 or 0.25	Long (4–6 hours)
Lidocaine	1	Intermediate (2 hours)
Mepivacaine	1	Intermediate (2 hours)
2-Chloroprocaine	1, 2, 3	Short (1 hour)

The local anesthetic agent is drawn up into two 20-ml syringes in an appropriate dosage, and then labeled. The extension tubing and syringes are attached to a stopcock and any air is removed. The extension tubing is utilized to facilitate needle placement and injection.

Prior to proceeding with the block the patient's full cooperation must be obtained. The importance of this cannot be overstated. If the patient is aware of what is to occur, success is more likely. Prior to administration of the block, an intravenous catheter should be inserted and appropriate fluid therapy initiated. The appropriate monitoring equipment, such as cardioscope, blood pressure cuff, and precordial stethoscope should be utilized.

After the appropriate monitoring equipment has been secured and checked, the patient's arm is abducted 90 degrees and the hand placed under his or her head. The artery is then identified by palpation and appropriate landmarks noted. Removal of axillary hair may be performed at this time. Using sterile technique, the area is prepared with a disinfectant solution. The disinfectant solution is removed with a sterile sponge and the axillary artery is palpated. It is useful at this point to have an assistant manage the syringe and stopcock assembly. The artery is retracted downward by the underfinger and the needle is introduced above the artery just under the greater pectoralis muscle. A skin wheal of local anesthetic is then raised and the needle is advanced toward the axillary sheath. An assistant must keep aspirating during needle insertion to detect if a blood vessel is entered.

When the axillary sheath is entered, a distinct "pop" will be felt. One should then advance the needle until paresthesia is elicited in an area close to the surgical site. The needle is then withdrawn slightly, digital pressure is applied distal to the needle site, and the local anesthetic solution is injected slowly. One must carefully monitor the patient for any symptoms of a toxic reaction during injection. The needle is then removed to the subcutaneous tissue of the axilla and the remaining solution is injected caudad to and cephalad from the insertion site to block the intercostal brachialis nerve (T2) supplying the upper axilla. This will help eliminate tourniquet pain.

If during insertion the axillary artery is penetrated, as revealed by aspiration, the needle may be advanced dorsally, through the artery, and one half of the anesthetic agent injected. The needle is then removed until it is located ventral to the artery and the remaining half of the anesthetic agent is injected. A T2 block is performed as previously described.

After the intercostal brachial nerve has been blocked, the arm should be adducted as soon as possible and gentle massage to the axillary area utilized to assist in spreading the anesthetic agent (Winnie et al, 1979).

Variations

As is true of most other anesthetic techniques, individual variations of this technique exist. Generally, variations are adopted as the anesthetist finds his or her success rate increasing with a particular variation.

One such variation is applying a tourniquet to the upper arm, just below the axilla. This prevents the local anesthetic from spreading distally and encourages its upward movement, although digital pressure may be just as effective (Winnie et al, 1979). Also, the use of a peripheral nerve stimulator has been advocated (Montgomery, 1973). It is set at a low voltage and attached to the needle. This may assist by detecting the location of specific nerves and provides a better perception of needle positioning. This variation can cause discomfort to the patient during testing (Smith, 1976).

Following administration of the block the anesthetist must constantly assess the patient's status. Onset time varies depending on the local anesthetic agent employed, but enough time must be allowed for onset to occur. Informing the surgeon of the time necessary for onset may prevent undue stress. The first sign of onset is characterized by a loss of proprioception in the arm as evidenced by an inability of the patient to touch his or her nose. Then usually motor blockade will develop, followed by sensory blockade, depending on the agent used (Winnie et al, 1977).

Management

Adequate sedation during the procedure will help ensure effective patient management and aid in making the operation a pleasant experience. Diazepam and fentanyl are useful agents to increase patient comfort. Diazepam offers the advantage of raising the seizure threshold.

As with any anesthetic technique, the anesthetist must be aware of the possible complications and their treatment. Although this technique is considered to be a very safe means of blocking the brachial plexus, there are still some possible complications that must be considered.

Formation of a hematoma due to axillary artery puncture is always a possible complication because the axillary artery lies in the axillary sheath with the plexus. Clinically, it usually has little significance and vigorous massage of the injection site will aid in avoiding its formation. Also, intravenous or interarterial injection must be avoided due to the toxic reactions and arterial damage that may result.

Aspiration while advancing and positioning the needle will help avoid this complication.

A spotty block is always a possibility and is due to incomplete blockade of all nerve fibers within the plexus. If this occurs, additional sedation and patient reassurance may be adequate to complete the operative procedure. If not, additional local infiltration or a specific nerve block may be administered to ensure that adequate anesthesia is present.

Whatever the route of administration, the local anesthetic eventually enters the bloodstream, and the possibility of a toxic reaction is always present. Prevention, of course, should be strived for. Toxic reactions can be prevented by limiting the dosage of local anesthetic, frequent aspiration, slow administration of the anesthetic, and close monitoring of the patient. Premonitory signs, such as anxiety, muscle twitching, headache, drowsiness, and slurring of speech, may indicate an impending toxic reaction. Should a reaction occur, 100 percent oxygen should be administered with assisted ventilation. Diazepam may help by decreasing limbic system excitability and precluding focal seizure generation. Also, sodium thiopental may be utilized as an anticonvulsant. The aim in the treatment of a toxic reaction is to prevent cerebral hypoxia.

INTRAVENOUS REGIONAL ANESTHESIA

Injection of a local anesthetic agent into a tourniquet-occluded arm is termed intravenous regional anesthesia (IV regional). It is one of the oldest forms of peripheral nerve blockade and is often utilized today due to its simplicity and relative safety.

Advantages and Disadvantages

Intravenous regional anesthesia offers distinct advantages. It is relatively easy to perform as long as a step-by-step process is followed. Also, the onset of anesthesia after injection is rapid (5 to 10 minutes) and the recovery time is short following tourniquet deflation.

A major disadvantage of the technique is the limited amount of time the tourniquet can remain inflated without causing tissue damage to the extremity. Generally, the tourniquet should not remain inflated for longer than 2 hours (Kessler, 1966; Bruner, 1951), after which time it must be deflated, resulting in a loss of anesthesia.

Anatomy

The technique of administering an intravenous regional anesthetic does not require specific anatomic landmarks, as is true of spinal or brachial plexus anesthesia. It is important to note that the local anesthetic, postinjection, is distributed throughout the extremity and is thought to work at three principal sites: (1) the peripheral nerve endings, (2) the neuromuscular junction, and (3) the nerve trunk (Reese, 1981). The primary site of action is controversial but appears to be on the small peripheral nerve branches (Holmes, 1980; Urban and McKain, 1982).

Indications and Contraindications

The indications and contraindications for an IV regional anesthetic are listed in Table 35–10. It is a very useful technique for soft tissue operations of the arm or hand (e.g., ganglia removals). The block provides a bloodless field and anesthesia with a relatively rapid onset and recovery of anesthesia.

If the surgery is expected to last more than 2 hours it is inadvisable to utilize this technique. After 2 hours, the tourniquet must be deflated to prevent tissue damage. It is possible to reinflate the tourniquet and reinject but, in actual practice, this is hard to accomplish.

Procedure

Administering an effective intravenous regional anesthetic requires specific attention to details. Table 35–11 emphasizes some of the important aspects in performing the block on a step-by-step basis.

Various local anesthetic agents have been used, but only lidocaine hydrochloride is presently approved by the U.S. Federal Drug Administration (Fisher, 1980). It is effective at low concentrations (0.5 percent) and relatively safe in large volumes. A dosage of 3 mg/kg lean body weight of 0.5 percent solution is recommended.

Before proceeding with the block the anesthetist must check all equipment for proper operation. This is true with any anesthetic technique but is particularly important with an intravenous regional anesthetic. Many unsuccessful blocks can be attributed to a leaky cuff or failure of the pressure system supplying the tourniquet. Prior to the block administration, the anesthetist must pressurize the tourniquet system to ensure that no leaks are present and identify that the connections are correct between the double-cuffed tourniquet and the selection switch.

The patient is placed in a supine position and cottonwool (Webril) and a double-cuffed tourniquet are applied to the proximal aspect of the extremity. The cottonwool (Webril) should be applied wrinkle free and in an adequate amount to prevent skin damage due to tourniquet pressure. The double-cuffed tourniquet should then be applied snugly to ensure that cuff pressure is applied to as large a surface area as possible upon tourniquet inflation.

An intravenous catheter is inserted into a good-sized

TABLE 35–10. INDICATIONS AND CONTRAINDICATIONS OF INTRAVENOUS REGIONAL ANESTHESIA

Indications
1. Suturing of lacerations
2. Reduction and manipulations of fractures
3. Amputations
4. Minor external operations (e.g., ganglion removal, cyst)

Contraindications
1. Severe peripheral vascular disease
2. Infections of the extremity
3. Patient refusal

TABLE 35–11. IMPORTANT POINTS IN THE ADMINISTRATION OF AN INTRAVENOUS REGIONAL BLOCK[a]

I. PREPARATION
  A. Equipment
    1. Resuscitation equipment and medications.
    2. Double tourniquet with switch valve and inflationary device.
    3. Esmarch bandage, roller gauze.
    4. IV catheter (20 gauge), extension tubing, 50-ml syringe.
  B. Patient
    1. Standard IV insertion.
    2. Explain procedure.
  C. Positioning
    1. Patient supine.
    2. Cottonwool (Webril) applied to upper arm.
    3. Double tourinquet applied.
II. PROCEDURE
  A. IV catheter inserted and connected to syringe assembly.
  B. Extremity elevated and wrapped tightly with Esmarch bandage.
  C. Proximal cuff inflated.
  D. Esmarch removed and extremity examined for blanching.
  E. Local anesthetic agent injected—monitor for toxic symptoms.
  F. IV catheter removed (optional).
  G. Distal cuff inflated—proximal deflated (to treat tourniquet pain).

[a] Refer to text for additional information.

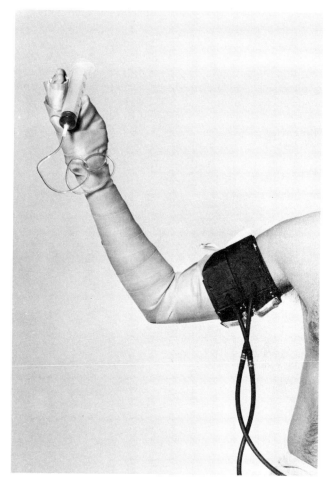

Figure 35–5. Application of double-cuffed tourniquet cuff on extremity wrapped with an Esmarch bandage.

vein using an appropriate aseptic technique. Individual opinion varies as to the best site for catheter placement but, generally, the closer the catheter site is to the operative field, the better the anesthesia will be in that specific area (Dunbar and Mazzee, 1967). Leaving the catheter in place can facilitate reinjection of the local anesthetic, but it makes placement near the operative site difficult.

One of the most important points in administering an intravenous regional block is to *ensure complete exsanguination of the extremity*. Early elevation of the limb and wrapping the extremity distally to proximally tightly with an Esmarch bandage should facilitate adequate exsanguination (Fig. 35–5).

The Esmarch bandage should be wrapped tightly up to the tourniquet and the proximal cuff inflated 100 to 150 torr above the patient's systolic pressure. A maximum pressure of 300 torr for the upper extremity should not be exceeded (Thorn and Alquist, 1971).

After the Esmarch bandage has been removed, the extremity should have a pale, blanched appearance with an absence of pulses. If this is not the case, it is advisable to rewrap the extremity to obtain better results. The presence of blood in the extremity will significantly decrease the action of the local anesthetic agent.

After the extremity has been exsanguinated adequately, the anesthetist slowly injects the local anesthetic agent while monitoring for signs of adverse reactions. After injection, the intravenous catheter may be removed and the disinfecting solution applied, in preparation for the surgical procedure. The onset of anesthesia should occur approximately 5 to 10 minutes after injection.

Management

The management of an intravenous block is similar in many respects to other regional anesthetic techniques.

Adequate sedation and effective communication will alleviate patient anxiety and help to ensure a pleasant experience.

Tourniquet pain may occur after prolonged tourniquet occlusion (Cole, 1952). Often, it can be eliminated by inflating the distal tourniquet and deflating the proximal one. This must be performed with caution. If at any time both cuffs become deflated, the block has been terminated. If this occurs one must monitor for signs of a toxic reaction caused by the bolus effect of the local anesthetic agent entering the bloodstream.

A local anesthetic toxic reaction may occur at any time but is more likely immediately after tourniquet release. The occurrence of a toxic reaction can be directly related to the duration of ischemia and the dosage and volume of medication administered. To help prevent the occurrence of a toxic reaction one should not exceed the recommended local anesthetic dosage, use a reliable tourniquet, and delay tourniquet release for 20 to 30 minutes following injection (Bier, 1967; Morrison, 1931).

To terminate the block, the anesthetist should use an inflation–deflation technique, especially if the time from injection is less than 45 minutes. The cycled deflation technique consists of deflating the tourniquet for 5 seconds followed by reinflating for 2 to 3 minutes (Merrifield and Carter, 1965). This procedure is then repeated two to three times. This will decrease the local anesthetic bolus effect associated with tourniquet release.

REFERENCES

Armstrong IA, Littlewood DG, Chambers WA: Spinal anesthesia with tetracaine—the effect of added vasoconstrictors. Anesth Analg 62:793–795, 1983.

Bier A: Concerning a new method of local anesthesia of the extremities. Arch Klin Chir 86:1007–1016, 1908. (English translation by Hellijas CS: Survey of Anesthesiology, Classical File 11: 294–300, 1967.)

Bruner JM: Safety factors in the use of the pneumatic tourniquet for hemostasis in surgery of the hand. J Bone Joint Surg 33A:221–224, 1951.

Ching D: Epidural space. Anatomical and clinical aspects. Anesth Analg 42:398, 407, 1963.

Cole F: Tourniquet pain. Anesth Analg 31:63–64, 1952.

Covino BG, Marx GF, et al: Prolonged sensory/motor deficit following inadvertent spinal anesthesia. Anesth Analg 59:399–400, 1980.

Dunbar RW, Mazzee RI: Intravenous regional anesthesia—Experience with 779 cases. Anesth Analg 46:806–813, 1967.

Fisher LB: Personal communication (Professional Information, Astra Pharmaceutical Products, Worcester, MA) 1980.

Freund FG, Bonica JJ, et al: Ventilatory reserve and level of motor block during high spinal and epidural anesthesia. Anesthesiology 28:834, 1967.

Greene NM: Uptake and elimination of local anesthetics during spinal anesthesia. Anesth Analg 62:1013–1024, 1983.

Greene NM: Present concepts of spinal anesthesia. Refresher Courses in Anesthiology 7:131, 1979.

Holmes CM: Intravenous Regional Neural Blockade in Clinical Anesthesia and Management of Pain. Philadelphia, Lippincott, 1980, pp. 343–354.

Kessler F: The brachial tourniquet and local analgesia in surgery of the upper limb. J Trauma 43–47, 1966.

Lanz E, Theiss D, Janicovic D: The extent of blockade following various techniques of brachial plexus block. Anesth Analg 62:55–58, 1983.

Lund PC: Reflections upon the historical aspects of spinal anesthesia. Reg Anaesth 8, 1983.

Macintosh R: Lumbar Puncture and Spinal Analgesia. Edinburgh, Livingstone, 1957.

Merrifield AJ, Carter SJ: Intravenous regional anesthesia—Lignocaine blood levels. Anaesthesia 20:287–293, 1965.

Montgomery SJ: The use of the nerve stimulator with standard unsheathed needles in nerve blockade. Anesth Analg 52:827–831, 1973.

Morrison JT: Intravenous local anesthesia, Br J Surg 18:642–647, 1931.

Moya F, Smith B: Spinal anesthesia for cesarean section: Clinical and biochemical studies of effects on maternal physiology. JAMA 179:609, 1962.

Reese C: Conduction anesthesia of the upper extremity—A literature and technique review. AANA J 269, June, 1977.

Reese C: Intravenous regional conduction anesthesia—A technique and literature review—Part I. AANA J 357–373, August 1981.

Reimann AF, Anson BJ: The spinal cord and meninges. Anat Rec 88:127, 1944.

Reisner LS, Hockman BN, Plumer MH: Persistent neurologic deficit and adhesive arachnoiditis following intrathecal 2-chloroprocaine injection. Anesth Analg 59:452–454, 1980.

Smith BL: Efficacy of a nerve stimulator in regional analgesia experience in a resident training programme. Anaesthesia 31:778–782, 1976.

Thompson G, Rorie D: Functional anatomy of the brachial plexus sheaths. Anesthesiology 59:117–122, 1983.

Thorn, Alquist AM: Intravenous regional anaesthesia—A seven year survey. Acta Anaesth Scand 15:23–32, 1971.

Urban B, McKain C: Onset and progression of intravenous regional anesthesia with dilute lidocaine. Anesth Analg 61:834–838, 1982.

Winnie AP, Tay C, et al: Pharmacokinetics of local anesthetics during plexus blocks. Anesth Analg 56:852–862, 1977.

Winnie A, Radenjic R, et al: Factors influencing distribution of local anesthetic injected into the brachial plexus sheath. Anesth Analg 58:225–233, 1979.

BIBLIOGRAPHY

Abouleish E: Pain Control in Obstetrics. Philadelphia, Lippincott, 1977.

Bromage PR: Epidural Analgesia. Philadelphia, Saunders, 1978.

Greene NM: Physiology of Spinal Anesthesia, 3rd ed. Baltimore, Williams & Wilkins, 1981.

Lund PC: The Principles and Practice of Spinal Anesthesia. Springfield, IL, Thomas, 1971.

Moore DC, Regional Block, 4th ed. Springfield, IL, Thomas, 1965.

Part VII
SPECIAL PROBLEMS

36

Malignant Hyperthermia

Jeanette Peter

Malignant hyperthermia (MH) is a rare but potentially fatal complication of anesthesia. It is an inherited condition involving the muscle. During an MH episode the skeletal muscle reacts abnormally to a triggering agent (usually an anesthetic drug) with an uncontrollable increase in muscle metabolism and heat production.

Historically, the first description of MH as a clinical syndrome appeared in 1960. The case report described a 21-year-old patient about to have surgery, who was extremely concerned about the risks of general anesthesia because several of his relatives had died as a result of ether anesthesia. The young man developed MH and survived. This report of the episode characterized by fever, tachycardia, tachypnea, and cyanosis focused the awareness of anesthetists on this rare syndrome. About the same time, Britt and Kalow became aware of a Wisconsin family in which 30 members had died in conjunction with general anesthesia. The Wisconsin area subsequently provided a large gene pool for Britt's study on the inheritance of MH.

It is likely that MH occurred prior to the sixties, but episodes were probably attributed to more commonly recognized causes of hyperthermia or misdiagnosed as "anesthetic convulsions."

The term malignant hyperthermia came into use because of the tremendous heat production that may occur. Body temperature may rise as much as 1C every 5 minutes. The use of the word malignant refers to the fulminating nature of the condition, which rapidly becomes fatal if vigorous therapy is not initiated.

INCIDENCE

Malignant hyperthermia is the most common cause of anesthetic-induced death in North America. The incidence of MH is about 1 in 15,000 for children, to 1 in 50,000 for adults. The ages recorded range from 2 months to 78 years old. The highest incidence is between the ages of 3 and 30 years. All racial groups have been affected. Males are more commonly affected than females; but this statistic may reflect the greater number of males presenting for surgery related to trauma. The mortality rate, originally about 60 percent, has decreased to about 7 percent in the 1980s.

Britt attributes this 7 percent mortality to errors of management, stating that appropriate treatment of MH should result in 100 percent survival.

Malignant hyperthermia is a pharmacogenetic disorder. The clinical manifestations follow the administration of a depolarizing muscle relaxant (usually succinylcholine) or any potent inhalational agent. Sympathomimetics and parasympatholytics increase the severity of already established reactions. There have been a few reports of large volumes of amide local anesthetics triggering MH reactions, usually in conjunction with a sympathomimetic (Table 36–1).

Wingard, in reviewing MH susceptible (MHS) families, found a higher incidence of sudden death and an increased incidence of automobile accidents in MHS families. (In one family the MHS child always became rigid when riding in a car.) Wingard proposed that stress and its associated sympathetic responses may induce human MH. He made the following observations:

1. MH is not always associated with a fulminant fever.
2. Most MHS patients can at one time be anesthetized with the so-called contraindicated drugs without developing MH.
3. Sometimes cases of MH are not recognized until the postoperative period when the major effects of anesthesia are no longer an important consideration.

Gronert, et al, reported a patient, confirmed to be MHS by muscle biopsy, in whom they recognized an MH-like stress-induced reaction. The patient was never hospitalized, never anesthetized, and was not taking drugs. Gronert successfully treated the patient with dantrolene, which relieved the symptoms. The above inconsistencies and observations led Wingard to suggest that one of the additional factors involved in triggering MH is stress.

A condition similar to human MH was recognized by swine breeders in certain strains of pigs. The stresses related to slaughter caused accelerated metabolism and deterioration of the muscle of these pigs, resulting in the production of pale, soft exudative (PSE) pork. The incidence of PSE animals increased with inbreeding designed to develop fast-

TABLE 36–1. ANESTHETIC AGENTS ASSOCIATED WITH MALIGNANT HYPERTHERMIA

Halothane (60% of cases)
Succinylcholine (77% of cases)
Enflurane
Isoflurane
Methoxyflurane
Trichloroethylene
Chloroform
Diethyl ether
Ethylene
Cyclopropane
Ethyl chloride
Lidocaine (large volumes)
Mepivacaine (large volumes)

Adapted from Ryan, JF: ASA Refresher Courses in Anesthesiology, 1976. Courtesy of the author.

growing, heavily muscled pigs. Any stress to which these pigs were subjected, such as separation, weaning, shipping, fighting, coitus, or slaughter resulted in increased metabolism, acidosis, muscle rigidity, high temperature, and death. This led to the term porcine stress syndrome (PSS).

In 1966, Hall described the development of fatal hyperthermia with muscle rigidity after the administration of succinylcholine to pigs. Since this time, strains of Landrace, Poland China, and Pietrain pigs have provided a suitable animal model for the systematic study of MH. Although there are some minor differences between porcine and human MH, the study of porcine MH has provided valuable information relating to the pathophysiology and clinical management of human patients with MH.

INHERITANCE

The inheritance of MH is more complicated than originally thought. MH is a complex genetic disease with phenotypic variations. It is triggered by environmental stress factors, anesthetic agents, and some muscle relaxants.

The variety of malignant hyperthermic responses has led those studying the inheritance of MH to propose the possibility of several routes of genetic transmission. The pattern of inheritance seems to range from dominant to recessive with graded variations in between, possibly involving more than one gene or more than one allele.

Multifactorial inheritance involving more than one gene has been supported by familial studies. Investigators found patterns of inheritance (confirmed by muscle biopsy) to affect both sexes of each generation, some as autosomal dominant. Studies of other families showed multifactorial inheritance involving more than one gene. These individuals tend to be the average of their parents, with gradations of susceptibility among family members.

Kalow and Britt compiled data supportive of genetic complexities. They correlated the severity of MH reactions with muscle specimen contracture tests. They found that the muscle specimen of those who had the most severe clinical episode reacted to halothane alone; the muscle of those who had less severe reactions reacted to caffeine alone but not to halothane; and in those who had the least severe

MH episode, the muscle reacted to a caffeine-halothane mixture but not to either alone. These same investigators used the pig model to study patterns of inheritance by conducting a breeding program over three generations. They identified susceptible pigs by responses to halothane in vivo and by responses of skeletal muscle fascicles to caffeine and caffeine-halothane in vitro. The following observations were made: (1) The trait occurred in all animals of the second generation, in contradiction to earlier theories that MH is transmitted by a single recessive gene. (2) The offspring of both the second and third generation reacted like the mean of their parents, thus ruling out transmission by a single Mendelian trait (single dominant gene). (3) Five rather than three genotypes were identified, thus demonstrating inheritance involving at least two abnormal genes, each represented by two different alleles. Studies such as these have provided support for the idea of a multifactorial inheritance.

ETIOLOGY

The clinical manifestations of MH, such as increased heat production, generalized muscular rigidity, increased glycogenolysis, and severe lactic acidosis can all be explained by an abnormally raised calcium ion concentration in the cytoplasm of the muscle cell (myoplasm). To facilitate understanding this explanation, a description of the basic muscle structure and of the mechanism of muscle contraction follows.

The cell membrane of the muscle fiber is called the sarcolemma. The muscle fiber itself is composed of several thousand myofibrils, suspended in a matrix called sarcoplasm. Each myofibril has about 1500 thick filaments called myosin and about 3000 thin filaments called actin. Myosin is a protein whose molecules have long, rod-shaped tail regions with enlarged heads that contain adenosine triphosphatase (ATPase) and actin-binding sites. Cross bridges extend along the myosin filaments and form linkages between the heads of the myosin molecules and the actin molecules. The thin filament, actin, is composed of roughly spherical molecules that form a double helix, which runs parallel to the myosin filaments.

The actin and myosin interdigitate, forming light and dark bands. The light bands, which contain only actin filaments, are called I bands. This is because they are isotropic to light (have equal refraction). The dark bands, which contain overlapping actin and myosin filaments, are called A bands (A bands are anisotropic to light, having different optical properties).

The point at which the actin filaments are attached to each other is called the Z-line or Z-membrane. Part of the actin filaments extend on either side of the Z-membrane to interdigitate with the myosin filaments. The portion between the Z-lines is called a scarcomere (Fig. 36–1).

Two other protein molecules, troponin and tropomyosin, are positioned along the actin strand. Troponin is made up of three subunits, TnT, TnI, and TnC. TnT binds strongly to tropomyosin, which covers the sites where the myosin heads bind to actin. TnI binds to actin, and TnC binds to calcium. Thus, the troponin-tropomyosin complex re-

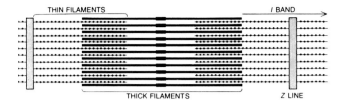

Figure 36–1. The myofibril, composed of interpenetrating arrays of thin filaments composed of actin, troponin, and tropomyosin and thick filaments composed of myosin. (*From Cohen C: The protein switch of muscle contraction. Sci Am 223:36–45, 1975.*)

presses the interaction of myosin and actin and maintains the muscle in a resting state (Fig. 36–2).

In the sarcoplasm there is also an extensive endoplasmic reticular system called the sarcoplasmic reticulum. The sarcoplasmic reticulum is composed of longitudinal tubules, which end in enlarged terminal cisternae and lie parallel to the myofibrils. Another tubular system, the transverse, or T-tubules, runs perpendicular to the myofibrils. The T-tubules abut against two of the terminal cisternae of the sarcoplasmic reticulum. The T-tubule is open to the exterior of the cell and contains extracellular fluid that is continuous with fluid outside the cell (Fig. 36–3).

The muscle membrane is of limited permeability that varies with the functional state of the muscle. In the resting state, the electrical potential of the muscle interior is slightly negative (-60 to -80 mV) relative to the exterior. Sodium is actively pumped out and potassium is actively pumped in by reactions catalyzed by membrane ATPases. Thus, at rest the concentration of potassium within the muscle is high while that of sodium is low.

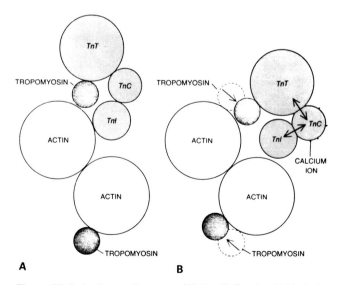

Figure 36–2. In the resting state (A) the TnT subunit binds to tropomyosin and the inhibiting subunit TnI binds to actin. In the active state, above a critical calcium level (B), linkages between troponin subunits are tightened and the link between TnI and actin is weakened. Tropomyosin moves deeper into the actin groove, exposing the site at which myosin can bind. (*From Cohen C: The protein switch of muscle contraction. Sci Am 223:36–45, 1975.*)

During relaxation, the level of calcium within the cytoplasm is low compared with that of the extracellular fluid. Calcium ions are actively extruded from the cytoplasm to the extracellular fluid across the surface membrane.

Calcium is stored in the terminal cisternae of the sarcoplasmic reticulum. The concentration of calcium within the terminal cisternae is about 1 to 3000 times that of cytoplasm. Such an enormous accumulation against a concentration gradient is brought about by reactions linked to ATP hydrolysis, catalyzed by a calcium-activated ATPase located in the terminal cisternae.

The process by which depolarization of the muscle fiber initiates contraction is called excitation-contraction coupling. The electrically excited sarcolemma is coupled to the calcium release from the sarcoplasmic reticulum. Depolarization of the cell membrane initiated by acetylcholine causes a sudden increase in the permeability of the membrane and inhibition of the membrane ATPases so that potassium ions leak out of the cell and sodium ions flow into the cytoplasm. The electrical potential of the cell interior is then converted from being slightly negative to being slightly positive.

The wave of depolarization flows along the sarcolemma, down the transverse tubules, and across the gap junctions to the sarcoplasmic reticulum. There the current flow in some way inhibits the ATPase of the sarcoplasmic reticulum and allows the calcium ions to follow their concentration gradient, rapidly flowing out of the terminal cisternae into the cytoplasm of the muscle fiber (Fig. 36–3).

The calcium ions released by the action potential initiate muscle contraction by binding to TnC. The linkage of TnC to troponin is strengthened and the linkage of TnI to actin is weakened, allowing tropomyosin to move laterally. This movement uncovers binding sites for the myosin heads (Fig. 36–2). The heads of the cross bridges of the myosin filaments immediately become attracted to the binding sites of the actin filaments. The cross bridges interact with the actin filaments and pull them toward the center of the sarcomere. This interaction causes the thin filaments to slide past the thick filaments and causes shortening as the Z-lines move closer together. Force is generated and the high-energy bonds of ATP are degraded to adenosine diphosphate (ADP), releasing heat and energy (Fig. 36–3).

Once calcium is released from the cisternae and has diffused to the myofibrils, muscle contraction will continue as long as the calcium ions are present in high concentrations in the sarcoplasmic fluid. However, shortly after releasing the calcium, the sarcoplasmic reticulum begins to reaccumulate calcium ions.

A continually active calcium pump is located in the walls of the longitudinal tubules and pumps calcium ions out of the sarcoplasmic fluid back into the cisternae for storage. Therefore, except immediately after an action potential, the calcium ion concentration in the myofibrils is kept extremely low.

Once the calcium ion concentration in the sarcoplasm has been lowered sufficiently, the calcium ions disassociate from TnC. This causes tropomyosin once again to block the sites of interaction of actin and myosin and the muscle relaxes (Fig. 36–3).

In the presence of a high intracellular calcium concen-

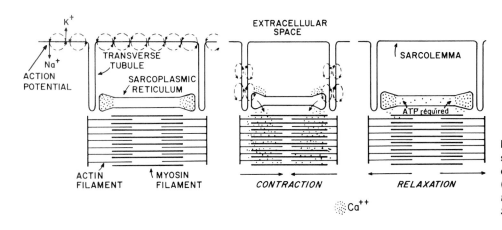

Figure 36–3. Diagrammatic representation of excitation-contraction coupling in normal skeletal muscle. (*After Hoyle G: How is muscle turned on and off? Sci Am 222:84–93, 1970.*)

tration, such as occurs in MH, the myofibrils remain locked together in a persistent contraction. There is a continuous and rapid production of heat as ATP is broken down by myosin-ATPase to ADP. Excessive amounts of ADP stimulate the various metabolic pathways as ADP is rephosphorylated to form new ATP. This results in further heat production, acceleration of oxygen consumption, carbon dioxide production, and lactic acidosis. The accelerated rate of ATP production is not, however, able to keep pace with the more rapid rate of ATP breakdown. There is insufficient ATP to provide energy for the various metabolic needs of the cell membrane, which then becomes permeable to myoglobin, potassium, and muscle enzymes.

Thus, many of the known changes present in MH syndrome could be accounted for by the theory that potent inhalational anesthetic agents and muscle relaxants in some way alter the calcium-storing properties of the cellular or intracellular membrane.

PATHOPHYSIOLOGY

The exact site of the defect in the muscle cell has been the subject of a great deal of investigation. Most studies have indicated skeletal muscle as the primary defective tissue in MHS subjects. Clinical indications of myopathy in MHS patients are substantiated by experimental data showing that agents that trigger MH in vivo also produce metabolic and contracture responses in MHS muscle in vitro. It has also been observed that MH muscle responds with an increased contracture when exposed to a wide variety of seemingly unrelated chemical stimuli such as halothane, caffeine, succinylcholine, potassium chloride, and the physiologic stimulus of temperature change. Such indiscriminate enhancement of the contractile response may therefore involve one of the basic regulatory mechanisms of muscle contraction.

It has been proposed that the excessive calcium present during the MH response could be due to a decreased reuptake of calcium ions by the sarcoplasmic reticulum from the myoplasm or to an increased release of calcium ions from the calcium-storing membrane of the cells, the sarcolemma, and the sarcoplasmic reticulum. Several groups have examined the reuptake of calcium by the sarcoplasmic reticulum in MHS muscle, but the results were conflicting and therefore no conclusive biochemical evidence is provided for this theory.

Accumulating evidence points to a defect in the mechanism leading to the release of calcium ions into the muscle fiber, a late step in the excitation-contraction coupling (ECC) pathway.

A very conspicuous abnormality in MH muscle is its marked sensitivity to caffeine, a drug that causes contraction of skeletal muscle by stimulating the release of calcium ions from the sarcoplasmic reticulum and by inhibiting reuptake of calcium by the sarcoplasmic reticulum.

It was discovered that dantrolene, a skeletal muscle relaxant, inhibited and reversed abnormal drug-induced contractures in MH muscle (Fig. 36–4). Dantrolene appears to exert its main effect by blocking the mechanism coupling depolarization of the sarcolemma membrane to calcium ion release from the sarcoplasmic reticulum, the ECC mecha-

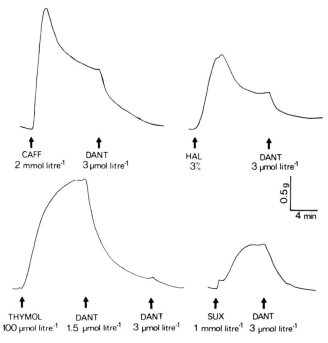

Figure 36–4. The effect of dantrolene sodium on caffeine-, halothane-, thymol-, and succinylcholine-induced contractures in MHS swine muscle. Caff = caffeine; dant = dantrolene; hal = halothane; sux = succinylcholine. (*From Okumura F, Crocker BD, et al: Br J Anaesth 52:377–383, 1980.*)

nism. The action of dantrolene suggests that the lesion is located at a link between the T-tubule system and the sarcoplasmic reticulum or the terminal cisternae of the sarcoplasmic reticulum or both.

Nelson, in 1978, compared human and pig muscle metabolism and pharmacology. He found that dantrolene is effective in blocking abnormal contracture responses in both humans and in the pig. Recently Nelson traced the source of the problem in pigs to calcium channels in the membrane of the sarcoplasmic reticulum. He postulates that a defective protein combines with the anesthetic drugs to keep channels open. Nelson is attempting to find a similar defect in muscle cells from patients with MH.

A lesion in the ECC mechanism provides a common pathophysiologic mechanism for MH inducers such as stress, depolarizing muscle relaxants, and anesthetic agents. An increased understanding of the etiology of MH has led to the realization that the most important aspect of treatment is to lower myoplasmic calcium ion content. Treatment has thus been centered around that approach.

Biochemical Changes

Although descriptions of MH episodes in humans exceed 1200 cases, a chronologic series of events has not been reported. Clinically, certain events have been observed consistently such as tachycardia, increased depth of ventilation, unstable blood pressure, increased body temperature, and muscle rigidity. Certain biochemical changes have been

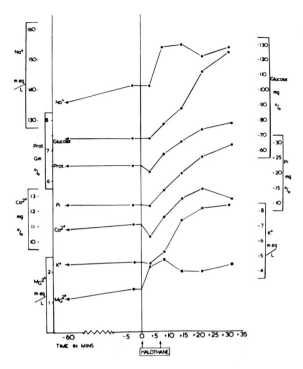

Figure 36–6. Changes in serum biochemistry determinations during an MH episode in the same animal as in Figure 36–5. (*From Harrison GG: In Gordon, Britt, et al (eds): The International Symposium on Malignant Hyperthermia, 1973, pp 271–286. Courtesy of Chas. C Thomas.*)

found to precede the increases in temperature and the development of rigidity so often associated with MH.

For obvious reasons, it is impossible to study MH in humans under controlled circumstances. Several studies inducing MH in swine have been done to systematically collect physiologic and metabolic data. (These data are similar to findings reported during episodes of human MH.)

Blood gas changes occur within minutes after initiation of the syndrome. These are the earliest objective signs of the development of MH. In the porcine studies, the venous hydrogen ion concentration increased within 5 minutes and the arterial hydrogen ion concentration increased in 10 minutes. Gross changes in oxygen consumption and increases in carbon dioxide production indicate a massive stimulation of aerobic metabolism (Fig. 36–5). There is a two- to threefold increase in whole-body oxygen consumption and an even greater increase in carbon dioxide production so that the respiratory quotient (RQ) exceeds one. (The normal RQ is 0.8 to 1.0.) This is a result of the early development of a severe lactic acidosis with the buffering of the increase in hydrogen ions by the plasma bicarbonate. Even with the large increase in oxygen consumption and the maintenance of a mean arterial P_{O_2} greater than 80 mm Hg, anaerobic glycolysis and lactate production are early features of porcine MH. A sevenfold increase in the plasma lactate concentration after the severe muscle stimulation of succinylcholine did not change appreciably until the terminal stages of the syndrome. In addition to anaerobic glycolysis and lactate production, serum potassium, magnesium, and phosphate increased significantly after 5 minutes (Fig. 36–6). This indi-

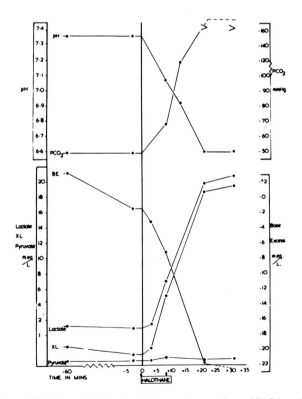

Figure 36–5. Arterial blood acid-base changes in an MHS Landrace pig during an MH syndrome provoked by halothane. (*From Harrison GG: In Gordon, Britt, et al (eds): The International Symposium on Malignant Hyperthermia, 1973, pp. 271–286. Courtesy of Chas. C Thomas.*)

cates a shift of these ions from the intracellular to the extracellular fluid and may be the result of an increase in the permeability of the sarcolemma membrane and the efflux of these ions from the liver. The most important changes in plasma electrolytes are the profound increases in potassium and inorganic phosphate concentrations. Although it is often assumed that the potassium is derived from the damaged striated muscle, Hall found that much of the potassium arises from the liver. The hyperphosphatemia is probably the result of the increased rate of hydrolysis of the adenine nucleotides (ATP, ADP, and adenosine monophosphate [AMP]) within the muscle. This increase in inorganic phosphates occurred 5 to 10 minutes after the administration of halothane or succinylcholine but still prior to the clinical diagnosis of MH.

Large increases in circulating catecholamines next occur during the hyperthermic response and are associated with tachycardia, arrhythmia, and an increase in cardiac output. The ability of the animal to increase its cardiac output to meet the metabolic demands in the presence of severe acidosis, hyperkalemia, and dehydration is an impressive feature of the porcine syndrome. Gronert and others have shown that myocardial metabolism was normal in hyperthermic pigs, although it has been suggested that cardiomyopathy is present in some susceptible human patients. Hall et al have postulated that the catecholamine stimulation of muscle metabolism is an integral part of the hyperthermic response. They also demonstrated that the increase in sympathetic activity is responsible for the severe tachycardia observed in MH by preventing the tachycardia with the administration of β-adrenergic blocking drugs to experimental pigs. They found a linear correlation between total plasma catecholamine concentration and plasma lactate concentration, providing supportive evidence for their contention that the catecholamine increase is associated with, if not directly attributable to, a product of metabolism. The metabolic and physiologic changes observed in porcine MH are essentially similar to those found after any severe muscle stimulation such as exhaustive exercise. In MH the problem arises from the subject's inability to control the severe catabolic (metabolic) state and enter a recovery phase.

Another common finding in porcine MH is hyperglycemia (Fig. 36–6). This results partly from the stimulating effects of the circulating catecholamines on hepatic glycogenolysis. Other factors contributing to the hyperglycemia include gluconeogenesis from the lactic acidosis and the inhibition of insulin secretion by the high circulating concentration of noradrenaline (Table 36–2).

An increase in heat production can be seen as early as 14 minutes after injection of succinylcholine, although the onset of hyperthermia and the temperature vary. The primary source of heat production is the skeletal muscle. The muscle temperature may increase as rapidly as 1C per 5 minutes. Total-body oxygen consumption accounts for only 50 percent of the heat produced during MH. Remaining sources of heat include glycolysis, hydrolysis of high-energy phosphates involved in ion transport and contraction-relaxation, and neutralization of hydrogen ions.

Assuming that MH primarily involves a sustained increase in the intracellular concentration of calcium, considerable and continuous amounts of energy are needed to transport calcium into the sarcoplasmic reticulum and the mitochondria. The immediate sources of this energy are creatine phosphate and adenosine phosphate, which are rapidly consumed. Heat is liberated during the continued synthesis and utilization of ATP during glycolysis. The lactic acid resulting from glycolysis is transported to the liver, where part is oxidized to provide the ATP necessary to convert the remainder to glucose, again causing the liberation of much heat. Glucose synthesized in this way, and from liver glycogen, is carried to the muscle. The cycle continues and the skeletal muscle and liver operate together as a giant ATPase.

Calcium taken up into the mitochondria uncouples oxidative phosphorylation, further increasing heat, carbon dioxide, and lactic acid production and oxygen consumption.

Under normal circumstances the body maintains a relatively constant core temperature by balancing endogenous heat production against heat loss. When the metabolic rate increases, compensatory cardiovascular changes occur to increase blood flow to tissues, eliminate waste products, and assist in heat dissipation. In malignant hyperthermia, however, the high rate of heat generation and concomitant retention of heat caused by intense peripheral vasoconstriction leads to a fulminating hyperthermic syndrome.

An additional source of heat may be accelerated substrate cycling of glucose-6-phosphate. This is a mechanism for heat generation in muscle that has been demonstrated

TABLE 36–2. MAIN METABOLIC, HORMONAL, AND ELECTROLYTE CHANGES DURING PORCINE MH. THE INCREASE OR DECREASE IN PLASMA ELECTROLYTE VALUES ARE RELATIVE TO THE OBSERVED HEMOCONCENTRATION

Metabolic	Hormonal	Plasma Electrolytes
↑ O_2 consumption ⎱ RQ > 1.0 ↑↑ CO_2 production ⎰	↑↑↑ Plasma noradrenaline	↑↑ Inorganic phosphate
↓↓ Arterial pH	↑↑ Plasma adrenaline	↑ Potassium
↑↑ Arterial P_{CO_2}	↑↑ Plasma glucagon	↔ Magnesium
↑↑ Blood lactate	↑ Plasma cortisol	↔ Calcium
↑ Blood pyruvate	↔ Plasma insulin	↓ Sodium
↑↑ Blood glucose		↓ Chloride
↑ Plasma glycerol		
↔ or ↓ Plasma FFA		

From Hall GM, Lucke JN, et al. Br J Anaesth 52:165–170, 1980.
FFA = free fatty acids; RQ = respiratory quotient.

in pigs that developed MH. The futile cycling mechanism causes hydrolysis of ATP with rapid depletion of cellular ATP and a high output of heat and lactate. The most likely mechanism is the rupture of mitochondrial membranes and inhibition of pyruvate dehydrogenation. This leads to the formation of lactate, decreased synthesis of ATP, and decreased restitution of phosphocreatine. The release of catecholamines and an increase in membrane permeability potentiate these effects and produce rigidity, hyperthermia, and acidosis. The consequence of the inhibition of mitochondrial respiration is decreased mitochondrial synthesis of ATP. Significant decreases in ATP are seen 5 to 10 minutes before death.

Hemoconcentration occurs early in the hyperthermic response secondary to a shift of water into the intracellular space. (This is not usually seen in humans because of massive amounts of fluid therapy.)

Although tachycardia is an early sign of the onset of MH, severe arrhythmias are also common, especially after the administration of succinylcholine or in the terminal stages.

Changes in arterial pressure during MH are not consistent as both hypertension and hypotension have been reported. Blood pressure changes can occur approximately 16 minutes after the initiation of the syndrome, as can the appearance of rigidity. When metabolic changes are extreme, as in the terminal stages of MH, cardiac output and the arterial pressure decrease rapidly and cardiac arrest occurs.

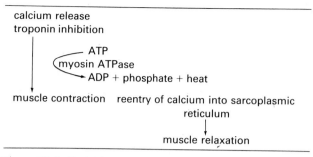

Figure 36–7. Excitation-contraction coupling in normal muscle.

Lastly, venous oxygen tension progressively decreases even when 100 percent oxygen is administered. This was seen approximately 57 minutes after the initiation of the syndrome. Acute sustained increases in venous carbon dioxide are seen at the same time (Figs. 36–7 and 36–8).

CRITERIA FOR DIAGNOSIS

Symptoms

At the present time there is no simple method for detecting patients who are susceptible to MH. Therefore early recognition and treatment of the syndrome are vital for a successful outcome. Any of the following symptoms should arouse suspicion during anesthesia unless another explanation is apparent: tachycardia, unstable blood pressure, cyanosis,

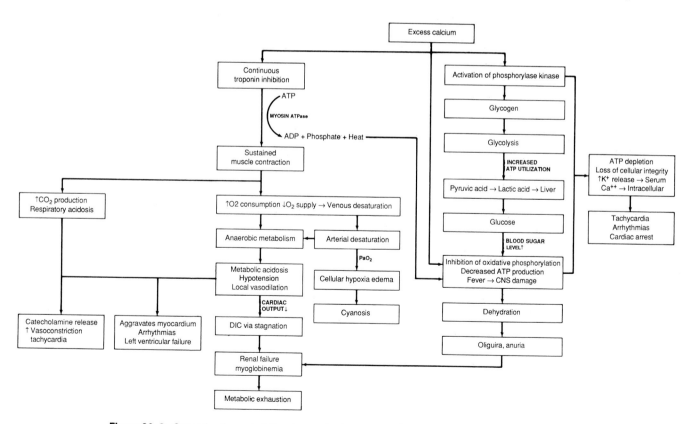

Figure 36–8. Cascade of events following excitation-contraction coupling in malignant hyperthermia muscle. ADP = adenosine diphosphate; ATP = adenosine triphosphate; CNS = central nervous system; DIC = disseminated intravascular coagulopathy.

TABLE 36–3. SIGNS AND SYMPTOMS OF MALIGNANT HYPERTHERMIA

1. Tachycardia (most consistent)
2. Tachypnea
3. Unstable blood pressure
4. Arrhythmias
5. Cyanosis
    a. Marked oxygen extraction → hypermetabolism
    b. Central venous desaturation
    c. Dark blood on surgical field
6. Muscle rigidity (not always present)
7. Profuse sweating
8. Mottling of the skin
9. Fever (late sign)

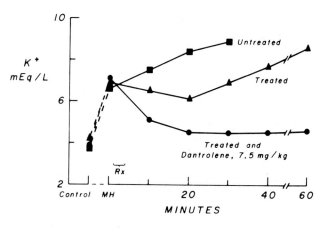

Figure 36–9. Arterial serum potassium during an MH episode in swine with no treatment, with supportive treatment only, and with supportive treatment plus dantrolene. (*From Gronert GA, Milde JH, et al: Anesthesiology 44:488–495, 1976.*)

dark blood on the surgical field, mottling of the skin, and excessive diaphoresis. Until recently, the most consistent early feature of an MH episode was tachycardia, often associated with an arrhythmia and tachypnea caused by metabolic and respiratory acidosis and hyperkalemia. However, with the end-tidal carbon dioxide analyzer now available, the earliest observable sign is a rising expired carbon dioxide tension.

Muscle rigidity, the unique sign of MH, may not develop until late, or may be slow developing. Most typically though, rigidity begins rapidly after administration of succinylcholine and is first perceived as masseter spasm. Masseter spasm, though a seemingly common event in children, should not be taken lightly. In mild or rapidly aborted MH reactions, masseter jaw spasm may be the only abnormality observed (Table 36–3).

Laboratory findings confirm signs of increased metabolism. Arterial blood gases should demonstrate hypoxemia and severe respiratory and metabolic acidosis. Excess lactate and pyruvate begin to accumulate almost immediately, resulting in a base deficit contributing to the acidosis. Suggested limits for the diagnosis of MH are a base excess of less than −5 mEq/L and an arterial P_{CO_2} greater than 60 torr without a reasonable explanation. Serum potassium and magnesium increase because of an increased permeability of the sarcolemma membrane. Serum phosphate increases, caused by the increased rate of hydrolysis of ATP, ADP, and AMP. Total serum calcium increases initially but later decreases precipitously. Late laboratory values are similar to the initial values, with the addition of hyperglycemia, myoglobinemia, myoglobinuria, hypocalcemia, and an elevated creatine phosphokinase (CPK), lactic dehydrogenase (LDH), and serum glutamic oxaloacetic transaminase (SGOT) (Table 36–4).

Fever is a later symptom. If the syndrome occurs after surgery has begun, an early sign may be the rapid heating of the anesthesia tubing and soda lime canister, or the patient's organs may feel hot to the surgeon. In particular, when the temperature is rising and there are signs of muscle stiffness and acidosis, the diagnosis is established and treatment must be instituted.

MANAGEMENT

MH can have a varied pattern of severity and symptomology. MH is triggered in relation to the susceptibility of the individual and to the concentration and duration of administration of the triggering agent. In many situations the full-blown, unmistakable picture of MH is not present. A tachycardia, occasionally with arrhythmias, accompanied by a gradual increase in temperature may not be impressive if the surgical procedure is brief. Some drugs, such as thiopental, appear to slow the development of MH so that the termination of the anesthetic may be sufficient therapy. The simple, yet important, treatment for rigidity after administration of succinylcholine is to terminate the anesthetic. The anesthetist must be alert to these abnormalities and obtain arterial and venous blood studies to document the hypermetabolism present with an MH episode.

When MH becomes fulminant (arterial blood P_{CO_2} greater than 60 torr and rising, mixed venous blood P_{CO_2} greater than 90 torr and rising, base excess less than −5 mEq/L and falling, and a temperature increase of at least 1 degree C per 15 minutes) rapid, vigorous therapy is necessary if the patient is to survive.

Dantrolene is a hydantoin derivative, representative of a new class of muscle relaxants that act directly on the

TABLE 36–4. LABORATORY FINDINGS IN MALIGNANT HYPERTHERMIA

Early	Late
Hypoxemia	Hyperglycemia
Hypercarbia	Myoglobinemia
Respiratory acidosis	Myoglobinuria
Metabolic acidosis	Elevated CPK, LDH, SGOT
Hyperkalemia	Hypocalcemia
Hyperphosphatemia	Hypokalemia
Hypercalcemia	
Hypermagnesemia	

CPK = creatine phosphokinase; LDH = lactic dehydrogenase; SGOT = serum glutamic oxaloacetic transaminase.

skeletal muscles. It acts by inhibiting calcium release without affecting uptake (see Appendix). Dantrolene is the only medication that will terminate MH in pigs after the onset of the syndrome. Numerous cases have been reported confirming its effectiveness in treating human MH. Dantrolene controls the abnormal metabolic responses and the associated acid-base imbalances, ion fluxes, and sympathetic stimulation more predictably than symptomatic therapy and is thus the drug of choice to treat MH (Fig. 36–9). The recommended intravenous dosage for humans is 2.5 mg/kg, which may be repeated every 5 to 10 minutes up to a total dose of 10 mg/kg.

Usually one or two doses will abort the reaction. If the temperature rises or if arrhythmias occur in the recovery period, dantrolene should be continued at the rate of 1 mg/kg/hr until the reaction is under control.

Dantrolene is stored as a lyophilized powder that contains 20 mg dantrolene and 3 g of mannitol per vial. Each vial requires 60 ml of sterile water to dissolve the powder. The drug and solvents should be stored in the anesthetic area, readily available for use.

TABLE 36–5. MALIGNANT HYPERTHERMIA PROTOCOL

1. Stop anesthesia and surgery immediately.
   Change rubber goods and anesthesia machine.
2. Hyperventilate with 100% oxygen.
3. As soon as possible, administer dantrolene sodium, mixed with sterile distilled water, 2.5 mg/kg intravenously. (Response to dantrolene should begin within minutes: if not, repeat up to 10 mg/kg total dose.)
4. Cool the patient using
   a. IV iced saline solution (not Ringer's lactate): 1000 ml/10 min for 30 min.
   b. Surface cooling with ice and hypothermia blanket.
   c. Lavage of stomach, bladder, rectum, peritoneal, and thoracic cavities with iced saline (3–6 L).
   d. If necessary, extracorporeal circulation and heat exchanger (femoral to femoral).
5. Correct acidosis and hyperkalemia (100 mEq sodium bicarbonate at once and up to 600 mEq total, guided by pH and Pco_2).
6. If arrhythmias persist after treatment of acidosis and hyperkalemia, procainamide 15 mg/kg IV can be given over 10 min.
7. Secure monitoring lines: ECG, temperature, Foley catheter, arterial pressure, central venous pressure. Monitor: ECG, temperature, urinary output, arterial pressure, blood gases, (Pco_2, Po_2), central venous pressure, electrolytes (K, Ca), pH, clotting studies.
8. Maintain urine output of at least 2 ml/kg/hr. Administer mannitol 12.5 g IV and furosemide 50 mg IV (up to four doses each).
9. If desirable, administer 10 units of insulin in 50% DW (10 ml) as an IV bolus to provide energy to cells and reduce hyperkalemia.
10. Monitor patient until danger of subsequent episodes is past.
11. Postcrisis follow-up therapy: administer oral dantrolene 1–2 mg/kg q.i.d. (for 1 to 3 days).

Ca = calcium; ECG = electrocardiogram; K = potassium.

Adapted from Diagnosis and Management of Malignant Hyperthermia, 1981. Courtesy of Norwich-Eaton Pharmaceuticals and the author.

Symptomatic Therapy

In addition to the administration of dantrolene, symptomatic therapy is important for successful treatment of MH. Certain items must be kept either in the operating room suite or the recovery room and be readily available. Most persons experienced in the management of MH recommend using an established protocol similar to the one prepared by John Ryan (Table 36–5). To deal effectively with an emergency situation, a sequence of actions such as the following should be defined prior to surgery and anesthesia:

1. Stop the anesthesia and surgery. First turn off all the agents except oxygen. (The patient usually will not regain consciousness until sometime postoperatively.) Change the soda lime and anesthetic tubing as soon as possible. Because of the rubber/gas solubility of the inhalational agents, some anesthetic remains in the tubing.
2. Hyperventilate with 100 percent oxygen. Hyperventilate using two to three times the minute ventilation. Hypoxemia, one of the early signs of the syndrome, will usually be corrected unless oxygen delivery has been delayed.

   Hyperventilation is often unsuccessful in lowering the Pco_2 to normal but must be maintained in an effort to control the severe respiratory acidosis present.
3. Give dantrolene. As soon as possible, administer dantrolene 2.5 mg intravenously. Response to dantrolene should begin within minutes. If not, repeat the dosage up to 10 mg/kg total dose.
4. Cool the patient. It is necessary to institute aggressive cooling to lower the temperature. Cooling should be stopped when the temperature falls to 38.3C (101F) to prevent inadvertent hypothermia. Resume cooling if the temperature starts to rise again.

   Surface cooling by packing the patient in ice is effective with small children because of their high surface area relative to body volume. In adults, iced intravenous saline (1000 ml every 10 minutes for 30 minutes) has been helpful in lowering body temperature. Additional cooling measures include iced saline lavage of the stomach, rectum, peritoneal cavity, and thorax. Lavage of the bladder, though recommended, should be avoided because of the need to monitor urine output. Cardiopulmonary bypass with a heat exchanger can be used, if available.

   Some authorities recommend peripheral vasodilation to aid in cooling the patient. Although not a part of Ryan's protocol, chlorpromazine, in small doses (2.5 to 5 mg IV) to avoid hypotension yet control shivering, and droperidol (2.5 to 5 mg) for its alpha-blocking effect have been reported to be useful.
5. Correct the acidosis. Administer sodium bicarbonate, 2 mEq/kg initially, then use the arterial blood gases as a guide for further therapy. Bicar-

bonate serves a dual function. It corrects the acidosis and also corrects the hyperkalemia. Increasing the pH drives potassium back into the cell.

6. Treat arrhythmias with procainamide. If arrhythmias persist after treatment of acidosis and hyperkalemia, procainamide 15 mg/kg IV can be administered over 10 minutes (1000 mg procainamide diluted in 500 ml isotonic saline). Lidocaine is *not* used because amides inhibit the transfer of calcium to the sarcoplasmic reticulum and therefore can aggravate the MH.

   Although cardiac glycosides have been used by some in the treatment of human MH without adverse effects, Britt, after reviewing statistical data, feels that cardiac glycosides may worsen MH by increasing myoplasmic calcium. Cardiac glycosides are currently considered hazardous to the MH patient.

7. Secure monitoring. Once these measures have been instituted, monitoring lines should be established to provide a guide to subsequent therapy. These include electrocardiogram, temperature, establishment of arterial line for blood pressure, arterial blood gases, electrolytes, a Foley catheter for urine output, and a central venous pressure line.

8. Administer fluids to maintain high urine output. Massive amounts of fluids are required to prevent dehydration and to maintain a high urinary output. Initial volume loading consists of 2 to 8 ml/kg of colloids and crystalloids, depending on patient response, determined by central venous pressure and urine output. A Foley catheter is mandatory. A urine output of greater than 2 ml/kg/hr prevents myoglobin from forming casts in the kidney, which can lead to renal failure. Furosemide 50 mg IV (up to four doses) and mannitol 12.5 g IV may be necessary to maintain urine output. Furosemide will also help start excretion of sodium if large amounts of sodium bicarbonate are necessary to control the acidosis.

9. Treat hyperkalemia. Standard protocol recommends giving 10 units of regular insulin in 10 ml of 50 percent dextrose and water as an intravenous bolus. This has a twofold purpose: (1) to reduce serum potassium by transferring potassium back into the cells; and (2) to provide an exogenous energy source and the transfer of glucose into the cells.

10. Additional therapy. Based on in vitro studies, Ellis has recommended steroids for the treatment of human MH. However, Britt, in a retrospective review, found the mortality rate higher with steroid use in the treatment of human MH. Conversely, Gronert feels that multiple factors contribute to MH-associated deaths and that steroids are probably helpful during these severe stresses.

Late Complications

If the aforementioned therapy is not instituted early or vigorously enough the following later complications may occur:

1. Consumption coagulopathy or disseminated intravascular coagulopathy (DIC). This may be caused by hemolysis, increased release of tissue thromboplastins resulting from increased permeability or overt tissue damage, shock secondary to inadequate capillary perfusion, to a defect in the red blood cell or platelet, or to some rare mechanisms related to the increased permeabilities present in fulminant MH. DIC usually occurs when the treatment has been too conservative and the patient has run markedly elevated temperatures over a prolonged period, with resultant dehydration and decreased peripheral blood flow. Various treatments reported to be useful include the administration of fresh-frozen plasma and clotting factors and heparinization.

2. Acute renal failure. Myoglobinemia and myoglobin casts in the kidney have been associated with renal failure, particularly in association with acidosis, hypovolemia, and hypotension. Therapy as previously outlined providing a high urinary output will help prevent renal damage.

3. Inadvertent hypothermia. Too vigorous cooling can result in inadvertent hypothermia. This can be prevented by careful temperature monitoring and termination of cooling when the patient's temperature reaches 101F (38.3C).

4. Skeletal muscle edema and muscle necrosis. Sustained tetanic muscle contraction causes an increase in muscle metabolism, produces local mechanical occlusion of the blood vessels, and decreases muscle perfusion. The resultant acidosis and hypoxia produce skeletal muscle edema and ischemia leading to necrosis. When cell damage occurs, enzymes such as CPK, SGOT, and LDH are released into the circulation. Ions follow their electrochemical gradient, with potassium leaving the cell and calcium entering the cell, producing hyperkalemia and hypocalcemia.

   During episodes of malignant hyperthermia, the muscle membrane wall changes in permeability, leaking various muscle constituents into the bloodstream. Myoglobinemia and myoglobinuria result.

5. Neurologic sequelae. Cerebral perfusion is essentially unchanged until the core temperature exceeds 103 F. However, the cerebral metabolic rate for oxygen increases linearly with temperature. Data indicate that cerebral hypoxia will occur during hyperthermia. Thus, cerebral hypoxia and acidosis can result in sequelae such as coma, paralysis, or decerebration.

6. Pulmonary edema. Pulmonary edema is usually reported after a cardiac arrest at the height of the syndrome. Treatment is the same as with other disorders.

7. Hyperkalemia. Hyperkalemia, caused by muscle cell damage, resolves with the return to normal temperature and stabilization of the patient. As potassium goes back into the cell, serum potassium values drop precipitously. For as long as 24 hours after MH, the patient is extremely sensitive to iatrogenic potassium administration. Potassium should therefore be given in very small amounts and only if electrocardiographic changes warrant.

Thus MH presents the following picture and related complications: tachycardia, tachypnea, arrhythmia, hypoxia, severe respiratory and metabolic acidosis, skeletal muscle rigidity, greatly increased metabolism, severe hyperthermia, reflected by a low Pao_2, high $Paco_2$, low pH, high lactic acid, hyperkalemia, hypercalcemia, then hypocalcemia, elevated plasma enzymes, and myoglobin in the plasma and urine.

Later complications include coagulation disorders, renal failure, muscle damage, left ventricular failure, and neurologic sequelae.

Follow-up for Malignant Hyperthermia

MH is an ongoing process that may last for days. Close patient monitoring is necessary even after the episode is over and must continue for 24 to 48 hours. This includes electrocardiogram, temperature, arterial line for blood pressure and blood gases, electrolytes (especially potassium, calcium), serum enzymes, coagulation studies, central venous pressure, and urine output.

Health care givers should be aware that as the initial dose of dantrolene is metabolized and excreted, retriggering can occur. Cases of recurrence of MH have been reported up to 30 hours after the initial episode. Intravenous dantrolene has a half-life of approximately 5 hours and should be continued for 12 to 24 hours. Oral dantrolene can be given as soon as the gastrointestinal system is functional (1 to 2 mg/kg q.i.d. for 1 to 3 days).

During the postoperative period there should be normal renal function, blood coagulation, bleeding time, and blood gases. The neurologic status must include absence of rigidity. The temperature and electrocardiogram findings must be normal.

Major indications of renewed trouble are rigidity, a slow rise in potassium, and mental agitation. Family counseling should be done during the recovery period. Families should be referred to the Malignant Hyperthermia Association of the United States (MHAUS), a patient self-help group that provides much support and information useful to MH families.

EVALUATION OF SUSCEPTIBILITY: PREANESTHETIC DIAGNOSIS OF MALIGNANT HYPERTHERMIA

If it were possible to identify the MH trait preoperatively, the mortality rate could be reduced to zero. However, at the present time, there is no one test that is inexpensive enough and noninvasive enough to use for all patients.

Studies of platelet aggregation, platelet ATP depletion, and blood type have thus far been inconclusive. Some recent tests using lymphocytes look promising, but there needs to be much work to confirm early results. Serum CPK studies are helpful in identifying the MH trait when CPK is elevated in conjuction with other criteria. But currently, the only certain method of detecting susceptibility is an in vitro study of muscle, which requires a muscle biopsy to obtain the specimen.

The usual preoperative evaluation of susceptibility to MH consists of obtaining a personal and family history of any myopathies or a history of any unusual reaction to anesthesia and a physical examination for the existence of any clinical muscle abnormalities.

All individuals who are susceptible to MH have an underlying disease of the muscle. Muscle and connective tissue have been found to be abnormal in 67 percent of all MHS patients and in 36 percent of their first-degree relatives. While some MHS patients are perfectly healthy, others complain of a wide range of physical abnormalities. These include short stature, club foot, webbing of the neck, ptosis, strabismus, kyphoscoliosis, lumbar lordosis, various hernias (inguinal, hiatus, umbilical), joint hypermobility, occasional repeated joint dislocations, winged scapulae, undescended testicle, calcium stones in the ureter or gallbladder, poor dental enamel, and misshapen and misplaced teeth. Some patients exhibit skeletal muscle hypertrophy that is occasionally asymmetric. In others, the myopathy is usually subclinical, although there is some muscle atrophy, particularly in the lower parts of the thigh. A few MHS patients are afflicted with mild forms of Duchenne's muscular dystrophy, limb girdle muscular dystrophy, or central core disease. MHS patients frequently complain of skeletal muscle cramps that range from mild to incapacitating, usually worse in the winter.

Britt believes MH to be a widespread membrane defect involving different types of cells including heart muscle. The electrocardiogram has been found to be abnormal in one-third of all MHS patients who have a positive muscle biopsy and in 15.4 percent of their first-degree relatives. The most common electrocardiographic abnormalities are ventricular or atrial hypertrophy, bundle branch block, or myocardial ischemia.

If any of the previously mentioned criteria are present, the patient should have a serum CPK test. Although the CPK test has received much criticism because many other muscle damaging conditions unrelated to MH can elevate the serum CPK, most experts still believe the test to be helpful in identifying families with suspected MH (Fig. 36–10). When CPK is elevated and the patient is a close relative of a known MHS individual, he or she can be considered to be susceptible. If the patient is a close relative of an MHS person but has a normal CPK on three occasions, then a muscle biopsy is necessary to determine susceptibility. The only confirmed diagnostic test, other than an unequivocal clinical episode, is the contracture response of muscle. This requires the excision of about 4 cm of thigh muscle under local anesthesia and should be performed at a center where muscle biopsies are done routinely. There are several types of tests on muscle to determine susceptibility to MH. These entail exposure of the muscle to varying concentrations of caffeine, succinylcholine, halothane, caffeine and halothane, or potassium. The abnormal muscle exhibits a contracture or a greater-than-normal contracture upon exposure to the pharmacologic agents (Fig. 36–11).

All patients who are considered susceptible to MH should wear Medic Alert bracelets and carry cards in their wallets warning against the use of potent inhalational agents, certain muscle relaxants, and amide-type local anesthetics. Patients and their families should be counseled as to the risks associated with exposure to triggering drugs and to excessive emotional and physical stress. However, these patients should also be reassured that when appropri-

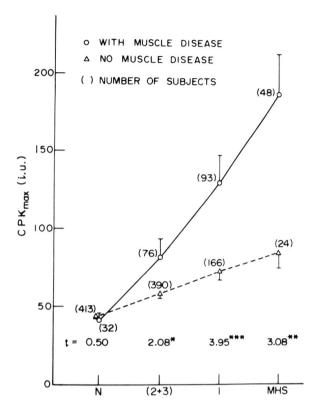

Figure 36–10. Maximum CPK levels in normal (N) individuals, MHS subjects, and their first-, second-, and third-degree (2 + 3) relatives. (*From Britt BA, Endrenyi L, et al: Can Anaesth Soc J 23:263–284, 1976.*)

ate precautions are taken, anesthesia can be administered to them safely.

A problem arises in evaluating patients who do not present a clear picture of MH susceptibility. These patients may have a vague history of anesthetic problems, have muscle problems such as intermittent cramping or weakness but nothing clinically demonstrable, or a serum CPK at the upper limits of normal. The anesthetist should be aware that a majority of the patients with muscle disease are not MHS. Conversely, many MHS patients have no clinical evidence of muscle disease. There are serious implications involved in assigning the MHS label to a person or family. One must have definitive evidence before doing so. When in doubt about MH susceptibility, however, a prescribed prophylactic anesthesia routine such as the one that follows should be employed.

Prophylactic Anesthesia Routine for MHS Patients

Preoperative Preparation. The patient may be admitted to the hospital 1 to 3 days preoperatively and placed on bed rest so as to reduce anxiety and avoid stress. During preoperative counseling the patient should be reassured about the special monitoring for MH and the treatment for MH should it develop.

Dantrolene sodium is recommended in doses varying from 4 to 6 mg/kg/day in divided doses. The patient must be observed for the possible side effects such as dizziness,

drowsiness, and muscle weakness. Vital signs and temperature should be recorded.

Preoperative assessment should include the usual history and physical examination as well as an electrocardiogram (regardless of age), a complete blood count, serum electrolytes, liver function tests, and coagulation studies. Sedation with a barbiturate or a benzodiazepine should be given the evening before surgery.

On the day of surgery patients may be given oral dantrolene 4 mg/kg 2 to 4 hours before the induction of anesthesia. The patient should be well premedicated in an effort to reduce anxiety and the associated catecholamine release. Phenothiazines, which may release calcium from the sarcoplasmic reticulum, and belladonna alkaloids, which appear to increase the likelihood of an MH reaction, should be avoided. An alternate approach is the administration of intravenous dantrolene immediately prior to anesthesia. Britt advocates a dose of 2 to 4 mg/kg IV over the last 1 to 4 hours prior to anesthesia and repeat doses during and after surgery. Flewellen et al maintain that acute administration of dantrolene will achieve MH prophylaxis. This group did a study and found that 2.4 mg/kg IV over 10 to 15 minutes rapidly achieves a predictable blood level, which they feel is prolonged enough for most surgical procedures.

Operating Room Preparation. In the operating room, routine monitoring equipment including electrocardiogram, temperature probe, cooling blanket, Doppler, and a vapor-free anesthesia machine (no vaporizer attached) with new tubings and soda lime should be ready for use. (A previously used anesthesia machine can be purged of vapor by replacing all porous parts and the soda lime canister and then running 100 percent oxygen through it for at least 12 hours.) Ice, lavage tubes, and an arterial line setup should be available. The emergency drugs and supplies listed in Table 36–5 should be available for use.

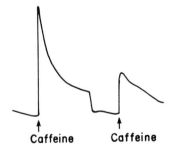

Malignant Hyperthermia Muscle

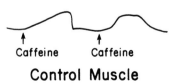

Control Muscle

Figure 36–11. Artist's representation of the response of human MHS muscle to caffeine contrasted with the response of normal human muscle to caffeine.

Anesthetic Agents. Anesthetic agents that have been used safely on MHS patients include nitrous oxide, thiopental, narcotics, droperidol, diazepam, pancuronium, atracurium, and vecuronium. All potent inhalational anesthetics, depolarizing muscle relaxants, and ketamine should be avoided.

If local or conduction anesthesia is preferred for a particular surgery, ester-type local anesthetics, such as procaine and tetracaine, appear to be safe. Amide local anesthetics, such as lidocaine or mepivacaine, are contraindicated because they can cause calcium release from the sarcoplasmic reticulum. Although it is unlikely that the systemic levels required to release calcium from the sarcoplasmic reticulum would be reached, amides have been implicated as possible triggering agents and are best avoided.

Although there have been a few reports of the successful use of spinal anesthesia in MH survivors, Wingard reported an episode of MH in the perioperative period in a patient who had received a spinal anesthetic.

The MH reaction triggered by anesthetic agents may be only part of an acute stress syndrome triggered by other factors as well. Because of this possibility, Ellis recommends general anesthesia for MHS patients even for muscle biopsy.

An MHS patient who is having local or conduction anesthesia should be well sedated. It should also be borne in mind that stimulation during light general anesthesia could trigger an MH response as well, an additional reason for very close patient monitoring.

Episodes of MH have occurred in the postoperative period. Therefore, monitoring of the MHS patient should continue for 24 hours.

APPENDIX

Dantrolene Sodium (Dantrium)

Dantrolene sodium, a hydantoin derivative (Fig. 36–12) is a muscle relaxant that acts specifically on skeletal muscle with no effect on cardiac or smooth muscle. It produces relaxation by acting directly on the skeletal muscle, affecting the contractile response at a site beyond the myoneural junction. Dantrolene blocks excitation-contraction coupling, probably by suppressing the amount of calcium ions released from the sarcoplasmic reticulum. Dantrolene selectively inhibits calcium ion release from the sarcoplasmic reticulum but does not affect sequestration of myoplasmic calcium back into the sarcoplasmic reticulum.

Dantrolene has a mean half-life of about 9 hours after an oral dose, and a half-life of 5 hours after intravenous administration.

Dantrolene is metabolized by hepatic microsomal enzymes. The metabolites are excreted in the urine. Metabolic patterns are similar in adults and children. Liver dysfunc-

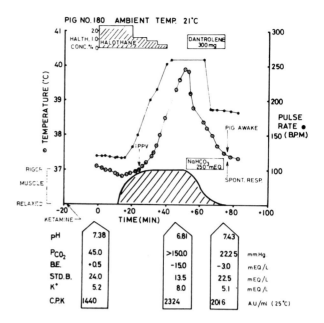

Figure 36–13. Temperature, heart rate, and biochemical values during an MH episode precipitated by halothane and after the administration of dantrolene in an MHS pig. BE = base excess; BPM = beats per minute; CPK = creatine phosphokinase; IPPV = intermittent positive pressure ventilation; K^+ = potassium ion; Pco_2 = pressure of carbon dioxide; STD B = standard bicarbonate. (*From Harrison GG. Br J Anaesth 47:62–65, 1975.*)

tion, as evidenced by blood chemistry abnormalities (liver enzyme elevation), hepatitis, seizures, and pleural diffusion with pericarditis have been reported as reactions occurring with chronic oral dantrolene use.

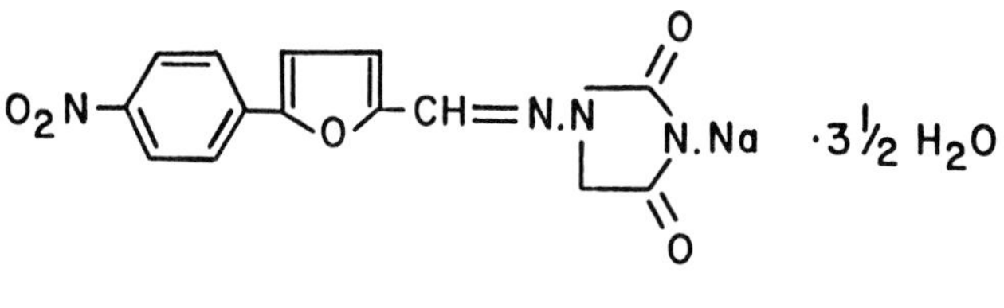

Clinically, dantrolene is used to control manifestations of spasticity resulting from upper motor neuron disorders, such as spinal cord injury, stroke, cerebral palsy, or multiple sclerosis.

In 1975 Harrison showed that dantrolene treatment would terminate the MH response of susceptible swine to halothane (Fig. 36–13). His observations were substantiated by numerous studies of MHS swine in response to MH induced by succinylcholine and halothane and by studies of isolated swine muscle strips with dantrolene producing relaxation of contractures induced by halothane and caffeine.

Oral dantrolene, having already been in use to treat spasticity in humans, was suggested for use as pretreatment in MHS humans. Denborough, at the Second International Symposium on Malignant Hyperthermia, reported a study comparing the effects of several drugs including procaine, procainamide, steroids, and dantrolene on the halothane-induced contractures of human muscle in vitro. He concluded that dantrolene was the drug of choice for treating malignant hyperthermia.

Harrison demonstrated that pretreatment of MHS swine with dantrolene would block the initiation of the MH response to halothane and succinylcholine. Wingard and Gronert, in experiments with swine, also substantiated this finding. Clinical reports of the effective use of dantrolene to reverse MH syndrome in humans when other supportive and drug therapies have proved ineffective have

Figure 36–12. The molecular structure of dantrolene.

established dantrolene as the drug of choice for the treatment of malignant hyperthermia. Furthermore, oral and intravenously administered dantrolene has been reported to be part of the successful prophylaxis for MH in patients undergoing surgery with known susceptibility.

In anesthetic-induced MH, evidence points to an intrinsic abnormality of the muscle tissue. In affected humans and swine, it has been postulated that "triggering agents" induce a sudden rise in myoplasmic calcium either by preventing the sarcoplasmic reticulum from accumulating calcium adequately or by accelerating its release. This rise in myoplasmic calcium ions activates the acute catabolic processes common to the MH crisis.

Dantrolene may prevent the increase in myoplasmic calcium ions and the acute catabolism within the muscle cell by interfering with the release of calcium ions from the sarcoplasmic reticulum to the myoplasm. Thus the physiologic, metabolic, and biochemical changes associated with the crisis may be attenuated or reversed.

As soon as the MH reaction is recognized, all anesthetic agents should be discontinued. An initial dantrolene intravenous dose of 2.5 mg/kg body weight should be given rapidly. Other supportive measures should also be instituted, for example, 100 percent oxygen, management of the metabolic acidosis, and institution of cooling measures. If the physiologic and metabolic abnormalities persist or reappear, this dose may be repeated up to a cumulative dose of 10 mg/kg. (Because of the high pH of the intravenous formulation, 9.5, care should be taken to prevent extravasation.)

It may be necessary to administer oral dantrolene in doses of 1 to 2 mg/kg q.i.d. for a 1- to 3-day period to prevent recurrence of the manifestations of MH.

Experience to date indicates that the dose for children is the same as for adults, with an initial intravenous dose of 2.5 mg/kg given rapidly.

Dantrolene should be available in the anesthetizing area of the operating suite and in the recovery room. It comes in ready to mix vials of 20 mg each. It should be reconstituted with sterile water for injection (USP) without a bacteriostatic agent. The contents of the vial must be protected from direct light and used within 6 hours after reconstitution. The expiration date should be routinely checked before reconstitution. Dantrolene has a shelf life of 3 years.

BIBLIOGRAPHY

Aldrete JA, Britt BA (eds): The Second International Symposium on Malignant Hyperthermia. New York, Grune & Stratton 1978.

Andersen IL, Jones EW: Porcine malignant hyperthermia: effect of dantrolene sodium on in-vitro halothane-induced contraction of susceptible muscle. Anesthesiology 44:57–61, 1976.

Britt BA (ed): Malignant hyperthermia. Int Anesthesiol Clin 17(4), 1979.

Britt BA: Dantrolene: a review. Can Anaesth Soc J 31:61–75, 1984.

Britt BA: Malignant hyperthermia. Can Anaesth Soc J 32:666–677, 1985.

Britt BA, Endrenyi L, et al: Screening of malignant hyperthermia susceptible families by creatine phosphokinase measurement and other clinical investigations. Can Anaesth Soc J 23:263–284, 1976.

Britt BA, Kalow W: Malignant hyperthermia: a statistical review. Can Anaesth Soc J 17:293–315, 1970.

Brownell AKW, Paasuke RT, et al: Malignant hyperthermia in Duchenne muscular dystrophy. Anesthesiology 58:180–181, 1983.

Clarke IMC, Ellis FR: An evaluation of procaine in the treatment of malignant hyperpyrexia. Br J Anaesth 47:17–21, 1975.

Denborough MA, Waine GL, et al: Insulin secretion in malignant hyperthermia. Br Med J 3:493–495, 1974.

Douglas JM, McMorland GH: The anaesthetic management of the malignant hyperthermia susceptible parturient. Can Anaesth Soc J 33:371–378, 1986.

Flewellen EH, Nelson TE: Masseter spasm induced by succinylcholine in children: contracture testing for malignant hyperthermia: report of six cases. Can Anaesth Soc J 29:432–449, 1982.

Flewellen EH, Nelson TE, et al: Dantrolene dose response in awake man: implications for management of malignant hyperthermia. Anesthesiology 59:275–280, 1983.

Gordon RA, Britt BA, et al (eds): The International Symposium on Malignant Hyperthermia. Springfield, Ill., Chas. C Thomas, 1973.

Gronert GA: Review: malignant hyperthermia. Anesthesiology 53:395–423, 1980.

Gronert GA: Controversies in malignant hyperthermia. Anesthesiology 59:273–274, 1983.

Gronert GA, Heffron JJA, et al: Porcine malignant hyperthermia: role of skeletal muscle in increased oxygen consumption. Can Anaesth Soc J 24:103–109, 1977.

Gronert GA, Milde JH, et al: Dantrolene in porcine malignant hyperthermia. Anesthesiology 44:488–495, 1976.

Gronert GA, Theye RA, et al: Catecholamine stimulation of myocardial oxygen consumption in porcine malignant hyperthermia. Anesthesiology 49:330–337, 1978.

Gronert GA, Thompson RL, et al: Human malignant hyperthermia: awake episodes and correction by dantrolene. Anesth Analg 59:377–378, 1980.

Hall GM, Lucke JN, et al: Malignant hyperthermia: pearls out of swine. Br J Anaesth 52:165–171, 1980.

Hall GM, Lucke JN, et al: Porcine malignant hyperthermia: VII. hepatic metabolism. Br J Anaesth 52:11–17, 1980.

Halsall PJ, Cain PA, et al: Retrospective analysis of anesthetics received by patients before susceptibility to malignant hyperthermia was recognized. Br J Anaesth 51:949–954, 1979.

Harrison GG: Control of the malignant hyperpyrexic syndrome in MHS swine by dantrolene. Br J Anaesth 47:62–65, 1975.

Henschel EO (ed): Malignant Hyperthermia: Current Concepts. New York, Appleton-Century-Crofts, 1977.

Kalow W, Britt BA, et al: The caffeine test of isolated human muscle in relation to malignant hyperthermia. Can Anaesth Soc J 24:678–694, 1977.

Lucke JN, Hall GM, et al: Porcine malignant hyperthermia: I. metabolic and physiological changes. Br J Anaesth 48:297–304, 1976.

Malignant Hyperthermia Association of the United States: The Communicator (newsletter) 4:4, 1986.

McPherson E, Taylor CA: The genetics of malignant hyperthermia: evidence for genetic heterogeneity. Am J Med Genet 11:273–285, 1982.

Merz B: Malignant hyperthermia: nightmare for anesthesiologists—and patients. JAMA 225:709–715, 1986.

Michel P, Fronefield H: Use of Atracurium in a known MHS patient. Anesthesiology 62:213, 1985.

Mitchell G, Heffron JJ, et al: Halothane-induced biochemical defect in muscle of normal and malignant hyperthermia-susceptible Landrace pigs. Anesth Analg 59:250–256, 1980.

Moulds RFW, Denborough MA: Biochemical basis of malignant hyperthermia. Br Med J 2:241–244, 1974.

Nelson TE: Abnormality in calcium release from skeletal sarcoplasmic reticulum of pigs susceptible to malignant hyperthermia. J Clin Invest 72:862–870, 1983.

Nelson TE, Austin KL, et al: Screening for malignant hyperthermia. Br J Anaesth 49:162–172, 1977.

Okumura F, Crocker BD, et al: Site of the muscle cell abnormality in swine susceptible to malignant hyperpyrexia. Br J Anaesth 52:377–383, 1980.

Ryan JF: Malignant hyperthermia. ASA Refresher Courses in Anesthesiology, 4:87–97, 1976.

Schwartz L, Rockoff MA, et al: Masseter spasm with anesthesia: incidence and implications. Anesthesiology 61:772–775, 1984.

Wingard DW: A stressful situation. Anesth Analg 59:321–322, 1980.

37

Anesthesia for the Thermally Injured Patient

David E. Beesinger, Colleen Lynch Beesinger, and Stephen Hays

*I*n the past decade, an increasing interest has been shown in the care of patients who receive thermal injuries. It is now well understood that such patients can best be cared for in major institutions with a formal burn unit. With this realization has come the development of burn teams, comprised of representatives of several different areas of expertise. Care of the thermally injured person requires input not only from physicians and burn nurses but also from physical therapists, occupational therapists, dieticians, clergy, anesthesiologists, and nurse anesthetists.

Major advances have occurred in the treatment of burn patients in this same decade that have decreased morbidity and mortality remarkably, to the point that people who have received burns of 60 to 75 percent of total body surface area are routinely discharged from the hospital and return to functional lives. New systemic and topical antibiotics have contributed significantly to this improved care. Increased nutritional support has progressed with expanded understanding of the physiology of the burn wound.

Another recent advance in burn care has been the development of early excision and grafting of the burn wound. Most major burn units pursue an aggressive, early surgical approach to the eschar formed by coagulation necrosis of the skin. The eschar is routinely removed as early as 2 to 3 days after injury, and skin grafts are placed at the time of excisional therapy. This aggressive surgical approach to the burn wound has proved to be very effective in decreasing morbidity and mortality but at the same time has created special problems for the anesthetist that are unique and variant to those encountered in general surgical cases. This chapter deals with the peculiarities encountered in the operating room when burn patients are subjected to operative procedures.

Because of the massive amount of fluid required for resuscitation of the patient in the first 24 hours, special attention must be paid to the cardiovascular hemodynamics at the time of surgery. In addition, burn wound sepsis is a continuous problem in these patients, and myocardial, renal, and pulmonary status require specific management.

Inhalation injuries often accompany thermal burns, especially when patients are injured in an enclosed space. Such patients may require ventilatory assistance and special efforts to prepare them for the operating room.

Patients with major thermal injuries have a poor body temperature maintenance ability, and several idiosyncrasies are encountered with the various anesthetic agents. Contractures or positioning problems may be encountered that require special consideration to avoid mechanical difficulties. The burn patient, therefore, must be considered as much more than just one who has a soft tissue injury. All organ systems must be considered, and functional abnormalities must be anticipated when a surgical procedure is required.

PREOPERATIVE CONSIDERATIONS

Evaluation of the Wound

Burn wounds are described as being first, second, or third degree according to the depth of coagulation necrosis caused by the thermal injury (Fig. 37–1). First degree burns are primarily equivalent to a sunburn, which is of no significance other than the discomfort caused to the patient.

Superficial second degree burns are similar to sunburns, although they are deeper. These burns extend into the superficial dermis but are associated with very few complications. They heal spontaneously because the dermis is intact, and they rarely become infected. Scarring is not associated with the superficial second degree burn unless it is converted to a deeper depth by infection. These wounds are generally not attacked surgically but are treated with topical antibiotics and allowed to heal without intervention.

Deep second degree burns, however, act more like full thickness or third degree burns. These injuries extend through the epidermis and into the deepest portions of the dermis. Nerve endings are intact so that sensation is present, and the wounds weep fluid. These wounds take approximately 3 to 4 weeks to heal and may well become infected. In addition, they scar excessively and may form contractures about the hands or other joints. For these rea-

Partial
thickness

Full
thickness

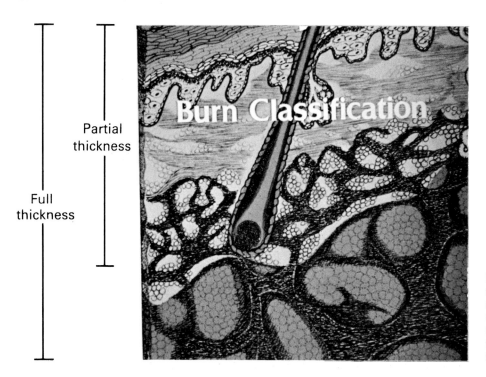

Figure 37–1. Partial thickness or second degree burns are those that cause injury extending into but not completely through the dermis. Full thickness or third degree burns extend through the dermis and into the subcutaneous tissue.

sons, deep second degree burns are often treated like third degree burns, that is, they are subjected to early surgical excision and split thickness skin grafting.

Third degree burns are those that cause necrosis that extends all the way through the dermis into the subcutaneous tissue. These wounds will not heal spontaneously, since all the dermis has been destroyed. They have no sensation and often have a dry, charred appearance. These wounds will require skin grafting at some point in the hospitalization. Third degree burns are treated surgically within the first 2 to 3 days, at which time excision removes devitalized tissue so that skin grafts can be placed.

In addition to determining the depth of the wounds, one must determine the size of the burn or extent of injury. This is commonly expressed as percentage of total body surface area injured, which can be determined in several ways, a very popular method being the rule of nines (Fig. 37–2).

Using this method, each area of the body is divided into 9 percent portions of the entire body surface area. Each upper extremity represents 9 percent, each lower extremity is 18 percent, the front and back of the torso are each 18 percent, and the head and neck represent 9 percent. One percent is added for the perineum and genitalia. With this technique, one can determine fairly accurately the extent of thermal injury. Another method for determining the extent of injury is the use of the Lund and Browder chart, which gives a more exact estimate of the percentage of the total body surface area made up by each area of the body.

Fluid Resuscitation

After measuring the patient's body weight in kilograms and knowing the percentage of surface area injured, one can determine the volume of fluid required for resuscitation in the first 24 hours (Fig. 37–3). The Parkland formula dictates that 4 ml of Ringer's lactate solution per kilogram of body weight per percent of total body surface area burned be given over 24 hours. Half of that volume is given in the first 8 hours, a quarter in the second 8 hours, and a quarter in the third 8 hours. The adequacy of resuscitation is then determined by hourly measurements of urine output, pulse rate, blood pressure, sensorium, and development of ileus.

In the second 24 hours, Ringer's lactate solution is discontinued, and colloid solution, usually in the form of plasma, is used to expand the intravascular volume. After plasma is administered, additional fluid, that is, 5 percent dextrose in water, in a daily maintenance volume is administered IV. If, during the second 24 hours, measurable parameters indicate that intravascular volume is not adequately expanded, additional plasma is given.

Because of the loss of fluid across the burn wound as well as the shift of interstitial fluid into the intracellular space that accompanies major thermal injury, the cardiovascular system may be very unstable in the first 48 hours. For this reason, general anesthesia should be avoided during this period whenever possible. However, a not infrequent exception is the need for escharotomy or fasciotomy during the first 24 hours. This procedure may be required when burns are full thickness and circumferential about an extremity or chest. Incision is made through the skin and subcutaneous tissue in the area of the burn in order to restore blood supply to an extremity distal to the area of circumferential burn. Similar escharotomies may be required on the chest to enable the thorax to expand for normal ventilation. Very few other surgical procedures are indicated during this critical period of burn care.

After the first 48 hours, fluid and electrolyte balance is not as critical but must be evaluated daily. The original resuscitation shifts from the intracellular space back into

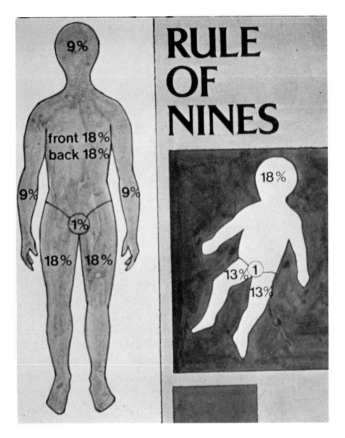

Figure 37–2. Regions of the body can be considered to represent multiples of 9 percent of total body surface area for rapid evaluation of the size of the thermal injury. The percentage represented by each region varies according to age.

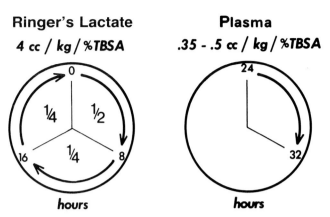

Figure 37–3. Large volumes of Ringer's lactate solution are required for resuscitation of the burn patient in the first 24 hours. In the second 24-hour period, plasma is administered and crystalloid is restricted.

the intravascular space, causing a diuresis after the first 2 days. During this time, the adequacy of cardiovascular hemodynamics is assessed by clinical examination as well as daily measurements of hematocrit, electrolytes, and serum creatinine. Valuable information is also gained from accurate recordings of intake and output and daily weights.

Inhalation Injury

If a patient was burned in an enclosed space, one must be suspicious of inhalation injury. The effects of heated air, carbon monoxide, and particulate products of incomplete combustion are injurious to the airways and tremendously complicate the care of the skin injury itself.

The patient should be examined for singed nasal hairs, erythema or swelling of the pharynx, and carbonaceous sputum. Arterial blood gas determination should be performed and the level of carboxyhemoglobin should be determined. Carboxyhemoglobin levels in the blood have a relatively linear relationship to the extent of inhalation injury. Carbon monoxide easily displaces oxygen from the hemoglobin moiety, creating a state of hypoxia at the cellular level. Determinations greater than 15 percent saturation are associated with significant and severe pulmonary insult. Carbon monoxide is easily displaced from hemoglobin, however, by the administration of high concentrations of

oxygen. The level determined in the emergency room, therefore, may not be indicative of the extent of inhalation injury, since most patients will have received oxygen therapy in transport to the hospital. Therefore, a level less than 15 percent should not lessen the index of suspicion.

Researchers at the Brooke Army Medical Center, Fort Sam Houston, Texas, have described another method of evaluating the extent of inhalation injury. Radioactive xenon is injected intravenously, and sequential scintiphotos are obtained. Delayed washout of the isotope on scans is associated with significant pulmonary injury.

When the index of suspicion of inhalation injury is high, bronchoscopy should be performed (Fig. 37–4). The flexible bronchoscope can be easily and quickly used to evaluate the status of the trachea and bronchi. Carbon or marked erythema lining the tracheobronchial tree is an indication of significant inhalation of noxious substances (Fig. 37–5). These patients usually develop adult respiratory distress syndrome (ARDS) and should be treated early with endotracheal intubation, high tidal volumes of 15 ml/kg, pulmonary toilet, and positive end-expiratory pressure (PEEP).

Inhalation injury creates a need for additional fluid replacement in the first 24 hours. Excess fluid administration, however, will increase the accumulation of pulmonary interstitial fluid and promote the development of respiratory insufficiency.

Arterial oxygen tension should be kept above 70 mm Hg, with the original efforts being directed toward elevation of PEEP instead of FIO_2. The respiratory rate should be controlled to keep the PCO_2 between 38 and 42. Bronchodilators are rarely indicated in treatment of inhalation injury unless wheezing, suggesting bronchoconstriction, is heard on examination. Intravenous steroids may be helpful if the pulmonary injury is not associated with significant dermal burn. When steroids are given on a long-term basis, the patient's immunologic response is further diminished, and burn wound sepsis is inevitable.

The anesthetist should always accompany the patient with pulmonary injury to the operating room for procedures. A life pack should be available for monitoring.

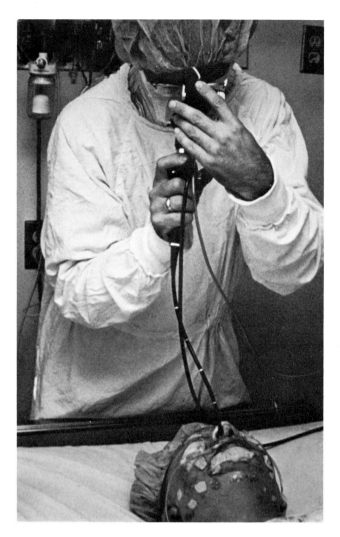

Figure 37–4. The patient suspected of having received an inhalation injury should undergo flexible bronchoscopy to evaluate the tracheobronchial tree for extent of injury.

Burn Wound Sepsis

Despite advances in topical antibiotics, systemic antibiotics, and the early surgical approach to the burn wound, infection is still the greatest cause of death in major thermal injuries. When colonization of the burn wound becomes excessive, invasion by microorganisms is inevitable. The result is septicemia, followed by septic shock and death. This progression of events creates special problems for the anesthetist when a surgical procedure is being considered.

Burn wound invasion is frequently monitored by doing quantitative wound biopsy cultures. These are routinely performed at least twice a week on wounds that are full thickness in depth. A small portion of the eschar is sent to the pathology laboratory, where the specimen is weighed, emulsified, and spread on culture media. After 24 hours, counts are performed and reported as the number of organisms per gram of tissue.

Within the first 5 to 7 days after injury, colony counts are generally less than 10^5 organisms per gram. This number is thought to be associated with superficial colonization of the eschar and is not indicative of burn wound sepsis.

After invasion of the wound and proliferation of organisms in the subdermal space, colony counts often go as high as 10^7 or 10^8 organisms per gram of tissue. Any count above 10^5 is considered to be consistent with invasive burn wound sepsis. Septicemia is usually not present at this point but will inevitably ensue if control of wound infection is not achieved.

At this point, several modalities are available to surgeons for wound treatment. If the patient has been treated with silver sulfadiazine (Silvadene) as a topical antibiotic for a prolonged period of time, a different antibiotic will be given. Mafenide acetate (Sulfamylon) is usually given as an alternative covering, since it penetrates the eschar more readily and disperses antibiotics deeper into the wound. Intravenous antibiotics are also instituted at this time. The choice of intravenous antibiotic is dependent on the appearance of the wound, the timing in the hospital course, and the organisms most prevalent in the burn unit.

Aminoglycosides, usually gentamicin or tobramycin, are most commonly used when invasive infection occurs. These antibiotics affect *Staphylococcus aureus* and most of the gram-negative rods. Carbenicillin or ticarcillin is commonly used for treatment of *Pseudomonas* infections. When septicemia occurs, the patient's intravascular volume usually becomes depleted, and the addition of aminoglycoside frequently brings about impairment of renal function. This consideration must be kept in mind in preparation for the operating room.

Subdermal clysis has also been advocated for the control of burn wound sepsis. Antibiotics are mixed in solution, generally with normal saline, and administered through IV lines and needles into the subdermal space. Concentration of the antibiotics in the area of greatest accumulation

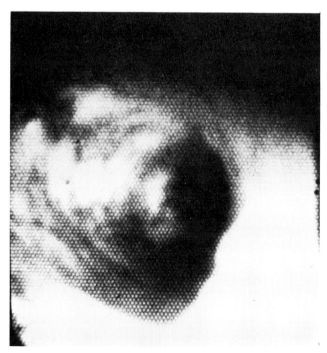

Figure 37–5. Finding of edema, erythema, and carbonaceous material in the bronchi indicates significant inhalation injury and dictates early treatment modalities.

of organisms is effective in reducing colony counts in quantitative burn wound biopsies.

A third modality available to the surgeon is excision of the infected eschar. It is at this point that the anesthetist becomes involved and must have an insight into the cardiovascular hemodynamic changes that accompany sepsis. Many different theories have been proposed to explain these changes, but several factors are found consistently. Cardiac output is uniformly elevated in burn patients at this point, with values of 10 to 15 L per minute being common. Pulse rates are uniformly elevated, and blood pressure may be normal or slightly depressed. Peripheral vascular resistance may be normal but is commonly depressed. The etiology of this finding is not clear, but it may be due to accumulation of lactic acid at the capillary level, causing dilatation of the vasculature. Another proposed etiology is the opening of arteriovenous shunts that prevent perfusion at the cellular level, causing hypoxia. In addition, it has been proposed that there is a myocardial depressant factor that accompanies major thermal injuries. This factor depresses cardiac function and limits myocardial reserve for stressful situations. The choice of an anesthetic agent, therefore, must fit these changes in cardiovascular hemodynamics and must not contribute further to myocardial depression or vasodilatation.

Burn wound infections require the anesthetist to be wary in mechanical areas as well as in those areas concerning physiology. Anesthesia equipment may be a source of cross-contamination in burn patients, and, therefore, disposable breathing circuits with bacterial filters should always be used. Strict aseptic technique should be adhered to when inserting catheters, and gloves should be worn by the anesthetist at all times during patient contact. All monitoring equipment that touches the patient should be either disposable or cleaned extensively between patients. Laryngoscopes, blood pressure cuffs, warming blankets, and all other apparatus should be similarly thoroughly cleaned.

Renal Insufficiency

Renal insufficiency is commonly associated with thermal injuries. There are generally two phases of this potential complication, the first occurring in the first 24 to 48 hours and being associated with intravascular volume depletion and acute necrosis of renal tubules secondary to hypoperfusion. With an understanding of the massive volumes of fluid required for resuscitation, this complication is now almost nonexistent.

Renal insufficiency also commonly accompanies administration of aminoglycosides as well as several other antibiotics. The combination of intravascular volume depletion, aminoglycosides, and diuretics very frequently precipitates acute tubular necrosis. More commonly, however, renal insufficiency is secondary to generalized septicemia. Again, the exact etiology is unclear, but the dysfunction may well be secondary to hypoperfusion or opening of arteriovenous shunting as is seen peripherally. In either case, acute hemodialysis may be necessary to prepare the patient for the operating room. Indications for hemodialysis are hyperkalemia and hyperosmolality. Peritoneal lavage has not been found to be effective in most centers for dialysis, since patients frequently have infected burn wounds of the abdominal wall, which make insertion of a catheter hazardous.

When acute hemodialysis is not available and hyperkalemia negates general anesthesia, potassium levels may be medically treated. Fifty grams of glucose and 25 units of regular insulin can be administered IV in addition to one to two ampules of sodium bicarbonate. Alkalinization and glucose–insulin administration will shift potassium into the intracellular space. It should be remembered that this is a temporizing measure but may save the myocardium from the catastrophic results of hyperkalemia.

Fever

Almost all burn patients with a significant mass of eschar tissue will have elevated body temperature. This is usually in the range of 100 to 101F, but it may well climb to 103F or 104F in the presence of active burn wound sepsis. Concomitant with the increased body temperature is an elevated pulse rate; therefore, atropine should not be given to these patients. Atropine is further contraindicated by its blockage of perspiration, thus taking away the patient's ability to dissipate body heat. A higher inspired oxygen content is required in the septic patient, and care should be taken to assure that the FIo_2 administered is at least equal to that which the patient was receiving before coming to the operating room.

Preoperative Medication

Preparing and transporting the patient to the operating room for a major surgical procedure may be as traumatic as the original injury. Any motion is uncomfortable for the patient, and anxiety levels are at a maximum during this period. The need for preoperative medication, therefore, should be anticipated and carefully considered.

Narcotics may be safely administered and generally should be the same drug the patient has been receiving for analgesia in the burn unit. Glycopyrrolate (Robinul) is a satisfactory agent in that it does not have the cardiovascular effects of atropine, it raises gastric pH, and it may not have the same effect on sweating. Tranquilizers are often useful for the diminution of anxiety, and many centers have found the oral administration of diazepam (Valium) to be very helpful as a preoperative medication.

It is of paramount importance that the anesthetist tell the patient the plan for anesthetic induction and maintenance. Anxiety is tremendously decreased when the patient understands what will happen to him or her on arrival in the operating room. The placement of IV lines and blood pressure recording devices should be planned well ahead of the procedure. Communication with the surgeon about these matters facilitates orderly procedures and prevents the two team members from competing for the same extremity.

INTRAOPERATIVE MANAGEMENT

Monitoring

The room temperature should be kept between 84F and 90F. This temperature is uncomfortable for team members but decreases the patient's body heat loss and maintains normothemia. Heating blanket and blood warmers should always be used, since major thermal injuries bring about increased body heat loss, and multiple transfusions tend to further decrease body temperature.

An automatic blood pressure monitoring device may be used, since it can be applied to any extremity and gives accurate systolic and diastolic pressures without invasion. The anesthetist's hands are freed, and constant readout of pressures is available.

Adhesive ECG leads frequently cannot be used on the burn patient because of the eschar and the use of irrigation fluid and topical antibiotic creams. In these instances, a 25-gauge needle can be placed subcutaneously, through normal skin or through eschar, and alligator clips can be attached for constant ECG monitoring. Precordial stethoscopes should be applied for induction and then replaced by an esophageal stethoscope. Temperature probes should be used to monitor body temperature throughout the procedure. Arterial lines are only seldom required except in patients with significant inhalation injuries who need serial arterial blood gas determinations. Placement of these lines should be correlated with the surgeon so that they will not be placed in areas that need to be excised or grafted.

Placement of IV lines may be difficult because, frequently, only small areas of unburned skin are available. A 16-gauge central line should be available for administration of blood and fluids as well as measurements of central venous pressure when indicated. Another large-bore peripheral IV catheter should be placed if possible to provide for rapid replacement of blood and fluids. Since maintenance of security of IV lines is always difficult in burn patients, the lines should be sutured or wrapped in multiple layers of Kerlex to avoid interruption. All IV fluids administered should be warmed.

Most burn patients with injury to greater than 50 percent of total body surface area will require IV hyperalimentation to obtain the required daily calories. Every effort must be made to keep these central lines from becoming contaminated during surgery. Hyperalimentation fluids should be stopped at the beginning of the surgical procedure, and 10 percent dextrose in water should be placed on the central line. This line should not be used for blood administration, nor should drugs be administered through it.

Blood Transfusion

As previously mentioned, blood loss is massive in patients being subjected to tangential excision and skin grafting. Cross-matched blood should, therefore, be in the operating room before surgery is begun. Transfusion should be started as soon as anesthesia induction is complete, since blood loss is rapid and voluminous upon starting eschar excision. This loss is compounded if two surgeons are operating on separate areas simultaneously. Pressure infusors are generally mandatory to regulate the rate of blood transfusion.

Blood replacement of approximately 250 to 300 ml per percentage of total body surface area excised should be anticipated. Weighing sponges used in surgery to determine blood loss may not be accurate in these patients, since a large amount of saline solution is used for irrigation and for hemostasis. Observation and measurement of field blood loss should be evaluated. Rapid infusion of blood should be continued until the cessation of eschar excision. After hemostasis has been obtained and skin grafts are being applied, blood loss is minimal. It is at this point that the anesthetist can measure hematocrit to determine if further transfusion is necessary. During the procedure, central venous pressure should be maintained between 8 and 15 cm of water, and urine output should be at least 0.5 ml/kg per hour in the adult and 1 ml/kg per hour in children.

Recovery

Special considerations are necessary after the patient's procedure is completed and he or she is taken to the recovery room. Strict isolation must be maintained in the recovery room to prevent contamination of burn wounds and to prevent cross-contamination from infected wounds to other patients in the recovery room. Warm blankets should be available to cover the patient on arrival, since excessive shivering on awakening from general anesthesia further increases metabolic demands and brings about a risk of dislodgement of the recently applied skin grafts. Whenever possible one should not reverse the effects of narcotics used during the operative procedure in order to further minimize shivering.

CHOICE OF ANESTHETIC AGENT

As each burn patient has a unique array of physiologic problems and possible complications, so must each patient's anesthetic regimen be unique and well planned. It is imperative to have close communication with the surgeon before a procedure so that problems with patient positioning, monitor placement, IV lines, and extubation will not be encountered.

Induction

Induction may be performed with either ketamine, inhalation agents, or short-acting barbiturates.

Ketamine is quick acting and allows for spontaneous respiration when administered IV at a slow rate. It will support the cardiovascular status of the patient, which may well exhibit an already depressed state. However, the anesthetist should anticipate excessive salivation and the possibility of laryngospasm, which may create airway problems.

The recommended dosage of ketamine is 2 to 4 mg/kg IV or 4 to 8 mg/kg IM. For lengthy procedures, it is helpful to use a 0.2 percent ketamine drip to maintain a desirable level of anesthesia. Smaller dosages of 1 to 2 mg/kg given IV are used at some institutions for dressing changes and small debridements within the burn unit. Such procedures have been found to be effective and safe when guided by the qualified anesthetist.

Short-Acting Barbiturates

The anesthetist has a choice of two commonly used short-acting barbiturates for induction. It should be remembered that these agents are short-acting not because of rapid metabolism but because of rapid redistribution. They then become long-acting when given in repeated doses.

Thiopental works very well for burn anesthesia induction. A test dose of 0.75 to 1.5 mg/kg should be given, after which dosages of 3 to 5 mg/kg can be used in the adult if no untoward effects on the cardiovascular system are seen with the test dose. Methohexital, another short-acting barbiturate, has the advantage of being able to be given rectally with good effects in pediatric patients.

Inhalation Agents

Several popular inhalation agents are available for induction of anesthesia in the burn patient. Halothane is an excellent inhalation agent for general surgery and trauma but has limited application in burns. Since halothane is a myocardial depressant and potent vasodilator, it should be avoided in general.

Enflurane has minimal hepatic toxicity and has more muscle relaxant activity than do other inhalation agents. A major disadvantage that must be considered in burn patients, however, is that there is a significant degree of myocardial depression associated with the drug. Its application in this area, especially in those patients with burn wound infections and poor myocardial reserve, is limited. Although isoflurane has not been fully tested in burn patients, it appears to be a satisfactory agent, since it maintains cardiac output by increasing heart rate at the possible expense of decreasing stroke volume.

Narcotics

Narcotics are commonly used for analgesia in burn units, and they make an excellent choice for the anesthetist in both induction and maintenance of anesthesia. Fentanyl is one of the more popular agents because it maintains blood pressure well and promotes cardiovascular stability. It is short-acting, although its duration is unpredictable after several doses. The suggested dose for fentanyl is 2 μg/kg on induction and 1 to 2 μg/kg every 20 to 30 minutes for maintenance.

Muscle Relaxants

It is now well accepted that succinylcholine is contraindicated for muscle relaxation in burn patients. This drug promotes release of potassium from muscle cells and is very commonly associated with cardiac arrest.

Nondepolarizing muscle relaxants may be used safely and effectively for anesthesia. Curare is relatively safe, but dosage requirements may be markedly elevated in these patients. An increase in gamma-globulin as a result of infection and septicemia is thought to be responsible for a partial resistance to the drug. Curare is associated with histamine release and ganglionic blockade, which may create hypotension when the patient is depleted of intravascular volume. In general, this drug should be avoided or used with extreme caution.

Pancuronium bromide is the generally preferred nondepolarizing muscle relaxant because of its ability to support the pulse rate, blood pressure, and cardiac output.

The recommended dosage is 0.07 mg/kg in the adult and 0.1 mg/kg in children. Vecuronium is a useful intermediate acting muscle relaxant. Less tachycardia is seen with administration of this drug when compared to pancuronium. Atracurium may be used satisfactorily in the burn patient but its use may be associated with histamine release and subsequent hypotension.

Recommended Regimen

With this knowledge, a rational approach to preoperative medication, induction, and maintenance can be recommended (Table 37–1). Lorazepam, 2 to 4 mg po or IM, and morphine, 8 to 10 mg IM, are an excellent preoperative combination. Patients generally do not remember being transported to the operating room and, upon awakening, do not know that they have undergone an operative procedure. This effect serves to diminish anxiety for subsequent surgery.

In the operating room, induction is started with a combination of 50 percent oxygen and 50 percent nitrous oxide. Fentanyl 150 μg and thiopental 50 mg are given IV. If the pulse rate and blood pressure remain stable, an additional 3 to 5 mg/kg of thiopental are given IV. Ventilation is slowly controlled, after which 0.07 to 0.1 mg/kg of pancuronium bromide is administered. After ventilation has been carried on for 3 to 4 minutes, intubation can be performed. An additional dosage of thiopental may be given during this induction time if blood pressure warrants.

Maintenance of the patient during the operative procedure is with 70 percent nitrous oxide, fentanyl, and pancuronium bromide if needed. Isoflurane or enflurane may be added if these agents are not satisfactory. The patient with circumoral or neck contractures that make intubation questionable should be preoxygenated with 100 percent oxygen. Muscle relaxants should be avoided, but induction can be carried out with spontaneous inhalation of isoforane or halothane.

If there is any doubt that the patient can be intubated, awake intubation after liberal use of topical anesthetics and cocaine should be performed.

SUMMARY

There is nothing magic about administering anesthesia to the burn patient. Special problems are encountered, however, that dictate considerations not necessary in general

TABLE 37–1. RECOMMENDED ANESTHETIC REGIMEN

Use	Agent and Dosage
Preoperative	Lorazepam 2–4 mg po or IV *or* Morphine 8–10 mg IM
Induction	50% O₂, 50% N₂O Fentanyl, 150 μg, thiopental 3–5 mg/kg Pancuronium bromide 0.07–0.1 mg/kg
Maintenance	30% O₂, 70% N₂O Fentanyl, pancuronium bromide Isoflurane or enflurane

surgery and trauma patients. These are primarily related to intravascular volume status, cardiovascular hemodynamics, infection, and idiosyncrasies of particular pharmacologic agents. Additional consideration must be given to positioning of the patient, placement of IV lines and monitor devices, and management of intubation in the patient with mouth or neck contractures.

With an understanding of the physiology of burn patients and the mechanical problems that may be encountered, the anesthetist can formulate a safe and effective plan for those patients who have sustained a major thermal injury.

BIBLIOGRAPHY

Agee RN, Long JM III, et al: Use of xenon in early diagnosis of inhalation injury. J Trauma 16(3):218–224, 1976.

Bevan DR, Dudley HAF, Horsey PJ: Renal function during and after anaesthesia and surgery: Significance for water and electrolyte management. Br J Anesth 45(9):968–975, 1973.

Bryce-Smith R: Complications. Int Anesth Clin 11(1):239–269, 1973.

Clarke AM, Solomon JR: The use of a new vasoconstrictor in the management of burns. Med J Aust 2(7):361–362, 1972.

Corssen G, Oget S: Dissociative anesthesia for the severely burned child. Anesth Anal 50(1):95–102, 1971.

Gunther RC, Schaner PJ, et al: Halothane for burn anesthesia. Anesth Analg 48(2):277–281, 1969.

Heath DF, Frayn KN, Rose JG: Effects of halothane on glucose metabolism after injury in the rat. Br J Anesth 50(9):899–904, 1978.

Henderson TR, Jones RK: Tyrosine aminotransferase induction in rat liver as a response to irradiation or flash burn injuries. J Trauma 14(4):317–324, 1974.

Howie CCM: Refrigeration anaesthesia for donor areas. Br J Anesth 43(6):616–619, 1971.

Howie CM: General anaesthesia in the adult burned patient. Postgrad Med J 48(557):152–155, 1972.

Lorthioir J: The early surgical treatment of burns. Panminerva Med 14(6):164–167, 1972.

Miller B, Srinivasagam N: A comparative study of general anesthesia versus droperidol and ketamine anesthesia in burned children. AANA J 42(3):236–240, 1974.

Packer KJ: Methoxyflurane analgesia for burns dressings. Postgrad Med J 48(557):128–132, 1972.

Patterson JF, Belton MK: Anesthesia experiences at a plastic surgery center in Vietnam. JAMA 215(5):777–782, 1972.

Phelps N: Intermittent inhalation in burns dressing. Nurs Times 68(31):970, 1972.

Pocta J, Simkova-Novotna M, Chvatlinova V: Treatment of burned patients by the anaesthesiologist. Acta Chir Plast (Prague) 13(2):71–77, 1971.

Sage M, Laird SM: Ketamine anaesthesia for burns surgery. Postgrad Med J 48(557):156–161, 1972.

Schaner PJ, Brown RL, et al: Succinylcholine-induced hyperkalemia in burned patients. Anesth Analg 48(5):764–770, 1969.

Sotornikova T, Leikep K, Adamkova M: Problems of anaesthesia and analgesia in burns. Acta Chir Plast (Prague) 19(3):228–232, 1977.

Ward CM, Diamond AW: An appraisal of ketamine in the dressing of burns. Postgrad Med J 52(602):222–223, 1976.

Wessels JV, Allen GW, Slogoff S: The effects of nitrous oxide on ketamine anesthesia. Anesthesiology 39(4):382–386, 1973.

Wilson RD: Anesthesia and the burned child. Int Anesthesiol Clin 13(3):203–217, 1975.

Zook EG, Roesch RP, Thompson LW, Bennett JE: Ketamine anesthesia in pediatric plastic surgery. Plast Reconstr Surg 48(3):241–245, 1971.

38

Care of the Cancer Patient

Hollis E. Bivens and Rebecca S. Williams

Anesthesia for the patient undergoing cancer surgery is no different from that administered to a patient having another type of surgery. Techniques and methods are, of necessity, those used for other types of surgery. The difference lies in the overall condition of the patient. The effects of previous surgery, chemotherapy, and radiotherapy, plus various disease states, alter the patient's response to anesthesia.

PREOPERATIVE EVALUATION

History and Physical Examination

As required for any diagnostic evaluation, a thorough history and physical examination are of utmost importance. A history of cardiac disease, including date of infarct, surgery, medication, ECG changes, and so on, is particularly significant. Consultation with a cardiologist who is familiar with the side effects of chemotherapeutic agents, radiation, and extent of surgery is necessary in all patients with abnormal heart functions. The cardiologist who visits the operating room frequently and is familiar with current techniques and problems of perioperative care can offer the most pertinent opinion of how the patient will respond to the planned procedures.

Cardiac disease in the cancer patient should be controlled to the greatest extent possible before anesthesia induction. The patient taking cardiac medication should be stabilized and continued on the appropriate dosage through the operative period.

Alcoholic patients frequently have hypertension, anemia, cardiac disease, cirrhosis, malnutrition, and dehydration in addition to cancer. Lesions of the alimentary tract may interfere with the patient's ability to eat (Figs. 38–1, 38–2, 38–3). A program of hyperalimentation may be required to correct protein and electrolyte imbalance. Lesions of the lips (Fig. 38–4), buccal mucosa, tongue, gingiva, pharynx, trachea, and lungs are associated not only with smoking but also with alcohol abuse. In these patients, it is not unusual to elicit a history of Guillain-Barré syndrome

or acute intermittent porphyria that will directly influence the selection of anesthetic agents.

Environmental history may be of significance in patient evaluation. Exposure to various chemicals, nuclear radiation, sunlight, dust, and other agents may create conditions that will affect the patient's response to anesthesia. These conditions include liver and kidney damage, serum cholinesterase deficiency, anemia, and pulmonary lesions, in addition to an increased incidence of cancer in patients exposed to such irritants.

Physical examination may reveal both unsuspected and grossly obvious variations or abnormalities that would interfere with placement of IV catheters, intraarterial catheters, endotracheal tubes, nasogastric tubes, ECG electrodes, temperature monitors, and other equipment (Figs. 38–5, 38–6).

Laboratory Examination

The laboratory examination should include, at the minimum, a sequential multiple analyzer battery (lactate dehydrogenase, serum glutamic oxalic transaminase, alkaline phosphatase, bilirubin, creatinine, albumin, total protein, and blood urea nitrogen determinations), a coagulation profile, measurement of hematocrit and hemoglobin, and urinalysis. In any patient taking antihypertensive medication, diuretics, cardiac medication, anticancer agents, or other medication, there may be a marked variation in serum electrolytes, especially potassium. Because these values may change within a few hours and electrolyte concentrations exert a profound influence upon myocardial function and drug action, the examination should be performed within 48 hours before anesthesia induction. This allows time for some corrective measures to be taken if they are necessary.

Obviously, liver function studies and enzymes are significant when a hepatic tumor or other disease produces abnormal values. Coagulation studies may indicate bleeding problems to be anticipated during surgery or that anticoagulants are being administered and not recognized. Hematocrit and hemoglobin values must be correlated with the patient's clinical status. Low values may indicate a need for preoperative transfusions, early replacement of blood

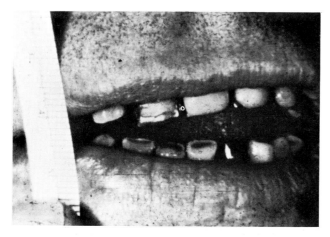

Figure 38–1. Lesion of temporomandibular joint restricts oral opening to less than 1 cm.

loss, or, if chronically low, careful monitoring of loss and minimal replacement.

Radiologic Examination

Radiologic examination frequently offers a synopsis of the extent of metastatic disease, allowing prior planning for surgery as a part of the overall plan of therapy or as the primary mode of treatment. Intracranial lesions require meticulous anesthetic management to prevent wide fluctuations in intracranial pressure. Intrathoracic tumors may show evidence in chest roentgenograms of obstruction, pulmonary effusion, pericardial effusion, or atelectasis that will have a direct influence on the administration of anesthesia. Bone lesions or pathologic fractures require careful patient movement and positioning.

As mentioned, complete cardiac evaluation is mandatory in all patients with histories of cardiovascular disease. This evaluation begins with a standard 12-lead ECG in such patients and in all patients older than 40 years of age.

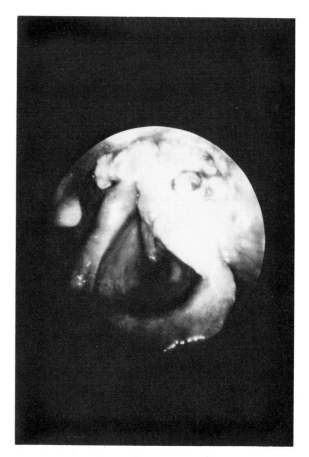

Figure 38–3. Lesion of the glottis.

Pulmonary disease in the cancer patient is not confined to a primary or metastatic tumor. Emphysema, chronic obstructive pulmonary disease, bronchitis, previous surgery, previous infection, and chemotherapy may produce varying degrees of respiratory insufficiency. Pulmonary function studies will provide an indication of the patient's ability to withstand the planned procedure, particularly if thoracic surgery is necessary. The additional data available from catheterization of the right side of the heart will be required in those patients with recent myocardial infarction, respiratory failure requiring positive end-expiratory pressure (PEEP) greater than 15 cm of water, and sepsis. In such patients, the pulmonary artery catheter should be used throughout the operative procedure.

Medication History

A thorough medication history may be very significant in the perioperative care of the cancer patient. Chemotherapy with doxorubicin (Adriamycin) may produce cardiotoxic effects: (1) early ECG abnormalities with multiple variations and (2) cumulative, dose-dependent, drug-induced cardiomyopathy. Most of the ECG changes are transient and will reverse to the original patterns within 1 to 2 months of discontinuation of treatment. The cumulative, dose-dependent, drug-induced cardiomyopathy produces congestive heart failure in patients receiving a cumulative dose

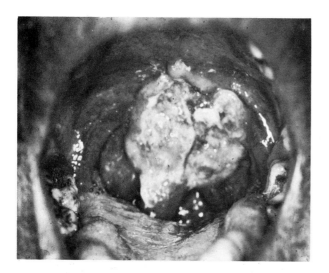

Figure 38–2. Lesion of the hard palate.

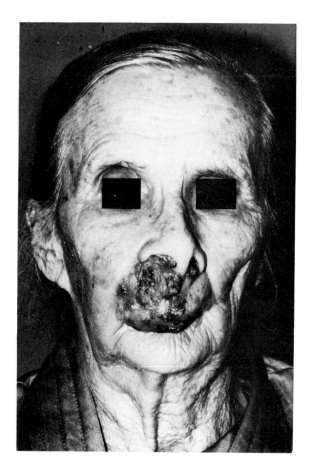

Figure 38–4. Nasal and lip lesion.

of more than 550 mg/M^2 surface area and has also been reported at lower doses. Patients with evidence of doxorubicin cardiotoxicity must be managed carefully, using central venous pressure, blood pressure, and urinary output to monitor appropriate fluid administration. Patients with severe alteration of left ventricular function or in whom massive blood loss is anticipated should have a pulmonary artery catheter inserted preoperatively.

Daunorubicin induces cardiomyopathy similar to that produced by doxorubicin but that is not amenable to early detection. The time from cessation of therapy to manifestation of cardiomyopathy varies from 2 to 1348 days, with the range usually 3 to 6 months after the first dose.

Bleomycin is frequently used in the therapy of testicular carcinoma and may produce pulmonary fibrosis, predisposing the patient to development of acute adult respiratory distress syndrome (ARDS) postoperatively. The tissue damage produced in the lung by bleomycin is very similar to that seen in oxygen toxicity. Patients known to have received bleomycin should be maintained at an inspired oxygen concentration of 30 percent or less.

Cisplatin, another frequently used agent, produces a persistent decrease in glomerular filtration rate. There are some reports of possible cardiotoxicity.

Cyclophosphamide, usually given in doses of 1 to 3 mg/kg per day or 10 to 15 mg/kg per week, has the major toxic effect of bone marrow depression. However, in some

patients, high-dose regimens of 120 to 240 mg/kg given over 1 to 4 days have resulted in severe hemorrhagic cardiac necrosis.

Some patients develop angina following the use of 5-fluorouracil (5-FU). In most reports, there were mild or no ECG changes, and the changes that were noted disappeared within a few hours after onset.

Most chemotherapeutic agents given IV produce fibrosis of the vessels used, sometimes making it very difficult to locate a patent, usable vein. A newly introduced agent, homoharringtonine, is reported to cause hypotension during anesthesia in patients being treated with the drug. Limited experience with this agent in the United States has shown no significant blood pressure variations.

Patients with cancer are also susceptible to other diseases that require chronic drug therapy. The patient's condition and therapeutic dosage level should be stabilized to the best degree possible before administration of anesthesia. Diabetics requiring insulin must be monitored carefully with urine and blood sugar testing and possibly arterial blood gas and electrolyte determinations. Crystalline insulin should be given IV during the procedure. A solution of 5 percent dextrose in water containing 15 units of crystalline insulin, given at a rate of 60 to 100 ml/hr, is a basic technique for control. Long-acting or intermediate-acting forms of insulin should not be given on the morning of surgery.

Steroid dosages should be increased during the periop-

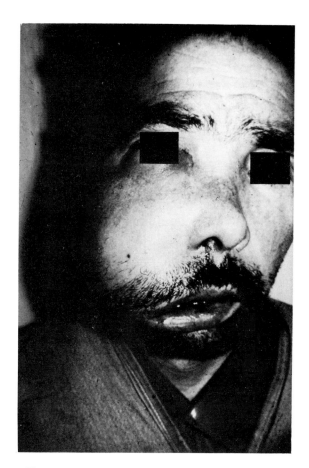

Figure 38–5. Maxillary lesion distorts entire airway.

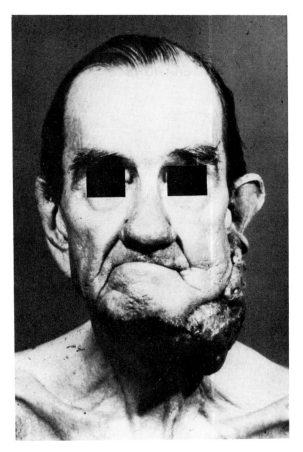

Figure 38–6. Lesion of neck and mandible obstructs airway.

erative period, with careful reduction in the postoperative phase. Cardiac glycosides, antihypertensives, diuretics, antiarrhythmics, and similar agents must be evaluated individually. Digitalis preparations should be continued, with serum potassium level monitoring. Diuretics and antihypertensives should be continued until the night before surgery, but long-acting diuretics (chlorthalidone, cyclothiazide, polythiazide) should be discontinued 2 to 3 days preoperatively. Beta-adrenergic blocking agents (propranolol) should be given until the night before surgery. Nitroglycerin paste applied to the skin before going to the operating suite is very helpful in patients who have angina.

Monoamine oxidase inhibitors should be discontinued 2 to 3 weeks before anesthesia administration because of the variable effects of their interaction with anesthetic agents. Although it is not necessary to discontinue alpha-methyldopa, blood bank personnel should be aware of its use when a type and crossmatch are requested. Many patients using this drug show a positive direct Coombs test.

Because of underlying infection, immunosuppression from chemotherapy and radiation, and the extent of surgery, prophylactic antibiotics are used frequently. A possible interaction between drugs used during anesthesia and certain of these agents makes awareness of the specific antibiotics significant.

The type and location of the patient's lesion plus the effects of radiation and chemotherapy frequently cause se-

vere malnutrition and dehydration. Obviously, such conditions can produce drastic alterations in hepatic, renal, and cardiovascular functions. The patient's response to anesthetic agents will be exaggerated. Hyperalimentation, blood component therapy, and fluid replacement should be instituted as far in advance of anesthesia administration as possible.

Drug-induced secondary anemia, leukopenia, and thrombocytopenia; pancytopenia from bone marrow metastases; anemia from gastrointestinal bleeding, hemolysis, or defective iron utilization in chronic disease; the effects of increasing age; underlying, low-grade infection; and, particularly, recent myocardial infarction must also be considered when assessing the patient's overall condition before anesthesia induction and surgery.

ANESTHESIA

Selection of the anesthetic should be related to the patient's overall condition, although the agent itself is not a major item in anesthetic management. Patients with abnormal liver function are not generally given halogenated agents. Inhalation agents should be considered in those patients who have chronic obstructive pulmonary disease. (At The University of Texas System Cancer Center M.D. Anderson Hospital and Tumor Institute, approximately 70 percent of anesthetics are performed with a fentanyl–nitrous oxide–muscle relaxant technique, and the remainder are done with enflurane, isoflurane, or halothane as the basic agent.)

Most cancer surgery is considered to be of a radical nature, and management of radical surgery patients requires continuous evaluation of alterations in the patient's condition. Continuous monitoring of the ECG, blood pressure, respiration, delivered oxygen concentration, heart rate, heart sounds, blood loss, muscle relaxation, and temperature is required in every patient. In those patients with cardiovascular abnormalities, pulmonary disease, renal disease, hepatic dysfunction, metabolic disorders, massive blood loss, and so on, it may be necessary to routinely monitor urinary output, central venous pressure, direct arterial pressure, cardiac output, arterial blood gases, serum electrolytes, urine and blood glucose, and coagulation parameters. During whole-body hyperthermia for solid tumors of the thorax, meticulous differential temperature measurement and control to at least 0.1C must be maintained. Routine electroencephalographic monitoring is practiced in some institutions for all major procedures.

As in any procedure, adequate ventilation must be maintained. A volume ventilator should be used in any procedure of more than 30 minutes' duration. Proper positioning and placement of support rolls aid ventilation.

Heating and cooling units should be used to maintain body temperature in all patients. Warm irrigating solutions, warm IV solutions, warm blood, and control of room temperature also assist in maintaining adequate patient temperatures.

Because of the altered physiologic condition of many cancer patients, it is important to position the patient properly, use adequate padding at pressure points, avoid excessive pressure when moving the patient, protect the eyes, and place protective barriers to prevent excess pressure from equipment or personnel during the procedure. Various arm, leg, chest, and head supports assist in proper positioning. Careful placement of the electrosurgery unit grounding pad is necessary to avoid excess pressure, burns, or cardiac effects. Positioning of the patient and equipment should be considered the responsibility of the entire operating team.

Large-bore IV catheters are mandatory during radical surgical procedures. Cannulation of the internal jugular or subclavian vein for monitoring central venous pressure or administration of fluids, or both, should be considered in most patients.

Although the admonition to administer anesthesia gently should be applied to every patient, it is particularly appropriate for cancer patients, since they are generally in poor physiologic condition and are highly susceptible to anesthetic agents. Their responses may be exaggerated and difficult to control. Slow induction progressing to an adequate depth of anesthesia for intubation and surgery is significant to avoid stress and its effects on the patient. Constant communication and cooperation among members of the operating team, the laboratory, and the blood bank must be maintained. Changes in ventilation, circulation, and stimulation should be discussed and planned for in advance. Unexpected, abrupt changes must be communicated immediately.

Fluid and blood replacement are determined by blood loss, intravascular volume, urinary output, central venous pressure, arterial blood pressure, and the specific procedure being performed.

To meet the need for continuous assessment of anesthetic administration, muscle relaxation, monitoring equipment data, laboratory examination results, and administration of blood components and fluids, more than one person must be available to manage a patient undergoing radical cancer surgery. During critical times of rapid blood replacement, severe alterations in cardiovascular stability, or changes in electrolyte and coagulation parameters, many members of the anesthesia care team may be required. Members of the anesthesiology staff should circulate through the operating suite constantly to assist with complex cases.

Reversal of narcotic and muscle relaxant effects must be monitored by the nerve stimulator and respirometer. If it is necessary to maintain assisted or controlled ventilation in the postoperative period, antagonism of these agents is undesirable. There must be satisfactory muscle strength and tidal volume if the patient is to be extubated in the operating room. Assisted ventilation by use of an Ambu bag, with accompanying oxygen, may be necessary during transportation to the recovery area. Continuous arterial blood pressure and ECG monitoring may be performed with a battery-powered portable monitor. Heating and cooling units plus warm blankets should be used during the immediate recovery period.

Routine care in the recovery room should include monitoring of the ECG, blood pressure, heart rate, respiratory rate and volume, temperature, urine output, rate of fluid administration, and administration of humidified oxygen. Monitoring of CVP, direct arterial pressure, and Swan-Ganz catheter pressures, plus mechanical respiratory assistance, may also be necessary. The patient's condition and care

must be followed by a staff anesthesiologist familiar with his or her status through the entire recovery phase and for at least 48 hours postoperatively.

SPECIAL CONSIDERATIONS

Cancer patients are highly susceptible to infection because of the immunosuppressive effects of radiation, chemotherapy, and frequently malnourishment. Therefore, all equipment and supplies used must be sterilized or cleaned as completely as possible. All invasive items must be sterile, and most of these items, such as endotracheal tubes, breathing circuits, intravascular catheters, IV fluid administration sets, blood filters, pressure transducer lines and domes, suction catheters, nasogastric tubes, esophageal stethoscopes, and regional block trays, are disposable after one use. Reusable items, such as oral airways, armored endotracheal tubes, endobronchial tubes, ventilator bellows, forceps, laryngoscope blades, and temperature probes, should be sterilized, preferably by ethylene oxide gas sterilization. Double-lumen endobronchial tubes, armored endotracheal tubes, and certain preformed, specialized tracheostomy tubes are now available in disposable form, and their use should be considered.

Adequate aeration of absorbent material must be accomplished before reuse. Fiberoptic laryngoscopes and bronchoscopes should be cold sterilized. Blood pressure cuffs, stethoscope chest pieces, and laryngoscope handles should be thoroughly cleaned after each use. Ventilators, warming blankets and units, anesthesia machines, monitoring units, tables, and other equipment should be cleaned with a disinfectant or detergent solution after each case.

The use of Bain and Mapleson D disposable breathing circuits should be considered in pediatric patients and some adult patients where nonrebreathing techniques are advisable.

The appropriate use of various blood components is obviously determined by their availability, communication with the blood bank, and the time required for transportation to the operating room. Packed red blood cells, diluted in the blood bank with saline, are generally given as replacement for blood loss. Fresh, whole blood may be required in some cases. All blood should be warmed before administration. Fresh frozen plasma should be used as necessary, generally 2 units with every 10 units of packed red cells. Plasma expanders, such as plasma protein fraction and hetastarch, may be useful. IV fluids given throughout the procedure, such electrolyte solutions as Plasmosol and Ringer's lactate, should be regulated by the patient's needs and not given on a purely routine basis.

Patients with rare blood types, those for whom blood is not readily available, or those who will not accept blood transfusions because of religious beliefs may benefit from the use of a blood cell separator. This machine is normally used in blood banks for the collection of platelets and white blood cells from donors. The blood cell separator allows blood to be removed from the body at one rate and simultaneously returned at another. The reservoir of red cells so formed is kept in constant contact with the body through a closed loop (Fig. 38–7) and returned as needed.

As in all operating rooms, waste gases should be evacu-

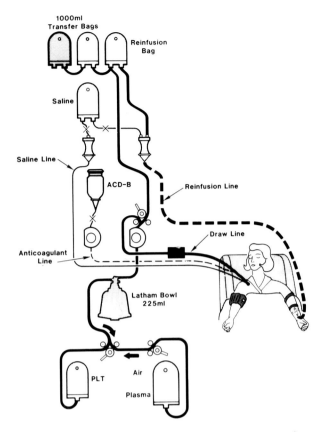

Figure 38–7. Diagram of the path used to draw, store, and reinfuse blood. ACD-B, acid citrate dextrose formula B; PLT, platelets.

ated to protect the operating team. Gases should be removed from the adjustable pressure limiting (APL) valve of the anesthesia machine and ventilator by an exhaust system separate from the vacuum used at the operating table. Air exchange within the room should be great enough to remove gases expelled when the machine is disconnected from the patient for a short time, for example, during intubation. Frequent inspection of all connections, with collection and analysis of air samples at various locations, must be made to maintain an atmosphere free of waste gases.

The body temperature of pediatric patients is more difficult to maintain at a normal level than is that of adults. It is frequently necessary to warm and humidify the operating room in addition to using a warming blanket on the operating table. For infants, it may be advisable to use an infrared warming unit.

Although standardization of equipment, supplies, and location is not restricted to cancer centers, such standardization is important in large operating suites. Standard equipment throughout the suite allows parts and modules to be interchanged. Specific locations for supplies and equipment in each room reduces confusion when personnel assignments are rotated and, especially, during emergency situations when time for obtaining supplies is critical. Familiarity with equipment throughout the operating suite is important in total patient care.

Whole-body hyperthermia, with or without radiation during the procedure, poses a unique, specific set of circum-

stances. Exact body temperatures must be monitored and controlled. Temperature measurements must be accurate to within 0.1C. Light anesthesia is adequate for extracorporeal heat exchange or noninvasive techniques for raising body temperature. Inspired gases are heated and humidified. Fluids must be carefully evaluated and replaced, particularly those lost through profuse perspiration. Serum electrolytes, arterial blood gases, and hematocrit and hemoglobin levels must be monitored constantly for fluctuations.

Regional perfusion with chemotherapeutic agents for nonmetastatic lesions is usually performed in patients in whom an early diagnosis has been made. This technique allows much higher doses of the agent to be applied directly to the tumor than can be tolerated by whole-body administration.

Subarachnoid alcohol block and celiac plexus alcohol block for control of intractable pain in advanced malignant disease should be considered in some patients. Alcohol blocks provide long-lasting relief without the need for frequent injections. Nerve blocks with local anesthetics are very useful as diagnostic aids and for temporary relief of pain. These procedures carry a minimal risk of mortality and complications and can be performed in debilitated patients.

Patients with cancer are a special group with unique characteristics and needs. All therapy, including anesthesia for surgery and specific nerve blocks for pain relief, must be structured to meet the individual patient's needs.

BIBLIOGRAPHY

Allen LM: Pharmacokinetic principles of antineoplastic drug therapy. Clin Pharmacol 23:71–81, 1983.

Ames M, Powis G, Kovach J (eds): Pharmacokinetics of Anticancer Agents in Humans. New York, Elsevier, 1983.

Balis F, Holcenberg J, Bliyer W: Clissical pharmacokinetics of commonly used anticancer drugs. Clin Pharmacokinet 8:202–32, 1983.

Belt R, Leite G, Haas C, et al: Incidence of hemorrhagic complications in patients with cancer. JAMA 239:2571–2574, 1978.

Chiu W: Diagnostic and therapeutic nerve block for cancer pain. Cancer Bull 33:93–98, 1981.

Dent R, McCall I: 5-Fluorouracil and angina. Lancet 1:347–348, 1975.

DeVita V, Hellwan S, Rosenberg S (eds): Cancer: Principles and Practice of Oncology, 2nd ed. Philadelphia, Lippincott, 1985.

Eyee H, Ward J: Control of cancer chemotherapy-induced nausea and vomiting. Cancer 54[Suppl 1]:2642–2648, 1984.

Hirsh J, Conlon P: Implementing guidelines for managing extravasation of antineoplastics. Am J Hosp Pharm 40:1516–1579, 1983.

Howland W, Goldiner P: Physiologic management of the cancer patient during surgery. Curr Probl Cancer 3:1–50, 1978.

Laszlo J (ed): Antiesmetics and Cancer Chemotherapy. Baltimore, Williams & Wilkins, 1983.

Marsoni S, Witter R: Clinical development of anticancer agents— A National Cancer Institute perspective. Cancer Treat Rep 68:77, 1980.

Minow R, Benjamin R, Lee E, et al: Adriamycin cardiomyopathy— Risk factors. Cancer 39:1397–1402, 1977.

Perry M, Yarbro J: Toxicity of Chemotherapy. New York, Grune & Stratton, 1984.

Seigel L, Lougo D: The control of chemotherapy–induced emesis. Ann Intern Med 95:352–359, 1981.

Slavin R, Millan J, Mullins G: Pathology of high-dose intermittent cyclophosphamide therapy. Hum Pathol 6:693–709, 1975.

Von Hoff D, Layard M, Basa P, et al: Risk factors for doxorubicin-induced congestive heart failure. Ann Intern Med 91:710–717, 1979.

Von Hoff D, Rozensweig M, Layard M, et al: Daunomycin-induced cardiotoxicity in children and adults: A review of 110 cases. Am J Med 62:200–208, 1977.

Walton B: Anaesthesia, surgery and immunology (Review article). Anaesthesia 33:322–348, 1978.

Wancho H, Pinsky G, Beattie E, et al: Immunocompetence testing in patients with one of the four common operable cancers—A review. Clin Bull 8:15–22, 1978.

Warfield M (ed): Routine machine solves the problem of transfusions for Jehovah's Witnesses. Newsletter (The University of Texas System Cancer Center M. D. Anderson Hospital and Tumor Institute) 26:2, 1981.

Winter P, Smith G: The toxicity of oxygen. Anesthesiology 37:210–241, 1972.

39

Anesthetic Management of the Patient with Neuromuscular or Related Diseases

Lida S. Dahm

Before the 1950s, patients with neuromuscular and spinal cord diseases were generally either left at home or placed in a nursing facility to die. With the launching of the first spinal cord centers in England by Guttmann, the long-time care of these patients gradually became an art. The availability of antibiotics and the increasing knowledge of pathophysiology gave the physician the ability to extend the life span into the chronic phase of the disease. Many of the children with birth defects or chronic debilitating disease who previously had died early in the course of their disease survived into adulthood and thus had an increasing number of general medical problems. This gradually led to the establishment of physical medicine and rehabilitation as a specialty.

With the neurologist making the diagnosis in many neuromuscular and spinal cord-injured patients and the rehabilitation specialist designing courses of management for the chronic phase of the disease, survival rates have increased markedly. Figure 39–1 compares the survival of quadriplegic patients during one 7-year period with that of the following 8-year period.

GENERAL PRINCIPLES

The general principles of management of the patient with neuromuscular disease follow those for any other patient with a chronic and potentially severely disabling disease. A good history is mandatory, especially a good family history, since susceptible patients may have devastating complications from malignant hyperthermia and hypoglycemia. An assessment of present activity gives an idea of respiratory and cardiovascular function. Some patients may be taking as many as 20 different medications that may have both antagonizing and potentiating side effects. Many of these medications affect the autonomic nervous system as well as electrolytes and the general metabolism.

An initial cardiac and respiratory baseline assessment is necessary when the patient is first seen by the surgeon. Many of these diseases are associated with chronically pro-

gressive disabilities; thus a return to baseline may never occur. This fact alone is of importance to the anesthesiologist in considering whether the patient had a smooth or difficult course postsurgery. It naturally follows that a patient whose general medical condition is worse at this time and who had a previous difficult postoperative course will have to be managed carefully throughout the perioperative period for any subsequent surgery.

Many of these patients are surviving with a narrow margin of function in the neurologic, respiratory, or cardiovascular systems. They may have poor tissue turgor and peripheral vascular disease. Possibly, they have been taking steroids or other long-term medication that changes coagulability and the turgor of the vessel walls. Their neuromuscular diseases may be associated with skeletal changes so that their heads cannot be moved, or their jaws may be fixed, making intubation difficult to impossible. One can list other similar abnormalities throughout the musculoskeletal system. If surgery has been frequent, the presence of tracheostenosis or malacia should be considered, especially if there is a tracheostomy scar.

Table 39–1 is a classification of neuromuscular and related diseases.

CLASSIFICATION AND SPECIFIC CHARACTERISTICS

Neuromuscular Diseases

Duchenne Muscular Dystrophy. This is one of the best-known of the neuromuscular diseases. Inheritance is through a sex-linked recessive gene, with the vast majority of patients being male. Parents of the index case may have no knowledge of the disease within their family.

The onset of muscle weakness occurs in the first decade, progressing to death in the late teens or early twenties. A pseudohypertrophy occurs, which is often followed by muscular atrophy. Pulmonary function is gradually decreased severely, and there is an increase in muscle weakness that

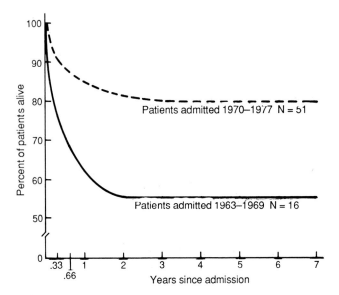

Figure 39–1. Survival curves based on two groups of acute spinal cord-injured patients with lesions of C-4 and above. (*Courtesy of RE Carter, M.D., The Institute for Rehabilitation and Research, Texas Medical Center, Houston, Texas.*)

is usually associated with scoliosis. The cardiopulmonary reserve is markedly reduced, which indicates to the anesthetist that these patients must be handled with care postoperatively. Laboratory findings include a greatly elevated creatinine phosphokinase (CPK), with ECG and echocardiographic manifestations of ventricular dysfunction. These

TABLE 39–1. CLASSIFICATION OF NEUROMUSCULAR AND RELATED DISEASES

  I. Neuromuscular diseases
    A. Muscular dystrophy
       1. Duchenne muscular dystrophy
       2. Central core disease
       3. Others
    B. Myasthenia gravis
    C. Myasthenic syndrome
    D. Myopathies
    E. Familial periodic paralysis
    F. Ataxias and other diseases
 II. Connective tissue diseases
    A. Rheumatoid arthritis
    B. Collagen diseases
    C. Granulomatous diseases
III. Skeletal problems
    A. Scoliosis
    B. Osteogenesis imperfecta
    C. Others
IV. Spinal cord trauma
    A. Acute phase
    B. Transition time
    C. Chronic phase
 V. Paralysis secondary to other etiologies
    A. Tumor
    B. Infection
    C. Vascular etiology

---

patients may have resting tachycardia and congestive heart failure secondary to the restrictive lung disease.

There is no specific treatment except for symptomatic care. Anesthesia may be required for muscle biopsies or orthopedic procedures early in the course of the disease. Minimal anesthetic and premedication agents should be used to avoid respiratory depression. Small doses of anticholinergics are used to minimize tachycardia. Special anesthetic considerations are directed toward the use of relaxants, since these patients may show an increased sensitivity to relaxants. On the other hand, there have been reports of muscle rigidity after succinylcholine administration in an occasional patient; thus, it is better not to use muscle relaxants. Intubation is facilitated in these patients because of their generalized muscle weakness. However, skeletal abnormalities secondary to long-term disease might create difficulty in intubating, and awake intubation would then be advisable.

Central Core Disease. This myopathy is associated with a weakness on exertion and an intolerance to high environmental temperatures. This is the one group of dystrophic patients who are definitely susceptible to severe hyperkalemia, which results in ventricular fibrillation and death after small clinical doses of succinylcholine. Central core disease should be considered in any patient who reports a history of difficulties with anesthetics and multiple deaths in the family associated with either heat or exercise intolerance. Often these patients have no other prodromata of any neuromuscular disease.

Other Myopathies. Other myopathies are varieties of other muscular dystrophies, such as fascioscapulohumoral dystrophy (FSH) and limb–girdle dystrophy, which are usually more benign than Duchenne muscular dystrophy. These dystrophies may create similar problems in anesthesia administration.

Malignant hyperthermia, which has overwhelming significance to the anesthetist, is considered in Chapter 36. Here, we emphasize that any patient with a history of vague or actual neuromuscular symptoms must be considered as a potential candidate for malignant hyperthermia. All of these patients must have an extensive history, physical examination, and laboratory workup.

Other Muscle Diseases. Other muscle diseases may create difficulties in anesthetic management. There are multiple disorders caused by one or more enzymatic defects in the pathways of glycogen storage and mobilization from the liver and muscle. Patients with these disorders may have relatively mild symptoms or associated severe cirrhosis or congestive heart failure and, thus, early mortality. Because of the difficulty in regulating blood glucose levels, the blood sugar must be followed carefully. Preoperative IV fluids are needed, since fasting produces profound hypoglycemia. Administration of succinylcholine may lead to myoglobulinuria; both hepatic and cardiac function may fail significantly in the perioperative period.

Myoneurojunctional Diseases

Myasthenia Gravis. This is probably the best known disease in this category. It is characterized by a fluctuating weakness that varies throughout the day and is worsened by exercise. This symptom appears to be more bothersome to the patient than the resultant fatigue. The ocular muscles generally are involved initially, and oropharangeal weakness occurs, with difficulties in swallowing and talking when other cranial nerves are involved. At this point, both limb and neck weakness may have occurred, but only during myasthenic crisis does one see severe respiratory weakness. These patients may be classified as very mild, with almost benign symptoms, to severe, with marked bulbar symptoms and severe generalized muscle weakness. Females are affected three times more frequently than males between the ages of 10 and 40; after age 40, the incidence is the same in males and females.

The causative event of myasthenia gravis is not known. Most patients have antibodies to muscle acetylcholine receptors, which are not bound directly to the site that binds acetycholine but are close to it. Because of this, binding is reduced between acetylcholine and the receptor. Involvement of the thymus gland in the disease process has led to thymectomy as the method of treatment. About 25 percent of patients may have complete remission, but those patients with a thymoma have a lower response.

The diagnosis of myasthenia gravis is made on the basis of clinical symptoms, a detailed history, and the characteristic electromyogram. Either edrophonium and neostigmine may be used as the anticholinesterase for diagnosis of the disease. The nonsurgical therapy of the disease consists of giving anticholinesterase agents, of which pyridostigmine and neostigmine, given orally, are most commonly used. The duration of action of pyridostigmine is longer and the drug has fewer side effects than does neostigmine. Patients with myasthenia gravis may also have been taking steroids.

An exacerbation of the symptoms occurs in myasthenic crisis, when severe respiratory weakness is associated with difficulty in swallowing. The increased secretions, respiratory infection, and muscle weakness produce a vicious cycle. Because of the lack of resistance to respiratory infections in these patients, respiratory support may be necessary through the crisis. The second crisis that may occur in the myasthenia patient is cholinergic crisis, which may be difficult to differentiate from myasthenic crisis. Cholinergic crisis is caused by overtreatment with anticholinesterase agents, which cause increased muscle weakness and secretions. A differential diagnosis can be made by the gradual injection of edrophonium to a maximum of 10 mg in a 70-kg patient. The patient who gets better is in a myasthenic crisis; the patient who becomes worse is in a cholinergic crisis.

The anesthetic difficulties arising in this disease are mainly those related to the muscle weakness; thus, whenever possible, avoid the use of muscle relaxants. These patients do not need muscle relaxants for thymectomies. Class 2–4 myasthenic patients need thymectomies. The need for postoperative ventilatory assistance is common. The biggest controversy in the anesthetic management of the myasthenic patient is about the use of anticholinesterase agents perioperatively. The general belief is that anticholinesterase agents should be given throughout the perioperative period to those patients who are already dependent on them. Those patients who have a relatively benign course may be watched and given the agents only as indicated. Complications of anticholinesterase agents include potentiation of the vagal responses and decrease in metabolism of ester local anesthetics. Also, muscle relaxation may be more difficult to produce. Patients with muscle weakness from whatever cause tolerate preoperative sedation poorly, and, therefore, preoperative and intraoperative depressant medications should be carefully monitored.

If the operative procedure can be performed under inhalation anesthesia alone, muscle relaxants often are not needed. The use of succinylcholine is controversial, since it has been said that myasthenics have less response to it than do normal patients. Most investigators have found that the usual intubating dose produces adequate relaxation and apparent rapid recovery. However, some patients have shown an early phase II block with an associated slow recovery. This phase II block may exist for several hours postsuccinylcholine. Thus, it is better to avoid the use of muscle relaxants. There have been various attempts to decide, in the preoperative evaluation which patients will need postoperative respiratory assistance. Generally, if the symptoms have continued for more than 5 or 6 years and anticholinesterases are needed, respiratory assistance postoperatively is required.

The Myasthenic Syndrome or Eaton-Lambert Syndrome. This syndrome is associated with carcinoma, and these patients' symptoms mimic the symptoms of myasthenia gravis except that they improve with activity. Although the bronchus is the most common site of the carcinoma, there may be thoracic tumors from prostate, breast, stomach, or rectum. At times, the weakness may occur 1 to 2 years before the diagnosis of carcinoma is made. Removal of the tumor does not affect the weakness.

Electromyography shows a reverse picture to that of myasthenia gravis. Although there is a reduced muscle response to single nerve stimulus, tetanic stimulation shows a progressive increase in muscle strength as the frequency in duration of the stimulation is increased.

These patients are extremely sensitive to nondepolarizing and depolarizing muscle relaxants, and weakness may last for many days after their use. Thus, muscle relaxants are to be avoided in these patients.

Atypical Plasma Cholinesterase. Patients with atypical plasma cholinesterase appear normal except for a history of profound and prolonged muscle relaxation after succinylcholine. Normal patients have muscular paralysis approximately 3 to 5 minutes after administration of 1 mg/kg succinylcholine, since the drug is hydrolyzed by plasma cholinesterase. Occasionally, a patient has an abnormal plasma cholinesterase that does not have the same rate of hydrolysis as the aceytylcholine. A local anesthetic inhibits the enzyme activities in the plasma of the patients. The percent of inhibition by dibucaine of the original hydrolysis is called the dibucaine number, or DN. The patient with normal enzymes has a DN greater than 80, the heterozygous patient has a DN of approximately 60, and a true homozygous patient with atypical plasma cholinesterase has a DN of approximately 20.

Patients with severe liver disease, malnutrition, burns, glycophosphate poisoning, or other debilitating conditions may also have lower plasma cholinesterase activity. Both pyridophosphate eyedrops and irradiation will lower the activity. The most common condition is during the latter portion of pregnancy, when, generally, no additional care is needed. Patients with a prolonged response to succinylcholine should be ventilated until adequate recovery of the myoneural junction occurs. Normally, pharmacologic agents are not needed, since the patient simply must be sustained with respiratory systems and monitored carefully.

Familial Periodic Paralysis. There are three distinct types of familial periodic paralysis—hypokalemia, hyperkalemia, and normokalemia—although certain characteristics are similar in all three. Generally, there is an autosomal dominant inheritance pattern. These patients may have attacks of quadriplegia that is related to the serum potassium level. The most common cause of death during these attacks is respiratory failure, often resulting from aspiration pneumonia or infection. Cardiac failure and shock have also been reported.

In patients with the hypokalemic form of familial periodic paralysis, the attacks may be increased by eating a heavy meal, and patients must, therefore, abstain from eating a heavy meal the evening before surgery. Potassium levels should be carefully managed. No matter what procedures are to be performed, the ECG should be closely monitored, since arrhythmias are common in this condition. A Swan-Ganz cathether or central venous pressure monitor should be used, since cardiac failure is also a problem in some patients. There is controversy in the literature about the use of muscle relaxants; therefore, it is advisable not to administer these relaxants if at all possible. Patients with the hyperkalemic form of periodic paralysis have acute attacks unrelated to high-carbohydrate meals. In fact, the attacks occur more often when the patients are hungry and may also be related to exercise. In general, the attacks last for a shorter period of time than in patients with hypokalemia. There is an outpouring of potassium from the muscles, and treatment of the hyperkalemic form is with insulin and glucose therapy. This type of treatment might precipitate an attack in hypokalemic patients.

Hyperkalemic patients are generally treated with diuretics, whereas hypokalemic patients are administered potassium supplementation. All of these patients, including those with normokalemia, must have their serum enzymes carefully monitored throughout the perioperative period.

Anesthetic problems occur mainly through small deviations in potassium levels, which may cause paralysis. Postoperative paralysis has been noted, and supplemental respiratory assistance should be available.

Neural Diseases

Ataxias, Demyelinating Diseases, and Other Diseases. The most prominent of the ataxias, Friedreich's ataxia, is a progressive disease associated with widespread conduc-

tive defects that strikes the male in the teenage period. The patient develops nystagmus and severe cardiac arrhythmia. The ECG must be carefully monitored throughout surgery, and cardiotoxic agents should be avoided if possible. In my experience, anesthesia has been tolerated well by these patients. They have a certain degree of muscle weakness and respiratory insufficiency during the latter stages of the disease, and, therefore, respiratory depression and excess sedative agents should be avoided.

Ataxias and athetosis from other conditions have been associated with an inappropriate response to atropine. In these patients, smaller doses of atropine are used than normally given to avoid a mild febrile response with oral temperatures of 38 to 39C. An increased incidence of malignant hyperthermia has been suspected in cerebral palsy patients with ataxia and athetosis, although this has not been fully documented.

Multiple sclerosis is the most common member of the demyelinating diseases. It is associated with exacerbations and remissions and typically occurs in three distinct forms: (1) rapidly progressive or malignant form, (2) slowly progressing with exacerbations and incomplete remissions over a long period of time, and (3) a relatively benign form that is very slowly progressive and is not associated with a shortened life span. There are very few patients who have one attack and then apparently are cured, with no subsequent attacks. The disease is associated with an exacerbation of weakness, visual symptoms, and numbness from paresthesias. Euphoria is general, and depression may occur. The patients are often given both steroids and ACTH, so they may require an increased amount of steroids at the time of anesthesia and surgery. Routinely, these are necessary if either drug is given within 3 months of surgery. Spinal anesthesia is contraindicated because of the nature of the disease and the resulting medicolegal implications. Temperature must be monitored carefully, since the onset of an infection or pyrexia may produce new symptoms. There have been reports of an exacerbation of attacks after anesthesia and surgery. In general, these exacerbations are shorter in duration and do not lead to permanent changes when compared to the expected exacerbation, which can signal a more progressive downhill course.

Patients with Down's syndrome have an increased sensitivity to atropine, and thus slightly lower doses than normal are administered. Neurofibromatosis is associated with increased bleeding when the neurofibromas are surgically excised, particularly during scoliosis corrections in which a neurofibromatous lesion is in the vertebral spine.

Connective Tissue Diseases

Rheumatoid Arthritis. Patients with rheumatoid arthritis may be children or adults. Children with rheumatoid arthritis have Still's disease and are often taking steroids as well as experiencing all of the pubertal changes occurring during growth. These patients progress in their disease and develop severe skeletal deformities. Intubation is particularly difficult, since very often the chin rests on the sternum, and these patients generally have compromised cardiorespiratory function.

Adult patients with rheumatoid arthritis generally have less severe skeletal deformities than do children. They are chronically ill, undernourished, and anemic, and most are polyarticular, with the small joints of the hand and foot affected. These patients may have lung involvement, with a diffuse infiltrate producing restriction and thus loss of compliance. One finds in both adults and children a markedly decreased ventilatory ability and low reserve due to the restrictive lung disease. Both pediatric and adult patients may have heart involvement in the valve leaflets, rings, myocardium, and endocardium, as well as the most common problem, amyloidosis, which involves the kidneys. Such patients may progress to renal failure, or the excretion of any drugs administered may be markedly diminished. The most constant finding is anemia of chronic disease, which is characteristic of patients with rheumatoid arthritis. This is usually not severe but is resistant to iron therapy.

Often, these patients have been taking acetylsalicylic acid, phenylbutazone, endomethizine, or steroids. Many of the new nonsteroid anti-inflammatory drugs have also been used in rheumatoid arthritis. One must be aware of the increased incidence of gastric disturbance and occult gastrointestinal bleeding in these patients, particularly if the hemoglobin is below 10 g.

Another disease with a similar pathology is ankylosing spondylitis, which involves particularly the sacroiliac joint and other end joints of the spine and hips, rather than the neck. There is a significant impairment of rotating motion and a limitation of binding. These patients may have a solid ridge of bone along the lumbar spine, making diagnostic spinal tap impossible. Because these patients may have been taking steroids or other drugs, a careful history and significant preoperative check for mobility of the jaw and other joints must be performed. These patients generally have surgery for corrective orthopedic procedures and for complications of corticosteroid therapy, as well as ordinary surgical procedures, such as appendectomy. Airway and respiratory management must be handled carefully in these patients, and they should be intubated before administration of anesthesia. In general, an awake intubation with a fiberoptic laryngoscope or bronchoscope is safer than is intubation after anesthesia induction. When blood loss is expected, one must be particularly concerned about both anemia and a decrease in platelet function secondary to steroidal or other therapy.

Collagen Diseases. The collagen diseases are systemic lupus erythematosus, scleroderma, polyarteritis nodosa, and dermatomyositis. Each of these diseases is discussed briefly, followed by a discussion of the general anesthetic management of each.

Systemic lupus erythematosus may be associated with pericarditis and other cardiac abnormalities as well as pleurisy. When a pericardial friction rub is present, the disease resembles rheumatic fever. There are multiple clinical problems occurring throughout the lungs and nervous system that may be associated with dysphasia, hemiplegia, and polyneuritis. The clinical course may be prolonged and characterized by exacerbations and remissions. This course may be induced by such drugs as hydralazine and isoniazid. Steroids are often used in these patients, and this must be considered in the perioperative management.

Scleroderma is associated with a brawny edema in the hands, feet, and face, followed by a second stage of a waxy, smooth, and tight skin. Secondary contractures occur and may make opening the mouth extremely difficult. Dysphasia, pulmonary complications, and a significant loss of weight with weakness, fever, and joint pains occur. Cardiac involvement can result from fibrosis and can produce heart failure in association with pulmonary hypertension. Renal complications are also seen. Again, steroids have been used in many of these patients.

Patients with polyarteritis nodosa are particularly susceptible to chronic and acute respiratory infections. Although early symptoms of fever and tenderness occur more frequently in the extremities, respiratory and renal symptoms occur as well; in fact, respiratory lesions may precede the other symptoms. Long remissions have resulted from steroid therapy, although no cures are reported.

Another collagen disease is dermatomyositis, which is a lesion of the skin wherein muscle fibers become vacuolated and degenerated. This is rare and extremely painful. Diplopia, dyspnea, and impaired sphincter control may be present; however, unlike the other collagen diseases, the lungs are generally not affected. When pulmonary disease does occur, it is related to the weakness, with resulting aspiration and respiratory insufficiency.

The anesthetist should consider a probable history of steroid therapy in planning the management of all these patients. Perioperative supplementation is often necessary. The presence of renal disease, and thus renal function, should be ascertained as should cardiopulmonary status. Tightening of the skin around the mouth in the patient with scleroderma means that regional anesthesia is generally preferred over general anesthesia. However, epinephrine in the regional anesthetic is contraindicated, since Raynaud's phenomenon exists. Because blood flow may be reduced in some patients with collagen diseases, determining blood pressure in the normal way can be difficult, and direct arterial monitoring would be advisable. In patients with polyarteritis nodosa, hypertension secondary to the renal disease may be present and should be considered so that hypotension does not occur, with its concomitant cerebral and cardiac problems. In the patients with dermatomyositis, the muscle weakness indicates that muscle relaxants are generally not necessary. A myasthenic response has been demonstrated in some patients with dermatomyositis, although this is not a consistent finding. Whenever relaxation is necessary, a small test dose should be used in these patients.

Thus, in all of these patients, close attention must be given to the cardiac, respiratory, and renal systems. The presence of vague and changing neurologic signs and symptoms plus the contractures due to skeletal, skin, and muscle deformities should all be thoroughly studied before the patient enters the operative suite.

Granulomatous Diseases. These diseases are considered a relatively rare group of clinical symptoms varying from a pure arthritis to diseases incorporating large vessels and granulomatous lesions in many areas. All of these diseases are chronic with insidious onset at varying times of life. Most of them are associated with a pulmonary infection that may progress to widespread consolidation.

The most important of these diseases is Wegener's granulomatosis, which is generally a triad of necrotizing giant cell granulomatosis of the upper respiratory tract and lungs, widespread vasculitis of the small arteries and veins, and focal glomerulonephritis. It progresses with gradual involvement of all the other symptoms and must be distinguished from tuberculosis, sarcoidosis, and mycotic infections. Of particular note is the severity of x-ray findings and the pulmonary symptoms. Symptomatic control occurs with steroids, but the disease is always fatal.

Sarcoidosis is a more benign disease. It is a systemic granulomatous disease with spontaneous incomplete remissions in the early stages and with a slowly progressive course when the disease persists. Particularly involved are the lungs, lymph nodes, and other reticuloendothelial tissue. The disease appears to resemble tuberculosis, but the tubercle or granuloma does not result in caseation and necrosis. Instead, healing takes place by fibrosis with scar formation. The patients are characterized by severe involvement of the tissues with very few symptoms, and they are generally treated with steroids. Thus, they come to the anesthetist as patients on long-term steroid therapy. They may also have lesions in the heart, particularly in the valves, as well as other organs of the body, but these are not as common as the lung lesions. From the anesthetist's standpoint, the pulmonary and cardiac manifestations are most important and should be carefully monitored throughout the course of the disease.

Skeletal Problems

Scoliosis. Neuromuscular diseases can result in the curvature of the spine known as scoliosis. Idiopathic scoliosis occurs during the developmental phase, particularly in young girls going through puberty. The potential exists for marked changes in respiratory and cardiovascular function when the scoliotic curve becomes severe. This may occur when idiopathic scoliosis is left untreated for many years or after other diseases, particularly such paralyzing diseases as polio or quadriplegia, in which the deformed spine and thoracic cage produce severe restrictive pulmonary disease. These patients need to be carefully evaluated preoperatively to assess their cardiopulmonary reserve. When the reserve is markedly decreased, they must be considered for respiratory care before correction of the scoliotic curve. This may even require such assistive ventilatory efforts as a tank respirator. Those patients with scoliotic curves greater than 110 degrees should be treated in centers particularly equipped to deal with multifaceted problems, where there are surgeons who can perform rapid and relatively bloodless surgery. Careful consideration of detail and

cooperation in surgical and anesthetic management can make this possible.

An association of idiopathic scoliosis and malignant hyperthermia has been questioned but has not been notable in centers dealing specifically with scoliosis. One can thus assume that these patients, as any patients, have the potential for malignant hyperthermia, but scoliosis is not a condition particularly associated with malignant hyperthermia.

The anesthetic management of patients with scoliosis has been simplified since somatosensory evoked potentials became clinically possible. This allows monitoring of sensory conduction from the lower extremities through the cerebral cortex throughout surgery. For this monitoring, it is necessary that the the patients not be deeply anesthetized with halothane, isoflurane, or enflurane, which would muffle the somatosensory evoked response. This may easily be accomplished with moderate doses of isoflurane and controlled ventilation. Careful attention to blood loss throughout the operative procedure is important. When blood replacement of more than 2 to 3 units is required, warmed blood is preferred to avoid hypothermia. The rapidity of the surgical technique is directly related to the blood loss (Table 39–2).

Osteogenesis Imperfecta. This is a disease in which the bone matrix is not properly laid down and results in weakened bones with repetitive fractures. When these patients need surgical correction, there is increased difficulty in positioning them, and the potential exists for new fractures in the course of operative and postoperative management. Other abnormalities associated with this disease include hyperthermia, hyperhydrosis, easy bruisability, and bleeding, with associated platelet cell dysfunction, kyphoscoliosis, cor pulmonale, and congenital heart disease or valvular heart disease. The kyphoscoliosis may cause severe restrictive pulmonary dysfunction, which can complicate the preexisting cardiac disease.

Anesthetic management should include careful attention to the positioning of the patient, being aware that mandibular fractures are a hazard. When face mask or laryngoscopy is performed, attention must be paid to the vulnerability of the mandible. Positioning and moving the patient is done with care. The increased bleeding tendency of these patients indicates that transfusions should be considered early in the course of surgery if bleeding is significant. Hyperthermia in these patients requires that the temperature should be carefully monitored throughout, and when the patient is febrile, elective surgery should definitely be postponed. A cooling blanket should always be available

TABLE 39–2. RELATIONSHIP OF BLOOD LOSS TO TOTAL PROCEDURE TIME IN 1726 IDIOPATHIC SCOLIOSIS PATIENTS OVER A 10-YEAR PERIOD

	Age in Years	Total Time of Procedure (Minutes)	Blood Loss (ml)	Transfusion (ml)
Average	17.98	116.49	754.40	494.00
Standard deviation	9.09	47.23	458.37	529.39
Range	2–74			

(From Idiopathic scoliosis surgery, 1970–1979, Baylor College of Medicine, Waco, Texas.)

for use. Anticholinergic drugs should be available but must be used with caution. One technique is to give the drug IV in small doses immediately before they are needed, such as before induction when intubation and an inhalation agent are to be used. Because of cardiopulmonary problems with kyphoscoliosis, careful cardiac and pulmonary evaluations are necessary both preoperatively and throughout the perioperative period.

Dwarfism. There are a variety of types of dwarfism; in all, 55 syndromes have been described. Some major abnormalities are atlantoaxial instability, spinal stenosis, airway and facial abnormalities, thoracic dystrophy, kyphoscoliosis or lordosis, congenital heart disease, and hydrocephaly (and possibly, associated mild retardation or seizure disorders). One or a combination of these may be present.

The variety of vertebral abnormalities should be carefully evaluated before elective surgery, with appropriate treatment when possible. The perioperative anesthetic evaluation should include this evaluation plus the potential difficulties in airway management. Patients may have hyperplasia of the mandible, micrognathia, or a relatively fixed jaw, creating difficulty in visualization at the time of intubation. Both the thoracic dystrophy syndrome, with a small, narrow, contracted chest cage, and kyphoscoliosis are associated with restrictive lung disease and must be considered preoperatively. Any of the congenital cardiac diseases are possible, although patent ductus arteriosus, atrial septal defects, and coarctation of the aorta are more common. CNS involvement usually appears as hydrocephalus, seizure disorders, and mental retardation.

The seizure disorders may be treated preoperatively with either diazepam or barbiturates, if the patient is not allergic to these, with follow-up barbiturate anesthesia. Special guidelines for anesthetic management include an avoidance, if possible, of regional anesthesia when neurologic deficits are evident. When there is paralysis or spinal stenosis, the potential for autonomic dysreflexia should be considered, and appropriate alpha blockers and beta blockers should be at hand. Cardiopulmonary status must be consistently monitored. There are no particular contraindications to any anesthetic agent as long as precise technique is used and anesthesia is not induced without ascertaining that good airway management is possible.

Other diseases in this category include the craniofacial dysostoses, Paget's disease of the bone, and fibrous dysplasia. In all of these conditions, careful positioning of the patient is mandatory. There must also be consideration given to neurologic disability secondary to lesions involving the vertebral bodies. The airway must be carefully evaluated preoperatively because of abnormalities in the facial bones, mandible, and neck. No particular drugs are recommended or disallowed, although careful attention to the ability to intubate is necessary before giving muscle relaxants in these patients. In all of these diseases, the use of regional techniques should be considered only when no skeletal lesions are in the area to be blocked. This avoids going through areas of the pathologic process and any associated bleeding or neurologic disability. Some of these patients may have endocrine abnormalities and increased bleeding secondary to the lesions. Thus, adequate blood should be immediately

available for replacement, and careful endocrine workup is necessary. Any associated neurologic disability should be documented before administration of anesthesia. When spinal cord injury has occurred in any of these patients, blood pressure must be carefully monitored to ascertain the potential problems of autonomic dysreflexia.

Spinal Cord Trauma

Etiology and Diagnosis. The etiology of spinal cord trauma is primarily motor vehicle accidents, with sports injuries, such as diving, as the second most frequent cause. Diagnosis must be made at the site of injury. Neuropathologists have demonstrated that inappropriate handling of these patients can result in worsening of the lesion and can convert a temporary insult into permanent paralysis. This includes the evaluation in the emergency room for isolated or multiple trauma and follow-up operative management. These patients must have necks and trunks maintained in a neutral position with appropriate traction throughout their period of instability. This is particularly important during the intubation process. Most spinal cord injury centers prefer to intubate these patients with the fiberoptic bronchoscope and thus avoid extension of the neck. There are three phases in the postspinal cord injury.

Spinal shock is the period that occurs immediately after injury (the first few hours after injury) to 1 to 6 weeks later. It is characterized by an areflexic and atonic stage, with loss of sphincter control, paralytic ileus, areflexic bladder, and loss of normal tendon reflexes. The specific danger is the cardiopulmonary instability, with marked hypoxia and hypotension occurring with slight changes in position. Postural hypotension is a definite problem when these patients are placed in any degree of tilt. Gradually, as their systems become adapted to the paralyzed state, the presence of postural hypotension is lessened. They may need to be treated with ephedrine or other agents to increase their tolerance of these positions. The duration of spinal shock depends on the severity of spinal cord injury, with the quadriplegic with a complete lesion having a longer phase of spinal shock and the patient with a transitory lesion showing a rapid progression through this stage.

Throughout this time, however, patients must be considered at risk for hypothermic conditions, since they are poikilothermic below the level of the lesion and, thus, in this area will reach a body temperature similar to the room temperature, and are unable to adapt to changing environmental conditions. Body temperature must be protected when the patients are in cold operating rooms to avoid hypothermia and an associated metabolic acidosis, especially in long operative procedures. During spinal shock, these patients are often taking steroids and have the potential for a stress ulcer. Also, there is an increased instance of thromboembolic phenomena; some of the patients are taking heparin and other anticoagulant therapy throughout the spinal shock phase and for the 6 months after injury.

The most noteworthy occurrence during the phase of spinal shock is a marked susceptibility to hyperkalemia after succinylcholine administration. After severe neurologic injury, burns, or massive trauma, the entire muscle acts as a myoneural junction in the area below the lesion.

This means that when a depolarizing muscle relaxant is given, there is a massive exodus of potassium from the entire muscle belly. The efflux of potassium into the central circulation will cause hyperkalemia, with serum potassium levels as high as 11 to 13 mg percent. As the serum potassium level progresses toward 7 to 8 mg percent, severe arrhythmias occur, with eventual ventricular fibrillation and death. Thus, succinylcholine is absolutely contraindicated in these patients. Presently, atracurium, vecuronium, or pancuronium, nondepolarizing muscle relaxants with onset of action within 2 to 3 minutes, are the muscle relaxants of choice in these patients.

Susceptibility to succinylcholine extends throughout the transitional phase, which may last as long as 18 months.

The transitional phase characteristics are a return to either the normal status in which neurologic recovery progresses or an adaptation to the paralyzed state. There may be a tingling sensation or other abnormal sensations that, to the patient, may be interpreted as pain. Patients should be carefully advised that this abnormal sensation is not necessarily pain and may signal a return of sensation and motor beginning, if indeed it is to begin. The cardiac condition stabilizes, with bradycardia remaining. It must be remembered that these patients are often athletic young men who have a basically slow heart rate. The onset of spinal cord injury just potentiates this, and heart rate levels in the 50 to 60 bpm range are not uncommon.

Autonomic dysreflexia is an unopposed massive sympathetic response or mass reflex response that occurs below the site of injury. This is most common in patients with a cervical or high thoracic lesion and is virtually never seen with patients paralyzed below the T8 level. Autonomic dysreflexia may occur postspinal cord trauma or after any other condition resulting in quadriplegia or high paraplegia. It is characterized by severe and extremely rapid hypertension, with associated sweating and bradycardia. The bradycardia may only be transient, lasting a couple of minutes, until it progresses to tachycardia, which is associated with painful headache that these patients may develop as the pressure reaches higher levels. The massive sympathetic outflow can lead to severe arrhythmias as well as CNS problems, with convulsions and cerebrovascular accidents. The preferred therapy for these patients is 5 mg of phentolamine IV immediately if blood pressure cannot be corrected rapidly by mechanical means. The most common cause of this is bladder and bowel distension; thus, simply emptying the bladder may correct the problem. Two surgical conditions in which autonomic dysreflexia occurs are transurethral procedures and plastic surgery on ischial and sacral ulcers. As the perisacral or perineal tissues are approached, there is an autonomic response similar to that of a full bladder, with the development of autonomic dysreflexia and the potential for arrythmias. These may be treated with lidocaine 1 mg/kg, which may be repeated in 5 to 10 minutes if arrythmia recurs. If arrythmia recurs or continues despite this treatment, propranolol (0.4 mg IV is the standard adult dose) may be necessary. Headaches may be treated with either a barbiturate, such as thiopental (in small doses of 50 to 100 mg), diazepam (5 mg IV in a normal adult), or midazolam (1 to 3 mg IV). Autonomic dysreflexia is certainly one of the most severe complications of quadriplegia and must be constantly considered in the operating room. The condition lasts throughout life and may appear suddenly many years after injury.

The adaptation of the respiratory system to the paralyzed state is most profound in the quadriplegic patient, who is suddenly without a voluntary intercostal function. In the ordinary patient with C5–6 quadriplegia, the diaphragm alone can account for approximately 1000 to 2000 ml for vital capacity. This is down from the 3000 to 4000 ml preinjury. Development of the accessory muscles of respiration over the few weeks to 1 month postinjury will gradually bring the vital capacity up to 2500 to 3000 ml. They will develop a cough mechanism as well as the use of the accessory muscles.

The bowel program needs to be carefully monitored to avoid obstipation and resulting autonomic dysreflexia. Regularity in habits, fluid management, and stool softeners are needed; thus, attention to diet and elimination are important perioperatively. In many patients, sphincter tone is increased during this phase and male patients particularly may need sphincterotomies to allow complete emptying. When stasis occurs and the bladder remains constant with a high postvoiding residual, there is a potential for reflux and thus degeneration of the upper tract as well as constant bladder infections. One of the prime causes of death in these patients is chronic renal disease. Intermittent catheterization has prevented many of the problems associated with chronic indwelling catheters. The best anesthesia for these patients for performance of sphincterotomies and other transurethral surgery is spinal or epidural anesthesia to avoid autonomic dysreflexia. Throughout this period, patients may have aberrant sensations and develop spasms. Clonus may occur secondary to minor sensory stimuli. These conditions need to be carefully monitored so that changes in the neurologic status may be ascertained.

After 18 months, the exaggerated reflexes have stabilized and reflexes now are related to altered neuronal spasticity of the reenervated neurons. The reflexes and functions are without the inhibitory, regulatory impulses from the brain. A continuation of the mass reflexes or autonomic dysreflexia as described above may appear. Plantar stimulation may evoke violent withdrawal of the lower extremities, or clonus may occur secondary to minor sensory stimuli.

The neurologic condition is generally stable. If the patient begins to show a degeneration of neurologic function, secondary complications, such as a syringomyelia (or cyst within the spinal canal) must be considered. The cardiorespiratory condition is generally stable. Patients who have had high lesions may have difficulty with the cough mechanism, and chronic pulmonary problems may occur. These must be carefully evaluated before surgery, and any infections must be treated. Some of these patients are treated with IPPB at home to successfully avoid pulmonary infections. The bowel and bladder generally are stabilized, and the patient is on a regimen to avoid distension of either.

Skin infections are a constant worry, and patients must turn frequently from side to side and avoid prolonged sitting to decrease skin irritation and subsequent ulceration. As much as 50 g/day of protein have been reported as lost from a deep decubitus ulcer. This is associated with the anemia of chronic disease, a wasting state, and progressive cachexia.

Some of these patients may have secondary or incomplete lesions and complain of pain in areas not thought to be clinically innervated. Neurophysiologic evaluation through somatosensory evoked potentials, polyelectromyography, and electrospinograms can diagnose whether conduction occurs from the peripheral to the cortex and from the cortex to the periphery.

Multiple drugs are used to reduce spasticity; dantrolene (Dantrium), baclofen (Lioresal), and diazepam (Valium) are the three most commonly used systemic agents. Regional techniques may be used, such as motor end-point injections under neurophysiologic control with 40 percent alcohol or peripheral nerve injections of 6 percent aqueous phenol. If there are massive spasms and contractures after 18 months, the potential for either a phenol/glycerine or radiofrequency rhizotomy must be considered in patients with complete spinal cord lesions. Patients may complain of pain due to the aberrant sensation. They must be fully counseled that this pain is secondary to the aberrant sensations and, if possible, try to live with it. When this is not possible, various mechanisms should be considered. However, the plasticity of the nervous system means various surgical techniques to cut the nerves are generally not effective and the pain will recur within a few months to a year.

The spinal cord injury may be associated with a head injury that occurs at the time of trauma or that occurs subsequently as part of any associated cardiopulmonary catastrophe. Any severe hypoxic episodes may result in brain stem lesions. One must constantly be aware that an unconscious patient may have an associated spinal cord injury as well as head trauma and must be handled gently from the time of injury, with a careful evaluation of neurologic function and careful attention to stabilization of the spine at all times.

The cauda equina syndrome, which occurs from a lesion to the lower end of the spinal conus medullaris and the nerves as they are leaving the spinal cord, is a lower motor neuron lesion. It is associated with flaccidity rather than spasticity and may occur in addition to the upper motor neuron lesion of a high spinal cord lesion. Approximately 10 percent of patients have an associated secondary spinal cord lesion below the lesion diagnosed. This must always be considered, both early in the postinjury course and later when symptoms are of a mixed lesion rather than only an upper motor neuron lesion. There may be pain, which is treated symptomatically.

Paralysis Secondary to Other Etiologies

Tumor. Any tumor may give rise to secondary metastatic disease in the spinal cord and associated areas, especially tumors of the lung and prostate. There can be both benign and malignant tumors arising in the spinal cord itself, as well as in the surrounding areas. These tumors may give rise to progressive neurologic defects or to severe symptomatology. Diagnosis of the underlying condition is surgical. The patient must then be treated as any other patient with an unstable spine, and the spinal column must be supported throughout the induction and perioperative phase. Often, these patients are given radiation treatment postoperatively; thus, they have the potential for all the secondary complications of radiation therapy. Pathologic fractures may occur secondary to both the radiation therapy and the original lesion.

Infection. The most common infection causing spinal cord disease is tuberculosis, with resultant paraplegia. Rarely does quadriplegia occur, since the lesions are most often in the thoracic and thoracolumbar spines. The patient may develop either acute or insidious onset paraplegia without evidence of pulmonary tuberculosis. It must be remembered that the progress of the disease is by hematologic spread to the vertebral column and spinal cord from the lungs. Any anesthetic given to these patients must be determined with an assumption of pulmonary tuberculosis.

Vascular Lesions. The Artery of Adamkowitz is the main supply to the anterior portion of the cord at the T8 level. After cardiac and particularly aortic surgery there may be hypotension or hypoxia of the cord secondary to inadequate blood supply during surgery. Thus, the patient may awaken to find him or herself partially or completely paraplegic. This may be a transient or a permanent condition, which may also occur secondary to trauma.

Anesthetic Management

Preoperative Evaluation. Table 39–3 lists the various requirements in the preoperative evaluation. As stated, a detailed history is probably the most important factor, followed by a physical examination with an extensive neurologic evaluation. The laboratory tests noted in Table 39–3 complement the history and physical but do not replace them. Of particular note are the numbers and types of medications that the patient is taking and the proper evaluation of their effects on the autonomic nervous system. All of these patients have a chronic disease and thus may have multiple causes for drug interaction.

For emergency surgery, one tries to have the patient in the best possible condition with an appropriate evaluation. For elective surgery, these patients must be in the optimal condition preoperatively, even if it means postponing surgery from weeks to months. This is particularly true for kyphoscoliosis surgery, in which the patient may be maintained for a period of time with respiratory assistance, as in the tank respirator. When the patient's condition is in a maximum state to tolerate both the surgery and immobilization of the postoperative period, surgery is performed.

TABLE 39–3. PREOPERATIVE EVALUATION FOR PROPER ASSESSMENT OF PATIENT STATUS IN PATIENTS WITH NEUROMUSCULAR DISEASES

1. Complete history and physical examination (especially drug history, neurologic examination, and study of neck mobility)
2. Anteroposterior and lateral chest x-ray, skeletal x-ray
3. Hemoglobin, hematocrit, urinalysis, prothrombin time, prothrombin plastin time, blood gas analysis
4. Where indicated, creatinine clearance, electrolytes, CPK, liver function tests, sedimentation rate, dibucaine number, occult blood in stools
5. Pulmonary function tests
6. Electrocardiogram, vector electrocardiogram where indicated
7. Myelogram in patients with myelodysplasia or other indications

Anesthetic Techniques. There is no special anesthetic technique that should always be used in these patients. Extensive monitoring of pulse, blood pressure, respiration, temperature, and ECG is mandatory whenever any standby, regional, or general anesthetic is contemplated. Other monitoring, such as a pulmonary artery catheter, central venous pressure, or direct arterial measurements, is helpful but not always mandatory in these patients. Particularly if extensive procedures are contemplated, direct arterial monitoring is required through the postoperative course for both arterial monitoring and arterial blood gases. The induction of anesthesia may be either through inhalation or IV agents or regional techniques. Absolute contraindications are two: (1) in the period of postmassive trauma or spinal cord injury, succinylcholine is absolutely contraindicated to avoid severe hyperkalemia which generally results in severe cardiac arrhythmias and potential death, and (2) the use of muscle relaxants or deep anesthesia in patients in whom an airway cannot be established is contraindicated. These agents must be avoided until it has been ascertained that an adequate airway is possible. Endotracheal intubation is often performed in an awake patient with a fiberoptic bronchoscope and local anesthesia. Otherwise, the induction of anesthesia is with the standard anesthetic agents.

It must be remembered that these patients often have a compromised cardiorespiratory system, and low-dose premedication and anesthetic medications are advisable. If the patient is taking ganglionic, alpha, or beta blockers or steroids, appropriate therapy must be undertaken throughout the perioperative period. The maintenance of anesthesia is as careful as possible to avoid any major shifts in blood pressure, pulse, or respiration. The compromised respiratory system must be carefully watched, and controlled ventilation during the time of surgery when deep anesthesia is necessary is preferable to allowing the patient to breathe alone.

Emergence from the anesthetic is again most carefully monitored to see that neither cardiac nor respiratory depression occurs. Even a short period of time in one position in the hypothermic, acidotic, or hypotensive state can lead to pressure necrosis of the skin and result in skin breakdown, particularly in a chronically disabled patient. Thus, careful attention to the patient's position is always necessary.

Postoperative Care. Postoperative care may be divided into cardiovascular, pulmonary, fluid and electrolytes, and neuromuscular systems.

Direct arterial pressure monitoring and an ECG are important for several days after major surgery. The pulmonary system must be carefully watched to avoid atelectasis and buildup of secretions. Therefore, IPPB is often used routinely when any surgical stress is contemplated. With minor operations, this is not necessary unless the patient is to be placed in unusual positions for an extended period of time postoperatively, particularly high cord-injured patients in whom decubitus ulcers are present and who need to be prone for an extended period postprocedure.

The quadriplegic is said to have a 10 percent decrease in total body water when compared to a normal patient, and there is an approximately 5 percent decrease in the paraplegic. When such patients are NPO before surgery, they may be in a marked dehydrated state. Therefore, preoperative hydration with IV fluids for 12 to 24 hours and continued careful monitoring throughout this period are absolutely mandatory to avoid increased breakdown of various tissues and any secondary problems. This is true whether general, regional, or monitored anesthesia is used. The neuromuscular condition must be carefully assessed both preoperatively and postoperatively to verify that no extension of the neurological lesion or no decrease of function has occurred.

Specific Problems. All the problems inherent in pediatric anesthesia plus neuromuscular disease must be carefully considered with the infant patient. If the mother has a condition, such as myasthenia gravis, the infant must be carefully assessed. Both maternal and infant histories are pertinent. The size of the infant mandates the amount of fluid and electrolyte replacement and drug dosage.

Geriatric patients present another challenge. They may have the primary lesion involving the neuromuscular system in addition to the associated cardiac and respiratory problems secondary to their general condition and age. It is important to remember the compromised situation of these patients and their lack of reserve.

Specific Techniques

1. Hypothermia is not indicated in the patient with acute postspinal cord injury. Although hypothermia is used in neurosurgery for aneurysms or similar conditions, not enough information is known about its use in acute spinal cord injury.
2. Hypotension may be used in extensive operations in a patient with an intact neurologic system. When there is a question of the vascularity or injury to the cord or in the patient who does not have a stable neurologic condition, hypotension is to be avoided. Hypotension is a good technique in a patient who is a Jehovah's Witness and is undergoing scoliosis surgery when there is no associated neurologic deficit.
3. Extracorporal circulation may be used to correct whatever cardiac condition or abnormality may be present, and the guidelines in the use of extracorporeal circulation should be followed. As with all the mentioned conditions, the patient has poor reserve and must be carefully monitored throughout the entire procedure.

SUMMARY

The diagnosis of neuromuscular diseases is in its infancy. Recent studies of normal and abnormal metabolism and function of the nervous system indicate a complexity of hormonal interactions. Anesthetic management must consider the basic pathology and functional reserve of the patient and the contemplated surgery. When it is believed that anesthesia induction cannot be performed safely, either the patient should be transferred to a center where it can be done or surgery should be postponed until the patient can tolerate the procedure. Strict attention to detail is mandatory.

BIBLIOGRAPHY

Carter RE: Medical management of pulmonary complications of spinal cord injury. Adv Neurol 22:261–269, 1979.

Dahm LS, Dickson JH, Harrison GH: Peri-operative and anesthetic management of the patient with scoliosis. Anesth Review 9:3–20, 1982.

Katz J, Benumof J, Kadis LB: Anesthesia and Uncommon Diseases, Pathophysiologic and Clinical Correlations, 2nd ed. Philadelphia, Saunders, 1981.

Quimby CA Jr, Williams RN, Greifenstein FE: Anesthetic problems of the acute quadriplegic patient. Anesth Analg 52:333–340, 1973.

Schonwald G, Fish KJ, Perkash I: Cardiovascular complications during anesthesia in chronic spinal cord injured patients. Anesthesia 55:550–558, 1981.

Stehling L, Zauder HL: Anesthetic Implications of Congenital Anomalies in Children. New York, Appleton-Century-Crofts, 1980.

Vandam LD, Rossier AD: Circulatory, respiratory and ancillary problems in acute and chronic spinal cord injury. In: ASA Refresher Courses in Anesthesiology. Philadelphia, Lippincott, 1975, Vol. 3, pp 171–182.

40

Anesthesia Pollution

Lawrence L. Ciccarelli and Benjamin M. Rigor

Approximately one quarter million health care professionals and employees are exposed to operating room hazards every year. These hazards or potentially dangerous conditions include such biologic agents as microorganisms, nosocomial infection, and contaminated needles; stress and pressure from hectic work schedules and conditions, noise and other extraneous factors; drug abuse or misuse; such physical agents as radiation, fire and explosion, electric shock or electrocution; and finally, medical gases and chemicals, such as ambient and trace levels of anesthetic gases, ethylene oxide fumes, and vapors of methylmethacrylate. This chapter has as its primary focus anesthesia pollution.

Before studies conducted in the last two decades, the possible harmful effects of trace anesthetic gases had not been appreciated, and most operating room personnel were not overly concerned about the venting of excess gases into the surrounding room air. One of the few antipollution devices in use involved the operating room air conditioning system, which allowed an average of 10 or more air changes in 1 hour. Although low flow techniques were used that allowed a minimization of the amount of excess anesthetic gas popped off into the operating room, their use was probably not for the purpose of pollution control but instead for economy and heat and humidity conservation.

POSSIBLE BIOLOGIC EFFECTS

When the possible toxic effects (Table 40–1) of trace anesthetic gases were realized, investigators began to make decisions about ways to monitor the concentrations of these gases and to remove the excess gaseous molecules from the operating room. With the development of sophisticated detection and monitoring techniques, leaks in the breathing circuit and in the anesthesia machine and its connections to the wall and to the breathing system began to be recognized. Hospital equipment workshops were provided with facilities for pressure testing components of anesthesia machines, and maintenance personnel were made aware of the importance of this work in an antipollution program.

Scavenging systems were developed to collect excess anesthetic gases from the popoff valve and dispose of them

outside of the building in many instances. Recognition and prevention of leaks in the breathing circuit and in the anesthesia machine and its connections were necessary before scavenging systems could be maximally effective. Major leaks in anesthetic equipment can render a scavenging system ineffective, and a program of equipment maintenance is an important part of pollution control.

It is evident that the reduction of anesthetic gas pollution can only be accomplished by the following measures:

1. Monitoring anesthetist exposure before and after an antipollution program is developed
2. Identification of leaks through monitoring
3. Removal of leaks through a preventive maintenance program
4. Adequate air conditioning system (preferably a non-recirculating system
5. Scavenging systems involved in the collection and disposal of gases
6. Modification of anesthesia techniques—low-flow, closed systems, use of regional anesthesia
7. Attention to detail

Before undertaking an antipollution program, one should know the metabolism of anesthetics and be aware of previous animal studies and epidemiologic studies on the possible effects of anesthetic gases.

There are four possible mechanisms of action of inhalational anesthetics:

1. Direct effect
2. Mediated effect on the immune response
3. Direct effect of metabolites
4. Mediated effect of metabolites

There have been many demonstrations of the metabolic breakdown of inhalational anesthetics by the liver enzymes. For many years it was assumed that the volatile inhalational anesthetics were either not metabolized or metabolized to a physiologically insignificant degree. Trace levels were thought to be harmless.

Cascorbi established that anesthetists have a faster rate

TABLE 40–1. ANESTHESIA POLLUTION: POSSIBLE ADVERSE BIOLOGIC EFFECTS

I. Behaviorial and other constitutional effects
  A. Learning deficits
  B. Perceptual, cognitive, and motor skills
  C. Russian anesthesia study
    1. Increased irritability (84.4%)
    2. Recurrent headaches (78.5%)
    3. Increased fatigability (75.5%)
II. Ultrastructural abnormalities
  A. Liver, kidney, and nerve tissues
  B. Decreased myelin synthesis and brain maturation
III. Reproductive organs
  A. Spontaneous abortions
  B. Premature delivery
  C. Teratogenesis and congenital malformations
  D. Infertility and genital prematurity
IV. Hemopoietic organs and systems
  A. Bone marrow depression and granulocytopenia
  B. Supression of immune process
  C. Neoplasm of the RES
V. Carcinogenesis

of halothane biotransformation than do non-operating room personnel. This observation apparently confirms that halothane can vary its own metabolism in humans. Animal experiments reveal that chronic exposure to one anesthetic can change the metabolism of another anesthetic.

One of the proposed mechanisms by which hepatotoxins and hepatocarcinogens induce lesions is by biotransformation to reactive intermediates. These intermediates can then interact with tissue macromolecules (DNA, RNA, protein, phospholipids). The high reactivity of these intermediates prevents their isolation and quantitation.

There is much evidence showing the bioactivation of xenobiotics, including inhalation anesthetics, to highly reactive intermediates. These intermediates covalently interact with tissue macromolecules and thus alter the integrity of the cells. Such alterations can lead to various tissue lesions, such as necrosis, hypertrophy, and carcinogenesis. It is, therefore, important to know to what extent anesthetic agents undergo bioactivation and the fate of the reactive intermediates produced.

Biotransformation of an anesthetic begins almost immediately upon its administration, thus introducing the potential of toxic metabolites. The similarities in structure between enflurane and isoflurane and certain known carcinogens, such as chloromethylmethyl ether, give circumstantial support to the theory that anesthetics have a potential for teratogenicity.

It has been proven that anesthetics have an effect on dividing cells. As early as 1878, ether was shown to affect the growth of plants. Mouse heteroploid cell growth has been slowed after exposure to 1 MAC concentrations of inhalational anesthetics. Several investigators showed that inhalational anesthetics slow cell growth but that DNA and RNA synthesis is unaffected. Cohen found that a decrease in cell growth occurred concomitantly with a decrease in mitochondrial respiration in animals.

Hematopoietic studies have shown severe bone mar-

row depression, granulocytopenia, and thrombocytopenia after weeks of continuous exposure of tetanus patients to nitrous oxide. However, a cause and effect relationship cannot be proven because other therapeutic agents were used in the study. It has also been shown that rats exposed to 80 percent nitrous oxide did not have abnormal blood counts until after 6 days of exposure.

Lymphocyte transformation is an important part of the human immune response, and it has been demonstrated that nitrous oxide inhibits lymphocyte transformation in humans. In another approach to anesthetic effects on immune response, inhibition of tumor cell killing by lymphocytes was measured. A 5 percent inhibition was reported for 0.5 percent halothane, and 44.7 percent inhibition for 2.5 percent halothane. Inhibition was found to increase from 15 percent to 42 percent as exposure time to 2 percent halothane increased from 1 to 4 hours. However, after Bruce and Wingard compared the effect on inhibition of tumor cell killing in those exposed to surgical trauma and nitrous oxide for 20 minutes to those exposed to surgical trauma and nitrous oxide for 3 minutes, they concluded that surgical trauma itself actually decreases the immune response. Another author concluded that anesthetics inhibit leukocyte action but only minimally when compared to surgery.

There are numerous animal studies to date. Ferstandig believes that these studies should be interpreted warily because diet affects tumor susceptibility, stress affects reproductive abilities, hypoxia causes congenital malformations, and low anesthetic concentrations affect animal behavior. Other physiologic or adverse conditions mimic biologic effects of pollution (Table 40–2).

Liver changes have been noted in animals that have been exposed to inhalational anesthetics. In one study, mice exposed to surgical levels of halothane for 1 hour per day for 30 days showed marked increases in liver weight. Another group of mice exposed to 0.7 percent halothane for 6 days per week for 29 weeks showed liver hypertrophy with fatty degeneration. Wallin exposed beagles to a "light plane" for 3 hours per day for 5 days per week for up to 7 weeks without any histopathologic changes in the liver. In another study, rats exposed to 0.25 percent halothane for 7 hours per day for 7 days developed ultrastructural changes in the rough and smooth endoplasm. These were considered to be normally occurring responses during metabolism of inhalational anesthetics. Chang noted changes in kidney and nerve tissue in addition to liver changes in exposed rats.

TABLE 40–2. OTHER PHYSIOLOGIC OR ADVERSE CONDITIONS MIMICKING BIOLOGIC EFFECTS OF ANESTHESIA POLLUTION

I. Diet—modification and carcinogenesis
II. Malnutrition
III. Stress and anxiety—reproductive problems
IV. Effects of hypoxia
  A. Congenital malformation
  B. Liver enzymes
  C. Teratogenic effect
V. Hypercapnia, hypotension, acidosis, and so on
VI. Atmospheric contaminants and pollutants

Rigor us has studied the changes in cyclic AMP and cyclic GMP levels in halothane-exposed rats. Whereas Nahrwold found a decrease in cyclic AMP levels in mouse brain exposed to halothane, the authors found that brain cyclic AMP levels of halothane showed a slight increase over control values. Cyclic GMP levels were increased significantly in halothane-exposed rats, and the response was directly related to the halothane concentrations. ATP levels were unchanged when compared to control values.

Because of the possible effects of trace amounts of inhalational anesthetics on human behavior, studies were undertaken by the authors and by others to study the effect of a drug on central nervous system activity in freely behaving rat brain. All of these researchers stated that the method of studying the effect of a drug on central nervous system activities is by behavioral testing, neurochemical assays, cytoarchitecture, and electrophysiology. In these studies, they chose the evoked field potential technique because it represents a method of studying the effect of a drug on the excitability of a neuronal population. The effect of halothane on the EEG of rats was also studied. It was found that after an initial decrease in electrical brain activity at 0.25 percent halothane, an increase was noted at concentrations of halothane at 0.5 percent and above.

IMPLICATIONS FOR OPERATING ROOM PERSONNEL

It must be kept in mind that during animal experimentation, laboratory animals are exposed to constant concentrations of anesthetics. It is probably not reliable to draw conclusions about the effect of trace amounts of anesthetics on humans from animal experimentation, since human exposure varies greatly in the operating room. The anesthetist moves between the recovery room, where the concentration is very low, and within a short distance of an expiratory valve where the concentration may be close to that being administered to the patient. Operating room personnel are not exposed to anesthetic agents to the same extent.

Animal studies, therefore, present difficulties in interpretation because the concentration of anesthetics and duration of exposure are frequently far in excess of what is used clinically and also because most studies are performed in lower animals.

Potential hazards of trace anesthetic concentrations in the operating room environment have been ignored in the past. By 1967, this apathetic complacency began to be shattered. Vaisman in a survey of 354 Russian anesthetists found that a wide variety of complaints were common. Headache and fatigue were the most commonly reported symptoms. Of 31 pregnancies among operating room personnel, he found that 18 ended in abortion. Ether was the most commonly used anesthetic in this survey. At present, Russian anesthetists receive a 10 percent higher salary than surgeons because of the hazardous nature of the job.

Whether or not anesthetists have a higher risk for cancer and/or a higher death rate than that found in the general population is a subject of interest. In a study published in 1968, Bruce et al made a comparison of statistics compiled by the American Society of Anesthesiologists and statistics from an insurance company. Both groups studied were

comprised of men only. There was no statistically significant difference between the two groups in this study. Although the frequency of tumors of the lymphoid and reticuloendothelial systems and suicides were similar in both groups, the incidence of lung cancer and coronary artery disease among anesthetists was less. However, the Ames test for mutagenicity and findings that infer that carcinogenicity is only positive for fluoroxene have provided a contradiction to this study. Also, laboratory studies to date have not proven that any commonly used anesthetics cause cancer in animals. Reports such as the one by Bruce et al have sustantiated the fact that anesthetists have a lower mortality rate than do physicians as a whole. While anesthetists have a significantly greater frequency of bone and joint disease and liver disease as well as arterial hypertension and peptic ulcer, there is subjective bias in reporting of the latter two making them difficult to assess.

In 1970, Askrog conducted a survey and found that the rate of spontaneous abortion increased for employees in the operating room, while the rate for the unexposed wives of male anesthetists rose from 7.6 percent to 20.4 percent. Corbett et al (1974) surveyed 621 female nurse anesthetists in Michigan. The survey revealed (1) an incidence of malignancy three times the expected rate, (2) an increased incidence of birth defects among offspring of the nurse anesthetists, and (3) an increased incidence of congenital abnormalities when the mother continued to work in the operating room during pregnancy. Since these and other studies used small population groups, the American Society of Anesthesiologists, with financial support from the National Institute of Occupational Health and Safety, undertook a study involving larger numbers of people. Fifty thousand operating room professionals were surveyed, with 24,000 unexposed medical and nursing professionals serving as controls. The results were that there was a 1.3 to 2 times greater incidence of spontaneous abortion in female operating room personnel. Women physician anesthetists suffered the highest risk, followed by nurse anesthetists. The incidence of congenital anomalies among liveborn offspring of exposed female physician anesthetists was double that among offspring of unexposed female physicians. Some hospitals warn female personnel who are pregnant that there is a possible risk of increased incidence of abortion and fetal malformation if they work in such an environment during their first trimester of pregnancy.

None of these epidemiologic studies have established a cause–effect relationship. It has been argued that causative factors could include long hours and the tension of the operating room, exposure to radiation, and exposure to patients with transmissible viruses. However, the American Society of Anesthesiologists concluded that an increase in disease rates was present in operating room personnel.

The effects of anesthetics on the fertility of animals has been studied. Bruce (1973) reported that male and female mice exposed to 16 ppm halothane for 7 hours per day 5 days per week for 6 weeks before mating showed no difference from control groups in the number of pregnancies, implants, resorptions, or live fetuses. There was no evidence of damage to the fertility process as a result of traces of anesthetics or repeated exposures.

The effects of anesthetics on abortion and teratology

has been studied in animals (Anderson, 1968). One study showed that 10 to 20 percent of chick embryos hatched when exposed to 80 percent nitrous oxide with 20 percent oxygen versus 60 percent nitrous oxide for controls. In general, these studies have shown that the chicken embryo is affected by anesthetics, but only when used in high concentrations. The same effect was seen no matter which volatile anesthetic was used. In summary, it appears that short exposure to even high concentrations of inhalational anesthetics has either no adverse reproductive effects or has statistically questionable effects. However, teratogenic effects have been shown for rats and hamsters exposed to nitrous oxide and for rats, mice, and hamsters exposed to halothane. One recent detailed study failed to show any teratogenic effects of halothane on the rat or rabbit.

In most animal studies, the first observable effects are decreased fertility and increased fetal death. With increasing doses, the number of surviving fetuses with anomalies begins to increase, the peak incidence of anomalies being at a dose that causes 50 percent fetal deaths. This stage is also important in the development of teratogenic effects. Although it is true that the most critical period of exposure is during organogenesis in the first trimester (15 to 56 days in women), there may be a particular sensitivity of the central nervous system to external factors during the period of myelination.

Extrapolation from animal data to humans would place the vulnerable period of the human brain from the seventh intrauterine month to the first few months after birth. However, there is no evidence to date that intrauterine exposure to anesthetics has long-term effects on the newborn. In fact, many of the common congenital malformations show a pattern of multifactorial inheritance.

Many of the commonly used anesthetics may or may not affect the human fetus. Nitrous oxide was initially found to cause leukopenia in patients with tetanus undergoing prolonged exposure to nitrous oxide. It was later shown that nitrous oxide inhibits hematopoiesis in rats, which led to widespread investigations showing that nearly all anesthetics and hypnotics are inhibitors of cell division and that the inhibition is concentration-dependent. One study demonstrated that inhalation of 50 percent nitrous oxide in oxygen and nitrogen by pregnant rats for 1 or 2 days, beginning on day 8 of gestation, produced profound effects on the offspring. There was a high incidence of intrauterine death, a significant frequency of skeletal and rib deformities, and a decrease in size of the embryo compared with controls. Exposure of pregnant rats to 0.8 percent halothane for 12 hours at various times during gestation increased the incidences of anomalous skeletal development and fetal death. Other studies have failed to demonstrate these teratologic effects in rats, rabbits, and mice exposed for brief periods to anesthetic concentrations of this agent. Mutagenicity has not been demonstrated to be caused by enflurane.

Considerable disagreement exists about the possible teratogenic effects of barbiturates. A more relevant practical aspect for the anesthetist is the possible protective effect of high doses of pentobarbital against asphyxial brain damage in the fetus. Central nervous system malformations have arisen after maternal administration of several narcotics in hamsters. In human studies on narcotic addicts or

persons in narcotic-dependent treatment programs, the focus of attention has been on morphine, heroin, and methadone. Offspring of such mothers have not shown abnormalities other than low birth weight. Several of the tranquilizing drugs have shown teratogenic properties in rats and rabbits (sometimes only in very large doses), but there has been no confirmation of such effects in humans. Several reports of a specific relationship between diazepam and oral clefts have been published. Although all of the commonly used muscle relaxants cross the placenta to some extent, there is no evidence that the normal clinical dose of such a drug used during a surgical procedure has any adverse effect on human fetal development. Also, there is no evidence available to define the teratogenic effects of these drugs.

The cytotoxicity of anesthetic agents is closely related to biodegradation, which in turn is influenced by oxygenation and hepatic blood flow. Thus, the complications associated with anesthesia, maternal hypoxia, hypotension, administration of vasopressors, hypercarbia, hypocarbia, and electrolyte disturbances may possibly be a greater cause for concern in causing teratogenesis than the agents themselves. The role of carbohydrate metabolism on embryonic development is very important.

Recent studies have attempted to relate operation and anesthesia during human pregnancy to fetal outcome, congenital anomalies, premature labor, or abortion. They failed to correlate congenital anomalies with anesthesia and surgical exposure. Premature labor, if it occurred, was more related to the disease necessitating the surgical procedure than to other factors, for example, the incidence was higher after appendectomy or other pelvic surgery than after other procedures. No particular anesthetic agent or technique seemed better. In these types of studies, the complicating factors are the frequency of maternal exposure to a multiplicity of drugs, the difficulty in separating the effects of the underlying disease and the surgical treatment from those of the drugs administered, the differing risks at different stages of gestation, and the variety, rather than the consistency, of anomalies that appear in association with one agent.

The effect of trace anesthetic gases on psychomotor skills has been studied. In 1974, Bruce found that nitrous oxide alone had worse effects on psychomotor skills than nitrous oxide plus halothane. These results fail to substantiate the findings of the previous study from the same laboratory in which the nitrous oxide plus halothane was associated with poorer performance on psychomotor tests when compared to the effect of nitrous oxide alone. Snyder et al studied operating room personnel for evidence of acute reversible or chronic cumulative cognitive dysfunction as measured by psychometric testing. In comparison with matched controls, no acute reversible deficits were noted in a relatively unpolluted operating room environment (six air changes per hour and venting of anesthesia machines at floor level).

There are many problems with epidemiologic studies that must be considered before analyzing any of the previously mentioned studies. First, the choice of cohort or control group is of critical importance because different age cohorts make for valueless conclusions. Different words can be interpreted differently by persons of different educational levels (words like abortion and abnormality). In addition, retrospective studies are inferior to prospective studies because the former depend on memory or records that were written without the knowledge that specific findings were to be reviewed at a later date. In a retrospective study by Bruce (1968), 441 deaths were reviewed and 17 lymphoid malignancies were found. This is a higher rate than that observed in the United States male population. In a later prospective study, Bruce did not observe this excess of malignancies. It appears that the questions asked, the cohorts chosen, and the size of the study may have given rise to fortuitous statistics. Epidemiologic studies to date have shown no correlation between anesthetics and cancer in men and only a dubious correlation in women. Also, no reproductive epidemiologic studies have shown a direct cause and effect relationship between trace anesthetics and reproductive disease. Possible flaws in reports and experimental designs exist (Table 40–3).

In summary, studies on humans and animal models have implicated volatile anesthetics as causes of decreased cell growth, bone marrow depression, immunodepression, liver changes, and cyclic AMP changes in brain tissue. Epidemiologic studies have implicated trace anesthetic gases as causes of headache, fatigue, malignancies, spontaneous abortions, and congenital malformations. The causes of these abnormalities are uncertain at this time. Anesthetic gases are believed to be the cause because they are tangible and measurable. Less tangible causes are increased risk of serum hepatitis, increased susceptibility to infection, stress and abnormal pregnancies, and stress and cancer.

PREVENTION AND SURVEILLANCE OF ANESTHESIA POLLUTION

Since trace anesthetic gases may cause problems in operating room personnel, it becomes mandatory to institute an effective antipollution program. The first important point in an antipollution program is the identification of leaks through monitoring. The first documentation of occupational exposure of operating room personnel to anesthetic gases was reported in 1969. Linde and Bruce described peak levels of 27 ppm halothane and 428 ppm nitrous oxide in the inhalation zone of the anesthesiologist when a nonrebreathing system was used. Another cause of concern involves hospital dental surgery operating rooms. Two studies of ambient gas concentrations during dental surgery indicate that the concentration of halothane in unscavenged

TABLE 40–3. ANESTHESIA POLLUTION: POSSIBLE FLAWS IN REPORTS AND EXPERIMENTAL DESIGNS

1. Sampling biases and errors
2. Vague definition of control
3. Posology differences
4. Technical and analytic problems
5. Investigator biases and preferences
6. Statistical errors and manipulations
7. Unreliable retrospective studies
8. No good prospective and epidemiologic studies

rooms may exceed 73 ppm. Indeed, significant segments of the dental profession and associated nurse anesthetist and dental assistants are occupationally exposed to trace concentrations of anesthetics.

There is no satisfactory evidence about the relation between anesthesia concentrations in the operating room environment and the real exposure of persons working in such an environment. Basically, three methods have been described to determine individual exposure to inhaled anesthetics.

Periodic or Multiple Spot Sampling

Air samples from the breathing zone are obtained in glass syringes. As early as 1969, Linde and Bruce used this method to determine the exposure of anesthetists. They reported nitrous oxide concentrations to average 130 ppm, with peak levels as high as 428 ppm, in the vicinity of the anesthetist. Unless measurements are made in the breathing zone and appropriately weighted, the real exposure can be seriously misjudged. In one study spot sampling was done from three points:

1. The breathing zone of the anesthetist 60 cm from the Heidbrink valve in the operating room
2. The periphery of the operating room about 1.8 m from the operating table; both samples were taken at a height of 1.5 m from the floor
3. At floor level near the anesthesia machine

Air was sampled by slow withdrawal into a clean, tight-fitting 100 ml glass syringe with a nylon tap. There were three results of spot sampling. First, halothane concentrations fell off with increased distance from the Heidbrink valve. Second, concentrations varied greatly in the anesthetist's breathing zone. Third, peripheral concentrations did not change much each time, that is, the level was a balance between contamination and ventilation.

Spot checks may give misleading information about the average exposure of personnel. Therefore it may be better to do continuous sampling to provide a time-weighted average concentration.

Continuous Sampling or Integrated Personal Sampling

This can be achieved by a portable infrared monitoring unit. In integrated personal sampling, samples may be collected in 250-ml glass bottles fitted with stoppers containing a springloaded valve. A simple vacuum regulator may be screwed into the stopper and a vacuum of about 0.9 atm is created so that constant flow can be obtained until the pressure in the bottle rises to atmospheric pressure. The regulator is fitted with a needle valve with which the rate of flow is adjusted to 15 ml/minute. The patient carries the bottle in a pocket, and a length of 1 mm nylon tubing is fitted with its open end attached to the outside of the face mask. Sampling is started by screwing in the regulator at the beginning of exposure and stopped at the end by unscrewing it. This method of sampling, using a continuous sampler carried on the person and sampling from the breathing zone, is a recognized but uncommon method of measuring exposure to gases and vapors. An advantage of this method is that it involves considerable saving of time and labor compared with taking and analyzing multiple end-tidal and spot samples. A major disadvantage is that it involves cumbersome and expensive apparatus.

Blood Sampling and End-Tidal Air Sampling

Sampling of the concentration of halothane in venous blood is performed to confirm the efficacy of scavenging systems. There is no doubt that exposed personnel absorb the anesthetic that they are exposed to. Blood samples showed halothane levels ranging from 4.1 ($\pm$2.0) μg/100 ml to 77.1 ($\pm$14.2) μg/100 ml after 3 to 4 hours of exposure. Even after 20 hours of freedom from exposure, blood levels were detectable. End-tidal samples when compared to blood samples can provide adequate information, and, furthermore, these are much simpler and easier to obtain from operating room personnel than are repeated blood samples. Corbett and Ball (1973) showed that nitrous oxide may be detected in the breath of an anesthetist for 3 to 7 hours after exposure, and halothane is detected in the breath of an anesthetist for 7 to 64 hours after cessation of exposure. Breath decay curves may show that the concentration of nitrous oxide is below 5 ppm in end-tidal samples 1 hour after the end of exposure.

In one study, anesthetic methods and the agents were controlled rigorously during spot sampling and integrated personal sampling. Identical anesthetic circuits were used with the same fresh gas flow. The concentration of nitrous oxide in the operating room increased immediately after the beginning of anesthesia. In addition, trace concentrations of nitrous oxide may still be present 12 to 18 hours after the end of the operating session in unventilated operating rooms. An unequal distribution of anesthetic gas is likely to occur in rooms that are not ventilated, with smaller rooms being generally less adequately ventilated than larger rooms. Variation in anesthetic concentration in the environment also depends on various factors, such as site and rate of gas leakage, the movement of personnel, the location of equipment, surgical drapes, and opening and closing of doors. The major areas of contamination include the area around the anesthesia machine, the area around the operating table, and certain pockets in the remainder of the room.

Different personnel are exposed to anesthetic gases to different extents. Without the use of scavenging in an unventilated operating room, the mean exposure of both the anesthetist and the scrub nurse in the operating room is identical, and the exposure of the circulating nurse is lower. Recovery room personnel exposure is negligible except if recovery room ventilation is poor or if the recovery room is near the operating room.

A program for reduction of operating room pollution depends for its success on the ability to measure the level of that pollution. The only successful way to do this is for major hospitals to possess their own equipment and to institute regular programs of checking and recording. Smaller hospitals may depend on the equipment of larger hospitals to save money. Discrete samples in glass syringes or other suitable containers may be analyzed by gas chromatography. These machines are very bulky and are not for operating room use. Halothane may be analyzed by an ionizing leak detector similar to those used for detecting refrigerant leaks in industry. This device, though, cannot be used for nitrous oxide. Nitrous oxide is used more often than halothane, and, therefore, a nitrous oxide measuring device is best. Nitrous oxide will leak from more places than will halothane. Halothane may be released by vaporizers, whereas nitrous oxide may leak from pipelines and cylinders under pressure. It has been demonstrated that halothane exists in the operating room atmosphere in the same proportion to nitrous oxide as it exists in the mixture being administered to the patient. A suitable analyzer for nitrous oxide is the continuous rapid infrared analyzer that costs approximately $3,000. One author stated that 14 operating rooms could be surveyed in 20 minutes. Individual anesthesia machines can be checked for leaks by probing about the machine, pipelines, wall sockets, and so on with the sampling hose of the analyzer. More expensive versions of the infrared analyzer (variable path length analyzers) can measure nitrous oxide and halothane and other volatile agents. Skill and care are needed in their operation, especially in the zeroing and calibration. When instituting a control program, the operating room should be monitored at no less than weekly intervals.

Hospital equipment workshops should have facilities for pressure testing components of anesthesia machines, and maintenance personnel should be aware of the importance of this work in the antipollution program. Push–fit connectors on pipelines should be checked regularly and repaired or replaced as necessary, as should any worn, cracked hoses, breathing bags, washers, and seals. Major leaks in anesthetic equipment can render a scavenging system ineffective, and a program of equipment maintenance is an important part of pollution control.

The high-pressure portion of the anesthetic machine is the part that is subjected to unregulated gas cylinder pressures. In this case, nitrous oxide leakage is of concern, although oxygen lines and cylinders should be checked for costly leaks. Major sources of waste gas in the high-pressure system are the nitrous oxide cylinder valves and hanger yokes. Washers may be absent or worn, or two washers may inadvertently have been placed in the yoke. Internal tubing and reducing valves may be leak sources. Therefore, levels of nitrous oxide should be analyzed on a regular basis.

The joints should be checked for leakage every 3 to 4 months by covering with soapy water. Clearly visible bubbles indicate a large leak, which may result from a defect in the crimped hose, a loose joint, or a faulty seal on the connector itself. Constant spillage can result in extremely high concentrations of nitrous oxide, which is expensive as well as being a health hazard.

Filling of vaporizers should be the final chore at the end of the day, when few people are about. Special pouring funnels prevent excess spillage when filling vaporizers, some of which have a pin-indexed system to prevent improper filling. Some authors recommend wrapping tissues around the bottle and discarding the tissues after the vaporizer is full. It must be kept in mind that if 1 ml of liquid halothane is spilled, it will vaporize to 200 ml of gas, which has a concentration of 1,000,000 ppm.

In addition to regular checking of anesthetic machines, ventilators, and vaporizer valves and seals, adequate air exchange in the operating room should be properly maintained and periodically assessed. For a given rate of leakage of an anesthetic agent into an operating room, the concentration in the room atmosphere is determined by the formula:

$$C = \frac{60L(10^6)}{nV}$$

where C = concentration of gas in room (ppm), V = room volume in liters, L = leak rate of gas (L/minute), and n = number of nonrecirculating room air changes per hour. From this formula it can be determined that in a room with a complete absence of ventilation (n = 0), a very high concentration of the agent would be theoretically possible. The greater the value of n, the lower the concentration. However, even well-ventilated operating rooms do not usually have a value greater than 25, and 10 is the usual number. When a proportion of the ventilation is recirculated, this modified formula applies:

$$C = \frac{60L(10^6)}{n(1 - R)V}$$

where R = fraction of air changes recirculated. Information on whether a hospital operating room uses a recirculating or a nonrecirculating air conditioning system can be obtained from the hospital engineer. A simplified rule-of-thumb is that in a normal sized operating room with 10 nonrecirculating air changes per hour, every 100 ml/minute leak of nitrous oxide leads to approximately 5 ppm in the atmosphere. The National Institute for Occupational Safety and Health Standards for Anesthetic Gases are shown in Table 40–4.

In addition to an adequate air conditioning system, scavenging also plays an important part in the reduction of levels of anesthetic gas concentrations in the operating room atmosphere. Scavenging is a general term that denotes all methods for the collection and disposal of the anesthetic agents that escape from the expiratory valve on the apparatus. There is a collecting and a disposal system, and the disposal system is divided into active and passive disposal systems.

Scavenging must conform to certain service and safety requirements:

1. Easy to operate.
2. It must not influence the pressure air currents of the anesthesia system.
3. It must allow the anesthetic apparatus to be freely movable around the operating room.
4. Safe from sparks.
5. Flammable gases must undergo sufficient dilution with ambient air and become nonflammable.
6. Possible failure in one or more parts of the anesthetic system should not influence the functioning of the anesthetic system.

TABLE 40–4. NATIONAL INSTITUTE FOR OCCUPATIONAL SAFETY AND HEALTH (NIOSH) STANDARDS

Anesthetic Gas	Criterion
Nitrous oxide	Not more than 25 ppm
Halogenated anesthetics + nitrous oxide	Not more than 0.5 ppm
Halogenated anesthetics	Not more than 2.0 ppm

Note: 100% of a gas = 1,000,000 ppm; 1% of a gas = 10,000 ppm; 0.00001% of a gas = 1 ppm.

Except for the pediatric T-piece, all patient breathing circuits have some form of expiratory valve. The collecting assembly delivers the excess anesthetic gases from the breathing machine to the interface. The interface is a portion of the scavenging system that provides positive and negative pressure relief and may provide reservoir capacity. Waste gases are directed to a single outlet that can be attached to the disposal system. The attachment should be of a diameter or shape different from the standard tapered 22 mm connectors of the patient's breathing circuit to avoid inadvertent incorrect connections. Most automatic ventilators designed for anesthesia have some built in provision for dumping excess gas. The dump valve is often, though not always, readily accessible, and a tube or similar collecting piece can be fitted to it. Such devices are often available from the manufacturers of the ventilator or, indeed, are an integral part on most new machines. Older machines may be difficult and a few types even impossible to scavenge. Such obsolete machines should probably be replaced. The collecting system now consists of two tubes, one leading from the ducted expiratory valve on the patient's breathing circuit and one leading from the dump valve on the ventilator. Provisions should be made so that the two tubes are connected independently to the disposal system. The exhaust tubing from the ventilator and breathing circuit must be able to accommodate large volumes of gas releases in a short time (for example, frequent dumping of the breathing bag). Tubing should be wide bore. A diameter smaller than ⅜ inch will offer too much resistance to gas flow.

Disposal systems are either active or passive. Active systems often are powered by suction. Early attempts at scavenging made use of the operating room vacuum system, but there are a number of disadvantages to this arrangement: it puts a constant load on the system (about 25 L/minute in each operating room), it may reduce the suction available to the surgeon and anesthesiologists, the anesthetic agents may in time damage the suction machinery, and, finally, the discharge may occur in an area where there are other personnel. A better system is one in which suction is generated by an independent device, which may be an electric blower, a diaphragm pump, or a venturi operated by compressed air. Gas may be removed by a fan, which must be explosion resistant because of the presence of oxygen. This type of system is much less expensive to install than a vacuum system. The discharge point of both of these systems should be to the outside atmosphere, preferably well away from any windows or air conditioning inlets.

With active suction disposal systems, there must always be provisions to prevent the application of suction to the patient circuit. This is usually accomplished by means of a reservoir bag or interface. A flowmeter in the suction line is desirable to enable control of suction and to give a visual indication that the system is working. A suction scavenger system should not maintain suction pressure above 7 cm of water pressure. Some disadvantages of active suction systems are that they are complicated and costly, as well as the fact that there may be mechanical failure and possibly additional noise if the switch is not turned on.

In the passive scavenging system, the gases are directed to the outside or into the outlet side of the operating room air conditioning. Some scavenging techniques channel the heavier than air anesthetic gases to the floor near the outlet side of the air conditioning. This technique is unsatisfactory because turbulence created by movement or air currents in the operating room soon spreads the vented gas to the operators' breathing zone. Ducting the gases to the floor level on the grounds that they are heavier than air has been shown to be virtually useless. One author reduces exposure to anesthetic gases by placing a banjo fitting over the Heidbrink valve to duct the gases through a single nozzle. Gases are then scavenged by disposal through tubing connected to the banjo fitting.

In older, poorly air-conditioned or nonair-conditioned operating rooms with passive scavenging, the duct can be led directly outside, preferably up to roof level, with a cowl to prevent entry of rain or dust. Such a system should be tested to ensure that reverse flow does not occur during high winds and examined regularly for blocking of the outlet by insect or bird nests.

If the passive scavenging system is used with an air conditioning system that uses partial recirculation, it becomes necessary for the ducted gases to enter the system downstream of the point of recirculation.

The reduction in trace anesthetic gas exposure is remarkable when scavenging is used. With adequate collecting systems and passive disposal, the anesthetist exposure can be reduced two- to fourfold. With adequate collecting systems and active disposal, the anesthetist exposure can be reduced another four- to sixfold. Use of the latter method in addition to an air-conditioning system that is effective will result in time-weighted averages for nitrous oxide of under 25 ppm (limit suggested by National Institute for Occupational Safety and Health). In most situations, control of nitrous oxide to a time-weighted average concentration of 25 ppm during the anesthetic administration period will result in levels of approximately 0.5 ppm of the halogenated agent.

In addition to monitoring, preventive maintenance, adequate air conditioning, and scavenging, it is very important that the anesthetist pay attention to detail:

1. Ensure that gas disposal lines are connected.
2. Avoid turning on the nitrous oxide flowmeter or the vaporizers before the patient is connected to the circuit. Turn them off when they are not in use.
3. Select the optimal size endotracheal tube for the patient and ensure that the cuff is adequately inflated.

TABLE 40–5. POSSIBLE SOLUTIONS TO ANESTHESIA POLLUTION

I. Use regional or conduction anesthesia
II. Use low-flow and closed systems
III. Engineering control procedures
   A. Air conditioning
   B. Scavenging or evacuation
IV. Modification of work practices
V. Leak testing and equipment maintenance
VI. Air monitoring and personnel surveillance

4. Disconnect the patient from the circuit as infrequently as possible. Brief periods of discontinuity in a breathing circuit result in marked rises of anesthetic spillage.
5. Empty the breathing bag into the scavenging system rather than into the room.
6. At the end of the surgical procedure, continue to administer oxygen for as long as possible, using high fresh gas flow rates to wash the anesthetic gases out of the circuit and the patient, leaving the patient attached to the circle for as long as it is convenient. This allows the anesthetic to be collected by the scavenging system, and it is good patient care to give oxygen on recovery.
7. Use low-flow anesthesia systems. It is possible to close an anesthetic circle by reducing fresh gas flows. In a circle system wherein oxygen is the only carrier gas, any fresh gas inflow greater than the patient's metabolic oxygen requirement is popped off as waste. A 70-kg man may require about 240 ml/minute of oxygen. For a fresh gas flow of 1 L/minute, 760 ml is unused. If the system has been carefully assessed as leak free, the adequacy of low fresh gas flow rates can be determined by monitoring distension of the breathing bag. However, without oxygen monitoring equipment, relatively high totals of fresh gas flow rates are necessary to ensure an inspired oxygen concentration of 50 percent when nitrous oxide is being used.
8. Use a mask that fits the contour of the face properly.
9. Perform high-pressure tests on the anesthesia equipment. *Test 1:* Turn on the nitrous oxide cylinders with the flowmeters off. Then turn the cylinder off and observe the time taken for the pressure gauges to fall. A good machine will hold its pressure for several hours; less than 1 hour is unacceptable. *Test 2:* Connect the outlet of the machine to a manometer. A rate greater than 100 ml/minute to main-

TABLE 40–6. WORK PRACTICE RECOMMENDATIONS

I. Functional waste gas disposal systems
II. Use of tight fitting masks
III. Tests for low and high pressure leaks
IV. Filling of vaporizers
V. No premature gas flow starts
VI. Awareness of disconnection
VII. Emptying of bags into scavenging system

TABLE 40–7. MEDICAL SURVEILLANCE PROCEDURES

I. Comprehensive medical and occupational histories
II. Placement and annual physical examination
III. Employee awareness and education
IV. Reporting of abnormal outcome of pregnancies
V. Record keeping and filing

tain a pressure of 30 mm Hg is unacceptable. Repeat the test, this time using the manometer connected to the Y-piece of the circle absorber. This will tell you if there is leakage in the machine itself or leakage in the breathing circuit.

Possible solutions to anesthesia pollution are shown in Table 40–5. Table 40–6 shows work practice recommendations, and medical surveillance procedures are shown in Table 40–7.

Before undertaking an antipollution program, one should be cognizant of the metabolism of anesthetics as well as previous animal studies and epidemiologic studies. The antipollution program itself should consist of monitoring, preventive maintenance, adequate air conditioning, scavenging, and attention to detail.

Acknowledgment. We express our special thanks to Mrs. Joyce K. Mills for typing the manuscript.

REFERENCES

Andersen NB: The teratogenicity of cyclopropane in the chicken. Anesthesiology 20:113–122, 1968.

Andersen NB: The toxic and teratogenic effect of cyclopropane in chicken embryos. In Fink BR (ed), Toxicity of Anesthetics. Baltimore: Williams & Wilkins, 1968, pp 294–307.

Askrog V, Harvald B: Teratogenic effect of inhalation anesthetics. Nord Med 83:498–504, 1970.

Bruce DL, Eide KA, Linde HW, Eckenhoff JE: Causes of death among anesthesiologists. Eksp Khir Anesteziol 3:44–49, 1967.

Bruce DL, Eide KA, Linde HW, Eckenhoff JE: Causes of death among anesthesiologists—A 20-year survey. Anesthesiology 29:565–569, 1968.

Bruce DL, Wingard DW: Anesthesia and the immune response. Anesthesiology 34:271, 1971.

Bruce DL: Murine fertility unaffected by traces of halothane. Anesthesiology 38:473–477, 1973.

Bruce DL, Bach MJ, Arbit J: Trace anesthetic effects on perceptual, cognitive, and motor skills. Anesthesiology 40:453–458, 1974.

Cascorbi HF: Factors causing differences in halothane biotransformation. Int Anesthesiol Clin 12:63–71, 1974.

Chang LW, Katz J: Pathological effects of chronic halothane inhalation: An overview. Anesthesiology 45:640–653, 1976.

Cohen PJ: Effect of anesthetics on mitochondrial function. Anesthesiology 39:153–164, 1973.

Corbett TH, Ball GL: Respiratory excretion of halothane after clinical occupational exposure. Anesthesiology 39:342, 1973.

Corbett TH, Cornell RG, Endres JL, Lieding K: Birth defects among children of nurse anesthetists. Anesthesiology 41:341–344, 1974.

Divakaran P, Rigor BM, Wiggins RC: Brain cyclic nucleotide and energy metabolite response to subanesthetic and anesthetic concentrations of halothane. Experientia 38:655–665, 1980.

Doenicke A, Wittmann R, Heinrich H, Pausch H: Abortive effect of halothane. Anesth Analg (Paris) 32:41–46, 1975.

Ferstandig LL: Trace concentrations of anesthetic gases: A critical review of their disease potential. Anesth Analg 57:328–245, 1978.

Linde HW, Bruce DL: Occupational exposure of anesthetists to halothane, nitrous oxide, and radiation. Anesthesiology 30:363–368, 1969.

Nahrwold ML, Cohen PJ: Additive effect of nitrous oxide and halothane on mitochondrial function. Anesthesiology 39:534–536, 1973.

Smith BE: Teratology in anesthesia. Clin Obstet Gynecol 17:145–163, 1974.

Synder BD, Thomas RS, Gyorky Z: Behavioral toxicity of anesthetic gases. Annals of Neurology 3:67–71, 1978.

Vaisman AI: Working conditions in surgery and their effect on the health of anesthesiologists. Eksp Khir Anesteziol 3:44–49, 1967.

Wallin RF, Napoli MD, Regan BM: Laboratory investigation of a new series of inhalational anesthetic agents: the halomethyl polyfluoroisopropyl ethers. In Fink BR (ed), Cellular Biology and Toxicity of Anesthetics. Baltimore: Williams & Wilkins, 1972, pp 286–295.

Part VIII
POSTOPERATIVE CONSIDERATIONS

41

Postanesthesia Care of the Surgical Patient

Cecil Drain

Total anesthesia care conceptually begins in the preoperative phase, moves into the intraoperative phase, and ends in the postoperative phase. Certainly, each phase of anesthesia nursing care is of utmost importance to ensure a positive outcome for the patient. Anestheisa care in the postanesthesia care unit (PACU) period has far-reaching implications for whether the patient will survive even the best administered anesthetic intraoperatively. The role of the nurse anesthetist in the PACU is one of collaboration. The nurse anesthetist has expertise that can enhance the quality of nursing care administered in the PACU.

Postanesthesia nurses are professional nurses who should be well versed in critical care nursing. Ideally the nurse:patient ratio in the PACU should be 1:1. PACU nursing is a recognized clinical specialty. The nurse anesthetist can collaborate with the PACU nurse on many administrative matters and provide expert input into the educational process in the PACU. This chapter discusses the basic care of the patient emerging from anesthesia, including oxygen therapy and mechanical ventilation.

POSTANESTHESIA CARE: ADMISSION PHASE

Postanesthesia care of the patient recovering from anesthesia is a critical part of the total anesthetic experience. It is imperative that the nurse skilled in PACU nursing and the nurse anesthetist communicate to facilitate a positive surgical and anesthetic experience for the patient.

Postanesthesia Report

Ideally, the surgeon and the anesthetist should accompany the patient to the PACU area, where the nurse anesthetist should give the following information to the PACU nurse: The patient's name, age, height, weight, and hospital number to identify the patient. The nurse anesthetist should describe the surgical procedure, including surgical and anesthesia time, and supply such preoperative information

as the patient's baseline vital signs, medications, allergies, medical and surgical history, mental status, presence of blindness or deafness, and drug addiction history. The nurse anesthetist should discuss the intraoperative anesthetic phase, covering preoperative medication, anesthetic agents including reversal agents, vital signs, arrhythmias, estimated blood loss, and fluid therapy. The nurse anesthetist should also discuss the postoperative management phase, including a mutual focus of nursing care required by patient, oxygen therapy, breathing exercises, coughing techniques, airway care, and mechanical ventilation. Finally, a mutual determination of the postanesthesia recovery score (PARS) should be made by the nurse anesthetist and the PACU nurse.

Postanesthesia Recovery Score

At the completion of the postanesthesia report, the PACU nurse and the nurse anesthetist should conduct a PACU assessment of the patient to determine the PARS. This score will aid both the PACU nurse and the nurse anesthetist in the collaborative effort to determine the focus of PACU care and to develop discharge criteria.

The PARS should be initiated when the patient is admitted to the PACU. Jointly, the nurse anesthetist and the PACU nurse who will be providing direct nursing care to the patient assess the patient. The nursing assessment using the PARS system should be repeated every 15 minutes by the same PACU nurse to verify the patient's improvement or deterioration. The five primary areas of assessment in the PARS are activity, respiration, circulation, consciousness, and color. A PACU patient can receive 0, 1, or 2 points in each area of assessment, with 2 being the best score. A total score of 10 indicates that the patient is in the best possible condition; scores of 8 or 9 are considered safe, and a score of 7 or less is considered unsafe (Fig. 41–1). A more specific discussion of the PARS system follows.

Name _____ Age _____ Sex _____ Date _____

Arrival Time to Recovery Room _____ Time of Discharge from Recovery Room _____

Type of Surgery _____ Analgesics Administered in Recovery Room

Anesthetic Agents (Including Muscle Relaxants) _____ Agent   DOSAGE   ROUTE OF ADMINISTRATION   TIME GIVEN

_____ _____

Preoperative Pain History _____ _____

_____

Preoperative Vital Signs BP ___ / ___ , P _____ R _____   Par Score at Discharge _____

Signs/Score		15-Minute Intervals											
		IN											
0 = Unable to lift head or move extremities voluntarily or on command 1 = Moves two extremities voluntarily or on command and can lift head 2 = Able to move four extremities voluntarily or on command. Can lift head and has controlled movement. *Exception:* Patients with a prolonged IV block such as bupivacaine (Marcaine) may not move affected extremity for as long as 18 hours. *Exception:* Patients who were immobile preoperatively	**Activity**												
0 = Apneic. Condition necessitates ventilator or assisted respiration 1 = Labored or limited respirations. Breathes by self but has shallow slow respirations. May have an oral airway 2 = Can take a deep breath and cough well, has normal respiratory rate and depth	**Respiration**												
0 = Has abnormally high or low blood pressure BP − 50 of preanesthetic level 1 = BP − 20–50 of preanesthetic level 2 = Stable BP and Pulse. BP − 20 of preanesthetic level (minimum 90 mm Hg systolic). *Exception:* Patient may be released by anesthetist after drug therapy	**Circulation**												
0 = Not responding or responding only to painful stimuli 1 = Responds to verbal stimuli but drifts off to sleep easily 2 = Awake and alert, oriented to time, place, and person. *Note:* After ketamine anesthesia the patient must have no nystagmus when released	**Consciousness**												
0 = Cyanotic, dusky 1 = Pale, blotchy 2 = Pink	**Color**												

Figure 41–1. Chart to Detail Postanesthesia Recovery Score (PARS).

Activity. Muscular activity is assessed by observing the patient's ability to move the limbs either spontaneously or on command. If the patient is able to move all four extremities, a score of 2 is given, if only two extremities can be moved, the score is 1, and if none of the extremities can be moved, a score of 0 is given. This evaluation is of particular importance when assessing patients who received subarachnoid, brachial plexus, Bier, or epidural blocks.

Respiration. If the patient can deep breathe or perform the sustained maximal inspiration (SMI) maneuver and freely cough, a score of 2 is given. If the respiratory effort is limited or if dyspnea is apparent, a score of 1 is given. If no spontaneous respiratory activity is evident, the patient receives a score of 0.

Circulation. Because this index is probably the most difficult to evaluate by a simple sign, blood presure is evaluated by comparing the reading derived in the PACU to the baseline preanesthetic systolic blood pressure value. When the systolic arterial blood pressure is between plus and minus 20 percent of the preanesthetic baseline level (as obtained by the Riva-Rocci method), the patient receives a score of 2. If the systolic blood pressure is within plus or minus 20 to 50 percent of the same control level, a score of 1 is given. When the PACU systolic arterial blood pressure is plus or minus 50 percent or more of the baseline reading, a score of 0 is given.

Consciousness. If the PACU patient is fully alert, as evidenced by the ability to answer questions, a score of 2 is given. If the patient is aroused only when called by name, a score of 1 is given. A score of 0 is given when the patient does not respond to auditory stimulation. For this particular assessment parameter, do not use painful stimulation because even decerebrated patients may react to the stimulus. Besides that, in such patients, it is difficult to develop a consistent, reliable, practical method.

Color. When patients obviously have a normal or pink skin color, a score of 2 is given. In patients in whom normal pigmentation of the skin prevents an accurate evaluation, the color of the oral mucosa should be assessed. If there is any alteration from the normal pink appearance that is not obviously cyanosis, the patient receives a score of 1. This includes pale, dusky, or blotchy discolorations as well as jaundice. When frank cyanosis is present, a score of 0 is given.

POSTANESTHESIA CARE: INTERMEDIATE PHASE

Maintenance of Physiologic Parameters

Respiratory System. Postoperative pulmonary complications are the single leading cause of morbidity and mortality in the postoperative period. An incidence of 4.5 to 76 percent, with an average of 11 percent, for pulmonary complications after abdominal operations has been reported. Most research has shown that the incidence of postoperative complications is highest after upper abdominal and thoracic surgery.

Atelectasis, or collapse of the alveoli, is a common postoperative pulmonary complication. Atelectasis accounts for more than 90 percent of the postoperative pulmonary complications. Normally, adults breathe regularly and rhythmically and spontaneously perform a maximal inspiration or sigh every 5 to 10 minutes. During anesthesia or in the postoperative period when there is an absence of these spontaneous deep breaths with an inspiratory hold, lung compliance decreases, resulting in lower alveolar volume. As these lung volumes decrease in the immediate postoperative period, transpulmonary pressure at resting lung volumes also decreases. Without periodic lung hyperinflations with inspiratory holds (sigh), the surfactant may not be allowed to form an appropriate layer about the terminal airways and alveoli. Ultimately, the surfactant will become bunched. Inappropriate surfactant function increases surface tension within the alveoli, which causes a higher lung recoil, or a stiff lung. One of the lung volumes reduced in the postoperative period is the functional residual capacity (FRC). When the FRC plus tidal volume falls below the closing volume (CV), the airways leading to dependent lung zones may be effectively closed throughout the respiratory cycle. Ultimately, atelectasis, hypoxemia, and pneumonia can result.

To reverse the events that lead to a reduction of the FRC alveolar collapse and hypoxemia, the patient should be encouraged to perform a sustained maximal inspiration (SMI) maneuver. This is a respiratory maneuver in which the patient is encouraged to take a deep inspiration and, at the peak of inspiration, to hold the inspired air for 3 seconds, then to exhale the air. The volume excursion and inspiratory hold obtained by the use of an incentive spirometer are similar to the SMI maneuver. This maneuver will increase the patient's lung volumes and, consequently, will reinflate the collapsed alveoli. The SMI is believed to inflate alveoli, increase lung compliance, and allow the surfactant to layer out, thus promoting an increase in lung volumes, specifically the FRC, with the end result being a decrease in the amount of atelectasis and hypoxemia.

Anesthesia, surgery, immobility, and the absence of an intraoperative cough maneuver are some factors that cause the patient to retain secretions. Research indicates that the forced expiratory volume in 1 second (FEV_1) is reduced in the immediate postoperative period. It is important for the PACU nurse to start the cough maneuver when the patient arrives in the PACU. The cascade cough is probably the most effective cough maneuver that can be used because the patient has a low FEV_1 in the immediate postoperative period.

To perform the cascade cough maneuver, the patient should be taught to take a slow deep inspiration, which will increase the lung volumes and tether or dilate the airways, allowing air to pass beyond the secretions. At the peak of inspiration, the patient is encouraged to perform multiple coughs at successively lower lung volumes. With each cough during exhalation, the length of the airways undergoing dynamic compression will increase, enhancing cough effectiveness. Between cough maneuvers, the patient should be encouraged to inhale deeply and close the glottis, which increases the pleural pressure, compressing the airways so as to milk them and move the secretions toward larger airways. Patients with pulmonary pathology that includes a history of retained secretions benefit from chest percussion and postural drainage to enhance the movement of secretions to larger airways, where they can be removed by coughing.

The original regimen of turn–cough–and–deep–breathe has been significantly modified. Clinical research demonstrates that the SMI maneuver and the cascade cough may be more effective in reducing the incidence of postoperative complications. The repositioning of the patient every 15 minutes during the immediate postoperative period aids in better matching of ventilation and perfusion ($\dot{V}_A/\dot{Q}$), and secretion clearance continues to be an important part of this regimen. Hence, the stir-up regimen, as described by Drain, is the SMI maneuver and cascade cough maneuver accompanied by the repositioning of the patient every 10 to 15 minutes.

Because patients recovering from anesthesia and surgery usually have some respiratory depression, low-flow humidified oxygen should be provided (see respiratory therapy section).

Cardiovascular System. The main anesthetic consideration in regard to the cardiovascular system in the immediate PACU period is to maintain the patient's cardiac output. The cardiac output (CO) is determined by the heart's effectiveness as a pump and the resistance to blood flow that occurs, mainly in the arteries. The systolic blood pressure reflects the amount of blood ejected during each left ventricular contraction, the speed of blood ejected, and the resistance of the aorta to blood flow. The diastolic pressure that occupies about two thirds of the cardiac cycle represents the rate at which the pressure in the aorta falls.

The methods of determining the systolic and diastolic blood pressures are direct and indirect. The direct method is an invasive technique that uses cannulation of an artery. The direct method is the most accurate way to determine blood pressure, but it carries a higher morbidity that does the indirect method. The indirect method is noninvasive and includes sphygmomanometry, ultrasonic detection, photoelectric, or manual palpation techniques. The sphygomomanometric method produces blood pressures values similar to direct methods of intraarterial pressures, especially when the pressure is within the range of 100 to 160 torr. Above 160 torr, indirect measurements tend to underestimate true systolic pressure. Below 100 torr, overestimation occurs. The Doppler or ultrasound devices are more accurate than standard sphygmomonometry in the hypotensive patient.

The rate of cardiac contraction also serves to determine the cardiac output. Depending on level, bradycardia may reduce the cardiac output. However, the slow rate will not inhibit the coronary artery filling time. Thus, the major clinical problem with bradycardia is reduced cardiac output. Tachycardia, besides increasing the cardiac oxygen demand, reduces the diastolic time needed for appropriate filling of the coronary arteries, and if severe, cardiac output may become ineffectual.

Cardiac arrhythmias, specifically supraventricular arrhythmias, will also reduce the heart's effectiveness as a pump. This is because cardiac arrhythmias can reduce the rate and force of contraction.

In the PACU, alterations in cardiac output can and do occur. This may be due to hypovolemia caused by such processes as dehydration, hemorrhage, or positive airway pressure. Cardiac dysfunction due to ischemia or depressant effects of anesthetic drugs and decreased peripheral vascular resistance due to sepsis and anesthetic drugs also produce alterations in cardiac output.

Bradycardia and arrhythmias can be due to hypoxemia, excess anticholinesterase drugs, or pain. Tachycardia can be due to hypovolemia, fever, shock, anxiety, hypoxemia, anticholinergic drugs, or pain.

Because many cardiovascular parameters of blood pressure, pulse, and electrical activities of the heart are affected by anesthesia and surgery, constant surveillance of the cardiovascular system is mandatory in the PACU. Monitoring equipment for the ASA I or II patient should include continuous ECG, blood pressure cuff, and chest auscultation. If there is any difficulty in hearing the Korotkoff or heart sounds, a Doppler device should be used. The Swan-Ganz pulmonary arterial catheter should be added to the monitoring armamentarium for the ASA III or greater patient. This method of monitoring enables the PACU nurse to assess the cardiac output, peripheral vascular resistance, and blood volume of the patient. In such a patient, urinary output should be monitored to provide an index of renal profusion and overall adequacy of cardiac profusion. A urinary output of 0.5 ml/kg per hour or more probably indicates adequate perfusion.

The PACU blood pressure and pulse readings should be compared to the baseline readings taken preoperatively to determine their significance. Interventions for hypotension should include the administration of oxygen and the institution of the previously described regimen to help eliminate the anesthetic gases and thus accelerate the emergence process. If indicated, the rate of IV fluid therapy should be increased, and the legs should be elevated. It should be noted that patients recovering from spinal or epidural anesthesia who experience hypotension in the PACU will usually resolve their hypotension episode when these interventions are performed. If the hypotension is still not resolved, vasoactive amines should be administered.

Bradycardia may be treated by the vigorous use of the described regimen and oxygen. If the bradycardia is due to anticholinesterase drugs, atropine or glycopyrrolate (Robinul) should be titrated intravenously to raise the pulse to acceptable levels. Finally, if the bradycardia is due to arrhythmias, the arrhythmia should be identified, documented, and treated vigorously.

In general, the patient with previously normal cardiac function can tolerate tachycardias up to 160 bpm without any deleterious sequelae. Tachycardia is a very important postoperative sign. It should be evaluated fully before treatment is instituted. The first intervention for tachycardia is oxygen administration. If an underlying problem, such as hypovemia, shock, fever, hypoxemia, or excess anticholinergic drug, is not present, the tachycardia is usually due to anxiety or pain. Then, a narcotic agonist is indicated.

COMMON PROBLEMS IN THE PACU

Hypoxemia

Hypoxemia, deficient oxygenation of the blood, is a relatively common entity in the PACU. Some possible causes of postoperative hypoxemia are a low inspired oxygen concentration, ventilation/perfusion mismatching ($\dot{V}_A/\dot{Q}$), increased oxygen consumption, decreased cardiac output, or hypoventilation.

The clinical signs of hypoxemia include hypertension, hypotension, tachycardia, bradycardia, cardiac arrhythmias, restlessness, diaphoresis, dyspnea, tachypnea, and hypoventilation. Cyanosis, which is defined as 5 g of reduced hemoglobin, is not a reliable sign of hypoxemia. Central nervous system symptoms of hypoxemia should be evaluated in the context of such other causes as pain, full bladder, and disorientation and restlessness due to postoperative excitement and somnolence.

Therapy for the hypoxemic patient begins with a positive assessment of hypoxemia. Objective assessment using arterial blood gases is the best documentation of hypoxemia. A Pa_{O_2} that is less than 60 torr indicates the presence of hypoxemia. Because anesthesia, surgery, and narcotics depress the respiratory mechanics and response to carbon dioxide, room air is insufficient for all patients recovering from general and high spinal or epidural anesthesia. Another justification for an increased inspired oxygen concentration is that many patients in the PACU may shiver, have a fever, and be disoriented or restless.

Consequently, the initial intervention to relieve hypoxemia is an increased $F_{I_{O_2}}$. Along with this, the patient may require interventions that are designed specifically to combat the specific cause of the hypoxemia. Patients suffering from $\dot{V}_A/\dot{Q}$ mismatching will respond to chest physiotherapy and the stir-up regimen described by Drain. Patients who demonstrate possible increased oxygen consumption by shivering should be warmed to near normal body core temperature. Patients demonstrating emergence excitement from general anesthesia will have an increased oxygen consumption. This phenomenon occurs frequently after scopolamine premedication. Physostigmine (1 to 3 mg IV) usually reverses the scopolamine-induced delirium and ultimately reverses the hypoxemia.

Hypercapnia

Elevated carbon dioxide tensions can occur commonly in the PACU period. Many factors contribute to the development of hypercapnia, including a depressed central response to carbon dioxide, inadequate muscular forces to move air, oversedation, or an increase in metabolic rate.

The pathophysiology leading to hypercapnia is centered on $\dot{V}_A/\dot{Q}$ mismatching or a blunting of the respiratory center's response to carbon dioxide. This is particularly important in the PACU when patients experience emergence excitement, shivering, or hyperthermia, all of which increase the metabolic rate that results in increased production. In this case, blunting of the carbon dioxide response occurs, and the respiratory system cannot adequately excrete the increased amount of carbon dioxide, hence, it is retained.

Assessment of hypercarbia may be difficult because of possible depression of other physiologic systems. The only definitive determinant of hypercarbia is direct blood gas analysis. However, objective signs of hypercarbia include low tidal volume and rapid respiratory rate, tachycardia, hypertension, and sternal retractions. Many hypercap-

nic patients will subjectively demonstrate restlessness, lassitude, and somnolence.

Preventive interventions for hypercapnia include aggressive implementation of Drain's stir-up regimen. If the patient continues to demonstrate objective and subjective signs of hypercapnia, reversal of the effects of anesthesia should be considered. If the residual anesthesia is due to excess narcotic depression, naloxone (Narcan), an opiate receptor antagonist, should be used. Because of the short duration of action of naloxone, both IV and IM routes of administration should be used simultaneously. The average adult dose is 0.2 to 0.4 mg IV and 0.4 to 0.8 mg IM. It must be remembered that naloxone will not reverse the respiratory depressant effects of barbiturates and tranquilizers. If the patient does not respond to the dose of naloxone, mechanical support of ventilation may be required.

Nalbuphine (Nubain), which is chemically related to both naloxone and the potent narcotic agonist, oxymorphone, has been studied in the PACU for its agonist–antagonist properties. Clinically, it has been demonstrated that 5 mg of nalbuphine administered IV to a patient who has narcotic respiratory depression will reverse much of the respiratory depression, yet the patient will remain analgesic.

If the residual effects of anesthesia are due to inadequate skeletal muscle relaxant reversal, an anticholinesterase and anticholinergic drug should be administered. Tests to determine if neuromuscular function is depressed are lift, hand grip strength, peripheral nerve stimulator, vital capacity of 10 to 15 ml/kg, and an inspiratory force of at least -20 to $+25$ cm H_2O. If the assessment determines that neuromuscular function is depressed, for the adult, neostigmine 2 mg and glycopyrrolate 0.4 mg should be given IV. Improvement in neuromuscular function should be observed in 2 to 5 minutes after injection of the reversal drugs.

Airway Obstruction

Obstruction of the upper airway (extrathoracic) may be caused by obstruction of the pharynx by the relaxed soft tissue or by partial or complete laryngospasm. Extrathoracic airway obstruction, such as a relaxed tongue on the posterior pharynx, can be reliably assessed. As the patient inspires, stridor can be auscultated over the partially obstructed area. Inspiratory stridor occurs because the airway pressure is more negative than atmospheric pressure during inspiration. During expiration, less stridor will be heard because the airway pressure will be greater than atmospheric pressure. Certainly, if a complete obstruction occurs, auscultation will reveal an absence of breath sounds, and sternal retractions will be seen.

As the patient is emerging from anesthesia in the PACU, the tongue may be relaxed and can occlude the pharynx, especially when the head is flexed while the patient is supine. Intervention for this type of airway obstruction is, first, to hyperextend the head. If the obstruction continues, the angle of the jaw should be lifted to move the tongue off the posterior pharynx. If more interventions are required, especially in the obtunded patient, an oral or nasal airway can be inserted. However, if the airway obstruction is due to masseter spasm and the jaws are clenched tightly, a nasal airway or nasotracheal tube placed into the nasopharynx should relieve the obstructed airway.

Laryngospasm, or adduction of the vocal cords, is commonly caused by secretions or manipulation of the vocal cords. Laryngospasm can be partial or complete. Partial laryngospasm is a partial adduction of the vocal cords. Upon assessment of the patient having a partial laryngospasm, inspiratory stridor over the larynx will be heard. Physiologically, this is because the obstruction is extrathoracic. Intervention for a partial laryngospasm is the administration of 100 percent oxygen under positive pressure by the use of a bag–mask system. High inflation pressures should be avoided, and the rate of ventilation should be timed to the patient's own rate. As the obstruction improves, careful oral suctioning should be implemented to prevent further laryngospasm.

Complete laryngospasm is characterized by complete absence of ventilation to the point of hypoxemia. At this point, a small dose of a rapid-acting depolarizing skeletal muscle relaxant (e.g., succinylcholine 10 to 20 mg) should be administered IV. Within 30 to 45 seconds postinjection, the vocal cords will begin to abduct. The patient should be ventilated gently via the bag–mask system using a 100 percent concentration. Once the succinylcholine is administered, the anesthetist should be prepared to perform an endotracheal intubation if the patient cannot be ventilated adequately or if regurgitation and aspiration of stomach contents are imminent.

In postintubation patients, especially in the pediatric age group, largyngeal edema and trauma may occur. This is a significant obstruction to the extrathoracic airway because the narrowest portion of the larynx in the pediatric age group is the cricoid ring. If untreated, this pathophysiologic process can progress to a complete obstruction of the airway. The obstruction is extrathoracic, and inspiratory stridor will be heard audibly or by auscultation. To differentiate between partial laryngospasm and largyngeal edema, administer 100 percent oxygen via the bag–mask system; the obstruction will progressively worsen if laryngeal edema is present. This assessment should be carried out rapidly. Once laryngeal edema is determined as the cause of the airway obstruction, the patient should be placed in an upright position and administered humidified oxygen and nebulized racemic epinephrine. Dexamethasone 8 to 10 mg IV should be administered to enhance the actions of the racemic epinephrine and to reduce the inflammation of the larynx.

In a younger patient, laryngeal edema can progress rapidly to complete obstruction. Hence, equipment for an emergency laryngotomy should be available. Oral or nasotracheal intubation should be attempted first. If this is unsuccessful, a laryngotomy should be performed by incising the cricothyroid membrane and inserting a tracheostomy tube or endotracheal tube into the airway.

Hypotension

One of the more common problems in PACU patients is hypotension; and it requires immediate corrective actions. If the hypotension is allowed to progress, severe damage can occur to the brain, the heart, and the kidneys. Because of the high metabolic activity in these organs, any sustained abnormal decrease in profusion pressure can result in ischemia or infarction.

In the PACU, many situations can lead to hypotension. Hypotension can be caused by decreased cardiac output or decreased peripheral resistance. A decreased cardiac output can result from hypovolemia. Hypovolemia can result from excess fluid loss or inadequate fluid replacement. If the patient is being mechanically ventilated, positive airway pressure, especially when the positive end-expiratory pressure (PEEP) mode is being used, can cause hypotension. This positive pressure will, if in excess, inhibit the preload and so reduce the cardiac output. Many anesthetic drugs, including halothane, isoflurane, enflurane, fentanyl, morphine, and meperidine, can cause myocardial depression, resulting in a reduced cardiac output. Finally, patients who have cardiac dysfunction, such as valvular disease, ischemia, or infarction, may have a reduced cardiac output.

Decreased peripheral resistance can result from several causes. Anaphylaxis and sepsis will reduce peripheral resistance. The anesthetic drugs noted as causes of decreased cardic output will also decrease the peripheral resistance.

Assessment for hypotension should begin with reaffirming the measurement. A blood pressure cuff improperly placed or of the wrong size will result in errors in blood pressure measurement. Also, if arterial transducer measurement is being used, calibration of the monitor should be rechecked or validated by a cuff blood pressure measurement on the same arm in which the radial artery was cannulated. Rapid bedside clinical assessment should include level of consciousness to determine brain ischemia resulting from reduced cardiac output. If urine output is less than 0.5 ml/kg per hour, hypovolemia or inadequate cardiac output is the most likely cause.

Once the assessment reveals the existence of hypotension, assessment of the possible cause or causes of the hypotension should be implemented. The assessment should focus on checking for continued blood loss, adequate blood replacement intraoperatively or postoperatively, myocardial ischemia or infarction through ECG confirmation, and observing for evidence of sepsis or adverse drug effects.

Interventions to return the patient to the normotensive state may include administration of oxygen, fluid infusion, reversal of depressant effects of the anesthetics, and treatment of arrhythmias or bradycardia. The first intervention should be the administration of oxygen to insure tissue oxygenation. If the patient is hypovolemic, blood or blood products or crystalloid solutions should be administered promptly. The type of fluid chosen may not be as crucial as adequate replacement in a timely manner with any fluid. Naloxone should be administered if it is determined that a narcotic is the cause of the hypotension. Vasopressors, especially with positive inotropic action, can be used occasionally to raise the blood pressue and prevent coronary hypoperfusion. If the etiology of the hypotension is decreased peripheral resistance, vasopressors that are agonists on the alpha-receptors should be administered.

Many patients arrive in the PACU with excess vagal tone, which results in bradycardia and hypotension. Anticholinergic drugs, such as atropine (0.2 to 0.4 mg) or glycopyrrolate (0.1 to 0.2 mg) given IV will reverse the increased vagal effects. Finally, if the hypotension is due to excess positive airway pressure, a reduction in the airway pressure is required along with administration of fluids.

Postoperative Pain

Acute pain is an unpleasant sensation and emotional experience usually caused by damage to tissue or by noxious stimulus. There are pain receptors, called "nociceptors," that are stimulated by noxious stimuli. They are located mainly in the skin, blood vessels, subcutaneous tissue, fascia, periosteum, and viscera. Nociceptors act as transducers and convert the painful stimulus into impulses that are transmitted along peripheral fibers to the central nervous system. The degree of nociceptor input from the periphery to the central nervous system is influenced by temperature, sympathetic function, vasculature, and the chemical environment.

More specifically, in the postoperative period, even as the effects of anesthesia disappear, the tissue injury continues, and liberation of pain-producing substances continues. These greatly reduce the high threshold of the nociceptors, leading to the production of pain. Moreover, stimulation of the cut ends of nerves further contributes to pain perception. For example, patients who have had thoracic surgery experience pain from the summation of sensory input from three sites of tissue injury: the skin, the deep somatic structures, and the involved viscera.

Once the pain stimulus reaches the central nervous system, a highly complex interaction of neural systems, psychological factors, and cultural factors is activated. These interactions of the sensory, motivational, and cognitive processes affect the motor system and initiate psychodynamic mechanisms that are translated physiologically into the affective responses characteristic of acute pain.

By activating the sympathoadrenal system, pain accelerates the cardiovascular system as observed in the parameters of pulse and blood pressure. If the patient has a significant degree of cardiovascular dysfunction, the pain should be lessened with appropriate interventions. It has been suggested that pain, especially from upper abdominal and thoracic surgical sites, will decrease or in fact eliminate the normal sighing mechanism. The absence of an appropriate sigh will lead to reduced lung volumes and, ultimately, to the atelectasis–pneumonia sequelae. Again, appropriate pain relief in these patients may reduce the incidence of atelectasis and pneumonia postoperatively.

Assessment of postoperative pain includes both behavioral and physiologic clues. Pain usually elicits an increased response by the sympathetic nervous system, which in turn, produces a high amount of catecholamines, which cause tachycardia, increased cardiac output, and peripheral resistance, ultimately increasing blood pressure. Other assessment parameters of excessive sympathoadrenal activity due to acute pain include respiratory changes, excessive perspiration, changes in skin color, nausea, and vomiting. Other objective and subjective signs include generalized or local muscle tension or rigidity, writhing, unusual postures, knees drawn up to abdomen, restlessness, rubbing, and scratching. Finally, pain may affect the behavioral affect of the patient, so that the patient in acute pain may be irritable, depressed, or withdrawn or have behavioral reverses, such as hostility in an ordinarily quiet person.

Once the assessment has been made and it has been determined that the patient is indeed experiencing acute postoperative pain, certain interventions are suggested. If the patient has received an inhalational anesthetic, such as isoflurane, enflurane, or halothane, and demonstrates objective and subjective signs of pain, postoperative pain relief by the use of narcotic agonists should be instituted early in the postanesthetic period. Similarly, patients receiving short-acting narcotic agonists intraoperatively, as in a nitrous oxide–narcotic technique, should be medicated early in the PACU period. If such narcotics as meperidine and morphine were used intraoperatively, the PACU patient should be administered narcotic agonists with caution to avoid respiratory depression due to synergistic actions of the intraoperative and postoperative narcotic agonists. Finally, if the PACU patient was administered droperidol (Inapsine) intraoperatively or preoperatively, great caution should be used because narcotic agonists as well as barbiturates are significantly potentiated by this butyrophenone tranquilizer. Therefore, the usual dosage of the narcotic agonists should be reduced by one-third to one-half during the first 8 to 10 hours postoperatively.

RESPIRATORY THERAPY IN THE PACU

Research indicates that no matter what type of anesthetic is administered intraoperatively (regional or general), lung volumes and cardiac output can decrease in the PACU. The site of the surgical incision does affect the degree of hypoxemia the patient may experience in the PACU. Patients who have had upper abdominal or thoracic surgical procedures performed will have a greater decrease in the FRC and hence will suffer a more significant degree of hypoxemia. Therefore, every patient who arrives in the PACU should receive supplemental oxygen therapy.

Oxygen Therapy

There are two types of oxygen therapy systems: high flow and low flow. When determining which system is better suited for the patient in the PACU, the comfort of the patient, humidification, and desired oxygen concentration should be considered.

A low-flow system for the administration of oxygen supplies less than the total inspired volume of gas needed by the patient. The additional volume of gas required to meet the patient's inspiratory demand is supplied by room air entrained during active inspiration. The actual concentration of inspired oxygen provided by a low-flow system will depend on four factors. The availability of a reservoir for the accumulation of oxygen will increase the inspired oxygen concentration. The larger the reservoir, the greater the resultant increase in inspired oxygen concentration. The nasopharynx and oropharynx act as an anatomic reservoir, with a volume of approximately 50 ml. The oxygen therapy device itself can also serve as a reservoir of varying volume, for example, the area under a facemask or the reservoir bag, which is a part of many oxygen systems. The oxygen flow rate provided will also vary the inspired oxygen concentration. In general, the greater the flow of oxygen into the system, the higher the inspired concentration. This effect will be limited by the volume of available oxygen reservoir. Once this reservoir is filled, the excess flow will escape into the atmosphere. In addition, the patient's ventilation pattern will affect the inspired oxygen concentration. A more rapid respiratory rate and a greater than normal tidal volume will reduce the inspired concentration. The degree to which this will occur will vary with the degree of change in the patient's ventilation pattern. Finally, the oxygen therapy device must fit properly to achieve the desired results.

The nasal cannula and catheter are classified as low-flow devices that deliver low to midrange oxygen concentrations. The nasal cannula is comfortable for the patient but is easy to dislodge from its proper position. Mouth breathing or any obstruction to the flow of oxygen through the nasal route will reduce the concentration of inspired oxygen. The nasal catheter is not as comfortable for the patient but offers greater stability. Both the cannula and the catheter, when used at excessive flow rates of oxygen, can cause considerable discomfort, such as drying of secretions, nasal bleeding, and gastric distension. The recommended flow rate for operation of the cannula and catheter is from 1 to 6 L/minute. Actual inspired oxygen concentrations will range from approximately 22 percent to 45 percent.

Oxygen masks offer slightly higher oxygen concentrations than nasal devices. With the addition of a reservoir bag, masks of various types can deliver very high concentrations of inspired oxygen. To deliver the highest concentration possible, the mask must have a tight fit, which may be uncomfortable for the patient. The oronasal facemask may be hazardous for patients at risk of regurgitation and aspiration. Oxygen masks should be operated at flow rates from 5 to 8 L/minute. The inspired oxygen concentration will range from approximately 40 percent to 60 percent. A concentration greater than 60 percent is difficult to achieve because of the limited reservoir available. Oxygen masks with an added reservoir bag can deliver very high inspired oxygen concentrations. This device must be operated at a flow rate great enough to prevent the reservoir bag from being emptied during inspiration. If this occurs, the patient will supplement the inspired volume with room air and dilute the oxygen concentration. Masks with a reservoir bag should be operated at a minimum flow rate of 6 L/minute. The maximum flow rate will vary depending on the patient's ventilation pattern. The concentration of inspired oxygen will range from approxiamtely 60 percent to very near 100 percent. Tracheostomy masks and T-tubes are similar to other masks in their oxygen delivery capabilities. However, since the upper airway is bypassed in the tracheotomized or intubated patient, the nasopharynx and oropharynx cannot be used as an oxygen reservoir. The loss of this reservoir will cause a slight decrease in the inspired oxygen concentration. The loss of the anatomic reservoir can be compensated for, if necessary, by using an oxygen therapy device with a larger reservoir.

The simple, clear plastic face tent is a low-flow oxygen therapy device. It is well tolerated by the patient recovering from anesthesia and does supply extra humidity to the patient. The recommended flow rate for the face tent is 4 to 8 L/minute through a bubble-through humidifier. The actual inspired oxygen concentration will range from approximately 30 percent to 55 percent.

A high-flow system for the administration of oxygen supplies a flow of gas in sufficient quantity to satisfy the total, or near total, inspired volume. An air entrainment principle is used to create this very high flow of gas. This type of system is capable of delivering both low and high concentrations of oxygen. The most common example of a high-flow system is the Venturi type mask, which uses a Venturi device to produce a high flow of a specific oxygen concentration. A relatively low flow of 100 percent oxygen is delivered through the Venturi device, creating a high velocity as it escapes. As a result of this high velocity, room air is entrained to mix with the 100 percent oxygen. This mixing, which is designed to occur at a specific ratio, produces a high flow with a relatively specific and consistent oxygen concentration. Depending on the manufacturer, various concentrations are available ranging from a low of 24 percent to a high of 50 percent. Because of the high flow created with this type of system, changes in the patient's ventilation pattern do not greatly affect the inspired oxygen concentration. In order to achieve the desired oxygen concentration, the manufacturers' guidelines pertaining to oxygen flow rate should be adhered to.

When a patient's drive to breathe is mainly due to the hypoxic or secondary drive, oxygen therapy in the PAR should not be omitted merely because of the fear that the patient will become apneic as a result of cessation of the hypoxic drive from high oxygen concentrations. The patient who is breathing on the hypoxic drive should receive oxygen in the PACU. In this case, a high-flow oxygen delivery system using the Venturi principle should be used. The minimal oxygen concentration for the patient can be dialed in on the Venturi principle mask. Arterial blood gases can be drawn after 10 to 15 minutes. For patients whose control of ventilation is by the secondary drive, a Pa_{O_2} between 60 to 70 torr is sufficient.

Mechanical Ventilator Support

The use of mechanical ventilatory support and the subsequent weaning of the patient from this support has evolved to include numerous techniques. A brief description of various techniques that are generally accepted methodology follows.

Spontaneous Modes of Ventilation. In certain circumstances when the muscles of ventilation are not capable of supporting the total ventilatory needs of the patient, ventilator assistance is necessary. However, it is commonly believed that spontaneous breathing is physiologically more effective in the distribution of ventilation than is positive pressure ventilation. For this reason, the patient should be permitted to breathe spontaneously to the extent possible. In situations where the patient has enough muscular power to ventilate adequately but an oxygenation problem exists, a ventilator is not necessary. Various techniques associated with spontaneous ventilation are available to improve oxygenation without the use of a ventilator. Each technique uses PEEP to improve the oxygenation level of the patient. It is, therefore, logical to begin the description of the various techniques with a definition of PEEP.

PEEP is the application of a pressure greater than atmospheric to the airway at the end of exhalation. This positive pressure is usually created by using some mechanical device that ends the exhalation phase of ventilation early. A certain volume of gas is maintained in the lung, over and above the normal volume, to achieve the desired airway pressure level. Basically, PEEP therapy improves oxygenation by expanding the gas-exchanging areas of the lung. Oxygenation can be improved without increasing the inspired oxygen concentration, and often the oxygen concentration can be reduced to nontoxic levels while maintaining an adequate oxygenation level.

The therapeutic range of PEEP suggested by Shapiro (1982) is 10 to 30 cm H_2O. An increase or a decrease in the applied level should be in increments of 5 cm H_2O. An appropriate PEEP level has been achieved when adequate arterial oxygenation and cardiac output have been realized at an inspired concentration of 40 percent or less. A PEEP level above 30 cm H_2O is referred to as "super PEEP." It is indicated in situations of extreme hypoxia when the patient's prognosis is extremely poor.

Expiratory positive airway pressure (EPAP) is the application of PEEP to the spontaneously breathing patient. Expiratory airway pressures are maintained above atmospheric pressure while inspiratory pressures occur at subatmospheric levels created during normal inspiration. EPAP is indicated in patients capable of performing all the work of breathing but requiring PEEP therapy.

Continuous positive airway pressure (CPAP) is the application of PEEP to the spontaneously breathing patient (EPAP). In addition, the inspiratory pressure is maintained at a level greater than atmospheric pressure. CPAP is clinically more effective when PEEP therapy is indicated. However, due to the CPAP, a reduced cardiovascular function may occur, and, therefore, EPAP may be more beneficial for the administration of PEEP.

Assisted Ventilation. This mode of ventilation augments the patient's spontaneous breathing efforts. The patient, by initiating a spontaneous inspiration, creates a subatmospheric pressure, which is sensed by the ventilator, triggering the inspiratory phase of ventilation. Once the ventilator initiates gas flow in response to the patient's breathing efforts, it takes control of inspiration, overriding the patient's efforts. The assisted mode of ventilation is commonly referred to as intermittent positive pressure breathing (IPPB). IPPB is used for both long-term ventilatory support and intermittent therapy. When it is used with a volume/time-cycled ventilator, the patient has control over the respiratory rate only. During intermittent therapy, a pressure cycled ventilator is usually used. In this situation, the patient not only controls the respiratory rate but also can influence the delivered tidal volume and inspiratory flow of the assist mode of ventilation but this has little physiologic advantage over the control mode of ventilation. It does, however, alleviate the need for pharmacologic assistance in controlling the patient's ventilation.

Intermittent Mandatory Ventilation. As with assisted ventilation, intermittent mandatory ventilation (IMV) is a method of augmenting the patient's spontaneous ventilation. IMV differs from assisted ventilation in that the patient's spontaneous breath does not trigger the ventilator into the inspiratory phase. The patient breathes spontaneously from a flow of gas from the ventilator circuit. Intermittently, the ventilator provides a mandatory volume of gas at a predetermined rate. The IMV rate is determined by the patient's capability of assuming a portion of the work of breathing. The patient's ventilatory pattern and delivery of the mandatory inspiration are independent of one another. In an attempt to synchronize the mandatory breath from the ventilator with the patient's ventilatory pattern, various techniques have been developed. Synchronized intermittent mandatory ventilation (SIMV), intermittent assisted ventilation (IAV), and intermittent demand ventilation (IDV) are all systems designed to provide the mandatory breath in response to a spontaneous inspiration at predetermined intervals. This is nothing more than assisted ventilation during the mandatory cycle. The use of IMV, SIMV, IAV, and IDV as a method of weaning has increased significantly in recent years. The patient may assume more of the work of breathing while reducing the mandatory ventilation rate. The patient is being weaned while remaining attached to the ventilator. Constant monitoring is not necessary during the weaning process, and the patient receives the same oxygen concentrations and humidification during both spontaneous and mandatory ventilation.

Controlled Ventilation. The use of intermittent positive pressure ventilation (IPPV) has decreased significantly over the past 10 years, primarily because of the use of intermittent mandatory ventilation (IMV) as a method of long-term ventilatory support. However, the use of controlled ventilation (CV) is still advocated in certain specific circumstances, such as central nervous system disorders or critically ill patients whose condition has not been stabilized. The respiratory rate, tidal volume, and inspiratory/expiratory flow rates may all be manipulated during controlled ventilation to obtain the desired physiologic effects. Total control of the patient's ventilatory pattern is the only advantage of IPPV as compared to other modes of ventilation.

Indications for Mechanical Ventilation

Basically, mechanical ventilation is instituted to correct one of three pathophysiologic processes: acute hypoventilation, high or low $\dot{V}A/\dot{Q}$. In the PACU, acute hypoventilation may be caused by inadequate skeletal muscle relaxant reversal, prolonged emergence from anesthesia, or overdosage of narcotic agonist in the PACU. The arterial blood gases of the patient with acute hypoventilation will demonstrate a decreased PaO_2 and an increased $PaCO_2$ and reduced pH. When acute hypoxemia is present, a volume-limited ventilator should be used. In this case, the intervention is intended to restore the patient's normal alveolar ventilation. Hence, the V_T should be set at 12 to 15 ml/kg range, with a range of 8 to 10 for respiratory rate. Sighs are usually not needed and the F_1O_2 should be ≤ 0.4. Twenty to thirty minutes after the institution of mechanical ventilation, arterial blood gases should be drawn and evaluated, and ventilator settings should be changed accordingly.

High $\dot{V}_A/\dot{Q}$ ($\uparrow$ dead space) is not particularly common in the PACU. Pulmonary embolis would be an example of a pathologic process causing high $\dot{V}_A/\dot{Q}$. The arterial blood gases of a patient with high $\dot{V}_A/\dot{Q}$ will demonstrate hypoxemia and a minimal hypercarbia. Another helpful test to determine the degree of dead space is the Bohr equation, commonly referred to as the V_D/V_T. If the V_D/V_T ratio is greater than 0.6, mechanical ventilation should be instituted. The same basic considerations in setting up the ventilator should be used for the patient with high $\dot{V}_A/\dot{Q}$ as for the patient with acute hypoventilation.

Low $\dot{V}_A/\dot{Q}$ (shuntlike states) is a more common pathophysiologic process that occurs in the PACU. Severe atelectasis is a common cause of low $\dot{V}_A/\dot{Q}$. Arterial blood gases in the patient with low $\dot{V}_A/\dot{Q}$ usually demonstrate hypoxemia with minimal hypercarbia and a low pH. Another helpful test to determine the amount of shunt is the $\dot{Q}_S/\dot{Q}_T$. The shunt formula can be used to determine the exact amount of right-to-left shunt. However, if the $F_{I}O_2$ and the Pa_{O_2} are known, the isoshunt line graph can be used to determine the approximate percentage of shunted blood. If a patient has a $\dot{Q}_S/\dot{Q}_T$ that is greater than 15 percent, mechanical ventilation should be strongly considered.

Because the FRC is low in patients with low $\dot{V}_A/\dot{Q}$, hyperinflation or PEEP may be required to return the FRC to normal levels. By returning the FRC to normal levels, the V_T will be taken out of the closing volume (CV) range, and ultimately alveolar ventilation will improve because there will be better matching of ventilation to perfusion in the lungs.

In patients who have undergone major operations and do not have underlying lung disease, mechanical ventilation may be required until the effects of anesthesia and surgery have dissipated. The patient initially should be provided with 100 ml/kg per minute of total ventilation. An IMV rate of 8 to 10 is usually acceptable, and a PEEP of 5 cm H_2O may be added to the expiratory limb of the ventilator circuit. The use of IMV has decreased the period of mechanical ventilatory support slightly and has probably made weaning safer.

Weaning from Mechanical Ventilation

While the patient receives mechanical ventilatory support, cardiovascular stability is of utmost importance. This is particularly true when the patient is being weaned from mechanical ventilation. Special attention to fluids and electrolyte balance should be given. The patient should be afebrile and in a good nutritional state before the weaning process is instituted.

The patient's respiratory status must be assessed before the weaning process can be started. The assessment parameters are usually grouped into three major categories: ventilation, mechanics, and oxygenation.

Assessment of ventilation centers around the arterial blood gas analysis. The Pa_{CO_2} should be within normal limits (35 to 45 torr). The V_D/V_T should be less than 0.6. If PEEP has been used, it should be 1 to 5 cm H_2O at the beginning of the weaning process.

As with ventilation, oxygenation is assessed by obtaining arterial blood gases. The Pa_{O_2} should be greater than 70 torr while on a $FI_{O_2} \leq 0.4$ and < 5 cm H_2O PEEP before attempting weaning.

The best tests for assessing the pulmonary mechanical function are the vital capacity (VC) and the maximal inspiratory force (MIF). Assessment of VC will reflect respiratory system compliance and mechanical muscle strength. The MIF will reflect neuromuscular strength. The VC should be 10 to 15 ml/kg, and the MIF should be more negative than 20 cm H_2O.

When the patient meets the three categories of assessment, the actual process of weaning can begin. It is important to restate that the patient must possess good cardiovascular stability, including adequate nutrition and blood volume. The patient should not receive any drugs that would sedate or depress the respiratory drive. During the weaning process, constant psychological and physiologic monitoring of the patient is mandatory. Vital signs, arterial blood gases, and mechanics should be recorded on a flow sheet. Once the patient is allowed to breathe spontaneously without the aid of mechanical ventilation, vital signs are recorded every 5 to 10 minutes for about ½ hour and then every 30 minutes after that. Arterial blood gases are checked 15 minutes after spontaneous breathing is begun and thereafter on an hourly basis. Mechanical ventilation is resumed if any of the following signs are shown: arrhythmia, hypertension or hypotension (change of 15 torr from baseline), tachycardia (> 120 bpm), pallor, cyanosis, agitation, increasing Pa_{CO_2} of greater than 1 torr/minute, pH less than 7.25 or Pa_{O_2} less than 70 torr.

Most of the postoperative patients who are receiving short-term mechanical ventilation can be weaned in several hours. Discontinuance of mechanical ventilation can be accomplished in one of two ways: periodic removal from the ventilator using the Briggs' T-piece or the use of IMV. If the method of weaning is to remove the patient periodically from the ventilator, a Briggs' T-piece can be used. The T-piece will ensure that the patient will be adequately oxygenated. The patient who received long-term ventilator care may only tolerate short periods (< 30 minutes) every 2 to 4 hours of the T-piece weaning process. As tolerated, these patients should spend less time receiving mechanical ventilation and more time using the T-piece. If it is anticipated that there will be a lengthy weaning process, the discontinuance from mechanical ventilation should be commenced in the morning when the patient has all his or her strength.

IMV is an acceptable method of weaning a patient from mechanical ventilation and offers many advantages. Some of the advantages are that it increases safety, decreases weaning time, preserves respiratory muscle strength and coordination by allowing ongoing spontaneous breathing efforts, and improves psychological adjustments to weaning. The focus of this method of weaning is that the number of breaths per minute is reduced and the patient takes over a greater proportion of his or her ventilation. Finally, the patient breathes spontaneously without the aid of mechanical ventilation. The weaning process with IMV is the same as with the T-piece regarding time off the ventilator.

Some patients develop an intolerance to the IMV

method of weaning. The intolerance may be due to increased resistance in the IMV circuit (as compared to the T-piece circuit), malfunctions of the ventilator setup, or overoxygenation during the weaning period. Patients who are difficult to wean via IMV may respond well to the T-piece method of weaning from mechanical ventilation.

POSTANESTHESIA CARE: DISCHARGE PHASE

Patient Teaching and Follow-up

Upon the patient's arrival in the postanesthesia care unit (PACU), nursing interventions are focused on the Drain stir-up regimen and monitoring the patient's physiologic parameters. Many studies indicate that the lung volumes, particularly in patients who have had upper abdominal or thoracic surgery, will remain decreased from 5 to 7 days postoperatively. Hence, the patient should be educated to continue using the SMI maneuver with or without the use of an incentive spirometer long into the postoperative phase. Accompanying this, the cascade cough and early ambulation should be emphasized to facilitate secretion clearance and better matching of ventilation to perfusion.

Follow-up should include postoperative visits to all patients who were in the PACU. The focus of the postoperative assessment should be on the patient's cardiorespiratory status. Again, those patients who were ASA grade III or greater or had upper abdominal or cardiothoracic surgery should be visited each postoperative day for 5 to 7 days.

Discharge Criteria

The use of the PARS system of scoring patients who are recovering from anesthesia is helpful in setting up discharge criteria from the PACU. When a patient arrives in the PACU, his PAR score may be 7 or 8. After a significant amount of time allowing for metabolism and excretion of the anesthetic agents, the PAR score may be 9 or 10, at which point, the patient may be discharged from the PACU. Many factors determine readiness for discharge; The use of regional anesthesia, the patient's prior condition, and the use of inhalational or IV anesthesia all have a significant impact on the decision to discharge the patient. Finally, if a patient has been medicated with a narcotic agonist in the PACU, he or she should not be discharged for 15 to 30 minutes postadministration of the drug so that the effects of the drug can be fully evaluated. Discharging patients from the PACU can be the responsibility of the patient's principal physician, the physician director of the PACU, or an anesthesiologist. The nurse or physician anesthetist who administered the anesthesia intraoperatively should be consulted during the discharge phase to enhance the decision-making process.

BIBLIOGRAPHY

Burrows B, Knudson R, Quan S, Kettel L: Respiratory Disorders: A Pathophysiologic Approach, 2nd ed. Chicago, YearBook, 1983.

Drain C: Anesthetic considerations of morbid obesity. AANA J 47:556–565, 1979.

Drain C: Postanesthesia lung volumes in surgical patients. AANA J 49:261–268, 1981.

Drain C: The anesthetic management of the patient: a broad view of the anesthetic considerations necessary regarding the respiratory system. AANA J 50:192–201, 1982.

Drain C: Managing postoperative pain—It's a matter of sighs. Nursing 14(8):52–55, 1984.

Drain C: Comparison of two inspiratory maneuvers on increasing lung volumes in postoperative upper abdominal surgical patients. AANA J 52:379–388, 1984.

Drain C, Cain R: The nursing implications of postoperative pain. Mil Med 146:127–130, 1981.

Drain C, Shipley-Christoph S: The Recovery Room: A Critical Care Approach to Post Anesthesia Nursing, 2nd ed. Philadelphia, Saunders, 1987.

Flynn J: Oxygen and retrolental fibroplasia: update and challenge. Anesthesiology 60(5):397–399, 1984.

Ganong W: Review of Medical Physiology, 12th ed. Los Altos, Lange, 1985.

Guenter C, Welch M: Pulmonary Medicine. Philadelphia, Lippincott, 1977.

Guyton A: Textbook of Medical Physiology, 7th ed. Philadelphia, Saunders, 1986.

Harper R: A Guide to Respiratory Care: Physiology and Clinical Applications. Philadelphia, Lippincott, 1981.

Hinshaw H, Murry J: Diseases of the Chest, 4th ed. Philadelphia, Saunders, 1980.

Levitzky M: Pulmonary Physiology, 2nd ed. New York, McGraw-Hill, 1986.

Miller R: Anesthesia, 2nd ed. New York, Churchill-Livingstone, 1985.

Murray J: The Normal Lung, 2nd ed. Philadelphia, Saunders, 1986.

Poulton T: Etiology and treatment of postoperative hypotension. Curr Rev Recovery Room Nurses 3:Lesson 11, 1981.

Shapiro B: Clinical Applications of Blood Gases, 3rd ed. Chicago, Year Book, 1982.

Traver G (ed): Respiratory Nursing: The Science and the Art. New York, Wiley, 1982.

Part IX
QUALITY ASSURANCE

42

Quality Assurance for Anesthesia

Jeffery M. Beutler

QUALITY ASSURANCE

The Process, the Trust, the Responsibility

Most anesthesia professionals are still attempting to deal with the question: What is quality assurance? To place QA into a general category would be to say that it is a prescribed process, which is a series of steps that are ongoing and that will result in desired outcomes. On closer examination, one must separately describe the terms *quality* and *assurance*. Quality can be simply defined as a degree of excellence or the essential characteristics of superiority. Assurance connotes trust; one may have confidence in a responsible person's performance. Defined as a single term, quality assurance is the act of making certain that prescribed standards of excellence are maintained.

Applied to anesthesia, QA becomes the cornerstone of the consumer's trust. The anesthesia practitioner must provide a service that is characterized by quality traits. The consumer, on the other hand, has confidence that the service provided will be quality in nature. The service provider must be aggressively involved in activities that will ensure that the degree of quality expected is the same as that delivered. Inherent to the trust component of QA is the social responsibility of health care providers to maintain a degree of quality that is commensurate with that trust. Anesthesia practitioners as health care professionals must be accountable for the quality of care delivered. Without a QA program, anesthesia practitioners are delinquent in the responsibilities and terms of the solemn patient–practitioner covenant.

Quality assurance is the new frontier for the Joint Commission on Accreditation of Hospitals. A QA program is used to mandate the quality of care provided. QA tends to exceed the previous limitations of prescriptive standards and is a comprehensive process through which health care providers can ". . . monitor the quality and appropriateness of care provided and improve care or clinical performance where needed" (JCAH, 1987).

Flexibility is built in to allow for the application of this standard in institutions and services differing in nature and scope. Likewise, the process can be applied to multiple and diverse patient care problems.

Quality assurance is the combination of two major processes, the problem solving technique and the managerial responsibility of control. Managerial control is a process by which important data is collected and analyzed to determine the degree that actual outcomes meet desired outcomes. When discrepancies between actual and desired outcomes exist, problems or opportunities to improve care are identified and resolved through the problem solving process. The end result is not a blanket answer to all health care problems, but rather it is a set of guidelines through which many diverse problems and concerns can be identified and resolved.

PROCESS COMPONENTS

There are five basic components to the QA process: ongoing monitoring, problem identification, development and implementation of solutions, reevaluation of the solution, and documentation of the process (JCAH, 1987).

MONITORING

The Hallmark of QA

To the anesthesia provider, monitoring is something that is done during the administration of an anesthetic. The patient's physical status is closely observed, and physiologic changes act as indicators of the patient's response to the type and depth of anesthesia administered. Monitoring as applied to QA is not different in degree but only in kind. The indicators monitored are signs of the overall quality of anesthesia provided at a given institution. QA suggests then that anesthesia practitioners must look beyond the patient-by-patient delivery of anesthesia care provided and monitor those criteria-based indicators that reflect the overall quality of anesthesia care provided by practitioners holding anesthesia privileges at a given health care facility.

Monitoring the quality and appropriateness of anesthesia care provided should be nothing new to the anesthesia practitioner. The symbol of quality anesthesia practice has always been vigilance. The concept of vigilance has only been expanded to include all aspects of anesthesia care from the preanesthetic visit to the patient's return to a preanesthetic level of health. The emblem depicting Morpheus, the Greek god of dreams, has greater implications today than ever before. Monitoring the quality and appropriateness of anesthesia care provided must be ongoing. Monitoring is composed of five primary components: major clinical activities, care indicators, measurement criteria, data collection, and data analysis.

The first step in establishing a monitoring program is to identify the major clinical activities performed by those individuals holding clinical privileges in anesthesia. This may include certified registered nurse anesthetists, physician anesthesiologists, surgeons, and obstetricians. A sample list of clinical activities includes (1) general anesthesia, (2) spinal anesthesia, (3) epidural anesthesia, (4) anesthesia for obstetrics, (5) placement of central venous lines, (6) intubation, (7) blood component therapy, (8) placement of arterial lines, (9) controlled ventilation, and (10) outpatient anesthesia. It is the responsibility of department members to develop a complete list of clinical activities specific to the individual department. All clinical activities must then be monitored to determine the quality of care provided.

The next step in the process is to establish indicators of care for each major clinical activity identified. Indicators are specific events, occurrences, or outcomes that are to be monitored. They are observable and measurable. Numbered indicators—corresponding to the numbered list of clinical activities in the previous paragraph—are (1) recall, (2) spinal headache, (3) wet tap, (4) 5-minute Apgar score less than 6, (5) pneumothorax, (6) trauma to teeth, (7) transfusion reaction (wrong patient), (8) collateral circulation checked preoperatively, (9) postoperative atelectasis, and (10) unscheduled admission to hospital.

One or more indicators should be developed for each major clinical activity. Some indicators, of course, can apply to multiple clinical activities. For example, neurological deficit could be an indicator of appropriateness of care for both regional and general anesthesia.

The indicators just listed are specific indicators of care because they relate to specific clinical activities. Generic screens or indicators should also be developed. Some examples are (11) death in the operating room, (12) death in the postanesthesia care unit or within 24 hours, (13) myocardial infarction in the operating room or within 24 hours of the procedure, (14) neurologic deficit, (15) unscheduled admission to the intensive care unit, (16) mechanical trauma, (17) infections, and (18) length of stay in postanesthesia care unit. Generic screens should always be ongoing monitors. All reported generic screens should be reviewed for quality and appropriateness of anesthesia care provided.

Once indicators of care have been identified and accepted by department members, measurement criteria should be established. Criteria are the standards against which the indicators are measured or compared. Criteria should be objective and explicit in nature. Criteria should be established based upon current accepted standards of care. The scope of criteria should be attainable and yet narrow enough to allow for problem identification. The following list of criteria represents examples of how criteria should be established and does not necessarily represent currently accepted standards of care.

Clinical Activity Indicator	Criteria (% Occurrence)
1. Recall	0
2. Spinal headache	Less than 3
3. Wet tap	Less than 1
4. 5-Minute Apgar score less than 6	0
5. Pneumothorax	Less than 1
6. Trauma to teeth	0
7. Transfusion reaction (wrong patient)	0
8. Collateral circulation checked preoperatively	100
9. Postoperative atelectasis	0
10. Unscheduled admission to hospital	Less than 1
11. Death in operating room	0 related to anesthesia
12. Death in the postanesthesia care unit or within 24 hours	0 related to anesthesia
13. Myocardial infarction in operating room or within 24 hours of procedure	0 related to anesthesia
14. Neurologic deficit	0 related to anesthesia
15. Unscheduled admission to the intensive care unit	0 related to anesthesia
16. Mechanical trauma	0 related to anesthesia
17. Infections	Less than 3
18. Length of stay in postanesthesia care unit	less than 2 hours average

Perhaps one of the most difficult tasks facing the clinicians is that of planning, organizing, and implementing a data collection system to facilitate monitoring. The clinician is advised to explore what systems for data collection already exist within the institution. For example, the medical record department may already have a data collection system and the addition of new information fields may not be a problem. The employment of an individual to do nothing but data collection for QA may be feasible in large anesthesia departments. Small departments of one to five people might consider collecting data after each case and hiring a part-time assistant to enter this data into a personal computer for the purpose of generating monthly QA monitoring reports.

Whatever method is used, the outcome of a data collection system should be significant information that establishes trends or identifies specific problems. Both the numerator and denominator of specific indicators must be given to establish the degree of compliance with the standard. For example, a monthly report may show that three patients had postspinal headaches. However, since 100 spinals had been administered, this represents 3 percent. Three percent is the established nominally acceptable criteria. Each indicator would be represented in the data report and compared to the number of clinical activities or the denominator. Effective data collection and management systems will also cross reference indicators with the specific practitioner associated with the event or outcome. This information will be invaluable in determining the need for training and education for specific department members. This information can also be used in the institution's clinical privileges renewal process.

The better the data collection and management system, the easier it is to analyze the data for problems, trends, or opportunities to improve patient care. Data analysis or review of the indicators should be done at least monthly. Sophisticated data collection and management systems could produce weekly or even daily reports to be reviewed. Problems identified should be managed through normal channels and reported at least monthly to the department at large and through the institution's QA program.

Instituting and maintaining monitors are essential components to monitoring. There is no single method for either component. However, several guidelines may assist in implementing both.

1. Involve department members in the selection of indicators and in data collection to gain their support and cooperation.
2. Select indicators that are meaningful.
3. Computerize data collection whenever possible. When not possible, systematize the collection procedure to make collection easier.
4. Use existing sources of data to prevent duplication of services.
5. Maintain a calendar outlining monitor start times, durations, and ending dates.
6. When planning to monitor a specific area of concern in the future, place a memo on the calendar about a month before the start time as a reminder.
7. Maintain a weekly or monthly file to serve as an organizer of activities to be accomplished on a perpetual basis.
8. Meet monthly to address QA functions and plan activities.
9. Use hospital-based departments that will aid in the collection and review of data, e.g., hospital QA department, infection control department, medical audit committee, utilization review, risk management or medical record department.

There is no one data source that can be used in problem identification. The more sources that are monitored, the greater the likelihood that significant problems will be identified and hopefully resolved. Table 42–1 is a partial list of suggested data sources from the JCAH manual entitled *Making Quality Assurance Work For You*.

PROBLEM PRIORITIZATION

Problems identified must be assigned a priority level based on the nature of the problem and the degree of impact expected on the quality of patient care provided. Priority can be grouped into levels, such as immediate, as soon as possible, or even deferred action. Problems may be assigned ordinate or temporal positions relating to the order in which they will be addressed. After identification of the problem, priority assignment for problem assessment and resolution is the next essential step in the problem resolution process.

TABLE 42–1. MULTIPLE DATA SOURCES FOR PROBLEM IDENTIFICATION

Morbidity/mortality reports
Tissue review
Blood use review
Medical record review
Safety committee findings
Infection control committee findings
Profile analysis
PSRO regional data
Incident reports
Laboratory reports
Radiology reports
Financial data
Liability claims data
Utilization review
Staff surveys
Patient surveys
Third party payer data
Direct observations
Clinical anesthesia conferences
Surgical committee meetings
Product evaluation committee

OBJECTIVE ASSESSMENT AND ANALYSIS

Once a problem or potential problem has been identified, steps must be taken to determine the cause or causes of the problem. Causes are not always obvious. Further assessment of the problem may be needed to allow the investigator to determine the scope of the problem and to establish the degree of impact this problem has on the patient care provided. Three forms of assessment are used: retrospective, concurrent, and prospective. The appropriate type is selected depending on the problem identified.

Retrospective assessment usually involves the review of standard medical documents. The documents are reviewed, and data are accumulated based on specific criteria established by the investigator. Standard records used in retrospective studies include anesthetic records, preanesthetic evaluation sheets, recovery room records, nurses' notes, doctors' order sheets, progress notes, incident reports, and other institutional records that contain pertinent patient care information.

Concurrent assessments are performed on an ongoing basis as care is being provided. Problems and causes are not only looked for, but corrective actions may be instituted at the same time. For example, cardiopulmonary resuscitation teams may be observed by a team of experts during an actual arrest, and corrective actions are instituted immediately as problems are identified. From those observations will come further plans for continuing education and changes in policies and procedures. Problems that need immediate attention can be handled in this manner.

Prospective studies involve the collection of specific data over a period of time, which will give clues about the frequency and cause of the problems. Prospective studies can take many forms. Some types of studies include informal observation based on specific criteria, interviews, and clinical studies based on explicit protocols. These studies are used to assess specific problems and can be tailored to collect all necessary data.

It is important to remember that the same rules are to be followed in conducting these studies as when performing any research studies. The study should be as simple and cost effective as possible and still allow for a significant contribution to resolution of the problem. The activity of QA, including studies, should be integrated so that patient care will not be hindered.

Choosing the type of audit or study is sometimes difficult, but usually the type of audit selected is determined by the type of problem identified. An area of general concern among health care practitioners has been one of selecting the type and size of the sample to be studied. Sample types fall into two general categories: probability and nonprobability samples (JCAH, 1980).

Probability is the most meaningful type of sampling, and the results will express a ratio of expected events for the whole population. Nonprobability sampling allows for the selection of a sample based on typical or expected sample characteristics. This type of sampling is usually not representative of the whole population and should not be used except when occurrence of a problem is expected to be frequent. The rule of thumb to apply to sample size is as follows:

1. Select the smallest meaningful sample.
2. "The sample should comprise a minimum of twenty (20) cases or five percent (5%) of the total population, which ever is greater" (JCAH, 1980).

Further description of statistical sampling and analysis exceeds the limitations of this chapter. The important point here is that audits and studies can be made more meaningful and less time consuming when the appropriate statistical principles are applied (Duke University, 1980).

After the data have been collected by either formal or informal means, objective analysis is essential to focus on the cause of a problem. It may be easy to accept the results of a study if the cause of a problem is the result of someone else's action, either a group or an individual. It is somewhat more distressing to the ego if the problem identified is the result of one's own action. The intent of QA is not punitive but corrective in nature. In order for objectivity to be maintained, all persons involved must be cognizant of the corrective nature of QA. QA is a process by which change can be instituted to improve patient care. It is for this reason that objectivity must be maintained in the collection and analysis of data.

CORRECTIVE ACTION

Planning and Implementation

Before this step, problems have been identified and assessed as to their causes. Once the cause of a problem is identified, a plan to resolve or correct the situation is relatively easy to develop. The plan for resolution should, whenever possible, be developed by those closest to the situation, providing the problem is within their abilities to solve it. At times, outside help or consultation is required. However, most

problems can be resolved within individual areas or departments. The JCAH strongly recommends that problem resolution be carried out through appropriate and existing mechanisms within the organization. Every new problem does not require a new committee. Problems identified should be referred to the appropriate individual or committee within the organization. Again, it must be emphasized that decisions should be made by those closest to the problem. For every problem there exists a multitude of solutions. Solutions, however, are usually not the problem in change. The problem is usually implementation of the solution. Plans developed by those who must implement them tend to be (1) more appropriate, (2) problem specific, and (3) more successful. Successful change is the object of QA. Therefore, those who will be involved in implementation must be involved in plan development.

Selection of outcome criteria should be a function of the professional members of the anesthesia service. The criteria should be based on nationally accepted standards, scientific knowledge, and collective clinical experience. The criteria selected as expected outcomes become the measure of quality in the delivery of patient care. The attainment of specified criteria will signify successful problem resolution.

Monitoring plans may include observation, time studies, medical record review, or other clinical studies. Any of these plans should produce data that give some indication of the degree of success in problem resolution. A plan that calls for an improvement in preanesthesia visits may have an implementation period of 4 weeks. During this period of time, preanesthetic activities would be monitored to assure that the plan is implemented appropriately. At the end of the implementation period, an appropriate study would be conducted to determine if the plan resulted in an improvement in preanesthetic care based on outcome criteria. If outcomes are different from what is expected, reevaluation of the problem will have to be instituted.

Essential components of the QA process are outlined in Figure 42–1. The left side of the diagram represents the process components, and the right side is a list of sources to aid in accomplishing each step of the process.

DOCUMENTATION

Documentation provides for continuity within a QA program. Problem-solving activities can be followed through from identification to resolution. QA activity documentation is required not only for accreditation purposes but also to provide for an organized QA program that is consistent over time. It aids in the prevention of wasteful duplication and poor follow-through. Documentation can also be used as a basis for QA program evaluation.

What then can be used as documentation of QA involvement? Many forms of documentation of QA activities may already exist within a given anesthesia service. Committee meeting minutes, policy and procedure manuals, intradepartmental and interdepartmental memos, continuing education records, departmental meeting minutes, and other printed media may validate the performance of QA activities. Each anesthesia service unit must inventory existing department practices and determine which can be con-

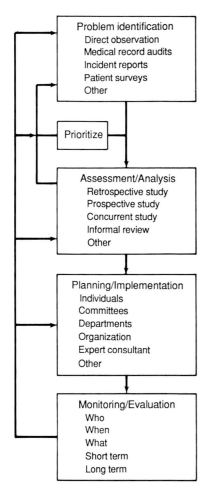

Figure 42–1. Essential components of the problem resolution process.

sidered as contributors to QA. It is important to use as many preexisting mechanisms as possible in performing QA activities. Utilization of existing mechanisms will help prevent duplication of activities and streamline the overall QA program. A QA program should be as integrated as possible to allow maximum time for delivery of anesthesia care. It is not the intent of QA or the JCAH to saddle health care providers with tasks that are so burdensome that health care delivery is hindered. Each departmental activity must be reviewed and assessed for activities that perform one or more of the following QA functions:

1. Problem identification
2. Problem prioritization
3. Establish cause (assessment and analysis)
4. Plan for resolution
5. Implementation of plan
6. Monitoring

Table 42–2 shows a sample list of departmental activities and identifies those QA functions performed by each activity. An X in the appropriate box indicates the type of function performed by the corresponding departmental activity.

Through normal meeting minutes and data collection reports, many of the existing QA activities can be documented. However, I recommend a single QA activity form that will assist in providing continuity in the overall QA program. A form of this nature should contain the following information:

1. Problem identified
2. Priority assigned
3. Identified by whom or which monitor
4. Probable cause(s)
5. Corrective action planned
6. Reevaluation: Include date expected, expected outcomes, and monitoring technique
7. Person or group preparing report
8. Reevaluation findings and date

It is extremely helpful to have a form of this nature made in duplicate so that one copy will remain in the department and the second copy may be sent to the hospital-wide QA department as evidence of ongoing QA activities.

DEVELOPING A QA PROGRAM FOR ANESTHESIA

Where to start is many times the most difficult question to answer. The following section provides loosely defined guidelines to aid in planning and implementing a QA program for anesthesia services.

As a leader of a QA program, it is essential to be as knowledgeable as possible about the subject matter. The first step in developing a QA program is to read as much material as possible about QA. Recommended are the sources at the end of the chapter as well as the many publications provided by the JCAH. The hospital QA director should be an excellent resource person and may be able to recommend other applicable readings.

The support of the medical director and other members of the department must be elicited. The support must be contributory in nature. The greater the personal involvement in developing the program, the greater will be the involvement in program implementation and maintenance. This support can be enlisted most readily by a plea to each member's commitment to quality. If that does not work, the fact that QA is required may have some motivational influence.

Educate the department members about what QA is. Encourage discussion of the subject in preliminary meetings and allow members to exchange ideas about the form and direction the program should take. Establish the format through which QA activities should be implemented and maintained. Some departments have created quality circles or QA committees or have opened the QA meeting to the department at large.

At least annually, the department members along with the medical director should evaluate the overall effectiveness of the program. The hospital QA department will assist in this endeavor and provide criteria to use in the evaluation.

The essential steps to be followed are

1. Identify all major clinical activities performed by those holding anesthesia privileges.

TABLE 42–2. INVENTORY OF QUALITY ASSURANCE FUNCTION

Departmental Activities	Problem Identification	Problem Prioritization	Assessment and Analysis	Plan for Resolution	Implementing	Monitoring
Clinical anesthesia conference	X	X	X	X	X	X
Morbidity and mortality conferences	X	X	X			X
Unit meetings	X	X	X	X	X	
Departmental meetings	X	X	X	X	X	
A.M. Conference	X			X	X	
Inservice meetings					X	
Anesthesia staff meetings	X	X	X	X	X	
Education committee meetings	X	X	X	X		
Statistical report	X	X	X			X
Peer review	X	X	X	X		X
Chart audits	X	X	X			X
Suggestion box	X		X			X
Surgery committee	X	X	X	X	X	
Laboratory QA	X	X	X	X		
Equipment preventive maintenance program	X	X	X	X	X	
Microbiologic surveillance	X	X	X		X	X
Patient survey forms	X	X	X	X		X

2. Identify one or more indicators of care for each activity.
3. Establish criteria against which the indicators will be measured.
4. Identify what institutional sources are available to assist your department.
5. Plan and implement a data collection system.
6. Establish a process by which indicators will be reviewed monthly.
7. Determine a method by which identified problems will be reported and resolved.
8. Develop a system for documentation of all QA activities within the department.
9. Establish a mechanism by which the department QA activities will be integrated with hospitalwide QA activities.

SUMMARY

The scientific process of QA has been reviewed from problem identification to problem resolution. Monitoring has been described as the cornerstone of anesthesia practice as it relates to ensuring the quality and appropriateness of anesthesia care provided. Each step of the QA process was outlined in detail. However, there is a great deal more to the process than just a scientific type of application. The responsible anesthesia practitioner must develop not only the plan but the art of being involved and committed to the patients receiving anesthesia care. QA, when applied effectively, provides the mechanism for professional commitment and personal involvement in providing anesthesia care at the highest degree of excellence.

REFERENCES

Duke University Hospital Nursing Service: Quality Assurance: Guidelines for Nursing Care. Philadelphia, Lippincott, 1980.

Joint Commission on Accreditation of Hospitals: Accreditation Manual for Hospitals. Chicago, 1987, p 123.

Joint Commission on Accreditation of Hospitals: The Q.A. Guide: A Resource for Hospital Quality Assurance. Chicago, 1980, pp xii, 104, 107–108.

Joint Commission on Accreditation of Hospitals. Making Q.A. Work for You. Chicago, 1981, p 51.

Joint Commission on Accreditation of Hospitals: Accreditation Manual for Hospitals—Anesthesia Services. Chicago, 1987, pp 8–9.

BIBLIOGRAPHY

Dewar DL: The Quality Circle Guide to Participative Management. Englewood Cliffs, NJ, Prentice Hall, 1980.

Greenspan J: Accountability and Quality Assurance in Health Care. London, Charles Press Publishers, 1980.

Healey TG, Gunn JP: Creating a quality assurance program in the anesthesia department. CRNA Forum 2:2–12, 1986.

Joint Commission on Accreditation of Hospitals: Quality and Appropriateness Review (audio cassette package). Chicago, 1984.

Joint Commission on Accreditation of Hospitals: Quality Review Bulletin (monthly publication). Chicago, 1980–1987.

Ouchi WG: Theory-Z. New York, Avon Books, 1981.

Walczak RM: JCAH Perspective: Quality Assurance in Anesthesia Services. AANA J 50:462–464, 1982.

Index

Italicized page numbers indicate tables and figures.